# SCIENCE

NEW SERIES. VOLUME XC

JULY-DECEMBER, 1939

NEW YORK
THE SCIENCE PRESS
1939

THE SCIENCE PRESS PRINTING COMPANY
LANCASTER, PENNSYLVANIA

# CONTENTS AND INDEX

NEW SERIES. VOL. XC—JULY TO DECEMBER, 1939

THE NAMES OF CONTRIBUTORS ARE PRINTED IN SMALL CAPITALS

ABRAHAMSON, E. M., Blood Serum, 598
Academy of Sciences, National, 23, 401, 403; of Arts and Sciences, 30, 610; of Medicine, New York, 359; of Ophthalmology and Otolaryngology, 437; of Science, Alabama, 111; North Carolina, 212; Indiana, 593; Virginia, 586; Swedish, Royal, 152
ADAMS, R., W. A. Noyes Laboratory of Chemistry, 71
Adsorption of Antibodies, A. ROTHEN and K. LANDSTEINER, 65
After-image and Judgment of Size, R. M. SUTTON, 616
Air, Population of, T. D. A. COCKERELL, 353; Compressor, G. J. RALEIGH, 598
Alcohol, Research Council on Problems of, 389; Formation of Bead of, C. F. WINANS, 394
Aldol Condensation, H. FRAENKEL-CONRAT, 114
ALLARD, H. A., Vocal Mimicry of the Starling, 370
American, Association for the Advancement of Science, Southwestern Division, V. C. KIECH, 38; Milwaukee Meeting, F. R. MOULTON, 45; Darwinian Ethics, S. J. HOLMES, 117; Stanford Meeting of the Pacific Division, J. M. LUCK, 123; Standards of Living, S. A. RICE, 167; Science and Social Pioneering, I. BOWMAN, 309; Grants-in-Aid of Research, 349; Columbus Meeting, F. R. MOULTON, 499; Public Relations of Science, W. C. MITCHELL, 599
Ames, Joseph S., and Committee for Aeronautics, 368
AMIS, E. S. and V. K. LAMER, Brom Phenol Blue, 90
AMMUNDSEN, E., Hemoglobin in Normal Individuals, 372
ANDERSON, B. G., Culture Medium for Paramecia, 448
ANDERSON, K., Herpes Virus, 497
ANDERSON, T. F. and B. M. DUGGAR, Yeast and Ultra-Violet Light, 358
Anesthesia by Chilling, G. H. PARKER, 63
ANSON, M. L., Egg Albumin, 142; Proteins, 256
Antibody Production, J. FREUND and M. A. BEHAN, 185
APGAR, C. S., JR., Operating Stand, 22
Apples, Color in, R. B. DUSTMAN and I. J. DUNCAN, 233
Archeology, American, C. E. GUTHE, 528
ARNOW, L. E. and J. C. OPSAHL, Adenocarcinoma Protein, 257
ASCHAM, L., M. SPEIRS and D. MADDOX, Iron in Dried Peas and Beans, 596
ASHLEY-MONTAGU, M F, Conscience of the Past, 180; Scientific Invention and Social Consciousness, 592
Astronomers Association, Amateur, Exhibition, 103
ASTRUP, T., Heparin and Blood-clotting, 36
Atkinson, Harry Victor, E. H. SHAW, JR., 55
Atmospheric Contamination, A. H. PFUND, 326
Aurora, Noteworthy, S. S. BERRY, 490
Australian National Research Council, 388
Authority, Education by, O. F. CURTIS, 93
Awards: of Geographical Society, 11; Milton, 31; Mead Johnson and Company, "B-Complex," 322; Charles T. Main, James R. Bright, 486; Undergraduate Student, David T. James, 486; Francis Amory Centennial Prize, 610

BAKER, R. H., David Todd, 8
BALDWIN, J. T., JR., Chromosomes from Leaves, 240
BARBOUR, H. G. and F. S. HAMMETT, Longevity, 538
BARKAN, G. and O. SCHALES, Pseudomethemoglobin, 616
BARR, C. G., H. W. REUSZER and F. THORP, JR., Chemical Composition of Suckleyana, 497
BATEMAN, H., Electromagnetics, A. O'Rahilly, 300
BATSON, O. V., Human Vascular Preparations, 518
BAUGH, R. H., Compound Words, 156
Beans, Disease of Snap, W. A. JENKINS, 63
BEARD, J. W., D. BEARD and H. FINKELSTEIN, Equine Encephalomyelitis Virus, 215
BEARDSLEY, N. F., Teachers of Physics, 618
BEHRMANN, V. G. and M. FAY, Blood pH, 187
BENNETT, A. A., Theoretical Mechanics, C. J. Coe, 111
BEQUAERT, J., Burgmeier's Revista de Entomologia, 540
BERGER, J. and C. F. ASENJO, Pineapple Juice, 299
Beriberi, F. H. LEWY and OTHERS, 141
BERRY, S. S., A Noteworthy Aurora, 490
BHASKARAN, T. H. and S. C. PILLAI, Fixed Nitrogen and Crop Production, 595
Bio-electric Potentials of Hen's Egg, A. L. ROMANOFF and C. L. COTTRELL, 471
Biological, Laboratory, Fisheries, 11, 265, 365; *Abstracts*, 293, 559; Survey of New Hampshire, 389; Edmund Niles Huyck Preserve, 534; Societies, American, Union of, 560; Citric Acid Synthesis, N. HALLMAN and P. E. SIMOLA, 594; Experiments, Radioactivity in, S. GOUDSMIT, 615
Biology and Education, A. D. MEAD, 241
BIRKHOFF, G. D., Theory of Numbers, C. H. Hardy and E. M. Wright, 158
BLOMQUIST, H. L., N. C. Academy of Science, 212
Blood, pH, Determination of, V. C. BEHRMANN and M. FAY, 187; Vessels and Liquid Latex, D. L. GAMBLE, 520; Serum, E. M. ABRAHAMSON, 598
Blossom-inducing Stimulus, R. H. ROBERTS and B. E. STRUCKMEYER, 16
BLUMENFELD, C. M., Epidermis of the Albino Rat, 446
BOGERT, M. T., Uses of Chemicals, T. C. Gregory, 422; International Union of Chemistry, 491
Bone Marrow, H. N. HOLMES and R. E. CORBET, 518
*Botanica, Chronica*, and the War, R. F. GRIGGS, 418; D. T. MACDOUGAL, F. E. LLOYD and H. S. REED, 566
Botanical Garden, N. Y., Tropical Flower Garden, 413
Botany in Italy, F. RAMALEY, 81
BOUSFIELD, W. A., Conditioned Response, 70
BOWMAN, I., Science and Social Pioneering, 309
BRAGG, W., Medals of the Royal Society, 580
BRAMLEY, A. and A. K. BREWER, Gases and Isotopes, 165
BRAND, A. R. and P. P. KELLOGG, Hearing of Canaries, 354
BRINK, R. A. and D. C. COOPER, Somatoplastic Sterility, 545
BRINKHOUS, K. M. and OTHERS, Heparin and Blood Clotting, 539
British: Association for the Advancement of Science, 83; Dundee Meeting, 132, 202; A. SEWARD, 189; E. K. RIDEAL, 217; I. BOWMAN, 309; Royal Society, 9, 580; Rothamsted Experimental Station, 56; Neurologic Research Institute, 57; Leverhulme Fellowships, 103; Natural History Museum, 131; Non-ferrous Metal Research Laboratories, 173; Forests, 200; Societies and the Community, H. L. HAWKINS, 261; London University, 292; Bird Protection, 364; Association in War Time, 387
BRITTON, S. W. and R. F. KLINE, Deslothing the Sloth, 16
BROH-KAHN, R. H., Sulfanilamide, 543
Brom Phenol Blue, E. S. AMIS and V. K. LAMER, 90
BROMLEY, S. W., New England Hurricane, 15
BROWN, F. C., History of Electricity, D. C. Miller, 234; Physics, E. G. Richardson, 566; R. M. Sutton, 567
BROWN, H. P. and J. A. AUSTIN, Microfilm Records, 573
Brown, William Henry, E. D. MERRILL, 531
Brucella antiserum, I. F. HUDDLESON and R. B. PENNELL, 571
BRUCKNER, J. H. and F. B. HUTT, Linkage in Fowl, 88

Brues, C. T., Food, Drink and Evolution, 145
Burrell, R. C. and H. A. Miller, Vitamin C Content of Spring Greens, 164

C., J. H., "Stars" in "American Men of Science," 252
Cadmium Poisoning, R. H. Wilson and F. DeEds, 498
Calingaert, G., Reaction in Organic Chemistry, 430
Canadian National Research Council, 468
Canaries, Hearing, A. R. Brand and P. P. Kellogg, 354
Cancer, Congress, International, 151; and the Public Health, T. Parran, Jr., 427
Cannon, W. B., Physiological Phenomena, J. J. Izquierdo, 516; Chemical Mediation of Nerve Impulse, 521
Cantarow, A., Urine Chloride Concentration, 375
Carnegie, Institution of Washington, 586; and Dr. Merriam, W. K. Gregory, 466; Corporation, Grants, 587
Carotene, Determination of, G. Kernohan, 623
Carpenter, G. D. H., Entomological Survey, 252
Carr, L. G., Plasmodium of Hemitrichia vesparium, 329
Carter, W., Prontosil a Dye for Insects and Plants, 394
Chalcedony, Artifacts Made from, L. L. Ray, 372
Chemical, Expedition, 103; Imports of the United States, 292; Industries, Exposition, 412; Society, American, Boston Meeting, 58, 132, Officers, 267, 611; Cryogenic Research, 348, Nominations, 414; Composition of Suckleya Suckleyana, C. G. Barr, H. W. Reuszer and F. Thorp, Jr., 497; Mediation of Nerve Impulse, W. B. Cannon, 521
Chemistry, Organic, Reaction in, G. Calingaert, 430; International Union of, M. T. Bogert, 491; of Insulin, E. J. Cohn and Others, 183
Chemists, Literature Service for, N. E. Gordon, 330
Chewing for Relaxation, H. L. Hollingworth, 385
Childers, N. F., D. C. Kiplinger and H. W. Brody, Gas Analysis, 447
Chlorazol Fast Pink BKS, R. E. Rose, 252
Cholodny, N. G. and A. G. Gorbovsky, Photosynthesis, 41
Christiansen, J. B., J. C. Halpin and E. B. Hart, Manganese and Hatchability of Hen's Eggs, 356
Chromosomes, from Leaves, J. T. Baldwin, Jr., 240; Bird and Mammalian, T. S. Painter, 307
Church, R., Center of Population, 418
Cilia, Shape of the, in Motion, A. M. Shanes, 259
Citations, One-man Authority, C. H. Muller, 207
Clark, G., Horsley-Clarke Instrument and Rat, 92
Claude, A., Chicken Tumor I, 213
Clausen, R. E., Sixth Pacific Science Congress, 449
Cockerell, T. D. A., Nomenclator Zoologicus, 178; Population of the Air, 353; Publications of British Museum, 395; Henry Clinton Fall, 609
Cohn, E. J. and Others, Insulin, 183
Coker, R. E., Naples Zoological Station, 206
Columbia University, 267, 322
Colvin, J. W. and C. A. Mills, Infection Resistance, 275
Compound Words, S. B. Talmage, 155; R. H. Baugh, 156; O. Raber, 157; M. Fuller and J. McMasters, 157
Conditioned Response, Demonstration, W. A. Bousfield, 70
Conscience of the Past, M F Ashley-Montagu, 180
Conservation, Health, 458; Soil, 611
Cook, O. F., A Household Palm, 298
Coolidge, H. J., Jr., Science in Africa, E. B. Worthington, 180
Corn, Glycogen in, D. L. Morris and C. T. Morris, 238
Correspondent, Museo Poey, of Havana, 490; Fred William Tinney, 608
Cortin, Excretion of, P. Weil and J. S. L. Browne, 445
Cosmic Rays, Allowed Directions of, I. Opatowski, 463
Cowles, Henry Chandler, G. D. Fuller, 363
Cowles, R. B., Reptilian Thermal Tolerance, 465
Cox, G. J. and Others, Mottled Enamel in Rat Molars, 83
Crafts, A. S., Solute Transport in Plants, 337
Cummins, H., Heinrich William Poll, 172
Curtis, O. F., Education by Authority, 93
Cushing, H., The Mayo Brothers' Clinic, 225
Cushing, Harvey, J. F. Fulton, 443; E. C. Cutler, 475
Cytochrome C, Spectrum, C. H. Theorell and Å. Åkesson, 67

Dale, H., Physiology of the Nervous System, 393
Dallenbach, K. M., Margaret Floy Washburn, 555
Daniels, L. B., Potato Disease in Colorado, 273
Davenport, C. B., Frederick Adams Woods, 607
Dawes, C. L., Arthur Edwin Kennelly, 319
Dawson, R. F., Protein Metabolism, A. C. Chibnall, 330
de Gara, P. F., Agglutination of Pneumococci, 378
Densitometer, X-ray, H. E. Webber, 115
Dental Symbols, B. Oetteking, 464
Deuber, C. G. and J. L. Farrar, Norway Spruce, 109
Diabetes insipidus, H. G. Swann, 67
Diehl, W. W., Endogone as Animal Food, 442
"Distinction" in "Science," C. S. Gager, 209
Diving, Oxygen Store in, D. Robinson, 276
Dodge, B. O., Genetics of the Fungi, 379
Dorfman, A., S. A. Koser and F. Saunders, Nicotinamide and Respiration of Dysentery Bacilli, 544
Dryer, Precipitate, A. Lowman, 143
Dublin, W. B., W. M. Boothby and M. M. D. Williams, Velocity of Sound in a Gas, 399
Duck Sickness and Selenium, A. C. Twomey, S. J. Twomey and L. R. Williams, 572
Durand, W. F., Robert Henry Thurston, 547
Dustman, R. B. and I. J. Duncan, Color in Apples, 233
Dye, Black, of the Navajos, D. T. O'Connell, 272
Dystrophy, N. Shimotori, G. A. Emerson and H. M. Evans, 89; Muscular, Nutritional, S. G. Morris, 424

Edington, W. E., Academy of Science, Indiana, 593
Edwards, E. A. and S. Q. Duntley, Skin Pigment, 235
Egg Albumin, M. L. Anson, 142
Eichelberger, L. and Others, Hemoglobin, 443
Electrochemical Society, 58, 202
Embryonic Tissue and Parturition in the Rat, A. Taylor, 472
Encephalomyelitis, Equine, Virus, V. Kubes and F. A. Rios, 20; J. W. Beard, D. Beard and H. Finkelstein, 315
Endogone as Animal Food, W. W. Diehl, 442
Engineering, Science, R. V. Southwell, 27; Marine, 226; Degree in, 267; College, 436; Education, 533; R. H. Thurston, Celebration, W. F. Durand, 547; Profession, Status of, 609
English, J., Jr., J. Bonner and A. J. Haagen-Smit, Plant Wound Hormone, 329
Entomologia, Borgmeier's Revista de, J. Bequaert, 540
Entomological Survey, C. D. H. Carpenter, 252
Esters, Desoxycorticosterone, R. F. Loeb and Others, 496
Evans, H. M. and Others, Pituitary Growth Hormone, 19; Role of Vitamin E in the Prevention of Dystrophy in Guinea Pigs, 89; Action of Ketene on Hormone, 140; Lactogenic Hormone, 376, 622; Vitamin $B_2$, 377
Evolution, Food and Drink and, C. T. Brues, 145
Expedition, Field Museum, 10, 102, 266, 388, 438, 610; Antarctic, 131, 366; Pacific Islands, 173; Ornithological, 246; to Canada, 347; Fahnestock, 437; National Geographic, 437; Hudson Bay, 458
Exudates, Inflammatory, V. Menkin, 237

Fall, Henry Clinton, T. D. A. Cockerell, 609
Farrand, Livingston, T. Parran, Jr., 583
Farris, E. J. and G. Engvall, Exercising Rats, 144
Fellowships, Guggenheim, 77; Lalor, 347
Felt, E. P., Pasture Insects, H. Osborn, 302
Ferguson, J. H., Heparin and Blood Clotting, 272
Fernholz, E. and S. Ansbacher, Vitamin K, 215
Fertilizer, Boron as, W. L. Powers, 36
Field Museum, 10, 102, 266, 388, 438, 610
Film Reactions and Biology, E. K. Rideal, 217
Firefly, "Spinthariscope," R. W. Wood, 233
Fisher, L. W., New England Geologists Conference, 593

Fisheries, Gulf Coast Laboratory, 11; Puerto Rico, 265; New Milford, 365; Alaska, Experimental Commission, 533; Bureau of, 76, Research Vessel, 227
Fishes, Viviparous Cyprinodont, C. L. TURNER, 42
FLANDERS, S. E., Adaptation Insects, 82
Flasks, Carrel, H. SHAPIRO, 308
FLEXNER, J., M. KNIAZUK and J. NYBOER, Gastric pH in Situ, 239
FORBES, A., Nervous System, J. F. Fulton, 17
FORBES, E. B., Physiology of Adult Ruminant, 270
Foreign Books and Periodicals, 459
FORTUYN, A. B. D., Origin of the Human Races, 352
FRAENKEL-CONRAT, H., Aldol Condensation, 114
FRAMPTON, V. L., Tobacco Mosaic Virus Protein, 305
Franklin and his Times, 484
French Association for the Advancement of Science, 254
FREUND, J. and M. A. BEHAN, Antibody Production, 185
Friction, Nature of, G. W. HAMMAR and G. MARTIN, 179
FRIEDEMANN, T. E. and W. D. SUTLIFF, Fermentable Polysaccharide in the Blood, 335
FULLER, G. D., Henry Chandler Cowles, 363
FULLER, M. and J. MACMASTERS, Compound Words, 157
FULTON, J. F., Physiology of the Nervous System, 110; Biography of Dr. Harvey Cushing, 443
Fungi and Fungous Diseases, J. G. HOPKINS and J. S. KARLING, 303
FUNK, C. and I. C. FUNK, Hormones, 443

GAGER, C. S., "Distinction" in "Science," 209
Galactic and Extragalactic Structure, O. STRUVE, 85
GAMBLE, D. L., Liquid Latex and Blood Vessels, 520
GARDNER, F. E., P. C. MARTH and L. P. BATJER, Spraying Apples, 208
Gas, Velocity of Sound in, W. B. DUBLIN, W. M. BOOTHBY and M. M. D. WILLIAMS, 399; Analysis, N. F. CHILDERS, D. C. KIPLINGER and H. W. BRODY, 447
Gases, and Isotopes, A. BRAMLEY and A. K. BREWER, 165; Respiratory, J. M. LITTLE and H. S. WELLS, 425
Gastric pH, J. FLEXNER, M. KNIAZUK and J. NYBOER, 239
GAW, H. Z. and L. H. KUNG, Fresh-water Medusae, 299
Gay, Frederick Parker, C. W. JUNGEBLUT, 290
Genera, Two Rare, T. K. RUEBUSH, 617
Geneticists, Mathematical, H. R. HUNT, 354
Genetics, International Congress of, 228; Mouse, 247; of the Fungi, B. O. DODGE, 379
Geodesy and Geophysics, International Union of: Addresses: R. M. FIELD, C. HULL, S. CHAPMAN, C. H. MARVIN, F. B. JEWETT and D. LACOUR, 339
Geological, Survey, U. S., 438, 508; Society of America, 611
Geologists Conference, L. W. FISHER, 594
Geology, Central Andes, 10; Historical, R. H. MITCHELL, 441; and Geography, Lectures, C. R. LONGWELL, 514
Geometry, Metric, K. MENGER, 38
Germany, Public Health in 1938, 321
GESELL, R., Warren Plimpton Lombard, 345
Glutathione, H. WAELSCH and D. RITTENBERG, 423
GOLDBERG, L., Stars in Space, B. J. Bok, 110
GORDON, N. E., Literature Service for Chemists, 330
GOUDSMIT, S., Radioactivity, 615
GOWEN, J. W. and A. M. LUCAS, Vaccine Virus and Röntgen Rays, 621
GRAHAM, C. L. and R. H. LAMBERT, Discharging of Liquids and Washing of Solids, 280
Graham, Evarts Ambrose, In Honor of, 414
GRAHAM, R., H. R. HESTER and N. D. LEVINE, Listerella, 336
GRANICK, S., L. MICHAELIS and M. P. SCHUBERT, Methylene Blue, 422
GRAY, I. E., Entomology, R. Matheson, 593
GREGORY, W. K., Carnegie Inst. and Dr. Merriam, 466
GRIGGS, R. F., The War and *Chronica Botanica*, 418
Grinnell, Joseph, W. E. RITTER, 75
GROSS, E. G. and I. H. PIERCE, Oscar Henry Plant, 557
Group Theory, G. A. MILLER, 234
Growth, Symposium, 32; and Lactation, J. R. HAAG and L. D. WRIGHT, 158; Quantitative, L. WALP, 597
GUDGER, E. W., A Whale Shark, 138
GUSTAFSON, F. G., Transport of Minerals through Stems, 306
GUTENBERG, B., Pacific Basin and Earthquakes, 456
GUTHE, C. E., American Archeology, 528

HAAG, J. R. and L. D. WRIGHT, Growth and Lactation, 158
HALLMAN, N. and P. E. SIMOLA, Citric Acid Synthesis, 594
HAMMAR, G. W. and G. MARTIN, Nature of Friction, 179
HARRINGTON, H. D., Identifying Plants, 157
HARRISON, R. G. and A. L. BARROWS, Activities of the National Research Council, 1938–39, 575
Harvard University, 31, 174, 323
HARVEY, E. N., Luminescence of Sugar Wafers, 35; Deep-Sea Photography, 187
HAWKINS, H. L., Scientific Societies, 261
Health, Conservation Contest, 458; Public, at Harvard, 174; Association, American, 248; in Germany, 321
HEIDT, L. J., Isolation of Monochromatic Light, 473
HEMMING, F., Rules of Nomenclature, 420
Hemoglobin, in Blood of Normal Individuals, E. AMMUNDSEN, 372; L. EICHELBERGER and OTHERS, 443
Heparin and Blood Clotting, T. ASTRUP, 36; J. H. FERGUSON, 272; K. M. BRINKHOUS and OTHERS, 539
Herbarium Specimens, C. S. SEMMENS, 624
Herpes Virus, K. ANDERSON, 497
HERRICK, G. W., William R. Perkins, 291
Hibernation of Anopheline Eggs, W. S. STONE and F. H. K. REYNOLDS, 371
HILDEBRAND, J. H., Pure Liquids and Solutions, 1
HIMWICH, H. E. and OTHERS, Cerebral Metabolism, 398
HOAG, J. B., Radio Waves in Water, 277
HOBBS, W. H., A Polar Mirage, 513
HOLLINGWORTH, H. L., Chewing for Relaxation, 385
HOLMES, H. N. and R. E. CORBET, Bone Marrow, 518
HOLMES, S. J., Darwinian Ethics, 117
HOLT, A. C., Medical Library Association, 255
Homeostatic Adjustment, A. S. MARRAZZI, 251
HOPKINS, J. G. and J. S. KARLING, Fungi and Fungous Diseases, 303
Hormones: Pituitary Growth, H. M. EVANS and OTHERS, 19, Lactogenic, H. M. EVANS and OTHERS, 376; Ketene, Action on, C. H. LI, M. E. SIMPSON and H. M. EVANS, 140; Generator, C. H. LI, 143; Lactogenic, C. H. LI, W. R. LYONS and H. M. EVANS, 622; Neuro-, Respiratory, T. KOPPANYI and C. R. LINEGAR, 141; Ovarian, U. J. SALMON, R. I. WALTER and S. H. GEIST, 162; Plant Wound, J. ENGLISH, JR., J. BONNER and A. J. HAAGEN-SMIT, 329; as Dietary Constituents, C. FUNK and I. C. FUNK, 443
HRDLIČKA, A., Paleolithic Find in Asia, 296
HUBBARD, G. D., Marking Specimens, 624
HUBERT, E. E., An Electric Sterilizer, 377
HUDDLESON, I. F. and R. B. PENNELL, Brucella antiserum, 571
HUNT, H. R., Mathematical Geneticists, 354
HUNTINGTON, E., Medical Climatology, C. A. Mills, 540
Hurricane, New England, S. W. BROMLEY, 15; Warnings, 266; '38, Ozone in, C. A. PETERS, 491
HUTCHINGS, B. L. and D. W. WOOLLEY, Hemolytic Streptococci, 41
Hydrogenation of 3-Methylxanthine, T. B. JOHNSON and J. C. AMBELANG, 68

Indian Tribes, Index, M. W. STIRLING, 514
Infection, Resistance, J. W. COLVIN and C. A. MILLS, 275
Insects, Adaptation of, S. E. FLANDERS, 82; Embalming, C. C. SMITH, 116
Insulin, Physical Chemistry, E. J. COHN and OTHERS, 183
Invention, Scientific, M F ASHLEY-MONTAGU, 592
Ionosphere, Ionization in, F. L. MOHLER, 137
Iron in Dried Peas and Beans, L. ASCHAM, M. SPEIRS and D. MADDOX, 596

JEFFREY, E. C. and E. J. HAERTL, Seeds in Trillium, 81
JENKINS, W. A., Disease of Snap Beans, 63
JEWETT, F. B., Remarks of the President at the Dinner of the National Academy of Sciences, 401

JOHNSON, T. B. and J. C. AMBELANG, Hydrogenation of 3-Methylxanthine, 68
JUNGEBLUT, C. W., Frederick Parker Gay, 290

KEITT, G. W., Toxicity of Sodium Salt, 139; Plant Pathology, I. E. Melhus and G. C. Kent, 331
KENNARD, E. H., Floyd Karker Richtmyer, 530
Kennelly, Arthur Edwin, C. L. DAWES, 319
KERNOHAN, G., Carotene, 623
Ketene, Action on Hormone, C. H. LI, M. E. SIMPSON and H. M. EVANS, 140; Generator, C. H. LI, 143
KIECH, V. C., Southwestern Division of the American Association for the Advancement of Science, 38
KOPPANYI, T. and C. R. LINEGAR, A Respiratory Neurohormone, 141
KRAATZ, W. C., Zoology for Pre-medical Students, 592
KRAMER, J., Root and Root-hair Structure, 140
KRAUS, C. A., Non-aqueous Solutions, 281
KUBES, V. and F. A. RIOS, Equine Encephalomyelitis, 20
KUNITZ, M., Crystalline Protein, 112

Labeling Museum Specimens, V. E. SCHEID, 69
Laboratory, Fisheries, Gulf Coast, 11; Puerto Rico, 265; New Milford, 365; Conference, 413; Galton, 436
LEAKE, C. D., Popularization of Science, 84; Books on Medicine, 180
LEVINE, S. Z., E. MARPLES and H. H. GORDON, Role of Vitamin C, 620
LEVITZ, M., D. PERLMAN and M. T. BOGERT, Synthesis of Spirocyclohexane-1, 1-Indanone-3, 114
LEWY, F. H. and OTHERS, Pellagrins with Beriberi, 141
LI, C. H., Ketene Generator, 143; and M. E. SIMPSON and H. M. EVANS, Action of Ketene on Hormone, 140; and W. R. LYONS and H. M. EVANS, Lactogenic Hormone, 622
Light, Monochromatic, Isolation of, L. J. HEIDT, 473
Lindgren, Waldemar, W. H. NEWHOUSE, 584
LINDSAY, R. B., Philosophy of Physics, W. H. Watson, 302
Linkage in Fowl, J. H. BRUCKNER and F. B. HUTT, 88
Liquids, Pure, and Solutions, J. H. HILDEBRAND, 1; Discharging of, and Washing of Solids, C. L. GRAHAM and R. H. LAMBERT, 280
Listerella, R. GRAHAM, H. R. HESTER and N. D. LEVINE, 336
LITTLE, J. M. and H. S. WELLS, Respiratory Gases, 425
LOCKE, A. and R. R. MELLON, Sulfanilamide, 231
LOEB, R. F. and OTHERS, Desoxycorticosterone Esters, 496
LOEHWING, W. F., Phasic Development, 552
Lombard, Warren Plimpton, R. GESELL, 345
Longevity, H. G. BARBOUR and F. S. HAMMETT, 538
LONGWELL, C. R., Lectures in Geology and Geography, 514
LOWMAN, A., Precipitate Dryer, 143
LUCK, J. M., Meeting of the Pacific Division, 123
LULL, R. S., Presentation of Danial Giraud Medal, 24
Luminescence of Sugar Wafers, E. N. HARVEY, 35
LYON, C. J., Preserved Wood, 419

MACDOUGAL, D. T., F. E. LLOYD and H. S. REED, *Chronica Botanica*, 566
MACDUFFEE, C. C., Elementary Matrices, R. A. Frazer, W. J. Duncan and A. R. Collar, 253
Mammals of the Great Plains, V. E. SHELFORD, 591
Manganese and Hatchability of Hen's Eggs, J. B. CHRISTIANSEN, J. G. HALPIN and E. B. HART, 356
MANNING, W. M., Collected Works, G. A. Miller, 593
Marking Specimens, G. D. HUBBARD, 624
MARRAZZI, A. S., Homeostatic Adjustment, 251
Mastodon Remains, W. J. SUMPSTINE and B. R. WEIMER, 539
Mathematical, Society of America, 175, 366; Errors in Encyclopedia Britannica, G. A. MILLER, 512
Mathematicians, Summer Meetings, 32
MATHER, K. F., Recent Books in Geology, 492
MATZKE, E. B., Botanical Books, 65
Mayo Brothers and Their Clinic, H. CUSHING, 225
MEAD, A. D., Biology and Education, 241
Mead Johnson and Company "B-Complex" Award, 322
Medals: *Daniel Giraud Elliot*, R. S. Lull, 24; *Agassiz*, H. U. Sverdrup, 24; *Chandler*, T. H. Chilton, 175; *William H. Nichols*, J. M. Nelson, 367; *John Fritz*, C. F. Hirshfeld, 460; *Melville*, L. M. Goldsmith, 485; *Mechanical Engineers*, J. E. Gleason, 486; *Holley*, C. E. Johnson, 486; *Worcester Reed Warner*, R. Eksergian, 486; *Pi Tau Sigma*, J. I. Yellott, 486; *Willard Gibbs*, V. N. Ipatieff, 486; *Egleston*, W. H. Aldridge, E. H. Armstrong, M. T. Bogert, G. Dunn, A. S. Dwight, H. Krumb, I. Langmuir, L. S. Moisseiff, R. Peele, S. J. Pigott, R. C. Stanley, A. L. Walker, 509; *Penrose*, W. B. Scott, 560; Royal Society: *Copley*, T. H. Morgan, 580; *Royal*, P. A. M. Dirac, D. Keilin, 581; *Davy*, J. W. McBain, 582; *Hughes*, G. P. Thomson, 582
Medical, Library Association, A. C. HOLT, 255; Society, Chicago, 293; School of the University of Minnesota, 323; M. B. VISSCHER, 494; Education at Chicago, 349; Association, American, Platform, 507; Climatology, C. A. Mills, E. HUNTINGTON, 540
Medicinal Products of the United States, 150
Medicine, Horizons, W. OVERHOLSER, 359; History of, 389
Medusae, Freshwater, H. Z. GAW and L. H. KUNG, 299
MENGER, K., Metric Geometry, 38
MENKIN, V., Inflammatory Exudates, 237
Merriam, Dr., and Carnegie Institution, W. K. GREGORY, 466
MERRILL, E. D., William Henry Brown, 531
Metabolism, Cerebral, H. E. HIMWICH and OTHERS, 398
Meteorite, Australian, 201
Meteorites, Where do They Come from?, C. C. WYLIE, 264
Methylene Blue, S. GRANICK, L. MICHAELIS and M. P. SCHUBERT, 422
Microbiology, International Congress, 228; Inter-American Society of, 508
Microfilm Records, Filing of, H. P. BROWN and J. A. AUSTIN, 573
Microorganisms and the Soil, S. A. WAKSMAN and J. P. MARTIN, 304
MILLER, G. A., Group Theory, 234; Mathematical Errors in Encyclopedia Britannica, 512
Mimicry, Vocal, of Starling, H. A. ALLARD, 370
Minerals, Transport through Stems, F. G. GUSTAFSON, 306
Mirage, Polar, W. H. HOBBS, 513
MITCHELL, R. H., Historical Geology, 441
MITCHELL, W. C., Public Relations of Science, 599
MOHLER, F. L., Ionization in the Ionosphere, 137
MONTGOMERY, C. G., Magnetism, 374; Radio-activity, 374; Physics, 514, 515
MOORE, D. H., J. VAN DER SCHEER and R. W. G. WYCKOFF, Antipneumococcus Horse Sera, 357
MORRIS, D. L. and C. T. MORRIS, Sweet Corn, 238
MORRIS, S. G., Nutritional Muscular Dystrophy, 424
Mosquito Larvae, C. M. WILLIAMS, 21
MOULTON, F. R., Milwaukee Meeting of the American Association, 45; Columbus Meeting, 499; Non-Technical Books on Science, 590
MULLER, C. H., One-Man Authority Citations, 207
MULLINS, L. J. and S. C. BROOKS, Living Protoplasm, 256
MURLIN, J. R. and OTHERS, Tumor Growth, 275
Museo Poey, Havana, CORRESPONDENT, 490
Museum, National, of Canada, 32; Thomas R. Baker, Rollins College, 365
Museums, American Association of, 247

Naples Zoological Station, R. E. COKER, 206
Nerve, Tissue Sections, Mounting, R. SPOERRI, 260; Impulses, Chemical Mediation of, W. B. CANNON, 521
Nervous System, J. F. FULTON, 110; H. DALE, 393
NEWHOUSE, W. H., Waldemar Lindgren, 584
Nicotinamide and Dysentery Bacilli, A. DORFMAN, S. A. KOSER and F. SAUNDERS, 544
Nitrogen, Fixed, and Crop Production, T. H. BHASKARAN and S. C. PILLAI, 595
Nomenclator Zoologicus, T. D. A. COCKERELL, 178
Nomenclature, G. A. MILLER, 207; F. HEMMING, 420

NORRIS, E. R. and D. W. ELAM, Crystalline Pepsin, 399
Noyes, William Albert, Laboratory of Chemistry, R. ADAMS, 71; Response, W. A. NOYES, 73
Nucleic Acids, Sensitizing Properties of, W. L. WICKENWERDER, M. V. BUELL and J. E. HOWARD, 356
Nutrition, Canine, W. C. ROSE and E. E. RICE, 186

O'CONNELL, D. T., Black Dye of the Navajos, 272
OETTEKING, B., Dental Symbols, 464
OPATOWSKI, I., Allowed Directions of Cosmic Rays, 463
Operating Stand, C. S. APGAR, JR., 22
Ophthalmology and Otolaryngology, Academy of, 437
Ornithological, Expedition, 246; Collection, Bishop, 347
Ornithologists' Union, American, 78
OSTERHOUT, W. J. V. and J. W. MURRAY, Water in Nonaqueous Solutions, 397
OVERHOLSER, W., Horizons of Medicine, 359
Oxidation, Red, Products of Tocopherols, L. I. SMITH, W. B. IRWIN and H. E. UNGNADE, 334

Pacific Islands, Expedition, 173; Science Congress, R. E. CLAUSEN, 449; Basin and Earthquakes, B. GUTENBERG, 456
PAINTER, T. S., Bird and Mammalian Chromosomes, 307
Paleolithic Find in Asia, A. HRDLIČKA, 296
Palm, Household, O. F. COOK, 298
Paramecia, Culture Medium for, B. G. ANDERSON, 448
PARKER, G. H., Anesthesia by Chilling, 63
PARRAN, T., JR., Cancer and the Public Health, 427; Livingston Farrand, 583
PAUL, J. R., J. D. TRASK and C. S. CULOTTA, Poliomyelitic Virus in Sewage, 258
PEARCE, L., Tryparsamide and Sleeping Sickness, 39
Pepsin, Crystalline Salmon, E. R. NORRIS and D. W. ELAM, 399
Perkins, William R., G. W. HERRICK, 291
PERLMAN, E., A Spectrocolorimeter, 279
PETERS, C. A., Ozone in the '38 Hurricane, 491
PEUGNET, H. B., Vitamin C and Frog Heart, 162
PFUND, A. H., Atmospheric Contamination, 326
Phasic Development, W. F. LOEHWING, 552
Philosophical Society, American, Grants, 568
Photography, 150; Deep-Sea, E. N. HARVEY, 187
Photosynthesis, N. G. CHOLODNY and A. C. GORBOVSKY, 41; S. RUBEN and OTHERS, 570
Phymatotrichum omnivorum, G. M. and M. O. WATKINS, 374
Physicians, College of, Philadelphia, Lectures, 349
Physicists, Visiting, Cornell University, 367
Physics, Teachers of, N. F. BEARDSLEY, 618
Pineapple Juice, J. BERGER and C. F. ASENJO, 299
Plant, Oscar Henry, E. G. GROSS and I. H. PIERCE, 557
Plants, Identifying, H. D. HARRINGTON, 157; Solute Transport in, A. S. CRAFTS, 337
Plasmodium of Hemitrichia, L. G. CARR, 329
Pleuropneumonia-like Microorganisms, A. B. SABIN, 18
Pneumococci, Agglutination of, P. F. DE GARA, 378
Poliomyelitis Virus in Sewage, J. R. PAUL, J. D. TRASK and C. S. CULOTTA, 258
Poll, Heinrich William, H. CUMMINS, 172
Pollen Germination, P. F. SMITH, 163
Polysaccharide, Fermentable, in the Blood, T. E. FRIEDEMANN and W. D. SUTLIFF, 335
Population Centers, C. B. READ, 61, 419; R. CHURCH, 418
Potato Disease in Colorado, L. B. DANIELS, 273
POULTER, R. W., Wound Healing in Red Clover, 108
POWERS, W. L., Boron as a Fertilizer, 36
Press and Scientists, 333
Prontosil, Dye for Insects and Plants, W. CARTER, 394
Protein, Crystalline, M. KUNITZ, 112; Adenocarcinoma, L. E. ARNOW and J. C. OPSAHL, 257
Proteins, Denaturation of, M. L. ANSON, 256
Protoplasm, L. J. MULLINS and S. C. BROOKS, 256
Pseudomethemoglobin, G. BARKAN and O. SCHALES, 616
Puerto Rico, Inter-American University, 201; Research Laboratory in Fisheries, 265

RABER, O., Compound Words, 157
Races, Human, Origin of, A. B. D. FORTUYN, 352
Radio Waves, J. B. HOAG, 277; and Plant Growth, J. VAN OVERBEEK, L. R. BRANTLEY and G. W. POTAPENKO, 470
RALEIGH, G. J., Air Compressor, 598
RAMALEY, F., Botany in Italy, 81
Rat, Molars, Mottled Enamel in, G. J. COX and OTHERS, 83; and Horsley-Clarke Instrument, G. CLARK, 92; Albino, Epidermis of, C. M. BLUMENFELD, 446
Rats, Exercising, E. J. FARRIS and G. ENGVALL, 144
RAY, L. L., Artifacts Made from Chalcedony, 372
RAZRAN, G. H. S., Conditioned Salivary Technique, 89
READ, C. B., Centers of Population, 61, 419
Research, Council, Canada, 30, 468; Biochemical, at Pittsburgh, 151; National, R. G. HARRISON and A. L. BARROWS, 575; in Venezuela, G. G. SIMPSON, 210; and Manufacturing, Courses, 247; Cryogenic, 348; on Problems of Alcohol, 389; in Industry, 535
Richtmyer, Floyd Karker, E. H. KENNARD, 530
RIDEAL, E. K., Film Reactions and Biology, 217
RITTER, W. E., Joseph Grinnell, 75
ROBERTS, R. H. and B. E. STRUCKMEYER, Blossom-inducing Stimulus, 16
ROBINSON, O., Oxygen Store in Diving, 276
ROBLIN, R. O., JR., and P. H. BELL, Sulfanilamide, 327
Rochester Athenaeum and Mechanics Institute, 150
ROMANOFF, A. L. and C. L. COTTRELL, Bio-electric Potentials of Hen's Egg, 471
Root and Root-hair Structure, J. KRAMER, 140
ROSE, R. E., Chlorazol Fast Pink BKS, 252
ROSE, W. C. and E. E. RICE, Canine Nutrition, 186
ROTHEN, A. and K. LANDSTEINER, Adsorption of Antibodies, 65
Royal, Society, and Kaiser Wilhelm Gesellschaft, 9; of Canada, 159; Swedish Academy, 152
Rubber, Vulcanization of, 273
RUBEN, S. and OTHERS, Photosynthesis, 570
RUEBUSH, T. K., Two Rare Genera, 617
Ruminant, Adult, Physiology of, E. B. FORBES, 270

SABIN, A. B., Pleuropneumonia-like Microorganisms, 18
Salivary Technique, Conditioned, G. H. S. RAZRAN, 89
SALMON, U. J., R. I. WALTER and S. H. GEIST, Ovarian Hormone, 162
Salt, Sodium, Toxicity of, G. W. KEITT, 139
SCHEID, V. E., Labeling Museum Specimens, 69
SCHMELKERS, F. C., Vitamin B Complex, 113
Science, Museum, London, 102; and Standards of Living, S. A. RICE, 167; Relations to Society, 294; The Voice of, 300; and Social Pioneering, I. BOWMAN, 309; Non-Technical Books on, F. R. MOULTON, 590; Public Relations of, W. C. MITCHELL, 599
Scientific, Societies, H. L. HAWKINS, 261; Congress, 485
SCOTT, W. B., Presentation of Daniel Giraud Medal, 23
SEALOCK, R. R. and H. E. SILBERSTEIN, Vitamin C, 517
Seeds, Germination of, I. V. SHUNK, 565
Seismological Society of America, A. J. WESTLAND, 183
SEMMENS, C. S., Herbarium Specimens, 624
Sera, Horse, Antipneumococcus, D. H. MOORE, J. VAN DER SCHEER and R. W. G. WYCKOFF, 357
SEWARD, A., The Western Isles through the Mists of Ages, 189
SHANES, A. M., Shape of the Cilia in Motion, 259
SHAPIRO, H., Carrel Flasks, 308
Shark, Whale, E. W. GUDGER, 138
SHAW, E. H., JR., Harry Victor Atkinson, 55
SHELFORD, V. E., Terrestrial Animals, 564; Large Mammals of the Great Plains, 591
SHORTLEY, G. H., Quantum Mechanics, V. Rojansky, 420
SHUNK, I. V., Germination of Seeds, 565
Sigma Xi, Society of the, 57
SIMPSON, G. G., Research in Venezuela, 210
Skin Pigment Changes and Sunlight, E. A. EDWARDS and S. Q. DUNTLEY, 235
Sleeping Sickness and Tryparsamide, L. PEARCE, 39

Sloth, Deslothing, S. W. BRITTON and R. F. KLINE, 16
SMITH, C. C., Embalming Insects, 116
SMITH, L. I., W. B. IRWIN and H. E. UNGNADE, Red Oxidation Products of Tocopherols, 334
SMITH, P. E., Physiology of the Pituitary Body, H. B. van Dyke, 355
SMITH, P. F., Pollen Germination, 163
SMITH, S. C., Alabama Academy of Science, 111
SNODGRASS, R. E., Insect Physiology, V. B. Wigglesworth, 159
Social Pioneering and Science, I. BOWMAN, 309
Solar Activity, H. T. STETSON, 482
Solutions, Non-aqueous, C. A. KRAUSS, 281
SOUTHWELL, R. V., Outlook of Engineering Science, 27
Spectrocolorimeter, A. E. PERLMAN, 279
Spirocyclohexane-l, l-Indanone-3, Synthesis of, M. LEVITZ, D. PERLMAN and M. T. BOGERT, 114
SPOERRI, R., Mounting Nerve Tissue Sections, 260
Spraying Apples, F. E. GARDNER, P. C. MARTH and L. P. BATJER, 208
Spruce, Norway, C. C. DEUBER and J. L. FARRAR, 109
"Stars" in "American Men of Science," J. H. G., 252; S. S. VISHER, 252
Sterility, Somatoplastic, in Medicago sativa, R. A. BRINK and D. C. COOPER, 545
Sterilizer, Electric, E. E. HUBERT, 377
STETSON, H. T., Solar Activity, 482
STIRLING, M. W., Index to "Indian Tribes," 514
STONE, W. S. and F. H. K. REYNOLDS, Bacteria-free Cultures of Trichomonas hominis, 91; Hibernation of Anopheline Eggs, 371
Stone, Witmer, 434
Stratosphere, Balloon Flights into, 246
Streptococci, Hemolytic, B. L. HUTCHINGS and D. W. WOOLLEY, 41
STRUVE, O., Galactic and Extragalactic Structure, 85
Sulfanilamide, A. LOCKE and R. R. MELLON, 231; R. O. ROBLIN, JR., and P. H. BELL, 327; R. H. BROH-KAHN, 543
SUMPSTINE, W. J. and B. R. WEIMER, Mastodon Remains, 539
Surface Currents, D. L. WEBSTER, 107
SUTTON, R. M., After-image and Judgment of Size, 616
SVERDRUP, H. U., Presentation of the Agassiz Medal, 26
SWANN, H. G., Diabetes insipidus, 67
SWANN, W. F. G., Matter and Light, L. de Broglie, 373; Wavelength Tables, G. R. Harrison, 373
Systematics, Association for Study of, 227

TALIAFERRO, W. H., Malaria, J. S. Simmons, 211
TALMAGE, S. B., Compound Words, 155
TAYLOR, A., Embryonic Tissue and Parturition in the Rat, 472
Terrestrial Animals, V. E. SHELFORD, 564
TERRY, R. J., A Thoracic Window, 43
THEORELL, H. and Å. ÅKESSON, Absorption Spectrum of Cytochrome C, 67
Thermal Tolerance, Reptilian, R. B. COWLES, 465
Thoracic Window, R. J. TERRY, 43
Thurston, Robert Henry, Hundredth Anniversary, 152; W. F. DURAND, 547
Tinney, Fred William, CORRESPONDENT, 608
Tobacco Mosaic, Virus Protein, V. L. FRAMPTON, 305
Todd, David, R. H. BAKER, 8
Trichomonas hominis, Bacteria-free Cultures of, W. S. STONE and F. H. K. REYNOLDS, 91
Trillium, Unfertilized Seeds in, E. C. JEFFREY and E. J. HAERTL, 81
Tuberculosis Association, National, Grants, 77
Tumor, I, Chicken, A. CLAUDE, 213; Growth, J. R. MURLIN and OTHERS, 275
TURNER, C. L., Viviparous Cyprinodont Fishes, 42
TWOMEY, A. C., S. J. TWOMEY and L. R. WILLIAMS, Selenium and Duck Sickness, 572
TYLER, A. and S. W. FOX, Sperm Agglutination, 516

Urine Chloride Concentration, A. CANTAROW, 375

Vaccine Virus and Röntgen Rays, J. W. GOWEN and A. M. LUCAS, 621
VAN OVERBEEK, J., L. R. BRANTLEY and G. W. POTAPENKO, Radio Waves and Plant Growth, 470
Vascular Preparations, Human, O. V. BATSON, 518
VAUGHAN, T. W., Presentation of Agassiz Medal, 24
VILLELA, G. G. and A. M. LEAL, Vitamin $B_1$, 179
VISHER, S. S., "Stars" in "American Men of Science," 252
VISSCHER, M. B., Celebration of the Medical School of the University of Minnesota, 494
Vitamin, B, F. C. SCHMELKES, 113, Mead Johnson and Company, 322; Vitamin $B_1$, G. G. VILLELA and A. M. LEAL, 179, G. E. YOUNGBURG, 566; Vitamin $B_2$, H. M. EVANS and OTHERS, 377; Vitamin C, H. B. PEUGNET, 162; R. C. BURRELL and H. A. MILLER, 164; R. R. SEALOCK and H. E. SILBERSTEIN, 517; S. Z. LEVINE, E. MARPLES and H. H. GORDON, 620; Vitamin E, N. SHIMOTORI, G. A. EMERSON and H. M. EVANS, 89; Vitamin K, E. FERNHOLZ and S. ANSBACHER, 215

WAELSCH, H. and D. RITTENBERG, Glutathione, 423
Waite Institute, School in Soil Science, 31
WAKSMAN, S. A. and J. P. MARTIN, Microorganisms and the Soil, 304
WALP, L., Culture Technic for Growth Studies, 597
Washburn, Margaret Floy, K. M. DALLENBACH, 555
Water in Non-aqueous Solutions, W. J. V. OSTERHOUT and J. W. MURRAY, 397
WATKINS, G. M. and M. O. WATKINS, Phymatotrichum omnivorum, 374
WEBBER, H. E., An X-ray Densitometer, 115
WEBSTER, D. L., Surface Currents, 107
WEIL, P. and J. S. L. BROWNE, Excretion of Cortin, 445
Western Isles through Mists of Ages, A. SEWARD, 189
WESTLAND, A. J., Seismological Society of America, 183
WICKENWERDER, W. L., M. V. BUELL and J. E. HOWARD, Sensitizing Properties of Nucleic Acids, 356
WIGGERS, C. J., Physiology, J. M. Luck, 332
WILDER, R. L., Plant Topology, M. H. A. Newman, 354
WILLIAMS, C. M., Mosquito Larvae, 21
WILSON, C. L., Plant Life, C. J. Hylander, 331
WILSON, R. H. and F. DEEDS, Chronic Cadmium Poisoning, 498
WINANS, C. F., Formation of Alcohol Bead, 394
Wood, Preserved, C. J. LYON, 419
WOOD, R. W., A Firefly "Spinthariscope," 233
Woods, Frederick Adams, C. B. DAVENPORT, 607
World's Fair, Hall of Man, 321
Wound Healing in Red Clover, R. W. POULTER, 108
WYLIE, C. C., Where do Meteorites Come from?, 264

Yeast and Ultra-Violet Light, T. F. ANDERSON and B. M DUGGAR, 358
YOUNGBURG, G. E., Color Reaction for Vitamin $B_1$, 566

Zoological Station, Naples, R. E. COKER, 256
Zoology, at Cornell University, 76; for Pre-medical Students, W. C. KRAATZ, 592

# SCIENCE

VOL. 90 FRIDAY, JULY 7, 1939 No. 2323

*Order and Disorder in Pure Liquids and Solutions:* PROFESSOR JOEL H. HILDEBRAND 1

*Obituary:*
*David Todd:* PROFESSOR ROBERT H. BAKER. *Recent Deaths* 8

*Scientific Events:*
*Exchange of Visits between the Royal Society and the Kaiser Wilhelm Gesellschaft; Survey of the Geology of the Central Andes in Peru; The Magellanic Expedition of the Field Museum; A Fisheries Biological Laboratory on the Gulf Coast; Awards of the American Geographical Society* 9

*Scientific Notes and News* 12

*Discussion:*
*Factors Influencing Tree Destruction during the New England Hurricane:* DR. STANLEY W. BROMLEY. *The Point of Origin of the Blossom-Inducing Stimulus:* PROFESSOR R. H. ROBERTS and B. ESTHER STRUCKMEYER. *On Deslothing the Sloth:* PROFESSOR S. W. BRITTON and R. F. KLINE 15

*Scientific Books:*
*Physiology:* DR. ALEXANDER FORBES 17

*Special Articles:*
*Mice as Carriers of Pathogenic Pleuropneumonia-like Microorganisms:* DR. ALBERT B. SABIN. *The Preparation of Pituitary Growth Hormones Free from Lactogenic and Thyrotropic Hormones:* PROFESSOR HERBERT M. EVANS and OTHERS. *The Causative Agent of Infectious Equine Encephalomyelitis in Venezuela:* VLADIMIR KUBES and FRANCISCO A. RIOS 18

*Scientific Apparatus and Laboratory Methods:*
*A Method for Studying Living Mosquito Larvae and Other Small Aquatic Invertebrates:* CARROLL M. WILLIAMS. *A Practical Operating Stand:* DR. CHARLES S. APGAR, JR. 21

*Science News* 10

*Index to Volume LXXXIX* i

SCIENCE: A Weekly Journal devoted to the Advancement of Science, edited by J. MCKEEN CATTELL and published every Friday by

THE SCIENCE PRESS

New York City: Grand Central Terminal
Lancaster, Pa. Garrison, N. Y.
Annual Subscription, $6.00 Single Copies, 15 Cts.

SCIENCE is the official organ of the American Association for the Advancement of Science. Information regarding membership in the Association may be secured from the office of the permanent secretary in the Smithsonian Institution Building, Washington, D. C.

# ORDER AND DISORDER IN PURE LIQUIDS AND SOLUTIONS[1]

By Professor JOEL H. HILDEBRAND
UNIVERSITY OF CALIFORNIA

THE only fault I can find with an occasion such as this is its effect upon my character; I shall doubtless emerge shorn of every shred of modesty I may have possessed on arrival. You will hardly expect me, however, not to feel, and therefore to express, several sources of satisfaction. I am, of course, greatly honored, not only by the action of the Jury of Award, but also by the presence this evening of so many fellow chemists, former students and old friends. Again, my heart is warmed by the kind things that have been said of me by Dr. Harned and Dr. Eyring. Harned was my first research student, and we did together the first work published in this country on the use of the hydrogen electrode to follow the course of a chemical reaction. I can claim only this credit for his subsequent notable scientific career that I did not spoil his natural instinct for research. As for Eyring, I claim a little credit for having helped to create the bracing atmosphere which he breathed as a graduate student in Berkeley and much more credit for having urged him to take the plunge into the liquid state which has resulted in his bringing up some brilliant results.

Further satisfaction is lent by the fact that the award of the Nichols medal is based upon having stimulated research. The problems involved in the theory of solubility are so numerous and complex that it became evident long ago that to catalyze their solution on a broad scale would be a finer achievement than to cultivate only a little of the large field which, years

[1] William H. Nichols Medal Address before the New York Section of the American Chemical Society, March 10, 1939.

ago, only a few of us occupied. I have endeavored, therefore, to analyze the problems, to point out the main hurdles that I was not equipped, myself, to surmount, and to gather the kind of data which would provide honest and crucial tests for any theories, whether my own or those of others.

It is highly gratifying, therefore, to see to-day a wide-spread interest in the liquid state and a number of brilliant investigators devoting attention to it. Symposia on liquids and solutions held recently by the Faraday Society and by our own division of physical and inorganic chemistry have been truly exciting. In my discussion this evening of "Order and Disorder in Pure Liquids and Solutions," I am presenting ideas credit for which I am pleased to share with a number of others, including Bernal, Butler, Debye, Eyring, Fowler, Guggenheim, Kirkwood, Lennard-Jones, London, Menke, Prins, O. K. Rice, Scatchard, G. W. Stewart and, I am eager to add, my own young collaborators.

In discussing order and disorder we shall find it convenient to make frequent use of the term "entropy," a word which is sometimes a bit terrifying. A student once asked me, "What is entropy?," saying that his instructor in engineering thermodynamics had answered that question by saying that "nobody understands entropy, you just use it." Now as a matter of fact, that is rather a gloomy view, and I should like, for my purposes, to review the background of this concept in a very elementary way. Entropy is a term occurring, as you know, in certain thermodynamic equations to account for the fact that heat can not be transformed quantitatively into work, and kinetic theory indicates that it is rather simply related to molecular disorder. The amount of disorder depends upon the number of possible arrangements. In a pure, monatomic, crystalline solid at absolute zero there is no disorder, and therefore no entropy. The molecules are in the position of checkers on a board whose spaces just fit them. However, a solid solution, say of two isotopes, would have entropy, due to the fact that there are a great many ways in which molecules of the two species might be arranged. It comes out that the entropy change in forming a mole of solution from its pure crystalline components is

$$-R(N_1 \ln N_1 + N_2 \ln N_2),$$

where $N_1$ and $N_2$ are their respective mole fractions in the solution.

As a pure solid is heated, it is as if the squares on the checkerboard increased in size, and the pieces, although remaining within the squares, could acquire a certain degree of disorder. Melting would correspond roughly to abolishing the squares, so that a given piece could be anywhere on the board where it could find space with, consequently, a considerable increase in the possibilities of disorder. Vaporization would correspond to spilling the checkers over a large floor space, where a given piece could be almost anywhere within the area, and the possible disorder dependent on the available area, diminished only by the relatively insignificant space occupied by the pieces themselves. The change of entropy of a dilute gas in expanding from $V_1$ to $V_2$ is $R \ln \frac{V_2}{V_1}$, *i.e.*, it is a function of volume only.

Let us return now to a closer examination of the degree of order existing in liquids, and begin with the simplest cases—those liquids whose molecules are effectively spherical. A crude model for such liquids could be a number of tennis balls in a box about 25 per cent. larger than the minimum that would hold them, and violently agitated by vibrating walls. Such an assemblage may be assumed to be in the maximum permitted state of disorder.

If instead of tennis balls we should use sausage-shaped balloons, a certain amount of order would be imposed solely by the fact that the balloons would tend to arrange themselves in parallel array. Again, if each ball or balloon, as the case might be, had a magnet somewhere just beneath the surface, these magnets would encourage some degree of order, however small. Since there are many substances whose molecules are linear, such as carbon dioxide and pentane, or flat, like benzene, we may suspect their liquids of some degree of order. The presence of electric dipoles in molecules such as ethyl iodide should have a similar orienting effect. Any chemical combination should likewise reduce the amount of disorder.

Now there are at least two distinct kinds of evidence available concerning orderly arrangement in the liquid state, one, the well-known diffraction of x-rays, the other, which I am presenting here for the first time, the change in entropy on vaporization. I shall deal first with the latter. All chemists are doubtless familiar with a useful rule discovered long ago by Trouton, which states that the heat of vaporization per mole divided by the boiling point on the absolute scale has the same value, about 21 cals. per degree, for a large number of liquids which we have come to distinguish as "normal." This quotient turned out to be not a constant but to have a slow upward drift with increasing boiling point. Several investigators published empirical formulas to take this into account. In 1915 I noted that a graphic plot of the logarithm of vapor pressure against the logarithm of absolute temperature, as in Fig. 1, indicated that the entropy of vaporization, which is given by the slope of the tangent to such a curve, is approximately the same if the liquids are compared, not at their boiling points, where the pressures are the same, but at temperatures so selected that the final volume of vapor is always the same. This substitute for Trouton's rule is a rather good approximation for normal liquids all the way from nitrogen to silver. We can perhaps see why equal volumes rather than equal pressures should be chosen simply by inspecting the thermodynamic equation, $\Delta S = \Delta V(dp/dT)$. The value of $\Delta S$ depends in part upon $\Delta V$, which in turn depends mainly upon the volume of the vapor.

Since all normal vapor pressure curves, when plotted as in Fig. 1, can be superimposed by sliding along a

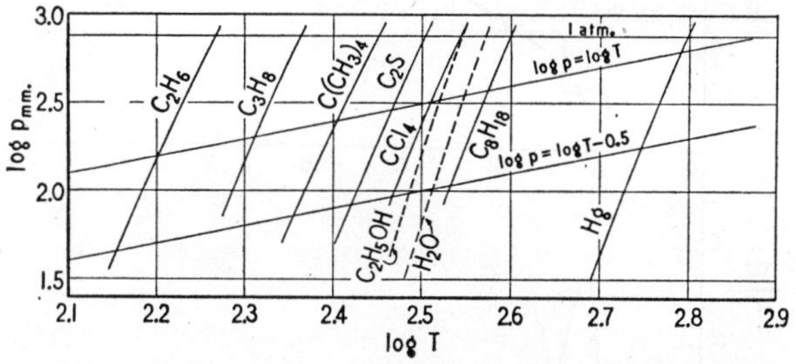


FIG. 1. Uniformity of entropy of vaporization of normal liquids at identical vapor concentration.

line of unit slope, we need only a single point, such as the boiling point, to enable us to draw a good approximation to the entire vapor pressure curve.

This rule should, of course, be true only for liquids in which there is the same amount of disorder. One way to insure this is to compare liquids in which the disorder is a maximum, which should be the case with liquids whose molecules are spherically symmetrical. Such molecules, however, are in the minority. More numerous are those which, as suggested above, have geometrical shapes tending to pack in some sort of ordered array. Still others are electrically polar and this also gives rise to more or less orientation. Now both of these effects show up quite clearly in increasing the entropy of vaporization to constant volume. Table 1 gives the entropy of vaporization at a concentration arbitrarily chosen as 0.0153 moles per liter, corresponding to log $Rc = 0.1$, together with the excess of each over the value for neopentane, a substance whose structure is so symmetrical that it has been selected as a standard of reference for all the others. Let us notice first the figures for the three isomeric pentanes.

TABLE I

STRUCTURAL ENTROPY OF LIQUIDS

| | | | |
|---|---|---|---|
| Hg | 0.0 | $CCl_4$ | 0.6 |
| $C(CH_3)_4$ | 0.0 | $SiCl_4$ | 1.1 |
| i–$C_5H_{12}$ | 0.1 | $SnCl_4$ | 1.7 |
| n–$C_5H_{12}$ | 0.6 | $C(NO_2)_4$ | 2.5 |
| n–$C_6H_{14}$ | 1.4 | $C_6H_6$ | 1.1 |
| n–$C_7H_{16}$ | 1.4 | $C_6H_{12}$ | 1.0 |
| n–$C_8H_{18}$ | 1.1 | $(C_2H_5)_2O$ | 1.7 |
| i–$C_6H_{14}$ (Di-isopropyl) | 0.2 | $(CH_3)_2CO$ | 2.4 |
| | | $C_2H_5OH$ | 6.9 |

The isopentane, with its branched chain, shows a slight excess, while the linear normal pentane shows a much larger excess, 0.6. Going to longer hydrocarbons, with their greater orienting effect, we see a still further increase, while comparing hexane with its much more symmetrical isomer, di-isopropyl, we see a drop from 1.4 to 0.2.

Carbon tetrachloride, although tetrahedral and rotating, has been shown by Menke through x-ray scattering to have some slight degree of structure and in harmony with this we find an excess entropy of 0.6 unit. Silicon and tin tetrachlorides, with their progressively larger, more open structures, show further increases to 1.1 and 1.7, respectively. Tetra-nitro-methane, with distortable nitro groups, shows evidence of still more structure.

Benzene and cyclohexane are free from dipole moment, but their flat rings are doubtless responsible for a marked degree of structure. Their rather high freezing points may be regarded as contributory evidence.

Ether has a moderate dipole, but this is fairly well buried, as shown by the fact that its electric polarization in solution varies only slightly with concentration. In harmony with this, its entropy of vaporization gives evidence of only moderate structure, for which its geometrical form is doubtless to a large degree responsible. To vaporize acetone, which has a larger and more exposed dipole, involves a much greater increase in entropy. Ethyl alcohol shows a greatly enhanced value due to the hydrogen bonds which give the liquid a pronounced structure, confirmed by x-ray scattering. We shall see later that each of these three sources of structure may influence the entropy changes occurring when different liquids are mixed.

The evidence then for the non-polar liquids in Table I indicates that most of them possess some degree of structure and are, therefore, not completely normal in the sense of possessing the most complete randomness of molecular distribution. It is true that if we omit neopentane and mercury, a number of others would differ but to a small extent from their mean value. It is only when we select the comparatively rare substances possessing complete symmetry that we bring to light the different degrees of approach to so-called normal behavior. My colleague, Dr. Pitzer, proposes, quite appropriately, to call liquids such as neopentane "perfect liquids." The fact that perfect liquids are rare does not destroy the usefulness of the concept. Ideal cases are almost as rare in physical science as in human behavior, but whenever a number of instances occur in which the departure from the ideal are small, as with normal liquids, it pays to analyze the implications of the ideal and thus approach more or less closely to an understanding of the actual cases.

What we have called completely random liquid structure does indeed possess a certain kind of structure, due to the fact that no two molecules can occupy the same space simultaneously. Their centers must always remain about one molecule diameter apart. If, therefore, we consider the distribution of molecular centers around any one molecule selected as an origin for polar coordinates, we may imagine a series of thin concentric shells of thickness $dr$ and radius $r$ from the central molecule, as in Fig. 2. It is evident that no such shell could contain any molecular centers until $r$ equaled the molecular collision diameter, which would, of course, vary slightly with the force of the collision and therefore with the temperature. As $r$ increases, the number of molecular centers in a shell would go through a minimum and reach a second maximum when a second layer of molecules is reached. This maximum would, of course, be less pronounced than the first, and so on for successive maxima. When $r$ is large compared to the molecular diameter, the ordering effect of the central molecular disappears and the number of molecular centers in the shell is simply the product of the volume of the shell, $2\pi r^2 dr$, by the molecular density, $N/v$,

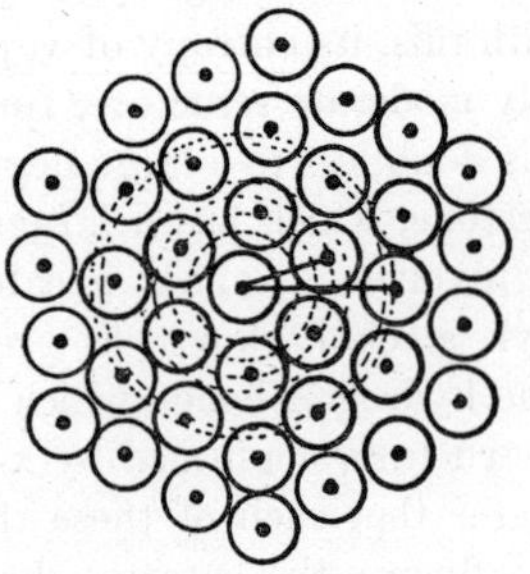

FIG. 2. Structure of a "perfect" liquid.

where $N$ is Avogadro's number and v, the volume per mole. For small values of $r$ this must be corrected by the factor, $W$, which is a function of $r$, as previously explained, whose form is represented in Fig. 3 and which expresses in a most useful way the structure of such a liquid. The form of this function was first determined by Menke for mercury and gallium, and more recently by Gingrich and coworkers for sodium and potassium. As might be expected, the form of the function, expressed in terms of molecular diameter, is essentially the same for these four substances; *cf.* Fig. 4. It varies slightly with the temperature, as one might expect, since thermal agitation and expansion tend to smooth it out to approach unity. My coworker, Dr. W. E. Morrell, was able to construct a model liquid with gelatin balls for molecules, which gave a distribution function of the same form, with a similar temperature dependence.

Having at hand such an expression to describe the structure of a perfect liquid it has been possible to solve an important problem, which is to connect the potential energy between pairs of molecules with the

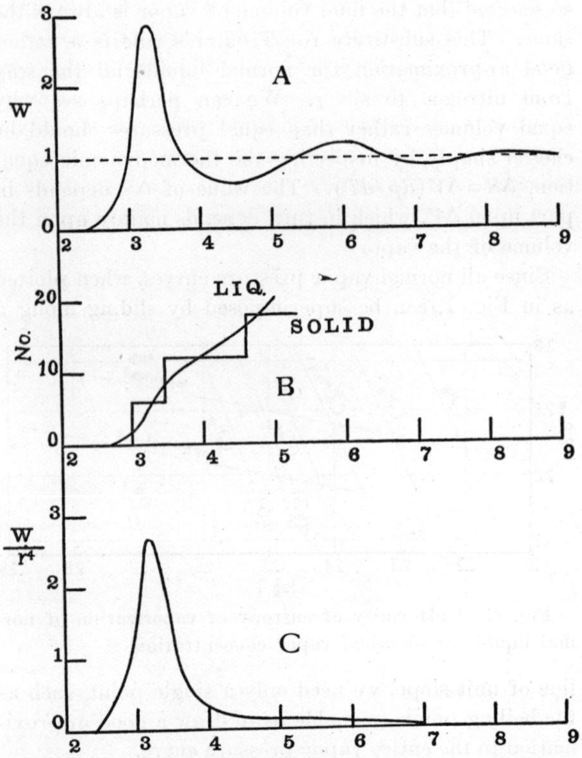



FIG. 3. A. Distribution function for mercury. B. Number of molecules around a central one at distance $r$. C. Potential function, area under which indicates small contribution by molecules beyond first layer to heat of vaporization.

potential energy of a mass of liquid E. This equation is

$$E = \frac{2\pi N^2}{v} \int \varepsilon W r^2 dr. \qquad (1)$$

The important theoretical study by London of the forces between non-polar molecules which result from

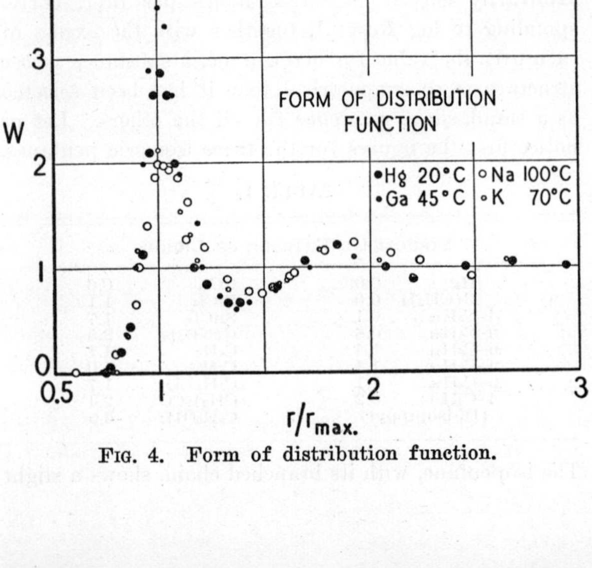



FIG. 4. Form of distribution function.

an interaction between their moving electrons shows that this potential varies inversely with sixth power of the distance, *i.e.*, $\varepsilon = -k/r^6$. If we substitute this expression for attractive potential in the preceding equation and neglect the repulsion we obtain the following expression, which throws light upon the energy of vaporization of a liquid.

$$\Delta E = \frac{-2\pi N^2 k}{V} \int \frac{W}{r^4} dr \qquad (2)$$

The value of the integral can be obtained by the aid of the curve in Fig. 3A and is represented by the area under the curve in Fig. 3C. (Curve B compares the structures of liquid and solid.) This curve shows what a small proportion of the energy of vaporization of a liquid is contributed by the molecules more than one diameter apart.

Again, the function plotted in Fig. 3A varies but slightly with temperature. The value of the integral determined graphically in the case of potassium drops off by some 5 per cent. in this range of temperature. We have known for some time that the energy of vaporization in a normal liquid is almost, but not quite, inversely proportional to its molal volume. We can see from equation (2) that it would be exactly proportional if the value of the integral were constant. As a matter of fact, I have shown recently that the drop of 5 per cent. in the value of the integral, together with the increase in molal volume for potassium when heated from 70° to 395°, accounts quite accurately for the decrease in the energy of vaporization of potassium in going from the lower to the higher temperature. Their ratio was calculated to be 1.154, while the measured values were in the ratio of 1.155. Moreover, I found that when benzene is expanded by the same amount, which in this case occurs between 0 and 72.5°, its energy of vaporization falls off in the same proportion as for potassium through the much longer temperature interval.

Turning now to solutions, let us begin again with the simplest conceivable cases, which will be solutions of spherical molecules of the same size and same molecular field strength. When such species are mixed an individual molecule has the same tendency to escape into a vapor phase as if it were surrounded entirely by its own kind. The number of molecules which so escape into a given vapor space will therefore be proportional to their percentage in the solution, and the solution obeys Raoult's law, the law of an ideal or perfect solution. The increase in free energy is $-RT \ln N_1$ and the increase in entropy is $R \ln N_1$, when one mole of component 1 is transferred from the pure liquid state to a large amount of solution in which the mole fraction is $N_1$.

If the molecules of the second species have not the same size but consist, say, of two normal paraffins of different length, we may expect them to be arranged in some approach to parallel array. An analysis of the number of arrangements possible in such a case shows it to be identical with the number in the preceding case, where molecules were spherical. In both cases, therefore, the degree of disorder is unchanged on mixing the two species, and hence the increase of entropy is the same, *i.e.*, $-R \ln N_1$ for each component. If the two species were as alike as two paraffins, we should expect little or no change in energy on mixing, *i.e.*, there should be no heat of mixing and therefore the free energy of mixing, which determines the vapor pressure, is dependent only on the entropy, hence the solution of long paraffin molecules, like the solution of spherical molecules, should obey Raoult's law, which is indeed the case, even for molecules of such different length as hexane and hexadecane.

Let us next consider spherical molecules of the same size but differing in strength of molecular field, as indicated by different energies of vaporization. In spite of the fact that the molecules with the larger attractive forces tend to squeeze out the molecules of the other component, we may choose temperatures sufficiently high so that thermal agitation may frequently overcome this tendency to segregation and give the same sort of random arrangement as exists in a pure liquid. For such a solution, the entropy of mixing will be the same as for an ideal solution; however, since the different attractive forces give rise to a heat or energy of mixing, the free energy change in forming the solution will not be ideal and the solution will not obey Raoult's law. Nevertheless, the fact that the entropy is ideal yields certain regularities in behavior which induced me to designate such solutions as "regular." If we can discover a satisfactory method for calculating the energy of mixing we can then get the free energy and hence vapor pressures and all other solubility relations. An extension of equation (2) to the case of a solution of two components of identical size, aided by the assumption, which is approximately true in the majority of cases, that the attractive constant between unlike molecules is the geometrical mean of the constants for the like species, gives the equation,

$$\bar{E}_1 - E_1^0 = [(\Delta E_1^0)^{1/2} - (\Delta E_2^0)^{1/2}]^2 N_2^2, \qquad (3)$$

for the energy of transferring a mole of component 1 from the pure state to a solution in which component 2 has a mole fraction, $N_2$. From this we can calculate the free energy and hence vapor pressures and solubilities.

When the molecules of the two species differ in size, the energy of mixing $n_1$ and $n_2$ moles of the components is

$$E = \frac{2\pi N^2}{V} \left[ n_1^2 \int (11) + n_2^2 \int (22) + 2n_1 n_2 \int (12) \right],$$

where $\int (11)$ is an abbreviation for $\varepsilon_{11} W_{11} r^2 dr$, etc. We have to make certain approximations in order to derive from this an equation containing nothing but terms easily accessible to experiment. The resulting approximate equation for regular solutions in general is

$$RT \ ln \ (a_2/N_2 = v_2 \left(\frac{N_1V_1}{N_1V_1 + N_2V_2}\right)^2 \left[\left(\frac{\Delta E_1}{V_1}\right)^{1/2} \left(\frac{\Delta E_2}{V_2}\right)^{1/2}\right]^2 \quad (4)$$

This equation is extremely useful and makes it possible to calculate with a fair degree of accuracy solubilities of substances even in cases where the deviation from Raoult's law is enormous.

A number of the factors discussed above, as well as others, are illustrated strikingly by the solubilities of iodine plotted in Fig. 5. The ordinates are logarithms of the mole fraction of iodine in solution and abscissas

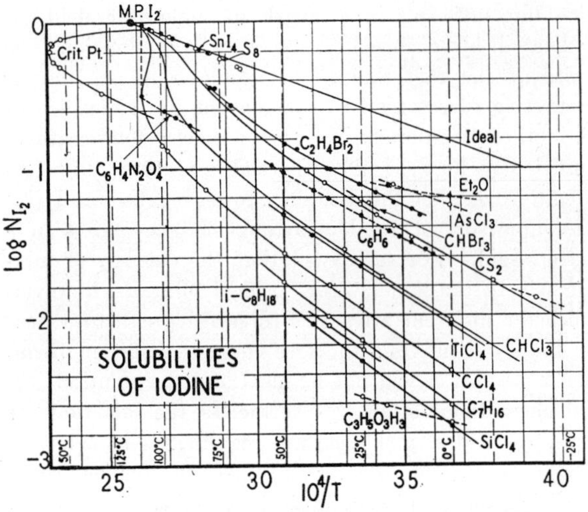


FIG. 5. Solubilities of iodine.

the reciprocal of the absolute temperature. The solid lines represent solutions whose color is violet, like iodine vapor; the broken lines represent red or brown solutions. The former obviously constitute a family of curves and indicate that these solutions are more or less regular; the latter are irregular. The ideal solubility is calculated by aid of the heat of fusion of iodine and difference between the specific heats of the solid and liquid.

Iodine has a high attractive field. Sulfur and stannic iodide do not differ from it much in this respect and are therefore able to mix with iodine in obedience to Raoult's law. As we descend the plot we encounter solvents of steadily diminishing internal pressures which are, therefore, progressively poorer solvents. The spacing of these curves corresponds rather closely to the difference between the internal pressure of iodine and that of the solvent in question. All we need to know in order to calculate the solubility of iodine in a solvent which gives a violet solution, where effects that we may call chemical are absent, is its energy of vaporization per cc. Of course, if we have one point on the solubility curve it is still better, for the general parallelism of the whole family of curves is quite evident.

An interesting extension of the curve for carbon tetrachloride was invited by the S-shape near the melting point, resulting from plotting the equation which fitted the observed points at lower temperatures. This S-shape indicates that there are two solutions of different composition in equilibrium with each other at the same temperature and that on raising the temperature iodine should melt to give a liquid incompletely miscible with carbon tetrachloride. It was estimated that these two liquid phases should have a critical solution temperature somewhat under 180° at a composition of about 71 mole per cent. of iodine. It was impossible to detect the presence of two phases by visual observation because of the opacity of iodine, consequently, a method was devised depending on the difference in density between the two liquid phases. The result was the determination of the liquid liquid-solubility curve shown in the upper left-hand portion of the figure, with a consolute temperature of 161° and a composition of 67 mole per cent. of iodine. This experiment constitutes a striking example of the value of the concept of regular solution. It is the more remarkable because in the region near the critical temperature there is undoubtedly an opposition between the mixing effect of thermal agitation and the segregating effect of different molecular attractions, which gives rise to clustering and departure from the randomness assumed in deriving the equation. Experiment shows, however, that this clustering is fortunately not sufficiently serious to introduce any serious error. This experimental conclusion has been recently brilliantly confirmed by Kirkwood by statistical mechanical analysis.

To recapitulate, there are but very few perfect liquids. There are many normal or approximately perfect liquids; still more which are abnormal due to pronounced lack of symmetry either of shape or of electrostatic field, and there are a number which are highly abnormal due to the presence of hydrogen bonds or other chemical bonds.

Similarly, there are but very few solutions which are ideal or perfect with any high degree of accuracy, at least through any considerable range of composition. A much larger number are approximately regular, *i.e.*, they show ideal entropy of mixing, although their free energy of mixing is not ideal. They may be regarded therefore as approaching a considerably lower, more easily attainable ideal.

Let us now turn our attention to solutions which show marked departure from regularity. Solutions of iodine in ethylene bromide, whose solubility curve is shown in Fig. 5, present an interesting example. The slope of the curve does not correspond to the family of curves for violet solutions, in spite of the fact that these solutions alone among all the divergent solutions are violet in color, indicating absence of any type of solvation. The polar character of ethylene bromide does not suffice to explain this anomaly, for chloroform, which has almost as large a dipole moment, gives regular solutions. The explanation seems rather to lie in a change in the structure and hence in the entropy of the ethylene bromide caused by changing temperature and iodine content. The dipole moments of ethylene chloride, and doubtless also of ethylene bromide, are highly dependent upon the particular inert solvent used in measuring them. It is evident that the rotation possible about the carbon to carbon bond introduces possibilities of structural change in the liquid which we may, at least at present, regard as responsible for the regular entropy of the solutions of iodine in this solvent.

The dotted curves in Fig. 5 all correspond to solutions which are brown in color and whose absorption bands shift with temperature, indicating changes in structure attending changes in degrees of solvation and, in certain cases also, of degree of association of the solvent.

An interesting departure from regularity has been recently reported by Scatchard and Wood for a solution that might have been expected to behave quite regularly, namely, benzene and cyclohexane. It was shown, however, that the heat and free energy of mixing are different, indicating an increase of entropy upon forming the solution. If we turn back to the evidence presented in Table I that both benzene and cyclohexane possess some structure, we can see that a decrease in the amount of structure when the two components are mixed would account for the increase in entropy. Since benzene rings are flat while cyclohexane rings are puckered, it is easy to see how the two slightly different kinds of structure would tend to interfere with each other and give rise to an increase in the general disorder.

This point of view has suggested itself so recently that not many cases have been examined to test its general validity. However, the cases so far examined give great promise that the theory will prove useful.

The large deviations, not only from ideal but also from regular behavior that accompany chemical combination are highly specific, and often strain our skill in predicting the strength of chemical union. We are assisted, however, by a large body of knowledge regarding the relative strengths of acids and bases and can safely predict that the stronger the union between a basic and acidic substance the more strongly will their solution deviate from regular behavior in the direction of increased solubility.

Again, there are only a few types of strong hydrogen bonds, since strong union through hydrogen occurs only with nitrogen, oxygen and fluorine. There is considerable hope that we may be able to set up approximate values of the strength of the bond between the like and unlike combinations of these three elements, which values will be subject to modification depending upon the rest of the molecule. We may hope that in many cases this modification may prove to be small, *e.g.,* the strength of the bond in alcohol can not be changed very much by the size of the alkyl group. The amino acids and proteins, despite their almost infinite variety, contain but a few types of hydrogen bonds, and we may hope to arrive at a good deal of understanding of their solubility relations by the aid of this simplification.

I should like to conclude by emphasizing a particular liquid structure which has a greater practical importance for us than any other, namely, the structure of water. We are still under the spell of an over-simplified theory of solution, which regarded the solvent mainly as affording space in which the solute could masquerade as a gas. It is true that we have now ascribed to this space a dielectric constant, but most papers dealing with aqueous solutions, particularly those of electrolytes, ascribe no further physical properties to the water than this. Any deviation from the laws of perfect solution, which for such substances can at best be true only at high dilution, are often "explained" by subtracting some of the water from its role as solvent and calling it water of hydration. What this can mean, physically, is often obscure, for all the water molecules are linked together by hydrogen bonds except in so far as they are momentarily disturbed by thermal agitation and, if the solute is chemically bound to some of the water and this is in turn chemically bound to water molecules farther removed, I do not see how one can draw a definite boundary between the water which is acting as solvent and that which is acting as water of hydration.

It seems to me that if we were not so influenced by the accident of the particular historical approach to the theory of solution upon which most of us have been brought up, we would not find it so difficult to approach an aqueous solution from the opposite point of view, which is to think of water as a chemical substance whose role in the solution is just as dignified as that of the solute and which is, moreover, a substance having a high degree of structure. We may then inquire what might be expected to happen if we would introduce into this structure solutes of different types, including, first, ions, small and large, with single or multiple charges; second, molecules with dipoles or, third, molecules which themselves can participate in the formation of hydrogen bonds. Latimer, in a series of important studies, has already shown that the entropy of solution of ions can be explained on the basis of alterations in the structure of the water. I venture to assert that the fruitfulness of such an approach is far from being exhausted.

For a long while we were satisfied with the classification of liquids into normal liquids, polar liquids and fused salt solutions. It became evident, however, that the mere fact of dipole moment was inadequate to account for solubility relations. We find, on the one hand, that iodine dissolves in chloroform, which is polar, and in carbon tetrachloride, which is non-polar, to give approximately regular solutions in both cases. Again, naphthalene, with zero dipole moment, dissolves in nitrobenzene, with a very large moment, to give an almost perfect solution. The polar character of the nitrobenzene causes little or no tendency for it to associate with itself rather than with the non-polar solute. We find, moreover, that although solubility in water has usually been regarded as proportional merely to the polar character of the substance in question, dipole moment alone is actually a very misleading guide. A striking illustration of this is given in Table II.

TABLE II
SOLUBILITY OF LIQUIDS IN WATER, 20°

| | Per cent. | $\mu \times 10^{18}$ |
|---|---|---|
| Benzene | 0.06 | 0. |
| Nitrobenzene | 0.19 | 4.19 |
| Aniline | 3.49 | 1.51 |
| Phenol | 8.2 | 1.70 |
| Ethyl iodide | 0.40 | 1.66 |
| Ethyl alcohol | ∞ | 1.70 |
| Propyl chloride | 0.27 | 2.0 |
| Propyl iodide | 0.11 | 1.6 |
| Propyl alcohol | ∞ | 1.7 |
| Water | ... | 1.85 |

We see that the solubilities of benzene and its three substitution products in water do not at all follow their dipole moments. These solubilities do, however, accord with the amount of hydrogen bond formation that may be expected in solutions of water with aniline and phenol, respectively. A similar difference exists between ethyl and propyl halides and alcohols. It is the ability of the hydroxyl of the alcohol or the phenol or the amino group in aniline to enter more or less into the structure of the water which accounts for their solubility. The structure of ice is an open, continuous structure, like that of trydimite, and contains no permanent individual molecules. The structure of water at lower temperature is the same, more or less broken down by thermal agitation. Hydroxyl containing substances such as the alcohols are similar except for the fact that the substituted groups diminish the number of hydrogen bonds. The profound difference between liquids containing ordinary dipoles, such as acetone and chlorobenzene and liquids containing

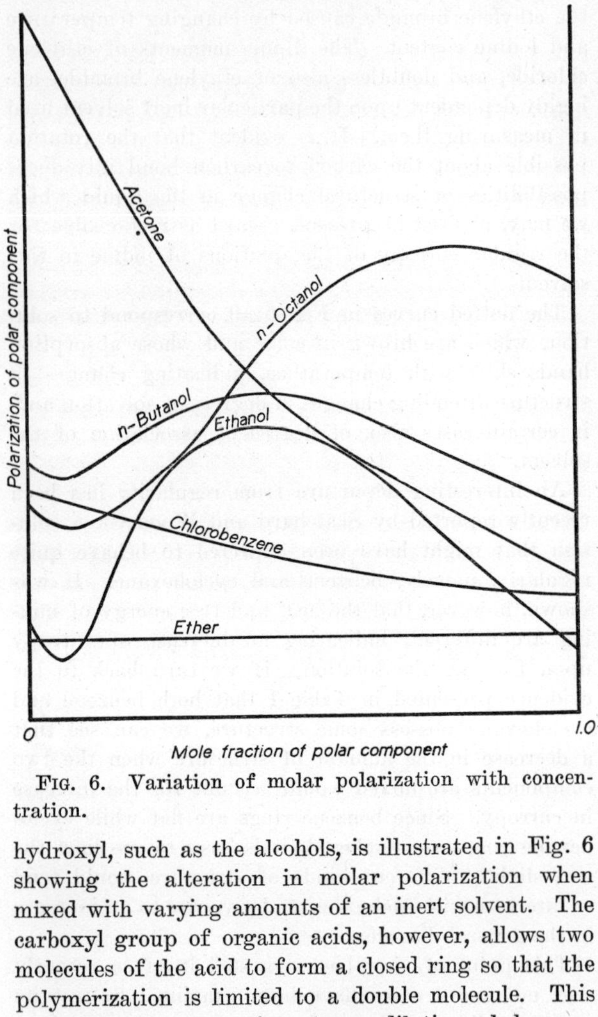


FIG. 6. Variation of molar polarization with concentration.

hydroxyl, such as the alcohols, is illustrated in Fig. 6 showing the alteration in molar polarization when mixed with varying amounts of an inert solvent. The carboxyl group of organic acids, however, allows two molecules of the acid to form a closed ring so that the polymerization is limited to a double molecule. This molecule may, except in extreme dilutions, behave as a constituent of regular solutions.

# OBITUARY

## DAVID TODD

WITH the passing of David Todd, on June 1 in Lynchburg, Virginia, at the age of 84, Amherst College lost another of the distinguished group of professors who added much to its prestige around the beginning of the century. The names of Tyler, Emerson, Olds, Loomis, Todd and the others were well known and respected both within and without the walls; and the last named of these was likely to receive the vote of the graduating class as the best known of all.

David Todd was born on March 19, 1855, in Lake Ridge, New York, the son of Sereno Edwards and

Rhoda Peck Todd, and a descendant of Johnathan Edwards. He enrolled in Columbia College, New York, in 1870, and entered Amherst College in 1873, where he received the A.B. degree in 1875, with membership in Phi Beta Kappa. He received the honorary Ph.D. degree from Washington and Jefferson College in 1888. After an absence of six years, in which he served under Simon Newcomb at the U. S. Naval Observatory in Washington, he returned to Amherst, in 1881, to take the new chair of astronomy. He was appointed professor of astronomy in 1892; he also served as secretary of the faculty of the college from 1891 to 1909, and was professor of astronomy and higher mathematics in Smith College from 1882 to 1887. He became professor emeritus in 1920.

More than a hundred technical and popular articles were contributed by Dr. Todd to various periodicals; they relate to solar eclipse problems, the solar parallax as derived from the transit of Venus, the orbits of the four bright satellites of Jupiter, the search for a trans-neptunian planet and other subjects. He contributed to Webster's Dictionary and to the Encyclopaedia Britannica. His best-known book is the "New Astronomy," first published in 1897, which has gone into many editions and is translated into Hungarian, Turkish and Chinese. He was a fellow of the American Association for the Advancement of Science, a member of the American Astronomical Society, the Washington Philosophical Society, the Astronomische Gesellschaft and honorary fellow of the Sociedad Geografica de Lima, Peru. He designed and supervised the construction of the Observatory of Smith College, and was instrumental in procuring funds to build the Amherst College Observatory, completed under his supervision in 1905, and to equip it with the excellent 18-inch refracting telescope by the Clarks.

Dr. Todd's interest in solar eclipses led him to many parts of the world. He was in charge of the National Academy of Sciences expedition to Japan in 1887, the U. S. Scientific Expedition to West Africa in 1889, and the Amherst expeditions to Japan in 1896, to Tripoli in 1900, to the Dutch East Indies in 1901, to Tripoli again in 1905 and to Russia in 1914. He invented an automatic device for photographing eclipses, and his misfortune with clouds on some of these occasions led to the keeping of meteorological records at selected stations for several years in advance of the eclipse. In addition, he was invited to direct the observations of the transit of Venus of 1882 at the Lick Observatory, then under construction on Mount Hamilton, California, and he cooperated with the astronomers of the Lowell Observatory in an expedition to Chile to photograph the planet Mars around the favorable opposition of 1907.

Dr. Todd's hobby was aviation, beginning as early as the 1880's. He took part in a number of balloon flights. He was founder member of the Aero Club of America, a member of the Board of the National Advisory Association of Aeronautics and of the Board of Governors of the Aerial League of America. In 1908, he founded at Amherst one of the first college aviation clubs, the Amherst Aero Club, the forerunner of the present Amherst College Flying Club.

Dr. Todd married Mabel Loomis, in 1879, who died in 1932. He is survived by his daughter, Mrs. W. V. Bingham.

ROBERT H. BAKER
HARVARD OBSERVATORY

## RECENT DEATHS

DR. CHARLES ADDISON ELLIOTT, professor of medicine at the Medical School of Northwestern University, chief of the medical service of Passavant Hospital, Chicago, died on June 26 at the age of sixty-six years.

DR. HARRY VICTOR ATKINSON, professor of physiology and pharmacology at the School of the Medical Sciences of the University of South Dakota, died suddenly on May 7 at the age of fifty-two years.

GUY PINNER, chief engineer of the American Cyanamid Company, died on June 26 at the age of fifty-one years.

EMMA SAREPTA YULE, pioneer in educational work in Juneau, Alaska, and in the Philippines and for fifteen years editor of the *Philippine Agriculturist*, died in Los Angeles on April 16.

PROFESSOR HARRY HUNTINGTON BARNUM, head of the department of mathematics at Robert College, Istanbul, Turkey, has died at the age of sixty-one years. He had been a member of the college faculty for thirty-nine years.

# SCIENTIFIC EVENTS

## EXCHANGE OF VISITS BETWEEN THE ROYAL SOCIETY AND THE KAISER WILHELM GESELLSCHAFT

IN the autumn of 1938, following a suggestion of the president of the Kaiser Wilhelm Gesellschaft, arrangements were made by the president of the Royal Society of London, Sir William Bragg, and representatives of the Kaiser Wilhelm Gesellschaft, for an exchange of visits between these two bodies. The Kaiser Wilhelm Gesellschaft, founded in 1911 at the suggestion of the Kaiser Wilhelm II, has at its aim the encouragement of the natural and human sciences, primarily by establishing and maintaining research institutes for natural science in Germany.

This exchange of visits was welcomed by the Royal Society, which, since its foundation in 1662, has always sought to maintain, irrespective of race or politics, the liveliest interest in the work of men of science throughout the world. Consequently, arrangements were made for two fellows of the society, Professor F. G. Donnan, emeritus professor of chemistry in the University of London, and Professor A. J. Clark, professor of materia medica in the University of Edinburgh, to visit Germany in March; at the express wish of the Kaiser Wilhelm Gesellschaft for a lecture on a non-scientific subject, Professor Dover Wilson, the eminent Shakespearean scholar, was invited by the Royal Society to visit Berlin to lecture. The visits, which took place in March and April, were highly successful. The visitors were most hospitably entertained by their German colleagues and were afforded facilities for visiting laboratories and research institutes.

The Royal Society is entertaining during this month four German men of science. They are Freiherr von Verschuer, of the University of Frankfort-on-Main; Professor R. Kuhn, of the Kaiser Wilhelm Institut für Medizinische Forschung, Heidelberg; Professor F. Wever, of the Kaiser Wilhelm Institut für Eisensforschung Forschung, Düsseldorf, and Professor Otto Hahn, of the Kaiser Wilhelm Institut für Chemie, Berlin-Dahlem. Freiherr von Verschuer and Professor Kuhn delivered lectures before the Royal Society on June 8 and 9, respectively; Professor Wever spoke on June 22 on metallurgical research, and Professor Hahn spoke at the Royal Institution on June 23 on the fission of uranium nuclei by neutrons.—*Nature*.

## SURVEY OF THE GEOLOGY OF THE CENTRAL ANDES IN PERU

DR. J. V. HARRISON, university demonstrator and lecturer in the department of geology at the University of Oxford, who is leading an expedition to Peru, is reported by a correspondent of the London *Times* to have sailed from Liverpool on June 17, to study and map the geology of a part of the Central Andes of Peru in the region between Canta, Huaauco and Huancayo. Dr. Harrison, who was in the same part of Peru in 1925, is accompanied by J. D. Weir, of University College, London, and Saskatoon University, who is a Rhodes scholar and a Burdett-Coutts scholar and who is working in the department of geology; C. H. Kearny, of the Queen's College, who is a Rhodes scholar from Princeton, and M. H. Donald, of Mealsgate, Cumberland, who has previously collected for the British Museum.

The expedition will collect fossils and specimens of rocks from the region for the British Museum (Natural History). Its plans have been approved by the Royal Geographical Society. The area to be mapped is part of an equilateral triangle, the apices of which are Tarma, Cerro de Pasco and Canta, with the center of the triangle roughly 80 miles northeast of Lima.

How much will be achieved depends entirely upon the weather, which in August and September can not be relied on. The altitudes range from 15,000 feet to 18,000 feet, and the region is subject to violent storms during the break-up of the settled July (winter) weather. Much of the time will be spent under canvas, and the expedition will rely on mule transport, with native muleteers.

Mr. Weir was with survey parties of the Canadian Geological Survey in two successive summers before he went to Oxford, and he has this year been awarded a third part of the Daniel Pidgeon Fund by the Geological Society. The first recipient of this award, in 1908, was the present professor of geology at Oxford, Professor James A. Douglas, who himself did much of his early field work in Peru and is an authority on the geology of that country.

Mr. Kearny, who collected archeological material in northwestern Mexico for a year before going to Oxford, will join the party at Lima. The expedition will return in October.

## THE MAGELLANIC EXPEDITION OF THE FIELD MUSEUM

THE "Magellanic Expedition" of Field Museum of Natural History, sponsored by Stanley Field, president of the museum, which will largely retrace in the farthest reaches of South America the steps of the early Spanish explorer for which it is named, planned to sail from New York for Lima, Peru, during the first week in July. Those sailing include Karl P. Schmidt, curator of amphibians and reptiles, his son, John Schmidt, field assistant, and Colin C. Sanborn, curator of mammals. They will be joined, probably in September, by Dr. Wilfred H. Osgood, chief of the department of zoology.

The expedition will attempt to complete the fragmentary knowledge of the fauna of the southern half of South America. All classes of animals will be sought—mammals, birds, reptiles, fishes, insects, marine invertebrates, etc. It is planned to explore the shores of the Straits of Magellan and the Island of Tierra del Fuego to the extreme southern tip of the continent.

Upon arrival in Lima, Mr. Schmidt and his companions will cross southern Peru by rail to Arequipa and Lake Titicaca, where collecting will begin. Crossing the lake by steamer, collections will be made in Bolivia. Further penetration into the interior of South America will be made variously by airplane, rail, boat, pack animals and afoot. After the arrival of Dr. Osgood the expedition will proceed through Chile down to the southernmost tip of the continent. It is in the region of the Straits of Magellan and Tierra del Fuego that it is expected the most important research will be conducted.

Dr. Osgood has made the following statement:

This region has not been scientifically explored by zoologists for more than one hundred years. In 1834, Darwin collected in this region, during the famous cruise of the *Beagle*. Since that time it has been neglected. Although Darwin made excellent collections of the fauna, which are still preserved in the British Museum, there are many gaps which remain to be filled in available knowledge of the natural history of the region. The Darwin collections are not satisfactory from to-day's standards because, naturally, facilities and techniques for the collecting and preservation of specimens had not been developed in his time to the point since achieved. On the Field Museum expedition it is expected that data will be obtained which will make possible the completion and revision of present knowledge based on the Darwin collections. It may be confidently expected further that we shall obtain examples of many species of animals still unknown or hitherto unrepresented in any collections.

Although the expedition will be concerned primarily with assembling specimens for research collections of the museum, specimens will be sought also for addition to the public exhibits and for one or two habitat groups showing animals in scenes reproducing their natural environments.

## A FISHERIES BIOLOGICAL LABORATORY ON THE GULF COAST

THE need has long been felt for an adequate marine biological laboratory on the Gulf Coast. To achieve this end the Bureau of Fisheries took possession of the abandoned Pensacola, Florida, Quarantine Station in September, 1937. Since that time, with the aid of grants from the Public Works and Works Progress Administrations, much has been accomplished toward enlarging existing facilities and adapting them to the needs of biological research. While the program of construction is not yet completed it is sufficiently far advanced to merit a statement of the facilities which will soon be available for biological research related to fisheries.

The station is located on a ballast rock island of 14 acres about seven miles from Pensacola. The island is about a half mile from the highway, but construction of a bridge and road to the station is under way. The location is one of the most favorable on the Gulf Coast, for it is relatively central and the marine fauna and flora are characteristic of the coast as a whole. The island is in Santa Rosa Sound, protected from storm damage by the 45-mile long Santa Rosa Island. The water of the sound is almost always clear and of a salinity generally ranging from 20 to 25 parts per 1,000 save in times of extreme precipitation, when it may fall to about 15 p.p. 1,000. Within a few miles are various bays, bayous and rivers offering any type of marine habitat. The gulf beach, where the water is always remarkably clear, is only a mile away. In the immediate vicinity an extensive fishery is carried on for red snapper, grouper, mackerel, mullet, flounder, pompano, shrimp, oysters and crabs. Within a mile of the laboratory one may find any type of bottom from firm sand to soft mud. The island itself, consisting of ballast rock, attracts a wide variety of marine life.

The laboratory building has been considerably enlarged and consists of the following rooms: a general research room 23 feet wide by 45 feet long, five private research rooms, a chemical research room, a dark room for experimental and photographic purposes, a stock room, an office, a large library and reading room, and a specimen room or museum 34 feet wide by 60 feet long. Running salt water will be provided wherever required. On the grounds are two concrete experimental tanks 15 by 30 by 5 feet deep, and two 10 by 20 feet by 5 deep. These will be supplied with running seawater.

Accommodations for a limited number of investigators are provided in a dormitory building which consists of five 2-bed rooms, a bath, a kitchen and a large combination dining and living room. In addition there is a large room, which will accommodate four beds, and a separate bath. Also on the island are a work shop, boat house and residence buildings for the accommodation of the regular staff. Two motor boats and several skiffs with outboard motors are available.

Those interested in obtaining further information may address the director, Dr. A. E. Hopkins, Bureau of Fisheries, P. O. Box 1456, Pensacola, Fla.

## AWARDS OF THE AMERICAN GEOGRAPHICAL SOCIETY

THE American Geographical Society of New York has announced the award of the Cullum Geographical Medal for 1938 to Emmanuel de Martonne, professor of geography at the University of Paris. The Charles P. Daly Medal for 1939 has been awarded to Herbert John Fleure, professor of geography at the University of Manchester, and the David Livingstone Centenary Medal for 1939 has been awarded to John R. Rymill in recognition of his scientific achievement and exploration in the southern hemisphere. Presentations of the medals will be made later in the year.

Professor de Martonne's special field is physical geography, a subject on which he has written many volumes, including "Europe Centrale" and the standard manual "Traité de géographie physique." He is president of the International Geographical Union and is one of the editors of the *Annales de Géographie*. In 1916–17 he was visiting professor at Columbia University. Among previous recipients of the Cullum Medal have been Robert E. Peary, Robert F. Scott, Sir Ernest H. Shackleton and Albert I, Prince of Monaco.

Professor Herbert John Fleure is known for his work on human geography. He is honorary secretary of the British Geographical Association and honorary editor of the magazine *Geography*, published by the association, and has taken an active part in the Regional Survey Movement in Great Britain. He is the author of several books and a number of articles, some of which have appeared in *The Geographical Review*, and is the joint author of "The Corridors of Time." Among those who have received the Charles P. Daly Medal in the past have been Roald Amundsen, Vilhjalmur Stefansson, Sir Francis Younghusband, Robert A. Bartlett and Roy Chapman Andrews.

John R. Rymill, to whom the David Livingstone Centenary Medal has been awarded, served as surveyor on two British Arctic air route expeditions led by H. J. Watkins. When, in 1932, on the second of these expeditions, Watkins died, Mr. Rymill succeeded him as leader. In 1935 he organized the British Graham Land expedition, which from January of that year to March, 1937, carried on, under his leadership, highly important, accurate, detailed survey work in Graham Land on the Antarctic Continent. The David Livingstone Centenary Medal has been awarded in the past to Theodore Roosevelt, Richard Evelyn Byrd, Hjalmar Riiser-Larsen and Lincoln Ellsworth.

Honorary membership in the society has been awarded to Sir Wilfred Grenfell for his contributions to geographical knowledge concerning the Labrador Peninsula; Henri Baulig, geomorphologist and professor of geography at the University of Strasbourg, and Giotto Dainelli, professor of geology and physical geography at the University of Florence.

Corresponding memberships have been awarded to: Ernst Antevs, research associate of the Carnegie Institution of Washington; Ludwig Leonhard Mecking, professor of geography at the University of Münster; William E. Rudolph, a civil engineer who has carried out extensive explorations in South America; Paul Gerhard Schott, retired section chief of the Deutsche Seewarte and honorary professor at the University of Hamburg, and Laurence Dudley Stamp, a reader in economic geography at the University of London and director of the Land Utilization Survey of Great Britain.

# SCIENTIFIC NOTES AND NEWS

THE University of St. Andrews will confer the honorary degree of doctor of laws at a graduation ceremonial to be held in Dundee during the visit of the British Association for the Advancement of Science to that city, on the following: William Boyd; Broughty Ferry; Frederick Tom Brooks, professor of botany at the University of Cambridge; William Graham Campbell, lecturer in orthodontics at the Dental School of the university; Charles Galton Darwin, director of the National Physical Laboratory; Alexander McKenzie, professor of chemistry emeritus at University College, Dundee; Sir Albert Charles Seward, until 1936 professor of botany at the University of Cambridge, president of the British Association; Professor Richard Vynne Southwell, professor of engineering science at the University of Oxford, and Sir Aurel Stein.

THE degree of doctor of science was conferred by the University of Pittsburgh at the commencement exercises on June 14 on Dr. Davenport Hooker, professor and head of the department of anatomy in the School of Medicine.

THE honorary degree of doctor of science was conferred by the Ohio Wesleyan University at its commencement on June 12 on Dr. C. E. Ferree, director of the research laboratory of physiological optics of the Johns Hopkins University.

THE honorary degree of doctor of science was conferred upon Admiral Leo Otis Colbert, director of the U. S. Coast and Geodetic Survey, by Tufts College, Massachusetts, at its eighty-third commencement exercises, by President Leonard Carmichael. The citation read: "The world has never needed maps more than it does to-day. Leo Otis Colbert, gifted investigator and cartographer-in-chief of our coasts, I confer upon you the degree of Doctor of Science."

THE annual award of the American Pharmaceutical Manufacturers' Association was presented to Dr. Nathan B. Eddy and Dr. Lyndon F. Small, of the U. S. Public Health Service, at the recent annual meeting, in recognition of the "fundamental and outstanding studies of the chemistry, pharmacology and therapeutics of morphine derivatives for the alleviation of human suffering."

FOR his paper presented at the 1938 annual meeting of the American Society for Testing Materials on "Drying Shrinkage of Concrete as Affected by Many Factors," R. W. Carlson, associate professor of civil engineering at Massachusetts Institute of Technology, has been awarded the Charles B. Dudley Medal of the society. This medal, which commemorates the name of the first president of the society, is awarded "to the author of the paper which is of outstanding merit constituting an original contribution on research." The presentation was made at the annual meeting on June 28.

THE Andrew Carnegie Gold Medals of the British Iron and Steel Institute for 1938 have been awarded to Dr. James White, of Glasgow, for his paper on "Equilibrium at High Temperatures in Systems Containing Iron Oxides," and to Dr. W. Ruff, of Wetzlar-Lahn, Germany, for his paper on "The Running Quality of Liquid Malleable Iron and Steel," published in 1936.

A PORTRAIT of Dr. Edward Lee Thorndike, professor of educational psychology and director of the Division of Psychology of the Institute of Educational Research at Teachers College, Columbia University, has been presented to Wesleyan University, from which he graduated in 1895. The portrait, which was painted by Howard L. Hildebrandt, was placed on public view on June 18 in the Honors College of the university.

VISCOUNT NUFFIELD and John Davison Rockefeller have been elected fellows of the Royal Society in accordance with the terms of Statute 12, which provides for the election of persons who, in the opinion of the council, "either have rendered conspicuous service to the cause of science, or are such that their election would be of signal service to the society."

DR. ALBRECHT PENCK, professor of geography at Berlin, has been elected a foreign member of the Vienna Academy of Sciences. The honorary doctorate of the University of Berlin has also been conferred on Dr. Penck.

M. LÉON BINET, professor of physiology in the Paris Faculty of Medicine, has been elected a member of the Académie de Médecine in the section of biological sciences, in succession to the late Dr. Antoine Béclère.

DR. HANS SPEMANN, professor of embryology at Freiburg in Breslau, celebrated his seventieth birthday on June 27; Dr. Walther Nernst, professor of physics at Berlin, celebrated his seventy-fifth birthday on June 25, and Dr. Max Planck, professor of physics at Berlin, celebrated the sixtieth anniversary of his doctorate on June 28.

DR. G. DONALD HUDSON has been appointed professor of geography at Northwestern University. For the past five years he has been with the Tennessee Valley Authority, first as chief of the Section of Geography and later of the Land Planning Division.

DR. MALCOLM BRUS KILDALE, of Salt Lake City, Utah, has been appointed successor to Cyrus Fisher Tolman, who retired from the chair of economic geology at Stanford University in 1938.

DR. LEO HESS, privat-docent in the department of internal medicine at the University of Vienna, arrived on June 27 in Waltham, Mass., to take up his work in the School of Medicine of Middlesex University.

DR. OWEN HERBERT WILLIAMS, lecturer in clinical surgery, honorary surgeon to the Royal Liverpool United Hospital and honorary surgeon to the Liverpool Radium Institute, has been appointed professor of surgery at the University of Liverpool, in succession to Professor R. E. Kelly, who is retiring on reaching the age limit.

DR. J. F. MCCLENDON has resigned as professor of physiological chemistry at the Medical School of the University of Minnesota, in order to accept the research professorship of physiology at the Hahnemann Medical College, Philadelphia.

DR. WINIFRED GOLDRING, assistant state paleontologist of the New York State Museum at Albany, has been promoted to the position of state paleontologist to succeed Dr. Rudolf Ruedemann, who retired on November 1, 1937. Dr. Goldring has had a provisional appointment since August 1, 1938.

DR. WILLARD M. HOEHN, research associate in biochemistry, Mayo Foundation and Mayo Clinic, has resigned to become endocrinological chemist at George A. Breon and Company, Inc., Research Laboratories, Kansas City, Mo.

DR. WILLARD C. RAPPLEYE, dean of the College of Physicians and Surgeons of Columbia University, was elected president of an advisory council established at a meeting held on June 24 at Chicago, by representatives of the Association of American Medical Colleges, the American Hospital Association, the Catholic Hospital Association, the Federation of State Medical Boards of the U. S. A., the Advisory Board for Medical Specialties, the National Board of Medical Examiners, the American College of Physicians, the American College of Surgeons, the Association of American Universities, the American Association for the Advancement of Science and the American Public Health Association. The purpose of the council is to correlate the efforts of universities, hospitals, licensing bodies, public health associations and boards of specialists.

*Nature* reports that the British Medical Research Council has appointed the following committees to advise and assist in promoting investigations into problems of preventive medicine: Sir W. Wilson Jameson, dean of the London School of Hygiene and Tropical Medicine, *chairman,* J. H. Brincker, J. Fenton, J. Ferguson, W. M. Frazer, L. H. R. Harries, A. Bradford Hill, W. D. Hood, J. R. Hutchinson, R. A. McCance, A. S. M. MacGregor, R. H. Parry, Professor R. M. F. Picken, W. M. Scott, J. C. Spence, Professor W. W. C. Topley, D. K. M. Chalmers, of the National Institute for Medical Research, *secretary.*

PROFESSOR ERNEST B. BABCOCK, head of the Division of Genetics of the College of Agriculture of the

University of California, has been invited to serve as a vice-president of the seventh International Botanical Congress, which will be held in Stockholm in July, 1940.

THE John and Mary Markle Foundation of New York recently made a grant of $3,000 for studies of liver poisoning in the department of chemistry at the Medical College of Virginia. This project will be under the direction of Dr. J. C. Forbes, associate professor of biochemistry at the college. The Dazian Foundation for Medical Research has also made a grant of $700 to the college for research in preventive medicine.

THE Committee on Scientific Research of the American Medical Association has made a grant to Dr. Max Schnitker, junior attending surgeon of the neurosurgical service of Toledo Hospital, Ohio, for investigations on the Berger Rhythm to be carried out in the department for medical research. A grant has been made to the department of surgery of the University of Chicago for aid in continuing work on the problem of ascertaining the mechanism of the recovery of blood pressure on completely sympathectomized dogs.

PROFESSOR G. D. HALE CARPENTER, who succeeded Sir Edward Boulton as head of the Hope department of zoology (entomology) of the University Museum, Oxford, has accepted an invitation from the chairman of the National Research Council in Washington, D. C., to attend the Pacific Science Congress in California, which will be held from July 24 to August 12. In California, he will be met by E. P. Mumford, an official member of the congress, now at Columbia University, on leave of absence from Oxford.

STANLEY D. WILSON, dean of the College of Natural Sciences and professor of organic chemistry at Yenching University, Peiping, China, is returning to the United States for a year's furlough beginning this July.

THE officers, executive committee and members of the Division of Geology and Geography, National Research Council, for the year beginning July 1, 1939, are as follows: *Chairman,* Chester R. Longwell; *Vice-chairman,* Preston E. James; *Executive Committee,* Chester R. Longwell, Preston E. James, Edson S. Bastin, Stephen R. Capps, Charles C. Colby, George Tunell; *Representatives of Societies,* Stephen R. Capps and John L. Rich, Geological Society of America; George Tunell, Mineralogical Society of America; Charles E. Resser, Paleontological Society; Preston E. James and C. Warren Thornthwaite, Association of American Geographers; Charles B. Hitchcock, American Geographical Society; Edson S. Bastin, Society of Economic Geologists; Robert B. Sosman, American Ceramic Society; F. H. Lahee, American Association of Petroleum Geologists; *Members at Large,* Norman L. Bowen, Charles C. Colby and Chester R. Longwell.

FOR some time past it has been occasionally impossible to accommodate investigators from other universities at the Biological Laboratory of the Atkins Institution, Soledad, Cienfuegos, Cuba. This difficulty has usually arisen from the fact that a good many visitors from Cambridge, both zoological and botanical, use Harvard House at Soledad during the summer months. This situation now is entirely changed. A new building has been erected with comfortable sleeping accommodations for sixteen persons so that there should be no question whatever, in the future, of overcrowding. Harvard University, therefore, will welcome inquiries concerning the facilities which are offered at the Cuban Station, where board and lodging are provided at $2.50 a day. Inquiries concerning the station may be addressed to Thomas Barbour, Custodian, Museum of Comparative Zoology, Cambridge, Massachusetts.

THE department of geology of the University of Kansas plans an enlarged program for the coming year. New curricula leading to the degree of B.S. in geology are to be introduced, with provision for options in general, petroleum, mining or geophysical work. On the graduate level, new courses in stratigraphy, ground water geology and geologic interpretation of aerial photographs will be offered by Dr. R. C. Moore, Dr. K. K. Landes and Dr. H. T. U. Smith, respectively. Dr. Robert M. Dreyer will be added to the instructional staff, and Dr. Landes will begin serving as chairman of the department, succeeding Dr. Moore, who has withdrawn in order to devote more time to the expanded program of the State Geological Survey.

THAT the leaders of science in Czecho-Slovakia have made every endeavor to continue scientific investigations during the past fateful year is indicated, according to *Nature,* by the fifteenth annual report of their National Research Council. At the annual general meeting in March, Professor B. Němec referred to the interruption of scientific work occasioned by the country's loss of territory and institutions. Research activities were therefore upon a restricted basis, though, he emphasized, it is necessary for a small nation to maintain its cultural activities at the highest possible level. He urged that renewed efforts be made to utilize all the country's remaining scientific institutions and resources for the continuance of all programs of research. Dr. Ulrich, secretary of the council, stated that donations were received from industries, corporations and private individuals so that as many students as funds permitted are being supported in the continuance of their work. Investigations in all branches of the natural sciences are still in progress at the universities and at approved institutes.

# DISCUSSION

## FACTORS INFLUENCING TREE DESTRUCTION DURING THE NEW ENGLAND HURRICANE

COMPARED to hurricanes in the South, the New England hurricane of September 21, 1938, was extraordinarily destructive to trees, both shade and forest, in its path. This seems all the more startling, since the great storms on the South Atlantic or Gulf coast frequently rage for 15 to 20 hours longer, while the high wind velocity of the New England catastrophe covered a period of only about 4 hours.

As it had been the privilege though not the pleasure of the writer to witness, at various times, five different hurricanes in the southern states, the contrast between the results of these so far as trees are concerned and those of the northern hurricane of last fall seemed the more striking and stimulated interest in determining the factors which may have been responsible for the greater tree damage in New England.

In the great Caribbean pine areas in South Florida, which were comparatively untouched by turpentining or lumbering, the great hurricane of 1928 did not affect the contour of these woods, as seen from a distance, to any great extent. True, there were trees blown over here and there, but there was not the picture of annihilation that was represented by the New England woods after the hurricane.

Apart from the obvious thought that the forests of the South, buffeted so frequently by great storms, represent the survival of the fittest to endure these conditions, there are six factors which seem paramount in explaining the greater susceptibility of the northern trees to the gale. These are here enumerated.

(1) *Extremely high wind velocities in local areas.* During the storm there were local gusts of great intensity, taking everything before them, the largest and strongest trees as well as the weakest. There are very few weather instruments in New England for the recording of gust velocities, but the Blue Hill Observatory recorded a gust of about 187 miles per hour and on Mt. Washington, 163 miles per hour. These compare with the strongest gusts of the southern storms. Over the broad path of the hurricane, however, the storm crushed the weak trees, the strong surviving.

(2) *The type of tree prevalent.* This undoubtedly had some bearing. The hard pines of the South are more gale-resistant than the white pines, Norway spruces, willows, poplars, locusts and soft maples of the North. In New England the types of trees standing the storm best were sycamores, oaks, old well-rooted elms and sugar maples, and beech.

(3) *Tree ages.* The age class was very important. The very youngest (under 20 years for white pines, under 30 for hardwoods) and the very oldest survived the gale. The younger trees were more supple, giving with the wind, and were comparatively better anchored in the soil by the tap root, while the very oldest trees were tougher, had deeper and stronger root systems and, due to natural branch spacing, offered less resistance to the wind in their tops. Casualties were greatest in the age range of 30 to 90 or 100 years. Inasmuch as a number of our dominant trees, such as white oak, hemlock and white pine, are known to exceed 500 years in age, a 100-year-old tree may be considered as "young."

(4) *Man-made conditions.* This was an important factor not only in regard to shade trees, but to woodlands as well. Cutting of roots of shade trees in construction of sewers, pipe lines, curbings and the like, thus depriving trees of anchorage, was probably the one most important factor in the destruction of street trees. The loss of shade trees on lawns, greens and commons by overthrow was also disproportionately great. This in many cases may be traced to the giving of lawns precedence over shade trees in regard to treatment, for example—the application of fertilizer for the benefit of the grass over the surface, which tended to stimulate surface root growth of trees, resulting in shallow root systems, poor anchorage and consequent wind-throw.

The nature of the woodlands in the path of the hurricane was important. Most of the woodlands in this area were composed of young trees, usually about 20 to 60 years old, an age range very susceptible to wind damage. This condition had resulted from the excessive and constant cutting of older trees for lumber and fuel. On the other hand, in many places near manufacturing centers, woods were repeatedly cut for fuel when scarcely double the size of broomsticks and, interestingly enough, these young sprout growths under 20 years of age were little damaged by the storm.

Just as the wind damage is greatest in the pine woods of the South, where the trees have been weakened structurally by turpentining or thinning out by lumbering, the destruction to New England woods was greatest where lumbering and thinning had taken place, and to sugar maple groves which had been weakened from various sources, ultimately traceable to the activities of man.

(5) *Insect and fungus trouble to trees.* There has been in many parts of the hurricane area during the past few decades excessive defoliation of shade trees by insects, such as the gipsy moth, elm leaf beetle and cankerworms. The cumulative result of years of this damage was decided weakening of the trees. Borers and bark beetles gained a foothold leading to infection by wood rot fungi. A large proportion of the hurricane-damaged trees had been structurally weakened by borers and wood rot fungi, prior to the storm.

(6) *Soil conditions.* Tree damage was particularly

great where hardpan or underlying rock restricted root growth, while the wetness of the soil due to four days of rain prior to the storm was an important factor in weakening the anchorage of shallow-rooted trees.

There has been a lesson to be gained from the hurricane by every one interested in trees. While New England may not be visited again by so great a storm for another hundred years or more, the factor of wind destruction to trees is always with us to a greater or lesser extent and the planting of sturdy varieties and proper care of our valuable shade trees should lessen and restrict to a considerable degree storm damage in the future.

STANLEY W. BROMLEY
BARTLETT TREE RESEARCH LABORATORIES,
STAMFORD, CONN.

## THE POINT OF ORIGIN OF THE BLOSSOM-INDUCING STIMULUS[1]

THE use of such techniques as grafting,[2] defoliation and the exposure of different parts of the plant to unlike photoperiods[3] has given rise to the belief that a "flower-forming hormone" originates in the foliage near the tip of the plant. The classical experience of inducing plants to flower by girdling would suggest that the leaves may not be the exclusive means of control of the blossom-inducing stimulus.

To observe the response of some plants to the transfer of the flower-forming substance by grafting, flowering and non-flowering plants of *Cosmos sulphureus* var. Klondike, morning glory, var. Heavenly Blue, *Petunia,* poinsettia, soybean var. Biloxi, stock (*Matthiola incana*) var. Xmas pink, tobacco var. Maryland Mammoth and *Xanthium echinatum* were grafted by the approach method, a modified tongue being used. Positive results were secured with morning glory, *Petunia,* soybean and *Xanthium,* the "donor"[3] plants stimulating the "receptors" to produce blossoms. The state of growth of the plants as well as the cultural environments appear to affect the results secured from grafts. For example, deflorating the *Xanthium* donors increases their influence. Flowering was not initiated by grafting in the case of plants of *Cosmos,* poinsettia, stock and tobacco.

It appears that a successful transfer of the flower-forming stimulus by a graft contact depends upon whether the species being used will give a systemic or local response to a photoperiod treatment of only a part of the plant. Exposure of a part of a morning glory, *Petunia,* soybean or *Xanthium* plant to the proper environment induces flowering throughout the plant. *Cosmos,* poinsettia[4] and tobacco, on the other hand, give local responses, as the part being exposed to the proper photoperiod comes to flower and the remainder stays vegetative.

The older receptor branches of *Petunia* in a warm environment blossomed in short days before the younger donor branches which were exposed to long days. That is, it appears that the presence of flowers is not essential to the functioning of branches as donors of the stimulus to flower.

Poinsettia and tobacco plants were induced to blossom in a warm, short-day location, contrary to their habit,[5] by the application of a current of cool air to a short length of the stem some three to four inches below the tip of the plant. These species were also stimulated to blossom in warm, short days by wrapping a taut rubber band about the stem a few nodes below the tip to constrict it.

The variable responses to grafting and to donor branches depending upon the flowering habit of the species and the effects of a "temperature girdle" and banding in causing blossoming indicate that the stem of the plant plays a part in the appearance of blossoms as well as does a leaf-formed hormone-like substance.

R. H. ROBERTS
B. ESTHER STRUCKMEYER
UNIVERSITY OF WISCONSIN

1 Published with the approval of the director of the Agricultural Experiment Station.

2 M. Ch. Cajlachjan, *Compt. Rend. Acad. Sci. U. R. S. S.,* 18: 606–612, 1938.

3 K. C. Hamner and J. Bonner, *Bot. Gaz.,* 100: 388–431, 1938.

4 R. H. Roberts, J. E. Kraus and N. Livingston, *Jour. Agr. Res.,* 54: 319–343, 1937.

5 R. H. Roberts and B. E. Struckmeyer, *Jour. Agr. Res.,* 56: 633–678, 1938.

## ON DESLOTHING THE SLOTH

DURING several visits to Panama and while making other observations, the possibility of raising the level of activity of the sloth made an interesting appeal. Considered academically and also to test the action of certain substances or conditions, this animal makes an excellent subject. Its basal level of movement is exceedingly low, and increments may readily be observed. Other features make it almost ideal for study, including its ease of handling and training and the plentiful supply in the tropics. Tests were made on both two-toed and three-toed species, the experimental work having been carried out mainly at Barro Colorado Island Laboratory, Canal Zone, and Gorgas Memorial Laboratory, Panama. It may be said that several ways were found of speeding up their activities.

Recognition that the body temperature of the sloth is normally much lower than that of other mammals suggested a temperature test. Mere exposure to the tropical sun for an hour or two raised the rectal temperature 4° or 5°, and thereupon the activity of the animal became much greater. This was evidenced by its rate of travel along the under side of a twelve-foot horizontal pole, timed by stop-watch. Again, setting up an emotional reaction in the sloth, by simple feints and passes before it, augmented its speed very markedly. Extract of the adrenal cortex made in this laboratory, when given in moderate doses (5 cc or so every hour or two), also provided an adequate stimulus to increased activity. Two other substances, adrenalin and prostigmin, were also found to be effective in raising the sloth from its (anthropomorphically considered) sluggardy. Several other preparations which were tested over several days (thyroid and pituitary, also benzedrine and strychnine solutions) gave negative results.

Raising the body temperature appeared to be the best stimulator; on the average the increments in rate of walking on warming approximated 50 per cent., and several cases showed increases of over 100 per cent. Cortico-adrenal extract was observed to maintain the increased rate of upside-down travel by the sloth for some ten or twelve hours after injection. This is in keeping with the earliest observations on the influence of the cortical hormone in augmenting activity.[1] Prostigmin as well as emotional excitement appeared to bring out the fighting instinct in sloths, along with the greater ability to "run" away.

The rate of progress of the sloth may be given interestingly on a mileage basis. It appeared from several hundred tests that the two-toed sloth normally averaged a little over three hours to the mile, and three-toed animals almost four-and-a-half hours. The slowest individual tardigrades, however, took over six hours for the distance. Under excitation such as that noted above, the mile was possible in about two hours, and in a burst of speed by one animal only, a mile an hour was accomplished.

It is likely that in the wild the higher rates of progress indicated would not obtain, because of difficulties of arboreal travel, lack of stimulus, etc. In some cases the sloth rests, indeed, for weeks on end, in the same place in the same tree. Beebe has written very engagingly on its habits.[2] It may be recalled that the sloth possesses only about one half the amount of muscle (percentally) found in other mammals, and that about one quarter of its weight is made up of stomach and contents—both serious handicaps to fast movement.[3] The present observations indicate, nevertheless, that several fairly effective methods of deslothing the sloth may be employed.

S. W. Britton
R. F. Kline
Physiological Laboratory,
University of Virginia

# SCIENTIFIC BOOKS

## PHYSIOLOGY

*Physiology of the Nervous System.* By J. F. Fulton. London, New York, Toronto: Oxford University Press, 1938. Pp. xv + 675.

In this extensive work the author has pursued his declared intention of serving the study of clinical medicine and of meeting the needs of the medical student. From this point of view the work has, in the main, been well done, and much valuable material for the student or clinician is included. To the reviewing physiologist, it seems that the book should rather be called "physiological anatomy." By far the greater part of the book is given to anatomical details, and indeed much of the fundamental physiology of the nervous system is so sketchily treated, with important parts of the subject omitted altogether, that a sense of unbalanced emphasis is left in the reader's mind. The entire fields of conditioned reflexes and electrophysiology—the latter a topic of rapidly expanding interest—are omitted; and, though it is explained that their omission is intentional, the book is thereby rendered an incomplete treatment of the subject indicated in the title. There are several evidences of haste in preparation, but this is to be expected in so large an undertaking by such a busy worker.

An admirable feature of the arrangement is the beginning of each chapter with a historical note and the conclusion of each with a concise, well-worded summary. The historical notes are both interesting and instructive, serving to enhance the understanding of present knowledge. The sequence of chapters, beginning with receptors, motor units and elementary reflexes and then proceeding upward through the spinal cord to the cerebrum, is logical and in the main clear, but it involves some repetition, as in the case of postural reflexes.

The author's interest lies in organization and integration, rather than in basic principles and constituent mechanisms. This is frankly stated in the following sentence (p. 71): "The problem of organization is the principal subject of the present volume; the nature of synaptic transmission, important though it always remains, must here be relegated to a few brief paragraphs." The major foundation stone of the physiology of the nervous system is that well-known but little understood event which we call the nerve impulse. There is scarcely a reference to the vast body of research which for a century has been directed to elucidating this phenomenon, and hardly a word of the results of these researches, beyond a brief, but excellent statement of the all-or-nothing principle.

The influence of the author's great teacher, Sher-

[1] E. Eagle, S. W. Britton and R. F. Kline, *Am. Jour. Physiol.*, 102: 707, 1932.

[2] W. Beebe, *Zoologica*, 7: 1, 1926.

[3] S. W. Britton, R. F. Kline and H. Silvette, *Am. Jour. Physiol.*, 123: 701, 1938.

rington, is much in evidence, and indeed the chief merit in the book is the broad, philosophical view of organization and integration which emanates from that influence. The minutely detailed account of the researches on stretch reflexes and other features of spinal cord physiology, which occupied the author during his years in Sherrington's laboratory, seems to involve over-emphasis of a specialized topic at the expense of other more fundamental matters, which suffer a corresponding neglect.

In a footnote (p. 73) is described how the author once espoused a chemical theory of central nerve function and disposed of rival electrical theories with arguments which, it may be noted, failed to consider the possibility of "reverberation," which was suggested in 1923 and for which a strong case has since been made by Lorente de Nó. The footnote goes on to explain how the author has now abandoned the chemical theory and with equal vigor espoused the electrical theory, just when cogent evidence for a chemical theory is becoming well-nigh overwhelming, without even a reference to experiments which have raised almost insuperable obstacles in the way of the electrical theory.[1] He prematurely accepts the evidence of Eccles, which seemed to rule out the synaptic action of acetylcholine, but which has since been convincingly answered by the work of Rosenblueth and Simeone.[2] In support of the electrical theory he makes dogmatic assertions concerning events in the cell membrane, including reiterated insistence on the unproved assumption that an antidromic impulse causes a discharge which sweeps through the entire nerve cell. This unfortunate bias reaches a climax on page 96, where he takes up the once ignored explanation of after-discharge by reverberating circuits and then states, "it seems unnecessary to discuss alternative hypotheses."

These adverse criticisms impress a reviewer to whom the basic questions appeal as standing at the portal of rational inquiry into the mechanism of conscious life. Not being qualified to pass expert judgment on the anatomical survey, which constitutes the greater part of the book, the reviewer is impressed with the quantity of material which is marshalled to provide an understanding of integration in the nervous system.

ALEXANDER FORBES

HARVARD MEDICAL SCHOOL

[1] W. B. Cannon and A. Rosenblueth, *Amer. Jour. Physiol.*, 119: 221–235, 1937.

[2] A. Rosenblueth and F. A. Simeone, *Amer. Jour. Physiol.*, 1938, 122: 688–707, 1938; *ibid.*, 708–721.

# SPECIAL ARTICLES

## MICE AS CARRIERS OF PATHOGENIC PLEUROPNEUMONIA-LIKE MICROORGANISMS

Two distinct strains of filtrable pathogenic microorganisms of the pleuropneumonia group have recently been isolated from the brains of mice and shown to possess tissue affinities of such a nature that they can produce in mice two experimental diseases which bear some resemblance to certain phases of rheumatic fever and rheumatoid arthritis in man.[1] Strain A induces a transitory, migratory polyarthritis, multiplies in the brain and in mesothelial cells of the pleura, pericardium and peritoneum, and produces a typical exotoxin which gives rise to choreiform signs. Strain B produces no such toxin, but has an almost specific affinity for the joints in which it gives rise to a chronic, progressive, proliferative, ankylosing arthritis. These two strains are biologically and immunologically distinct from each other, from *Pleuropneumonia bovum* and from pleuropneumonia-like microorganisms that have been isolated from rats in pure culture or in association with *Streptobacillus moniliformis*.[2] These findings clearly suggested the necessity of determining whether or not similar microorganisms could be isolated from patients with rheumatic fever and rheumatoid arthritis, and following this indication, Swift and Brown[3] reported the isolation of pleuropneumonia-like microorganisms from acute rheumatic fever material.

The chief purpose of the present communication is to record certain experiences which indicate the inadvisability of using mice in attempting to isolate such microorganisms from human material. While studying exudates and tissues from patients with rheumatoid arthritis or rheumatic fever, it was found that inoculation of such material, normal synovial fluid or sterile broth into the eyes (vitreous) of mice, yielded positive pleuropneumonia-like cultures with great regularity. In a typical test, material under investigation was injected into both eyes of six 3-weeks-old mice; six days later the eyes were removed with separate, sterile instruments, immersed in anesthetic ether for one to two minutes (this was sufficient to bring about adequate sterilization of the exterior of the eye), incised, and streaked across 30 per cent. ascitic fluid agar. In most instances, innumerable, typical, microscopic, pleuropneumonia-like colonies appeared within two days. With the Rockefeller Institute Swiss stock, at least four or five mice out of each group of six yielded positive cultures from one or both eyes in ten different experiments. The colonies on solid medium resembled those of Strain A; after several transfers on fluid

[1] A. B. Sabin, SCIENCE, 88: 575, 1938; *ibid.*, 89: 228, 1939.

[2] E. Klieneberger, *Jour. Hyg.*, 38: 458, 1938.

[3] H. F. Swift and T. M. Brown, SCIENCE, 89: 271, 1939.

medium the cultures were found to be agglutinated in high titre by anti-A serum and to produce a neurotoxin which was completely neutralized by the "A" strain antitoxin. Further studies revealed that these microorganisms were inhabitants of the external surface of the eye, from which they could be cultured with great regularity, and frequently in large numbers unassociated with any bacterial colonies. It was apparent that as a result of the intraocular injection some of these microorganisms were carried into the eye, where they multiplied in the course of a few days. Similar studies carried out with mice of the Rockefeller Institute albino stock and of another Swiss strain (Freed) originating from the Institute stock but bred elsewhere for the past six to seven years, revealed the same condition, but the carrier rate was lower; it was thus possible to encounter groups of six mice from which these microorganisms could not be obtained, while in other groups of six, either all or a varying number yielded positive cultures of the same type. Evidence was also obtained that these microorganisms inhabit the mucosa of the nose and accessory sinuses from which they may be carried into the lungs in the course of nasal instillation under anesthesia.[4] It may be of interest to note here that in one test in which six mice were given nasal instillations under ether anesthesia and intraocular injections of pericardial fluid from a patient who succumbed to acute rheumatic carditis, three different types of pleuropneumonia-like microorganisms were isolated: a Type A from the eyes, a Type B from the lungs of one mouse, and a new type (to be called "C") which produced arthritis in mice but no toxin and was immunologically distinct from all the others studied. Two pleuropneumonia-like strains producing pneumonia in mice (isolated by Dr. Dienes in the course of passaging two human rheumatic heart muscle suspensions through the lungs of mice) were submitted to me for study[5]; they were found to be immunologically identical with Strain A and to produce neurotoxin in cultures which was neutralized by "A" antitoxin. Of three cultures isolated by Drs. Swift and Brown from pneumonic lungs of mice inoculated with rheumatic fever material, one was found to be a Type A, one a Type B and the third the same as the newly isolated Type C.

It is apparent, therefore, that the presence or absence of pleuropneumonia-like microorganisms in rheumatic fever and rheumatoid arthritis exudates and tissues will have to be established primarily by cultural methods, and not by passage through mice or other animals. Using a large variety of solid and fluid media and "passaging blindly" six or more times, I have been unable thus far to grow pleuropneumonia-like microorganisms from thirteen rheumatoid arthritic exudates (twelve patients), four rheumatoid subcutaneous nodules (three patients), rheumatoid synovial tissue (two patients), acute rheumatic blood, pleural fluid, pericardial fluid and heart muscle (two patients),[6] but many more cultivation experiments will have to be performed with suitable specimens before a final decision can be reached.

ALBERT B. SABIN
LABORATORIES OF THE ROCKEFELLER INSTITUTE FOR MEDICAL RESEARCH, NEW YORK, N. Y.

[4] This finding suggests that viruses, such as that of influenza, which are passaged by nasal instillation in mice, should be cultured periodically to determine whether or not they have been contaminated by microorganisms of the pleuropneumonia group.

[5] Dr. L. Dienes informs me that he was able to isolate a similar strain by passaging normal mouse lung.

[6] I am deeply indebted to Dr. Edward F. Hartung, of the New York Post-Graduate Hospital, for supplying most of these specimens.

## THE PREPARATION OF PITUITARY GROWTH HORMONE FREE FROM LACTOGENIC AND THYROTROPIC HORMONES

THE knowledge that the anterior hypophyseal growth hormone is comparatively stable to alkali led us to assume that this protein would be free from disulfide linkages (–S–S–) and therefore resistant to cysteine reduction. Therefore a 5 per cent. solution of growth hormone in its purest form[1] was treated with double the amount of cysteine at pH 8.0. The reduction which resulted caused a precipitation of one half the total protein, whereas the supernatant contained most of the growth hormone when tested in normal plateaued female rats. (Table 1.)

TABLE 1

RETENTION OF GROWTH HORMONE POTENCY AFTER TREATMENT OF ANTERIOR HYPOPHYSEAL EXTRACTS $DAP35_2$ AND $DAP74_1$ WITH CYSTEINE

| Preparation | | Daily dose of total protein | Daily dose of soluble protein | Number of rats per group | Grams grain per rat* |
|---|---|---|---|---|---|
| | | mg | mg | | |
| $DAP35_2$ | Untreated ....... | 1 | 1 | 9 | 39 |
| | Cysteine treated .. | 1 | 0.43 | 6 | 39 |
| $DAP74_1$ | Untreated ....... | 1 | 1 | 12 | 51 |
| | Cysteine treated .. | 1 | 1 | 5 | 43 |

* Average gain of normal plateaued female rats by 17 daily injections over a period of 20 days.

We tested the above-mentioned cysteine-treated growth hormone for its lactogenic and thyrotropic activity. Up to the very high levels tested, these hormones were found to be absent.[2] (Table 2.)

[1] Prepared by modification of the method published by Evans, Uyei, Bartz and Simpson (*Endocrinology,* 22: 483, 1938).

[2] As regards gonadotropic hormones: the follicle-stimulating hormone was known to be nearly completely absent from the untreated solutions, so tests for this substance were not considered necessary; inactivation of ICSH did

TABLE 2

DECREASE IN POTENCY OF LACTOGENIC AND THYROTROPIC HORMONES IN GROWTH HORMONE AFTER CYSTEINE TREATMENT

| Preparation of growth hormone | | Lactogenic M.E.D.* squab crop intramuscular | Thyrotropic M.E.D. squab thyroid intramuscular |
|---|---|---|---|
| | | mg | mg |
| $DAP35_2$ | Untreated .... | 20 | < 1 |
| | Cysteine treated (total protein). | > 45 | > 45 |
| $DAP74_1$ | Untreated ...... | 10 | 0.75 |
| | Cysteine treated (soluble protein) | > 52 | > 52 |

* Minimal effective dose.

From these results the following calculations can be made: 100 units[3] of untreated growth hormone contained from 5 to 10 units of lactogenic and from 100 to 150 units of thyrotropic hormone, whereas 100 units of cysteine-treated growth hormone contained less than one unit of either of these hormones.

Lactogenic, thyrotropic and gonadotropic hormones were next subjected to the same treatment with cysteine. Crude thyrotropic and gonadotropic hormones were found to be inactivated under the same conditions. The reduction of lactogenic hormone was accompanied by a precipitation. In a concentration above 0.1 per cent. this precipitation was almost quantitative, and no activity could be recovered from the precipitate or supernatant if a 40:1 ratio of cysteine to lactogenic hormone was allowed to react for two days at room temperature. Below 0.02 per cent. lactogenic hormone concentration, no precipitate was formed and no inactivation occurred under these same conditions. We are inclined to believe that the –SH form of the lactogenic hormone is as active as the native hormone and that its apparent inactivation is due only to its extremely low solubility.[4]

It has long been known that many organs which depend upon the pituitary for normal functioning may influence the body weight of animals. It is believed by others[5,6,7] that stimulation of these organs is essential for growth promotion by pituitary extracts or that growth is dependent upon synergism or addition of these effects. That the pituitary growth hormone has now been freed from two more (and possibly others) of the specific stimulating hormones of the pituitary seems of the greatest importance in establishing the individuality of this hormone.[8] A more detailed analysis of the action of cysteine on pituitary hormones and of the biological and chemical properties of the growth hormone obtained by this method will be published in the near future.

DONALD L. MEAMBER
HEINZ L. FRAENKEL-CONRAT
MIRIAM E. SIMPSON
HERBERT M. EVANS
UNIVERSITY OF CALIFORNIA

not appear to be quite as complete as inactivation of the other hormones. It is, however, true that fifty times the M.E.D. found in the untreated solution gave only a doubtful response.

3 Growth unit defined in reference 1.

4 While this work was in progress, it was learned from a remark by Bates in the discussion in the Cold Spring Harbor Symposium for Quantitative Biology (1938, p. 271) that he too had observed the inactivation of lactogenic, thyrotropic and gonadotropic hormones by cysteine.

5 O. Riddle, Sigma Xi Lectures for 1936–7, Ohio State University Symposium on Hormones, p. 450.

6 O. Riddle, *Endocrinology*, 19: 1, 1935.

7 O. Riddle and R. W. Bates, *Endocrinology*, 17: 689, 1934.

8 H. M. Evans, *Proc. Assn. Res. Nerv. and Mental Dis.*, 17: 175, 1938.

## THE CAUSATIVE AGENT OF INFECTIOUS EQUINE ENCEPHALOMYELITIS IN VENEZUELA

THE writers have been engaged in the study of the causative agent of infectious equine encephalomyelitis since the year 1936, when it made its appearance in Venezuelan Goajira. In this work, particular attention has been devoted to the etiological angle, which is, of course, of the utmost importance in the control of this disease. Some of the results obtained up to this date are briefly stated below.

(1) From the brain of animals which died of this infection in rural areas, a filterable virus has been isolated.

(2) This virus was found to be highly pathogenic to guinea pigs, whatever the mode of inoculation (intracerebral, intraperitoneal, intramuscular, subcutaneous), and caused them to die in from 48 to 72 hours after inoculation.

(3) Rabbits also proved to be very susceptible; they succumbed in from 72 to 96 hours after intracerebral inoculation.

(4) The disease could not be artificially transmitted to cattle, and this is in accordance with observations in rural localities, where bovines are refractory to the infection.

(5) The virus, carried again into horses, induces an acute condition with a clinical and anatomopathologic picture identical with that observed in animals attacked under natural conditions in rural areas. From the brain of horses thus inoculated, the original virus has been isolated.

(6) The virus is easily grown in chick embryos, which die in about 18 hours following inoculation. By means of successive passages, such a concentration was achieved that dilutions of 1:5.000.000 proved lethal to guinea pigs.

(7) The production of protective vaccine has been based on chick-embryo culture of the virus. Laboratory animals immunized with it withstand successfully

thousands of lethal doses, a fact which proves the efficacy of the vaccine. For three months the Laboratories of Veterinary Bacteriology and Parasitology have been supplying the Ministry of Agriculture and Animal Husbandry of Venezuela weekly with considerable quantities of this autochthonous vaccine in order to combat the disease in rural areas.

(8) To determine the immunobiological characteristics of encephalomyelitic virus isolated in this country, the following has been employed:

(a) U. S. eastern strain virus;
(b) U. S. western strain virus;
(c) vaccine made in this country from the virus under observation (autochthonous);
(d) bivalent vaccine made from U. S. eastern and western strain viruses;
(e) encephalomyelitic serum made from autochthonous virus;
(f) U. S. bivalent encephalomyelitic serum made from both eastern and western strain viruses;
(g) U. S. monovalent encephalomyelitis serum made from western strain virus;
(h) Argentine encephalomyelitic serum made from Argentine virus.

From these comparative researches, carried out both *in vivo* and *in vitro,* it is to be inferred: (1) That the Venezuelan encephalomyelitic virus is wholly different both from the American western virus and from the Argentine virus, with which it has no immunobiological connection. (2) That it also differs immunobiologically from the American eastern strain virus, with which, however, it has some connection on account of its high virulence, pathogenicity, etc. (3) That the immunizing power of the protective vaccine made from autochthonous virus surpasses by far that of the American bivalent vaccine, prepared from both eastern and western viruses. (4) That the Venezuelan encephalomyelitic serum neutralizes the corresponding specific virus, not only *in vivo,* but also *in vitro.*

(9) As a result of these studies, the causative agent of infectious equine encephalomyelitis has been isolated for the first time in Venezuela. It is assumed that the agent in question constitutes a *sui generis* strain, different from the encephalomyelitis viruses described up to now.

(10) Venezuela should be given full credit for being perhaps the first South American country where the production of encephalomyelitic vaccine from embryo-cultured virus has been undertaken.

(11) The writers are about to finish a complete report on these researches which will be published in due course.[1]

VLADIMIR KUBES
FRANCISCO A. RÍOS
LABORATORIES OF VETERINARY BACTERIOLOGY
AND PARASITOLOGY, MINISTRY OF
AGRICULTURE AND ANIMAL HUSBANDRY
OF VENEZUELA, CARACAS

# SCIENTIFIC APPARATUS AND LABORATORY METHODS

## A METHOD FOR STUDYING LIVING MOSQUITO LARVAE AND OTHER SMALL AQUATIC INVERTEBRATES

A VERY real problem in attempting to study small, living, aquatic animals under the microscope is to keep them in the field of vision without continual change of focus. The usual practices of entangling the animal in cotton threads or of treating the preparation with various drugs are generally undesirable, since the question naturally arises as to whether one is still dealing with a "normal" animal. There are, likewise, numerous objections to imprisoning the animal beneath a coverslip, because of the possible crushing of the preparation and the equally serious matter of cutting off its oxygen supply.

After numerous attempts to remedy this situation, the following very simple solution was found: A piece of thin copper wire (about No. 22 B. and S. gauge), six inches long, was bent at one end into a small circle one quarter inch in diameter, the ring of wire thus formed being made secure by several turns of the end of the wire around the stem of the loop. The other end of the wire was twisted around a small, square block of lead, such as is commonly used by histologists. The lead served as support for the wire pedicel and ring, as shown in Fig. 1.

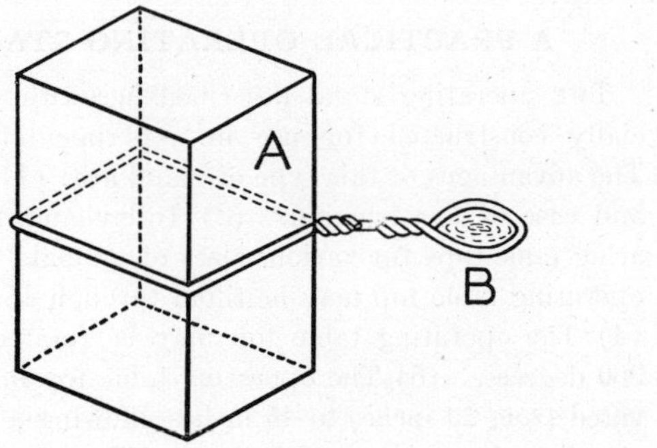


FIG. 1. Device for studying small, living, aquatic animals. *A,* lead block; *B,* wire loop with inclosed film of water.

[1] An already studied stock culture of our virus, with its virulence increased by consecutive passages through susceptible animals, has been supplied, for the sake of cooperation, to Lederle Laboratories, Pearl River, N. Y. C. E. Beck and Ralph W. G. Wyckoff, of these laboratories, published a communication on the subject in SCIENCE, 88: 2292, 530.

Now to use the device the wire ring is simply dipped into water momentarily and a film of liquid imprisoned across the ring. The animal is then placed in this film and is automatically retained therein by the action of the surface tension on the two sides. The lead weight serves to hold the ring on the stage of the compound or dissecting microscope in any position desired.

The device has the advantage of confining the animal to a small area and, essentially, to a single plane so as to eliminate the necessity of continual change of focus. The animals so far studied by this method show surprisingly little tendency to struggle, but, to the contrary, go about their feeding and regular body movements within the fluid layer in what appears to be a normal manner. Furthermore, the large area for gaseous diffusion eliminates any respiratory difficulties.

The method has proved of exceptional value in studying mosquito larvae and their relations to the surface, but, presumably, is to be recommended for vital preparations of other aquatic invertebrates. The films last for considerable lengths of time, depending, of course, upon the relative humidity of the laboratory air. A number of them were timed at over an hour. Loss of thickness due to evaporation, however, may be readily remedied from time to time by addition of a drop of water to the film without disturbing the preparation.

The film may be varied in thickness to accommodate animals of different sizes by adding more or less water with an eye-dropper or by using various sizes of wire in the loop.

A further advantage is the ability thus offered to study the ventral side of the animal by simply turning the lead block over on its other end.

CARROLL M. WILLIAMS
HARVARD UNIVERSITY

## A PRACTICAL OPERATING STAND

THE operating stand described herewith was especially constructed for use in experimental surgery. The advantages of this type of stand are: (1) Low cost and ease of construction. (2) Interchangeable operating table tops for various sizes of animals. (3) The operating table top may be tilted through 180 degrees. (4) The operating table top may be rotated through 360 degrees. (5) The operating table top may be elevated from 29 inches to 45 inches allowing a sitting or standing operating position. (6) The single column allows maximum leg room and the entire stand occupies little laboratory space.

The entire column (1) is constructed of pipe and pipe rail fittings. A is a 2-inch pipe rail base, B is a piece of 2-inch pipe 20 inches long drilled and tapped at C for the locking bolt, D is a piece of $1\frac{1}{2}$-inch pipe 20 inches long and E is a $1\frac{1}{2}$-inch pipe rail adjustable base. The brace F and H is of strap iron and is attached to the operating table top by means of an awning bracket G.

The operating table top is of the size that will accommodate the animal being studied and is made mainly of wood, held together by strap iron. The cross sec-

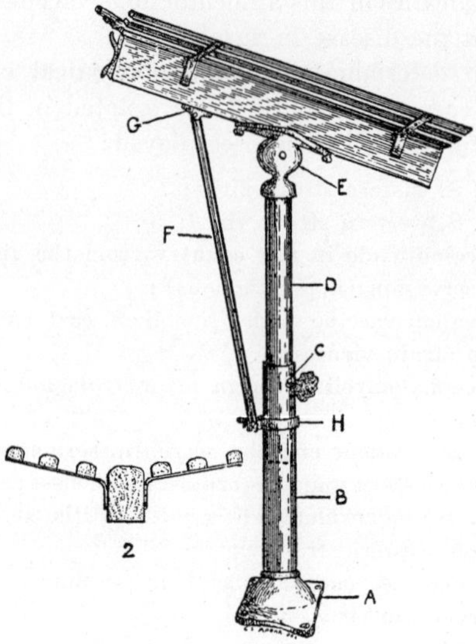


1
FIG. 1

tion (2) shows the manner of construction. A ready means of interchanging table tops is provided by threaded lead sockets in the wood base of the top; thumb screws in these hold the top securely to the column. In use the stand is securely bolted to the floor.

CHARLES S. APGAR, JR.
CORNELL UNIVERSITY MEDICAL COLLEGE,
NEW YORK, N. Y.

## BOOKS RECEIVED

*Annual Review of Biochemical and Allied Research in India, Vol. IX, 1938.* Pp. 165. Society of Biological Chemists, Bangalore. Rs. 3, or 6 sh.

BALAREW, D. *Der Disperse Bau der Festen Systeme; Allgemeine Theorie der Verunreinigung Fester Systeme.* Pp. vi + 240. 45 figures. Steinkopff, Dresden. RM 8.62.

*Bollettino del Centro Volpi di Elettrologia; October, November, December, 1938, XVII, No. 4.* English edition. Pp. 124. 7 figures. Volpi Centre of Electrology, Venice. L. 30.

BORING, EDWIN G., HERBERT S. LANGFELD, HARRY P. WELD and others. *Introduction to Psychology.* Pp. xxii + 652. 128 figures. Wiley. $3.00.

BRUNT, DAVID. *Physical and Dynamical Meteorology.* Second edition, revised. Pp. xxiv + 428. 119 figures. Macmillan. $6.75.

COWDRY, E. V., Editor. *Problems of Ageing; Biological and Medical Aspects.* Pp. xxx + 758. 121 figures. Williams and Wilkins. $10.00.

DUBOIS, H. M. *Monographie des Betsileo (Madagascar); Travaux et Mémoires de L'Institut D'Ethnologie, University of Paris, XXXIV.* Pp. xvi + 1510. 191 figures. 10 plates. The Institute, Paris. 275 fr.

GRIAULE, M. *Masques Dogons. Travaux et Mémoires de L'Institut D'Ethnologie, University of Paris, XXXIII.* Pp. viii + 896. 261 figures. 32 plates. The Institute, Paris. 275 fr.

SCIENCE

Vol. 90 — Friday, July 14, 1939 — No. 2324

*Medals of the National Academy of Sciences:*
*Presentation of the Daniel Giraud Elliot Medal:* Professor W. B. Scott. *Response:* Professor Richard Swann Lull ... 23
*Presentation of the Agassiz Medal:* Dr. T. Wayland Vaughan. *Response:* Dr. Harald Ulrik Sverdrup ... 24
*The Changing Outlook of Engineering Science:* Professor R. V. Southwell ... 27
*Scientific Events:*
*Scholarship Awards of the Canadian National Research Council; The Permanent Science Fund of the American Academy of Arts and Sciences; Awards from the Milton Fund of Harvard University; Winter School in Soil Science at the Waite Institute; The Field Program of the National Museum of Canada; Symposium on Growth and Development; Summer Meetings of Mathematicians* ... 30
*Scientific Notes and News* ... 33
*Discussion:*
*The Luminescence of Sugar Wafers:* Professor E. Newton Harvey. *Heparin and the Inhibition of Blood-clotting:* Tage Astrup. *Boron as a Fertilizer for Western Oregon Soils:* W. L. Powers ... 35
*Societies and Meetings:*
*The Southwestern Division of the American Association for the Advancement of Science:* Veon C. Kiech. *A Symposium on Metric Geometry:* Karl Menger ... 38
*Reports:*
*Tryparsamide in the Control of African Sleeping Sickness:* Dr. Louise Pearce ... 39
*Special Articles:*
*Effect of Indole-3-Acetic Acid on Photosynthesis:* Drs. N. G. Cholodny and A. G. Gorbovsky. *Growth of Some Hemolytic Streptococci on a Chemically Defined Medium:* Brian L. Hutchings and Dr. D. W. Woolley. *Foetal Structures in Viviparous Cyprinodont Fishes:* Professor C. L. Turner ... 41
*Scientific Apparatus and Laboratory Methods:*
*A Thoracic Window for Observation of the Lung in a Living Animal:* Professor Robert J. Terry ... 43
*Science News* ... 6

SCIENCE: A Weekly Journal devoted to the Advancement of Science, edited by J. McKeen Cattell and published every Friday by

THE SCIENCE PRESS

New York City: Grand Central Terminal

Lancaster, Pa. — Garrison, N. Y.

Annual Subscription, $6.00 — Single Copies, 15 Cts.

SCIENCE is the official organ of the American Association for the Advancement of Science. Information regarding membership in the Association may be secured from the office of the permanent secretary in the Smithsonian Institution Building, Washington, D. C.

# MEDALS OF THE NATIONAL ACADEMY OF SCIENCES[1]

## PRESENTATION OF THE DANIEL GIRAUD ELLIOT MEDAL AND HONORARIUM TO RICHARD SWANN LULL

Though I was not a member of the committee that made this award, I heartily concur in the propriety of it, and am especially glad that the long-continued and admirable labors of Professor Lull are receiving recognition which, though belated, will undoubtedly be welcome.

The award is made especially for the monograph on "The Horned Dinosauria or Ceratopsia," which is a very comprehensive and thorough piece of work. After an introduction on the stratigraphy of the formations in which remains of these incredible monsters have been discovered, and a section on their geographical distribution, which ranges from Mongolia to South America, the body of the work is given up to a description of the material scattered through the various museums of the United States and Canada. Then follows a description of the habitats and manner of life of these great reptiles, upon the problems of which much light was thrown by the Mongolian discoveries, the American Museum expeditions having collected several nests of *Protoceratops,* a small dinosaur of this group, in which many eggs were found just as they had been left by the mothers. Some of these were near to hatching and contained recognizable embryonic skeletons. Then finally there is a discussion of the evolution of this group throughout the Upper Cretaceous period, in which the great quantity of material is marshalled in an orderly way and their mutual systematic relations admirably discussed.

It should be added that the committee also had in mind the great body of Professor Lull's work on fossil mammals and his artistic achievements in the way of restoring these long-vanished creatures.

It is to me a particular pleasure to recognize the fine Yale tradition in vertebrate paleontology, which

[1] Presented at the annual dinner, Washington, D. C., April 25, 1939.

began with the work of Professor Marsh in 1859 and has continued with distinguished success and fine results until the present day, a period of 80 years. For a long time vertebrate paleontology in North America was practically confined to Philadelphia and New Haven; and in 1880 Sir Archibald Geikie published in *Nature* an article headed "Yale College and Palæontology," which was an enthusiastic description of the marvels that he had seen during a visit to Professor Marsh.

Another aspect of this work which deserves to be emphasized is the gratifying cooperation it indicates between all the museums of the country, such an infinite improvement over the state of more or less declared hostility and warfare in the days when the famous Marsh-Cope feud overshadowed all the paleontological work of the country.

W. B. SCOTT

## RESPONSE BY THE MEDALIST

To paraphrase part of a note recently received from Japan: It is with "the greatest honour and unutterable throb of heart I feel in offering you this word of thanks."

I am in a sense a successor of Othniel C. Marsh, for twelve years president of this august body, whose vast collections at Yale and the United States National Museum have not only greatly enriched our science but given those of us who followed him a duty and a privilege beyond compare.

Marsh's collections were made with a view to monographing in succession great groups of animals. Of his projected memoirs but two were completed in his lifetime—the Dinocerata and the Toothed Birds. For the others beautiful lithographic plates were prepared and many species described in a great number of papers published in the *American Journal of Science.* Upon Professor Marsh's death in 1899 my own preceptor, Henry F. Osborn, succeeded him as vertebrate paleontologist to the United States Geological Survey and proposed to carry out Marsh's original plan. He realized that this was too great a task for any one man to accomplish, and, while reserving for himself the Brontotheres or Titanotheres, the Proboscidea and the Sauropod Dinosaurs, he delegated other problems to his associates.

One of these, the Ceratopsia, was entrusted to J. B. Hatcher, to whom Marsh had given the task of collecting Ceratopsian material from the famous locality in the Lance formation of old Converse County, Wyoming. Hatcher succeeded so well that he secured 30 odd skulls and much skeletal material now in the Yale Peabody and National Museum.

Hatcher worked diligently at his task and had finished the discussion of the history of discovery, the morphology and systematic descriptions when his hand too was arrested by death, leaving a bulky typescript but no further notes. My own connection with the work arose through having had some field experience in collecting Ceratopsia and in describing a skull which I had helped to collect, and as a consequence I was asked to complete the Marsh-Hatcher memoir. This was done, using so far as possible the conclusions of my predecessors, and the finished manuscript was presented to the United States Geological Survey for publication. A delay of one, two and finally three years made me begin to think that a strange fatality was in some way connected with the exploitation of these creatures of old, as in the case of King Tutankhamen's tomb, but by the grace of Providence I survived to see the memoir in its published form in 1906.

Since that time new discoveries have been made, especially in the Red Deer region of Alberta, where new forms came to light, dimly known in part from the earlier collections in the Judith River of Montana, but here displayed with such beauty and perfection of detail that one soon realized the incompleteness of the story as set forth in the memoir of 1906. Most of this new material was described by Lambe, Brown, Parks and others, but the need of assembling in memoir form the knowledge they had gained became more and more apparent. Having the facilities offered by a richly endowed chair at Yale and the courteous privilege of study in the several American and Canadian museums, we undertook the work, the result of which you have honored to-night.

It was fascinating to study the Ceratopsia, not as dry bones, but to visualize them as living creatures in an environment such as they may be found on earth to-day and to try to imagine their mode of life, their endowment of weapons and prowess, and why such apparent fitness availed them nothing when in the fullness of time their extinction came. Our task is that of a resurrectionist, for, as Robert Dick put it years ago,

> Hammers and chisels and a'
> Chisels and fossils and a'
> Resurrection's our trade
> For by raising the dead
> We've glory and honor and a'.

And when to this is added recognition by the National Academy of Sciences, one's cup is filled. For this culminating honor I thank you!

RICHARD SWANN LULL

## PRESENTATION OF THE AGASSIZ MEDAL TO HARALD ULRIK SVERDRUP

IT is an honor to introduce to you as the duly selected recipient of the Agassiz Medal of the National Academy of Sciences for the year 1938 Harald Ulrik Sverdrup, Knight of the First Class of the Order of St. Olaf, member of the Academy of Science of Oslo, honorary member of the Royal Meteorological Society of Great Britain, the German Meteorological Society and the geographical societies in many countries; the recipient of the Vega Medal in gold awarded by the Swedish Geographical Society, and of other medals and prizes; professor of geophysics in the Christian Michelsen Institute in Bergen, Norway, and director of the Scripps Institution of Oceanography of the University of California.

Before mentioning the accomplishments which constitute the basis of the award of the Agassiz Medal to Sverdrup a brief note will be made on the previous recipients of this medal. The medal was established in 1911 by Sir John Murray as a memorial to his friend, Alexander Agassiz. It was first awarded in 1913 to Johan Hjort. Between the establishment of the medal and 1938 it had been awarded sixteen times in thirty-four years. The countries of those to whom the awards had been made are as follows: Germany 1; Monaco 1; Netherlands 1; England 2; United States of America 3; Norway 4; Sweden 2; Denmark 2.

Prior to 1938 of the sixteen medals that had been awarded eight had gone to residents of Scandinavian countries, and four of the Scandinavians were Norwegians. We now add another Scandinavian, a Norwegian, to this list. Out of seventeen awards of the medal five have gone to Norwegians, giving clear evidence of the world leadership in oceanographic research of that country.

Before 1918, when Sverdrup took charge of the scientific work on the vessel *Maud* for Amundsen, although only thirty years of age, he had already published several important scientific papers. In fact, Sverdrup became an active producer of scientific papers as early as 1914, when he was only twenty-six years old, and he has since then, except while frozen in the ice on the north Siberian Shelf, had an unbroken record of important publications down to the present. In 1918 Sverdrup joined the *Maud* under Amundsen's general direction for a drift across the ice of the Polar Seas. The winters of 1918, 1919 and 1920 were spent frozen in the ice on the north Siberian Shelf. In 1921, however, the vessel needed repairs, and it went to Seattle, Washington, for reconditioning. During that time Sverdrup came to Washington, D. C., and spent his first winter here. The *Maud* left Seattle on June 3, 1922, and the winters of 1922, 1923 and 1924 were again spent frozen in ice in the Arctic Region. The expedition finally reached Nome on August 22, 1925, and the members of it were again in touch with civilization after an absence of three years and two months. On December 5, 1925, the party arrived at Seattle, Washington. Sverdrup spent, in the waters off the north Siberian Coast, six winters frozen up in the ice, except one escape. During this time he had many interesting experiences, some of which I trust that he will at least mention to you. During the winter of 1919, the one escape, he went from Ayon Island and joined the Chukchi tribe, with whom he spent seven months.

Sverdrup says in his general report on the expedition, "When the ship was underway under her own power, the scientific work was very limited and restricted to ordinary meteorological observations because the ship had no special crew, and we had all of us to act as sailors. My duties were, for instance, to take care of the navigation of the ship and of the cooking. When we were drifting with the ice the scientific work was, on the other hand, given much time and the scientists received assistance from every member of the expedition." It is not possible in the brief time allowable for this introduction to say more regarding the reports on the *Maud* expedition than that they contained numerous valuable contributions to different aspects of oceanography, particularly tides and currents, and to many aspects of geophysics.

In 1931 Sverdrup had charge of the scientific work on the submarine *Nautilus* with Sir Hubert Wilkins for an expedition to the Arctic, and he was author of the reports entitled, "Part I, Introduction and Narrative," and "Part II, Oceanography."

Sverdrup has prepared reports on the results of other expeditions such as the one conducted by Sir Douglas Mawson in Antarctic waters, and he contributed one chapter to the discussions of dynamical oceanography in the reports of the Discovery Committee on its operations in south Polar Seas.

Since going to the Scripps Institution of Oceanography at the end of August in 1936, Sverdrup has made many cruises in the waters within a few hundred miles of the California coast and has published a series of brilliant papers. During March of this year he organized and took part in an expedition to the Gulf of California which has given us the first really scientific information on the fundamental oceanographic features of that most interesting body of water.

From what has been said it is obvious that Sverdrup has taken part in many oceanographic expeditions. He has not only prepared reports on the results of these expeditions but has been one of the leading contributors to the theoretical aspects of oceanographic problems. He is also one of the world leaders in modern dynamical meteorology.

Enough has been said to make it clear that the Agassiz Medal is being awarded to the proper person, but before closing these remarks something should be said about Sverdrup the man. He has spent a great deal of time in America. It has already been mentioned that he was in Washington during the winter of 1921. It was then that I first became acquainted with him. He spent some time in Washington while he was preparing the scientific reports on the results obtained on the *Maud*. He was entrusted with the preparation of those parts of the report on the results of the *Carnegie* expedition in 1928 and 1929 that deal with dynamical oceanography and other physical and chemical aspects of the sea. While these reports were in preparation he was in Washington for some time. He was one of the advisers for the National Academy Committee on Oceanography and went to Woods Hole during the summer of 1928 and spent some time with the members of the committee. I well remember the pleasure I felt when my wife and I reached Bergen in October, 1932, and Sverdrup was standing on the pier to welcome us. Our first meal in Norway was in his house. Numbers of Americans not only know Sverdrup's scientific work, but have an intimate personal acquaintance with him. He is a man of the finest character in every way, who has made friends with every one in this country who has had the good fortune to know him.

Mr. President, in presenting the Agassiz Medal to Harald Ulric Sverdrup you give worthy recognition to scientific achievement of a very high order of merit and give pleasure to the friends of a man who has endeared himself to many in this country.

T. WAYLAND VAUGHAN

## RESPONSE BY THE MEDALIST

I WISH to express my deep appreciation of the honor which has been bestowed upon me by the award of the Agassiz Medal for contributions to oceanographic research. It makes me especially happy that the award has been made by the National Academy of Sciences of the United States, because it has been my good fortune to be associated with American institutions since my very first contacts with scientific work. As a graduate student I became in 1911 research assistant to Professor Vilhelm Bjerknes, who, thanks to a grant from the Carnegie Institution of Washington, was able to start young men on scientific careers. Thus, at that time I was already indirectly connected with that institution, which later on cooperated with the *Maud* Expedition, and of which I have been a research associate since 1928. Through my contact with the Carnegie Institution I have made friends in this country, and it is thanks to these friends that I now can take pride in being a member of the faculty of the University of California.

Dr. Vaughan has said too many kind words about my contributions. It is a somewhat doubtful pleasure to listen to a review of one's own merits, but for reasons which I should like to explain I am glad that Dr. Vaughan mentioned my work in the Arctic. Certain mental hardships of scientific Arctic exploration are rarely discussed. I am thinking of the feelings of uncertainty which often arise and which can not be dispelled because there is no adequate literature available for reference and no possibility for discussion with men of similar interest. On the *Maud* we started new investigations, we built new instruments, and I spent considerable time in theoretical studies of tidal currents. Although there were periods when I was so completely absorbed in the work that weeks and months passed quickly, there were other periods when I wondered and worried for fear I had made some elementary mistake, for fear the new investigations were suffering from systematic errors, for fear our new instruments did not perform as they should or that my theories were unsound. In such periods there was no one to consult, no literature to look up. Thinking back now I find myself again walking the deck of our vessel, turning the questions over in my mind, trying to find some flaw in my reasoning. In the end I always had to tell myself that, right or wrong, I was doing my best and would have to go on doing so, hoping that I was on the right track. Perhaps you will understand that an occasion like this brings ample compensation for all the hours of worry and uncertainty.

There is another matter I wish to mention to you. During the last winter in the Arctic, in 1924–25, we used to discuss what we wanted to do after returning to civilization. One of our party wanted to go to Peru, cross the Andes and, instead of drifting with the ice, to drift down the Amazon River on a raft. He did. I used to say that I should like an opportunity to do oceanographic work in the Pacific Ocean. It took me much longer to reach that goal. Although in 1930 I came into intimate contact with the problems of the Pacific through discussion of the excellent data collected by the *Carnegie,* it is only within the last three years that my wish has been actually fulfilled. In 1924–25 I thought of the Pacific Ocean as a pleasant contrast to the Arctic; now I am more than ever impressed by the tremendous amount of work as yet to be done in the Pacific Ocean, and by the fact that, in spite of the pioneering of Alexander Agassiz and Sir John Murray, large areas in the Pacific Ocean are still completely unknown from the point of view of the oceanographer. This fact has again and again been emphasized by Dr. Vaughan, who during his years as director of the Scripps Institution of Oceanography, greatly stimulated the interest in the exploration of the Pacific.

The Scripps Institution has a fortunate location and adequate resources for intensive studies of limited areas off the coast. While it can attack some of the many problems of the Pacific, a general exploration of the Pacific Ocean is an undertaking of such dimensions that no single institution can contemplate it.

Recently, Great Britain honored the memory of Sir John Murray by a "John Murray Expedition" to the Indian Ocean. It appears to me that the best manner in which the United States can honor the memory of Alexander Agassiz will be to organize a large-scale Alexander Agassiz Expedition for exploration of the Pacific Ocean.

HARALD ULRIK SVERDRUP

# THE CHANGING OUTLOOK OF ENGINEERING SCIENCE[1]

By Professor R. V. SOUTHWELL

PROFESSOR OF ENGINEERING SCIENCE, UNIVERSITY OF OXFORD

BRIEFLY, here too my thesis is that we should avoid undue humility! The times are out of joint, and having attained to command of nature greater than the world has seen before, because man has not learned to use his mastery wisely, illogically now (as it seems to me) he inclines to question the value of that mastery, and the labors that have given it. In particular I want to record my protest against what seems to be an implication in much that is written nowadays, that because the range of engineering includes guns, battleships, aeroplanes, tanks, therefore engineers are to be regarded as a class more than others responsible for the horrors of modern war.

Here are words spoken by Sir Alfred Ewing, in a presidential address to the association (1932) which I keep to read ever and again, for its showing of what at the best an engineer's outlook may be:

> An old exponent of applied mechanics may be forgiven if he expresses something of the disillusion with which, now standing aside, he watches the sweeping pageant of discovery and invention in which he used to take unbounded delight. It is impossible not to ask, Whither does this tremendous procession tend? What, after all, is its goal? . . .
>
> The cornucopia of the engineer has been shaken over all the earth, scattering everywhere an endowment of previously unpossessed and unimagined capacities and powers. Beyond question many of these gifts are benefits to man, making life fuller, wider, healthier, richer in comforts and interests and in such happiness as material things can promote. But we are acutely aware that the engineer's gifts have been and may be grievously abused. In some there is potential tragedy as well as present burden. Man was ethically unprepared for so great a bounty. . . . The command of Nature has been put into his hands before he knows how to command himself.

Here too are words spoken somewhat earlier, in his wonderful James Forrest Lecture, 1928, on "A Century of Inventions." In them still more clearly, as I read them, he seems to feel as engineer a sense of special responsibility:

> I used, as a young teacher, to think that the splendid march of discovery and invention, with its penetration of the secrets of Nature, its consciousness of power, its absorbing mental interest, its unlimited possibilities of benefit, was in fact accomplishing some betterment of the character of man. . . . But the war came, and I realized the moral failure of applied mechanics. . . . We had put into the hand of civilization a weapon far deadlier than the weapons of barbarism, and there was nothing to stay her hand. Civilization, in fact, turned the weapon upon herself. The arts of the engineer had indeed been effectively learnt, but they had not changed man's soul. . . .
>
> Surely it is for the engineer as much as any man to pray for a spiritual awakening, to strive after such a growth of sanity as will prevent the gross misuse of his good gifts. For it is the engineer who, in the course of his labors to promote the comfort and convenience of man, has put into man's unchecked and careless hand a monstrous potentiality of ruin.

To which I personally would answer: "Yes, for the engineer as much as any man, *but no more.*" And when, in more recent pronouncements, I find the charge so glibly formulated—"It is engineers who have given men these potent weapons of destruction: on them *more than others,* then, rests the responsibility for their use"—then, admitting the premise, I protest against the deduction. I would say rather: "On them as much as on others (but no more) rests the responsibility for their use." Do not think that I imagine the load thus shared will be light for all. I have no illusion about the weight of responsibility—it is appalling; but I hold that we must share it equally, as citizens, not look for scapegoats when we have been free either to choose our path or leaders to direct us.

I can conceive no subject in which, more than this, clear thinking is wanted to-day: the desire to hand on responsibility is so deep-seated, and the will to believe that we could have had the benefits of science without its risks and its temptations. But knowledge is of good and evil: it is of its essence that we can not know how to cure poison without knowing poison and its action, how to control and use explosives without acquiring power for harm as well as good. We may elect either to shun it or pursue, but we can not have it both ways. Either we must choose, deliberately, impotence as preferable to the power of doing evil, or we must accept knowledge for the double-edged tool it is, vowing to use it wisely. We may not say to the scien-

[1] The concluding portion of the address of the president of the Section for Engineering of the British Association for the Advancement of Science, Cambridge, 1938.

tist, "Keep searching, but let your discoveries be such as must benefit and can not hurt us"; or pretend that the use we make of science is something outside our responsibilities as citizens, a thing imposed upon us by science itself. *Knowledge is not moral:* good and evil are its opposite sides, inseparable in its very nature. I have no quarrel (though no sympathy) with the plea we sometimes hear, for a cessation of scientific activity: it is arguable that on balance knowledge is undesirable. But when men talk of "beneficent" and "destructive" science as though we were free to pick and choose, then I say that they have not even begun to understand what science is.

Holding these views, I find it matter for regret that so often our concern with the impact of science on the life of the community, which is good and healthy, is expressed in a manner that is neither. Too often we seem to be weakly apologizing for results that have followed our activities, as it were because we did not take sufficient care. Need the geneticist apologize for having increased the earth's fertility, because we have found no better use for plenty than to destroy food while thousands are in want? Ought doctors to regret that by coming to a fuller understanding of disease they have lengthened the span of life in a world where birth rates are falling? Here and in countless other instances, science impinging on the life of the community has set problems that will tax to the utmost its courage and intelligence; the hardest and clearest thinking will be wanted, and it is right that engineers and scientists should seek to contribute their share. But I think that we only confuse the issue when we intervene *as specialists* in discussions which concern us really not as specialists but as members of a community.

Whether in these days, when all but a small minority seem convinced of the necessity of rearmament, the engineer is still regarded as scapegoat or has (for a time) been transferred to the rôle of savior, I have no means of judging. But if any still reproach him for making what all men now seek to buy, I would answer that horror is not peculiar to modern war; all war is horrible, both in nature and by purpose, and wars are made not by engineers but by communities. No war is righteous, though it seem so at the time; or inevitable, except as a penalty of national sins: pride, greed and indolence; and those more contemptible because weaker sins, vacillation of purpose, persistence in shams, clinging to safety even at the loss of honor.

More and more frequently, in lectures and in editorials, the decline of international standards is noticed with consternation and lament. Naturally, perhaps, in this country we are apt to see it mainly as an increasing tendency towards "repudiation of law and order in favor of brute force,"[2] revealed most clearly in states that have abjured the democratic ideal. But I think that the malady is at once deeper and more general. Dare we claim that our own policy has shown no falling away from earlier belief in straight-dealing, generosity and the sanctity of contracts?

Increasingly, as it seems to me, nations incline to put trust in the adroitness rather than the sincerity of their statesmen. Ethics are out of fashion, and while as individuals we may still admit the moral imperative, the notion that motives recognizable as moral can have place in international affairs seems now to be rejected as impracticable idealism. Force and deceit, it appears, although unpleasant are held to have "survival value": the gangster compels our unwilling admiration, at least in the field of world affairs. But what if there should be something in the notion, that because success in the life-struggle can come not only by individual strength but also by ability to associate and combine, morality has survival value as being (thus regarded) one of the factors which make association possible? A bank may come to ruin not only through fraudulent or incompetent direction, but because its depositors, panic-stricken, seek each his own legitimate interests at the expense of the common weal: may not a less narrow concept of moral obligation be necessary to the continuance of our civilization, even as wider than national horizons are necessary in the spheres of economics and finance? Perhaps this "idealism" is not so impracticable after all?

Collective security attained by higher standards of fair dealing—it is an epitome of man's progress from the cave to association in the village, in towns and in nations, and I see no ground for believing that the notion can never transcend national barriers. Men write as though it were new—a product of post-armistice utopianism. That it is not new let these sentences, none written less than 100 years ago, bear witness (Guedalla, 1931):

Soyez sur qu'en politique il n'y a rien de stable que ce qui convient aux intérêts de tout le monde; et qu'il faut regarder un peu plus loin que soi-même.

. . . although the aggrandizement and security of the power of one's own country is the duty of every man, all nations may depend upon it that the best security for power, and for every advantage now possessed, or to be acquired, is to be found in the reduction of the power and influence of the grand disturber.

If we lose our character for truth and good faith, we shall have but little to stand upon in this country.

I would sacrifice Gwalior, or every frontier of India, ten times over, in order to preserve our credit for scrupulous good faith, and the advantages and honor we gained by the late war and the peace. . . . What brought me through many difficulties in the war, and the negotiations for peace? The British good faith, and nothing else.

If this be utopianism, then some of our historical

[2] Vide *Nature*, May 28, 1938.

judgments will need revision; for all were said or written by Arthur, Duke of Wellington—a man not lightly to be charged with saying what he did not mean.

You will say, now I am drifting perilously near to politics! It is precisely the point I want to make: I say that inevitably, when instead of science we discuss its impact on the life of the community, we *must* verge on politics, because what concerns the community *is* politics, both etymologically and in fact. The old convention, that science should have no politics, seems to me sane and wise: how to preserve it if as scientists we are to concern ourselves with the life of the community, that is a question I must leave to others more subtly-minded. For myself I see no reason why as scientists we should meet to discuss anything but science. Contrary to common belief, it is not our habit to pursue science throughout the whole of every day; and on all counts I hold it were better that we came to political discussions in hours of leisure, unlabelled, than give support to a notion that political problems will yield to something known as "the scientific attack." Talk to me of the scientific approach in physics, and I shall have an idea of what you mean, though you will easily bewilder me with detail: talk to me of "scientific approach" to problems of real life, I shall suspect you of indulgence in mere jargon.

This is not to assert that science unfits a man for political discussion: if only because by training men of science are prepared to believe that problems of urgency may yet be hard, I hold on the contrary that some scientific leaven is beneficial in almost any body of administrative humanists. It is a protest against our facile modern use of the word "scientific" (which if it means anything connotes a special kind of approach to special problems) where "trained common sense" is the faculty which is really needed. In science we seek to explain phenomena which we believe to be outside man's control: it is the faith in which our work is done—for if the facts were not inexorable, and could be altered at man's pleasure, how could we hope to find enduring "laws"? But politics is concerned with action in fields where we believe that we can influence results: I see no reason to believe that the same technique will serve.

Rather than seek to defend our activities from the charge that evil can come of knowledge misapplied, might it not be better that we undertook a harder task, trying to instill into the mind of the public a clearer notion of the aims with which real scientific work is done? For what is that notion now, in these days of "popular science"? At best, a picture of life lived monastically by men who care nothing for the world outside their laboratories, but spend their energies unceasingly in the quest for more and more knowledge of less and less. (Is it surprising if the public question the right of such men to leisure, seeing that by their carelessness, as it appears, forces are unleashed which may bring our civilization to utter ruin?) At worst, an uncomprehended picture of modern "wonders of science"—gifts which these same men have conferred upon their fellows, altruistically wrestling from nature the secrets of spiritual and material benefit; so that somehow, while the astronomer fosters humility by telling the vastness of interstellar space, Heisenberg's principle of determinacy is thought to bring mystic comfort to men oppressed by the notion of all-pervading law. Equally unfounded, it is, I believe, the other side to that sense of responsibility for the consequences of science, about which I have spoken already; and on a more material plane it is the mainstay of the patent medicine business! For it has given us a public superficially acquainted with "recent progress in science," yet in reality no less ignorant, and more gullible, than was the public of Victorian days.

Never have greater powers of exposition been devoted to the "popularization" of science: when, I wonder, shall we find like powers devoted to the harder task of a real *apologia*? To telling, not of the treasure found, but of the quest; to showing the true man of science (for it is the fact) neither as care-free *dilettante* nor as philanthropist, but seeking truth like the artist, because he must? That, I maintain, is the real spirit of science, be it pure or applied; a spirit that breathes in every book of science worth the name: to make of difficulty a stimulus, to be unwearied in determination to do good work. Is it not there, rather than on a favorable trade-balance of benefits conferred, that we who have chosen science should stand in our defence? Were it not better that the public be told plainly: This is our work, which we do because we must?

A lead has been given, and we may be proud that the giver was an engineer; for the gleam is seen in that noble presidential address by Sir Alfred Ewing from which I have quoted already:

> The quest of truth goes on endlessly, ardently, fruitfully. And yet with every gain of knowledge we realize more clearly that we can never really know. To understand, as Einstein lately said, is to draw one incomprehensible out of another incomprehensible. From time to time we discover a fresh relation between observed phenomena, but each of the things which are found to be related continues to evade our full comprehension; and that is apparently the only kind of discovery we can achieve. Our joy in the quest itself never fails; we are constantly learning that it is better to travel than to arrive.

That I say is the spirit! Let us have the courage of the artist to exalt our calling, and while deploring the folly that has led us and other men to misuse them, let us not weakly question that the gifts of science hold potential good. Fairly regarded, the record of engineering is not such that we need feel ashamed of our calling. Again, to quote Sir Henry Tizard (1938):

There is nothing new in the fact that experiment and invention are transforming the habits of men and are adding to their problems. What is new is that we are all more aware of it, because the rate of change has been steadily increasing. . . . Bad news is, as a rule, better copy than good news. But can it seriously be argued that any section of society is worse off and living under worse conditions than a hundred years ago? Broadly speaking, the natural result of all scientific discovery has been greatly to improve the conditions of life and all our social relations, in spite of—or possibly even because of—the fact that scientific workers have been too busy doing their own jobs well to worry about other people's.

So Dr. Johnson to Mr. Boswell: "My dear friend, clear your *mind* of cant. . . . You may say, 'These are bad times; it is a melancholy thing to be reserved to such times.' . . . You may *talk* in this manner; it is a mode of talking in society: but don't *think* foolishly."

# SCIENTIFIC EVENTS

## SCHOLARSHIP AWARDS OF THE CANADIAN NATIONAL RESEARCH COUNCIL

THE National Research Council announces that forty-one awards of scholarships have been made for 1939–40. These scholarships form part of the means by which the council stimulates postgraduate training and scientific research in Canada. The successful candidates this year are drawn from fourteen Canadian universities. One of the candidates will study dairy bacteriology at the National Institute for Research in Dairying at Shinfield near Reading, England; all the others will carry on postgraduate research at Canadian universities. Three holders of special scholarships will be in training at the National Research Laboratories in Ottawa, where they will acquire experience in the study of industrial and commercial problems. Two of these scholarships have a value of $1,000 each and the other one is worth $750; four fellowships at $750 each and thirty-four studentships at $650 each are tenable at the universities.

Of the successful candidates for awards twenty will work in the field of chemistry, eight in physics, two in geology and one in engineering. In the biological sciences two will work in bacteriology, one in entomology, one in plant biochemistry, one in genetics and cytology, two in general biology and three in biochemistry.

In addition to the fellowships and studentships announced above provision has been made for a number of bursaries at $250 which are to be held under cooperative arrangements between the National Research Council and the universities in which the graduate students will be enrolled. Particulars of these further awards will be announced at a later date.

## THE PERMANENT SCIENCE FUND OF THE AMERICAN ACADEMY OF ARTS AND SCIENCES

INCOME from the Permanent Science Fund, according to agreement and declaration of trust, shall be applied by the American Academy of Arts and Sciences to such scientific research as shall be selected ". . . in such sciences as mathematics, physics, chemistry, astronomy, geology and geography, zoology, botany, anthropology, psychology, sociology and economics, history and philology, engineering, medicine and surgery, agriculture, manufacturing and commerce, education and any other science of any nature or description, whether or not now known or now recognized as scientific, and may be applied to or through public or private associations, societies, or institutions, whether incorporated or not, or through one or more individuals."

Applications for grants under this indenture are considered by a committee of this academy on stated dates only. The next meeting to consider applications will be held on October 1. Applications should be made on special forms furnished by the committee. Correspondence, including requests for application blanks, should be addressed to the chairman of the Committee on the Permanent Science Fund, Professor John W. M. Bunker, Massachusetts Institute of Technology, Cambridge, Mass.

Grants-in-aid from this fund were voted by the academy on April 12, 1939, as follows:

To Professor Emil Bozler, of the department of physiology, the Ohio State University, for the purchase of apparatus to be used in a study of action potentials of smooth muscle, $250.

To Dr. Donald E. Cameron, professor of neurology and psychiatry, Albany Medical College, for the purchase or construction of apparatus, as specified, to study the change in response to repetition of an unpleasant situation in psychotic patients, $200.

To Professor William H. Cole, department of physiology and biochemistry, Rutgers University, for technical assistance, materials and special apparatus for the determination of the chemical composition of the bloods of invertebrates, $500.

To Professor Robert S. Harris, department of biology, Massachusetts Institute of Technology, for the purchase of a newly developed instrument for optical quantitation of vitamin $B_1$, for a study of the daily requirement of young and adult individuals in respect to this vitamin, $400.

To Dr. Caryl P. Haskins, Union College, Schenectady, N. Y., to aid in the construction of apparatus for studying the effects of proton bombardment of spores, $500.

To Professor Charles E. Lane, University of Wichita, Kansas, for technical assistance and materials in a study in the relationship between the pituitary, the ovary and the estrous cycle in rats, $300.

To Karl O. Lange, research meteorologist, Blue Hill Observatory, to aid in the construction and testing of automatic radio transmission of meteorological records to a central station, $300.

To Professor Willem J. Luyten, department of astronomy, University of Minnesota, as an aid in securing a supervisor for student measurements in his study of the proper motions of stars in the southern hemisphere, $500.

To Professor Hugh M. Raup, Harvard University, as a contribution toward general field expenses of a botanical survey of the southwestern part of the District of Mackenzie, contingent upon his securing necessary funds to assure the trip in the summer of 1939, $400.

To Professor Kenneth A. Siler, department of physiology and pharmacology, University of Arkansas School of Medicine, for the purchase or construction of necessary instruments in an investigation of the blood flow of the coronary system, $250.

## AWARDS FROM THE MILTON FUND OF HARVARD UNIVERSITY

AWARDS in the sciences from the Milton Fund have been made as follows to instructors in Harvard University, to enable them to conduct research or prepare publications in the fields mentioned after their names:

Henry Asbury Christian, Hersey professor of the theory and practice of physics, for a study of the clinical medical records of the Peter Bent Brigham Hospital accumulated in the period 1913–39 under his direction as physician-in-chief.

William Dameshek, instructor in medicine, to extend previous investigations and make new ones on the etiology and treatment of certain hemolytic syndromes, with particular reference to the rôle of the spleen.

Ralph Eigil Fadum, instructor in civil engineering, for research on the stress-deformation characteristics of clays.

Knox Henderson Finley, instructor in psychiatry, for experimental studies with insulin and metrozol used in the treatment of dementia praecox, and to continue a study of the capillary beds of the hypothalamus with the aid of a cerebral blood vascular injection technique.

Alden Buchannon Greninger, assistant professor of metallurgy, for the purchase of optical equipment to aid in studies of martensite transformation in alloy systems.

Frederick Vinton Hunt, assistant professor of physics and communication engineering, to extend the results of an earlier investigation of auditorium acoustics by means of steady-state measurements.

Arthur Edwin Norton, Gordon McKay professor of applied mechanics, to continue a study of certain lubricants at or near the condition known as ''apparent solidification'' due to high local pressure.

John Rock, assistant in gynecology and research associate in obstetrics, and Austin Moore Brues, associate in medicine and instructor in biochemical sciences, for a study of ovulation, fertilization, nidation and electrical potentials associated with ovulation.

Reinhold Rüdenberg, Gordon McKay professor of electrical engineering, to investigate the extinction of electric alternating-current arcs by influencing the external circuit.

Karl Sax, professor of botany, for research on the effect of x-rays and neutrons on chromosomes.

Theodore Eugene Sterne, lecturer on astrophysics, for a spare moving system for a Paschen galvanometer and for repairs to the old system.

Theodore James Blanchard Stier, assistant professor of physiology, to continue the study of carbohydrate and lipid assimilation in yeast.

Paul Anthony Vestal, instructor in botany, to obtain information and specimens of the important plants (both cultivated and native) used by the Ramah-Atarque Navajo Indians.

Robert Weston Vose, instructor in applied mechanics, for a study of the aeolotropy of elasticity accompanying shear strain.

Ralph Hartley Wetmore, associate professor of botany, for studies in development and differentiation in the angiosperms.

George Bernays Wislocki, Parkman professor of anatomy, for a study of the anatomy of the manatee.

## WINTER SCHOOL IN SOIL SCIENCE AT THE WAITE INSTITUTE

ACCORDING to *The Australian Journal of Science*, arrangements have been made for a Winter School for Soil Workers to be held at the Waite Agricultural Research Institute for ten days during the month of August. The school will be held under the auspices of the University of Adelaide and of the Council for Scientific and Industrial Research, and will open on August 14. Fees will not be charged, but all those attending must be accredited by their respective state departments, universities or other organizations.

It is believed that the school will be of value to soil workers, not only in the personal contacts that will be made and ideas interchanged, but that methods and procedures of established value will be brought to the notice of every one. These ends will be served by a series of lectures and demonstrations following a definite plan rather than by a conference of disconnected papers.

The lecturers and demonstrators will include Professor J. A. Prescott, C. S. Piper, Dr. A. Walkley, T. J. Marshall, C. G. Stephens, R. J. Best, T. H. Strong, J. S. Hosking and A. C. Oertel.

The following subjects have been chosen as likely to be of general interest. In most cases an introductory lecture will be followed by a practical demonstration:

climatology and soil classification, soil survey, texture, structure, color and water relationships of soils; minor elements in relation to plant growth; methods for the determination of trace elements, including chemical, spectrographic and polarographic methods; soil acidity and lime requirement, including use of the glass electrode; the conductivity method for the determination of soluble salts and the electrometric method for the determination of soluble chlorides; wet and dry combustion methods for the determination of soil carbon; soil-rhizobium relations; a one-day excursion through the country near Adelaide, with examination of several soil profiles.

Dr. A. Walkley, of the Waite Institute, is secretary to the school.

## THE FIELD PROGRAM OF THE NATIONAL MUSEUM OF CANADA

SIX parties have been placed in the field this year by the National Museum of Canada, according to an announcement made by the Mines and Geology Branch of the Department of Mines and Resources, Ottawa. The program includes biological investigations in British Columbia and New Brunswick; botanical studies in Ontario; ethnological researches in British Columbia and the Prairie Provinces, and archeological work in Ontario and Quebec. The work is directed toward the gathering of new information on Canadian fauna and flora and native races, and the acquiring of new specimens for the National Museum.

C. M. Barbeau will make ethnological studies of the Indians of the northern coast of British Columbia, in a resumption of work first undertaken many years ago.

J. D. Leechman will collect anthropological specimens from the tribes of Indians of the Prairie Provinces.

W. J. Wintemberg will make excavations of prehistoric village sites at Tadoussac and Chicoutimi, Quebec, and at Dunnville and Port Maitland, Ontario. Last year he established the site of the Mission of St. Ignace II, the scene of the martyrdom of Fathers Bréboeuf and Lalemant.

H. M. Laing will continue the biological survey along the Pacific coast of British Columbia which has been in progress for some years.

T. M. C. Taylor will make a botanical survey in the vicinity of Heron Bay on the north shore of Lake Superior, Ontario.

W. E. Godfrey will collect zoological specimens and record wild-life observations in the western part of New Brunswick.

## SYMPOSIUM ON GROWTH AND DEVELOPMENT

A SYMPOSIUM on "Growth and Development" will be held from August 7 to 11, sponsored by the editors of *Growth*, at Truro Central School, North Truro, Mass.

The announcement of the objects of the symposium reads:

> Biologists are finding themselves increasingly perplexed by the lack of an adequate conceptual framework with which to guide their own investigations and to bring the results of many specialized studies into a more coherent and meaningful relationship. There is an especially acute need for bridging the gap between genetics and embryology and examining the implications of highly diverse findings of experimental biology for an understanding of growth and development. The editors of *Growth* have therefore decided to inaugurate a Conference on Growth and Development at which discussions of these theoretical issues will be held in the hope of achieving some clarification and unification of thinking in these areas. Grants towards the cost of the conference have been received from the Macy and Rockefeller Foundations. Each session will be opened by a presentation of one paper, the discussion of which will be initiated by a designated leader for that topic, and during the course of the conference moving pictures related to growth and development will be shown. It is hoped that the last day of the conference may see some efforts at generalizing and synthesizing the outcome of the previous days' discussions. It is planned to issue proceedings of the conference, at least in summary form, as a supplement to *Growth*. It is expected that a society will be formed by persons interested in growth during the period of the conference.

The sessions will last from 9:30 in the morning to 3 o'clock in the afternoon, excepting on Friday, when there will be only a morning session.

The program follows:

*August 7*—"Cell Division and Differentiation," W. H. Lewis and P. W. Gregory.
*August 8*—"Genes and Development," Curt Stern and C. H. Waddington.
*August 9*—"Chemical Factors," J. Needham.
*August 10*—"Regeneration," O. E. Schotte; "Organization," E. W. Sinnott.
*August 11*—"Concept of Organism," J. H. Woodger.
*Discussion Leaders*—L. G. Barth, H. S. Burr, L. B. Clark, A. B. Dawson, O. Glaser, H. S. Greene, V. Hamburger, L. Rapkine, K. V. Thimann, Paul Weiss.

Members of the program committee are N. J. Berrill, C. B. Davenport and D. M. Whitaker. Those interested should write to Dr. Philip White, Rockefeller Institute for Medical Research, Princeton, N. J., or to Dr. F. S. Hammett, Provincetown, Mass., for specific invitation and for further information.

## SUMMER MEETINGS OF MATHEMATICIANS

THE summer meeting and colloquium of the American Mathematical Society and the twenty-second summer meeting of the Mathematical Association of

America will be held at the University of Wisconsin on Monday and Tuesday, September 4 and 5.

The meetings of the American Mathematical Society will begin on Tuesday afternoon. A series of three colloquium lectures to be delivered by Professor M. H. Stone, of Harvard University, on "Convex Bodies" will be given on Wednesday morning, on Thursday afternoon and on Friday. A second series of four lectures by Professor A. A. Albert, of the University of Chicago, on the "Structures of Algebras" are planned for Tuesday afternoon, Wednesday, Thursday and Friday mornings. Sessions for the presentation of papers will be held on Tuesday and Thursday afternoons and on Wednesday, Thursday and Friday mornings.

A joint dinner of the society and the association will be given on Thursday evening at 6:30 at the Loraine Hotel. The charge will be $1.25 per plate.

Wednesday afternoon will be left open for recreation. No formal excursions are being planned, but boat rides, picnics, visit to the Forest Products Laboratory of the United States Government, a visit to the Banta Publishing Company or visits to near-by scenic spots may be planned. There will be informal teas in the refectory building on Monday and Tuesday afternoons, following the meetings.

## SCIENTIFIC NOTES AND NEWS

AN oil painting of Dr. James B. Conant, president of Harvard University, previously Sheldon Emory professor of organic chemistry, has been presented to the university by the class of 1914, of which he was a member. The gift was made in connection with the twenty-fifth reunion of his class. It is planned to hang the painting in the faculty room of University Hall.

DR. JOSEPH SWEETMAN AMES, of the Johns Hopkins University, who became president-emeritus in 1935 and who, before his election to the presidency in 1929, was professor of physics, celebrated his seventy-fifth birthday on July 3.

MEMBERS of the American Committee for Democracy and Intellectual Freedom and others have signed a letter congratulating Dr. Franz Boas, professor emeritus of anthropology, Columbia University, on the occasion of his eighty-first birthday, which occurred on July 9. Messages have also been sent to him by President Roosevelt and Secretary Wallace.

A LUNCHEON in honor of Dr. Charles F. Kettering, president of the General Motors Research Corporation, will be given by the Chamber of Commerce of Los Angeles on July 18. Dr. Kettering will make an address entitled "Industry's New Horizons."

M. MARC TIFFENEAU, professor of pharmacology and materia medica in the faculty of medicine of the University of Paris, has been elected a member of the section of chemistry of the Paris Academy of Sciences, in succession to the late Professor G. Urbain.

THE degree of doctor of music was conferred at the commencement exercises of the University of Chicago on Dr. Carl E. Seashore, research professor of psychology and emeritus dean in the State University of Iowa, in recognition of "his contributions to the science of music."

THE honorary degree of doctor of science was conferred by Williams College at commencement on Dr. Louis Frederick Fieser, professor of chemistry at Harvard University.

BATES COLLEGE, Lewiston, Me., conferred on June 19 the degree of doctor of science on Dr. Herbert E. Walter, emeritus professor of biology at Brown University, and on Dr. H. O. Whitnall, professor of geology at Colgate University.

DR. GEORGE T. HARGITT, professor of zoology at Duke University, received the degree of doctor of science at the commencement exercises of Syracuse University.

TRINITY COLLEGE, Hartford, Conn., conferred on June 19 the doctorate of science on Dr. Willard Cole Rappleye, dean of the College of Physicians and Surgeons of Columbia University, who was the commencement speaker.

IN conferring the doctorate of laws on Dr. William Herbert Hobbs on June 17 at the University of Michigan the following citation was made by President Ruthven: "Professor of geology and director of the Geological Laboratory for twenty-eight years; since 1934 Professor Emeritus, whose achievements in science and influence in research will remain memorable in the annals of the University. To every task undertaken he brings an informed opinion and resolute will. His scholarly publications, many in number, range literally from pole to pole. Learned societies have elected him to office; mountains and glaciers bear his name; explorers buffeted by ice and storm value his share in their unending quest."

THE College of Physicians of Philadelphia awarded on July 14 the Alvarenga prize to Dr. Harry Goldblatt, professor of experimental pathology and associate director of the Institute of Pathology, of the School of Medicine of Western Reserve University, for his "contributions to the pathogenesis of hypertension." This prize was established by the will of Pedro Francisco daCosta Alvarenga, of Lisbon, Portugal, an associate fellow of the College of Physicians, to be awarded annually on each anniversary of the death of the testator, July 14, 1883, "to the author of the best memorial upon any branch of medicine, which may be deemed worthy of the prize."

Dr. William Washington Graves, director of the department of neuropsychiatry at St. Louis University School of Medicine, has received the St. Louis Medical Society award of merit "in consideration of the results of his studies on inherited variations in relation to the problems of the human constitution."

The Melchett Medal for 1939 of the British Institute of Fuel has been conferred on H. A. Humphrey, formerly consulting engineer to Imperial Chemical Industries, Ltd., for his work in "the development of fuel and appliances in connection therewith."

The retirement from the faculty of Princeton University is announced of Professor Ulric Dahlgren, who has been connected with the university since his graduation in 1894, since 1911 as professor of biology.

After serving for thirty-eight years as head of the department of chemistry of DePauw University, Dr. William M. Blanchard has relinquished his teaching duties, but will continue to serve for a time as dean of the College of Liberal Arts. Dr. Jesse L. Riebsomer has been appointed acting head of the department of chemistry for next year. Dr. J. C. Cowan, of the University of Illinois, has been appointed instructor in organic chemistry.

The title of Dr. R. M. Ogden, dean of the College of Arts and Sciences at Cornell University, has been changed from professor of education to professor of psychology, and he will be in future a member of the department of psychology. He remains dean of the college.

Dr. W. Halsey Barker, son of Dr. Lewellys F. Barker, of Baltimore, has been appointed to the newly established position of assistant dean of the School of Medicine of the Johns Hopkins University. He will aid Dr. Alan M. Chesney, dean, chiefly in the field of student relations. He will serve also as a member of the Committee on Admissions of the Medical School.

Edward Slater Sheiry, for six years head of the department of civil engineering in Robert College, Istanbul, has been appointed head of the department of civil engineering of Cooper Union, New York City, with the rank of full professor. He succeeds Professor Fred E. Foss, who retired in 1938 at the age of seventy-six years after serving for twenty-nine years. Assistant Professor Ray C. Brumfield has been acting head of the department during the past year.

M. G. Evans, lecturer in physical chemistry in the University of Manchester, has been appointed to the chair of physical chemistry at the University of Leeds, in succession to the late Professor H. M. Dawson.

Dr. James Wilfred Cook, professor of chemistry in the University of London, has been appointed Regius professor of chemistry in the University of Glasgow, to succeed the late Professor George Barger.

Professor Frank Horton, university professor of physics at Royal Holloway College and a member of the Senate of the University of London since 1925, has been elected vice-chancellor for the year 1939–40. Professor A. W. Reed has been made deputy vice-chancellor. Lord Dawson of Penn, who has hitherto been a representative of the faculty of medicine on the senate, has been appointed a coopted member in place of the late Sir Frank Dyson.

Dr. William W. Skinner has been appointed associate chief of the Bureau of Agricultural Chemistry and Engineering of the U. S. Department of Agriculture. In association with the chief of the bureau, Dr. Henry G. Knight, he will assist in the supervision and direction of all scientific, technical, engineering and administrative work, including the four Regional Research Laboratories authorized by the Congress to search for new and wider industrial outlets for agricultural commodities. Dr. Skinner has been a member of the Department of Agriculture since 1934.

Dr. Christian A. Ruckmick, formerly professor of psychology at the State University of Iowa, is now associated with the C. H. Stoelting Company of Chicago, for fifty-three years manufacturers of and dealers in psychological and physiological apparatus and supplies. He has been appointed to the position of secretary and general sales manager formerly held by W. C. Wideman.

Dr. Alexis Carrel, who is retiring as a member of the Rockefeller Institute for Medical Research, sailed for Europe on July 6.

Dr. Walter C. Lowdermilk, chief of the division of research of the U. S. Department of Agriculture, who was invited by the Palestine Government to investigate the situation of conservation, has spent some weeks in making observations, which have extended into the Negeb and to the Aqaba area of Transjordan.

Dr. Fred N. Briggs, associate professor of agronomy at the Agricultural College at Davis of the University of California, has sailed for Europe. He has leave of absence for six months which he will spend in visiting plant-breeding stations. He plans to attend the International Genetics Congress to be held this month in Edinburgh, Scotland.

Dr. E. I. White and W. N. Croft, both of the British Museum (Natural History), J. A. Moy-

Thomas, of Oxford, and J. Brough, of the University of Manchester, left England on June 24 to join the English, Norwegian and Swedish Geological Expedition to Spitsbergen. They expect to be away until towards the end of September. The expedition plans to collect remains of primitive vertebrate animals in the Wijde Bay area, from which little or nothing has hitherto been collected.

THE School of Medicine of the Johns Hopkins University and the Johns Hopkins Hospital will receive more than $1,000,000 by the will of the late Victor Morawetz, a New York attorney.

APPLICATIONS must be on file with the U. S. Civil Service Commission at Washington, D. C., on July 31 for the positions of meteorologist, at a salary of $3,800 a year; of associate meteorologist, at $3,200 a year, and of assistant meteorologist, at $2,600 a year. To become eligible, applicants must qualify in one or more of the following optional branches: eligibles are particularly desired who qualify in both Option 2 and Option 4, or who qualify in Option 2 and are trained in hydrology, or who qualify in Option 4 and are trained in oceanography: (1) Radiometeorography, (2) Synoptic Meteorology (Air Mass Analysis), (3) General Meteorology and Climatology, (4) Physical and Dynamical Meteorology, (5) Statistical Meteorology, (6) any other well-defined specialized branch of meteorology.

THE Cemenstone Corporation of Pittsburgh has established an industrial fellowship in Mellon Institute for conducting fundamental chemical and physical research on precast concrete units such as are being manufactured by the company. The main objective of the investigation is to develop practical methods and technics that will be of wide applicability in production. Donald R. MacPherson, for the past five years a member of the research staff of the Portland Cement Association in Chicago, has been appointed to the fellowship.

THE third International Congress for Microbiology will be held in New York at the Waldorf-Astoria Hotel from September 2 to 9. More than six hundred papers on a variety of subjects will be presented: for example, papers on bacterial variation and taxonomy, microbiological chemistry and physiology, viruses and viral diseases, rickettsiae and rickettsial diseases, fungi and fungous diseases (including bacterial diseases of plants), protozoology and parasitology, medical and veterinary bacteriology (including chemo- and serotherapy), industrial and agricultural microbiology and immunology. Any one interested in these subjects may attend the meetings. A registration fee of $5.00 will be charged. Those wishing to attend should communicate with the treasurer, Dr. Kenneth Goodner, Rockefeller Institute, York Avenue and 66th Street, New York, N. Y.

THE tentative program has been issued of the public health and nutrition section of the sixth Pacific Science Congress, of which Dr. K. F. Meyer is chairman, to be held from July 24 to August 12 at Berkeley, Stanford University and San Francisco, California. The program will be divided into four sections, as follows: Epidemiology of Diseases of the Pacific Basin; Nutritional Problems of the Pacific Basin; Industrial Hygiene; Health Education (to meet in joint session with the tenth annual meeting of the Western Branch of the American Public Health Association).

# DISCUSSION

## THE LUMINESCENCE OF SUGAR WAFERS

IF a "necco" wafer with a wintergreen flavor is broken in a dark room, a bright greenish flash of light appears, easily visible with dark-adapted eyes. This phenomenon is well known and is undoubtedly connected with the triboluminescence of sugar. The unusual aspect is the influence of the wintergreen flavor, for necco wafers with chocolate, liquorice and cinnamon flavors give no luminescence when broken and those with lemon, lime, clove and sassafras flavor give only a fair flash, about like that of lump sugar. The color of the wafer may be partly responsible for lack of luminescence, since dark-colored chocolate and liquorice-flavored wafers are not luminescent. However, the pink-colored sassafras-flavored wafer gives a fair luminescence, while the light orange cinnamon flavor gives none.

One necessity to obtain luminescence on breaking candy wafers is to have a mass of small sugar crystals, which are white, like snow. Thus, white "life savers" of wintergreen or clove flavor luminesce on breaking, but the mint, lime or cherry variety which are translucent and glass-like do not. Neither do "beechnut drops" of any flavor, also glassy, nor various taffies such as butter-scotch.

In a previous article[1] I pointed out that many triboluminescent crystals, such as salicylamid, salophen and uranyl nitrate, when crushed or shaken in a low pressure atmosphere of neon gas, still showed the bright greenish or colorless triboluminescent sparks with no trace of red which might indicate that the triboluminescence was an electrical discharge exciting the surrounding neon gas. Reddish electrical discharges can occur, however, when non-triboluminescent substances, such as chitin, diatomaceous earth or $KClO_3$ crystals, are broken in the neon atmosphere. Of special interest are sugar (rock candy) crystals, which

[1] SCIENCE, 89: 460, 1939.

gave a reddish luminescence when shaken in neon and some colorless triboluminescence also.

Longchambon[2] has observed the bands of nitrogen in triboluminescent sugar in air, and Wick,[3] in a thorough investigation of the general phenomena of triboluminescence, finds no triboluminescence of sugar when ground under xylol in a mortar. Both observations would indicate that sugar triboluminescence is mostly due to electric discharge in air. I have observed triboluminescence of sugar broken under various solvents, and additional experiments have led me to the belief that sugar molecules themselves can be excited to luminesce.

If a necco wafer with a wintergreen flavor is broken in a pure hydrogen atmosphere, in a vacuum (some air present, about 0.05 mm Hg) or in 10 to 20 mm neon there is always the greenish flash of light, of about the same intensity as in air. No red excitation of the neon occurs. Necco wafers and lump sugar will also luminesce if broken under water, 95 per cent. alcohol, acetone, toluol and xylol. Indeed, if soaked in alcohol, acetone, toluol or in xylol exhausted with an air pump for 5 minutes, to displace air between the sugar crystals, and then ground in a mortar, a triboluminescence appears in all solvents, brightest in the xylol and toluol and less marked in the acetone. I am therefore of the opinion that true triboluminescence of sugar (*i.e.*, excitation of luminescence in the sugar molecule) can occur as well as electrical discharges in the gas between sugar crystals. The reason the wintergreen-flavored necco wafer is particularly bright is because oil of wintergreen (methyl salicylate) is fluorescent and (1) excited to fluoresce by the triboluminescent light or (2) by electrical discharges when the wafer is broken. In ultra-violet light without the visible (mercury arc and Wood's filter), the wintergreen necco wafer is markedly bluish fluorescent, while lump sugar is practically non-fluorescent. The fluorescence of the wintergreen oil would add itself to the triboluminescence of the sugar when a necco wafer is broken.

E. NEWTON HARVEY

PRINCETON UNIVERSITY

## HEPARIN AND THE INHIBITION OF BLOOD-CLOTTING

IN 1936 Fischer,[1] using a purified fibrinogen solution, showed that the clotting of this solution with calcium chloride and thrombokinase was not inhibited by even great concentrations of heparin. Inhibition only occurred after the addition of minute amounts of serium or plasma (fresh or heated to 56° C.). He offered no definite explanation to these experimental results.

Experiments, performed to obtain further information on this process and which are to be published soon, have now shown: (1) The method used by Fischer in purifying the fibrinogen is not very reliable in obtaining a fibrinogen free from prothrombin. A pure prothrombin-free fibrinogen does not clot by the addition of calcium chloride and thrombokinase; (2) solutions containing purified fibrinogen and prothrombin, together with $CaCl_2$, clot readily by the addition of thrombokinase. On this process heparin is without any inhibitory action; (3) plasma and serum contain substances which are necessary for the inhibitory action of heparin.

Heparin alone is thus without any activity against the clotting process, and the activity is due to the presence, together with heparin, of yet unknown substances present in serum and plasma. These experiments thus confirm the recent work of Brinkhous, Smith, Warner and Seegers,[2] and it seems worth while to note such simultaneous and independent, but identical, new results, since this has not happened very often in the history of blood coagulation. The literature concerning this subject is for the most part confused by controversial statements.

TAGE ASTRUP

CARLSBERG FOUNDATION,
COPENHAGEN, DENMARK

## BORON AS A FERTILIZER FOR WESTERN OREGON SOILS

DURING the past decade studies have been conducted by the Oregon Experiment Station Soil Department with the aid of federal Adams funds to determine the value of the so-called minor elements in Oregon soil fertility and plant nutrition. Positive results have been secured with iodine, manganese, copper, zinc and boron. Response from iodine has been secured on Aiken silty clay loam and Deschutes sandy loam. Manganese and zinc have increased yields of certain crops on western Oregon peat. Copper has caused response with soils from the John Day and Illinois Valleys, while boron has been effective on most of the soil types used for alfalfa in northwestern Oregon.

Boron was shown to be essential to normal development of broad beans by Warrington in England in 1923. Boron has been used to control "top sickness" of tobacco, "brown heart" in turnips, "cork spot" in apples, "yellow top" in alfalfa and "crown rot" or "heart rot" of sugar beets, especially on soils of basic reaction. In the Pacific Northwest old soils, leachy soils or those derived from basaltic rocks seem more apt to be deficient in boron. Some unhealthiness in various plants formerly attributed to virus may be due to lack of boron. Soil reaction or lime and moisture

[2] *C. R. Ac. Sc.* 174: 1633, 1922; 176: 691, 1923.
[3] *Jour. Opt. Soc. Amer.*, 27: 275, 1937.
[1] A. Fischer, *Enzymologia*, 1: 81, 1936.

[2] K. M. Brinkhous, H. P. Smith, E. D. Warner and W. H. Seegers, *Am. Jour. Physiol.*, 125: 683, 1939.

contents, perhaps also temperature, may affect availability of boron.

In Oregon, recent experiments by the writer have demonstrated that yellow top of alfalfa can be controlled and yield strikingly increased on various soils by use of 30 pounds of boric acid an acre. Normal color was restored in the field within thirty days and with controlled conditions in the greenhouse within a few days. Bronzing and blighting of tops has been prevented and branching promoted.

Yellow top of alfalfa develops mainly under droughty conditions, although poor drainage may also lessen availability of boron. New leaves near the top of the stem become bronzed and then yellowish and tend to shatter off. The terminal bud and the blossoms may develop a blighted appearance. Application of boric acid or borax causes a lush green growth with branching of stems and, apparently, longevity of the alfalfa stand is promoted.

Boric acid has been used periodically in our experimental culture solutions for a decade to overcome a certain type of chlorosis or yellowing of foliage. One-half part per million has proven sufficient and may safely be used. The injurious effect of an excess is difficult to distinguish from that of a deficiency.

Chemical analyses of water, plant and soil profiles collected by the writer and made in our laboratories or by the U. S. Department of Agriculture show unfavorably low boron content in soils, waters and plants from affected areas. The use of boron to correct malnutrition has doubled boron content of plants, has slightly affected protein content and raised chlorophyll content 50 per cent. Boron content by the acid digestion method has ranged from 1½ part per million for peat to 7 parts per million for Willamette silty clay loam and is fairly uniform throughout the soil profile, though perhaps more available in the surface soil.

During the past three seasons in two dozen trials, use of boron on northwestern Oregon soils has controlled yellow top of alfalfa and trebled the yield for dry weather cuttings. Boron promises to be as profitable for western Oregon alfalfa land as sulfur has been in eastern Oregon. Similar symptoms have been observed and corrected on clovers and grasses.

Surface canker or "breakdown" of table beets has been controlled in the plant house and field in our experiments the past year perhaps for the first time. Canker caused rejection of whole fields of the 1937 crop.

Celery stem crack has been more completely controlled in field trials by Professor A. G. B. Bouquet and the writer where early applications were made. Assistance was given in treating some six acres.

Symptoms of boron "deficiency" disease, such as bronzing of tops and cracking at the nodes (or joints) with asters, broccoli and cabbage have led to boron applications to soil about these plants with promising results.

INDICATED EFFECTS OF BORON

(1) Boron may aid in the development of nodules on legumes.

(2) Apparently it is necessary for maintenance of elasticity and good condition of the conducting tissues and growing tip of the stem.

(3) It is apparently necessary for proper cell division and to the growing tip.

(4) Lettuce develops improperly in the absence of boron.

(5) May control nutritional deficiency diseases such as "heart rot" or surface "canker" of beets, "yellow top" of alfalfa and "stem crack" of celery.

(6) May aid availability of iron or of moisture.

(7) Boron may promote longevity and branching of alfalfa.

(8) Boron seems to improve keeping quality of apples.

There is less evidence of any deficiency of boron in eastern Oregon unless on neutral soils with rapid drainage. At the Hood River field station drought spot has been controlled with borax, and keeping quality of apples grown on Milton gravelly loam is reported by O. T. McWhorter to be improved. Use of boron with zinc is reported by Stephenson and Schuster to have been more effective in correction of little leaf of stone fruit trees near The Dalles.

While chemically pure boric acid was applied in dilute solution with a garden sprinkler in early, controlled experiments, the use of ordinary borax is usually cheaper for field use and will give similar results (unless on soils of basic reaction) if applied evenly and very early in the season. The boron treatment has been found to carry into the third season. Thirty pounds of borax may be evenly mixed with an equal amount of sandy loam or uniformly mixed with superphosphate or other fertilizer to dilute and aid evenness of application over each acre. The granular form has been successfully sown, as is clover seed. Slight temporary toxicity has followed application of 40 pounds of boric acid an acre to grass. Two pounds boric acid contain approximately as much of the element boron as does three pounds of borax. Borax may be secured of wholesale druggists or certain fertilizer dealers in Portland at about $3.25 per 100-pound bag. Several tons have been applied to western Oregon soils this 1939 season. It appears possible to increase the annual crop value in Willamette Valley at least $100,000 a year by the use of borax as fertilizer.

W. L. POWERS

OREGON AGRICULTURAL
EXPERIMENT STATION

# SOCIETIES AND MEETINGS

## THE ANNUAL MEETING OF THE SOUTHWESTERN DIVISION OF THE AMERICAN ASSOCIATION FOR THE ADVANCEMENT OF SCIENCE

THE Southwestern Division of the American Association for the Advancement of Science held its nineteenth annual meeting on May 2, 3, 4 and 5, in the extreme southeastern portion of its territory at Alpine, Texas, and the McDonald Observatory on Mt. Locke, forty miles from Alpine. Dates for the meetings were a week later than usual in order to make them coincide with the dedication of the new observatory. Inspection of the observatory, on May 2, and the dedication exercises, on May 5, were the unusual and distinctive features of the program. The attendance of the visiting astronomers who came to Alpine for the dedication ceremonies greatly enriched the meetings of the division. The delivery of the tenth John Wesley Powell Lecture by Professor Arthur H. Compton, on the topic "Physics Views the Future," was an outstanding event. The presidential address delivered by Dr. E. F. Carpenter, on the topic "The Revolt Against Thought," featured another evening of the sessions.

The attendance at the meetings was very good, particularly of those members who live in West Texas. The host institution, the Sul Ross State Teachers College, provided every facility possible for the comfort and entertainment of the visitors as well as presentation of the scientific features of the meetings. The exhibits at the museum of the West Texas Historical Society deserve special mention. In the business sessions the division voted to meet next year at Tucson, Arizona, with the University of Arizona, the Desert Laboratory and the Southwestern Forest and Range Experiment Station serving as host organizations. The meeting place for 1941 will be Lubbock, Texas, and for 1942, Las Cruces, New Mexico.

Officers of the division for the coming year, including those newly elected at the sessions, are as follows: *President,* J. R. Eyer, New Mexico State College, and *Vice-President,* C. V. Newsom, University of New Mexico. Dr. Emil Haury, University of Arizona, was elected as *Secretary-Treasurer* for the customary indefinite term of office. Members of the executive committee are as follows: E. F. Carpenter, University of Arizona, and S. B. Talmage, New Mexico School of Mines, who will serve until 1942; F. W. Sparks, Texas Technological College, and F. E. E. Germann, University of Colorado, who will serve until 1941; D. S. Robbins, State College, New Mexico, who will serve until 1940.

Section officers are as follows: Biological Section—*Chairman,* D. M. Crooks, University of Arizona, and *Secretary,* A. L. Hershey, New Mexico State College. Mathematics Section—*Chairman,* J. W. Branson, New Mexico State College; *Vice-Chairman,* E. J. Purcell, University of Arizona; *Secretary,* H. D. Larson, University of New Mexico. Social Science Section—*Chairman,* Emil Haury, University of Arizona; *Secretary,* Gordon C. Baldwin, University of Arizona. Physical Sciences Section—*Chairman,* C. W. Botkin, New Mexico State College; *Secretary,* O. B. Muench, New Mexico Normal University.

VEON C. KIECH,
*Secretary*

## A SYMPOSIUM ON METRIC GEOMETRY

IN ordinary analytic geometry each point of the space is characterized by coordinates (each point of an n-dimensional space by n coordinates), and the distance between any two points is a certain function of their coordinates. At the beginning of this century this concept of space was remarkably generalized by Fréchet. He did not make any assumption concerning the nature of points. Points are simply elements of some set, not necessarily defined by coordinates or in any other particular way. Fréchet merely assumed that with each pair of points a number, called the distance between the two points, is associated. This concept was introduced in order to unite several classical theories into one general theory, an aim similar to that of E. H. Moore's general analysis. Since their introduction much has been learned of the topology of Fréchet's metric spaces, *i.e.,* of their properties of density, connectivity, etc. But only during the last ten years has a systematic theory of the metric properties of these general spaces been developd, *e.g.,* of their convexity properties, their geodesics, etc. Recently L. M. Blumenthal summarized this theory in a book, "Distance Geometry," published in the University of Missouri Studies (Vol. XIII, No. 2).

This metric geometry was the subject of the third annual mathematical symposium held on April 12 and 13 at the University of Notre Dame. In the first meeting on April 12, Dr. L. M. Blumenthal, of the University of Missouri, spoke about the characterization of pseudo-spherical sets with application to determinant theory. A set is called pseudo-spherical if it can not be isometrically imbedded into the sphere though its subsets can. A set which can not be imbedded into the plane, though each subset can, consists of exactly five points, as it can be shown, and is called a pseudo-plane quintuple. Dr. P. M. Pepper, of the University of Notre Dame, presented some recent results on pseudo-plane quintuplets. He mentioned two surfaces slightly more complicated than the plane into which these quintuples can be imbedded. Dr. M. Sadowsky, of the Armour Institute of Technology, presented a new model of surfaces whose local metric is that of the Euclidean plane. Dr. L. M. Blumenthal gave a new metric characterization of the straight line.

On the following morning Dr. Marston Morse, of the Institute for Advanced Study, spoke about metric spaces related to the theory of critical points and applied in the calculus of variations. Dr. Karl Menger, of the University of Notre Dame, analyzed the minimum problem of the calculus of variations from the point of view of metric geometry. Dr. I. J. Schoenberg, of Colby College, dealt with the analytical aspects of isometric imbedding. The discussion was conducted by Dr. G. A. Bliss, of the University of Chicago.

The last meeting, directed by Dr. Marston Morse, dealt with the problem of imbedding metric spaces into Euclidean and more general spaces. Dr. Emil Artin, of Indiana University and the University of Notre Dame, dealt with the algebraic treatment of the question; Rev. B. J. Topel, University of Notre Dame, with imbedding into groups; Dr. A. M. Milgram, of the University of Notre Dame, with the imbedding of partially ordered sets into certain universal ordered sets. Dr. Karl Menger, of the University of Notre Dame, sketched a general theory of relation-preserving imbedding synthesizing these various theories.

KARL MENGER
UNIVERSITY OF NOTRE DAME

# REPORTS

## TRYPARSAMIDE IN THE CONTROL OF AFRICAN SLEEPING SICKNESS

RECENT reports on the progress of the extensive campaigns against African sleeping sickness (*T. gambiense* infection) indicate that the outlook for satisfactory control is much more promising than has heretofore been the case. This encouraging situation is directly associated with tryparsamide therapy, the effects of which were first demonstrated in the Belgian Congo in 1921.[1,2]

One of the major obstacles to a successful solution of the problem has been the failure of therapeutic agents in advanced cases, that is, those with involvement of the central nervous system. It is now known from the results of cerebrospinal fluid examination, moreover, that this involvement occurs much earlier than was formerly thought. Various drugs which are of benefit in the early phases of the infection are of little or no avail in later stages. Not only does the disease progress to a fatal termination, but the recurring presence of trypanosomes in the peripheral circulation constitutes a potential reservoir of infection. In marked contrast to these unsatisfactory results are those obtained with tryparsamide, the therapeutic action of which extends to the advanced stages. Because of this unique property, tryparsamide can be used in the routine mass treatment of both early and late cases.

Campaigns against sleeping sickness have long been a prominent feature of public health activities in the various colonies concerned, for control of the disease is a vital necessity to tropical Africa. A marked intensification of this work began some fifteen years ago, and it is significant that it was directly associated with the demonstration of the curative action of tryparsamide. An example of the notable results achieved is shown in the accompanying tabulation of official statistics of the Belgian Congo for the eleven-year period 1926–37, during which time tryparsamide has been increasingly employed.[3]

ELEVEN-YEAR RESULTS OF THE SLEEPING SICKNESS CAMPAIGN IN THE BELGIAN CONGO 1926–1937

| Year | Number of natives examined | Old cases under treatment | New cases | Index of new infections, per cent. |
|---|---|---|---|---|
| 1927 .... | 1,704,477 | 70,940 | 16,260 | 0.95 |
| 1928 .... | 2,126,356 | 46,372 | 24,440 | 1.16 |
| 1929 .... | 2,383,892 | 50,244 | 27,046 | 1.12 |
| 1930 .... | 2,779,448 | 70,423 | 33,562 | 1.20 |
| 1931 .... | 2,685,768 | 67,272 | 25,582 | 0.95 |
| 1932 .... | 2,832,083 | 77,268 | 21,346 | 0.75 |
| 1933 .... | 3,572,423 | 93,954 | 27,939 | 0.78 |
| 1934 .... | 3,824,097 | 86,147 | 24,101 | 0.63 |
| 1935 .... | 4,356,270 | 66,774 | 18,930 | 0.43 |
| 1936 .... | 5,282,646 | 53,429 | 18,708 | 0.36 |
| 1937 .... | 5,034,442 | 50,980 | 14,921 | 0.29 |

It will be noted that, although the number of natives examined annually for sleeping sickness was trebled in this period, that is, from 1,704,477 examined in 1926 to 5,034,477 in 1937, the index of new infections in 1937, 0.29 per cent., had fallen to one fourth the maximum figures of 1.16, 1.12, 1.20 per cent. in 1928, 1929, 1930, respectively. In addition, there was a marked decrease in the number of old cases continued under treatment from year to year, that is, from the high number of 93,954 in 1933 to 50,980 in 1937, a result of particular significance from the standpoint of efficiency of treatment.

Highly satisfactory results are reported by the Fonds Reine Elizabeth. This organization has had a wide experience in sleeping sickness work since 1931,

[1] L. Pearce, *Jour. Exp. Med.*, 24: 6, Supplement No. 1, 1921.

[2] L. Pearce, *Rockefeller Institute for Medical Research Monograph 23*, 1930, Science Press.

[3] L. Van Hoof, ''Rapport sur l'Hygiène Publique au Congo Belge,'' 1937.

first in the Bas-Congo and, beginning in 1935, in the adjacent Kwango area, two provinces in which the disease is a particularly serious problem. The intensive five-year campaign in the Bas-Congo resulted in a decrease of the total endemic index of 2.49 per cent. in 1931 to 0.59 per cent. in 1936.[4] During two and one-half years in the Kwango, 35,099 patients were under observation, of whom 28,008 were considered to have been satisfactorily treated, 4,451 were still under treatment, 1,225 had died and 1,415 had disappeared.[5] The conclusion was reached that with adequate treatment more than 90 per cent. of curative results could be obtained.

A typical course of treatment comprises 1 gram of moranyl (germanine or Bayer 205) followed by 12 to 14 weekly doses of tryparsamide.[4] The average dosage of tryparsamide is 1.0 to 3.0 grams. It may be necessary to prolong or to repeat treatment in advanced cases.[2]

In the Cameroons (French Mandate) a similar intensive campaign has likewise included the use of tryparsamide, particularly in cases known to be advanced. The official medical report for 1936[6] states that in this year 515,933 persons of a population of 572,910 living in seven severely infected districts were examined. There were 24,006 old and 2,107 new cases. Of the old cases under treatment, it was found that 23,362 patients no longer had trypanosomes in the peripheral blood, while in 644 patients organisms were still present. Of special significance, however, from the standpoint of satisfactory treatment was the fact that during the year 11,659 patients were considered cured upon the basis of blood and cerebrospinal fluid examination. The precise system of treatment employed is not given in this report, but it is known from other sources that tryparsamide enters largely into the therapeutic procedures followed. Additional evidence of the progress of the work in the entire colony is afforded by the decline in the index of "circulating virus," that is, the proportions of persons in whom trypanosomes are demonstrated in the peripheral blood: 1932, 1.43 per cent.; 1933, 0.82 per cent.; 1934, 0.8 per cent.; 1935, 0.8 per cent.; and 1936, 0.56 per cent.

Recent surveys carried out in colonies west of the Cameroons show that sleeping sickness occupies a more important place among diseases than was hitherto supposed. This is the case, for instance, in Nigeria, where a sleeping sickness service was established in 1931. The official medical report for 1936[7] states that the total number of cases diagnosed and treated since the initiation of this service is 240,900, while 24,033 patients have been treated at general medical stations. During the year 1936, examination of 417,495 natives in the northern provinces of the colony revealed 47,550 cases, an incidence of nearly 11.5 per cent. An additional 14,571 cases were diagnosed and treated at field dispensaries and general hospitals, making a total of 62,021 cases treated in this year. The standard treatment now comprises three 1.0 gram doses of antrypsol or Bayer 205, followed by five 2.0 gram doses of tryparsamide.

Finally, attention should be directed to the fact that the introduction of tryparsamide therapy has resulted in the gratifying response of native cooperation in the treatment of both old and new cases. This significant change in the point of view of the native population which has been emphasized in various reports is obviously a factor of the greatest practical importance in the control of the disease.

The immense scope of the sleeping sickness problem is shown in a report of the League of Nations dealing with the geographical distribution of the disease.[8] From official data for 1935 or in a few instances for 1934, the following conclusions are drawn:

> In the African territories situated between the tropics, the total population of which may be estimated at 65 millions, nearly 7 millions were examined in the course of a single year. 140,000 fresh cases were discovered and treated, besides a similar number of old cases. In territories where the campaign has been going on for a long time (Belgian Congo, French Equatorial Africa, Cameroons under French Mandate), out of nearly 15 million inhabitants, the number examined in the course of a year exceeds 6 millions.

An effective therapeutic agent is a crucial factor in sleeping sickness campaigns, but the importance of other measures can not be overlooked. Authorities are well aware of the necessity of communal clearings directed against the tsetse fly and of the control of the movement and concentration of populations. Nevertheless, under the conditions now obtaining in tropical Africa, the successful solution of the problem must necessarily include the mass employment of therapeutic agents which are capable of curing not only early, but advanced cases. Up to the present time the only drug which fulfils this double requirement is tryparsamide. Future accomplishments based upon its widespread administration throughout infected areas are clearly foreshadowed by the unprecedented results already obtained.

LOUISE PEARCE

ROCKEFELLER INSTITUTE FOR
MEDICAL RESEARCH,
PRINCETON, N. J.

4 De Brauwere, Fonds Reine Elizabeth. Rapport Annuel, 1936.

5 *Ibid.*, 1937.

6 Rapport Annuel du Territoire du Cameroun, 1936.

7 Annual Report of Medical Services of Nigeria, 1936.

8 Epidemiological Report (Sleeping Sickness) of the League of Nations, 1936, Nos. 10–12.

# SPECIAL ARTICLES

## EFFECT OF INDOLE-3-ACETIC ACID ON PHOTOSYNTHESIS

W. MITCHELL and CH. L. HAMNER[1] have recently shown that indole-3-acetic acid (heteroauxin) "stimulates plants to synthesize more solid matter, without causing a corresponding increase in leaf area." The authors' conclusion is based on experiments with young decapitated kidney-beans (*Phaseolus vulgaris*), where a lanoline paste containing indole-3-acetic acid was applied on the cut surface of the stem end. Such plants accumulated in the course of three days almost twice as much dry matter as did the control under identical environmental conditions. The control plants were also decapitated but treated with lanoline paste without heteroauxin.

The most probable explanation of the interesting fact established by Mitchell and Hamner is that heteroauxin from the paste on the cut surface penetrated into the green leaves of the experimental plants and intensified their photosynthetic activity. This assumption is supported by the experiments conducted by the authors during the summer of 1938.

Pairs of leaves were cut off from various plants (lilac, poplar, jasmine, hemp, hydrangea and others), care being taken to choose leaves as similar as possible in regard to age, size and position on the stem. The leaves were placed into two glass chambers, the lower ends of the leaf petioles being immersed in a Knop solution, and the intensity of photosynthesis determined. Electric lighting was employed. The surface of the chambers was cooled by a stream of running water in order to avoid overheating the leaves. The leaves were lighted for about one and three quarters of an hour. After several hours, a second determination was made of the quantity of carbonic acid decomposed by these leaves under the same conditions of lighting and in the course of an equal interval of time. These two determinations made it possible to estimate the photosynthetic activity of the leaves experimented on. It was expressed in milligrams of carbonic acid decomposed by one square decimeter of leaf surface in one hour.

One of the leaves was then immersed with the lower end of the petiole in a Knop solution containing 1 mg of heteroauxin per liter of water; while the other (control) was immersed in a Knop solution without heteroauxin. After several hours both leaves were again placed in the chambers and the intensity of assimilation was determined under the previous environmental conditions.

These experiments, repeated many times with various subjects, showed in the vast majority of cases a considerable intensification of photosynthesis under the influence of the indole-3-acetic acid introduced into the leaf. Thus, the hemp leaf, whose photosynthetic activity was expressed by figures of 10.00 and 9.60 mg in the first two determinations in the Knop mixture (with a four-hour interval between experiments), gave 19.24 mg and, in four hours, 18.00 mg of decomposed $CO_2$ after being kept in a Knop solution with heteroauxin (1 mg per liter) for nine hours. The control leaf gave the following values on parallel determinations: 12.10; 12.90; 14.73; 13.80. It should be noted that the photosynthetic activity in the control leaf kept in a Knop solution remained at the same level for the subsequent thirty hours; whereas, the experimental plant receiving the same solution with the addition of heteroauxin showed a considerable reduction of photosynthesis towards the end of the experiment (control, 14.83 mg; experimental leaf, 2.10 mg).

In another experiment on hydrangea, where the leaf was kept for 24 hours in a Knop solution with heteroauxin, the intensity of photosynthesis increased from 5.10 to 14.88 mg, while in the control leaf a decrease—from 3.34 to 2.14 mg—was observed.

Using higher heteroauxin concentrations (10 mg per liter) did not cause any changes in photosynthesis in our experiments.

Thus we arrive at the conclusion that indole-3-acetic acid causes a temporary intensification of photosynthesis on being directly introduced into the assimilating tissues of the green leaf in very low concentrations.

N. G. CHOLODNY
A. G. GORBOVSKY
LABORATORY OF PLANT PHYSIOLOGY,
ACADEMY OF SCIENCES OF THE
UKRAINIAN SSR,
KIEV, U. S. S. R.

[1] *Botan. Gazette*, March, 1938, p. 569.

## GROWTH OF SOME HEMOLYTIC STREPTOCOCCI ON A CHEMICALLY DEFINED MEDIUM

HEMOLYTIC streptococci have previously been grown in complex media containing tissue extracts and have not been successfully cultured on mixtures of pure chemicals. Many problems dealing with the metabolic activity of these organisms would be aided if it were possible to know all the constituents of the medium on which the bacteria were grown. We have been able to obtain luxuriant growth of a representative strain of hemolytic streptococci on a medium containing only pure chemical compounds. The organism used was one of the Lancefield type D group, *S. zymogenes* strain H-6905.

We have recently shown[1] that a wide variety of hemolytic streptococci require riboflavin, pantothenic acid and a suitable reducing substance such as "reduced" iron. In addition, protein hydrolysates and

[1] D. W. Woolley and B. L. Hutchings, *Jour. Bact.*, in press.

aqueous liver extract are also required. We have now found that the protein hydrolysate may be replaced by a mixture of pure amino acids mixed in such proportions as to simulate the composition of casein. The liver extract[2] was purified by adsorption on and elution from lead sulfide, followed by adsorption on and elution from fuller's earth. The resulting concentrate was active at a level of 1 microgram per cc. The properties of the active material revealed by these concentration procedures led us to try various basic growth factors, and it was found that crystalline vitamin $B_6$[3] was effective.

Representative data illustrating the response obtained on our chemically defined media are shown in Table 1. The amino acid mixture supplied the following amounts of material per cc of medium: glycine 0.1 mg, dl-alanine 0.4 mg, dl-valine 1.6 mg, dl-leucine 1.0 mg, d-isoleucine 0.5 mg, dl-serine 0.2 mg, l-proline 1.0 mg, l-hydroxyproline 0.1 mg, dl-phenylalanine 1.0 mg, l-tyrosine 0.7 mg, l-cystine 0.1 mg, d-arginine hydrochloride 0.8 mg, l-histidine hydrochloride 0.4 mg, d-lysine hydrochloride 1.0 mg, l-tryptophane 0.3 mg, dl-methionine 0.8 mg, l-aspartic acid 0.5 mg, d-glutamic acid 2.5 mg, dl-threonine 0.6 mg. Growth was measured by quantitative determination of turbidity, as previously described. The figures in Table 1 represent the per cent. of the incident light which was transmitted by the culture. The pantothenic acid was supplied as a highly purified concentrate, but a synthetic product derived from di-hydroxy caproic acid was previously shown to replace it.

TABLE 1

| Additions to glucose-salts medium | Photometer reading |
|---|---|
| (1) Riboflavin + reduced Fe + pantothenic acid | 100 |
| (2) (1) + amino acids | 74 |
| (3) (2) + vitamin $B_6$ (0.5γ/cc.) | 10 |

It was noted that slight growth usually occurred when the amino acids, but not vitamin $B_6$, were added. This may possibly be due to contamination of some of the amino acids with the vitamin. It was not possible to supply every amino acid as a synthetic product, and while those that were not synthesized were carefully recrystallized, it may be that they were still contaminated.

The amino acid requirements for *S. zymogenes* have been determined on our medium, and glutamic acid and tryptophane were found to be essential. Details of the work, together with observations on a variety of species, will be published elsewhere.

BRIAN L. HUTCHINGS
D. W. WOOLLEY
UNIVERSITY OF WISCONSIN

2 We wish to thank Dr. David Klein of Wilson Laboratories for generous gift of this material.

3 We wish to thank Dr. S. Lepkovsky for a sample of crystalline vitamin $B_6$.

## THE PSEUDO-AMNION, PSEUDO-CHORION, PSEUDO-PLACENTA AND OTHER FOETAL STRUCTURES IN VIVIPAROUS CYPRINODONT FISHES

OVOVIVIPARITY or viviparity occurs in all species of four families of the cyprinodont fishes. Most of the specializations for viviparity in embryos and ovaries found in other viviparous fishes occur in this single order, and in addition there are unique features not found elsewhere. Within two of the families (Poeciliidae and Goodeidae) different species show degrees of specialization varying from simple conditions similar to those of oviparous fishes to extremes involving the partial degeneration of the yolk sac, and the development of new structures (pseudo-amnion, pseudo-chorion, pseudo-follicular placenta, trophotaeniae and gut modifications). Simple adaptations occur in the early embryos of extremely specialized forms, but these are ephemeral and are replaced in later stages of gestation by newer and more specialized structures. In the families Jenynsiidae and Anablepidae the living species have become highly specialized and no species retains simple modifications, except in early stages of ontogeny. There are numerous parallel developments in the four families.

The development, function and history of these adaptational structures is parallel roughly to that of the foetal membranes and yolk sac in the amniotes as a whole in the following respects:

(1) The yolk supply is adequate for nutrition up to the time of birth or hatching in some cases, but the yolk sac becomes degenerate in more specialized groups and the function of nutrition is taken over by new structures.

(2) Membranes or specialized organs functioning as respiratory, nutritive and excretory devices are developed from the somatopleure of the pericardial or peritoneal spaces and from the gut. They become highly vascular.

(3) In cases of advanced viviparity the uterus (ovary in fishes) becomes greatly modified.

(4) Foetal membranes or specialized structures are temporary and are discarded at birth.

*Poeciliidae.* The embryos are retained in the ovarian follicles for the whole period of gestation. In some genera (Mollienesia and others) the yolk sac is large and furnishes an adequate nutritional supply for the whole period of gestation. The somatopleure of the extra-embryonic pericardial cavity becomes vascularized, thus augmenting the respiratory surface, and lateral extensions fuse dorsal to the posterior head region to form a continuous band, a unique feature in this family. Specializations within the family are of two types. (1) *Heterandria formosa* and others have very small yolk sacs. The lateral extensions of the somatopleure of the extra-embryonic pericardial cavity completely envelop the head, forming an outer vascular membrane (*pseudo-chorion*) and an inner non-vascular layer (*pseudo-amnion*) which is adherent to the embryo. The vascular membrane with its blood vessels derived from the old vitelline circulation is used as an organ for respiration and nutrition throughout gestation. The surrounding follicle becomes highly vascular and develops a layer of high, irregular columnar cells. (2) In Aulophallus and some species of Poeciliopsis which have small yolk sacs the lateral portions of the pericardial somatopleure are poorly developed, but the ventral portion becomes enlarged into an extensive vascular belly sac. The surrounding follicle develops on the internal surface an extensive system of anastomosing villi which are vascular and are covered with a secretory epithelium. The wall of the belly sac, together with the wall of the follicle with its villi, form a *follicular pseudo-placenta*.

*Anablepidae.* A more complicated and apparently more effective *follicular pseudo-placenta* has been developed in at least two of the three existing species of Anableps. The belly sac becomes very large and at an early stage takes over and expands the vitelline circulation. The blood vessels of the sac become expanded into rows of connected and projecting vascular bulbs. The surrounding follicle is covered on its inner surface with a mat of long vascular villi which are covered with a low epithelium.

The looped small intestine is everted into the cavity of the belly sac in *Anableps anableps*. In *A. dowei* the large intestine becomes a balloon-like sac which nearly fills the cavity of the sac. In both species there is a metamorphosis of the gut at birth involving shortening and reorganization. Follicular fluid is imbibed by the embryo and absorption takes place by means of specialized villi of the gut. The concentrated unabsorbed material is retained in the gut.

*Goodeidae.* In this family and in the Jenynsiidae the embryos are evacuated from the ovarian follicles into the ovarian cavity at early stages and develop in the ovarian cavity.

Goodeid species have various degrees of specialization in foetal structures. (1) In the primitive Ataeniobius the yolk sac is fairly large, and there is no expansion of the pericardial membrane. In late gestation the embryos imbibe ovarian fluid through an enlarged opercular opening and the mouth. (2) *Goodea luitpoldii* has a smaller yolk sac. The extra-embryonic pericardial sac is somewhat enlarged and vascular in early stages but recedes with the development of the trophotaeniae, ribbon-shaped outgrowths from the rectal lip which increase the absorbing surface. (3) Lermichthys, Neotoca and others have very small yolk sacs. Extensions of the pericardial somatopleure arise early but begin to recede at the thirty-five somite stage. A very extensive system of vascular trophotaeniae begins to develop at the twenty somite stage and with the recession of the extra-embryonic pericardial membrane takes over the functions of respiration and nutrition.

*Jenynsiidae.* In *Jenynsia* (*Fitzroya*) *lineata* the embryo augments the respiratory surface by expanding the vascular pericardial sac. The sac reaches the maximal size at the 6 mm stage at the point at which the yolk becomes exhausted. The pericardial sac begins to recede at this point, but in the meantime club-shaped vascular flaps grow out from the ovarian wall and extend into the branchial and mouth cavities through an enlarged opercular opening. Respiratory exchanges are accomplished by this device during the remainder of the gestational period, but nutritional materials are obtained by absorption from ovarian fluid imbibed through the mouth or opercular openings.

C. L. Turner

Northwestern University

# SCIENTIFIC APPARATUS AND LABORATORY METHODS

## A THORACIC WINDOW FOR OBSERVATION OF THE LUNG IN A LIVING ANIMAL

During my investigation of the presence of fluid in the pulmonary air sacs a number of techniques have been tried to make these chambers accessible for observation in the living animal. Whereas this is a simple matter in the case of amphibians, it is not so in dealing with mammals, as every investigator who has approached the provinces of structure or physiology of the terminal spaces of the lung has realized. In attempts to overcome the difficulty of maintaining the lung under natural physiological conditions and at the same time having it available for observation and experiment, an instrument has been devised which is simple in construction, easy to adjust and which has proved successful for observations of the superficial air sacs and alveoli in the cat's lung. The principle of the method seems to be sound and practicable; some changes in the construction of accessory parts and in the means of illumination may be found desirable.

The instrument, made of bronze, consists of a short hollow cylinder, at one end of which is mounted a small cover glass window and at its opposite or internal end is formed a quadrilateral plate or flange. When adjusted in the thoracic wall, the cylinder projects through an opening made in an intercostal space, the plate fitting against the internal surface of the wall and the instrument fixed in place by means presently to be explained. When the air has been drawn out of the pleural cavity by an exhaust tube, the surface of the lung comes in contact with the window and remains there in view during respiration. Details of the form and the dimensions of the principal parts of the instrument are shown in the accompanying figures.

The preferred points of opening the chest in an adult cat have been either the right second intercostal space or the right fifth intercostal space; the former because the movement there of the cephalic lobe is slight; the latter, chosen for manipulation of the ventral thin edge of the lung. In either case the pectoral muscles were divided and retracted (cat anesthetized with urethane), exposing intercostal muscles and the ribs. An opening barely large enough to admit the plate is made through the parietal pleura and the instrument, controlled by the handle, is introduced into the pleural cavity, then adjusted so that the cylinder stands between the two adjacent ribs. A piece of dental rubber dam somewhat larger than the plate and having a hole cut in the center to fit when stretched over the cylinder, is applied to the external face of the plate before the instrument is introduced into the chest. Fixation of the window in the thoracic wall is accomplished by screwing a flange upon the threaded cylinder down to the level of the ribs, thereby drawing the plate with its rubber mantle snugly against the internal surface of the thoracic wall. Two small lugs on the edges of the plate impinge upon the margins of the ribs, so that any tendency toward twisting of the window is prevented. By these means the window is incorporated in the chest wall, joints are sealed, and it moves with the movements of the wall in respiration, unless fixed, as it can be, by clamping the handle to the animal carrier.

Air that entered the pleural cavity when the window was inserted is removed by suction through an exhaust tube, whose bore opens internally immediately beneath the cover glass. When the last air is drawn out the surface of the lung strikes the glass with a noticeable clink. Clamping the suction tube maintains the vacuum. The cover glass, set in Canada balsam on a shoulder of the cylinder, is placed eccentrically in order to give room in the cylinder for the handle, the exhaust tube and a tunnel (Fig. 1, a). The latter goes very

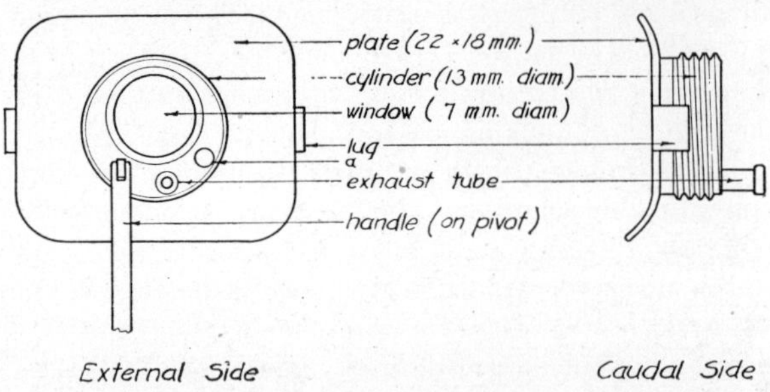


FIG. 1. Thoracic window.

obliquely to open beneath the cover glass and provides a way for experimental procedures, quartz rod lighting, etc.

Observations have been made with the binocular microscope and with a skin microscope; illumination for the former being an arc lamp, for the latter a 6-volt bulb. From both these sources of direct light the glare has been a disadvantage, controlled somewhat by the

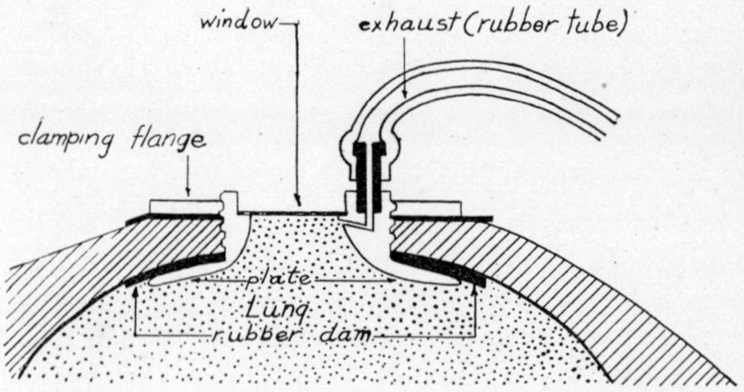


FIG. 2. Schematic transverse section of thoracic wall with thoracic window adjusted.

use of polaroid film. Experiments with quartz rod transmitted lighting are in progress. Good views of the superficial air sacs and alveoli have been obtained and a motion picture has recently been made recording such phenomena as could be brought forth with low power magnification and arc lamp illumination. With higher power lenses the capillary nets could be observed. Studies by means of the thoracic window are in progress and will be communicated in later publication.

ROBERT J. TERRY
WASHINGTON UNIVERSITY, ST. LOUIS

## BOOKS RECEIVED

*Accident Facts. 1939 edition.* Pp. 104. Illustrated. National Safety Council, Chicago. $0.50.

MATHER, KIRTLEY F. and SHIRLEY L. MASON. *A Source Book in Geology.* Pp. xxii + 702. 42 figures. McGraw-Hill. $5.00.

PAPPENHEIMER, ALWIN M., MARIANNE GOETTSCH and ERWIN JUNGHERR. *Nutritional Encephalomalacia in Chicks and Certain Related Disorders of Domestic Birds.* Monograph of the Storrs Agricultural Experiment Station. Pp. 121. Illustrated. Connecticut State College, Storrs.

PAULING, LINUS. *The Nature of the Chemical Bond and the Structure of Molecules and Crystals.* Pp. xiv + 429. Illustrated. Cornell University Press. $4.50.

RODALE, J. I. *Sleep and Rheumatism.* Pp. 130. 22 figures. Rodale Press, Emmaus, Pa. $1.50.

SHIVELY, LEVI S. *An Introduction to Modern Geometry.* Pp. xi + 167. 122 figures. Wiley. $2.00.

STURTEVANT, A. H. and G. W. BEADLE. *An Introduction to Genetics.* Pp. 391. 126 figures. Saunders. $3.25.

*Travaux de L'Association Internationale de Géodésie; Tome 13, Fascicule 2, Rapports Nationaux sur les Travaux Exécutés dans les Différents Pays, Edimbourg, September, 1936.* Illustrated. The Association, Paris.

VESTAL, PAUL A. and RICHARD E. SCHULTES. *The Economic Botany of the Kiowa Indians as it Relates to the History of the Tribe.* Pp. xiii + 110. Illustrated. Botanical Museum, Cambridge, Mass.

WADDINGTON, C. H. *An Introduction to Modern Genetics.* Pp. 441. 160 figures. Macmillan. $4.00.

YAPP, W. B. *An Introduction to Animal Physiology.* Pp. xv + 319. 46 figures. Oxford University Press. $3.00.

# SCIENCE

Vol. 90 — Friday, July 21, 1939 — No. 2325

*The Milwaukee Meeting of the American Association for the Advancement of Science:* Edited by Dr. F. R. Moulton ... 45

*Obituary:*
*Harry Victor Atkinson:* Professor Edwin H. Shaw, Jr. *Recent Deaths and Memorials* ... 55

*Scientific Events:*
*The Annual Field Day of the Rothamsted Experimental Station; English Neurologic Research Institute; The Society of the Sigma Xi; The Convention of the Electrochemical Society; The Boston Meeting of the American Chemical Society* ... 56

*Scientific Notes and News* ... 59

*Discussion:*
*Centers of Population of Learned Groups:* Professor Cecil B. Read. *A New Disease of Snap Beans:* Dr. Wilbert A. Jenkins. *General Anesthesia by Chilling:* Dr. G. H. Parker ... 61

*Scientific Books:*
*Recent Botanical Books:* Professor Edwin B. Matzke ... 63

*Special Articles:*
*Adsorption of Antibodies by Egg Albumin Films:* A. Rothen and Dr. K. Landsteiner. *Adsorption Spectrum of Further Purified Cytochrome C:* Professor Hugo Theorell and Å. Åkesson. *Sodium Chloride and Diabetes insipidus:* Dr. H. G. Swann. *The Attempted Hydrogenation of 3-Methylxanthine:* Professor Treat B. Johnson and Joseph C. Ambelang ... 65

*Scientific Apparatus and Laboratory Methods:*
*Labeling Museum Specimens:* Professor Vernon E. Scheid. *A Simple Demonstration of the Conditioned Response:* Professor W. A. Bousfield ... 69

*Science News* ... 10

SCIENCE: A Weekly Journal devoted to the Advancement of Science, edited by J. McKeen Cattell and published every Friday by

THE SCIENCE PRESS
New York City: Grand Central Terminal

Lancaster, Pa. — Garrison, N. Y.

Annual Subscription, $6.00 — Single Copies, 15 Cts.

SCIENCE is the official organ of the American Association for the Advancement of Science. Information regarding membership in the Association may be secured from the office of the permanent secretary in the Smithsonian Institution Building, Washington, D. C.

# THE MILWAUKEE MEETING OF THE AMERICAN ASSOCIATION FOR THE ADVANCEMENT OF SCIENCE

**Edited by Dr. F. R. MOULTON**

PERMANENT SECRETARY

For the second time in its history the American Association for the Advancement of Science held a meeting in Wisconsin. The first meeting in Wisconsin was held in Madison from August 17 to August 22, 1893; the recent meeting in Milwaukee was held from June 19 to June 24, 1939. The proximity of Milwaukee to Chicago with its several great educational institutions and its unsurpassed accessibility by railroads has obviously prevented its being selected hitherto as a meeting place for the association. It is delightfully located, however, on the shores of Lake Michigan and has ample facilities for a very large convention.

In 1893, at the time of the meeting in Madison, there were 1,982 members of the association; at the time of the meeting in Milwaukee there were 20,310 members. The attendance at the meeting in Madison was 290; at Milwaukee, about 700. There were 168 papers presented at Madison, and 264 papers and addresses at Milwaukee. In comparing these statistics of attendance and papers it should be remembered that the regular annual meeting of the association was held at Madison, while only a summer meeting was held in Milwaukee.

Although many of the programs presented in Milwaukee were of a very high order of excellence, the attendance was low, only about a third of that at the meeting in Ottawa a year ago. It is a question whether there are not so many meetings of scientists that general summer meetings of the association fail to justify their cost in effort and money. Possibly the association would better fulfil its purpose of advancing the interests of science and society if, instead of holding general summer meetings of all sections, it would arrange for those sections and affiliated societies which find it advantageous to have summer programs to hold special regional meetings in connection with universities and other organizations.

## REGISTRATION

Although about 700 persons were in attendance at the meeting, only 331 registered and secured the General Program of all sessions and events. The registrants were distributed as follows: Alabama, 1; Arkansas, 1; California, 5; Colorado, 1, Connecticut, 3; Washington, D. C., 18; Georgia, 1; Idaho, 1; Illinois, 58; Indiana, 4; Iowa, 8; Kansas, 2; Maine, 1; Massachusetts, 10; Michigan, 21; Minnesota, 17; Missouri, 13; Nebraska, 1; New Jersey, 6; New Mexico, 1; New York, 20; North Carolina, 1; North Dakota, 1; Ohio, 13; Oklahoma, 1; Oregon, 1; Pennsylvania, 7; Rhode Island, 1; South Dakota, 2; Vermont, 1; Wisconsin, 48; Milwaukee, 60; Foreign and Unknown, 4.

## GENERAL SESSIONS

On June 20 the eighth Hector Maiben Lecture was delivered by Dr. Victor G. Heiser, distinguished author of "The Odyssey of an American Doctor," on "The Influence of Nutrition on the Diseases of Middle and Old Age." A large and appreciative audience listened attentively to Dr. Heiser's exposition of some of the astonishing consequences of unbalanced diet.

On Wednesday evening, June 21, Dr. Heber D. Curtis, director of the observatories of the University of Michigan, delivered a lecture, illustrated by motion pictures, on "Solar Storms." The motion pictures, taken with the remarkable apparatus developed at the McMath-Hulburt Observatory, showed most astounding phenomena taking place on the sun. The large audience sat in awe before pictures of great masses of flaming gas, thousands of times greater in volume than the earth, shooting up from the surface of the sun tens of thousands of miles and, strangely, often shooting down with comparable velocities. Indeed, the photograph of one eruption was shown that ascended to a height of over 600,000 miles.

The third conference on "Science and Society" presented a program of four general sessions on "The Economic System in Relation to Scientific Progress." The program is given in the report of the Section on Social and Economic Sciences below.

## SYMPOSIA

Eleven symposia were presented at the meeting, in addition to a symposium at Madison under the sponsorship of the Division of Physical and Inorganic Chemistry of the American Chemical Society and the University of Wisconsin, in cooperation with the Section on Chemistry (C).

1. The Section on Geology and Geography (E) held a joint symposium with the American Society of Agricultural Engineers, the Section on Engineering, Association of American Geographers and the Geological Society of America on "Soil Conservation and Land Utilization in the Great Lakes Region," at which 14 papers were presented in two sessions. The contributions were by M. L. Nichols and Bruno Klinger, C. F. Stewart Sharpe, Eugene I. Roe, T. M. Bushnell, Otto E. Guthe, A. H. Paschall, Dallas E. Perfect, E. A. Norton, Paul M. Barrett, F. P. Struhsaker, W. F. Ramsdell, A. R. Whitson, L. B. Thomson and Louis A. Wolfanger.

2. The Section on Zoological Sciences (F) presented a symposium on "The Relation of Genetics to Geographical Distribution and Speciation," under the chairmanship of L. J. Cole, who opened the symposium with introductory remarks. The discussions were by Carl L. Hubbs, M. R. Irwin and R. W. Cumley, A. H. Sturtevant, L. R. Dice, and Alfred C. Kinsey.

3. The Section on Zoological Sciences (F) presented also a second symposium on "Regeneration," under the chairmanship of J. W. Buchanan, who opened the symposium. The papers of this symposium were presented by W. C. Curtis, Olin Rulon, William Balamuth, L. H. Hyman, and the session closed with a tribute to H. V. Wilson by W. C. Curtis.

4. The Section on Botanical Sciences (G) in a joint session with the Ecological Society of America, the Society of American Foresters and the Section on Agriculture (O) presented a symposium on "Socio-economic Approach to Land Use," under the chairmanship of L. R. Schoenmann. The participants were Aldo Leopold, K. C. McMurry, G. S. Wehrwein and Raphael Zon.

5. The American Society of Plant Physiologists in joint session with the Section on Botanical Sciences (G) and the American Phytopathological Society presented a symposium on "Photoperiodism," at which the speakers were W. F. Loehwing, Karl C. Hamner, R. H. Roberts and B. Esther Struckmeyer.

6. The Section on Psychology (I) presented a symposium on "Measuring Attitudes," one section of which was under the chairmanship of Stephen M. Corey and the other of which was under the chairmanship of Gilbert J. Rich. At the former, the speakers were Maurice Newburger, Louis D. Goodfellow, David A. Grant and Herbert I. Meyer, Delton C. Beier, and H. Wilkes Wright.

7. The Section on Psychology (I) presented also a symposium on "Neuromuscular Tension," under the chairmanship of Edmund Jacobson.

8. The Section on Social and Economic Sciences (K) presented a broad symposium on "Population

Problems and Programs in the Northern Lake States," under the direction of an organizing committee consisting of Warren S. Thompson, E. P. Hutchinson and Stanley D. Dodge. The first part on "The Settlement of the Northern Lake States" was presented in joint session with the Population Association of America and the Ecological Society of America, under the chairmanship of Stanley D. Dodge. Papers were presented by Glenn T. Trewartha, W. Bruce Dick and Guy-Harold Smith.

The second part, on "Population Capacity under Different Forms of Land Use," was presented in joint session with the Population Association of America and the Ecological Society of America. E. P. Hutchinson was chairman and the speakers were Charles M. Davis, Stanley D. Dodge and Raphael Zon.

The third part, on "State and Regional Planning," was presented in joint session with the Population Association of America, under the chairmanship of Warren S. Thompson. The contributors were Samuel Teper, George Wehrwein and M. W. Torkelson.

The fourth part, on "Population Adjustment through Migration," was presented in joint session with the Population Association of America, under the chairmanship of Conrad Taeuber. Papers were read by C. E. Lively, Ray E. Wakeley and J. F. Thaden.

The fifth part, on "Regional Differentiation of Culture Patterns," was presented under the chairmanship of C. E. Lively, at which A. R. Magnus, Philip Beck and George W. Hill presented papers.

The sixth part, on "Agricultural Policies and Programs of the Federal Government," was presented under the chairmanship of Warren S. Thompson. The participants were C. C. Taylor and H. R. Tolley.

The final session on "Evaluation of Federal Policies and Programs" was held under the chairmanship of R. C. Smith, and papers were presented by Lowry Nelson, T. W. Schultz and Noble Clark.

9. The Section on Medical Sciences (N) in cooperation with the American Neisserian Medical Society organized and presented a comprehensive symposium on "Gonococcus and Gonococcal Infection."

The first session was on "The Biology of the Gonococcus," at which papers were presented by Gaylord W. Anderson, Alden K. Boor, N. S. Ferry, Michael Wisengrad, C. Philip Miller, Wesley W. Spink and Alfred Cohn. The subject of the second session was "The Diagnosis of Gonococcal Infection." The contributors to the discussion of this subject were Christine E. Rice, Annis E. Thomson and Agnes C. Hamann, Charles M. Carpenter, Oscar F. Cox and William A. Hinton, Adolph Jacoby, Walter M. Brunet, J. Albert Key, Sara E. Branham, and C. L. Martin.

"Sulfanilamide and Related Compounds" comprised the third session, with papers by Ralph R. Mellon and Lawrence E. Shinn, Charles M. Carpenter and Gerald M. Barbour, Ruth A. Boak, Cassius J. Van Slyke, Percy S. Pelouze, J. F. Mahoney and Anna Nimelman, Nathaniel Jones and Stafford L. Warren, Reuel A. Benson, Roger W. Barnes and H. M. Elliott, and Russell D. Herrold.

At the final session on "Therapy and Control" the papers were by Ruth Boring Thomas, Rogers Deakin, Eleanor L. Adler, Arthur Steer and Irving Weinstock, N. A. Nelson, Robert S. Westphal, W. A. Brumfield, Jr., and R. A. Vonderlehr.

10. The Subsection on Pharmacy of the Section on Medical Sciences presented a symposium on "Vitamins with particular reference to their Standardization." The speakers were Aaron Arnold, P. H. Phillips, C. A. Elvehjem, W. D. Woolley, A. Black and Mrs. Flemintine P. Dann.

11. The Society of American Foresters presented a symposium on "Forest Rehabilitation in the Lake States," the first session being under the chairmanship of T. Schantz-Hansen, at which papers were read by Ray Bassett, H. Basil Wales, Russell N. Cunningham and George Banzhaf. At the second session, under the chairmanship of Henry Schmitz, papers were read by O. W. Swan, William Heritage, F. H. Eyre and D. M. Matthews.

## RADIO PROGRAMS

Radio programs were arranged by Dr. John D. Ball for all the three broadcasting stations located in Milwaukee. Paul B. Sears, in cooperation with John D. Ball, Jr., H. H. Remmers, Frank A. Thone and F. R. Moulton, delivered broadcasts over station W.T.M.J.; Otto Struve and J. J. O'Neill in cooperation with John D. Ball, over station W.T.S.N.; E. P. Hutchinson and F. R. Moulton, over station W.E.M.P.

## SCIENTIFIC SESSIONS

### SECTION ON PHYSICS (B): AMERICAN METEOROLOGICAL SOCIETY

*(From the program of the society)*

The American Meteorological Society, under the presidency of Robert E. Horton, held four sessions on Monday, June 19, and Tuesday, June 20, at which 22 papers were presented. The contributions at the first session were by Eric R. Miller, John G. Albright, Eugene D. Emigh, George W. Mindling, L. Walter Dick and Winston Manning. The first two papers were historical and biographical subjects. At the second session, which was devoted mostly to hydrographic problems, the speakers were R. H. Musser, William E. Barron, Albert D. Sanial and Norman A. Matson, Bertram S. Barnes, and LeRoy K. Sherman. The papers read before the third session were partly on relations of meteorology to airplane flights and partly on solar radiation. The contributors were Paul

A. Gareau, Homer W. Ball, Arthur M. Marks, Jr., Eugene D. Emigh, Irving F. Hand, L. F. Miller, and R. H. Roberts and B. Esther Struckmeyer. At the final session papers were presented by Charles F. Brooks and Leslie R. Bean, and two motion pictures were shown, one on forecasting floods on the Potomac and Ohio Rivers and the other on exploring the upper air.

### SECTION ON CHEMISTRY (C)

(*From report by Neil E. Gordon*)

Section C cooperated with the Division of Physical and Inorganic Chemistry of the American Chemical Society in a symposium on "The Kinetics of Homogeneous Gas Reactions," which was presented at Madison, Wisconsin, from June 20 to June 22, inclusive. The speakers at the first session, over which George Scatchard presided, were Everett Gorin, Walter Kaufmann, John Walter and Henry Eyring, Eugene P. Wigner, and J. A. Christiansen. At the second session, Farrington Daniels presiding, papers were presented by George Scatchard, K. F. Bonhoeffer, K. H. Geib and O. Reitz, F. O. Rice and K. F. Herzfeld, and H. A. Taylor and Milton Burton. Harold C. Urey presided at the third session, at which papers were read by O. K. Rice and Hallock C. Campbell, Guenther von Elbe and Bernard Lewis, and R. H. Crist and J. E. Wertz. At the fourth session, S. C. Lind presiding, the contributors were G. B. Kistiakowsky and W. W. Ransom; Richard A. Ogg, Jr., and W. J. Priest, Robert W. Pease, and Farrington Daniels and Preston L. Veltman. Philip A. Leighton presided at the final session at which papers were presented by W. Albert Noyes, Jr., and F. C. Henriques, Jr., G. K. Rollefson and D. C. Grahame, E. W. R. Steacie and Roger Potvin, and S. C. Lind. Each session was followed by a general discussion.

### SECTION ON ASTRONOMY (D)

(*From report by Harlan T. Stetson*)

Meetings of Section D were held on Wednesday and Thursday, June 21 and 22, at which the vice-president and chairman of the section, Everett I. Yowell, presided. At the session on Wednesday the contributions were on a variety of topics in several fields of astronomy and astrophysics. John A. O'Keefe, of the Yerkes Observatory, presented evidence that carbon dust periodically emitted from the star R Coronae Borealis causes the variation in brightness of that well-known variable, while Otto Struve, director of the Yerkes Observatory, discussed the chemical composition of interstellar gas. An unusual nebula with a cometary-like appendage was brought to the attention of astronomers by John Titus, of the Yerkes Observatory. Paul Herget, of Cincinnati, gave his recent results on the satellite system of Jupiter. These papers were typical of the program, which included altogether fourteen contributions in the fields of astronomy and astrophysics. About 60 persons were in attendance in Milwaukee.

On the invitation of Dr. Struve, about 70 persons gathered at the Yerkes Observatory on the shores of Lake Geneva, in Wisconsin, for the Thursday session. Dr. Struve addressed the assembly on the topic, "The Yerkes Observatory Looks to the Future," and Dr. Ross, of the observatory staff, spoke on the history and the development of optics in astronomy, including the solution of many problems in connection with the construction of the 100- and 200-inch telescopes in California. A very pleasant tea at the director's residence, by invitation of Dr. and Mrs. Struve, followed the scientific session in the observatory. Opportunity was afforded those who remained over into the evening to examine selected objects through the 40-inch Yerkes telescope. Participating in the program with the members of Section D were delegations from the Milwaukee and the Chicago Astronomical Societies.

### SECTION ON GEOLOGY AND GEOGRAPHY (E), GEOLOGICAL SOCIETY OF AMERICA AND ASSOCIATION OF AMERICAN GEOGRAPHERS

(*From report by Howard A. Meyerhoff*)

The Section on Geology and Geography (E), meeting jointly with the Geological Society of America, was in continuous session from June 15 to 24. Section activities started with a preconvention field excursion in northern Michigan under the able leadership of R. M. Dickey and Kiril Spiroff, of the Michigan College of Mining and Technology. Despite a comparatively small party and consistently bad weather, three effective days were spent examining the pre-Cambrian and Cambrian rock sections of the Marquette and Gogebic ranges and of the Keweenaw Peninsula. The relationships of rocks and mineralization to the mining activities of the Upper Peninsula received special attention, and brief stops were made at the museum of the College of Mining and Technology and at several mines and mills.

At the opening session in Milwaukee on Monday, June 19, Dr. Ira Edwards, of the Milwaukee Public Museum, presided over a short program devoted chiefly to papers on pre-Cambrian geology. Tectonic and glacial problems constituted the subjects for discussion on Monday afternoon, when Rollin T. Chamberlin, of the University of Chicago, occupied the chair. The glacial papers furnished an excellent background for the field excursion scheduled for Tuesday, when F. T. Thwaites, of the University of Wisconsin, led a small party over the moraines and outwash of southeastern Wisconsin. Problems of correlation and dating were stressed, and those participating were as much impressed with the details of glaciation, which must still be worked out, as with the vast amount of expert work already done.

Kirk Bryan, vice-president of the American Association and chairman of the section, presided over the two sessions held on Wednesday, June 21. Paleozoic stratigraphy and sedimentation furnished the theme of the morning meeting, and several of the papers dealt with new methods of attacking old problems in stratigraphic research and in sedimentary petrology. In the afternoon, the Section on Anthropology (H) met briefly with Section E to hear the paper by Kirk Bryan and Louis L. Ray on "Quaternary Chronology and the Antiquity of the Folsom Culture." W. C. McKern occupied the chair, while Dr. Bryan presented the geologic facts of correlation which have led him and Dr. Ray to date the Folsom Culture provisionally as 25,000 years old. Geomorphic and geographic papers filled in the balance of an interesting and varied afternoon, in which members of the Association of American Geographers officially participated.

As a sequel to the stratigraphic session on Wednesday morning, members of Section E were provided on Thursday with an opportunity to study the Silurian and Devonian formations of the Milwaukee region. Under the expert guidance of Ira Edwards, the field party discovered that the thick mantle of glacial drift has not buried all the rocks which form the foundation of southeastern Wisconsin.

On Friday the Section on Engineering (M) and the American Society of Agricultural Engineers joined with the geologists and geographers in a symposium on "Soil Conservation and Land Utilization in the Great Lakes Region." E. F. Bean, state geologist of Wisconsin, and L. R. Schoenmann, of Michigan State College, presided, respectively, over the morning and afternoon sessions, in which problems of soil conservation were analyzed from the point of view of the engineer, the geologist, the forester, the agronomist and the agriculturist. The fourteen speakers were drawn from federal, state and educational institutions in Ohio, Indiana, Michigan, Wisconsin, Minnesota and the Prairie Provinces of Canada; hence the problems were viewed from all geographic angles, as well as from all professional standpoints. The size of the audience was not commensurate with the significance of the symposium, but those present participated actively in discussions which prolonged the meeting considerably beyond the scheduled hour for adjournment.

Because of small registration and the geological interests of those registered, the post-convention field excursion under the leadership of E. F. Bean was considerably modified. The proposed itinerary was shortened to include the drift margin between Madison and Baraboo, the Cambrian and pre-Cambrian geology of the Baraboo Range and the erosional features of the Wisconsin Dells. The party disbanded on June 25 with genuine regret that the full field program had not been followed.

In developing the Section E program, the secretary was materially aided by John R. Ball, F. T. Thwaites, E. A. Norton, Louis A. Wolfanger, F. M. Feiker, E. F. Bean, Ira Edwards and others. In view of the quality of the papers, the attendance was somewhat disappointing, for only 90 persons were present at one or more meetings, and the attendance at individual sessions did not exceed forty.

### SECTION ON ZOOLOGICAL SCIENCES (F)

*(From report by George A. Baitsell)*

The program of the Section on Zoological Sciences (F) at the Milwaukee meeting was limited to two important symposia. One symposium, on "The Relation of Genetics to Geographical Distribution and Speciation," was under the chairmanship of L. J. Cole, of the University of Wisconsin, and the other one, "Regeneration," was under the chairmanship of J. W. Buchanan, of Northwestern University. Both of these symposia were of such interest as to attract unusually large audiences, the total attendance for the two days being somewhat over 100. It is expected that the papers presented in the two symposia will be published at an early date.

The papers presented were as follows:

*Genetics Symposium:*

1. Speciation in fishes. C. L. Hubbs, University of Michigan.
2. Some factors in the geographical distribution and speciation of Peromyscus. L. R. Dice, University of Michigan.
3. The geographical distribution of gall wasps. A. C. Kinsey, Indiana University.
4. Inter-racial crossing and mutation. A. H. Sturtevant, California Institute of Technology.
5. Speciation from the point of view of genetics. M. R. Irwin and R. W. Cumley, University of Michigan.

*Regeneration Symposium:*

1. The histological basis of regeneration and re-association in lower invertebrates. W. C. Curtis, University of Missouri.
2. The environmental control of regeneration in Euplanaria. Olin Rulon, Wayne University.
3. Regeneration in protozoa; a study of morphogenesis. William Balamuth, University of California.
4. Aspects of regeneration in Annelids. L. H. Hyman, American Museum of Natural History.

At the close of this symposium, Dr. Curtis presented a tribute to the late Dr. H. V. Wilson, of the University of North Carolina, in which he emphasized the outstanding quality of Dr. Wilson's personal character and scientific research.

SECTION ON BOTANICAL SCIENCES (G) AND AMERICAN SOCIETY OF PLANT PHYSIOLOGISTS

*(From report by W. E. Tottingham, W. J. Hamilton, Jr., and Berch Henry)*

The American Society of Plant Physiologists (F. P. Cullinan, *secretary*) cooperated with Section G of the association in conducting a symposium on "Photoperiodism," on Tuesday forenoon. A. E. Murneek, past president of the society, presided, and 50 persons attended. W. F. Loehwing presented an introductory statement of the current status of this concept, emphasizing the need of modification in ideas concerning "flowering" and its associated physiology. The significance of the appearance of flower primordia and differentiation of sexual parts was stressed. Differences of photoperiodic requirement for the inception of these developmental phases were noted and the inadequacy of the hormone concept to account for sexual differentiation was pointed out. Karl C. Hamner discussed the photoperiodic responses of several species in relation to the theory of hormone function in the flowering of plants. He presented evidence that, according to species, flower development may be initiated in either light or darkness or in combination of the two. Melcher's concept of the functioning of at least two hormones in the responses of Hyoscyamus was considered possibly applicable to the species here concerned.

R. H. Roberts reported that anatomical studies offer evidence for structural characteristics which follow blossom induction. He suggested that these may account for continuance of effects from short-term photoperiodic treatment. Inducing of blossoming by cooling a portion of the stem was interpreted as indicating that this organ may participate with the leaves in causing flowering.

A brief program of general papers was presented in the afternoon with W. F. Loehwing, president of the society, presiding. There was an attendance of 35. R. B. Harvey described procedure for determining ethylene in stored apples and pointed out the relation of this compound and associated products to the climacteric or tissue-breakdown phase of metabolism.

R. H. Landon described the preservation of strawberries and raspberries by addition of 20 to 30 per cent. carbon dioxide to the atmosphere of the storage room. In general the firmness and flavor of the fruit were retained to remarkable degrees.

Orville Wyss (sponsored by P. W. Wilson) presented a paper on the exudation of nitrogenous compounds from the root nodules of leguminosae. Illustration of the development of associated non-leguminous plants and findings from the determination of nitrogen in the tissue were shown as evidence.

On Wednesday the society convened with the Botanical Society of America, the American Phytopathological Society, the American Society of Plant Taxonomists and the Mycological Society of America at the University of Wisconsin in Madison. In the forenoon these groups were welcomed by President C. A. Dykstra and Dean E. B. Fred, with E. M. Gilbert presiding. Informal responses were made by representatives of the bodies concerned. In the afternoon an invitation program arranged by the Society of Plant Physiologists consisted of addresses by G. F. Thornton on "The Rôle of the More Abundant Mineral Elements," and by B. M. Duggar on "Aspects of Radiation as Applied to Some Physiological Problems." Forty persons were in attendance. The remainder of the afternoon was devoted to inspection of equipment in the research laboratories of the division of plant physiology of the university. At an informal dinner arranged by the Phytopathological Society colored and motion pictures of fungi and flora of Wisconsin were shown by a representative of the Wisconsin Conservation Commission. On Thursday afternoon the following program was presented before a largely attended joint session of the several societies, with I. E. Malhus presiding.

1. Physiological differentiation of sex in dioecious angiosperms. J. Fisher Stanfield, Chicago Teachers College, Chicago, Ill.
2. New species of plant microfossils from the Des Moines Series of Iowa. L. R. Wilson, Coe College, Cedar Rapids, Iowa.
3. Genetics of pollen tube growth in Datura. J. T. Buchholz, University of Illinois, Urbana, Ill.
4. Phylogeny of the Gramineae. Paul Weatherwax, University of Indiana, Bloomington, Indiana.

The remainder of activities through Friday consisted of field trips, inspection of laboratories and social gatherings. Effective arrangements for the entertainment of visitors had been arranged by a committee, of which N. C. Fassett was chairman. Abundant non-technical interests were provided for the ladies, a tea on Wednesday afternoon and picnic of all attendants of the several groups on Thursday being high spots among the events.

The Ecological Society of America (W. J. Hamilton, Jr., secretary) held its summer meetings in conjunction with the A. A. A. S. at Milwaukee, June 19 to 24, at which eight papers were presented. On Tuesday morning the society had one session, C. F. Korstian presiding, at which papers were presented by Edward Haskell, Eldon J. Strandine and Theodore M. Sperry. During the afternoon, members of the society met with the Section on Social and Economic Sciences in a symposium on "Population Problems and Planning in the Northern Lake States."

On Wednesday morning a symposium on "Socio-economic Approach to Land Use" was well attended.

Aldo Leopold presented a paper on "The Relation of Game Management to Land Use." The second paper was by K. C. McMurry on "Geography and Land Use." The third paper was given by George S. Wehrwein on "The Economist's Approach to the Problem of Ecology," while the final paper was presented by Raphael Zon on "The Broader Social Implications of Land Use in the Cutover Region." Discussion of the papers was led by L. R. Schoenmann, presiding officer.

The Thursday morning session, held jointly with the Section on Social and Economic Sciences (K), dealt with the status of population mobility and on the application of culture area concept and research studies.

A three-day joint field trip with the Society of American Foresters was participated in by about 100 persons. The field trip, covering a distance of approximately 600 miles, gave the ecologists and foresters opportunity to see forest plantings, commercial selective logging, some Forest Service salvage logging of cutover areas, a Forest Service nursery and the virgin timber and selectively logged area on the Menomonie Indian Reservation, which is one of the finest remaining hardwoods in the Lake States.

### SECTION ON ANTHROPOLOGY (H)

*(From report by Wilton Marion Krogman)*

At the Milwaukee meeting 17 papers were presented before the section, the attendance being about 15 persons. The major portion of the program centered about the theme of the pre-history of man in North America and subsequent acculturation. Earl Count stated that the earliest physical type of the American Indian was not basically Mongoloid, but contained elements more closely related to the present-day peoples of Australia-Melanesia. A series of papers was devoted to the analysis of presumed early material from Lake Pelican, in Minnesota. T. E. Evans reported on jaws, F. J. Borelli on teeth, P. B. Candela on blood-grouping, J. E. Hill on associated mammalian remains and Mrs. Gertrude S. Evans on associated artifacts. Certain "primitive" characters of jaws and teeth were pointed out; the blood-group was ascertained to be *A;* the mammalian remains were found to be identical with living forms of muskrat and pocket-gopher; the artifacts were very doubtfully related to "Yuma-Folsom" types. In all, there was no reason to consider the material as of any great antiquity. A. E. Whiting discussed the origin of Indian corn, concluding that it might have arisen from any wild-growing form within the area where corn was found at the time of the discovery of America. H. C. Shetrone reported on representations of the human form found in Ohio prehistoric art, giving some idea of physical type and of costume. Mrs. Gretchen Cutter outlined the archeological sequence at a specific site from Will County, Illinois, as Middle Mississippi in earlier levels, Woodland in later. Miss Frances Densmore showed how the ceremonies of the modern Indians demonstrate acculturation, in that they blend traits of aboriginal religion with Christian doctrines. At the Wednesday afternoon session the section met jointly with the Section on Geology and Geography to hear the paper by Kirk Bryan and L. L. Ray on the glaciology of the Southern Rockies with special reference to the antiquity of the Folsom culture at the Lindenmeier, Colorado, Site. The age was given as the third Wisconsin substage (Corral Creek Moraine), 25,000 years old, according to the Antevs chronology. Henry Field presented the results of his extensive study of the modern peoples of Persia: basically long-headed Mediterraneans, with evidence that roundheads (Proto-Alpines and Armenoids) came in at an early historic date. The section is indebted to Dr. S. A. Barrett and his staff for cordial hospitality and the opportunity to inspect the fine displays in the Milwaukee Museum, in which the sessions were held.

### SECTION ON PSYCHOLOGY (I)

*(From report by Hulsey Cason, secretary pro tem)*

The program of the Section on Psychology included two sessions of six papers each and two symposia. The sessions were of high quality, and the average attendance was about 30 persons.

Of special interest in the session on General Psychology was the strong paper by Dean Edward A. Fitzpatrick, of Marquette University, on "The Scholastic Self." This paper and the animated discussion which followed brought out in clear relief the shortcomings of our modern system of educational regimentation, the principal failing of the schools being in the direction of the psychological influences on the students themselves. The general conclusion reached by Laird T. Hites and Howard Becker on the family and marriage courses in universities was that these courses should include materials from various academic fields and that they should not be given from the limited point of view of a single university department.

A very profitable symposium on "Measuring Attitudes" was conducted by Stephen M. Corey. The discussion by Mr. Corey and H. H. Remmers brought out the need for a clearer concept of attitudes and for additional clarity in the use of statistical measures.

Of special interest and scientific value was the symposium on "Neuromuscular Tension," the speakers being Edmund Jacobson, Earl Fowler and Maurice H. Krout, of Chicago, and Walter B. Cannon, of the Harvard Medical School. Dr. Jacobson and the other participants in the symposium presented much evidence showing the intimate interrelation of various organic functions and the practical medical value of the method of progressive relaxation.

SECTION ON SOCIAL AND ECONOMIC SCIENCES (H)

(*From report by E. P. Hutchinson*)

The Milwaukee program of the section contained two separate sessions on economics, a luncheon meeting with Pi Gamma Mu and two symposia. Of these two latter, one dealt with "Population Problems and Programs in the Northern Lake States"; the other, the third in the Science and Society series, with "The Economic System in Relation to Scientific Progress."

The population symposium, held under the auspices of the Population Association of America, was designed to give an understanding of the nature and origin of the existing problems and to review the measures undertaken to meet them. A total of 20 papers, divided into seven sessions, were contained in the symposium. In the introductory session of Tuesday morning Glenn T. Trewartha traced the history of the settlement of Wisconsin, outlining the transition from exploitation to occupation of the area and the attendant changes in the pattern of population distribution. W. B. Dick identified the principal places of origin of the earliest settlers as the Genesee Valley, New York, and certain portions of the adjacent states, and traced the favored routes of in-migration. Using census data for the period 1850 on, Guy-Harold Smith demonstrated the growth and changing distribution of population in Wisconsin, emphasizing the clustering movement which succeeded the early occupation, and predicted a continuation of this trend.

Following this historical introduction, E. M. Davis interpreted the changes of population and its distribution in terms of the changing economy of the area, indicating the demographic concomitants of the rise and fall of the lumbering industry, of the coming of railroads, etc. Stanley D. Dodge indicated the dependence of the population capacity of an area on the prevailing form of land use or economy and means of estimating this capacity. Raphael Zon emphasized the undesirability of a lively exploitive economy in the northern cutover area, and the desirability of local utilization of revenues.

Following an outline of population trends in Wisconsin by Samuel Teper, George Wehrwein discussed the work of the Wisconsin State Planning Board, emphasizing the importance of rural zoning as a direct means of regulating population distribution and the necessity of such a means of preventing universal settlement. M. W. Torkelson presented the recommendations of the Regional Committee for the economic rehabilitation of the cutover area, these being for reforestation and for the relocation of the inhabitants into comfortable and efficient settlements.

The third of the projected series of conferences on "Science and Society" was on "The Economic System in Relation to Scientific Progress." It consisted of four general sessions, at the first of which George W. Edwards delivered an address on "The Capitalistic System and How it Evolved," followed by Rufus S. Tucker, who spoke on "Free Enterprise and Scientific Development." At the second session Charles F. Roos presented a paper on "The Application of Natural Science Methodology to Economic Studies," and H. G. Moulton delivered an address on "Economics and its Dynamic Aspects." The speakers at the third session were Leverett S. Lyon, on "The Role of Government in the Economic System," and James W. Bell, on "Government Finance and Economic Stability." The final session consisted of a paper by Charles H. Judd, on "Present Relations of Government to Science," and another by William F. Ogburn, on "Should the Government Finance Non-governmental Research Activities?"

SECTION ON MEDICAL SCIENCES (N) AND SUBSECTION ON PHARMACY

(*From reports by Malcolm H. Soule and Glenn L. Jenkins*)

Of the 50 papers prepared for the Section on Medical Sciences (Malcolm H. Soule, reporting) 18 were devoted to various subjects of general interest, ranging from such topics as the cause of cancer to the use of helium in encephalography, and 32 were contributions to a Symposium on "The Gonococcus and Gonococcal Infection." The first session, held on Monday afternoon, was introduced with a group of three reports on the problems of lead and arsenic in the body. Humanity living in a big city is always exposed to small quantities of lead from gasoline fumes discharged by automobiles; hence information as to its possible action is desirable. In one study the blood and urine of 165 lead workers were examined for the effects on the blood picture and the presence of the heavy metal, two thirds of these individuals having had continued exposure to inhalation of lead dust in the storage battery industry for periods of from 5 to 20 years. In the findings distinction was drawn between lead absorption and lead intoxication, the former being a warning of possible future lead intoxication; the latter condition, while an agonizing experience, being easily relieved by intravenous calcium treatment.

One of the benefits of microbic life to mankind was brought out in a paper dealing with the coagulation of the blood. Since newborn infants have no prothrombin in their systems, they are unusually susceptible to death from hemorrhage. Prothrombin is formed from vitamin K. Bacteria introduced into the body shortly after birth, in the ordinary course of exposure, synthesize vitamin K, which in turn is converted into prothrombin, and in this manner nature provides a real barrier against post-natal bleeding.

The activities of the Milwaukee Convalescent Serum Center, which is one of the outstanding units of its kind in the country, were described. During the past five years human convalescent scarlet fever serum has been prepared and used in the prophylaxis and treatment of scarlet fever. In a few instances this material has been employed in other infections caused by hemolytic streptococci. Patients with erysipelas have responded favorably in every instance following the administration of the serum.

The symposium, "The Gonococcus and Gonococcal Infection," was jointly sponsored by the American Neisserian Medical Society and Section N. Four sessions, which ran consecutively, were held on Tuesday afternoon, Wednesday morning and afternoon and Thursday morning, the average attendance being 60.

The program on Tuesday focused attention on the biology of the gonococcus. This micro-organism was discovered in pus from infected individuals just 60 years ago, and its causal relationship to one of the most wide-spread maladies of man was accepted, although it was some time before the germ was cultured on artificial media. During the intervening years the delicate nature and the fastidious requirements of the organism have been repeatedly confirmed, but little has been added to our knowledge of the mechanism by which the associated disease is produced. The discussion favored a belief in the synthesis of toxins, but the nature of these metabolites is enigmatical. Possibly the crux of the problem is that the technique of toxin production under artificial conditions is fraught with many difficulties, and all procedures with this end in view must be carefully standardized in order to obtain data that are in essential agreement. Research with this organism is complicated by the lack of a suitable susceptible laboratory animal. To date no investigator has produced, except in humans, an infection which simulates in a satisfactory degree the ordinary disease as it occurs in man. Such experiments are naturally limited and difficult to control. The existence of natural immunity in certain individuals is recognized, but the attempts at stimulating artificial immunity by the introduction of any of the biologicals available at present has been uniformly disappointing.

On Wednesday morning 9 papers were contributed to the problem of diagnosing gonococcal infection and the criteria for its cure. The disease in males lends itself to rather easy diagnosis, but in females the problem is complicated. The examination of stained smears of specimens from suspicious areas is of considerable aid, but cultural studies are recognized as essential for the diagnosis in doubtful instances and as a criteria for cure. Such procedures must be carried out at repeated intervals by well-trained workers. Three papers on gonococcal arthritis, meningitis and proctitis completed the morning program.

Sulfanilamide and related compounds received, as was to be expected, considerable attention in the symposium. It was agreed that in some types of gonococcal infection, such as ophthalmia neonatorum, the use of this drug is followed by almost miraculous cures. In other manifestations the results are good but not as striking. In a limited number of patients the use of the chemicals seems to delay therapeutic progress, possibly the strain of germ involved having become drug-fast. Encouraging reports were given following the administration of sulfapyridine, this compound having certain advantages over sulfanilamide. The mechanism by which any of these drugs exerts its beneficial action was discussed at great length, but the available data permitted of no conclusions. The final paper on the symposium was devoted to the administrative problems in the control of gonococcal infection.

The symposium, the most comprehensive ever held on this subject, was an outstanding success. The discussions afforded an opportunity for an interchange of experiences in using the present laboratory aids for diagnosis and served the very practical purpose of stimulating a most critical attitude in evaluating the reports of the results of treatment with the newer chemical compounds.

Two sessions of the Subsection on Pharmacy (Glenn L. Jenkins reporting) were devoted to a symposium on the vitamins with particular reference to their standardization.

Aaron Arnold, in his report on thiamin, pointed out that interfering substances limit the value of the chemical methods of determination and that the biological method based on growth is the most reliable procedure. Simpler and more rapid methods for the determination of thiamin and new criteria of its functions will make it possible to determine whether the level for optimum nutrition is appreciably above the requirement level. P. H. Phillips, in comparing the methods for the assay of riboflavin based on fluorescence, color and photolysis, and growth promotion, pointed out that the bio-assay method is the most accurate method now known, but that the colorimetric method offers much promise when applied to the degradation products of this vitamin. Methods using micro-organisms are economical, rapid and accurate for the determination of trace levels. Evidence has been obtained which indicates that riboflavin may be necessary for the deaminization of amino acids and the formation of urea in the liver. It plays an important rôle in nerve nutrition in chicks which exhibit neuromalacia on low riboflavin diets and recover rapidly when the deficiency is supplied by the administration of riboflavin. C. A. Elvehjem reviewed the procedures which led to the isolation of nicotinic acid fraction of the Vitamin B complex. He showed that while chemical procedures, bacterial growth methods and bio-assays offer possibilities, the most reliable assay procedure at present is the curative method applied to dogs in which black tongue has been induced by feeding a suitable nicotinic acid deficient basal ration. It was emphasized that a chemical method of assay is greatly needed so that our knowledge of the distribution of nicotinic acid, as well as other factors in foods, may be made known. When this knowledge is available it will be possible to modify the diet, particularly in areas where pellagra is prevalent, and fortify the diet with nicotinic acid if necessary to prevent the disease. W. D. Woolley discussed the chick antidermatitis factor and pantothenic acid of the vitamin B complex. The assay of the former is best carried out on chicks by noting the growth and prevention of dermatitis as compared to chicks on a basal diet. A method for the determination of pantothenic acid which is rapid, economical and accurate has been devised. It is based on the discovery that pantothenic acid is essential for the growth of a wide variety of hemolytic streptococci. An assay by this method can be completed in 24 hours and it excels the animal method in precision. All the authors of papers pertaining to the *vitamin B complex* emphasized the need for chemical methods of assay and for methods of assay which would permit the determination of the concentration of vitamins in the blood.

A. Black critically examined the factors which influence the accuracy of vitamin A assays. He pointed out that the biological methods measure the combined vitamin A activity of the various compounds which may become available as vitamin A to the rat and that the method is not specific for any particular kind of vitamin A. Methods based on the measurement of the absorption of light by means of spectrophotometers have been widely used and are the most accurate and give the most information about the sample.

Vitamin E, the anti-sterility vitamin, was reviewed as to its sources, isolation, chemistry, physiological activity and assay by Mrs. Flemintine P. Dann. The production of pure alpha tocopherol (Vitamin E) offers promise of leading to a more quantitative method than the present bio-assay.

### SECTION ON AGRICULTURE (O): SOCIETY OF AMERICAN FORESTERS

(*From report by Henry E. Clepper*)

The Society of American Foresters met in five sessions, one of which was a joint session with the Ecological Society of America. Twenty-two papers were presented covering research with chemicals in forest fire control, the utilization of forest products, forest recreation, reforestation, forest management, selective logging, land planning and land use, soil conservation, game management and a discussion of the social and economic problems of forestry in the Lake States.

The foresters' banquet was held at the Milwaukee Athletic Club.

Four days were devoted to field trips. Visits were made to the Forest Products Laboratory, Madison, Wis., to the Goodman Lumber Company operations, the Nicolet National Forest and the Menomonie Indian Reservation.

Approximately 100 members of the Society of American Foresters attended the sessions. In addition, about 20 non-members participated in the field trips.

### SECTION ON EDUCATION (Q)

(*From report by H. H. Remmers*)

The Section on Education (Q) held three sessions at which 17 papers were scheduled. Owing to unforeseen circumstances two of the speakers were unable to appear. The attendance at the meetings ranged from 20 to 46, with an average slightly over 30 for the various sessions. The general theme of the three sessions was the education of the emotions.

In the first morning session Miss Margaret Joseph, of Shorewood High School, Milwaukee, presented an interesting study on "The Factor of Interest in the Teaching of Mathematics." Her data indicated that if pupils in the lower fourth of the distribution on scores of a group intelligence test and a reading test were not required to take high-school mathematics, there would be practically no failing students in mathematics. A paper on "Interests and Attitudes of Junior High School Pupils," by W. Clark Trow, of the University of Michigan, presented an interesting longitudinal study of which the implications for guidance were made strikingly clear. H. Meltzer, of the Psychological Service Center, St. Louis, Mo., presented an important paper on "Educational Implications of a Study of Race Attitudes of School Children." In general, the data showed less differentiation of children's attitudes toward races than do those of adults, and also a significant change over the period from 1934 to 1938 in the same population of school children, the change being in general one of a relatively less favorable attitude toward totalitarian countries and a more favorable attitude toward the democracies. Numerous factors were shown to condition the racial attitude, such as home, neighborhood, companions, etc. Human tragedies as the result of inadequate sex education were delineated by Robert S. Drews in a paper under the title "Evaluation of Adult Neuroses in the Light of Inadequate Sex Education." In the discussion the relative inadequacy of both educators and physicians in terms of the training programs for each were brought out. The final paper in the first morning session was by Roy C. Bryan, Western State Teachers College, Kalamazoo, Michigan, on "Evaluation of Student Reaction to Secondary School Teachers." Dr.

Bryan stressed the importance of the emotional factors in all learning and the way in which emotionalized attitudes toward the teacher may condition the learning and adjustment of the pupil.

The first paper of the afternoon session was on "The Use of Music in an Educational Program of Mental Hygiene," by Dr. O. Irving Jacobson, of Shurtleff College, Alton, Illinois. Dr. Jacobson's experiment concerned a galvanometric study of 16 subjects subjected to different types of music. While no conclusions could be drawn from the relatively limited data, a number of very interesting leads for further research appeared. The second paper, "Some Educational Implications of the American Youth Commission Study of Civilian Conservation Corps Camps," by Kenneth Holland, associate director of the American Youth Commission, Washington, D. C., presented a picture of the uniqueness of the educational problems in CCC Camps and the relative emotional and educational adjustment which the enrollees make. The third paper, by Stanford C. Ericksen, University of Arkansas, on "An Experimental Investigation of Student Motives: Why Do Students Want to Make Good Grades?" showed that motivation in learning in college varies with sex of the student, the curriculum, the class, membership in Greek letter fraternities, etc. That more realistic and wholesome attitudes toward problems of marriage are being developed was shown in an interesting paper by E. F. Van Buskirk, of Stephens College, under the title, "Interests and Attitudes of College Women in Regard to the Biological Basis of Marriage and Some of its Social Implications." The final paper in the afternoon session was presented by Miss Mildred B. Mitchell, of the Psychopathic Hospital of the State University of Iowa, under the title, "The Revised Stanford-Binet Test for Adults." The tests were shown to be considerably more discriminative than the 1917 edition.

The final morning session was introduced by a paper by J. H. Farley, of Lawrence College, under the title "Modern Higher Education, Comprehensive Reflective Thinking and the Factors of Emotion, Interests and Ideals." This paper was a critical examination of the outcomes of modern higher education in terms of student thinking and emotional adjustment. The second paper, by E. I. F. Williams, of Heidelberg College, on "Constructive Emotions as Resources in Teaching," summarized in excellent fashion some of the more significant experimental findings with reference to the education of the emotions and brought out important educational implications of these findings. "Adjustment *vs.* Mental and Physical Health in Freshman Medical Students," by Leo P. Clements, of Creighton University, considered the unhygienic nature of the medical curriculum when viewed in the light of serious emotional and physical maladjustment of students. A paper by F. C. Dana, of Iowa State College, on "Engineering Problems Courses as Aid to Discovering Interests and Aptitudes of Students," reviewed the experience at Iowa State College over a period of more than 20 years with such a course, and described the methods and means of detecting the characteristics of students in the interests of their educational-vocational guidance by means of this course. The final paper on "General Semantics and the Control of Affective Processes in Education" was presented jointly by Miss M. Kendig, of the Institute of General Semantics, in Chicago, and by C. B. Congdon, psychiatrist at the University of Chicago. A growing interest in the problems of semantics as related to emotional adjustment made this paper particularly timely.

# OBITUARY

## HARRY VICTOR ATKINSON

### 1887–1939

ON May 7, 1939, at Vermillion, S. D., death from a cerebral hemorrhage cut short the career of Professor Harry Victor Atkinson in his fifty-second year. He was born at Van Wert, Ohio, on February 12, 1887. Fundamentally trained in chemical engineering at Ohio State University (B.S., 1911), he continued in that field only three years. Supported by an instructorship in physiological chemistry at the Northwestern University School of Medicine (1914–17), he undertook the study of physiology and allied sciences at that institution and at Rush Medical College. From 1917 to 1920, he was instructor of physiology at Cornell Medical College, a position that was interrupted by nine months' service overseas in the Chemical Warfare Service. Working under an instructorship in pharmacology, he completed his work for the doctorate degree in pharmacology at the Medical School of the University of Illinois (1922).

His academic career reflects the esteem in which he was held by the members of his profession. He was, successively, associate professor of pharmacology, Texas, 1922–24; professor of pharmacology, Texas, 1924–26; associate professor of pharmacology, Iowa, 1926–28; and professor of physiology and pharmacology at the University of South Dakota from 1928 until his untimely death. Of his nineteen publications, he will be particularly remembered for his work on the conversion of protein to fat in the dog and his studies on the chemical changes in the blood during anesthesia. He held membership in the American Society for Pharmacology and Experimental Therapeutics, the Society for Experimental Biology and

Medicine, the American Association for the Advancement of Science, the South Dakota Academy of Science and Sigma Xi.

Professor Atkinson made many lasting friendships among his colleagues, and was a continual source of help and inspiration to his students, many of whom he helped obtain financial support for the continuation of their studies. Although his life was short, his fundamental contributions in pharmacology and physiology assure his work a permanent place in the literature of these sciences. His widow, Bertha Hartmann Atkinson, and two daughters survive him.

EDWIN H. SHAW, JR.

UNIVERSITY OF SOUTH DAKOTA

## RECENT DEATHS AND MEMORIALS

DR. WARREN PLIMPTON LOMBARD, for thirty-one years professor of physiology at the School of Medicine of the University of Michigan, died on July 13 at the age of eighty-four years.

DR. FREDERICK P. GAY, since 1923 professor of bacteriology at the College of Physicians and Surgeons of Columbia University, died on July 14, aged sixty-five years.

DR. JOHN H. MCFADDEN, assistant professor of psychology at the University of Pittsburgh, died on May 28. He was in his forty-first year.

DR. DONALD CLINTON BARTON, since 1935 research and consulting geologist and geophysicist for the Humble Oil and Refining Company at Houston, Texas, died on July 8 at the age of fifty years. He was president of the American Association of Petroleum Geologists.

HAVELOCK ELLIS, author and sociologist, known for his researches in the psychology of sex, died on July 8 at the age of eighty years.

DR. E. KIDSON, since 1927 director of the Meteorological Services of New Zealand, has died at the age of fifty-seven years.

ACCORDING to the *Journal* of the American Medical Association a bronze plaque, the gift of an anonymous donor, has been presented to the St. Louis Medical Society in honor of the late Dr. Nathaniel Allison, at one time dean of the School of Medicine of Washington University. The bronze plaque is the work of Carl C. Mose.

*Nature* states that a portrait of James Watt was unveiled by Sir Nigel Gresley at the Institution of Mechanical Engineers during the course of a reception held on June 9. The portrait represents Watt at fifty-seven years of age; it was painted in 1792 by Charles Frederick von Breda, and was acquired by the institution from the family of John Rennie in 1936. During the reception, a formal announcement was made of the award of the James Watt International Medal to Henry Ford, and an address was delivered by the American Ambassador.

# SCIENTIFIC EVENTS

## THE ANNUAL FIELD DAY OF THE ROTHAMSTED EXPERIMENTAL STATION

ACCORDING to an article in *Nature* the annual field day and inspection of the laboratories was held at Rothamsted on June 28, with Lord Radnor, chairman of the Lawes Agricultural Trust Committee, presiding. There was a large attendance representing agriculture and the allied industries. Sir E. Kaye le Fleming, chairman of the Council of the British Medical Association, was the chief guest.

In his survey of the activities of the station, Sir John Russell mentioned that some work had already been carried out in the Dunn Nutritional Laboratories at Cambridge on certain aspects of the vitamin content of the produce of the Rothamsted plots. But so far there has been no confirmation of the view frequently expressed that the nutritive value of produce grown with organic manure is superior to that grown with artificial fertilizers. The produce of the classical fields should provide excellent material for settling points such as these.

An increasing amount of experimental work at Rothamsted is concerned with the action and value of organic manures. Studies are in progress with straw in its many forms, with turf obtained by the ploughing up of grassland, with green manures and with town refuse. An extensive investigation of poultry manure has been completed, and work on wastes and sewage sludge is in prospect. So far, yield determinations have been the chief measurements; but the much more difficult questions of quality and nutritional value can scarcely be ignored.

The tour of the farm, always an important part of the proceedings, affords an unrivalled combination of the oldest and the newest in field experimentation. Broadbalk, carrying an excellent crop of wheat this year, showed the striking effects of the manurial treatments begun by Lawes and Gilbert ninety-six years ago and continued ever since, the plots gaining rather than losing interest from the periodical bare fallows recently superimposed upon them. The field is studied now, not simply as a demonstration of manurial principles, but as a guide to the practical problems of corn growing under semi-continuous conditions.

Passing on to the modern experiments, the visitors inspected several of the new designs set out to measure fertilizer effects on a sequence of crops.

An indoor program followed. Investigations in the

laboratories link up with the farm work in many directions. Thus "take-all," one of the foot-rot diseases of cereals, is intensively studied in the Plant Pathology Department, where many of the conditions of the survival of the fungus in the soil have been worked out, and control methods are being beveloped. In the Entomological Department a technique for measuring the wire-worm population of the soil has been perfected and used to assess the value of the various soil insecticides tested in the plots. Various methods put forward for predicting the manurial requirements of soils on the basis of their chemical analyses are being examined in the Chemical Department. A wider range of soils than the Rothamsted Farm can provide is necessary for this work, and in recent years an increasing number of outside centers have been established, each providing the results of a precise and comprehensive fertilizer test and the corresponding sample of soil for laboratory examination.

The Rothamsted Centenary is due in 1943, and the committee proposes to celebrate it by putting the laboratories, farm buildings and other equipment into complete order for the work that awaits them. The director announced the present position of the Appeal Fund, and said that although good progress has been made in very difficult times, £7,000 is required to complete the first part of the scheme costing £60,000.

## ENGLISH NEUROLOGIC RESEARCH INSTITUTE

THE opening of a new well-equipped building for investigation into the causes of mental defects and abnormalities and borderline conditions which has been opened at Bristol by the secretary of state for the Dominions in the presence of a distinguished company of neurologists is described in the *Journal* of the American Medical Association. It is called the Burden Neurological Research Institute because it has been made possible by the cooperation of Mrs. R. G. Burden, warden of Stoke Park Colony for Mental Deficients, within the grounds of which the new building has been erected. Professor Golla is to be the director, and the staff will consist of Grey Walter, electrophysiology; Dr. Max Reiss, a Czech endocrinologist; N. S. L. MacLeod and A. Tingey, biochemists, and Dr. Wylie McKissock, visiting surgeon.

Among those present was Dr. P. O'Brien, representative in Paris of the Rockefeller Foundation, which has made a generous contribution to the neurosurgical department. The Medical Research Council has also made a grant in support of some of the research work. The director, Professor Golla, said that only those who had realized how the multiplicity of competing claims hampered the work of the large hospital clinics would fully appreciate the advantages of such a research institute, which was equipped in the very best way for the investigation not only of the functions of the nervous system but of the body as a whole. In the preoccupation with the brain there was some tendency to forget the bodily stratum of mental disease. It was intended to take a few carefully selected cases and investigate them by every means available to electrophysiologic and endocrinologic research. An immediate occupation would be the study of the varied group of pathologic states of the brain which were responsible for epileptic seizures. What the neurologist called epilepsy was the least understood of the common nervous diseases. It was hardly an exaggeration to say that our knowledge had received little addition since the time of Galen until certain researches, carried out chiefly in America and England, had given hints for further investigation. There were now good grounds for hoping that certain electrophysical methods would enable us to understand and combat this distressing disease.

## THE SOCIETY OF THE SIGMA XI

THE Case Chapter of the Society of the Sigma Xi held its annual initiation on the evening of June 2. Twenty-eight students were elected to full membership. Officers elected for the next year were Professor Francis Whitacre, *president;* Professor Robert Shankland, *vice-president;* Dean T. M. Focke, *treasurer,* and Professor Richard S. Burington, *secretary.* Following the ceremonies, at which Professor G. E. Barnes, retiring president, presided, Dr. Zay Jeffries, technical director of the Incandescent Lamp Department of the General Electric Company, spoke on "New Light Sources."

The Sigma Xi Club of Peking held its annual meeting on May 4. Dr. Eugene L. Opie, of Cornell University Medical College, was the guest speaker. He gave an address on "The Study of Tuberculosis." New officers were elected as follows: *President,* Professor K. P. Young, Peiping Research Institute; *Vice-president,* Dr. H.-C. Chang, Peiping Union Medical College; *Secretary-Treasurer,* Dr. Peter P. T. Sah, Fu Ren University. The printed membership list of the club gives the number of active resident members as twenty-nine with twenty-seven non-resident members.

A Sigma Xi Club of Hawaii has been formed, with a charter membership of fifty. The first officers are: *President,* Dr. C. J. Hamre; *Vice-president,* Dr. Martha Potgieter; *Secretary-treasurer,* Dr. S. S. Ballard; *Councillors,* Dr. H. E. Gregory and C. E. Pemberton. The first regular meeting of the club was held on June 7 at the University of Hawaii, when Dr. R. N. Perlstein, of Leahi Home, spoke on "Epidemiological Study of Tuberculosis Families in Hawaii."

## THE CONVENTION OF THE ELECTROCHEMICAL SOCIETY

THE fall convention of the Electrochemical Society will be held in New York City on September 11, 12 and 13. New York was selected by the Board of Directors in order to combine attendance at the convention with a visit to the New York World's Fair. It is planned that these take the place of the usual plant inspections. There will be three technical sessions, to be held at the Hotel Commodore. The Monday morning session will be devoted to papers on electrothermics and electronics. On Tuesday morning will be the symposium on "Recent Progress in Electro Analysis," in charge of Professor Hiram S. Lukens, of the University of Pennsylvania. The Wednesday morning session will be in charge of Dr. Robert B. Mears, of the Aluminum Company of America, and will be devoted to "The Influence of Cathodic Reactions on Corrosion." There will be at least six contributions at each of the three sessions. A special session will be held at the Fair Grounds on Monday afternoon in the Hall of Science. Professor Bradley Stoughton, of Lehigh University, will deliver the sixth Joseph W. Richards Memorial address. His lecture will be entitled "Modern Marvels of Electrochemistry." It will be profusely illustrated and open to the public.

The principal social function will be the medal dinner on Tuesday evening, September 12, at which the Edward Goodrich Acheson Gold Medal and the $1,000 prize will be presented to Dr. Francis C. Frary, director of the Research Laboratory of the Aluminum Company. Past President William G. Harvey is the chairman of the committee of arrangements for this dinner.

Monday evening, September 11, has been reserved for an informal supper get-together and meeting at one of the popular restaurants on the Fair Grounds. The supper and entertainment will be sponsored by the local chemical companies.

In view of the large number of visitors in New York this September, members are urged to make their hotel reservations as early as possible. The headquarters of the convention will be the Hotel Commodore, 42d Street and Lexington Avenue, New York City.

## THE BOSTON MEETING OF THE AMERICAN CHEMICAL SOCIETY

THE ninety-eighth meeting of the American Chemical Society will be held in Boston from September 11 to 15. Eighteen divisions will hold meetings, and papers and addresses reporting progress in every major sphere of chemical science will be presented at the sessions. Five thousand chemists, industrialists and representatives of allied fields are expected to participate.

Dr. James Bryant Conant, president of Harvard University and holder of the William H. Nichols Medal for achievement in chemical research of the New York section of the society, has been appointed honorary chairman of a convention committee of nearly a hundred members. Dr. Gustavus J. Esselen, president of Gustavus J. Esselen, Inc., and a director of the society, has been named general chairman.

Executives of leading industrial corporations and educational institutions will deliver addresses at a special celebration on Wednesday, September 13, of the centenary of the discovery of the vulcanization of rubber by Charles Goodyear, when numerous papers describing the progress of rubber research and manufacture in the United States will be read at a general meeting in the afternoon and at a dinner meeting in the evening.

The evening speakers and their topics are: W. S. Knudsen, president of General Motors Corporation, "What the Rubber Industry Has Meant to the Automobile Industry"; P. W. Litchfield, president of Goodyear Tire and Rubber Company, "The Rubber Industry"; Dr. Karl T. Compton, president of Massachusetts Institute of Technology, "Vulcanization from the Physicist's Standpoint"; Dr. Conant, "Vulcanization from the Chemist's Standpoint." Dr. Charles A. Kraus, of Brown University, president of the American Chemical Society, will preside and make a speech of welcome.

Speakers in the afternoon will be E. B. Babcock, chief chemist of the Firestone Tire and Rubber Company, "What is Vulcanization?"; A. B. Newhall, executive vice-president of the B. F. Goodrich Rubber Company, "Work of Thomas Hancock"; R. W. Lunn, managing director of the Leland and Birmingham Rubber Company, "Work of Charles Goodyear"; W. A. Gibbons, director of research of the United States Rubber Company, "The Rubber Industry Since 1839."

A Symposium on Vulcanization will be held on Thursday, September 14, under the auspices of the Division of Rubber Chemistry, the chairman of which is George K. Hinshaw, of the Goodyear Tire and Rubber Company.

Thirteen other divisional symposia are planned. The Chemical Education Division will discuss "The Training and Opportunities for Women in Chemistry." "Vitamins and Nutrition" will be discussed by the Divisions of Agricultural and Food, Medicinal and Biological Chemistry. Fields to be dealt with in other symposia include plant hormones, nitrogen-free extracts, methods in protein chemistry, sterols and related compounds, x-ray studies of substances of high molecular weight, the combustion of solid fuels, industrial wastes, unit processes, resins and plastics from hydrocarbons, low-temperature research and compounds with elements in unusual states of valence.

Dr. Kraus will deliver the annual presidential address before a joint session of the Divisions of Organic and Physical and Inorganic Chemistry, on Thursday, September 14, at 2 P.M. Professor Frederick G. Keyes, of the Massachusetts Institute of Technology, will give an experimental lecture on "Properties of Matter at Very Low Temperatures" on Thursday afternoon during "open house" by the institute to members of the society.

Technical sessions will be held by the Divisions of Cellulose, Agricultural and Food, Colloid, Biological, Fertilizer, Gas and Fuel, Industrial and Engineering, Inorganic, Rubber, and Water Sewage, and Sanitation Chemistry, and of Microchemistry, Chemical Education, History of Chemistry and Sugar Chemistry and Technology.

Professor Ernest H. Huntress, of the Massachusetts Institute of Technology, who is chairman of the Northeastern Section of the society, is vice-chairman of the general convention committee. Professor Arthur R. Davis, of the institute, is secretary, and Frederick S. Bacon, of Boston, is treasurer. Chairmen of subcommittees are announced as follows: R. R. Stevens, accommodations; Kenneth E. Bell, entertainment; Grinnell Jones, ladies' entertainment; A. A. Vernon, student chemists; W. F. Twombly, publicity; J. M. Bierer, finance; E. O. Holmes, equipment for technical sessions; A. A. Ashdown, publications; H. J. Skinner, group meetings; L. F. Hamilton, registration; W. L. Jennings, reception; Mrs. F. C. Sargent, women chemists; L. A. Pratt, C. V. Briggs and J. J. Healy, Jr., trips; H. O. Kulberg, signs; H. L. Sherman, parking arrangements.

# SCIENTIFIC NOTES AND NEWS

DR. LAWRENCE J. HENDERSON, Lawrence professor of chemistry at Harvard University, has accepted an invitation by the Royal Society to deliver the next Pilgrim Trust Lecture in London.

A CERTIFICATE of honorary membership in the American Society of the History of Medicine was presented at the recent annual dinner of the society to Dr. Rudolph Matas, professor emeritus of general and clinical surgery at Tulane University, in recognition of his work in having "preserved and passed on to generations of students the best traditions of medical humanism."

A DINNER in honor of Dr. Victor J. Chambers, of the University of Rochester, who is retiring from teaching, but will continue as dean of the Graduate School, was given on June 15 by his students and friends, two hundred of whom were present. A fund of $2,000, to be known as the Chambers Memorial Fund, was presented to the university to be used for loans to students of chemistry. Professor Chambers was presented with a suitably engraved gold watch.

COLLEAGUES of Dr. Isaac H. Manning, of the University of North Carolina, who is retiring with the title of Kenan professor emeritus of physiology, recently gave a dinner in his honor at which he was presented with a silver pitcher. A second testimonial dinner was given by alumni of the school. Dr. Manning has been for thirty-eight years a member of the faculty of the university, for twenty-eight years as dean of the School of Medicine.

AT a meeting of the Mexican Society of Natural History held in Mexico City on June 16, Dr. Robert Hegner, professor of protozoology in the Johns Hopkins University, was made an honorary member, and Dr. Redginal Hewitt, instructor in protozoology in the Johns Hopkins University, a corresponding member. On this occasion, Dr. Hegner delivered an address on "The Natural History of Parasitic Protozoa."

DR. ALEXANDER WETMORE, assistant secretary of the Smithsonian Institution, has been made an honorary member of the "Magyar Kiralyi Madartani Intezet."

AT the recent commencement exercises at Franklin and Marshall College the degree of doctor of science was conferred on Dr. Mitchel Carroll, professor of biology and head of the department, and on Dr. H. Justin Roddy, professor of geology and executive curator of the museum.

THE doctorate of science has been conferred by the University of London on Professor Niels Bohr, of Copenhagen, and on Sir Robert Robinson, Waynflete professor of chemistry at the University of Oxford.

AT a congregation of the University of Birmingham on July 1 the doctorate of science was conferred on Dr. Edward Battersby Bailey, director of the Geological Survey of Great Britain and of the Museum of Practical Geology, London; on Dr. Niels Bohr, professor of physics at the University of Copenhagen, and on Sir William Bragg, director of the Royal Institution and president of the Royal Society.

THE honorary degree of doctor of music recently conferred by the Chicago Musical College on Dr. Carl E. Seashore, of the State University of Iowa, was reported incorrectly in SCIENCE as having been conferred by the University of Chicago.

THE French League against Cancer has awarded the Amerongen prize of 160,000 francs to Professor A. H. Roffo, director of the Institute of Experimental Medicine for the Study and Treatment of Cancer at the University of Buenos Aires.

THE Royal College of Surgeons, England, has awarded the John Tomes prize for the years 1936–38 to Dr. Arthur Bullerd, for his researches into the bacteriology of the mouth. Professor Ernst W. Hey Groves has been appointed Moynihan lecturer for the current year.

AT the Milwaukee meeting of the American Neisserian Medical Society, which met in conjunction with the American Association for the Advancement of Science, the Francis Amory research award for 1940 was given to Dr. P. S. Pelouze, assistant professor of urology at the University of Pennsylvania School of Medicine.

THE American Radium Society awarded at the recent St. Louis meeting its Janeway Medal for 1939 to Dr. Gioacchino Failla, physicist to the Memorial Hospital for the Treatment of Cancer and Allied Diseases, New York City.

WITH the close of the academic year, Dr. Laetitia M. Snow, Susan M. Hallowell professor of botany at Wellesley College, retired from active service with the title emeritus. At the annual meeting of the Alumnae Association of the college she was elected to honorary membership. She will make her home in Pacific Grove, Calif., where she will continue her research at the Hopkins Marine Station of Stanford University.

PROFESSOR REGINALD PATRICK LINSTEAD, of the University of Sheffield, England, has been appointed professor of chemistry at Harvard University and a member of the University Committee on Pharmacotherapy. Professor Linstead has been at Sheffield for the past year, and for more than ten years previously was at the Imperial College of Science, London.

DR. THOMAS B. TURNER, of the International Health Division of the Rockefeller Foundation, has been appointed professor of bacteriology at the Johns Hopkins University School of Hygiene and Public Health.

Dr. C. E. NEEDHAM, associate professor of geology and mineralogy of the New Mexico School of Mines, has been elected president of the school. Other appointments are: Dr. M. L. Thompson, to be assistant professor of geology and paleontology, and Dr. N. P. Peterson, to be assistant professor of mining and metallurgy. Dr. Needham is also director of the New Mexico Bureau of Mines and Mineral Resources, and Drs. Thompson and Peterson are geologists on the staff of the bureau.

GORDON M. CAIRNS, of Ithaca, N. Y., has been made head of the department of animal industry in the College of Agriculture of the University of Maine. He succeeds Professor L. S. Corbett, who has been head of the department for the past twenty-six years. Professor Corbett retains his work as dean of men.

DR. DAVID F. SMITH, professor of chemistry at the University of Buffalo, has been placed at the head of the work on agricultural motor fuels at the Northern Regional Research Laboratory. He will undertake research intended to develop methods of producing gaseous, liquid and solid motor fuels from agricultural materials.

DR. ALBERT B. SCOTT, formerly of the Research Department of Parke, Davis and Company and for the past two years associated with The General Chemical Company, in New York City, has become connected with The Norwich Pharmacal Company. He is in charge of organic research in the new laboratories of the company at Norwich, N. Y.

DR. ELBERT C. COLE, professor of biology at Williams College, has been elected an alumni trustee of Middlebury College for a term of five years beginning on July 1.

THE Committee on Scientific Research of the American Medical Association has made grants to Dr. Felix Saunders, of the University of Chicago, for the continuation of studies on growth factors for bacteria; to Drs. Hugh J. Morgan and George P. Vryonis, of the School of Medicine of Vanderbilt University, for the study of bacterial infections in the chick embryo; to Dr. William C. Langston and Dr. Paul L. Day, of the School of Medicine of the University of Arkansas, to be used in their experiments on nutritional cytopenia in the monkey, and to Dr. Marion Fay, professor of physiological chemistry at the Woman's Medical College of Pennsylvania, for a continuation of experiments on the physiological effects of strontium.

DURING the summer Dr. John T. Stark, chairman of the department of geology of Northwestern University, is studying the volcanoes of the South Seas, with headquarters in Tahiti; Dr. John R. Ball, professor of geology, is making a study of the geology of the Tennessee Valley, which soon will be flooded by the Tennessee Valley Authority. Dr. William E. Powers, assistant professor of geology, is spending some time in Hawaii studying evidences of glaciation in the Hawaiian mountains. Dr. Arthur L. Howland has been commissioned by the U. S. Geological Survey to search for strategic mineral deposits in the Northern Rockies. A similar expedition will occupy Dr. C. H. Behre, Jr., after the summer term closes. Dr. Edward C. Dapples will be in central Illinois searching for oil deposits.

DRS. PAUL H. HARMON, director of the Division of Handicapped Crippled Children of Illinois; Thomas D. Masters, internist in diseases of metabolism in the Springfield clinic, and F. J. Phillips, assistant in chest surgery of the University of Chicago Clinics, gave a series of lectures and held clinics in their respective specialties before the Tampico Medical Syndicate of Tampico, Mexico, from June 14 to 18.

The thirteenth International Congress of Zoology, which was to have been held this year in Rio de Janeiro, has been postponed. It will be held at Paris in July or August, 1940. The address of the general secretary is 55 Rue de Buffon, Paris (V^e).

The twelfth International Congress of Psychology will be held in Edinburgh from July 22 to 27, 1940. When the Committee of Organization is fully constituted formal invitations will be issued. Subjects for symposia, general discussion and lectures are under consideration by a preliminary arrangements committee. A volume of proceedings, containing abstracts of papers read, will be published, the cost of which is included in the congress fee for active members, which has been fixed at thirty shillings; the fee for associates is fifteen shillings. Arrangements are being made by which a large proportion of the members can be accommodated in university hostels.

The sixteenth National Colloid Symposium met at Stanford University from July 6 to 8. The registration was one hundred and sixty, five foreign countries being represented. The papers will be published in the autumn in *The Journal of Physical Chemistry.*

The Committee on Research Grants of the Illinois State Academy of Science announces that requests for small grants to aid research will be received up to February 1, 1940. Requests should be accompanied by detailed statements of preceding background, general purpose and estimated expenses, and supported by three letters of recommendation sent directly by the writers. Individual grants can probably not exceed $75 per project. It is the custom to make grants only to those connected with smaller institutions within the state. Correspondence should be directed to C. H. Behre, Jr., department of geology and geography, Northwestern University, Evanston, chairman of the committee.

The University of Minnesota Expedition to Richmond Gulf (Province of Quebec, Canada) left Senneterre, P. Q., on June 25 on the first leg of its flight to Richmond Gulf on the east coast of Hudson Bay. The objectives of the expedition are primarily botanical. The great variety of habitats, both from the physiographical point of view and the variety of soils associated with differing geological formations, make the region a promising one for a study of local factors affecting the distribution of plants in a region apparently glaciated recently. Associated problems, such as geochronology and tree ring chronology, will also be studied. The region being in a zone transitional to the barren grounds makes tree-line studies also possible. The personnel consists of Ernst C. Abbe, assistant professor in the department of botany of the University of Minnesota, organizer of the expedition; Mrs. Lucy B. Abbe and John Marr, assistant in the department of botany. The expedition is supported by grants in aid of research from the Graduate School of the University of Minnesota, the Bache Fund of the National Academy of Sciences, the American Academy of Arts and Sciences, the American Philosophical Society (Penrose Fund), the Smithsonian Institution and the Minnesota Academy of Sciences.

*Museum News* reports that the administration of the Blaskley Botanic Garden has been separated from the Santa Barbara Museum of Natural History and that the garden is now being conducted independently under the name of Santa Barbara Botanic Garden. Title to the property, however, remains in the name of the museum. The endowment provided by Mrs. William H. Bliss in memory of her father, Henry Blaskley, and heretofore adequate for the garden's maintenance, is no longer sufficient because of the decline in income from investments. In order to carry it on a group of those interested has formed the Santa Barbara Botanic Garden, Incorporated, and is appealing for contributions. Officers of the new corporation are William Lassiter, *president;* Mrs. Anne Stow-Fithian, *vice-president;* Frederick B. Kellam, *secretary;* and Frank J. McCoy, *treasurer*. Elmer J. Bissell, formerly director of the garden, is honorary president. Maunsell Van Rensselaer continues as director of the garden.

# DISCUSSION

## CENTERS OF POPULATION OF LEARNED GROUPS

A few years ago one of the learned societies announced that in response to requests for an annual meeting held in the Far West, the next meeting would be in Richmond, Va. To the members residing many miles west of the Mississippi River, this statement seemed ludicrous. However, some one raised the question: With respect to the membership of the organization, could it be possible that Richmond is *far west*?

The study reported is an attempt to determine the center of population for the membership of certain of the learned societies in the United States. The method used is essentially that of the Bureau of the Census in determining the center of population of the United States, as described on page 20, Volume II, 15th Census of the United States:

> The center of population may be said to represent the center of gravity of the population. If the surface of the

United States be considered as a rigid level plane without weight and the population distributed thereon, all individuals being assumed to have equal weight, the point on which this plane would balance would be the center of population. This pivotal point would be the center of gravity of the hypothetical plane; and its location would be affected not only by the numbers of persons on the different parts of the plane, but also by the distance of each individual from the "center."

In making the computations for the location of the center of population it is necessary to assume that the center is at a certain point. Through this point a parallel and a meridian are drawn, crossing the entire country. In making the computations for 1930, the same point was selected as in 1920; this intersection is assumed to be where the parallel of 39 degrees north latitude intersects the meridian of 86 degrees west longitude, which lines were taken as the axes of moments.

The product of the population of a given area by its distance from the assumed parallel is called a north or south moment, and the product of the population of the area by its distance from the assumed meridian is called an east or west moment. In calculating north and south moments the distances are measured in minutes of arc; in calculating east and west moments it is necessary to use miles, on account of the unequal length of the degrees and minutes in different latitudes. The population of the country is grouped by square degrees—that is, by areas included between consecutive parallels and meridians—as they are convenient units with which to work. The population of the principal cities is then deducted from that of the respective square degrees in which they lie and treated separately. . . . The population of each square degree north and south of the assumed parallel is multiplied by the distance of its center from that parallel; a similar calculation is made for the principal cities; and the sum of the north moments and the sum of the south moments are ascertained. The difference between these two sums, divided by the total population of the country, gives a correction to the latitude. In a similar manner the sum of the east and of the west moments are ascertained and from them the correction in longitude is made.

In this study, no attempt was made to use square degrees; rather the latitude and longitude of the stated post-office address of each member were determined as accurately as possible. In the absence of other figures, the data were estimated from a large-scale atlas. This task was in itself no slight one, in one case it required determination of the latitude and longitude of over 2,000 towns and cities.

The selection of the groups studied was somewhat arbitrary. The first group studied was not one of the learned societies, but consisted of all college students in the United States, as listed in the *World Almanac.* In the selection of societies to be studied a very important factor was the availability of a fairly recent membership list. The growing tendency toward stability of the respective centers made it seem probable that the study of other societies of a non-specialized nature would not show marked differences from the results here reported.

In the case of the American Chemical Society, the secretary advised that a complete list of the individual membership was not available for the purposes of this study. The society has 84 local sections scattered throughout the United States. It was assumed that a fair approximation would be obtained by assuming the entire membership of a local section concentrated in the city or at the center of the region for which the section takes its name, and this method was used in this situation. It should be emphasized that this method neglects altogether approximately 2,700 members, who are unattached to any section. This might produce a definite change in the center of population.

Table 1 summarizes the available information regarding the various centers of population studied. The nearest city was interpreted to mean a city of 150,000 or more.

TABLE 1

| Organization | Number of individuals | Center of population: Latitude | Center of population: Longitude | Nearest city |
|---|---|---|---|---|
| College enrolment | 885,282 | 39°19′ | 84°45′ | Cincinnati |
| American Chemical Society by sections | 17,469 | 40° 5′ | 83°49′ | Dayton |
| Geological Society of America | 562 | 39° 1′ | 87°32′ | Indianapolis |
| American Historical Society | 2,926 | 39°54′ | 82°13′ | Columbus |
| Mathematical Association of America | 1,928 | 39°32′ | 84°57′ | Cincinnati |
| American Association of Petroleum Geologists | 2,448 | 35° 6′ | 98°12′ | Oklahoma City |
| American Physical Society | 2,653 | 40° 1′ | 83°23′ | Columbus |
| American Psychological Association | 2,269 | 40°15′ | 83°35′ | Columbus |
| American Association of University Professors | 11,165 | 39°30′ | 84°27′ | Cincinnati Dayton |
| American Association for the Advancement of Science | 17,141 | 39°41′ | 84°10′ | Dayton |
| American Speech Correction Society | 206 | 40°44′ | 87° 7′ | Chicago Indianapolis |
| American Society of Zoologists | 797 | 40° 5′ | 83°39′ | Columbus Dayton |

Obviously, the effect of the western oil fields is felt upon the center of population for the American Society of Petroleum Geologists. For the other groups, however, there is a definite tendency for the centers of population to cluster. In fact, all are found within a rectangle about 200 miles from east to west and about 100 miles from north to south.

It is interesting to note that with the single exceptional case noted, these centers of population tend to be slightly north and very definitely east of the center of population of the United States, which in 1930 was 39°3′45″ north latitude and 87°8′6″ west longitude. On the other hand, it seems hard to find any national group for which Richmond, Va., or even Pittsburgh could be considered "far west." Quite possibly some eastern members fail to realize the size of the United States as a whole.

From one point of view, the ideal place for an annual meeting of one of these societies would be the nearest city to the center of population, for the total number of miles of travel necessary for every member to attend would thus be a minimum. From this point of view, it would certainly seem that Columbus and Cincinnati are excellent convention cities.

The writer wishes to acknowledge his indebtedness to students working under the National Youth Administration, without whose help in the routine details this study would have been impossible.

Cecil B. Read
University of Wichita

## A NEW DISEASE OF SNAP BEANS

In June of 1938 while the writer was making a disease survey of his hybrid progenies and varieties of snap beans in connection with a bean-breeding program, he discovered a very destructive disease which has not previously been described. During the present growing season the disease has again appeared and is even more destructive than during 1938.

The end result of this disease is a severe chlorosis followed by wilt and death of the host. Perhaps the most characteristic symptom of the disease throughout its course is a pronounced deep brown to black discoloration of the inner phloem and outer xylem of the entire plant. Of course, the extent of vascular discoloration varies with the extent and severity of infection.

When severely infected, the roots appear dark gray to black on the exterior, due to the intense discoloration of the vascular elements. Symptoms on the upper hypocotyl and stem appear as longitudinal streaks or stripes of varying width, varying in color from brown to brownish purple due to the masking effect of the chlorenchyma. The only external symptoms on infected pods is the presence of a brownish purple discoloration of one or both sutures, which might easily be mistaken for a slight anthocyanescence. In cross sections of infected pods few to all the vascular bundles are discolored, depending on the extent of infection. The chlorenchymatous pulp of severely infected young pods often presents an "inky" appearance.

This disease takes its greatest toll about blossoming time. Although some less severely infected plants survive and mature seed, fatalities are extremely high.

Numerous attempts to isolate a causal organism in culture have consistently failed. This fact, combined with other data at hand, indicates that the disease is caused by a virus. Certain experiments indicate that the virus has a long incubation period, since plants from seed taken from infected pods remain apparently healthy until about blossoming time.

Further work on the etiology of the disease is in progress. From our records we find indications that the disease was brought in on western-grown seed. This note is being published with the hope that persons noting a disease with the above described syndrome will report to the writer.

Wilbert A. Jenkins
Georgia Experiment Station

## GENERAL ANESTHESIA BY CHILLING

The use of ether, chloretone and other drugs as anesthetics preparatory to operating on lower animals is often objectionable because of the after-effects of the drugs. This difficulty can be overcome by the use of low temperatures for stupefaction. Fishes, amphibians and reptiles may be conveniently and fully anesthetized by immersion in water and cracked ice or simply in cracked ice. After ten to fifteen minutes in the cooling mixture the animals are fully stupefied and, if they are laid out on cracked ice, they may be subjected to an extended and uninterrupted operation. Recovery is quick and satisfactory at the ordinary temperature of the laboratory, and the animals so treated may be almost at once tested in a particular way without waiting for the gradual disappearance from their systems of an anesthetizing drug. This method has been applied with success in the Harvard Laboratories to salt-water and fresh-water fishes, to amphibians and to reptiles. Wiesner (1935) appears to have been the first to use it. Both he and Pfeiffer have applied it to new-born rats. Whether it will have any operative significance for adult, warm-blooded vertebrates remains to be seen. Press reports of a kind of cold hibernation induced in human beings by a slight lowering of their bodily temperatures is suggestive of such a step.

G. H. Parker
Harvard University

# SCIENTIFIC BOOKS

## RECENT BOTANICAL BOOKS

*The Stapelieae*. By Alain White and Boyd L. Sloane. 3 vols. xvi + 1186 + 23 + 23 pp. 1,233 + figs. + xxxix plates + 2 maps. 2nd edition. Pasadena: Abbey San Encino Press. 1937. $12.50.

Since the Stapelias are found only in the eastern

hemisphere, they have hardly received due consideration in our general concepts of xerophytic plants. Extending from India and Ceylon to Spain, and south to Cape Province in southern Africa, this group of twenty genera is widely spread, though South Africa is spoken of as "the broad paradise of the Stapelieae."

The treatment of the distribution of this tribe of Asclepiads, the discussion of the history of previous work on the group, the descriptions of the twenty genera and all the known species, the copious and beautiful illustrations, thirty-nine in full-page color plates, and the mass of pertinent data assembled about these plants make these three volumes a monumental compendium of information on this unique alliance. They will prove invaluable to the specialist. In *Caralluma* 105 species are given, in *Stapelia* 99, in *Huernia* 45, while *Frerea, Drakebrockmania, Stapeliopsis, Diplocyatha, Hoodiopsis* and *Luckhoffia* are monotypic.

The normal tremor that accompanies the opening of a volume essentially taxonomic is rightly lacking in the case of "The Stapelieae." The general botanist as well as the layman can read this work with pleasure and with profit. Even a partial study and an examination of the excellent figures leave the reader with a distinct impression of the group, with its succulent, rather spiny, photosynthetic stems—only the genus *Frerea* has fleshy leaves—its striking, mottled, showy, flesh-colored, rather complex flowers and its silky-haired seeds. The authors tell us that "the ability of Stapeliads to attract desert flies and a predisposition to succulence were doubtless principal factors in enabling the tribe to dwell in the semi-arid societies they frequent."

Those who study "The Stapelieae" should gain a knowledge and an appreciation of these Asclepiads. Most of us will never have an opportunity of finding them in their native habitats, and many of the genera and species are not often seen in cultivation. These books therefore fill a real need; reading them is almost as satisfactory as studying the plants in the field, though the reader will wish all the more that he might do both.

It is also distinctly refreshing to come upon a work that seems so free of the usual restrictions on pagination and on quality of reproduction. These three volumes give every indication of being exactly what the authors wished them to be; neither effort nor expense has been spared. Such books are lasting.

*A Textbook of General Botany.* By RICHARD M. HOLMAN and WILFRED W. ROBBINS. xvii + 664 pp. 482 figs. 4th edition. New York: John Wiley and Sons. 1938. $4.00.

FOUR years have elapsed since the publication of the third edition of this justly popular book, and although a number of changes have been made in the new edition, they are not really basic alterations. In format, in style and in contents—even to most of the details—the fourth edition parallels the third closely, and thus maintains the high standards and effectiveness of its predecessors.

The first half of this book deals with the structure and physiology of seed-bearing plants. In this the usual material on stem, root, leaf and flower is presented, along with a concise treatment of the functions of each. In the second half the groups of the plant kingdom are taken up; theories of evolution, heredity and fossil plants are also ably discussed.

In the fourth edition certain changes have been made. There is greater emphasis on active solute absorption, the part on conduction has been altered, the tissue classification has been revised. In the previous edition the plant kingdom was divided into the Thallophyta and Embryophyta; the new book suggests also an alternative grouping in which the vascular plants or Tracheophyta are composed of Psilopsida, Lycopsida, Sphenopsida and Pteropsida. A glossary has been added, and the list of books for reference and collateral reading has been brought up to date.

The new edition has 482 figures, compared with 463 in the third; the additional illustrations are largely half-tones of photographs or of photomicrographs, and some of the old figures have also been replaced. Most of the original excellent drawings and diagrams have been kept, however.

This text is outstanding in the ease with which it can be studied and in the diagrammatic clarity with which the material is presented. It is still the answer to a freshman botanist's prayer.

*An Introduction to Botany.* By ARTHUR W. HAUPT. xii + 396 pp. 278 figs. New York and London: McGraw-Hill Book Company. 1938. $3.00.

A NEW text-book of botany, added to the volumes recently printed, some of which are still moist, should bear certain marks of distinction to warrant its publication; these are happily not wanting in "An Introduction to Botany."

The author has digested and presented clearly and concisely the rich botanical heritage of the past several generations. There are adequate discussions of the structure, physiology, reproduction and heredity of plants, while six chapters, covering 113 pages, are devoted primarily to their evolutionary development. Thus the usual material of botanical texts is included, though the sequence in certain cases departs from the traditional.

More striking for an elementary book is the chapter on environmental relations, which reflects the growing emphasis of the biological sciences on ecology. Here the elementary student can gain an acquaintance with the floristic regions of North America, as well as a conception of the characteristic associations and successions. Structural adaptations to the factors of the environment are not neglected, and such time-honored topics as saprophytism, parasitism and symbiosis are given due consideration.

Indicative of the modern trend to consider biological science from some of its broader aspects—from without as well as from within—are three chapters, one on "The Principles of Evolution," one on "The Causes of Evolution" and one on "Plant Life of the Past." These cut across the subject-matter of various fields and leave the reader with an inkling, at least, of the magnitude of the organic world.

Some will wish, perhaps, that the author had entrusted to his students more of the choice bits of the results of modern research, even though such findings may not be destined for eternity; but that is largely a matter of individual preference, and this book, intended primarily for a one-semester course, is necessarily limited in length.

The illustrations are superior—clear and convincing, artistically prepared and largely original.

The author aims "to introduce the college student to the science of plant life"; this he does, admirably.

*General and Economic Botany.* By ERNEST ELWOOD STANFORD. xxix + 675 pp. 436 figs. New York and London: D. Appleton-Century Company. 1937. $4.00.

SINCE the subject-matter of botanical science continually increases, the text-book extract prepared for student consumption tends to become more and more concentrated. There is a feeling of luxury, therefore, in opening a volume like this, that exceeds somewhat the usual limitations on length and that offers the reader a glimpse of some of the more interesting and humanly important features of this field of endeavor.

"General and Economic Botany" covers the subject-matter included in the standard texts somewhat more fully than usual. There are chapters on cells and tissues, the morphology of leaves, stems, roots and flowers; the functions of these parts of the plant are largely woven into these same chapters, although fifty-seven pages are set aside for "The Seed Plant and Its Environment."

The plant kingdom is divided into the Thallophyta and the Embryophyta, the former being subdivided into the Schizophyta, Phycophyta and Mycophyta, while the latter includes the Bryophyta, Pteridophyta and Spermatophyta.

The seed plants are obviously the author's forte, as might be expected in a book placing emphasis on the economic aspects of the subject. One hundred and forty-four pages are devoted to the groups of the Angiosperms alone. Our more common and important orders and families are considered carefully, along with a considerable number of those more characteristic of the tropics.

Within the covers of this volume information is assembled on a wide variety of botanical topics. Most of our other general texts, for example, contain little or nothing on such items as glutathione, phyllodia, kapok, marihuana, dulse, rainfall and erosion areas of the United States and countless other subjects here included.

The broad basis on which this work is fashioned is reflected also in the 436 illustrations, not a few of which are original, though many have been culled from a wide variety of sources. The lack of uniformity in the figures is more than offset by their diversity of origin and by the scope of the subjects that they portray.

Specialists in particular fields will undoubtedly find shortcomings and inaccuracies. They are almost inevitable in a book of this breadth prepared by one man. From its very scope it lacks the unity of a more compact treatise—it suggests the banyan tree rather than the Colorado blue spruce.

The author writes that his aim is "to introduce the student to one great area of the biological world as a larger place to live in, rather than to train botanists to join an overcrowded profession." If those who study this book are willing to contribute some leisure and some meditation, he will succeed, and they will profit.

EDWIN B. MATZKE
COLUMBIA UNIVERSITY

# SPECIAL ARTICLES

## ADSORPTION OF ANTIBODIES BY EGG ALBUMIN FILMS

THE possibility of demonstrating immunological reactions with films on a water surface, or those transferred on to metal plates by the Langmuir technique has been dealt with in several recent papers.[1] We have carried out experiments with solutions of crystallized hen egg albumin and anti-egg albumin rabbit sera. Films were deposited under a pressure of 12 dynes/cm on chromium-plated slides covered with 37 to 51 layers of barium stearate. Increments of thickness were followed optically as described by Blodgett and Langmuir.[2] Polarized sodium light was used as source of illumination and the value 1.495 was assumed for the index of refraction of the proteins. When a 1 per

[1] *Cf.* E. F. Porter and A. M. Pappenheimer, *Jour. Exp. Med.*, 69: 755, 1939; M. F. Shaffer and T. H. Dingle, *Proc. Soc. Exp. Biol. and Med.*, 38: 528, 1938.

[2] K. B. Blodgett and J. Langmuir, *Phys. Rev.*, 51: 964, 1937.

cent. solution of ovalbumin was applied to two monolayers of immune serum (thickness of double layer 25A) there was an increase in thickness of about 35A, but the same increase was seen with normal rabbit serum. Experiments were also made with plates coated with monolayers of sera on which monolayers of ovalbumin were deposited, or *vice versa*. Here likewise no difference was found in the behavior of immune and normal sera. On the other hand, when the slides were first coated with one or two layers of spread ovalbumin and then (undiluted) immune serum applied to the plate for 3 minutes, a specific effect was observed (see Table 1) as in the work of Porter and Pappenheimer with pneumococcus polysaccharide. In the experiments summarized in Table 1, made with various immune and normal rabbit sera, an interval of 20 minutes was observed between initial spreading and transfer of the film, in order to allow time for unfolding. The increase in thickness following the application of an immune serum was the same whether there were two layers or one layer of egg albumin. The differences between the adsorbed layers of various heterologous antisera call for further investigation.

TABLE 1

| Number of layers of ovalbumin | Total thickness ovalbumin | Serum applied | Increase in thickness |
|---|---|---|---|
| | (A) | | (A) |
| 2 ......... | 20 | Anti-ovalbumin, No. 1 | 50 |
| 2 ......... | 18 | " " No. 2 | 58 |
| 2 ......... | 19 | " " " " | 49 |
| 1 (down) .. | | " " " " | 50 |
| 2 ......... | 16 | " " No. 3 | 41 |
| 2 ......... | 16 | " " " " | 41 |
| 2 ......... | 14 | " " No. 4 | 40 |
| 2 ......... | 18 | " " " " | 55 |
| 1 (down) .. | 9 | " " " " | 45 |
| 1 (down) .. | 9 | " " " " | 46 |
| 2 ......... | 17 | " horse serum No. 1 | 5 |
| 2 ......... | 19 | " " " " " | 7 |
| 2 ......... | 21 | " " " No. 2 | 5 |
| 2 ......... | 15 | " chicken serum | 14 |
| 2 ......... | 16 | " " " | 14 |
| 2 ......... | 22 | " Pneumococcus I | 7 |
| 2 ......... | 15 | " " " | 7 |
| 2 ......... | 17 | " guinea pig red cells | 6 |
| 2 ......... | 18 | " " " " " | 12 |
| 2 ......... | 15 | " horse red cells | 15 |
| 2 ......... | 10 | " " " " | 15 |
| 2 ......... | 22 | normal No. 1 | 4 |
| 2 ......... | 16 | " " " | 7 |
| 2 ......... | 20 | " No. 2 | 2 |
| 2 ......... | 21 | " No. 3 | — |
| 2 ......... | 17 | " No. 4 | 7 |

It would appear therefore that thin films (9 A) of protein are still capable of reacting with antibodies while, as has been reported by Danielli, Danielli and Marrack,[3] the reactivity of antibodies is destroyed by unfolding of the molecule. The experiments of these authors, unlike ours, were made with purified antibody and are free from the objection, prevailing in the case of whole antiserum, that the films may contain too small a proportion of antibody.

[3] J. F. Danielli, M. Danielli and J. R. Marrack, *Brit. Jour. Exp. Path.*, 19: 393, 1938.

The available observations on antibody films and inactivation of antibodies by denaturing agents lend support to the view that the specific reactivity of antibodies is to a large extent dependent upon structures different from those which mainly determine the specificity of antigens.[4, 5]. In this connection reference ought to be made to the theory of Mirsky and Pauling[6] on the structure of proteins, according to which proteins owe characteristic specific properties to the folding of the polypeptide chain "into a uniquely defined configuration . . . held by hydrogen bonds. . . ." Pointing in the same direction as the above evidence is the puzzling fact that an unlimited number of different antibodies can be produced, all having the same chemical characteristics of serum globulins; one idea to be considered among others is the possibility of different ways of folding of the same polypeptide chain.

In experiments made with plant haemagglutinins (*cf.* 7), it was seen that monolayers of bean agglutinin (phasin) of a thickness of 9 A, or double layers dipped for a short time in a suspension of washed horse blood, became covered with red cells in a homogeneous single layer which was not removed by repeated rinsing with saline solution. The agglutinin used was a purified preparation showing only a single boundary when examined by the method of Tiselius.[7] A similar result was obtained with a partially purified agglutinin of castor beans, swine blood being used. For reasons not yet known this conspicuous reaction was not regular, the coating with blood cells being often sparse or spotty. If the plant agglutinins actually are relative in the unfolded state, in apparent contrast to antibodies, this might be connected with the low specificity of these reactions.[8] However, no definite conclusions can as yet be drawn from these observations, particularly in view of the possibility of errors in the interpretation of this sort of experiments, recently emphasized by Langmuir and Schaefer.[9] After this communication had been completed there appeared a paper by L. A. Chambers[10] concerning films of a nucleoprotein antigen.

A. ROTHEN
K. LANDSTEINER

THE ROCKEFELLER INSTITUTE FOR MEDICAL RESEARCH, NEW YORK, N. Y.

[4] K. Landsteiner and J. van der Scheer, *Jour. Exp. Med.*, 67: 709, 1938.

[5] J. R. Marrack, IV Congresso Internazionale, Rome, 1939, Vol. I, p. 347.

[6] A. E. Mirsky and L. Pauling, *Proc. Nat. Acad. of Sciences*, 22: 439, 1936.

[7] L. G. Longsworth and D. A. MacInnes, *Chem. Rev.*, 24: 282, 1939.

[8] K. Landsteiner, "The Specificity of Serological Reactions," 1936, Chas. C Thomas, Springfield, Ill.

[9] J. Langmuir and V. J. Schaefer, *Chem. Rev.*, 24: 199, 1939.

[10] L. A. Chambers, *Jour. Immunology*, 36: 543, 1939.

## ABSORPTION SPECTRUM OF FURTHER PURIFIED CYTOCHROME C

As shown previously,[1, 2, 3] cytochrome c may be prepared from beef heart with an iron content of 0.34 per cent. This product, arrived at by different methods, was till now considered as pure. However, a thorough investigation of the cytochrome c by means of *Tiselius* electrophoretic apparatus revealed the possibility of a further purification. If electrophoresis experiments are carried out at pH = 10.5 (*i.e.*, higher than the isoelectric point of the cytochrome) two moving boundaries on each side of the U-tube appear, a colorless component migrating faster than the cytochrome. After complete removal of the colorless component, the cytochrome c had an iron content of 0.41 per cent. A further purification by means of electrophoresis at pH 7.3 raised the iron content to 0.43 per cent., corresponding to a molecular weight of 13,000. This value is definitely lower than one fourth of the molecular weight of the hemoglobin. The purified cytochrome c, contrary to the unpurified one, migrated in the electrical field as a homogeneous substance at all pH values investigated.

The purification had no influence upon the absorption spectrum in the visual region. The oxidized cytochrome shows different absorption bands, depending on the pH of the solution.[2] A reinvestigation of the visual part of the spectrum now revealed some new absorption bands and the existence of *four different forms* of the ferri-cytochrome c:

TABLE 1

| Type | pH | Bands, mμ | Color of the solution | Dissociation constant, pK′ |
|---|---|---|---|---|
| I .. | 1 | 627; (540–490) | brown | I– II: 2.5 |
| II .. | 4–8 | 695; 560; 540–515 | brownish red | II–III: 9.5 |
| III .. | 11 | 507–545 | red | III– IV: 12.7 |
| IV .. | 14 | 570; 530 | brownish red | |

The different types change reversibly one into another by changing the pH. A quantitative investigation, carried out by means of photoelectrical light absorption and pH measurements, showed that the different types go over one into another along common dissociation curves.

Solutions of an intermediate pH, types I and II both being present, were analyzed by means of the difference in light absorption at 530 mμ, $\beta_{I,\,530} = 1.82 \times 10^7$; $\beta_{II,\,530} = 2.68 \times 10^7$. The other curves were determined in an analogous manner at 650 mμ. The relative amounts of the different types were plotted against the pH (Fig. 1).

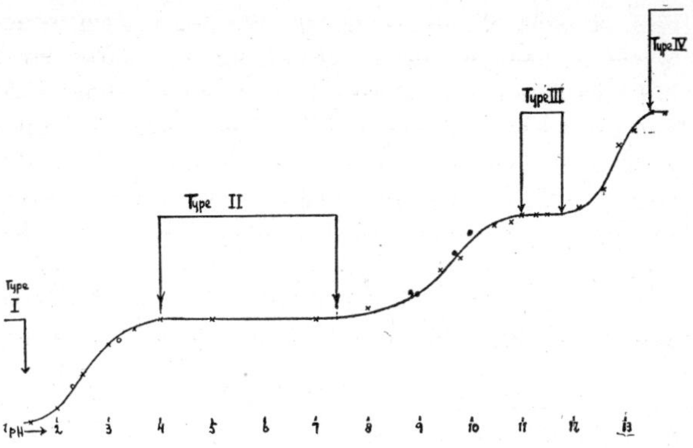


FIG. 1

The great stability of the cytochrome c, even at extreme pH values, depends very probably on the strong linkage of the protein component to the 2- and 4-standing side chains of the hemin.[4, 5] The authors hope that determinations of the magnetic properties of the iron atom in the four different types of the ferri-cytochrome c will give further evidence on the constitution of the cytochrome c.

HUGO THEORELL
Å. ÅKESSON
MEDICAL NOBEL INSTITUTE, STOCKHOLM

[1] Theorell, *Biochem. Zeits.*, 279: 463, 1935.
[2] *Ibid.*, 285: 207, 1936.
[3] Keilin and Hartree, *Proc. Roy. Soc., London*, B, 122: 298, 1937.
[4] Theorell, *Biochem. Zeits.*, 298: 242, 1938.
[5] *Ibid.*, in press.

## SODIUM CHLORIDE AND DIABETES INSIPIDUS

IT has been noted that the abnormally large fluid exchange of experimental diabetes insipidus (d.i.) varies directly with the amount of food the animal ingests.[1] In fasting and in sickness (and therefore probably anorexia), d.i. largely subsides.[2, 3, 4] By varying the NaCl intake of rats, in which d.i. had been experimentally produced by removal of the posterior hypophysis, we have found that the severity of the condition varies directly not with the intake of food in general but rather with the intake of the NaCl in the food. An NaCl-low diet[5] was used alone or to it were added known quantities of NaCl. Reduction of the daily NaCl intake (but not the total intake of food) from 250 mgms to 1.3 mgms caused a reduction of the daily fluid intake from the d.i. level of 60 cc to 25 cc. Equivalent results are obtained by fasting d.i.

[1] C. P. Richter, "The Pituitary Gland," Baltimore, 1938.
[2] P. Bailey and F. Bremer, *Arch. Int. Med.*, 28: 773, 1921.
[3] G. M. Curtis, *Arch. Int. Med.*, 34: 801, 1924.
[4] C. Fisher, W. R. Ingram and S. W. Ranson, *Arch. Neurol. and Psychiat.*, 34: 124, 1935.
[5] E. Orent-Keiles, A. Robinson and E. V. McCollum, *Am. Jour. Physiol.*, 119: 651, 1937.

rats. Conversely, in both types of experiment it is possible to cause a full return of the d.i. by giving 250 mgms of salt per day without any food. Similarly, excess NaCl administration is well known profoundly to aggravate an existing d.i.[6] All the above experiments were done with rats in the permanent phase of d.i. We have found, however, that the transient phase is not dependent on the rate of NaCl ingestion; it occurs even though the NaCl content of the diet has been previously reduced or, as is well known, in fasting.

Although the rate of ingestion of NaCl greatly influences the permanent phase of d.i., we do not think it exclusively responsible for the condition. If the NaCl intake is reduced to zero by fasting, a degree of d.i. still recurs at the time of the onset of the permanent phase. At this time, the fluid exchange of the d.i. animals rises to about three times normal, as contrasted with seven times normal when such animals are fed. In d.i. rats, therefore, a large portion of the abnormal fluid exchange which commences with the permanent phase can be ascribed to the return of the animal's appetites with consequent ingestion of NaCl in the animals' food.

Using Richter's[7] technique for determining appetites in the rat during deficiencies of various kinds, we have also found that there is in d.i. in the rat a considerable appetite for salt. Diabetic rats ingest approximately three times the quantity of salt that the normal rat ingests when given a choice between water and physiological saline to drink.

*Summary:* The severity of permanent diabetes insipidus in the rat is directly related to the amount of NaCl ingested; if little or no NaCl is taken in, the condition exists in only a mild form. The effect of fasting on diabetes insipidus can be attributed to the withdrawal of NaCl rather than to the withdrawal of food in general. Also, the diabetic rat shows a considerable appetite for NaCl. These findings, coupled with the fact that the diabetic animal is abnormally sensitive to NaCl administration, suggest that in diabetes insipidus the primary defect is some abnormality in NaCl metabolism.

H. G. SWANN

UNIVERSITY OF CHICAGO

## THE ATTEMPTED HYDROGENATION OF 3-METHYLXANTHINE[1]

THE observation by vanVeen and coworkers that *toxoflavin* $C_6H_6O_2N_4$ (I), the highly toxic substance produced by the bacterial action of *Bacterium cocovenenans* on certain food products originating in the commercial production of cocoanut oil in Java,[2] is reduced catalytically in the presence of platinum oxide to a purine containing a saturated glyoxaline ring (II), stimulated the authors to investigate the behavior of 3-methylxanthine (IV) on catalytic reduction.

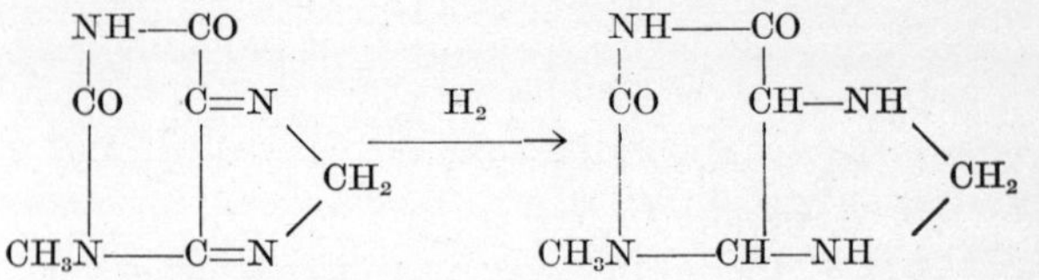


I II

The graphical formula (I) proposed by vanVeen to express the structure of *toxoflavin* is isomeric with that of 3-methylxanthine (IV), and is the first representative of the desmotropic formulation for purine (III) to be described in the chemical literature.

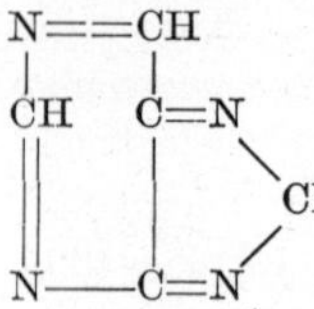


III

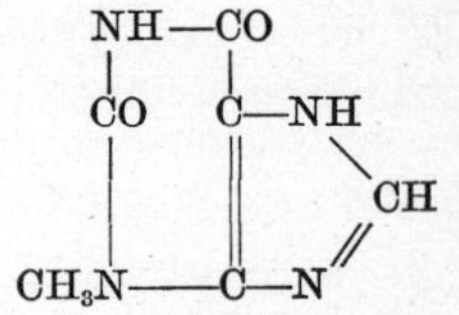


IV

It is a well-known fact that xanthine (V), 3-methylxanthine (IV) and several other alkylated xanthines undergo reduction electrolytically[3] with absorption of hydrogen at the 6-position of the purine cycle. This treatment leads to the hydrogenation of the carbonyl group (CO) to a methylene radical ($CH_2$) and formation of a desoxypurine derivative (VI). There was no attack by hydrogen on the imidazole cycle of the purine nucleus of the various xanthine compounds subjected to this electrolytic technique of reduction. Uric acid is also reduced in a similar manner.[4]

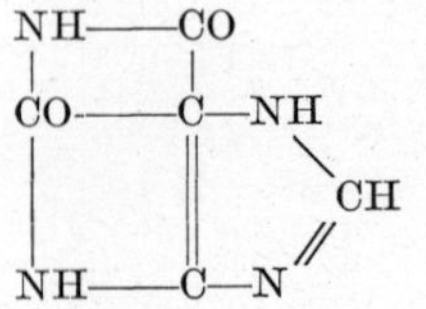


V

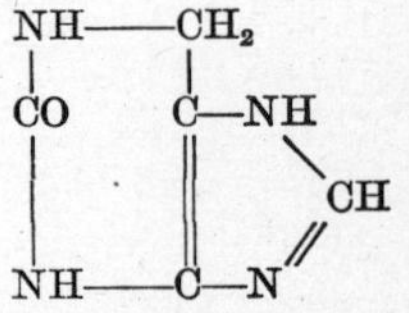


VI

The authors now desire to report that it has been their experience that both xanthine (V) and 3-methylxanthine (IV) are extremely resistant to structural changes when subjected to hydrogenation in the pres-

[6] H. G. Swann, *Endocr.*, 24: 253, 1939.

[7] C. P. Richter, *Endocr.*, 21: 50, 1937; *ibid.*, 22: 214, 1938.

[1] Researches of pyrimidines, CLXII.

[2] vanVeen and Mertens, *Rec. trav. chim.*, 53: 402, 1934; vanVeen and Baars, *Kononklijke Akad. Wetenschappen Amsterdam*, 40: 6, 1937; vanVeen and Baars, *Rec. trav. chim.*, 57: 248, 1938.

[3] Tafel and Weinschenk, *Ber.*, 33: 3370, 1900; Tafel and Ach, *Ber.*, 34: 1166, 1901. See also Johnson, "The Chemistry of Pyrimidines, Purines and Nucleic Acids," Gilman's "Organic Chemistry," Volume II. John Wiley and Sons, Inc., New York City, New York, 1938.

[4] Biltz, *Jour. pr. Chem.*, 145: 83, 1936.

ence of certain catalysts. Both purines, suspended in glacial acetic acid, were recovered unaltered after exposure to hydrogen gas for 8 hours in the presence of Adam's platinum catalyst and under 1.5–2.0 atmospheres pressures. Reduction experiments were also applied by substituting absolute alcohol for glacial acetic acid as solvent and shaking in an atmosphere of hydrogen gas in presence of Raney nickel as the catalyst, under 160–200 atmospheres pressure at 200° for 10 hours. Both purines were partially destroyed by this treatment. In the case of 3-methylxanthine 60 per cent. of the purine was recovered unaltered. Its identity was established by the results of analysis (calc. for $C_6H_6O_2N_4$: N, 33.72 per cent. Found, N, 33.60 per cent.) and by conversion to caffeine by alkylation according to the directions of Emil Fischer.[5]

Exposure of xanthine (V) to catalytic hydrogenation at different hydrogen pressures and temperatures in the presence of copper-chromium-oxide catalyst led to such extensive decomposition of the purine that this reduction technique proved to be of no value and consequently was not applied with 3-methylxanthine. In none of our experiments did we obtain any evidence of the reduction of carbonyl to methylene in position —6, or any hydrogenation of the unsaturated imidazole nucleus of the xanthine molecule. These results are in marked contrast to those reported for *toxoflavin* (I) when exposed to the action of hydrogen under similar experimental conditions.

The resistance of hydrogenation of 3-methylxanthine (IV) is in accordance with the behavior of imidazoles which have previously been investigated. Although 2,4,5-triphenylimidazole[6] (lophin) is reduced with difficulty in the presence of platinum black[7] to 2,4,5-tricyclohexyl-4,5-dihydroimidazole, and 2,4,5-triphenyl-4,5,-dihydroimidazole to this same dihydro-derivative and finally to 2,4,5-tricyclohexylimidazoline, the same experimental conditions were ineffective when applied to imidazole itself, 2,4,5-trimethylimidazole, histidine, lysidine and to benzimidazole. The authors were also unable to hydrogenate benzimidazole-benzimide with Adam's platinum, Raney nickel or copper-chromium-oxide catalysts. It will be of interest to determine whether isomers of the xanthine (VII) and isoxanthine (VIII) types will differ in their behavior on catalytic reduction.

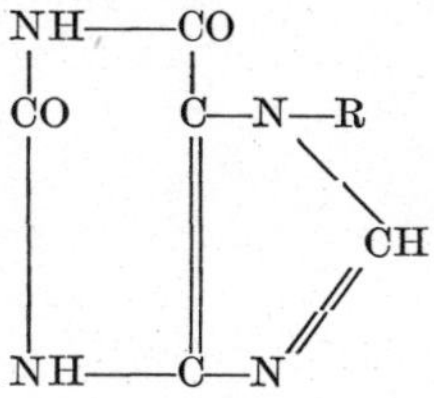
VII

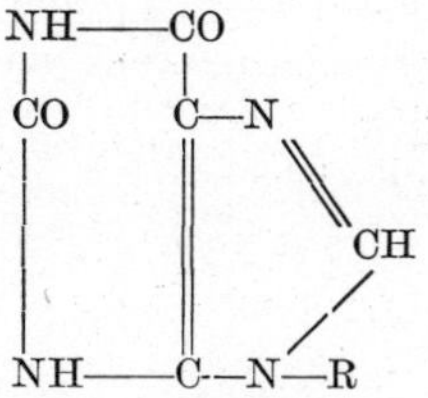
VIII

TREAT B. JOHNSON,
JOSEPH C. AMBELANG,
*Sterling professorship of chemistry research assistant, 1938–39*
YALE UNIVERSITY

# SCIENTIFIC APPARATUS AND LABORATORY METHODS

## LABELING MUSEUM SPECIMENS

To workers engaged in museum or natural science activities the labeling of specimens is generally a necessary but time-consuming task. A quick and efficient method is always sought. The writer has developed a method which has proved to be very satisfactory.

The complete series of symbols to be used are hand-printed with black drawing ink or typed on strips of tough white or brown gummed paper. Brown or Cellophane "Scotch" tape may be used if the symbols are to be hand-printed, but the tape does not make as satisfactory a label as the gummed paper. Sufficient space is left between the symbols to permit cutting to the desired size. When completely marked the individual labels are cut from the strips. The single label is moistened on the gummed side and fastened to the specimen by a little pressure. A perfect attachment at this stage is not necessary as it serves only to hold the label while the "varnish" is being applied. By the time a number of labels have been attached to their respective specimens the first ones are entirely dry and are ready for the "varnish." A coating of Cenco Label Varnish[1] is applied so as to cover the paper label and to overlap about one sixteenth to one eighth of an inch on the adjacent portion of the specimen. The overlap serves as a seal of attachment. The dauber that is attached to the stopper of the bottle is too large and clumsy for this purpose. A small sliver of wood cut to a chisel end about one eighth of an inch across serves as the best means of application; although a small brush may be used. The "varnish" dries sufficiently upon application to prevent running so that it is not necessary to place the labeled portion of the specimen in better than an approximately horizontal position while drying. The specimens are ready for use in less than an hour but are generally let stand over night.

Recently two articles in this journal[2] described other

[5] Fischer and Bromberg, *Ber.*, 30: 221, 1897.

[6] Waser and Gratsos, *Helv. Chim. Acta.*, 11: 944, 1928.

[7] Willstatter and Waldschmid-Leitz, *Ber.*, 54: 113, 1921; Waser and Gratsos, *Helv. Chim Acta.*, 6: 200, 1923.

[1] This may be obtained in small bottles from the Central Scientific Company, Chicago, Ill.

[2] E. E. Jacobs and Mary Auten, SCIENCE, 84: 210, 1936; I. P. Tolmachoff, SCIENCE, 84: 464, 1936.

methods of labeling specimens. The first requires the use of an electric stylus and transfer paper. The second employs the more usual materials of quick-drying enamel, turpentine and a fine brush. Although both are excellent methods the author considers the one herein described to have many additional merits to recommend it. The printing or typing of the symbols is done on paper under normal conditions of a typewriter or smooth table top; thus assuring that they will be well formed and legible. All printing or typing can be done at one time. The label and "varnish" are both easily and simply applied. The "varnish" does not smear the symbols. The "varnish" is acid, alkali, alcohol and waterproof, thus permanently preserving the surface of the label in addition to holding it to the specimen. The equipment and materials employed are simple, cheap and easily obtained. The surface of a specimen needs no previous preparation, such as filing a rough surface or etching glass, as the "varnish" will stick to anything.

This method has been in use in the author's laboratory for a number of years. The labels on specimens of fossils and rocks, some with rough and porous surfaces, in constant use in student exercises show no signs of damage after several years' handling.

VERNON E. SCHEID

UNIVERSITY OF IDAHO

## A SIMPLE DEMONSTRATION OF THE CONDITIONED RESPONSE

WHILE the technique of establishing a conditioned response is theoretically simple, laboratory manuals usually omit this important principle in their experiments on learning. The reason for the omission is probably to be found in the difficulty encountered in securing unequivocal results within a short space of time by means of equipment ordinarily available.

The writer has regularly employed the following procedure in demonstrating conditioning to groups of students. Because of the ease and speed of the technique, it has been a useful adjunct to lectures on learning. The necessary apparatus includes a golf ball, a screen, consisting of an 8- by 10-inch cardboard clamped to an 18-inch support, and a "clicker" (any device capable of making a sharp click). The subject seats himself by a table upon which he extends his right arm palm downward. The experimenter holds the golf ball in full view about 14 inches above the extended hand and instructs the subject to avoid inhibiting his natural response to the falling ball. Having dropped the ball several times, allowing the subject to withdraw his hand to avoid being hit, the experimenter next drops the ball from behind the screen which is fixed at about the same height. It is important to have the screen so adjusted that the subject has just time enough to respond to the sight of the falling ball. This is the response to be conditioned. The experimenter now makes several clicks from behind the screen as the subject's hand lies extended, and all may observe that the sound by itself elicits no visible withdrawing reaction. At this point the experimenter gives eight to twelve simultaneous presentations of the original and substitute stimuli. This is accomplished by holding the "clicker" in one hand and the ball in the other, both hands being behind the screen. The coordination may take a small amount of practice, but it is easily learned. The click alone is then capable of eliciting the withdrawing reaction. By repeatedly presenting the click without reinforcement from the falling ball, it is possible to demonstrate extinction. A few additional reinforcements can then re-establish the conditioning. Should the subject voluntarily inhibit the conditioned response, the fact may be revealed by dropping the ball without the accompaniment of the auditory stimulus. In this case the ball will strike the extended hand.

W. A. BOUSFIELD

CONNECTICUT STATE COLLEGE

## BOOKS RECEIVED

BENT, ARTHUR C. *Life Histories of North American Woodpeckers;* U. S. National Museum Bulletin 174. Pp. viii + 334. 39 plates. Smithsonian Institution, Washington. $0.50.

BON, FRED. *Ist Es Wahr Dass 2 × 2 = 4, Ist? Dritter Band, Von den Mathematischen Grundbegriffen.* Pp. 80; *Zweiter Band, Von den Kriterien der Wahrheit.* Pp. 83. The Author, Leipzig.

BOYD, WILLIAM C. *Blood Groups;* reprinted from *Tabulae Biologicae, Vol. XVII, Part 2.* Pp. 113–240. 13 figures, 4 plates. W. Junk, Den Haag, Holland.

GALÉ, JULIÁN A. *Catalogo Descriptivo de las Orquideas Cubanas; Boletin Técnico No. 60, Estacion Experimental Agronomica, Santiago de las Vegas, June, 1938.* Pp. 221. Secretaria de Agricultura, Cuba.

GREGORY, THOMAS C., Editor. *Uses and Applications of Chemicals and Related Materials.* Pp. vi + 665. Reinhold. $10.00.

HARTNACK, HUGO. *202 Common Household Pests of North America.* Pp. 319. 380 figures. Hartnack Publishing Co., Chicago. $3.75.

Imperial Bureau of Dairy Science. *Dairy Science Abstracts; Vol. 1, No. 1, May, 1939.* Pp. 113 + v. The Bureau, Shinfield, England. 25/– per volume of four numbers.

KLEITMAN, NATHANIEL. *Sleep and Wakefulness as Alternating Phases in the Cycle of Existence.* Pp. xii + 638. 33 figures. University of Chicago Press. $5.00.

LHERMITTE, JEAN. *L'Image de Notre Corps.* Pp. 254. Nouvelle Revue Critique, Paris.

LOBECK, A. K. *Geomorphology; an Introduction to the Study of Landscapes.* Pp. xii + 731. Illustrated. McGraw-Hill. $4.50.

*Rapports Generaux, Travaux de L'Association de Geodesie, Tome 14, 1938.* Illustrated. The Association, Paris.

*Report of the First Scientific Expedition to Manchoukuo under the Leadership of Shigeyasu Tokunaga, June–October, 1933; Section V, Division I, Parts V, VII, IX, XI, XIII, Insects of Jehol.* Illustrated. Waseda University, Tokyo.

STURTEVANT, A. H. and G. W. BEADLE. *An Introduction to Genetics.* Pp. 391. 126 figures, 3 plates. Saunders. $3.25.

# SCIENCE

VOL. 90 FRIDAY, JULY 28, 1939 No. 2326

*Dedication of the William Albert Noyes Laboratory of Chemistry at the University of Illinois:* PROFESSOR ROGER ADAMS; PROFESSOR WILLIAM A. NOYES ... 71
*Obituary:*
*Joseph Grinnell:* PROFESSOR WM. E. RITTER. *Recent Deaths and Memorials* ... 75
*Scientific Events:*
*Transfer of the Bureau of Fisheries; Reorganization of the Work in Zoology at Cornell University; Grants of the National Tuberculosis Association; Guggenheim Fellowships for Brazil, Canada, Peru and Uruguay; American Ornithologists' Union* ... 76
*Scientific Notes and News* ... 79
*Discussion:*
*Present-day Botany in Italy:* PROFESSOR FRANCIS RAMALEY. *The Production of Unfertilized Seeds in Trillium:* PROFESSOR EDWARD C. JEFFREY and EDWIN J. HAERTL. *The Role of Arrhenotoky in the Adaptation of Insects:* DR. STANLEY E. FLANDERS. *Mottled Enamel in Rat Molars:* DR. GERALD J. COX and OTHERS ... 81
*Quotations:*
*The British Association for the Advancement of Science* ... 83
*Scientific Books:*
*Popularization of Modern Science:* PROFESSOR CHAUNCEY D. LEAKE ... 84
*Reports:*
*Astronomical Symposium on Galactic and Extragalactic Structure:* PROFESSOR OTTO STRUVE ... 85
*Special Articles:*
*Linkage of Pea Comb and Blue Egg in the Fowl:* DR. J. H. BRUCKNER and PROFESSOR F. B. HUTT. *Role of Vitamin E in the Prevention of Muscular Dystrophy in Guinea Pigs:* NOBUKO SHIMOTORI, GLADYS A. EMERSON and DR. HERBERT M. EVANS. *A Quantitative Study of Meaning by a Conditioned Salivary Technique:* DR. G. H. S. RAZRAN. *The Gelatin of Brom Phenol Blue:* DR. EDWARD S. AMIS and PROFESSOR VICTOR K. LA MER ... 88
*Scientific Apparatus and Laboratory Methods:*
*A Practical Method of Obtaining Bacteria-free Cultures of Trichomonas hominis:* DR. WILLIAM S. STONE and MAJOR FRANÇOIS H. K. REYNOLDS. *The Use of the Horsley-Clarke Instrument on the Rat:* DR. GEORGE CLARK ... 91
*Science News* ... 6

SCIENCE: A Weekly Journal devoted to the Advancement of Science, edited by J. MCKEEN CATTELL and published every Friday by

THE SCIENCE PRESS
New York City: Grand Central Terminal
Lancaster, Pa. Garrison, N. Y.

Annual Subscription, $6.00 Single Copies, 15 Cts.

SCIENCE is the official organ of the American Association for the Advancement of Science. Information regarding membership in the Association may be secured from the office of the permanent secretary in the Smithsonian Institution Building, Washington, D. C.

## DEDICATION OF THE WILLIAM ALBERT NOYES LABORATORY OF CHEMISTRY AT THE UNIVERSITY OF ILLINOIS

By Professor ROGER ADAMS
HEAD OF THE DEPARTMENT OF CHEMISTRY, UNIVERSITY OF ILLINOIS

OUR meeting to-day is to honor Dr. William Albert Noyes, formerly head of this department. This is a rather unusual occasion; first, because there is probably a larger proportion of the graduate students and faculty in chemistry gathered here to-day in a group than at any time since I have been associated with the department, and second, because we are naming a building, one half of which is thirty-seven years old and the other half twenty-three years old.

The older members of the staff know Dr. Noyes and his accomplishments. The younger men who are so busily engaged in their studies toward advanced degrees know too little of him. I shall, therefore, outline briefly his career.

Dr. Noyes was born in Iowa and took his undergraduate degree at Grinnell College in 1879. He then went to Johns Hopkins for graduate work. In those days Johns Hopkins was the leading institution for graduate work in chemistry in the country. There he studied under Professor Remsen, whose name is known to all of you, and received the doctor's degree in 1882. His first scientific publication with Professor Remsen appeared that year.

Dr. Noyes served as instructor at the University of Minnesota in 1882–1883 and then accepted a professorship at the University of Tennessee, where he stayed until 1886. The probability is (though I do not have the facts) that at this institution he acted not only as professor of chemistry, but assistant in the laboratory, purchasing agent, janitor and possibly even stenographer as well. In 1887, he became professor at the Rose Polytechnic Institute, where he remained until

1903. The Rose Polytechnic Institute is considered a small school, but before 1900 it was relatively larger in comparison with the other technical schools of that day. During this period Dr. Noyes devoted his time to teaching and research, with facilities inadequate for either. He had a very heavy teaching schedule and in addition was required to do much of the laboratory assisting and other work of the chemistry department usually assigned to others. The necessity of doing all these things would discourage the average individual. Few men, under such circumstances, are able to get ahead and succeed.

During those seventeen years Dr. Noyes not only wrote two text-books but published regularly the results of his investigations in the field of organic, inorganic and analytical chemistry. Because of his accomplishments he became nationally recognized by all American chemists as an outstanding figure. As a consequence, in 1903 he was called to one of the choicest positions in the country as the first chief chemist of the Bureau of Standards, a position which offered opportunity and facilities for scientific research.

The University of Illinois was fortunate in its choice when, in 1907, Dr. Noyes was selected to head the department of chemistry. He continued in that capacity until 1926, when he became *emeritus*.

After this brief survey of the positions he has held I shall speak of some of his specific accomplishments. Dr. Noyes has written two texts and a laboratory manual in inorganic chemistry, a text-book in qualitative analysis, a text and a laboratory manual in organic chemistry. He has likewise completed significant investigations in the three fields of organic, inorganic and analytical chemistry. Few men have combined such a breadth of knowledge.

His researches include the determination of the atomic weight of oxygen, of hydrogen and of chlorine, the values for which were accepted by the Committee on Atomic Weights. The average of the hydrogen-oxygen ratio which he found is essentially the average of all the other values reported by other investigators. In analytical chemistry he developed methods for the determination of phosphorus, of sulfur and manganese in iron. His earlier researches in organic chemistry were on the oxidation of benzene derivatives with potassium ferricyanide and on the structure of camphor. Dr. Noyes was one of the first to recognize the significance of the electron theory and to apply it to ions. His interest in valence and polarity has continued ever since, and much of his research time in the last twenty-five years has been devoted to this field, in which he has made important contributions. Dr. Noyes's ability as a teacher is demonstrated by the prominent men of science trained under his tutelage.

He devoted much of his energy and ability to the American Chemical Society. Not only did he give unsparingly of his time to the formulation of the successful policies of the society, but he did more than any one else in developing the publications of the society. From 1903 to 1907 he was secretary of the society. He was editor of the *Journal of the American Chemical Society* from 1902 to 1917. Because of his successful editorship this journal became one of the leading chemical periodicals of the world. Dr. Noyes played a major role in the establishment of *Chemical Abstracts* and acted as its first editor. The groundwork which he laid resulted in the *Chemical Abstracts* as we know it to-day, the leading abstract journal of the world. His editorial ability led to his being chosen as the first editor of *Chemical Reviews*. Since 1919 he has been editor of *Scientific Monographs* of the American Chemical Society. It would be difficult to find another individual who has contributed as much to the success of the American Chemical Society.

The importance and significance of his accomplishments can best be recognized by the honors he has received from his scientific colleagues. He holds three honorary degrees; he has been the recipient of the Willard Gibbs Medal, the Nichols Medal and the Priestley Medal. This latter is given every three years by the American Chemical Society to a man who has contributed much to American chemistry. He is a member of the three leading honorary societies open to scientists, the American Academy of Arts and Sciences, the American Philosophical Society and the National Academy of Sciences. The American Chemical Society honored him by electing him to its presidency.

In addition to his teaching, editing and scientific work, he has been interested in many other things and has found time for extensive writing. His articles on international affairs, on economics, on peace and on religion are numerous. Many have been printed in foreign languages.

The facts I have given you are, for the most part, a matter of public record. His value to the chemistry department at the University of Illinois can only be known in full by his colleagues and students. He came here in 1907. In the period from 1890 to 1904 the man at the head of the chemistry department was Professor Arthur William Palmer, a scholar and scientist, who understood how chemistry should be taught and who was an investigator at heart. He was severely handicapped, however. With inadequate housing for chemistry and meager funds for supplies and equipment, he was unable to develop the department as he could have done with better support. He did, however, organize the department in such a way that the stage was set for expansion when the opportunity offered. Dr. Noyes, with his resourcefulness, energy, experience and judgment was able to start the department on a rapid and healthy growth. When he arrived in 1907 the senior staff numbered eleven and the graduate students seventeen. In 1926, when he became emeritus, there was some seven-fold increase in the number of graduate students and the staff had increased to twenty-five. The graduate assistants had trebled or quadrupled in number.

It is pertinent to point out to the younger members of our group the situation of chemistry in the universities from 1900 to 1922. Among university men chemistry was recognized as one of the basic sciences and its importance was not minimized, but in a state institution of the Middle West it is necessary also that it must be so recognized by the general public (and I include legislators as "general public"). In those days the layman looked upon a chemist as an analyst or a dispenser of drugs. Dr. Noyes, with his doggedness, persistence and insistence, was able to convince the administration of the university that it was essential to have increased funds to expand and build a strong department. He recognized also that he must have efficient staff members. Dr. Noyes found a capable group of men in the department when he came here. Among his colleagues were many whose names are familiar to all of you, such as Professor Edward Bartow, now head of the department of chemistry at the State University of Iowa, Dr. A. T. Lincoln, lately retired as head of the department of chemistry at Carleton College, and the late Professor Samuel Wilson Parr.

Dr. Noyes exercised infinite care in the selection of newcomers to his staff. He received the concerted opinion of many individuals before appointing a prospective instructor. He was able to get capable men, and if they left for better positions he sought just as carefully again to find progressive individuals interested in teaching and scholarly work. The administrative and teaching policies of the department were worked out with equal care. As a result, in 1926 when he retired he had a large department which was recognized nationally and internationally.

If I were to close my remarks here, I would omit an important factor in Dr. Noyes's success, his personal characteristics. He has always been absolutely fair; he instilled confidence into his staff members which resulted in a department cooperative and striving for its success. He showed kindliness toward every one, and never lacked time to help and advise a student or staff member.

In closing, let me say that it is a rare individual whom we are honoring to-day. On behalf of the chemistry department, the administration and the trustees of the University of Illinois, I take pleasure in dedicating this building as "The William Albert Noyes Laboratory of Chemistry." We are all happy in the realization that this name will be associated in perpetuity with the chemistry department of the University of Illinois.

## RESPONSE BY PROFESSOR NOYES

I THINK I need hardly say how greatly I appreciate the honor which has been bestowed upon me by the university, and especially I appreciate the honor coming from my colleagues of this department and of the university.

In speaking further I thought you might be interested to know something of the background from which I have grown (I suppose I am justified in saying "have grown") to the position which I have held here. I was a country boy born on a farm near Independence, Iowa. One of my early memories as a small boy was that my mother once had lighted a scrap of paper and put it into a wine glass and then clapped the palm of her hand over the glass and showed how, on account of the rarefied air, the glass was held by the pressure of the air to her hand. That was perhaps the earliest physics experiment that I noticed. After that, I became interested especially in physics and chemistry, though with some interest in other sciences as well. A short time after that when my older sisters were reciting their lessons in natural philosophy (we should call it elementary physics), I always stopped and listened, I was so much interested in what they were saying. Then in the years to follow, with the very few advantages I could find in a country farmhouse, with a few additions from the village drug-store, I began to try experiments in physics and chemistry. I read the scientific books not only in those subjects but in others which were available to me, so that I acquired quite a knowledge of these sciences very early in life. I made up my mind while still quite young to go to college, and I learned the elements of Latin from an older sister. Most of my preparation for college, with the exception of three months in Grinnell Academy, was acquired by personal study by myself without a tutor. I learned the Greek alphabet one day while I was cutting corn. I spent in this preparation and later in college four years in the study of Latin and Greek, for the classical course at Iowa College was very much the strongest and best course at that time. I have never regretted the time spent on those languages and the ability to speak which came in that way and in other ways in the years which followed. As I went on the members of the classical course took chemistry in the junior year. When the class went into the laboratory and lecture room of chemistry I went with them, but from that time on, for the last two years at Grinnell, I spent my afternoons in the chemical laboratory studying qualitative and quantitative analysis.

I paid my way through college by going out each winter to teach a district school for three or four months, keeping up my work in college by studying during the evenings so that I completed the work in Grinnell in four years. Not only that, but for the work in chemistry which I had done, with a little extra study I received at the end of the four years both the A.B. and the B.S. degrees. The following year I taught in the Academy of Iowa College thirty hours a week. In my spare time I did what I think is properly called "graduate work" in the laboratory. I did some more analytical work, but mostly work of a different type. In fact, when I went to Johns Hopkins in 1881 Professor Remsen looked over my notebook of analytical chemistry and said, "You do not need to study analytical chemistry here"; although the majority of the graduate students who went to Johns Hopkins at that time were required to take a course in analytical chemistry before they began their work for a degree. That work at Grinnell included, among other things, the determination of graphite and combined carbon in cast iron, using an old Liebig combustion furnace of sheet iron and heated with charcoal. I presume I am the only chemist living in America who ever used a furnace of that type.

The second year after graduation Professor Herrick, the head of the department, wished to go back to Yale for some graduate work and I was asked to take charge of the department of chemistry that fall, 1880, which I did, and went on doing some further chemical work in the direction of study myself.

I went to Johns Hopkins in January, 1881. After I had worked for nearly three months, Professor Remsen called me into the balance room one day and asked me if I would undertake a study of the Frankland method of water analysis for the National Board of Health, for we did at that time have a National Board of Health, although it disappeared long ago. This work was done not under Remsen but under Professor Mallet, of the University of Virginia, and through that summer I received from him three bottles daily containing water and other materials, but chiefly water, gathered over the country, especially where there was reason to suspect that the water had caused disease. I made analyses by carefully evaporating with the addition of sulfurous acid to expel carbon dioxide, evaporating to dryness in that way, scraping the residue from the dish, mixing it with copper oxide and burning it in a tube exhausted with a Sprengel pump of my own construction to get carbon dioxide and nitrogen from the residue. The carbon dioxide and nitrogen I measured in a small narrow tube which I had myself made at Grinnell, graduating it with a millimeter scale by the old Bunsen method and which served my purpose better than the Frankland apparatus which had been provided.

I can not dwell further on details. My training in mathematics at Grinnell had been rather deficient, and instead of taking the regular mathematical course in electrical measurements, I took work in experimental physics under the direction of Professor Rowland. Some of you know that he gave to the world the best determination of the mechanical equivalent of heat which had been made up to that time, and also invented, while I was at Johns Hopkins, the concave grating which has proved so useful in the determination of spectral lines. I took my degree in 1882, three years after I had taken my A.B. and B.S. degrees at Grinnell. You would not allow that sort of thing here, I know, after teaching thirty hours a week for a year in the Grinnell Academy and taking charge of the department for a term.

Professor Adams has spoken of my going to Minnesota as instructor. That was my title, but for two thirds of that year my time was spent in making analyses for the Minnesota Geological Survey and I gave only one short course in organic chemistry toward the close of the year. In September, 1883, I was notified by wire that I had been appointed professor of chemistry at the University of Tennessee, where I spent three years. I am always interested, as I look back, to remember that I was the only Northern man on the faculty, and many of my colleagues had been officers in the Confederate army. We got on beautifully together. In many of my classes I had young men with the initials J. D. (Jefferson Davis) or S. J. (Stonewall Jackson). Those were successful years, and I continued during that time the researches on the oxidation of benzene derivatives with potassium ferricyanide which I had begun at the University of Minnesota.

After that I went to the Rose Polytechnic Institute, where I continued for seventeen years. We had there a course in chemistry. I had to give the whole of it, not only general, but analytical and organic, for those who were going into chemistry, and afterwards, also, the thesis work in the last year of the course. I may say that the researches for at least three or four of the theses carried out by seniors under my direction at the Rose Polytechnic were among the important things which I have done in the way of research in chemistry. During those years I also became interested in the atomic weight of oxygen, as we called it in those days, and made a determination which convinced me that the value for the atomic weight was considerably below the 15.96 which was generally accepted at that time. Professor Morley completed his almost lifelong work on the study of the densities of the two gases, and after he had published his results I took occasion to go over my work and concluded that because I had applied a correction in what I was convinced was the wrong way, my results, if properly calculated, were the same, or very nearly the same, as Morley's. I said nothing about it except to friends, nor did I publish anything. I was waiting to do that until I could complete the work. I might add, the opportunity given by the facilities at the Bureau of Standards for doing this work was one reason for my going to Washington from the

Rose Polytechnic Institute. In the new determination my value or the mean of my value and Morley's was about one part in 5,000 different from either. I have just a little pride in the fact that the value which is now most generally accepted in the tables comes a little closer to my value than to that of Morley. His was a fine piece of work carefully done.

Then came the offer here. I first learned, through Professor Parr and Professor Bartow, that the University of Illinois was looking for a head of the chemistry department. They asked me at a meeting of the American Chemical Society in New Orleans to consult with them about a suitable candidate. I, of course, consented and talked with them for some little time. As I talked I saw the possibilities which lay before the head at Illinois and I finally asked if they would consider me. (I learned afterwards that they had undertaken the conversation with the intention of offering me the headship). Then President James asked me to come here and look over the field. I did so. One of the questions which President James asked me was, "Is it possible to build a strong graduate department of chemistry here in the Middle West?" I must admit that I was just a little in doubt, but I did think it was worth trying.

The work here has succeeded beyond my hope and expectation. I wish to repeat what has already been said with regard to the foundation laid here by Professor Arthur W. Palmer, that, to my mind, gives him perhaps more right than me to the honor of having the chemistry building bear his name. Not only that, I had two magnificent colleagues, Professor Parr and Professor Bartow, who stood by me through the years that followed (Professor Parr until the end of my term) and were always with me helping in the work of the department. In addition, the department was so well organized and we had such able men as the heads of the divisions that I could delegate to them a large part of the work being done. The growth of the department depends upon this cooperation between a group of men who worked together and succeeded.

Again, let me thank my colleagues and the board of trustees of the University of Illinois for the high honor which has been given me.

# OBITUARY

## JOSEPH GRINNELL

FORTUNATELY the editor of SCIENCE requests of me an "obituary notice" of Joseph Grinnell. This frees me from any attempt at a biography, even a sketchy one, of the man.

First, then, as to the great loss to family, friends, the University of California in general and its Museum of Vertebrate Zoology in particular, and to the realm of knowledge to which he devoted his life—the loss to all these is heavy indeed, the more because of its untimeliness. At the very climax of his usefulness general and scientific, one's first impulsion is toward the old fatuous query: "Why? But the second, more deliberate impulsion is toward consideration of the man—his personality and achievements—with little regard for the number of years involved.

Born (February 27, 1877) on the fringe of civilization, of parents both naturalists by innate qualities, what cultural influences would be likely to thwart his naturalistic tendencies?

The father, Dr. Fordyce Grinnell, was a government physician to the plains Indians at Fort Sill in the then Indian Territory. The family moved to Pasadena when the boy was seven years old. Here the home became famous as "The Bird's Retreat."

With maturing years in such a home, these following upon the first years as a frontiersboy with Indian children as playmates, little wonder what happened later.

Graduation from the Pasadena High School, A.B. from the Throop Polytechnic Institute (now the California Institute of Technology) and A.M. and Ph.D. from Stanford were unquestionably important happenings. But his "field work," covering so large a portion of Western North America, from far into Alaska to well into Lower California, judged by the time spent at it, by his publications and by the part it played in his classroom teaching and his guidance of graduate students would, I am sure, warrant a judgment about him similar to that passed by Darwin on what the voyage of the *Beagle* did for him: "The first real training or education of my mind."

Grinnell never sacrificed the scientific study of nature to popular or practical or literary interests. This is shown by the 550 or more published works, several of them sizable books sufficiently technical to satisfy any reasonable demand in this direction; and by the men and women who earned advanced degrees by more or less of their work with him and who now are widely scattered over North America in responsible positions of research, administration, teaching in institutions of learning or in government service. But not for a moment should his interest and efforts in general education and the great matter of conservation be forgotten. Some specific information about these interests are shown by his class work as a university teacher, his leadership in the Cooper Ornithological Club and his editorship of its journal, *The Condor*.

More specific information about his achievements comes from a look at the Museum of Vertebrate Zoology. A half hour's inspection of it by anybody at home in such a place is enough to bring expressions like: What an admirable example of an institution with a plan in process of execution! And the plan—what is it?

Though never coached or even authorized by Grinnell to answer the question, I venture an answer that I think would please him and I hope would be agreed to by all closely connected with the institution. The museum is an important adjunct to an endlessly intensive study of the land vertebrates of a limited geographic region designatable as the Western Slope of North America.

The function of the museum is to serve as a sort of post-mortem laboratory and conservatory for studying such aspects of the creatures as can not possibly be studied while they are alive. Grinnell always subordinated work indoors on dead animals to work out of doors on living ones.

Fortunate indeed for the scholar, no matter what his realm, of whom it may be so honestly said at the end of his life, as of Joseph Grinnell, Well done, good and faithful servant! Long and in manifold ways may your labors go on bearing fruit in their own right and by the labor of others.

Wm. E. Ritter

University of California
July 4, 1939.

## RECENT DEATHS AND MEMORIALS

Dr. Edmund Heller, the explorer, since 1935 director of the Fleishhacker Zoological Park in San Francisco, previously director of the Milwaukee Zoological Gardens, died on July 18. He was sixty-four years old.

Dr. John Mellanby, Waynflete professor of physiology at the University of Oxford, died on July 15 at the age of sixty-one years.

Dr. Heinrich Poll, for many years director of the Anatomical Institute in Hamburg, died on June 12 in Lund, Sweden.

Eight new dormitories, recently erected at the University of Wisconsin, have been named after former distinguished members of the faculty and scholars who have been connected with the university. These include: Chamberlin House, named after Thomas C. Chamberlin, who was president of the university from 1887 to 1892, when he became head of the department of geology in the then newly established University of Chicago; the Refectory has been named Van Hise Hall, after Dr. Charles R. Van Hise, a graduate of the university, from 1886 to 1903 professor in the department of geology and from 1903 until his death in 1918 president of the university.

# SCIENTIFIC EVENTS

## TRANSFER OF THE BUREAU OF FISHERIES

Effective as of July 1, the Bureau of Fisheries became a bureau in the Department of the Interior. For the present, its Washington offices will remain in the Department of Commerce Building.

Secretary Ickes has, for several years, advocated the benefits of grouping conservation activities in the Department of the Interior, and the shift of the Bureau of Fisheries in accordance with the President's reorganization plan fulfils that policy. The bulletin issued by the bureau points out that there is every reason to believe that the bureau will continue to grow and render greater service to the public and that there is no reason to believe that the change will in any way affect the status of employees of the bureau. It will involve changes in procedure to a limited extent, and copies of all regulations or administrative orders concerning employees will be brought to their attention from time to time as occasion requires.

The Bureau of Fisheries, originally an independent commission, was established pursuant to a joint resolution of Congress approved on February 9, 1871. Until July 1, 1903, it retained its independent status and was known as The United States Commission of Fish and Fisheries.

Upon organization of the Department of Commerce and Labor in 1903, it became a bureau in that department, and, in 1913, when separate Departments of Commerce and Labor were established, it became a bureau in the Department of Commerce. The transfer of the Bureau of Fisheries to the Department of the Interior marks an additional step in the evolution of the bureau.

## REORGANIZATION OF THE WORK IN ZOOLOGY AT CORNELL UNIVERSITY

A reorganization and expansion of the work in zoology at Cornell University became effective on July 1. The changes brought about have been contemplated for a number of years, but have been precipitated by the closing, on June 30, 1938, of the Ithaca Division of the Cornell University Medical College. Most of the former members of that division are included in the new department of zoology. As a result of various shifts of personnel and interests over the past three decades, the work in vertebrate zoology and ornithology had become attached to the department of entomology. These fields have now been transferred to the new department of zoology.

As a result of these changes, the staff of that department and their fields of specialization are as follows:

*General Zoology and Invertebrates:* Assistant Professor B. P. Young; Dr. W. E. Heming and Dr. Amy G. Mekeel, instructors.

*Histology and embryology:* Professor Emeritus S. H. Gage, Professors B. F. Kingsbury and H. B. Adelmann; M. N. Bates, instructor.

*Physiology:* Assistant Professor J. A. Dye.

*Biochemistry:* Professor J. B. Sumner and Dr. A. L. Dounce, instructor.

*Comparative neurology:* Professor J. W. Papez and W. A. Stotler, instructor.

*Vertebrate taxonomy, ecology and anatomy:* Professor A. H. Wright and Assistant Professors G. M. Sutton and Paul Kellogg and H. L. Kutz, instructor.

*Ornithology:* Professor A. A. Allen, Assistant Professors G. M. Sutton and Paul Kellogg, and H. L. Kutz, instructor.

*Animal Genetics:* Professor F. B. Hutt.

*Parasitology:* Professor R. Matheson.

*Limnology:* Associate Professor C. McC. Mottley.

The two men last named remain members of the department of entomology, but are also members of the department of zoology. Dr. L. A. Maynard, professor of animal nutrition, and Dr. H. H. Dukes, professor of veterinary physiology, are members of the department for three years, serving in an advisory capacity as liaison officers between the department and the Agricultural and Veterinary Colleges. Dr. F. B. Hutt, professor of animal genetics and head of the department of poultry husbandry, is chairman of the department of zoology for the year 1939–40.

The new department is supported by contributions of personnel, equipment and funds for maintenance from both the College of Arts and Sciences and the College of Agriculture. Its headquarters is in Stimson Hall, formerly occupied by the Ithaca Division of the Cornell Medical College, but some members of the department will retain their present quarters in McGraw Hall pending alterations necessary for their accommodation in Stimson Hall. The work in ornithology will remain in Fernow Hall, which in recent years has been specially equipped for studies in that field.

## GRANTS OF THE NATIONAL TUBERCULOSIS ASSOCIATION

THE National Tuberculosis Association has announced that the following grants for medical research from July 1, 1939, to June 30, 1940, have been renewed:

For chemistry of the tubercle bacillus, under the direction of Professor R. J. Anderson, of the Sterling Laboratory of Chemistry, Yale University.

For physiological study of the fractions of the tubercle bacillus, under the direction of Professor M. C. Winternitz and Robert M. Thomas, of the laboratory of pathology, Yale Medical School.

For chemistry of carbohydrates and antigenic properties of the fractions of the tubercle bacillus, under the direction of Professor Michael Heidelberger, of the department of practice of medicine, Columbia University.

For microbiology of the living tubercle bacillus, under the direction of Professor M. C. Kahn, Cornell University Medical School.

For relationship between diabetes and tuberculosis, under the direction of Dr. M. Maxim Steinbach, of the department of bacteriology of Columbia University.

For chemistry of tuberculin, under the direction of Dr. Florence B. Seibert, of the Henry Phipps Institute of the University of Pennsylvania.

For improvement of x-ray technique, under the direction of Professor Charles Weyl and S. Reid Warren, Jr., of the Moore School of Electrical Engineering of the University of Pennsylvania.

For clinical studies in association with tuberculin and x-ray researches, under the direction of Drs. Stiehm, McCarter and Lundegren, of the University of Wisconsin.

For a study of the lysis of the tubercle bacillus, under the direction of Dr. Charles Weiss, Mt. Zion Hospital, San Francisco.

New grants were announced:

For study of tubercle bacilli in animals by making them radioactive, under the direction of Drs. I. L. Chaikoff and J. Traum, of the University of California.

For study of intraperitoneal inoculations of tubercle bacilli in animals, under the direction of Dr. H. S. Willis and Dr. C. E. Woodruff, of the Wm. H. Maybury Sanatorium at Northville, Mich.

For a study of the relationship of tuberculosis and adrenal insufficiency, under the direction of Dr. George W. Thorn, Raybrook Sanatorium, New York.

## GUGGENHEIM FELLOWSHIPS FOR BRAZIL, CANADA, PERU AND URUGUAY

THE extension of the fellowships of the John Simon Guggenheim Memorial Foundation to four additional countries of the Western Hemisphere has been announced. Brazil, Peru and Uruguay are brought within the Latin American fellowship plan, and Canada is added as a separate unit. These extensions increase the number of countries in which the Guggenheim fellowships are granted to eight. The fellowships offered to Canada will also be available to the Crown Colony of Newfoundland. Puerto Rico also is included.

During the past ten years the foundation has granted eighty-seven fellowships in Argentina, Chile, Cuba, Mexico and Puerto Rico. These Latin American fellowships and the fellowships offered to Canada are all on approximately the same basis as those granted in the United States. Men and women, married and unmarried, of every race, color and creed are eligible on equal terms. The income of the foundation is devoted to its fellowships, which aim to provide opportunities for men and women of the highest ability to further their work in all fields of knowledge and all branches of the fine arts. Fellows are usually between the ages of twenty-five and forty years. They are appointed solely on the basis of the quality of their accomplishments, past and prospective, with no thought of distributing fellowships by fields of work, by colleges or universities, according to geographical considerations within the countries included in the plans of the foundation, or with regard to any factors extraneous to the question of quality. Thus, funds available for Latin American fellowships will be granted to the most highly qualified candidates regardless of the countries of their origin.

When former United States Senator and Mrs. Simon Guggenheim established the Latin American fellowships as a part of the activities of the John Simon Guggenheim Memorial Foundation, earlier set up in memory of a son and now endowed by them with more than $7,000,000, they said:

We regard it as necessary that the republics of America should draw nearer to each other in ascertaining for the common benefit what advances have been made by each nation in knowledge, including the solution of common problems, and in the understanding and appreciation of each other's deepest culture. It is our conviction that this may best be accomplished by aiding scholars and artists of proven abilities to carry on research and creative work in contact with the scholars and artists of other lands. Such aid should be afforded under the freest possible conditions to men and women devoted to science and liberal studies, great teachers, creators of beauty, and generally to those devoted to pursuits that dignify, ennoble and delight mankind.

It is with no nationalist or propagandist intent that we desire to make available such assistance. Men and women devoted to pushing forward the boundaries of knowledge and to the creation of beauty, reared with the impress of the same republican institutions and principles of progress, must of necessity approach nearer and nearer together in scientific and artistic respect for each other's attainments and culture. There is, moreover, a republic of learning and art which knows no boundary lines, and we desire only that scholars and artists from the American republics should meet and learn and teach what to them is Truth. For better understanding among the citizens of the American republics nothing is needed but more knowledge—a knowledge of the other's culture that yields nothing in zeal for one's own.

While, during the past ten years, the foundation has granted eighty-seven Latin American fellowships to assist research and creative work in the United States, an almost equal number of citizens of the United States have been granted fellowships for work in Latin America. This is in accordance with Senator and Mrs. Guggenheim's conviction in establishing the Latin American fellowships "that we have much to learn in those countries that are our elder sisters in the civilization of America and much to give their scholars and creative workers."

Under a clause authorizing the appointment of "permanent residents" of the United States twelve scholars of Canadian origin who are members of the faculties of American universities have already been the recipients of Guggenheim fellowships, and two fellows from the United States are now professors in Canadian universities.

The foundation awards an average of sixty fellowships annually in the United States and, in the same ratio of fellowships to the total population of the country, contemplates granting approximately six fellowships a year to Canadians. The stipends of the Canadian fellowships, as those for the United States, will normally be $2,500 a year.

## AMERICAN ORNITHOLOGISTS' UNION

THE fifty-seventh annual meeting of the American Ornithologists' Union was held at the Museum of Vertebrate Zoology, University of California at Berkeley, and at the California Academy of Sciences at San Francisco, Calif., from June 19 to 24, with a registered attendance of 248. Thirty scientific papers were read, many illustrated by color slides or films. The three days of sessions included a like number of evening entertainments, open house at the museum, the annual dinner and business meetings of various sections. On Friday, one hundred and eight ornithologists visited Point Reyes to study nesting colonies of aquatic birds on rocky islands along the Pacific Coast. On Saturday and Sunday, forty-two visitors traveled to Point Lobos and the Hastings Research Area.

Officers elected for the new year were as follows: *President,* Dr. James P. Chapin, New York City; *Vice-presidents,* George Willett, Los Angeles, and Dr. J. L. Peters, Cambridge, Mass.; *Secretary,* Dr. Lawrence E. Hicks, Columbus, Ohio; *Treasurer,* Rudyerd Boulton, Chicago; *Council,* P. A. Taverner, Ottawa; Ludlow Griscom, Cambridge, Mass., and Dr. Alden H. Miller, Berkeley, Calif.

The Brewster Medal Award was awarded posthumously to Dr. Witmer Stone for his two volumes on "The Birds of Old Cape May." Two fellows, Dr. Alden H. Miller, Berkeley, and George Willett, Los Angeles; one honorary fellow, Oskar Heinroth, Berlin, Germany, and two corresponding fellows, G. C. A. Junge, Leyden, and David Lack, London, were elected.

In addition to 532 new associate members, seven new members were named as follows: Paul Kellogg, Ithaca, N. Y.; Wesley F. Kubichek, Washington, D. C.; Joseph A. Hagar, Marshfield Hills, Mass.;

Emmet R. Blake, Chicago; Ivan R. Tomkins, Savannah, Ga.; Louis W. Campbell, Toledo; Owen J. Gromme, Milwaukee.

The meeting in 1940 will be held at Boston in October; the following meeting will be held in Denver. The 1942 meeting will be a joint meeting with the eleventh International Ornithological Congress in Philadelphia in May, 1942.

# SCIENTIFIC NOTES AND NEWS

A PORTRAIT of Dr. H. Gideon Wells, professor of pathology and director of the Otho S. A. Sprague Memorial Institute of the University of Chicago, has been presented to the university. The portrait, which was painted by Wayman Adams, was placed on public view on June 23, in the auditorium of the Pathology Building.

THE City of Ithaca has presented to Dr. Emile M. Chamot, professor emeritus of chemistry of Cornell University, an engrossed scroll expressing appreciation of his services to the city since 1905 as advisory chemist of the water department. He resigned on June 1.

AT the commencement exercises of Purdue University the degree of doctor of laws was conferred on Josiah K. Lilly, Indianapolis, chairman of the board of the Eli Lilly Company, a trustee of the university from 1927 to 1938. The doctorate of science was conferred on Dr. George N. Hoffer, of West Lafayette, director of the mid-west office of the American Potash Institute, and for many years a member of the teaching staff in the School of Science and of the research staff of the Agricultural Experiment Station, and on Dr. Rodney B. Harvey, professor of plant physiology at the University of Minnesota and head of the section of plant physiology at the Experiment Station.

THE South Dakota School of Mines at its commencement exercises on June 1 conferred the honorary degree of doctor of engineering on Dr. Harrison E. Howe, of Washington, D. C., editor of *Industrial and Engineering Chemistry*.

AT the graduation ceremony of the University of Aberdeen held on July 6, the honorary degree of doctor of laws was conferred on Dr. C. L. Burt, professor of psychology in the University of London, and on Dr. A. Low, from 1925 until 1938 professor of anatomy in the University of Aberdeen.

THE University of Oxford has conferred the honorary degree of doctor of science on Sir Edward Mellanby, secretary of the Medical Research Council.

It is reported in *Nature* that the following have been elected to the physical mathematical class of the Prussian Academy of Sciences: Professor A. Butenandt, director of the Kaiser-Wilhelm Institut für Biochemie in Berlin; Professor K. Meyer, director of the Institut für Ackerbau und Landbaupolitik, Berlin; Professor A. Ludin, professor of hydraulic and agricultural hydraulic engineering, Berlin; Dr. F. Seewald, director of the Deutsche Versuchsanstalt für Luftfahrt, Berlin, and Professor J. Bartels, professor of geophysics, Berlin.

DR. DONALD C. BALFOUR, of the Mayo Foundation, and Professor Peter Bull, of Oslo, were admitted as honorary fellows of the Royal College of Surgeons, England, at the quarterly meeting of the council on July 13.

DR. CARL CORI, professor of zoology at the German University at Prague, celebrated the fiftieth anniversary of his doctorate on July 7.

THE Goethe Medal for art and science has been conferred on Dr. Eugen Fischer, professor of anthropology at Berlin.

THE following members of the faculty of Cornell University have retired with the title of professor emeritus: Vladimir Karapetoff, electrical engineering; Heinrich Ries, geology; Albert E. Wells, mechanic arts, and Edward A. White, floriculture and ornamental horticulture.

DR. FRANK A. WAUGH, for thirty-seven years professor of landscape architecture and horticulture at the Massachusetts State College, retired with the title of emeritus at the end of the academic year. A dinner was recently given by his friends and former students at which it was announced that a fund had been established in his honor to provide financial aid for students in the department. Assistant Professor Raymond H. Otto has been made head of the department.

DR. RAYMOND B. ALLEN, since 1936 dean of the Wayne University College of Medicine, has been appointed executive dean of the Chicago colleges of the University of Illinois. He will coordinate the educational and research activities of the medical, dental and pharmacy units.

DR. HARVEY E. JORDAN, professor of histology and embryology and assistant dean of the department of medicine of the University of Virginia, has been appointed dean to succeed the late Dr. James Carroll Flippin.

HARRY J. REED, acting director of the Agricultural Experiment Station of Purdue University, a member of the staff for twenty-two years, has been appointed dean of the School of Agriculture and director of the Agricultural Experiment Station and of the Department of Agricultural Extension. He succeeds Director J. H. Skinner, who has been on leave for some months because of illness and who has retired.

DR. R. T. CRAWFORD, chairman of the astronomical department of the University of California at Berkeley, has been made director of the Students Observatory.

DR. JOSEPH HINSEY, professor of physiology and head of the department at the Cornell University Medical College, New York City, has been appointed professor of anatomy and head of the department of anatomy.

DR. EDMOND J. FARRIS, associate in anatomy in charge of operations at the Wistar Institute of Anatomy and Biology, Philadelphia, has been named executive director. He succeeds Dr. Milton Jay Greenman, who died on April 7, 1937.

MORRIS E. LEEDS, founder and president of the Leeds and Northrup Company, Philadelphia, known for his work in the development of electrical and heat measuring apparatus, has become chairman of the board of the company. He is succeeded in the presidency by C. S. Redding, vice-president in charge of engineering research. Mr. Leeds is president of the Board of Education of Philadelphia and of the Board of Managers of Haverford College.

PROFESSOR LELAND E. WEAVER, of the extension department of poultry husbandry at Cornell University, will spend next year at the University of Hawaii, in an exchange of professorships with Professor C. M. Bice.

DR. FRANKLIN S. HARRIS, president of Brigham Young University, has been given a leave of absence to accept a commission of the Government of Iran to reorganize its Department of Agriculture and to plan for the rehabilitation of the agriculture of the country. Prior to becoming president of Brigham Young University in 1921, Dr. Harris was director of the Utah Agricultural Experiment Station and was earlier professor of agronomy at the station. During his absence Dr. Christen Jensen, dean of the Graduate School, will serve as acting president of the university.

AMONG the investigators stationed this summer at the Scripps Institution of Oceanography at La Jolla, Calif., and the subjects on which they are working are: W. C. Jacobs, U. S. Weather Bureau, possible relations between slow changes in sea level and variations in meteorological conditions; Dr. F. P. Shepard, University of Illinois, and his assistant, Kenneth Emory, analyzing data on submarine geology and obtaining new facts; Dr. Victor Schechter, the College of the City of New York, marine biological problems; Dr. Roy W. Drier, Michigan College of Mining and Technology, the possibility of spectrographic analysis of bottom sediments; Dr. R. H. Tschudy and W. F. Whedon, studying for the United States Navy the organisms which cause fouling growth on ships' bottoms; Otis Barton, inventor of the bathysphere; Granville Ashcraft, University of Southern California, analysis of sea water; Dr. D. W. Johnson, Columbia University, study of old shore lines; H. B. Holmes, U. S. Bureau of Fisheries, temperature distribution in reservoirs and lakes, and E. Palmer, Federal Bureau of Fisheries, Stanford University.

DR. CARLOS E. CUMMINGS, director of the Buffalo Museum of Science, New York, who is chairman of a committee to make a special report to the Rockefeller Foundation on the scientific and educational exhibits of the world fairs in New York and California, recently visited San Francisco to make a survey of the Golden Gate Exposition. He was accompanied by Chauncey J. Hamlin, president of the Buffalo Society of Natural Sciences; Trevor Thomas, Liverpool, England; Dr. Hu, Shanghai, China; Francis Young, Boston, Mass.; Harry Geiger, Los Angeles, and Stanley Stubbs, New Mexico.

PROFESSOR ERNEST B. BABCOCK, of the College of Agriculture of the University of California, has been invited to serve as president of the section of genetics of the seventh International Botanical Congress.

DR. B. J. C. TE HENNEPE, bacteriologist of the State Serum Institute at Rotterdam, arrived in New York on July 21 as the head of a European delegation to the World Poultry Congress to be held in Cleveland, Ohio, from July 28 to August 7. The delegates were from Holland, Belgium and France.

SIR THOMAS LEWIS, physician to the University College Hospital, London, specialist in heart disease, has been appointed to the annual Edward K. Dunham Lectureship for the Promotion of the Medical Sciences in the Harvard Medical School for the coming academic year.

PROFESSOR J. BJERKNES, director of the Geophysical Institute, Bergen, Norway, will give a series of lectures and seminars on various phases of modern meteorology at the Meteorological Office, Toronto, from August 10 to 26. These lectures will be given daily, and all meteorologists are invited to attend and take part in the discussion. A number of rooms are available in one of the university residences at a nominal rate on application to J. Patterson, controller, Meteorological Service of Canada, 315 Bloor St., W., Toronto. These lectures are made possible by a grant from the University of Toronto.

APPLICATIONS must be on file with the United States Civil Service Commission at Washington, D. C., not later than August 14 for the positions of senior engineer with a salary of $4,600 a year; of engineer, with a salary of $3,800 a year; of associate engineer, with a salary of $3,200 a year, and of assistant engineer, with a salary of $2,600 a year. Vacancies in these positions in Washington, D. C., and in the field, and in positions requiring similar qualifications will be filled from these examinations, unless it is found in the interest of the service to fill any vacancy by reinstatement, transfer or promotion. The salaries given above are subject to a deduction of 3½ per cent. toward a retirement annuity.

THE National Research Council has continued for the fiscal year 1939–40 its subscription to a table in the Naples Zoological Station. Qualified investigators wishing to enjoy the facilities of the Naples Laboratory should make application to the office of the Division of Biology and Agriculture, National Research Council, 2101 Constitution Avenue, Washington, D. C.

# DISCUSSION

## PRESENT-DAY BOTANY IN ITALY

A MUCH-BELATED number of the *Nuovo Giornale Botanico Italiano* (Vol. 45, No. 1) celebrates the fiftieth anniversary jubilee meeting (1938) of the founding of the Italian Botanical Society and the two hundredth anniversary of the death of the distinguished Florentine botanist, Pier Antonio Micheli (1679–1737). Addresses by the president of the Botanical Society, Professor Napoleone Passerini, and by the secretary, Professor Alberto Chiarugi, describe the founding of the organization and its fifty years' accomplishments. The society now has 209 members, most of them in the neighborhood of Florence and Pisa and in northern Italy, but some in every province of the kingdom. The published "commemorative oration" by Professor Giovanni Negri is an appreciative twenty-five-page account of the life and work of Micheli, "father of mycology," author of "Nova Plantarum Genera."

The publication includes about thirty contributions in various fields, as: morphology, anatomy, physiology, mycology, ecology and geographical botany. Among the longer articles is one by Rodolfo P. Sermolli, describing and illustrating with three full-page plates some features of the vegetation in higher mountain districts of Italian East Africa. Adriano Fiori lists the plants of a number of the Italian Aegean Islands. Raffaele Ciferri gives an account of the rediscovery of *Emericella variecolor* (Eurotiaceae), a fungus on rotting olive fruit. Ciferri and Giglioli propose a "formula"—based on a definite schedule of description—for describing varieties and forms of wheat. Roberto Corti reports upon collections of plants from Cufra and other oases in southeast Libya and farther south in Tibesti.

This jubilee publication gives some idea of present-day botanical activity in Italy, although it must not be forgotten that there are other Italian botanical journals, besides special publications of some of the universities. The work of Italians in horticulture, agriculture and forestry is somewhat well known in the United States, but their botany has generally received less attention from Americans than it deserves.

FRANCIS RAMALEY
UNIVERSITY OF COLORADO

## THE PRODUCTION OF UNFERTILIZED SEEDS IN TRILLIUM

TRILLIUM has always been used as an admirable object for cytological investigations on account of the huge size of its chromosomes. This genus, which is found in North America and in Asia, presents cytological peculiarities in both continents. The descriptions of its meiotic divisions reveal extreme irregularities and a large amount of sterility. It has been supposed that these abnormalities were due to the intolerance on the part of the genus to cultivation. The present authors have satisfied themselves that this is not the cause of the irregularities, since they are present just as strikingly in material gathered from normal wild plants as in those under cultivation. As a result of the investigations of the processes leading to the formation of the embryo, in certain species of the genus it became clear that in contrast to the dandelions and hawkweeds (Hieracium) apomixis rather than parthenogenesis is present. The reduction division in the embryo sac mother cell is quite normal in contrast to the situation in the pollen mother cells, and five chromosomes are present. One of the derivatives of the mother cell survives, as is usually the case, and gives rise to an embryo sac. Ordinarily this contains only four nuclei, a situation paralleled by the Onagraceae and allied forms, as well as by certain orchids. Of the four nuclei one becomes the egg and another an abortive synergid. The remaining two nuclei fuse together and form the endosperm nucleus. The pollen tubes usually do not penetrate the ovary and in the rare cases that this happens, they do not effect fertilization. There is as a consequence no fecundation of either the egg or the endosperm as a result of fusions effected by nuclei from the pollen-tube. In spite of the absence of fertilization the egg develops into an abortive embryo in which the divisions show five chromosomes; in other words, the embryo is haploid. This embryo does not attain any considerable size and ultimately aborts. The endosperm, which is diploid as a result of its method of origin, forms in the usual manner and first contains a large central cavity around which are rapidly dividing cells. After the abortion of the haploid embryo and after the endosperm has reached considerable degree of development, a diploid embryo makes its appearance in the micropylar region of the endosperm and is continuous with the endosperm tissues. This is the embryo which perpetuates the plant. Frequently with the abortion of the haploid embryo the whole seed aborts. In other cases the seeds may reach a certain size without any embryos in them at all and in a number of instances what appear superficially to be seeds, even when relatively mature, do not contain an embryo. In certain cases all the seeds in an ovary may be in this condition. In all the mature seeds examined by the present writers in the following species of Trillium embryos produced from the endosperm were found to be present: *T. grandiflorum, T. erectum, T. undulatum* and *T. sessile.*

It would appear from the abnormal method of reproduction in Trillium that too great importance can not be attached to the reproductive chromosomes of the anthers and their behavior.

EDWARD C. JEFFREY
EDWIN J. HAERTL

HARVARD UNIVERSITY

## THE ROLE OF ARRHENOTOKY IN THE ADAPTATION OF INSECTS

THE sperms of Hymenoptera appear to be only female-producing. The lack of male-producing sperms is correlated with the production of males from unfertilized eggs, a form of parthenogenesis known as arrhenotoky. Since the production of females in arrhenotokous Hymenoptera only takes place after mating and since oviposition in many species occurs as readily before as after mating, a preponderance of males might be expected. Actually, however, arrhenotokous Hymenoptera as a rule produce more females than males.

This preponderance of females is possible because of the presence in insects of a mechanism for the storage and conservation of sperms. This mechanism consists of a spermatheca (sperm reservoir), the spermathecal gland, the sperm duct and associated nerves and muscles. The primary function of this mechanism is to discharge a limited number of activated sperms upon each egg as it passes down the oviduct. When a species produces males from unfertilized eggs this mechanism automatically becomes the means of controlling the proportion of the sexes. When it functions females are produced; when it fails to function males are produced.

The fact that, in the Hymenoptera in general, there is a preponderance of females shows that mating usually occurs before oviposition and that the spermatheca contains sufficient sperms to fertilize most of the eggs. Since male progeny also are produced by the female before its supply of sperms is exhausted, it is evident that some stimulus other than the mere passage of the egg through the oviduct is needed to cause the discharge of sperm in Hymenoptera. This operation appears to be dependent on two sets of reflexes: one involving the spermathecal gland (the stimuli originating externally); the other the spermathecal muscles (the stimuli originating internally with the movement of the eggs through the oviduct). The glandular reflex apparently serves to activate the stored sperms; the muscular reflex apparently synchronizes the discharge of sperms with the expulsion of the egg. Lack of fertilization results either from inadequate stimulation, an excessive rate of oviposition or lack of sperm.

Since in the Hymenoptera the activation of sperms is a result of environmental stimulation, it is evident that the environment controls the sex ratio in most species. As a result of such control extreme variability characterizes the sex ratio in this group of insects.

The fact that, in general, there exists a preponderance of females indicates a remarkable adaptation to environment.

In this connection it is interesting to note a phenomenon which occurs in a few species of Hymenoptera and is correlated with the preponderance of females. This is intra-specific hyperparasitism: a phenomenon also dependent on arrhenotoky. In this type of parasitism all the males, in most species, are the progeny of unmated females and in pure cultures are obligatory parasites of the immature stages of the female. The females are obligatory parasites of scale insects and mealy bugs. Male hyperparasitism, however, is not necessarily entirely intra-specific. In at least one species the male appears to be an obligatory inter-specific hyperparasite, rarely, if ever, parasitizing the immature female of its own species. Such a species would be unable to reproduce in pure cultures. The hyperparasitic males develop under diverse environmental conditions. In extreme cases the males develop only ectoparasitically in a dry environment, whereas the female develops endoparasitically in a fluid environment. The adults of both sexes frequent like environments.[1]

STANLEY E. FLANDERS

UNIVERSITY OF CALIFORNIA
CITRUS EXPERIMENT STATION,
RIVERSIDE

[1] *Ann. Ent. Soc. of Amer.*, 32: 11–26, 1939; *Univ. of Calif. Publ. in Ent.*, 6: 401–422, 1937.

### MOTTLED ENAMEL IN RAT MOLARS

IN an experiment planned to learn the conditions for producing mottled enamel in rat molars, we have fed members of unreduced litters of albino rats, born and suckled on a sucrose-casein type of ration, graded daily doses of fluorine as sodium fluoride by pipette. The amounts given were 0, 1, 2, 4, 8, 16, 32 . . . micrograms each, respectively, to as high as 256 micrograms to a single rat, the tenth in its litter. The rats were weaned at 21 days and fluoride feeding was discontinued. The animals were then placed on a ration of yellow corn meal 66, whole milk powder 30, alfalfa powder 3 and sodium chloride 1, for eight weeks and sacrificed.

The first and second molars of both the maxillae and mandible of the rat which had 256 micrograms of fluoride showed dull white, deeply corroded enamel. Particularly the cusps of the upper molars appeared denuded of enamel. The third molars appeared normal. Two rats which received 128 micrograms of fluorine daily showed a diffuse milkiness of the enamel at the gingival line of the first two molars and some rounding of cusp edges. Other rats, 34 in all, receiving less than 128 micrograms of fluorine, had apparently normal molars.

The high dosage of fluorine required to produce mottled molars is more evidence that the rat is less sensitive to fluorosis than man.

The successful production of mottled enamel in the permanent teeth of an animal in which dental caries can also be induced permits direct experimentation of the interrelations of these two diseases. It also provides a means of study of the time relations of the formation of normal and mottled enamels.

GERALD J. COX
MARGARET C. MATUSCHAK
SARA F. DIXON
W. E. WALKER
NUTRITION FELLOWSHIP OF
THE BUHL FOUNDATION,
MELLON INSTITUTE

## QUOTATIONS

### THE NEED FOR EXTENSION OF MEMBERSHIP OF THE BRITISH ASSOCIATION FOR THE ADVANCEMENT OF SCIENCE[1]

IN 1931, the centenary year of the British Association, the General Treasurer's Report stated that the activities and liabilities of the association had increased to such an extent that further endowment would be essential in order to consolidate the position which it had attained at the close of its first century.

During the past few years the British Association has not hesitated to extend in fresh directions its activities for the advancement of science.

A new Division for the Social and International Relations of Science was established in 1938. It is charged with coordinating work that deals with these relations both at home and abroad, and with carrying out inquiries and research; and it is empowered to hold meetings not only during the annual meeting of the association, but also independently. The division is in full activity: its organization necessarily involves expenditure; and the fields of inquiry already opened to view indicate that with more ample resources the association will be able to undertake, through the division, new work of national and international importance.

As from October, 1939, the association will cease to publish its report in an annual volume, which is felt to be no longer the most effective medium of publication. Instead, a quarterly periodical will be issued under the title of *The Advancement of Science*. It is confidently expected that this new quarterly will assure a more adequate record of the transactions of the association and engender a wider interest in them; but in order to give full effect to this expectation the association must be in a position to restrict itself less severely than hitherto in the matter of printing costs.

In 1937–38 the association broke new ground by sending a representative scientific delegation to India to join the Indian Science Congress Association in celebrating the jubilee of that body. The practice of organizing such delegations to overseas territories, especially those in which normal meetings of the association could not be expected to take place, is regarded as an imperial service of first importance, and one which the association is peculiarly qualified to render. Proposals for more than one such delegation overseas are under consideration now. But in order to further the extension of this principle, it is obviously desirable that the association should be able to bear out of its own funds a larger share of the cost of delegations than is possible at present.

A happy development of international contacts has recently been inaugurated by the establishing of more intimate relations between the British and the American Associations for the Advancement of Science. It has been agreed that in alternate years the British Association shall invite an American lecturer, and the American Association a British lecturer, to their respective annual meetings. Grants will be made to cover the expenses of the lecturers.

Increased financial resources are essential if the asso-

[1] An appeal signed by P. G. H. Boswell, General Treasurer of the Association, Burlington House, London.

ciation is to take fuller advantage of its opportunities in the directions indicated above, as well as in various other ways. For instance, the practice, adopted in recent years, of offering exhibitions to young students nominated by universities and colleges, enabling them to attend meetings of the association without cost to themselves, is obviously capable and worthy of extension. The presence of distinguished scientific visitors from overseas has always been encouraged at the annual meetings: in present world-conditions it is less easy than formerly for such persons to come at their own expense, and the association is without funds to assist them. The possession of Charles Darwin's house, Down House, in Kent, which is maintained as a national memorial open to the public, offers opportunities which could be realized if the association had means to supplement the endowment which accompanied Sir Buckston Browne's gift of this property.

These wider potentialities in the association's sphere of work have all emerged in recent years; but there must also be borne in mind the field of scientific research and inquiry in which the association has honorably labored almost since its foundation. The ability to make grants for research is of the essence of its being, and to maintain and strengthen this activity is one of the first tasks of every successive general treasurer.

At each of the last seven annual meetings (1932–38) the attendance of members has exceeded 2,000, the average number being 2,375. That average had not been attained in any similar period previously. Here, then, is evidence of growing interest in the work of the association. But of those who attend the annual meetings (apart from life members), only a small proportion—about one quarter—are regular annual subscribers. The remainder subscribe only for the year of any particular meeting which they attend. I need hardly emphasize the difficulties that arise in attempting to budget on a membership income which fluctuates annually as widely as that of the association. The financial position of the association will be greatly strengthened by a substantial increase in the numbers both of regular yearly subscribers and of life members; and this appeal is issued in the hope that such an increase may be achieved. It is addressed to all who appreciate the benefits which science confers, and would wish to aid the association in discharging its function of the advancement of science.

# SCIENTIFIC BOOKS

## POPULARIZATION OF MODERN SCIENCE

*The Wisdom of the Body*. By WALTER B. CANNON, George Higginson professor of physiology in the Harvard Medical School. Revised and enlarged edition. 333 pp., with 40 illustrations. W. W. Norton and Company, New York, 1939. $3.50.

*The Science of Health and Disease: A Text-book of Physiology and Hygiene*. By HOWARD W. HAGGARD, director of the laboratory of applied physiology of Yale University. Revised edition. xiii + 594 pp. with 10 plates and 89 figures and 16 tables. Harper and Brothers, New York, 1938.

*The Stuff We're Made of*. By W. O. KERMACK, research laboratory, Royal College of Physicians, Edinburgh, and P. EGGLETON, lecturer in biochemistry, The University, Edinburgh. viii + 342 pp. with 8 plates and 55 figures. Longmans, Green and Company, New York, 1938. $3.20.

*You're the Doctor*. By VICTOR HEISER. 300 pp. W. W. Norton and Company, New York, 1939. $2.50.

*Health, Hygiene and Hooey*. By W. W. BAUER. 322 pp. The Bobbs-Merrill Company, Indianapolis, 1938.

A CHARACTERISTIC feature of scientific endeavor during the past decade has been the earnest effort on the part of reputable scientists to popularize current scientific ideas and to promote public appreciation of how science may profitably be applied in everyone's daily life. Naturally this effort concentrates along biological lines with special attention to individual and public health. The publication of Paul de Kruif's "Microbe Hunters" in 1926 set an example which a host of followers have tried to imitate.

Some of the current efforts to popularize new scientific ideas are included in the books reviewed here. These range in style from the dignified and often technical presentation of Professor Cannon to the smart fast-moving wisecracks of Dr. Bauer.

Professor Cannon's volume brings up to date his 1932 exposition of the same title. It also adds a new chapter on the effects of age on homeostatic mechanisms. For the coordinated physiological processes which maintain the complex steady states in the organism peculiar to living beings, involving, as they may, all organs and parts working cooperatively, Professor Cannon suggests the special designation, *homeostasis*. He introduced this term in order to differentiate these steady physiological states, characteristic of living things, from the relatively simple physico-chemical states in closed systems where forces are balanced and where the constant condition may be termed equilibrium. In this volume Professor Cannon considers "first, what may be regarded as the fundamental condition of stability, then the various physiological arrangements which serve to restore the normal state when it has been disturbed, and finally, the narrowing limits of adaptation imposed by age." The book, of course, is a classic and is already one of the most influential in the development of fundamental theory of modern physiology. That its popular presentation is appreciated widely enough to require a revised second edition, is clear testimony to the skill and clarity with which Professor Cannon has developed his idea.

In his introduction to Professor Haggard's volume, Professor Yandell Henderson, brilliant and blunt as always, says it is designed "for employers and engineers in charge of labor," as "a text-book for college students," and that "every educated man should see it." It clearly and convincingly develops the thesis that modern medicine is almost entirely a matter of applied physiology. As a text-book, it could be considerably improved by the inclusion of references to significant articles or reviews. It might also be improved by some degree of personalization, that is, by indicating who some of the scientists have been who have contributed to the gathering of the information which Professor Haggard reports so impersonally.

Dr. Kermack and Dr. Eggleton's book is the first to make a consistent effort to interpret biochemistry to the public. It is admirably designed and clearly developed. These Edinburgh scientists begin by placing living things in proper proportion to the rest of the universe. They next discuss the limitations of the scientific method and go on to explain how the complex molecules of living things are built up from a relatively small variety of atomic bricks. The discussion of foodstuffs is from the standpoint of "the biological motor car." In connection with growth, repair, reproduction and special functional adaptations, the authors make illuminating observations on such matters as the economics of forced labor, the proper design of bicycles and Olympic champions. Vitamins, enzymes and hormones are entertainingly discussed. Even the no-man's-land where what is living is not to be clearly distinguished from what is not living, is bravely probed. It is in every way a beautiful work. It could, however, be improved by judicious bibliographical references to readily available original sources.

Dr. Heiser's program for personal health is a remarkable combination of clever organization, hard horse sense born of much wisdom and experience and entertaining personal anecdotes. As in the case of "An American Doctor's Odyssey," Dr. Heiser's "You're the Doctor" gives evidence of professional journalistic organization. These are some of the chapter titles: "The All-devouring Gut," "Brother Rat," "Diet and Health with Key to the Vitamins," "How Now, Brown Cow," "A Little Poison Now and Then," and "Wher'er I Roam." The general point of the whole volume is summarized in the last chapter, headed "A Merry Heart Doeth Good Like a Medicine."

Frankly journalistic is Dr. Bauer's "Health, Hygiene and Hooey." To those familiar with the medical quackery exposés in *Hygeia* and the *Journal of the American Medical Association,* Dr. Bauer's technique is well known. The information is essentially sound, and its presentation is entertaining. Dr. Bauer wisely remarks: "The best safeguard against exploitation is a knowledge of principles. Individual exploiters come and go; nostrums rise, flourish and vanish; quackery is different every day and yet, fundamentally, the same. A person who understands the characteristics of charlatanism will not be fooled by the individual exploiter. Therefore, I have not chosen to 'name names,' but rather to set up principles. . . ." Some of the chapter headings illustrate his method: "Wim, Wigor and Witamins (pinpricks in the vitamin inflation)"; "Soft Soap and Skin Games (facts and nowhere-near facts about the skin you love to retouch)"; "A Fake for Every Ache (common symptoms pay dividends to the quack and charlatan)"; "Life Begins Before Birth (we will grow old—why not gracefully?)"; "Common Sense, Preferred (how to be happy though healthy)." The book contains much factual information, but again fails to document more readily available sources.

Popularization of modern science may become a socially beneficial procedure. The success of the effort depends largely upon its sincerity. Journalistic tricks are justifiable if they stimulate attention, provoke entertainment and supply the essential information. Science popularizers should write simply without condescension and clearly, without emphasizing the obvious. When prepared by a master in his own right, as in the case of Professor Cannon, the result is likely to become not only a classic in science, but in general literature as well.

CHAUNCEY D. LEAKE

UNIVERSITY OF CALIFORNIA,
SAN FRANCISCO

# REPORTS

## ASTRONOMICAL SYMPOSIUM ON GALACTIC AND EXTRAGALACTIC STRUCTURE

IN connection with the dedication on May 5 of the W. J. McDonald Observatory of the University of Texas—a joint project of the University of Texas and the University of Chicago—an astronomical symposium was held at the observatory. The purpose of this symposium was to bring together the leading experts in the various fields of astronomy directly or indirectly working on the general problem of galactic and extragalactic structure, and to present, in the form of a series of connected lectures and discussions, a unified picture of the present views concerning the structure of the universe. The symposium was sponsored by the Warner and Swasey Company—the builders of the 82-inch McDonald telescope—and through the generosity of this famous firm many astronomers from this country and from abroad were invited to participate in the symposium. The general character of the symposium may well be described by quoting the words of one of the participants, Dr. J. H. Oort, of the University Observatory, Leiden, Holland:

> The question of the general dimensions of the galactic system, which preoccupied astronomers around the beginning of this century and which stimulated Kapteyn, in 1906, to develop the plan of selected areas, can no longer be considered as one of the burning problems of to-day. We might venture to say that another group of problems, *viz.*, those connected with the spiral structure of stellar systems, is now generally coming to the foreground. The great majority of, and possibly all, stellar systems of great flattening show such a structure, and it is natural to conclude that the galactic system would exhibit similar structure if looked at from a suitable position. This is evidently an important problem, as it may well be expected that the study of possible spiral structure in the galactic system may help to elucidate the character of spiral structure in general.

In order to elucidate the spiral structure of galaxies, we must systematize our knowledge of the various units of which these galaxies are composed: the stars, the cosmic dust clouds and the gaseous nebulae. In the discussions frequent reference was made, especially by Professor H. N. Russell, of Princeton, to the possibility that an additional unit may ultimately be found in the form of "chunks," ranging in size from meteoric particles to Jupiter, but there is as yet no direct observational evidence of such "chunks" outside the solar system.

In order to estimate the mass of our galaxy we must know the masses of the individual stars. Professor Russell's paper was devoted to the problem of determining the masses of the stars from observations of binary motion. While, in principle, the problem is simple, there are many serious difficulties in practice, and a large part of the discussion was devoted to the elimination of accidental and systematic errors in the parallaxes, etc. The data obtained by Professor Russell yield a new expression for the mass-luminosity relation (in solar units):

$$\text{Log L} = 3.82 \log \overline{\text{m}} - 0.24$$

Professor G. P. Kuiper, of the Yerkes Observatory, discussed a little-known group of stars which are somewhat less luminous than ordinary dwarfs, but which can not be identified with the true white dwarfs. For these stars Dr. Kuiper suggests the name of subdwarfs. Two dozen of these stars were discovered by him during the first six weeks of regular use of the 82-inch McDonald reflector. In addition, Dr. Kuiper announced the discovery of two new white dwarfs.

The problem of stellar colors and stellar spectra is of particular importance for the interpretation of the structure of our galaxy, because only after we have determined the colors and the spectra can we estimate the effect of the absorbing dark clouds in interstellar space upon the apparent distribution of the stars in the Milky Way. This problem was discussed by Mrs. Cecilia Payne Gaposchkin, of Harvard Observatory. Of particular importance is her discussion of the systematic errors of the Potsdam system of spectral classification and the conclusion that "the negative density gradients for blue stars that have been derived by others for the area in Carina (S.A. 193) are partly a result of the systematic errors of spectral classification."

A powerful new method for the determination of star colors was outlined by Dr. W. W. Morgan, of the Yerkes Observatory. When these colors are combined with spectroscopically determined luminosities they serve to give us reliable values of selective interstellar absorption. Several excessively red B stars were discovered in this work, and it was pointed out that an excessively red star may be either of type N or of type B—the latter, of course, being reddened by interstellar absorption.

The problem of space reddening was discussed by Professor Joel Stebbins, of the Washburn Observatory, University of Wisconsin, who, together with Drs. Huffer and Whitford, has determined photoelectric colors of 1,300 B-type stars. The main conclusions of the paper are: ". . . the dark clouds of interstellar material are located close to the main plane of the Milky Way; they are irregularly distributed and do not make up a thin uniform layer. The absorption of light is much greater for stars toward the center than toward the anticenter of the galaxy, and even the brightest parts of the Milky Way are only half as bright as they would be if we could see them in the clear."

The effects of interstellar reddening are so conspicuous and there are so many excessively red stars of early spectral type that it is difficult to understand how the effect could have remained controversial until less than ten years ago. The profound influence of our recognition of interstellar absorption upon theories of galactic structure is one of the most significant advances of recent years.

Professor Harlow Shapley, of the Harvard Observatory, discussed the importance of variable stars in the measurement of great distances. A large number of cluster-type Cepheids in high galactic latitudes has been used to determine the thickness of our galaxy and the law of galactic concentration for cluster-type Cepheids. Important applications of variable stars have also been made at Harvard to the determination of distances of external galaxies.

The problem of diffuse, reflecting matter in space was discussed by Dr. C. T. Elvey, of the McDonald Observatory. Elvey and Rudnick have discovered a new faint glow in the Milky Way which comes from star light that is reflected by large numbers of very small particles. The existence of this "galactic light" has recently been confirmed by Henyey and Greenstein at the Yerkes Observatory.

The composition of the interstellar gas was the topic of a paper by Dr. O. Struve, of the Yerkes and McDonald Observatories. The principal result is the very large abundance of hydrogen.

Dr. Bart J. Bok, of the Harvard Observatory, gave an account of important investigations which are now being carried on under his direction at Harvard. The work is based upon accurate star counts which are used to determine first the interstellar absorption and then the space distibution of the stars in our galaxy. The presence of considerable negative density gradients in stellar distribution was discovered for several Milky Way regions.

The importance of galactic clusters in problems of Milky Way structure was stressed in a paper by Dr. R. J. Trumpler, of the Lick Observatory of the University of California. "When the known galactic star clusters are projected on the galactic plane, their arrangement shows no relation to the generally accepted structure of the galactic system, but indicates a grouping with the sun near its center. . . . The possibility that star clusters are confined to outer regions of our stellar system and are missing in its central condensation is indicated by the examination of extragalactic nebulae. A large number of undiscovered distant clusters, however, should be expected in galactic longitudes 0°–70° and 220°–290°. In the former region the strong obscuration marking the dark division of the Milky Way is probably responsible for the scarcity of known clusters. It is suggested that the search for distant clusters should be made by photographs utilizing red light, as the latter has a greater penetration of absorbing (scattering) material."

Dr. J. H. Oort finds that the

> star densities indicate a curious distribution: a region of relatively small density near the sun is found to be surrounded in all longitudes by extensive regions where the density is two or more times higher; this is a large-scale structure, showing equally on both sides of the galactic plane. The plausible comparison with spiral structure presents, however, a difficulty in the unexpected increase of density found when proceeding from the sun in the two opposite longitudes perpendicular to the direction of the center. This warns us not to accept these results without reserve. The principal assumption involved could, however, be verified to some extent by the color-excesses. One of the most urgent needs appears to be the further study of color-excesses, also in low latitudes, so that the density distribution may also be determined in regions near the galactic plane. An essential but difficult point is the determination of the relation between color-excesses and total absorption.

An accurate photometric study of the extragalactic system IC 1613, a member of the local group of galaxies, was presented by Dr. Walter Baade, of the Mount Wilson Observatory. Astronomers will especially welcome the extension of the photographic scale to magnitude 21.0. This has enabled Dr. Baade to determine accurate light curves of 20 Cepheid variables with periods between 146 days and 3 days and to determine a new period-luminosity curve from his data.

Dr. Harlow Shapley spoke on the distribution of external galaxies made at the various stations of the Harvard Observatory. Attention was called to the uneven distribution of the external galaxies in different regions. The structural features of extragalactic nebulae were reviewed by Dr. Edwin Hubble, of the Mount Wilson Observatory. The photographs secured by him with the large reflectors at Mount Wilson suggest "the segregation of material already distributed through the nebulae rather than the ejection of material into previously unoccupied regions. The patterns appear to develop inside the central lenses or within the surrounding envelopes. In early barred spirals (SBa), however, incipient spiral structure is generally found at the rims of the central lenses or of the surrounding envelopes. The further development of spiral structures progresses smoothly, along several closely parallel lines, to the familiar late type patterns (Sc and SBc)."

The theoretical interpretation of spiral structure was the subject of a paper by Dr. Bertil Lindblad, of the Stockholm Observatory (Sweden).

> In the case of nebulae with thin spiral arms, as exemplified by the nebula M 81, the arms can be well represented by the asymptotic orbits extending from a spheroidal central mass. The tidal effects of ejected matter on the matter moving at the edge of the central system may lead to a successive dissection of the original central system and in favorable cases to a heavy spiral structure like that of M 51. From the point of view of this theory the abundance of spiral nebulae of a fairly uniform type concerning essential features like the form of the arms, the number of turns of the spiral whorls around the center, etc., seems possible to understand. The theory favors the opinion that the direction of rotation of the system agrees with the direction in which the

spiral arms wind around the center when followed outwards from the nucleus.

Dr. S. Chandrasekhar, of the Yerkes Observatory, presented a new theory of stellar motions which is applicable to various types of stellar systems, and which will doubtless revolutionize stellar dynamics.

Professor E. A. Milne, of the University of Oxford (England), gave a lecture on "Cosmological Theories," in which he begins,

> with a logical analysis of the large-scale universe of matter and motion as it appears to observation, avoiding any appeal to laws or concepts derived from smaller-scale phenomena. . . . Starting from the individual's awareness of the passage of time, it is possible to set up a system of congruent timekeeping in different places, to construct in turn a kinematics and a dynamics, hence to give a logical meaning to "uniform time," to give accounts of gravitation and electromagnetism, and finally to show how to identify the various logical constructs so encountered in the physically observed universe. . . . The stimulus for the development of this logical structure has arisen from the great American discoveries of the phenomena associated with the extragalactic nebulae. Such discoveries have justified us in formulating our deepest questionings, and have helped to separate questions which are genuine questions from those which have merely conventional answers.

OTTO STRUVE

YERKES OBSERVATORY,
WILLIAMS BAY, WISCONSIN

# SPECIAL ARTICLES

## LINKAGE OF PEA COMB AND BLUE EGG IN THE FOWL

RECENT studies in this laboratory show that the dominant gene causing blue shells on eggs of the domestic fowl is closely linked with that for pea comb. During the last two decades a number of fowls that lay blue eggs have been introduced into this country and to Europe from South America. These vary considerably in color of plumage and in structural characteristics. In most cases they resemble Dark Brown Leghorns in color but have pea combs. They are generally called "Araucanas" after that region in Chile in which they are most abundant.

Unlike the brown pigments of hens' eggs, which are applied on the surface only, the blue color is found all through the shell and is quite evident on the inside. When the blue is combined with varying shades of brown (as in egg-shells of Rhode Island Reds and other breeds) the result is a series of green and olive colors, varying with the intensity of the brown color. The ability to lay blue eggs results from a unifactorial dominant autosomal mutation.[1]

In February, 1938, the writers obtained a male Araucana descended from stock imported from South America and mated it with a number of females, including "testers" for two autosomal linkage groups. This male had a pea comb, and all but one of the females had single combs. Among 35 laying daughters from single-combed dams, the following combinations were found:

| | |
|---|---|
| *Parental combinations* | |
| Single comb, white egg: | 18 |
| Pea comb, blue egg: | 15 |
| *Cross-overs* | |
| Single comb, blue egg: | 0 |
| Pea comb, white egg: | 2 |
| | 35 |

Such a distribution could not occur by chance. The possibility that one gene is responsible for both type of comb and color of egg-shell seems very unlikely, because Brahmas, Sumatras and Cornish Indian Games, all pea-combed breeds, do not lay blue eggs. Evidently the Araucana male was heterozygous for pea comb and for blue egg, carried in the coupling phase. Since in 35 gametes only two cross-overs occurred, the amount of crossing over between the two genes is apparently not more than 6 per cent. Tests to measure this figure more exactly are in progress.

Hertwig[2] found 32.8 per cent. crossing over between pea comb and marbling (a pattern in the down of chicks) and 45.6 per cent. between marbling and naked neck. Confirmation of the latter association is desirable because of the long map distance involved. Though the gene for blue egg is now added to this group, its usefulness for further mapping of the chromosome is likely to be somewhat limited because it is manifested only in one sex and even there not until the birds lay. Moreover, its close linkage with pea comb would necessitate large numbers in any linkage test where these two genes were to be separated.

A tentative map[3] for chromosomes of the fowl, published in 1936, showed 18 genes in five linkage groups. Since then the "naked" gene has been added to the sex chromosome[4] and the addition of blue egg makes a total of 20 genes in the five groups. Some of these, as well as one or two other loose linkages that have been suggested, need further study.

J. H. BRUCKNER
F. B. HUTT

CORNELL UNIVERSITY

[1] R. C. Punnett, *Jour. Genet.*, 27: 465–470, 1933.

[2] P. Hertwig, *Verhandl. Deutschen Zoolog. Gesell.*, pp. 112–118, 1933.

[3] F. B. Hutt, *Neue Forschungen in Tierz. u. Abstammungslehre (Duerst Festschrift)*, Bern, pp. 105–112, 1936.

[4] F. B. Hutt and P. D. Sturkie, *Jour. Hered.*, 29: 370–379, 1938.

## ROLE OF VITAMIN E IN THE PREVENTION OF MUSCULAR DYSTROPHY IN GUINEA PIGS REARED ON SYNTHETIC RATIONS

MADSEN *et al.*[1] were the first to attain any notable success in inducing the guinea pig to eat synthetic rations. In the course of their experiments they observed the relatively early appearance of severe muscular dystrophy not unlike the lesions first extensively studied by Goettsch and Pappenheimer.[2]

When the cod liver oil was removed from the diet, being replaced by other substances which satisfied the A and D requirements, the dystrophies were not prevented but were very notably delayed. It was hence apparent that the dystrophies were not actually caused by the cod liver oil, although they were precipitated and exaggerated in some unknown way by it.

Some three years ago we began the study of the nutritional requirements of guinea pigs with synthetic rations. With a slight modification of the diet of Madsen *et al.*, we have had no difficulty in producing the early severe dystrophies of these observers. This animal material, with the particular diet employed—a diet in which the increased proportion of cod liver oil seems responsible for particularly early and severe dystrophy—appeared ideally adapted for experiments attempting evaluation of the possible role of vitamin E in the prevention of such dystrophies.

A year was spent demonstrating that the administration of 0.75 cc or even of 0.5 cc of wheat germ oil daily to guinea pigs on this diet prevented the development of dystrophies up to the 355th day of life, when the experiment was discontinued. The muscle creatine values in these animals were normal. The controls (without wheat germ oil) all developed typical early dystrophies and in each case were sacrificed when practically moribund at times varying from the end of the first to the end of the third month.

These encouraging results with wheat germ oil led us to a repetition of the experiment employing the pure substance, alpha tocopherol, instead of wheat germ oil. In the midst of this work, several important papers appeared, reporting the employment of alpha tocopherol. Barrie,[3] as well as Goettsch and Ritzman,[4] have shown that alpha tocopherol prevents the development of muscular dystrophy in suckling rats from mothers reared and held on low E—facts which we can confirm. Mackenzie and McCollum[5] have also reported that alpha tocopherol cures the dystrophy which develops in rabbits maintained on the Goettsch and Pappenheimer diet, supplemented with 10 per cent. ether extracted wheat germ.

Since Cummings and Mattill[6] have shown that oxidative reactions initiated by the auto-oxidation of cod liver oil are destructive to vitamin E, we fed the cod liver oil (1 cc per os) and alpha tocopherol (3 mg per os) on alternate days. These guinea pigs likewise remained free of evidence of muscular dystrophy and have now been sacrificed on the 200th day of life, showing normal values for muscle creatine.

It is therefore apparent that in another animal form and with a particular dietary regimen in which an early severe dystrophy of the striated musculature invariably appears, alpha tocopherol acts effectively to prevent the dystrophy.

NOBUKO SHIMOTORI
GLADYS A. EMERSON
HERBERT M. EVANS
UNIVERSITY OF CALIFORNIA, BERKELEY

[1] L. L. Madsen, C. M. McCay and L. A. Maynard, Cornell Univ. Agric. Exp. Sta. Memoir No. 178, 1935; L. L. Madsen, *Jour. Nutr.*, 11: 471, 1936.

[2] M. Goettsch and A. M. Pappenheimer, *Jour. Exp. Med.*, 24: 145, 1931.

[3] M. M. O. Barrie, *Nature*, 142: 799, 1938.

[4] M. Goettsch and J. Ritzman, *Jour. Nutr.*, 17: 371, 1939.

[5] C. G. Mackenzie and E. V. McCollum, SCIENCE, 89: 370, 1939.

[6] M. J. Cummings and H. A. Mattill, *Jour. Nutr.*, 3: 421, 1931.

## A QUANTITATIVE STUDY OF MEANING BY A CONDITIONED SALIVARY TECHNIQUE (SEMANTIC CONDITIONING)

IF a human subject has acquired a conditioned reaction to some specific verbal stimulus, let us say the sight of the word "cent," what will be the course of the generalization or the transfer of the conditioning to other words similar in meaning or in visual-auditory form? Will there be more transfer of conditioning to a word like "penny" than to a word like "scent" or will the reverse be true? A number of experimenters have established conditioned responses to verbal stimuli,[1] and most of them have noted transfer from conditioned sensory stimuli to their verbal correlates and *vice versa.*[2] But in no case was there any attempt to separate the semantic—or meaning-content—factor of the verbal conditioning from its mere visual-auditory form. It is clear, however, that such a separation lies well within the limits of the conditioning technique. By using, for instance, in the transfer tests one series

[1] O. P. Kapustnik, in "Fundamental Mechanisms of Conditioned Reflex Activity in Children" (edited by A. G. Ivanov-Smolensky), Moscow-Leningrad, 1930, 11–22 (Russian); N. N. Traugott, E. P. Smolenskaya, N. N. Traugott and V. K. Fadeyava, L. E. Khozak, T. V. Kovsharova, L. I. Kotliarevsky, in "Studying the Highest Forms of the Neurodynamics of Children" (edited by A. G. Ivanov-Smolensky), Moscow, 1934, 273–450 (Russian); C. V. Hudgins, *Jour. Gen. Psychol.*, 8: 3–52, 1933; G. H. S. Razran, *Arch. Psychol.*, 28: 1–124, 1935; R. Menzies, *Jour. Psychol.*, 4: 75–120, 1937; K. Diren, *Jour. Psychol.*, 3: 291–308.

[2] Kapustnik, Traugott, Smolenskaya, Traugott and Fadeyeva, Khozak, Kovsharova, Kotliarevsky, Diren and Razran, *loc. cit.*

of words that are similar to the conditioned word in meaning but differ from it in verbal form and another series that are similar in form but differ in meaning, the conditioning values of the two factors may be readily compared and the amount of pure semantic—or meaning—conditioning easily determined.

A preliminary study of this rather significant problem was thus undertaken by the writer with the aid of a list of homophones and synonyms and with the use of salivation as the conditioning technique. Four simple words—*style, urn, freeze* and *surf*—were flashed on a screen at random order before three subjects who were chewing gum, sucking at lollipops or eating small tea-sandwiches. The subjects' individual eating periods lasted three minutes, in the course of which each word-to-be-conditioned was flashed fifteen times, and altogether five eating periods were made in each experimental session. After each eating period came an eight-minute testing period, during which the subjects' salivations to the exposed words were determined. The determinations were made by means of the writer's "cotton" technique that consists in ascertaining increments in weights of dental cotton rolls inserted under the subjects' tongue for periods of one minute. (With the use of proper control and rotation this technique is highly satisfactory and reliable.) The subjects were not aware of the attempts to condition them and were told that the purpose of the experiment was "to study the effect of eye-fatigue upon digestion." They became conditioned rather quickly, after two or three eating periods, but the tests with the transfer words were begun only on the second experimental session. The transfer words were: *stile, fashion; earn, vase; frieze, chill; serf, wave.*

TABLE 1

CONDITIONED SALIVATIONS OF 3 ADULT HUMAN SUBJECTS TO 4 WORDS, THAT HAVE BEEN FLASHED ON A SCREEN WHILE THE SUBJECTS WERE EATING, AND TO 4 HOMOPHONES AND 4 SYNONYMS OF THESE WORDS*

| Words | Experimental session | | | | Mean |
|---|---|---|---|---|---|
| | 2 | 3 | 4 | 5 | |
| Style | 234mg. | 276 | 293 | 218 | 255 |
| Stile | 57% | 51% | 43% | 49% | 50% |
| Fashion | 64% | 76% | 66% | 69% | 69% |
| Urn | 186 | 199 | 234 | 223 | 211 |
| Earn | 41% | 34% | 26% | 34% | 34% |
| Vase | 50% | 54% | 48% | 44% | 49% |
| Freeze | 268 | 308 | 314 | 246 | 284 |
| Frieze | 38% | 32% | 45% | 46% | 40% |
| Chill | 43% | 56% | 68% | 72% | 60% |
| Surf | 190 | 230 | 240 | 310 | 243 |
| Serf | 24% | 20% | 18% | 28% | 23% |
| Wave | 46% | 52% | 68% | 58% | 56% |
| Mean for conditioned words | 220 | 253 | 270 | 249 | 249 |
| Mean for homophones | 40% | 34% | 33% | 39% | 37% |
| Mean for synonyms | 51% | 60% | 63% | 61% | 59% |

* Each entry is a mean of 9 determinations and represents milligrams of net conditioned salivation (minus control salivation) in one-minute periods (the entries for the homophones and synonyms are given in percentages of the main conditioned salivation).

The results are presented in Table 1. The entries in this table are means of nine determinations, three for each of the three subjects. The entries for the conditioned words, or the words that have actually been associated with the eating, are given in milligrams of net conditioned salivation (minus control salivation) per one-minute periods. The entries for the transfer words are in percentages of salivation of the conditioned words. As seen from the table, by far the greater portion of the transfer conditioning went to the synonyms rather than to the homophones. The average transfer to the former was 59 per cent. and to the latter only 37 per cent., quite a pronounced difference. Furthermore, there was also some evidence that, as the conditioning progressed, the homophones lost some of their transfer and the synonyms gained. Again, while the amount of transfer for different synonyms varied considerably, ranging from 43 per cent. for *freeze-chill* in the first experimental session to 76 per cent. for *style-fashion* in the second experimental session, still in no case was the transfer for any homophone greater than that for its corresponding synonym. Within the limits of the present study the conclusion seems thus to be warranted that verbal conditioning is primarily semantic.[3] A subject gets more conditioned to the meaning of a word than to its mere visual-auditory form (although this pure form conditioning is, as seen from the table, by no means negligible). At any rate, the experiment provides an objective method for an experimental attack of a problem that heretofore could be discussed only in the light of subjective introspection or, at best, in the light of gross clinical observation.[4]

G. H. S. RAZRAN

COLUMBIA UNIVERSITY

## THE GELATIN OF BROM PHENOL BLUE[1]

WHILE investigating the kinetics of the fading of brom phenol blue (tetrabromophenolsulfonphthalein) in dilute alkali, we[2] observed that the completely faded solution, on acidification, became progressively more viscous and in a few minutes set to a clear lemon-colored gel. Although gel formation is not an unusual phenomenon with high molecular weight solutes, the concentration sufficient to produce a stiff jelly is so low as to merit further study from those interested in the mechanism of gelation. Although only a few dyes of its series have been investigated, brom phenol blue appears to be unusual in forming a gel. Phenolphtha-

[3] The possibility that the conditioning to the synonym was only indirect, through first recalling the actual conditioned word, was ruled out by a "free association" test.

[4] Salivation is of course not the only suitable response for dealing with this problem. The galvanic skin response, the pupillary and wink reflexes and indeed any response that is readily conditioned and quantified should, as far as we know, be equally good.

[1] Contribution from the Chemistry Department, Columbia University.

[2] Amis and LaMer, *Jour. Am. Chem. Soc.*, 61: 905, 1939.

lein fades in alkali and can be regenerated by acidification but does not gel. The time of gelation after acidification is dependent upon the initial concentration of the dye (Table 1).

TABLE 1

| Molar concentration of dye | Gelation time |
|---|---|
| $1.0 \times 10^{-2}$ | 1 min. |
| $4 \times 10^{-3}$ | 35 min. |
| $1.7 \times 10^{-3}$ | only viscous liquid |

The fading process consists in a high dielectric solvent like water of the rate-determining addition of a univalent negative hydroxyl ion to the divalent negative ion of brom phenol blue forming a colorless carbinol. In solvents of dielectric constant less than 64.5, the kinetic process involves the univalent $(NaBr\phi B)^-$ ion. On acidification the colorless carbinol reacts with hydrogen ion forming the yellow acid form of brom phenol blue, since the addition of alkali sufficient to neutralize the acid added regenerates the characteristic blue color of the dye in intensity dependent upon the length of time lapsing after acidification. The kinetics of this process is being investigated.

It is suggested that the gel formation is dependent upon hydrogen bond formation. The gel gives evidence of being thixotropic. It is stable for only a few hours, after which time brown crystals, presumably the acid form of the dye, appear and grow steadily throughout the gel.

A solution $10^{-2}$ M in dye and 0.2 N in NaOH was not completely faded in 27 days. When heated to 60–70° for 20 minutes to hasten the fading we observed that the blue color of the original solution was regenerated. After 4 hours at room temperature the color faded, approximating that of the original on the 27th day. Gelation occurred both before and after heating.

EDWARD S. AMIS
VICTOR K. LAMER
COLUMBIA UNIVERSITY

# SCIENTIFIC APPARATUS AND LABORATORY METHODS

## A PRACTICAL METHOD OF OBTAINING BACTERIA-FREE CULTURES OF TRICHOMONAS HOMINIS

*Trichomonas hominis* has been isolated in bacteria-free culture by using the following procedure: 6 mm Pyrex tubing 8 inches in length is plugged with cotton in each end, wrapped in paper and then sterilized by dry heat. The paper is removed from the sterile tube and, using a micro-burner, a capillary tube 16 inches long is drawn from one end of the tube. The distal tip is then broken off with a sterile forceps (great care must be exercised throughout the remainder of the procedure not to contaminate the terminal 4 inches of the capillary until it has been sealed). The tube is grasped in one hand and the proximal portion of the capillary tube in the other hand; then, by working on the edge of a very low flame, a series of loops or traps 3 or 4 mm in height are made as shown in the illustration.

Using a rubber tube (portion of an 18-F catheter) attached to a 10-cc syringe, the butt end is slid on the cotton-plugged end of the tube. Suction is then applied and the tube filled to within one inch of the top with sterile liquid medium. (Ringer 1 part, horse serum 8 parts.) Great care must be taken to see that no air bubbles are introduced into the capillary portion of the tube. The distal end of the capillary is sealed in a flame so that very little if any air is trapped in that portion of the tube. For stability and protection the capillary end of the tube is now slipped into a clear Cellophane envelope and the envelope fixed to the tube by adhesive tape. The tube is then incubated in a vertical position in a special rack (using pinch clothes pins for holders), for 48 hours and then observed for sterility. If no turbidity develops, for practical purposes it can be considered sterile. The liquid suspension of protozoa and bacteria is then carefully inoculated by layering into the top of the tube. The inoculated tubes are kept vertical and incubated at 37° C. From time to time the migration of the protozoa can be observed under the microscope by mounting the microscope on a platform so that the stage can be held in a 45 to 90° angle to the horizontal plane and using a mechanical stage prepared as illustrated. Trichomonas migrate slowly, and it usually takes 48

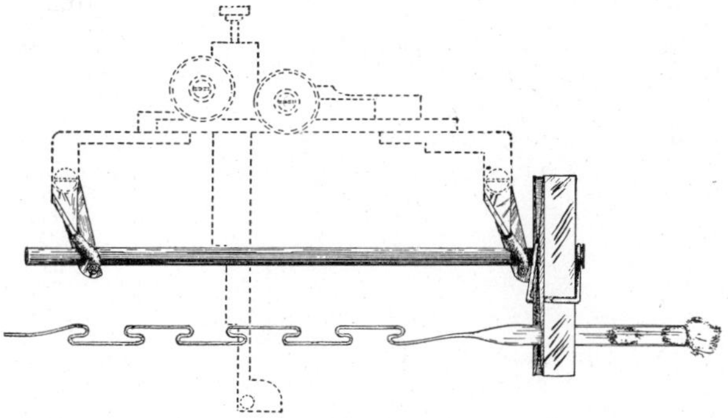

FIG. 1

hours or longer for the organisms to reach the bottom of the tube.

When the protozoa have reached the bottom of the tube the distal end of the capillary is cut off and sealed at the same time by applying a small flame to the area of the last trap. The severed sealed capillary is again observed for actively motile protozoa (usually many present) and is then submerged in tr. iodine (7 per cent.) for one hour. At the end of this time the capillary is removed from the iodine by using a sterile forceps. The last sealed end is then carefully grasped by the fingers and the capillary held in a vertical position. The iodine drains toward the fingers, and when the outside of the tube is dry, segments from the distal end of the tube are broken off, with a sterile mosquito forceps, into selected culture media. *Trichomonas hominis* has been repeatedly isolated bacteria-free by using this technique.

DISCUSSION

Our observations on the migration of motile protozoa seem to indicate that, with the exception of the free living phototactic organisms, their migration in liquid media is greatly influenced by the force of gravity. Very little progress is made against the force of gravity unless currents in the liquid support this movement. Currents in the liquid contents do not occur in capillary tubes, whose outside diameters do not exceed 0.8 mm. Migration of organisms in the liquid of the capillary apparently is influenced only by the motility of the organisms and the force of gravity, which result in gradual migration down the capillary. Motile bacterial organisms seem to be unable to make progress beyond the second trap and practically all of them are held back by the first trap.

The apparatus should be adaptable to the isolation of other actively motile flagellates and perhaps ciliates. However, we have not had the opportunity to test it using other organisms.

WM. S. STONE
FRANCOIS H. K. REYNOLDS
ARMY MEDICAL RESEARCH BOARD,
ANCON, CANAL ZONE

## THE USE OF THE HORSLEY-CLARKE INSTRUMENT ON THE RAT[1]

SINCE the reintroduction[2] of the Horsley-Clarke instrument[3] its use on the cat and monkey has become quite popular. A recent modification[4] has proved of considerable value. Lately it has been found possible to utilize the same instrument on albino rats by employing a few easily constructed special parts.

Ear plugs were dispensed with since the ear bars on the machine can be seated directly into the external auditory meatuses of the rat. Then, in order to center the animal, a c-shaped clamp is fastened to the ear bars. This makes it possible to loosen the screws holding the ear bars in position on the frame of the instrument and to move the animal back and forth, although the ear bars themselves remain rigidly seated in the rat's ears. A transverse bar and a light nose clamp were substituted for the usual mouth and eye clamps. After the ear bars are seated and the animal centered the nose-piece is adjusted so that the rat's long upper incisors rest just in front of the transverse bar. The nose clamp is then lowered. This centers and immobilizes the nose and holds the maxillae firmly against the transverse bar. No exact dimensions of these parts need be given, for they should be built so as to fit in the Horsley-Clarke machine with which they are to be used. Any machinist having the Horsley-Clarke instrument before him and with photographs of these parts which will be furnished on request should have no difficulty in making the special parts.

The operative procedures are quite simple. Under Evipal anesthesia (0.1 gm/kg. intraperitoneal) the hair is cut off the top of the head, the animal placed in the machine and an incision 1.5 to 2.0 cm long made through the skin in the midline. The electrode carrier is then set at the zero midsagittal plane and the electrode slowly lowered. If the tip of the electrode does not come to rest exactly upon the interparietal suture the animal is improperly placed in the machine and must be removed and replaced properly. The tip of the electrode is then raised and an opening in the skull made with the aid of a dental drill. Then the electrode is lowered to the desired point and the lesion made.

In working with rats it is very necessary that animals of uniform size and age be used. We have found it convenient to select animals weighing between 90 and 100 gms. If animals of more widely varying size are used little uniformity can be expected in the location of the lesions.

It would be desirable to produce chart sections of the rat's brain for the determination of coordinates of nuclei and fiber tracts, as has been done in the case of the cat and monkey. So far, however, such chart sections have not been made, since by the sacrifice of a few animals the location of any desired point in terms of the coordinates of the instrument can be determined by the method of trial and error.

GEORGE CLARK

[1] From the Institute of Neurology, Northwestern University Medical School.

[2] S. W. Ranson, *Psychiat. en neurol. bl.*, 38: 534, 1934.

[3] V. Horsley and R. H. Clarke, *Brain*, 31: 45, 1908.

[4] Frank Harrison, *Arch. Neurol. and Psychiat.*, 40: 563, 1938.

## BOOKS RECEIVED

BERRY, EDWARD W. *Contributions to the Paleobotany of Middle and South America; Johns Hopkins University Studies in Geology, No. 13; Edward B. Mathews, Editor.* Pp. 168. 3 figures. 23 plates. Johns Hopkins Press. $2.00.

GUTENBERG, BENO, Editor. *Internal Constitution of the Earth; Physics of the Earth—VII.* Pp. x+413. 27 figures. McGraw-Hill. $5.00.

*South African Journal of Science; Report of the South African Association for the Advancement of Science, Pietermaritzburg, Vol. XXXV, December, 1938.* Pp. xx+514. Illustrated. The Association, Johannesburg. 30 s. net.

# SCIENCE

Vol. 90 — Friday, August 4, 1939 — No. 2327

*Education by Authority or for Authority? Are Science Teachers Teaching Science?*: Professor Otis F. Curtis ... 93

*Scientific Events*:
*Future of the Science Museum, London; Expeditions of the Field Museum, Chicago; The Leverhulme Research Fellowships; The Seventeenth Chemical Exposition; Exhibition of the Amateur Astronomers Association of New York City; Recent Deaths and Memorials* ... 102

*Scientific Notes and News* ... 104

*Discussion*:
*Surface Currents in Deep Tidal Waters*: Professor David L. Webster. *Problems of Wound Healing in Red Clover Stems*: Dr. Robert W. Poulter. *Rooting Norway Spruce Cuttings without Chemical Treatment*: Professor Carl G. Deuber and John L. Farrar. *Physiology of the Nervous System*: Professor J. F. Fulton ... 107

*Scientific Books*:
*The Distribution of the Stars in Space*: Dr. Leo Goldberg. *Theoretic Mechanics Treated Vectorially*: Professor Albert A. Bennett ... 110

*Societies and Meetings*:
*The Alabama Academy of Science*: Professor Septima C. Smith ... 111

*Special Articles*:
*Isolation from Beef Pancreas of a Crystalline Protein Possessing Ribonuclease Activity*: Dr. M. Kunitz. *Isosterism in the Vitamin B Complex*: Dr. F. C. Schmelkes. *A Reversed Aldol Condensation*: Dr. Heinz Fraenkel-Conrat. *The Products of the Cyclizing Dehydration of 1-beta-phenylethylcyclohexanol-1 and the Synthesis of Spirocyclohexane-1,1-Indanone-3*: Meyer Levtiz, David Perlman and Professor Marston T. Bogert ... 112

*Scientific Apparatus and Laboratory Methods*:
*An X-Ray Densitometer for Measuring Relative Densities of Muscle, Bone and Other Tissues*: Hugh E. Webber. *Method of Embalming Large Insects*: Dr. Charles Clinton Smith ... 115

*Science News* ... 10

SCIENCE: A Weekly Journal devoted to the Advancement of Science, edited by J. McKeen Cattell and published every Friday by

THE SCIENCE PRESS
New York City: Grand Central Terminal
Lancaster, Pa. Garrison, N. Y.

Annual Subscription, $6.00 Single Copies, 15 Cts.

SCIENCE is the official organ of the American Association for the Advancement of Science. Information regarding membership in the Association may be secured from the office of the permanent secretary in the Smithsonian Institution Building, Washington, D. C.

# EDUCATION BY AUTHORITY OR FOR AUTHORITY? ARE SCIENCE TEACHERS TEACHING SCIENCE?[1]

By Professor OTIS F. CURTIS
CORNELL UNIVERSITY

I find it rather difficult to discuss the teaching of science as I wish to discuss it without first discussing some of the more general aspects of teaching and education. So perhaps by way of introduction we should first consider the question as to what constitutes an education and what are to be its aims. This may be a controversial topic, but it is necessary to formulate at least tentative objectives before one can effectively discuss attainment or methods.

With some of the many subjects taught in the elementary schools, as well as in the trade and technical schools, the answer as to purpose and accomplishment may seem relatively obvious. The pupil learns to read, to write and to do simple problems in arithmetic. He obtains information and rules that he uses in daily routine. But in increasingly large numbers, young people are taking high-school and college subjects for, as they say, their "general educational or cultural values," not fitting themselves specifically for a vocation or trade. But why should a high percentage of the population study higher mathematics, ancient languages, modern languages, English literature, history, economics, chemistry, physics, geology, botany, zoology, etc.? Are these subjects or fields of general educational or cultural value? If so, why? And are they of equal value? Is a man educated or cultured because he has spent one to four years in studying or can read or speak a half dozen or more languages? Is he educated because he can solve intricate problems in mathematics, or can determine the chemical composition of a rock or a plant, or can synthesize some important compound? Is he educated because he can

[1] Condensed from the address of the retiring president of the American Society of Plant Physiologists, at Richmond, Va., December 28, 1938.

accurately describe the structural minutiae of a cat or a corn plant?

To some people an individual is considered educated if he has had a certain amount of formal schooling in any subject. Each of us, however, can call to mind several individuals who have had extensive and intensive formal schooling, but whom we should not consider as soundly or broadly educated. Probably no one subject is peerless as a subject for educational purposes, because we can find no relation between the subject of one's specialty and what we might consider his standard of educational attainment.

I doubt if we can agree as to what subjects are best for a general education, or even as to what constitutes an education; unless we agree that mere attendance at school for a given number of years will insure an education. Nevertheless, let us try to formulate an objective which, although it may fall short of what one might wish to include, still is not beyond hope of attainment. I think we can agree that the training of a person, if he is to be considered broadly educated, should be such as to give him understanding of himself, of the world about him and of his relationship to that world. It should give a foundation for further advancement and an ability to appreciate values and distinguish between the true and the false. It should prepare him to live with satisfaction in the present world; to meet without panic and without prejudice various problems as they arise; and he should be able not only to grow with, but also to help in improving, a growing world and changing civilization.

Our present civilization has developed the extensive school system which to-day gives an opportunity for large numbers of individuals to take advantage of the knowledge and experience of their contemporaries as well as their predecessors. In this school system are offered courses over a wide range of subjects and at levels suited to almost any age and ability. In the secondary schools, colleges and universities there are made available to students a vast array of courses for giving special training in almost any field one could wish to study. It seems surprising, however, that, of the students from these schools, so many of them seem to lack just what one would expect educated people to possess. They have such strong prejudices, political prejudices, social, religious, class and racial prejudices. They are so easily influenced and controlled by slogans, by propaganda and by dogma. They are so lacking in critical judgment, in poise, and so little given to looking for, and critically evaluating the evidence on both sides of a question. In fact, it often seems that people who have had a formal education are likely to have stronger prejudices, are less eager or less willing to hear both sides of a question than are those with less schooling. They are often more smug, more self-satisfied and less reasonable. This may be due to the fact that their training has made them complacent by giving them a false confidence and over-assurance. It has failed to make them more cautious and more humble. In short, it has failed to give them understanding. That it has failed in giving understanding is indicated by evidence of many sorts. For example, large numbers of our people, although they have literally spent years in school and are also exposed on all sides to developments of astronomy and related sciences, and have thus had opportunities far beyond those available even to the most privileged of a few generations ago, yet they believe in astrology and are swayed by the most impossible beliefs and superstitions as regards the influence of the stars on their individual lives. It is a disgrace to our civilization that it has gone so far in science as to develop the radio, and yet one can hear over this same radio the drivel of so-called "professors of astrology" whose pronouncements are on a level of thought comparable to that of primitive peoples or those of ancient or medieval times who had no contact with scientific method or thought.

It seems strange that in this day and age states can pass laws against the study or teaching of evolution: that other states can pass laws dictating what can be presented in books on history (to say nothing of the complete control over all fields of teaching as is practiced in many foreign countries); that laws are passed prohibiting the discussion of communism in schools: that states with the richest and perhaps the best-developed school systems in the world can pass or nearly pass ridiculous and even vicious laws. In the past two decades legislatures have passed or nearly passed laws against sanitation, against vaccination and against scientific investigation with living organisms. In such states with these richly supported school systems there are strongly organized groups of Anti-vivisectionists, Anti-evolutionists, Theosophists, Faith Healers, New Thoughtists, etc. It is my impression, though I have seen no data, that a high proportion of the people that make up these groups are from the so-called "more educated" classes. There are some grains of truth in the propositions of most of these organizations, but their adherents go to the greatest extremes and appear entirely lacking in understanding and in common sense, in judgment and in ability to evaluate critically. They fail to distinguish truth from the partly true or the false, to recognize values; and yet these people, many of them, have had the opportunities of higher education, including college and graduate schooling.

Not many years ago a professor in a university of high standing, a professor in a science department, let his son die of appendicitis without even consulting a physician. He knew there was something wrong with his son, but he had become a Faith Healer. When asked by a doctor why he had not called in a physician when his child was in such a condition he replied, "Even you doctors sometimes lose your cases." There is no doubt but that one's mental attitude may have a great influence on his health, but one must use judgment as to when certain rules of procedure apply and when they are not adequate. This man's education, although it was in a so-called science subject, had not gone deep enough to enable him to recognize that one individual can not cure appendicitis in another by thinking high thoughts or by refusing to recognize acute and obvious signs of physical ill-health. It is true of course that many individuals imagine symptoms where none exist and may thus, through nervous control, actually bring on physical disturbances. But why go to such extremes? An educated person should be capable of using judgment and not merely blindly follow rules. Another professor with a national reputation in the field of economics, one who has had a fair amount of training in science, not long ago made the statement that "Vaccination and serum treatments are all bunkum." Within a few years I have received chain letters from two men, each holding the degree of doctor of philosophy. Each letter promised good luck if forwarded, and bad luck if the chain was allowed to be broken. The superstitious fears of these doctors of philosophy made them uneasy or perhaps even afraid to break the chain. No doubt each of you can think of comparable cases of individuals who have had extensive schooling but who seem to fail to show understanding or even "common sense." The medicine man, the believer in witchcraft and the voodoo priest are practicing right in our midst to-day, although they call themselves by more high-sounding names.

Is this failure of so-called educated people to come up to the standards we wish and have a right to expect, is this due to the weakness of the students themselves? Is it due to the failure to give training in the proper subjects? Is it due to incompetence of the teachers? Is it perhaps due to the fact that teachers may be placing the emphasis in the wrong place, that is, to wrong methods in teaching?

As for this matter of the method of teaching, a fact which has not been sufficiently recognized in some of our educational institutions is that there is often very little of the so-called transfer of training. That is, a very thorough training in one subject does not make one better able to judge in another, except in so far as the two have points in common, and it is often necessary that these points be very similar. I was talking with an Englishman who had just received his degree of doctor of philosophy in botany from a leading English university. His sister was going to India as a missionary. I asked him what her subject of specialization was and he said, "French; it makes no difference what subject she takes so long as she gets an education." But one may wonder what relation a training in French literature and language would have to missionary work in India. It is true that educators in recent years have been emphasizing this lack of transfer of training, but it seems that in many departments of education, instead of teaching a few basic courses in such a manner as to favor transfer, they merely multiply courses. By so doing they hope to give specific information on methods of teaching each and every subject a teacher may wish to teach. To obtain a teacher's certificate in some states it seems more important that the prospective teacher has a separate course in the method of teaching each subject to be taught than that he has thorough knowledge in the subject he proposes to teach.

To me this trend is entirely in the wrong direction. No schooling can ever hope to give the answers to all the problems that might arise, whether they be problems in teaching or in any other field. I am of the opinion that there is much more transfer of the right sort than is commonly recognized. I have reference to one's attitude or method of approach to a problem in hand; that is, approach with an open mind, without prejudice; an attempt to ascertain all possible facts bearing on the matter; a search for opposing evidence; a critical weighing of the evidence; a recognition of what constitutes evidence; a readiness to recognize possible complexities and contradictory evidence; and perhaps that all the evidence is not yet at hand. Such training in critical method may be given in many different subjects and fields. But much of the schooling even in colleges and universities is not of such a nature as to give this training.

Mathematics and ancient languages are often cited as "excellent for training the mind, tending to make one think clearly and accurately." It is true that to a certain extent mathematics does require a critical and analytical attitude, but its relation to everyday problems is often remote. In one sense mathematics may be too rigid and straightforward, too much given to rules and formulae, too exact for education towards a more satisfactory life, because the problems of living are not so definite as problems in mathematics. Mathematics starts with clearly verifiable assumptions or arbitrarily makes its own rules, and is therefore likely to lead to over-confidence when one comes to deal with subjects in which the premises themselves are questionable or indefinite.

This tendency toward over-confidence is often apparent in those who have had a formal schooling and introduces a serious problem in the field of teaching and education. The old saying "A little learning is a dangerous thing" has a real basis in fact. If one acquired a smattering of information, especially if the teacher presented it with great confidence and an air of authority, with no cautions or qualifications and with no indications as to degree of certainty or uncertainty, an individual is likely to act on it without real understanding; whereas one without this superficial training feels less confident and is likely to be more cautious in acting. When trained dogmatically to follow directions or apply rules without understanding the underlying principles, there is always a danger of misapplying them, as did the professor who thought he could cure appendicitis in his son by mental treatments.

It seems that much of the training in our grade schools and high schools and even in universities is of this authoritative or dogmatic type. The pupil is not trained to think for himself, for the major emphasis is placed on learning so-called facts. Day by day, more and more information is drilled into the minds of our students. They are led to accept some text or individual as authority and are not encouraged to form their own opinions or to use their own judgment. However, to accept blindly the opinions and statements of others, to accept authority, does not lead to understanding by the pupil. In fact, the teacher who teaches authoritatively teaches answers, and is not helping the student to learn for himself or to arrive at a real understanding. Such a teacher is likely himself to accept authority from others, and the matter he presents tends to become more and more unrelated to the truth and to lose real significance. Vitality leaves a subject when it is carried on by authority, no matter what the subject.

In the minds of many people "teaching" and the indoctrination of dogma are synonymous. At least this appears to be the interpretation of many legislators when they pass laws prohibiting the discussion by teachers of evolution or of cummunism; or of private citizens who write denunciatory letters to school superintendents or college presidents if they hear that some teacher has discussed socialism, communism or evolution. To them a teacher's only function is dogmatically to instill doctrines or "facts" into the minds of pupils; to tell them *what* to think, not *how* to think. I am not defending those teachers who are advocating the adoption of communism or any other "ism." These self-styled intelligentsia are often more dogmatic and more dangerous than the unthinking and dogmatic conservative. I say more dangerous because, with an abrupt adoption of untested schemes there is the likelihood of upsetting natural balances to which civilization has become gradually adjusted, and this sudden change may lead to entirely unsuspected and violent disturbances.

On the other hand, I am defending those teachers who are trying to encourage their pupils to think for themselves, to examine controversial topics in the hope that better understanding may lead to improvement. Although there may be marked disagreement concerning what constitutes improvement or just where changes should be made, few, if any, will maintain that no improvement of any sort is possible in political, scientific, social, religious or economic practices. It follows of necessity therefore, especially in a democracy, that the citizens should have training in evaluating the evidence that is offered in support of, or in opposition to, proposals of various sorts. If, however, teachers by choice or coercion merely pass on accepted information, education becomes static and there can be no progress; and yet many of our citizens, including also by far too many teachers, consider that the major function of an education consists in forcing the pupils to accumulate a mass of information, or in indoctrinating them with certain beliefs.

Advances in the various fields of the sciences during the past one hundred years or less have profoundly affected our physical well-being, and have also had a marked influence on thought not only in science but in the fields of philosophy, religion, economics and social relations. Because of a recognition of these great achievements in the fields of science, increasing attention has been given to the teaching of sciences in our schools. Usually, however, the main emphasis, and often the only emphasis in the teaching of science, is placed on the presentation of a formidable array of facts and information which the pupil is supposed to store in his memory. But is this memorization of facts the most important function of an education in science? If not, what should a student get from his course in science?

He certainly should get some idea as to the method and view-point of science. By method I do not mean the details of technique but the broader principles.

He should become acquainted with the methods of discovering facts, of obtaining evidence, and he should have experience in critically evaluating this evidence.

He should have some training in what constitutes evidence, and learn to distinguish between what is, on the one hand, mere assumption, dogma or opinion based on prejudice or on fragmentary evidence that is open to several alternative explanations, and, on the other hand, knowledge based on verifiable proof that is not open to alternative interpretations. To the man who bases his conclusions on dogma handed down from generation to generation, it may seem a new and revolutionary idea when he comes to realize that totally independent investigators can arrive at the same truth, even though they use different methods and start perhaps with different premises. The student should appreciate that something is true, not because some great individual said so, but the man discovered it because it is true. Neither apostolic succession, a controlled school system, nor an inspired press is necessary to carry on truth. On the contrary, these are likely to prevent progress, not promote it.

The student in science should learn to evaluate evidence and draw his own conclusions, and not merely accept an answer given by a book or a teacher. I am afraid we teachers too often discourage independent thinking. We expect correct answers or answers in the same words as we ourselves have formulated them, and pay too little attention to the type of reasoning which leads to the answer. Often a minor slip leads to an unsatisfactory answer when the main line of reasoning is the student's own and is perfectly sound. In attempting to get the answer satisfactory to the teacher, the student is often forced to learn by rote. He may then present a suitable answer but have no clear idea as to the underlying principles. I knew of a high-school teacher of geometry who forced her students to use the same lettering as the text in proving a theorem. If the letters were changed she could not prove it herself. She had learned by authority, had memorized the formula, and was passing it on verbatim. She did not herself understand the proof.

The student in science should learn to use the principles he has been studying in solving problems for himself. He should be encouraged to make frequent applications of these principles to every-day happenings. This will favor the transfer of training and make the training of greater value.

The student of science should appreciate the willingness and keen desire of the true scientist to reconsider his former conclusions; to look for evidence opposing his conclusions, not only for that supporting them, so that all weaknesses may be discovered and removed from the foundation of the structure he is building; to change his opinion if necessary; or to reserve his conclusion and suspend final judgment if the evidence seems inadequate or contradictory.

Is it not true that commonly the chief emphasis, if not the only emphasis in teaching science especially in the elementary courses, is devoted to the imparting of information, presenting the results of scientific investigations? Even in many of the more advanced courses and in the texts at all levels, the method of presentation in the text, the questions asked in the text and by the teachers deal largely with information and not interpretation. When interpretation is called for, the student is often asked merely to recall or recite the interpretation given in the text or by the teacher. It may be useful to know the answers to questions concerning simple definitions, the dates of specific happenings, the conclusions of specified individuals, the descriptive characteristics of various structures or substances, lists of the names of things, etc. A teacher can ask and correct answers to such questions without great mental exertion. Perhaps that is why so many teachers have settled into their little ruts and are satisfied with that type of testing and teaching. Answers to a high proportion of such questions usually merely involve memorization and recall. Some of the facts asked for may be useful or necessary, but many are of no real significance. It would seem better to set problems that involve an understanding of the principles and their applications, problems that involve a critical evaluation of the evidence bearing upon interpretations. To solve these problems they must not merely recall a few facts but must understand them and be able to use them in their thinking.

Instead of placing the major emphasis upon memorization of facts and information, therefore, would not our science teaching be much more meaningful if we emphasized these other phases that I have just mentioned? Do not the same points apply also, though perhaps with differing degrees of emphasis, in all teaching, whether it be science, history, literature, economics or religion?

As I have just said, one really interested in the truth should be constantly on the lookout for possible flaws in his conclusions or in the supporting evidence, and should actively search for possible opposing evidence to make sure that he has not overlooked something. Unfortunately most humans in their desire to prove themselves correct are prone to shut their eyes to opposing evidence or belittle it when it is brought to their attention. This undesirable trait finds many illustrations in most fields of education, and its fallacies and dangers should be stressed in our teaching. One might wish that this weakness would not appear in the field of science, but of course all scientists are human and show the same trait in varying degrees. It was not long ago that I learned of the following episode. One individual who was engaged in teaching and research in a given field of science had found several questionable statements in a publication of a second individual engaged in the same type of work. The first wrote to the other offering to send him a list of the points which he questioned. He was astonished to learn, however, that the writer of the article was not interested even in finding out what evidence or what interpretations were being questioned. How a scientist could be so sure of himself that he isn't interested in learning what mistakes another investigator working in the same field may think he has made, or what alternative interpretations he may have to offer, is beyond my comprehension.

One might think that the increased teaching of science subjects in our schools, and a recognition of the marvelous advances resulting from the use of the scientific method would have valuable educational effects, giving training in more independent and critical thinking and in avoiding superficiality, inexactness and sensationalism. But in much of our teaching, perhaps especially in our science subjects, the teacher or text supplies a systematic array of so-called "facts" which the pupil is supposed to store in his memory. We are trying to make walking encyclopedias, not intelligent beings. Where laboratories are used, the student is given a chance to familiarize himself more thoroughly with these facts, and to fix them more definitely in his mind. They also give experimental proof of the fact, which is certainly better than trusting entirely to teacher or text, but at the same time the experiment proves that the teacher and text are right. Usually the simpler and more dependable experiments are selected for the student to repeat. They are therefore almost certain to come out right. If not, the student becomes discouraged. The expected results, however, are usually obvious, so if the student does not get them he often "fakes" them. Have the experiments therefore been as valuable as we thought?

A university professor in a science subject not long ago told me that most of his laboratory experiments were "fool proof." He said, "They are bound to come out right even if the student is careless." His course is highly systematized; students are well satisfied; things behave as expected. A high-school science teacher told me recently that most of his demonstration experiments were "faked." I know of another university professor who doesn't hesitate to "fake" demonstrations at science meetings or to slip into the laboratory after the students have gone and add products to their experimental flasks to make the experiments come out "right." But does this give training in science? Will this training help the student when he meets everyday problems and must make his own decisions? Does not this lead to over-confidence, to a false confidence and eventually to disillusionment and bitterness? No wonder students after they leave school become discouraged when their theories do not work. No wonder children as well as older people, who have been trained by authority and dogma, in the home, in schools and in church, become so severely upset, or revolt against all their early training—the true and false alike—when some of the so-called facts, so dogmatically taught them, are eventually found to be false or based on no foundation of evidence. What training have they had in distinguishing the true from the false; in meeting and solving problems for themselves?

Personally I prefer to set up experiments that will not come out as the student expects, and I am occasionally pleased if they come out "wrong." If the student knows the answer, why do the experiment? If it comes out as he expected, what has he learned? It is true that he may remember the point more easily and if it is highly important—well and good. He may learn something also of the techniques of experimental science. If, on the other hand, the results are not those expected, he has something to explain. If his original idea was correct he may not learn much by proving it. If it was wrong he must modify his idea. More often the expectation was correct, but there was some slip in the manipulation, or some complicating factor that was overlooked. If he finds what it is, he has learned something. In attempting to square his results with his expectations he will learn something of science and scientific method. If the experiment is "fool proof" or the data are "faked" the student gains nothing and may lose much. Of course if too many experiments come out "wrong" a student is likely to get discouraged and blame the teacher, the equipment, his partner or the subject.

As our knowledge of facts and laws of science increases, I am afraid it is becoming increasingly true that so-called "science" is being taught more and more dogmatically. In physics, for example, or in chemistry or in biology, there are so many laws and facts that are known and well established that it requires most of the available time of a course to present a survey of these facts, and little or no time is left for considering seemingly contradictory evidence, that is, for training in scientific methods and attitudes. It is true that in these days the texts are being constantly revised so that the information is more nearly up to date than formerly. But many teachers using such texts complain because of the necessity of change. I know of one teacher in a field of science who prefers to use a text written in 1896 to those written more recently. It is easier of course to learn once for all time and not have to change. Perhaps such teachers would prefer to have their own subject as static as medicine was between the second and sixteenth centuries. Galen's writings on anatomy and medicine, which were written in the second century, were used as authoritative texts for one thousand four hundred years. Galen and his writings were used not as an example, not as a step toward a better understanding, but as a final authority; instead of a new beginning in medical advancement it was the end of advancement for 1,400 years. An inflexible text or creed or formulation of a principle or hypothesis, if fixed in its details so as not to allow for growth or change, although useful and an improvement at the time of its formulation is likely to interfere with progress. Vesalius about 1543 questioned some of the statements ascribed to Galen and began to investigate for himself. His teachings and his studies were considered sacrilegious, and he was persecuted for them and narrowly escaped death at the hands of the Inquisition. One of the students of Vesalius said that his teacher not only demonstrated new truths to him, but "so taught that the student could discover new truths for himself," could develop beyond what he was taught. *Is not that the test of sound teaching?*

When new interpretations or conclusions are presented in our revised texts or revised lectures are the old ones displaced and the new merely substituted for the old? Would it not be much better occasionally to present some of the old conclusions with the supporting evidence, then give the new evidence showing why it was necessary to change our conclusions? Some students, however, resent having to decide for themselves, perhaps because from childhood they have been told what to believe.

I was developing contradictory evidence of this sort one time when a student, who was carefully taking notes, slammed his notebook with disgust, saying, "You tell us one theory and then contradict it." Another time I was giving contradictory evidence and pointed out how I was not sure myself which interpretation was correct. A student asked, "Why bother about these things when you do not know yourself?" "Why bother about outworn, discarded theories?" "Give us the things you do know about and let the rest go." Give answers; give the "latest dope." I pointed out, of course, that some texts and some teachers do give one side only as the truth, others the opposite side, and I hoped that, by considering both sides they would have a better understanding of the real truth. I well remember the case of a student who dropped a course in plant taxonomy because the professor said he could not tell for certain to which of two species a given plant belonged. It was intermediate and had characteristics of both species. This student "refused to study under a professor who did not know his subject." I have also heard of another professor in the same field of botany, a member of an organization in which much of the teaching is by authority. This professor, when he found such intermediate plants that could not be definitely classified, destroyed the plants, remarking that "they were the product of the devil."

To present only clearly established information, leaving out all the uncertainties, gives the students an entirely wrong view-point. It is not training him in science nor does it give him understanding. A professor in a department of horticulture at a well-known college of agriculture was greatly liked by his students. He was clear-cut and definite in his teachings, telling the students just what to do. Several years later some of his students reported that this course, which as students they had thought the "best" in their university course, was really the "worst." The rules did not work and they had no training in meeting problems. I think it was Mark Twain who said that after a long life full of many experiences he had found that it wasn't the things that he did not know that gave him most trouble, but the things he knew that weren't so.

Another case that came to my attention was that of a girl who had taken courses in a department of home economics where the latest findings were presented, but with no training in evaluating the evidence. When she returned to the university two or three years after graduating, she attended a lecture in which the conclusions were in direct contradiction to those of her previous training. She had been taught facts and conclusions and had not been trained to draw conclusions from evidence. She was greatly disturbed and at a loss to decide what to do. With such methods of teaching information only, one would need to return to school every few years to keep up with the information. Perhaps our college degrees should be labelled "good for five years only." Why not teach in such a way that the student can carry on, as did Vesalius and some, but too few, of our teachers to-day? Not long ago there was an article by Christian Gauss[2] which bore the title, "Why Don't College Graduates Stay Educated?" In my opinion the answer is that we have not really been educating them. We have been merely giving them conclusions, answers to specific questions, and have not been training them in evaluating evidence, in the methods of solving problems for themselves, in methods of continuing education.

I was speaking along this line before a small group a few years ago when one of the professors (one whom I admire and one who is, I think, a stimulating teacher for advanced students) remarked that, contrary to his usual custom, he was that year using a text. The text made statements which he knew were wrong. He hated to let them go unchallenged, but since he was teaching from the text he said nothing. But of what value is the teacher if he merely drills his pupils on information, false and true alike, which is already available in the text? This same professor said, "Surely you do not bring contradictory evidence into an elementary course?" I replied, "Of course, I welcome an opportunity to bring controversial material into an elementary course, especially if it is of such a nature that the student can easily appreciate the evidence." Then the student can get some feeling for the method of science, a truer idea of the real state of things, a truer understanding. If one attempts to present controversial material in an elementary course or text it is likely to make the course too long or the text too bulky, or it may necessitate the omission of important material. But, on the other hand, I sometimes wonder if we don't try to make our courses too complete and thereby lose depth. By depth I do not refer to more detail. Detail is often unnecessary padding.

If time is limited, why not leave out of the lectures or discussions much of the well-known material? Of course the student must have some basic information, but that is available in the text or reference books and original articles. What he needs from his teacher is

[2] *Saturday Evening Post,* 208: 26, December 7, 1938.

not more information, but where to find it when he needs it; and still more how to evaluate it, and how to use it. In some elementary courses it may be better to use the historical approach and show how at one time the available evidence supported a given conclusion, but how new evidence has led to the necessity of change. Then by definite comparison one can show how some of our present-day conclusions may need revision in the light of new evidence not now apparent. With many of our students, most of them in fact in colleges of arts and sciences, an elementary course or two is all they will ever get in science, so if they do not get a truer picture in this elementary course, where will they get it?

That many college-trained people have little or no appreciation of scientific principles is indicated by the frequent appearance in current monthly and weekly magazines and newspapers of supposedly serious articles purporting to deal with science, and yet the writers demonstrate abysmal ignorance of some of the most elementary scientific principles. This is partly due, I think, to poor teaching in our elementary science courses, especially that in the biological sciences, and in part to the fact that only a small proportion of the students who receive the A.B. degree from colleges of arts and sciences have had more than one or two freshman courses in some science. From a preliminary study that I have been making, it appears that a large number of those students taking their major work in English, foreign languages, history, philosophy and such have had less than 6 per cent. of their college work in the sciences, including both biological and physical sciences, while about 50 per cent. of these students have had no biological science whatever. Yet it is from this group that a large proportion of secondary school teachers, writers and journalists probably come. These writers and teachers perhaps shudder at mistakes in spelling or grammar, and we all enjoy the "howlers" in student papers in history, geography and such; but too few have had adequate training in the sciences to recognize the frequency of the ludicrous mistakes in these fields as they appear in writings in supposedly reputable magazines and newspapers. There is little difference between many college graduates and those who have not gone beyond the eighth grade in so far as their mental attitudes or judgments in the fields of science are concerned. Recent articles like "Chemistry Wrecks the Farm," "The Chemist Conquers Agriculture," "Civilization Faces a Joke," and a host of similar supposedly serious articles, merely demonstrate the vast ignorance of the field of biology of many writers, journalists and editors. Newspaper editors would hardly dream of sending a reporter who had never seen a football game to write up such a game for his paper, yet they expect reporters who have had no training whatever in science to write on the work of scientists.

It seems to be assumed by many writers and editors that the only things that will interest the general public in science is the spectacular, the miraculous, the colossal or the seemingly impossible at last come true. Of course it is more difficult to make clear and interesting the more critical aspects of science and the scientific method, but opportunities for doing so are not utilized. That many people are interested in following the development of seemingly contradictory evidence and the unfolding of hidden clues is indicated by the wide-spread interest in detective stories. One wonders whether a similar interest in science might not be awakened.

The public is becoming so accustomed to startling and even revolutionary discoveries in the fields of science, to such sudden apparent shifts in conclusions, that there seems to be developing a rather dangerous attitude among certain people. It is true that some individuals are over-conservative, over-prone to decide once for all on a subject and never reopen it for new light. But others go to the opposite extreme, become so accustomed to change that they have no convictions, no basic theories of life; are so afraid of being considered behind the times that they go to the other extreme and blindly follow every new fad. This "open-mindedness," as they perhaps call it, might better be described as "empty-mindedness." Our public school system ought to combat this tendency and not foster it. The sophisticated and disillusioned youth who has no convictions and becomes skeptical of all things may have been forced into such an attitude because he has been dogmatically taught one contradiction after another, and has been given no solid foundation training for forming his own judgments. But here again, is it not the emphasis on the findings of scientific investigations, findings that have led to frequent changes in practices, which have given the appearance of insecurity? Is it not the failure to emphasize the method and attitude of science that is at fault? The emphasis has been put in the wrong place, on the seemingly miraculous result rather than on the rigorous discipline that led to the new discovery. Truth and the underlying methods of discovering truth do not change.

The public has become so accustomed to the seemingly miraculous accomplishments in the fields of science that instead of using the scientific method and examining evidence critically, building on a solid foundation, many people merely become more gullible and accept any claim, no matter how fantastic. You will all recall the recent excitement over the supposed invasion from Mars. The astonishing developments in the field of the radio seem on the surface highly miraculous and, to many who have no understanding of the underlying physical principles, it seems but a simple step to telepathy, and from that to communication with the spirits of the dead. I have heard college-trained people cite the radio as proof for spiritism. It may be amusing at times to let one's imagination run riot, and sometimes giving free rein to unchecked imagination, fanciful thinking or appeal to superstition may have no dangerous outcome. But, for example, if the faith healers could gain complete control over medical and sanitary procedures and practices, the unchecked plagues of smallpox, typhus, cholera, yellow fever, typhoid and such would decimate a large part of the population of the world, and what are now only isolated tragedies resulting from the failure of misguided and ignorant individuals to make use of proven remedies would become devastating conflagrations.

Is there not something wrong with our educational systems when in this so-called scientific age we find, among our high-school, college and university graduates, many who believe nothing definite and have no convictions, while many others will believe anything, no matter how fantastic? Is there not something wrong when so many join the ranks of the fundamentalists, fighting the teaching of truth about evolution and progress as it applies to biology? When so many others join the ranks of the "one hundred percenters" opposing the recognition of truth in history, in economics, or in government? When many are so gullible as to be deceived by the most faulty and superficial reasoning? Has not the teaching of science failed when so many taking these high-school and university courses join the ranks of the faith healers fighting sanitation and health measures, degrading both religion and science? It is clear that some of the most elementary principles of science are disregarded by those graduates of our best universities who go to fortune tellers and astrologers for advice, or for spirit messages from the dead; who feel uncomfortable unless they knock on wood; are superstitious about so many things, about lucky or unlucky numbers, about black cats or walking under ladders; who rely on charms or "lucky" pieces of one sort or another, or who forward chain letters for fear of bad luck.

When we recognize these weaknesses of those who are the products of our institutions of higher learning, weaknesses typical of primitive peoples or those with but few educational opportunities, we must recognize that part of it must be due to weaknesses in our educational system and methods. Part, I am convinced, is due to the fact that large numbers of students, as well as teachers, have had little or no training in science, especially in those phases of the biological sciences that bear upon one's everyday thinking and behavior. Part, I feel, is certainly due to the emphasis on teaching *what* to think rather than *how* to think; to a tendency to teach by authority, by dogma, rather than for authority, for understanding.

One of the more telling points in an article by Dallas Lore Sharp on "Education for Authority"[3] was his free translation of the Biblical passages as follows: "The people were astonished for He taught them as one having authority and not as those who had gone to college." Is not too much of our teaching to-day like that of the scribes of old, too much like that of the followers of Galen, a mere passing on of information, with little or no training in understanding? Are we not failing in helping our students to gain a real understanding, to gain an attitude of mind which aids in solving problems, in the discovery, unfolding and appreciation of truth and a recognition of values? Are we building a foundation that will lead to further growth and to a more satisfactory living?

As I look at it, science is successfully taught only as its teachers can get their pupils to appreciate how advancement in knowledge is accomplished only gradually and by the critical examination and reexamination, the testing and retesting, of each step in a fabric of evidence; and how the truth is clarified only after the many possible weaknesses or alternative interpretations are critically examined and tested from all angles and by many workers. Training in science should make the individual more critical, not more credulous, should lead him out of superstition and not sink him deeper into the attitudes of the superstitious.

I have been contrasting methods of teaching science, that is, teaching by drilling the students to memorize the conclusions of others, a mere accumulation of information, as contrasted with training in evaluating evidence, in understanding and in solving problems for themselves. Is not a training for real understanding, for authority, immensely superior to teaching by authority or by dictation? Do not the principles apply to all ages from the first grades in school to old age? Do not the same principles apply also to each of us as individuals, not as teachers, but as students continuing our education? Are we as individuals meeting problems by attempting to understand them or are we accepting authority, either from our former or present teachers or from our own past conclusions which perhaps were based on incomplete evidence? Are we as individuals growing, or are we static? In all fields of education, whether it be art or music, literature, religion, sociology, history, government, economics or one of the sciences, we need education for appreciation not by dictation, for understanding not by indoctrination, for authority not by authority.

[3] *Atlantic Monthly*, 128: 13–21, 1921.

# SCIENTIFIC EVENTS

## FUTURE OF THE SCIENCE MUSEUM, LONDON

THE future of the Science Museum, South Kensington, is discussed in the report of the Advisory Council and summarized in the London *Times*. It is recalled that in the report last year the council gave a brief résumé of its recommendations for the future of the museum as an integral part of a general project for the development of the South Kensington site. They afterwards issued a full report, and subsequently Lord Stanhope, then president of the Board of Education, received a deputation of the council.

Lord Stanhope, the present report states, expressed his sympathy and agreement with the council's recommendations as to the floor space needed for exhibition galleries, library and ancillary accommodation. "He expressed his doubts, however, as to whether the site area . . . would be available in its entirety without jeopardizing the whole project, and suggested that it might be necessary to confine the museum to a smaller site and erect a loftier building with exhibition galleries on four more floors."

The Advisory Council have expressed their "profound concern" at such a policy. "They understand that the site area which they require for the Science Museum only affects the project to the extent of precluding the location of another new museum on this already crowded site, and that the project is based on a tentative plan prepared early in 1937 before the needs of certain institutions were known.

"They reaffirm their opinion that it is unwise to erect a museum with several stories of exhibition galleries. Two, or at the most three, such stories should be the maximum, for the public are averse voluntarily to mounting higher, and upper galleries remain unvisited mausoleums. The modern practice in museum buildings in other countries confirms our opinion."

The council considers that the site area they request for the Science Museum in the future falls short of the areas now occupied by the other major national museums. While maintaining its function of preserving historical records of science and industry, it should be in a position to serve a wider educational purpose in connection with the national industries.

## EXPEDITIONS OF THE FIELD MUSEUM, CHICAGO

THE paleontological expedition of the Field Museum of Natural History, under the leadership of Assistant Curator Bryan Patterson, has begun operations in western Colorado. Mr. Patterson is accompanied by James H. Quinn, also of the department of geology, and a corps of volunteer workers will be recruited in the vicinity of the excavations.

The expedition will remain in the field for about three and a half months. The field of operations lies in Mesa, Garfield and Gunnison Counties, where an extensive series of formations belonging to various periods and eras in the earth's history is exposed. Important collections of fossil animals and notable additions to knowledge have already resulted from previous expeditions conducted in this general region during 1932, 1933 and 1937. This program will be continued by the present party, which will carry on work mainly in late Paleocene and early Eocene deposits (the opening epochs of the Age of Mammals), with some attention also being paid to the late Cretaceous formations (the closing period of the Age of Reptiles).

The main objective of the expedition is to collect fossil mammals from the Paleocene and Eocene. Specimens from these early horizons are of great interest to students of mammalian evolution. The dinosaurs and other reptiles that had previously dominated the earth were but a short time extinct (geologically speaking), and the mammals were just getting well under way. Many groups that no longer survive were flourishing, and several of the dominant mammalian types of the present time were represented by exceedingly primitive ancestors.

In addition to the work on vertebrates, attention will be paid to geological observations and to the collecting of fossil plants. It is hoped that by means of the latter it will be possible to make somewhat more precise age determinations and correlations of the late Cretaceous formations than has hitherto been done.

The expedition which has been collecting marine animals and other invertebrates along the Atlantic and Gulf coasts of Florida since early in May has completed its work. Dr. Fritz Haas, curator of lower invertebrates, and Staff Taxidermist Leon L. Walters, who conducted the expedition, have returned to the museum. More than 6,000 specimens, representing the most important features of the invertebrate life forms native to the region, were collected. On Sanibel Island, Dr. Haas conducted researches on the relationships between the various types of fauna and the environmental conditions in which they are found. He also investigated the rôle of molluscan life in building up land through the accumulation of shells.

One of the main objectives of the expedition was the collecting of material and data for a proposed habitat exhibit of the loggerhead turtle. This material was collected on Sanibel Island, and plaster molds were made which will form the basis for lifelike reproductions. Mr. Walters was fortunate in being able to observe the entire nesting procedure.

## THE LEVERHULME RESEARCH FELLOWSHIPS

The Advisory Committee for the Leverhulme Research Fellowships has recommended, and the trustees have approved, the following awards, tenable for varying periods up to two years:

W. H. B. Court, M.A., lecturer in economic history, University of Birmingham, "India and British Economic Policy in the Past Century."

W. Cule Davies, D.Sc., Ph.D., lecturer in chemistry, University College, Cardiff, Leverhulme Research Fellow, "Studies of the Organic Compounds of Nitrogen, Phosphorus and Arsenic."

R. M. Davies, D.Sc., lecturer in physics, University College, Aberystwyth, "Experimental Investigations on Turbulent Flow in an Air-tunnel."

R. Dennell, M.Sc., assistant lecturer in zoology, Imperial College of Science and Technology, London, "The Structure and Physiology of the Luminous Organs of Atlantic Deep-sea Crustacea."

R. W. Firth, M.A., Ph.D., reader in anthropology, University of London, "The Social Structure and Economic Organization of Rural Malays."

D. Ll. Griffiths, F.R.C.S., clinical assistant, Orthopedic Department, Manchester Royal Infirmary, "The Comparison of Radiological and Histological Features in Bone Tumors."

A. E. Ingham, M.A., university lecturer in mathematics, Cambridge, "The Analytical Theory of Numbers."

B. Jones, B.Sc., Ph.D., lecturer in chemistry, University of Sheffield, "A Study of Reaction Kinetics in Solution."

E. B. Maxted, D.Sc., Ph.D., special lecturer in catalysis, University of Bristol, "Studies in Catalyst Poisoning."

D. A. O'Duffy, B.Sc., research and development assistant, Bahrein Petroleum Company, Leverhulme Research Fellow, "Lubrication Problems at High Temperatures and Pressures.

L. F. Taylor, M.A., I.E.S. (Ret.), late research lecturer in Indo-Chinese ethnography and linguistics, University College, Rangoon, "An Ethnographical and Linguistic Survey of Burma."

Miss M. L. Tildesley, chairman of the Comité de Standardisation de la Technique authropologique, London, "The Definition, Measurements and Classification of Anthropometric Characters."

W. A. Waters, M.A., Ph.D., lecturer in chemistry, University of Durham, "Mechanisms of Reactions Involving Free Organic Radicals."

E. L. E. Wheatcroft, M.A., professor of electrical engineering, University of Leeds, "The Mechanism of Development of Electric Sparks with Reference to Lighting Discharges."

## THE SEVENTEENTH CHEMICAL EXPOSITION

The seventeenth Chemical Exposition will be held in the Grand Central Palace, New York City, during the week beginning on December 4, when it will celebrate the completion of its twenty-fifth year of service to the chemical and allied industries. Many of the exhibitors in the first exposition, which was held in 1915, have engaged space this year. It is now established on a biennial basis.

Three floors of the Grand Central Palace have been reserved for the exposition, which will include chemicals and chemical products, laboratory equipment and supplies, instruments of precision, materials handling equipment, brewing, distilling and bottling equipment, industrial chemical machinery and materials, containers and packaging machinery and materials of construction. At the last exposition more than 46,000 visitors attended, representing 45 states in the United States and 130 cities and towns in 47 foreign countries. Members of the Advisory Committee include the presidents of the principal chemical organizations. Its chairman is Dr. M. C. Whitaker, long a leading figure in the chemical industry. Charles F. Roth, who has been similarly responsible for the preceding expositions, will be personally in charge.

The student course in chemical engineering which has become an established feature of the exposition, will again be presented. Professor W. T. Read, dean of chemistry of Rutgers University, who has served as director in previous expositions, will this year again be in full charge. This course enables the selected college students who enroll to coordinate lectures by leading authorities with actual examination of the materials and chemical engineering equipment discussed.

Unit processes of chemical engineering will be represented by a broad range of exhibits. Combustion processes include furnaces, kilns, refractories and the recording instruments essential for regulation and control. Crushing, grinding and mechanical separation will be represented by sifters, agitators, classifiers and ball mills. Classification of materials based on magnetic properties also will be demonstrated. Advances in the processes of filtration, evaporation and drying will be illustrated by many exhibits. Apparatus will include filters of every type and evaporating equipment applicable not only to the chemical industries but also to the food industries. Drying equipment will be shown in its relation to every phase of the pharmaceutical industry, and there will be special reference to the processing of foods.

## EXHIBITION OF THE AMATEUR ASTRONOMERS ASSOCIATION OF NEW YORK CITY

The first national exhibition of the work of amateur astronomers was opened in the American Museum of Natural History on July 30 and will close on August 20. The exhibition is sponsored by the Amateur Astronomers Association of New York City and by other societies in the metropolitan area. It includes exhibits from more than two hundred amateur astronomers belonging to more than thirty clubs throughout the country.

A national convention of amateur astronomers, with sessions at the museum and the New York World's Fair, will be held on August 19 and 20, the closing days of the exhibition. August 19 will be Amateur Astronomers Association Day at the New York World's Fair. An address "Astronomy in the World of To-morrow" will be given on that day at the fair by Dr. Harlow Shapley, director of Harvard College Observatory.

A nine-inch reflecting telescope made by school students in Flint, Mich.; star photographs from an amateur in New Brunswick, Canada; lens-making tools from Lewiston, Maine, and a home-made spectroscope from Norwalk, Conn., are among the exhibits. The Alabama Astronomical Association shows photographs; Earl C. Witherspoon, of Sumter, S. C., is displaying a home-made Herschel wedge for use in solar telescopic observations. A Schmidt camera, the new type of telescope now being widely used by professional astronomers, difficult of design and construction, is being exhibited by Stanley Brower, of Plainfield, N. J., with samples of stellar photographs. A celestial globe, complete with automatic electric motions, is being shown by E. C. Stanton, of Bethesda, Md. The Cook Observatory of Wynnewood, Pa., is exhibiting photographs of its equipment and samples of its work. Exhibits from members of the National Capital Amateur Astronomers Association in Washington, D. C., are also on view. The New Haven Astronomical Society includes in its exhibit tools and devices used in the production of telescope mirrors, grinding machines, testing apparatus and the like. Donald S. Kimball, president of the group, is showing a series of forty-four auroral photographs taken from his home in Hamden, Conn.

Visitors are invited also to visit the workshop of the optical division of the association in the basement of the Hayden Planetarium, where they may watch the making of telescopes, mirrors, lenses, mountings and other equipment. The Junior Astronomy Club is represented by photographs and the paintings made on its 1932 eclipse expedition to Peru, as well as by instruments constructed by its members.

Honorary life membership in the association will be presented during the convention to Leslie C. Peltier, of Delphos, Ohio, who has to his credit the discovery of several comets and novae. A special performance will be given at the Hayden Planetarium and at "Time and Space," the special exhibit of the museum at the World's Fair. The exhibition will be open on week days and Saturdays from 10 A.M. to 5 P.M. and on Sundays from 1 P.M. to 5 P.M.

## RECENT DEATHS AND MEMORIALS

DR. WILLIAM JAMES MAYO, of the Mayo Foundation and the University of Minnesota, surgeon and chief of staff of the Mayo Clinic, died on July 28 at the age of seventy-eight years.

DR. WILLIAM ARTHUR TARR, professor of mineralogy and geology at the University of Missouri, died on July 28. He was fifty-eight years old.

DR. HARTLEY BURR ALEXANDER, professor of philosophy at Scripps College, Claremont, Calif., previously professor of philosophy at the University of Nebraska, died on July 27 at the age of sixty-six years. In addition to his publications in philosophy and psychology Dr. Alexander is known for his work in Indian anthropology.

DR. ALFRED HARKER, emeritus reader in petrology at the University of Cambridge, a fellow of St. John's College, died on July 29 at the age of eighty years.

*Nature* announces the death of Dr. W. A. Jolly, professor of physiology in the University of Cape Town, and of Brigadier-General the Hon. C. G. Bruce, leader of the Mount Everest Expeditions of 1922 and 1924.

As a permanent recognition of the contribution of the late Professor Charles Sumner Plumb, the animal husbandry building of the Ohio State University will be called "Plumb Hall," on the recommendation of the College of Agriculture, in which Professor Plumb served as professor of animal husbandry for thirty-seven years. At the same time the board of trustees recorded its "profound appreciation and the gratitude of the university for the gift of the priceless library" of Professor Plumb, whose death occurred in March. The library consists of more than 1,600 items.

# SCIENTIFIC NOTES AND NEWS

THE "golden jubilee" of David Fairchild, formerly chief of the Division of Plant Exploration and Introduction of the U. S. Department of Agriculture, author of "The World is My Garden," who joined the department fifty years ago, was marked on July 24 at Glenn Dale, Md., when Secretary Henry A. Wallace presented him with the Frank N. Meyer Medal. This was the sixteenth award of the medal, which was established by the will of Mr. Meyer, who was also a plant explorer of the Department of Agriculture.

THE Southern Minnesota Medical Association has presented its annual gold medal to Dr. Vernon L. Hart, professor of surgery at the medical school of the University of Minnesota, for the best scientific exhibit at the recent meeting of the Minnesota State Medical

Association. Dr. Hart's subject was "Fracture Problems."

The senate of the University of Glasgow announces the award of the Struthers Gold Medal and Prize to Dr. George M. Wyburn for a series of embryological studies embodied in papers published in the *Journal of Anatomy*. The Harry Stewart Hutchison Prize has been awarded to James Holmes Hutchison for his dissertation entitled "The Iron-deficiency Anemia of Childhood."

It is stated in *Nature* that Dr. Emil Abderhalden, professor of physiology at Halle, and Dr. Max Planck, professor of theoretical physics at Berlin, have been elected honorary members of the Société Philomathique of Paris.

The University of Leeds has conferred the degree of doctor of science on Dr. W. L. Bragg, Cavendish professor of physics at the University of Cambridge.

The University of Tasmania has conferred the degree of doctor of science on John William Evans, government entomologist of the Department of Agriculture, Tasmania.

Dr. Marjorie S. Harris, professor of philosophy at the Randolph-Macon Woman's College, Lynchburg, Va., has been elected president of the Southern Society for Philosophy and Psychology; Dr. Norman L. Munn, professor of psychology, Vanderbilt University, has been elected secretary and treasurer.

Dr. Frank Brawley, of Chicago, has been made president-elect of the American Academy of Ophthalmology and Otolaryngology. He succeeds Dr. Albert C. Snell, of Rochester, N. Y., who has resigned because of ill health.

The following members of the faculty of the Ohio State University are among those who will retire with the title professor emeritus on September 1: Dr. Clair A. Dye, dean of the College of Pharmacy, who has been on the faculty for forty-nine years; Charles W. Foulk, professor of chemistry, and Christopher E. Sherman, professor of civil engineering, for forty-three years; Frank C. Caldwell, professor of electrical engineering, for forty-six years; Horace Judd, professor of mechanical engineering, for thirty-seven years, and Elmer G. Horton, professor of medicine, for thirty-seven years.

Dr. Bienvenido M. Gonzalez, from 1927 to 1939 dean of the College of Agriculture, has been elected president of the University of the Philippines. Dr. Leopoldo B. Uichanco, professor of entomology and head of the department of entomology, will take his place as dean of the College of Agriculture.

Adelbert Diefendorf, for the last nine years professor of civil engineering at the University of Pittsburgh, has been made head of the department of civil engineering at the University of Utah.

Dr. R. D. Haworth has been appointed to the chair of chemistry in the University of Sheffield in succession to Professor R. P. Linstead, who has resigned. Dr. Wilson Smith has been appointed professor of bacteriology in succession to the late Professor J. W. Edington.

B. L. Goodlet, professor of electrical engineering in the University of Cape Town, Union of South Africa, has been appointed to the chair of electrical engineering at the University of Birmingham to succeed the late Professor W. Cramp.

Dr. K. N. Kaul, of the University of Lucknow, has become a member of the staff of the Royal Botanic Gardens, Kew, England.

Professor Francis Colin Minett, director of the Research Institute in Animal Pathology at the Royal Veterinary College, London, and professor of pathology at that college, has been appointed director of the Imperial Veterinary Research Institute of the Government of India. He will leave for India late in August.

Dr. David F. Smith, professor of chemistry at the University of Buffalo, has been placed at the head of the work on agricultural motor fuels at the Northern Regional Research Laboratory of the U. S. Department of Agriculture at Peoria, Ill. He plans to study methods of producing gaseous, liquid and solid motor fuels from agricultural materials.

By action of the house of delegates at the annual meeting of the Ohio State Medical Association, a bureau of public education has been established in the executive offices of the association in Columbus. Richard A. Aszling, recently a member of the staff of the Dayton *Daily News*, has been appointed director of the bureau.

Dr. Vern O. Knudsen, professor of physics and dean of the graduate division of the University of California at Los Angeles, has been named a member of the Los Angeles Building Commission. Dr. Knudsen has specialized in acoustical problems and in 1935 won the $1,000 prize of the American Association for the Advancement of Science for his research on the absorption of sound by gases.

Dr. Harry F. Olson, director of acoustical research for the Radio Corporation of America, will inaugurate work in electrical acoustics at Columbia University. A study will be made of the possibility of improvement in the quality of sound reproduction in radios and motion pictures. The course is part of a program undertaken by the School of Engineering to enable practicing engineers of the metropolitan area to enroll for specialized academic studies. It is parallel with, and complements, two other courses in sound production, one on communication electronics given by Dr. Eugene Peterson, of the Bell Telephone Laboratories, and the other on the acoustical properties of rooms and buildings conducted by Dr. V. A. Schlenker, of the department of physics.

HERBERT HOOVER has been named a member of a committee of the board of trustees of Stanford University to recommend a successor to President Ray Lyman Wilbur, who will retire on January 1, 1942. The trustees' committee will cooperate in the selection with an advisory committee of the Stanford Academic Council, composed of Dr. Eliot Blackwelder, professor of geology; Edwin A. Cottrell, professor of political science; J. P. Mitchell, registrar; Dr. C. V. Taylor, dean of the School of Biology, and Dr. Lewis M. Terman, professor of psychology. Dr. Wilbur's term was recently extended by the board of trustees beyond the retirement age of sixty-five in order that he might be president of the university when it celebrates its fiftieth anniversary.

HENRY LUNZ, in charge of the Seed and Weed Control Section of the Wisconsin State Department of Agriculture, was elected chairman of the Seed and Weed Council at a recent joint meeting with the Wisconsin Seed Dealers Association at Madison. He succeeds O. S. Aamodt, chairman of the department of agronomy at the College of Agriculture. The council is an organization of groups in Wisconsin interested in seed and weed problems, including the Wisconsin Experiment Association, the State Department of Agriculture, Wisconsin Seed Dealers Association, State University College of Agriculture, State Extension Workers Association, the Central Retail Feed Dealers, Wisconsin Bankers Association, Wisconsin Crop Reporting Service, the Association of Agricultural Instructors, the Wisconsin Council of Agriculture, and others.

ACCORDING to *The Australian Journal of Science* elections representing the States and the Australian Capital Territory on the Executive Committee of the Australian National Research Council have been made as follows: Australian Capital Territory: Dr. B. T. Dickson, Dr. W. G. Woolnough; New South Wales: Professor R. D. Watt, Professor W. J. Dakin; Victoria: Professor E. W. Skeats, Mr. W. E. Wainwright; South Australia: Sir Douglas Mawson, Sir William Mitchell; Queensland: Professor H. C. Richards, Dr. D. A. Herbert; Western Australia: Professor E. de C. Clarke, Dr. G. L. Sutton. Professor R. D. Watt has been elected deputy chairman.

DELEGATES to represent the United States at the seventh International Congress of Genetics at Edinburgh from August 23 to 30 have been appointed as follows: Dr. Hugh C. McPhee, of the U. S. Department of Agriculture, *chairman;* Dr. Albert F. Blakeslee, of the Carnegie Institution, Cold Spring Harbor, N. Y.; Dr. Lewis J. Stadler, of the University of Missouri, and Dr. Sewall Wright, of the University of Chicago.

PROFESSOR E. C. SLIPHER, of the Lowell Observatory, is visiting the South African Observatory of the University of Michigan at Bloemfontein in the Orange Free State for special observations of the planet Mars.

DR. N. H. DARTON is spending the summer in central Europe. He plans to visit Berlin, where he will read the proofs of his contributions to the American volume on the "Geology of the Earth," now in press in Berlin.

A PUBLIC meeting of the Chicago branch of the American Association of Scientific Workers held on July 18 at the University of Chicago was addressed by J. D. Bernal, professor of physics at the University of London, who spoke on the subject of his recent book, "The Social Function of Science."

THE American Astronomical Society will hold its sixty-second meeting at the University of California at Berkeley on August 7, 8 and 9.

THE twenty-fourth annual meeting of the Optical Society of America will be held at the Lake Placid Club, Essex County, New York, on October 12, 13 and 14. In addition to the usual program of contributed papers, a special program of invited papers is being arranged on the general topic of the "Optics of Vision." Papers are being prepared on the following subjects: Comparison of Structures of the Eyes of Humans and of Other Animals, Neural Connections between the Retinas and the Brain and Binocular Vision; Chemistry of Visual Systems, Recent Researches in Color Vision, Aniseikonia, Luminosity Methods and Results, Vision and Highway Accidents, the Supra-Threshold Realm of Seeing. The program committee is attempting to leave afternons free for recreation, except as this time may be required for committee meetings and similar activities. The annual dinner will be held on Friday evening, October 13, when the award of the Frederic Ives Medal will be made.

THE sixteenth annual meeting of the History of Science Society will be held in conjunction with the American Association for the Advancement of Science at Columbus, Ohio, from December 27, 1939, to January 2, 1940. The headquarters of the society will be at the Chittenden Hotel. Members wishing to appear on the program should communicate with Professor Louis C. Karpinski, department of mathematics, University of Michigan, Ann Arbor, Michigan. Dr.

Henry R. Viets, 8 The Fenway, Boston, Mass., is secretary of the society.

THE regular summer meeting of the Pennsylvania Academy of Science will be held at Laporte, Pa., on August 11 and 12. Field trips in botany and geology are planned. For further information, address the Secretary, Dr. V. Earl Light, Lebanon Valley College, Annville, Pa.

THE American Institute of Physics, New York City, has announced that it will conduct from November 2 to 4 a symposium on temperature. It is planned to coordinate the treatment of the subject of temperature in the several branches of science and engineering, to review principles and record recent work, to accumulate contributions for a comprehensive text to be published after the symposium, to emphasize the importance of temperature as a branch of physics and to improve technical curricula through making available up-to-date information.

# DISCUSSION

## SURFACE CURRENTS IN DEEP TIDAL WATERS

IN a recent article in SCIENCE, Shepard, Revelle and Dietz[1] report the discovery of unexpectedly strong bottom currents well out on the rugged continental shelf off the coast of Southern California. They note that these currents can not be explained as tidal currents of the regularly alternating type usually recognized, but must be due primarily to large eddies having no direct relation to the state of the tide.

Since some observations of my own during several summer vacations have led me to a similar conclusion about many surface currents in the deep water of the Inside Passage along the coast of British Columbia and since the importance of such eddies is only beginning to be recognized, I venture to present the results of these observations, even though they are only those of an amateur.

So far as I have observed, the times and heights of high and low water in the Inside Passage and its tributaries follow the predictions in the tide tables remarkably well, indeed so accurately that I have sometimes set my watch by them and later found it right within five minutes. The same is true of the times of turning of the current in the tidal rapids, of which there are at least ten on this coast strong enough to make white water. On the other hand, there are passages such as Welcome Pass, about 40 miles NW of Vancouver, where I have observed the current many times, and where there is no way to predict it at all. Thus on consecutive days with but little difference in the heights of the highs and lows, one may observe the current at corresponding tidal intervals and find it running in opposite directions on the two days, often with a strength of one or two knots, which is about as strong as the current gets in this pass. This pass differs from ones where the current can be predicted, however, in running parallel to a much wider alternative passage between the two bodies of water which it connects and in having only a moderately strong current.

[1] F. P. Shepard, R. Revelle and R. S. Dietz, SCIENCE, 89: 488, May 26, 1939.

Similarly along the shores of the Strait of Georgia, in the calm, clear weather that justifies the local steamship company in calling it "The Sunshine Belt," one may often observe currents of a knot or so, either alongshore or toward the shore or boiling up out of the bottom near the shore or meeting one another and sinking along a line made visible from afar by a thick accumulation of driftwood. Such currents all show a similar unpredictability.

My guess on the origin of these currents has been that they are eddies broken off from the strong tidal currents entering the Strait of Georgia through the relatively narrow Rosario and Haro Straits and Discovery Passage. With the configuration of the shore and bottom as it is, any such eddy, formed in the flood, can easily become detached from the current of the narrow strait and wander about aimlessly all over the Strait of Georgia. The observation of these unpredictable currents at places 60 or 80 miles away indicates that the eddies may persist for many days after detachment.

A similar effect occurs in the narrow fjords, such, for example, as Jervis Inlet. In this inlet the chart reports tidal currents of one knot, both ebb and flood, in places where calculations from the cross-sections of the fjord and the areas inland of those places would not indicate as much as one tenth of a knot, and where there are no big currents of fresh water like that of the St. Lawrence River. In some of those places at least, the currents are unpredictable. This I have observed especially in Jervis Inlet; and likewise in Alaska, in Le Conte Inlet. In the latter fjord I have observed the eddies only once, but that time with considerable detail owing to the fact that the eddies unexpectedly packed the small icebergs from Le Conte Glacier in around me and almost crushed my boat. On that occasion, with the boat unable to make her usual speed, the slow milling around of the icebergs gave a clear picture of the big, slow eddies.

My general conclusion from these observations, then, is that in deep waters of this type, aside from narrows or straits carrying exceptionally strong currents, the current at any point is most likely to be primarily due to eddies having their origin in stronger and more strictly tidal currents at other places.

In this respect the deep waters of British Columbia and Alaska show a marked contrast to such shoal waters as Nantucket Sound, Massachusetts, where the currents are almost entirely strictly tidal. As a physicist I feel sure that the difference is due primarily to the great influence of viscosity in the shoal waters and the lack of it in the deep. In the same capacity, I would guess that there would be still less influence of viscosity in such larger and deeper waters as Shepard, Revelle and Dietz have been studying. Therefore we may expect their conclusions to apply very generally in deep waters with rugged bottoms.

DAVID L. WEBSTER
STANFORD UNIVERSITY

## PROBLEMS OF WOUND HEALING IN RED CLOVER STEMS

FORAGE legumes, like other herbaceous plants having no protective covering other than an epidermis, are subjected to injury by grazing animals and insects. In particular, the mowing of fields is a severe test both because of the wounds and also through the loss of the plant body including most of the buds. In spite of such injuries these plants are usually able to continue growth though frequently with some modification of form and size.

The stems of three important herbaceous legumes—*Trifolium repens* L., white clover, *Medicago sativa* L., alfalfa, and *Trifolium pratense* L., red clover—were studied with respect to the time and the nature of their wound responses. While primary interest centered in the healing processes, attention was given to various conditions, interrelated with lesion, which may cause the death of these legumes.

In connection with the healing of wounded herbaceous stems considerable credit must be given to the preliminary barrier or pseudocicatrice,[1] formed by death and collapse of tissue following injury. This, in itself, is protective in considerable degree and by checking the dying back of tissues permits certain underlying cells to develop a permanent barrier of wound cork, the cicatrice, which effectively heals the wound. Ultimately, in the three legumes studied, a region of solid living pith at some point in the injured stem permits the protective structures to be formed.

The pith in white clover generally remains alive and completely fills the central zone. Following a transverse cut a continuous pseudocicatrice quickly covers the injured surface. Suberin is demonstrable in the walls of the outermost living cells underneath the pseudocicatrice within thirty-six to forty-eight hours after lesion. By the sixth day suberization has extended from two to four cells further into the underlying tissues. About this time mitoses begin in subjacent cells, and this phellogen forms two to five additional layers of cork, which completes the cicatrice. Its development requires about fifteen days, and in final form it extends entirely across the stem, interrupted only by the vascular tissue.

However, in certain stems of white clover the central region of the pith dies and spaces develop. Following a cut across one of these hollow stems the pseudocicatrice can not be completed across the pith region, and water loss by way of this cavity causes the stem to die back to the nearest node. There a block of living parenchyma furnishes a foundation upon which a continuous pseudocicatrice is built. Four to five days may be required for the stem tissues to die back to this node, and both initiation and completion of the barriers are correspondingly delayed. Ultimately a cicatrice is always developed in the firm tissue of the node, similar to that which is built at the plane of injury in stems having solid living pith.

The pith of alfalfa stems is dead and broken throughout all internodes, but at the nodes there is usually a continuous living tissue. Consequently its healing processes correspond closely with those of white clover stems having dead pith. Dying back to the node takes five to ten days, but in the nodal zone the cicatrice is quickly formed. In general, mature alfalfa stems are safely healed within twenty-one days.

In red clover the pith is larger and makes up over half of the stem's diameter, relatively more than in white clover or alfalfa. Because this pith normally dies within two cm of the meristem, growth of the internodes breaks down the central tissue, leaving hollow stems. The nearest lower zone of solid living cells is at the junction with the crown, unless there is a growing lateral branch with sufficient living pith at the junction to permit the formation of protective barriers. The defective pith causes the whole axis to die downward to where a platform of living cells makes possible the establishment of the pseudocicatrice, which is quickly followed by the cicatrice of wound cork.

Due to this prolonged dying back of all wounded red clover stems there is necessarily a considerable delay in healing processes. When cut as low as four inches from the base there is a lapse of two to three weeks, even in midsummer, between the time of injury and the earliest evidence of healing. This means an interval of at least a month between the date of injury and completion of the cicatrice. This dying back of stems slows down later in the growing season and during the autumn months the development of healing tissues is greatly retarded or entirely inhibited. Rarely does a cicatrice reach completion before winter if a stem is cut across after early September. Successful healing takes place in the autumn only when

[1] Robert B. Wylie, *Bot. Gaz.*, 90: 260–278, 1930.

the lesion is very close to the crown in a region of living pith. Under no other circumstances has suberin been found in stems wounded as late as October.

While no growth responses are possible during the colder months the dying back of wounded stems continues even through the winter. During late autumn and early spring the unprotected junctions of these dead stems with the living crown are attacked by organisms which undoubtedly enter through the open hollow stubs. This infection leads to breakdown of tissue which extends into the crown and when spring growth is resumed the plants can not wall off these diseased parts. Consequently, as early as July the central region of the crown and the upper part of the tap root have largely decayed, leaving usually only a thin shell of living tissue. Such plants may look normal during the spring, but they are definitely less able to withstand the later periods of summer drought and nearly all of them die before autumn. In a general way these difficulties are commonly related to the hardships of the previous winter, but they go back instead to autumn injuries. The considerable time that elapses in red clover between the lesions of autumn and their effects the following summer has concealed the disastrous results of late wounding.

The nature of the pith on these legumes is a determining factor both with respect to the location of wound barriers and the promptness with which they are formed. In stems having solid living pith the cicatrice is developed quickly near the wound surface under the pseudocicatrice. But if there are dead or broken portions of pith the location of the barriers is necessarily shifted and stems die back to a plane of solid living pith. This long lag between injury and cicatrization is the critical period for red clover.

Since the summer of 1934 hundreds of clover fields throughout Iowa and neighboring states have been studied not only with respect to the immediate results of wounding, but also as to ultimate effects of cutting and pasturing. It is a common practice of long standing to clip or pasture red clover during the first fall after spring seeding. Careful check on large numbers of fields shows that there is a striking correlation between fall treatment and the percentage of infected plants at intervals during the following summer. These fields were selected at random from those having fair stands of clover and for which the cultural history could be obtained. A summary of these records shows, (1), that if the fields were heavily clipped during the late autumn the proportion of diseased plants during the following summer ranged from 50 to 95 per cent., and (2), that fields if left uninjured after the first of September had only 1 to 10 per cent. of infected plants by midsummer of the following year.

Apart from the effects of lesion, clover plants frequently die as a result of "winter-killing." This is especially true if crowns are exposed either by mowing or heavy pasturage late in the season. The death of such plants is undoubtedly caused by winter hazards other than those related to wounds. Nevertheless, it can not be stressed too strongly that late cutting or pasturing not only promotes this winter-killing, due to increased exposure as a result of removing plant cover, but, even if fields survive the winter, most of the plants inevitably suffer from crown infection the following growing season as a result of their inability to heal the wounds of the previous autumn.

It is not uncommon in eastern Iowa for entire fields of red clover to live through three growing seasons, and several cases are on record of four-year-old fields. But, in all the instances investigated where fields lived more than the second summer, the plants were neither cut nor pastured after the first of September and so went into the winter with considerable ground cover and with all wounds safely healed at or above the crown level.

It seems clear from study that in this region late-season treatment, apart from certain winter hazards, largely determines the fate of red clover in a given field.

Robert W. Poulter

State University of Iowa

## ROOTING NORWAY SPRUCE CUTTINGS WITHOUT CHEMICAL TREATMENT

At the New Haven meetings of the New England Section of American Plant Physiologists, held on May 12 and 13, a method was described by which cuttings of 39-year-old Norway spruce trees were successfully rooted in large numbers during the past winter. Vegetative propagation of this economic forest and ornamental species permits establishing clones with desirable growth characteristics. One of our immediate objects will be the propagation of Norway spruce trees that have a natural immunity to the spruce gall aphid.

The results of the rooting tests were based on 3,200 cuttings collected at monthly intervals from October to January, inclusive. The factors tested included (1) month of collection; (2) length of cuttings, short (5 to 10 cm) and long (10 to 20 cm); (3) cuttings with and others without a heel of two-year-old wood; (4) no preliminary treatment, standing in water 24 hours or in indole butyric acid solutions with 2.5, 5, 10, 20, 40, 60, 80 and 100 mgms of the chemical per liter. The cuttings were planted in builders' sand in an open greenhouse bench with day temperatures around 70° F. and night temperatures never lower than 55° F. Analysis of the data is based upon the examination of the bases of the cuttings 14 weeks after planting.

Detailed analysis of the influence of the several factors investigated must await subsequent publication.

The two outstanding results appear to be, first, that the season at which the cuttings are taken governs to a large degree the percentage of rooting, and second, that treatment with indole butyric acid seems to retard rooting. The greater the concentration of this chemical the more rooting was retarded. In addition, long cuttings were superior to short cuttings and cuttings without heels rooted in greater numbers than those with heels. Placing the bases of the cuttings in tap water for 24 hours prior to planting in sand retarded rooting somewhat.

Terminal and lateral twigs of lateral branches located between six to eight feet from the ground were used when making the cuttings. Best rootage was secured from plain cuttings 10 to 20 cm long made in December and planted directly in the sand bench. In 14 weeks 90 per cent. of these cuttings were rooted. Both the December and January cuttings had larger roots and more advanced top development by May 1 than cuttings collected in October or November. In May more than a thousand rooted cuttings were planted in a tree nursery outdoors and in pots so that tests of their degree of immunity to spruce gall aphids could be conducted in the late summer.

CARL G. DEUBER
JOHN L. FARRAR
YALE UNIVERSITY

## PHYSIOLOGY OF THE NERVOUS SYSTEM

IN his painstaking appraisal of my book, "Physiology of the Nervous System," which appeared in SCIENCE for July 7 (the anniversary of its publication), Dr. Forbes has suggested that I deliberately omitted treatment of the nerve impulse and certain basic problems of neuromuscular transmission. The statement is true and lest misconception should arise from the review, it must be pointed out that the book deals primarily with the *central* nervous system, including the autonomic division. Dr. Ralph Gerard will describe the special physiology of peripheral nerve, *i.e.*, the nerve impulse and neuromuscular transmission, in a separate monograph of this series, which will appear in the near future. This will also deal with the principles of electrophysiology.

Since Dr. Forbes likewise offers a friendly accusation of prejudice with regard to the humoral theory of synaptic transmission, may I take this opportunity of stating once again that I know of no evidence fit for critical examination that would place the liberation of acetylcholine as a *primary* event essential for synaptic transmission, in any division of the nervous system, central or peripheral. The work of Rosenblueth and Simeone cited by Dr. Forbes was published after my book had left the press. A full statement of the evidence for the electrical concept of synaptic activity will appear in a series of five papers by Drs. Gasser, Erlanger, Bronk, Lorente de Nó and Forbes in the September number of the *Journal of Neurophysiology*, which is now in the press. It seems therefore unnecessary to offer here any further defense of my position in this interesting and important controversy.

Save for those points, which might mislead the uninformed reader, Dr. Forbes's review is fair, generous and much appreciated.

J. F. FULTON
YALE UNIVERSITY

# SCIENTIFIC BOOKS

*The Distribution of the Stars in Space.* By BART J. BOK, associate professor of astronomy, Harvard University. xvi + 124 pp. Chicago: University of Chicago Press, 1937. $2.50.

THE editors of the *Astrophysical Journal* are currently engaged in sponsoring a series of astrophysical monographs, which are designed to bring up to date the state of knowledge in the various fields of stellar astronomy. The first volume in the series, by Dr. Bok, is a critical exposition of the information available in 1937 on the distribution of the stars in the galactic system. A truly amazing number and variety of researches have been carried out in this field during the past fifteen years. To organize and discuss critically the results of these multitudinous investigations is an imposing task, and one which the author accomplishes with clarity and dispatch.

The fundamental problem of stellar statistics is to deduce the true stellar distribution in the galaxy from observational data on the apparent numbers, brightnesses, colors, spectral types and motions of the stars. Chapter I of "The Distribution of the Stars in Space" deals with the many statistical methods, both analytical and numerical, that have been devised for this purpose. Methods for detecting deviations from random stellar distribution in any area of the sky are valuable for promoting the discovery of inconspicuous dark nebulae. With regard to the problem of the determination of space densities, Dr. Bok discusses the relative merits of analytical and numerical methods and presents strong arguments in favor of the latter procedure. Simple analytical formulae are inadequate to represent the complex variations in stellar distribution over the sky. The most serious obstacle in the path of attaining a complete understanding of the details of stellar structure is the presence of clouds of obscuring material in the galaxy. The author describes how stellar statisticians have been attempting to cope with this vexatious problem, with encouraging results.

Chapter II gives the present available sources of information on star counts, spectral types and the distribution of dark nebulae. A gratifying feature of Dr. Bok's discussion of the observational material is the manner in which he points out where new observations are most sorely needed. This feature, which is characteristic of the entire monograph, should prove highly stimulating to future research.

The third and final chapter deals with the general problems of galactic structure. Studies of the distribution of stars in directions perpendicular to the galactic plane are not complicated by the bogey of interstellar absorption, and considerable progress has been achieved in those directions, particularly by Oort. The author makes a critical survey of the arguments for and against the hypothesis of a local system of stars in which the sun is approximately central, and concludes that the hypothesis may at least be accepted as a working model. The monograph concludes on a highly optimistic note. Although only the most general features of galactic structure are now well established, Dr. Bok feels that the current rapid accumulation of observations will soon begin to reveal the finer details of stellar structure, and suggests that, as a working model, the galactic system may be regarded as a rather open spiral system, similar in form to Messier 33. On this basis, and accepting the hypothesis of a local system, the sun would be located in a spiral arm about two thirds of the distance from the center to one edge.

"The Distribution of the Stars in Space" is an extremely important contribution to the field of galactic structure, invaluable alike to both students and research workers in the field.

LEO GOLDBERG

## THEORETICAL MECHANICS TREATED VECTORIALLY

*Theoretical Mechanics, a Vectorial Treatment.* By CARL JENNESS COE. New York: The Macmillan Company, 1938, 13 + 555 pages. Price, $5.00.

THIS text-book combines effectively an introduction to theoretical mechanics with training in the notation and methods of three-dimensional vector analysis (Gibbs's notation). Save for some words of caution in view of modern developments in relativity theory and quantum analysis, the selection of topics follows the classical tradition of such authors as Appell, Love, Routh, Webster and Whittaker. Rarely do mere physical facts intrude. Damped motion and sliding friction are touched upon, but the notions of elastic limit, atom, fluid, Young's modulus, oscillograph, viscosity or other commonplace terms of the physical laboratory find no place in this theoretical mathematical study. Included are chapters on the general principles of mechanics, on vector calculus and on potential theory (using three-dimensional vector calculus). But no attempt is made to introduce a generalized vector-space or tensor methods. Some prior training in calculus is assumed on the part of the student. An abundance of numerical exercises is provided which should give him facility and power in working with concepts which thereby can not but acquire clear significance.

ALBERT A. BENNETT

BROWN UNIVERSITY

# SOCIETIES AND MEETINGS

## THE ALABAMA ACADEMY OF SCIENCE

AT Montgomery, the capital, in the shadow of the spot where Jefferson Davis took the oath of office as president of the Confederacy, the Alabama Academy of Science held its sixteenth annual meeting, on April 14 and 15, with Huntingdon College as host. P. H. Yancey, of Spring Hill College, Mobile, presided. The historic background of this beautiful old southern "city of homes," together with the burst of bloom which is characteristic of the season, and the gracious hospitality of the college and of the Montgomery members, made this a memorable occasion. Eighty members, a number of visitors and over a hundred members of the Junior Academy, representing twenty-one schools, which met at the same time, registered. A certificate of award for the best paper and four certificates for the best exhibits in the various scientific fields were given the juniors by the senior academy. P. P. B. Brooks, head of the science department, Sidney Lanier High School, counselor at the place of meeting, assisted by James Holt Starling, head of the biology department, Troy High School, counselor to the president of the Junior Academy, had charge of arrangements for the Junior Academy, for which James H. Kassner, associate professor of chemistry, university, is acting permanent counselor.

Two symposia featured the program of the academy, which included forty-eight scientific papers, presented in four sections at Flowers and Bellingrath Halls and the Haughton Library on Friday afternoon and Saturday morning. Section I held a symposium on "The Biological Control of Malaria." This was presented by members of the health and safety department of the Tennessee Valley Authority, Wilson Dam, and the Alabama State Departments of Public Health and of Conservation. Section II held a symposium on the "Chemistry of the T.V.A. Phosphate Fertilizers," given by the chemists of that division. Both created a great deal of interest and discussion.

The Academy Award from the American Association for the Advancement of Science was voted to J. Allen Tower, assistant professor of geography, Birmingham-Southern College, Birmingham, for "Preparation of an Atlas of Alabama and a Geography of Alabama." Birmingham-Southern College was selected as the next meeting place, the date to be set by the college in collaboration with the academy president.

Social features of the meeting included a tea for the visiting ladies at the home of Mr. and Mrs. E. D. Emigh. Other hostesses for this function were Mrs. Patrick H. Smyth, Mrs. Peter A. Brannon and Mrs. Haygood Paterson. The annual academy banquet was held at the Jefferson Davis Hotel on Friday night, with Haygood Paterson, commissioner of agriculture and industry, as toastmaster. The presidential address, "Science and the World Crisis," given by P. H. Yancey, featured the banquet. This was preceded by the address of welcome, made by Dr. Hubert Searcy, president of Huntingdon College, with response by Walter B. Jones, director of the State Department of Conservation. A motion picture, "The River," given through the courtesy of the National Park Service, closed the banquet, which was followed by an informal social in the ballroom of the hotel. On Saturday morning a geology field trip to old Fort Toulouse and Wetumpka was conducted by W. B. Jones and J. Y. Brame. Other attractions open to visitors were the State Health Laboratories, U. S. Weather Bureau, Montgomery Museum, and Seeing Montgomery Trip. Luncheon was served on both days at Pratt Hall, the college dining room.

Officers for 1939–1940 were elected as follows: *President,* George D. Palmer, associate professor of chemistry, University (elected last year); *President-elect,* C. M. Farmer, head of the biology department, State Teachers College, Troy; *Vice-Presidents and Chairmen of their respective sections:* Samuel Reed Damon, director of the Bureau of Laboratories, Alabama State Department of Health, Section I, Biology and Medical Sciences; Ingomar M. Hostetter, associate professor of mathematics, Howard College, Birmingham, Section II, Physics, Chemistry and Mathematics; A. J. Westland, seismologist, Spring Hill College, Mobile, Section III, Geology, Anthropology and Archeology; and E. D. Emigh, Weather Bureau, Montgomery, Section IV, Industry, Economics and Geography; *Editor of the Journal,* E. V. Jones, Birmingham-Southern College, re-elected for three years; councilor of the American Association for the Advancement of Science, J. H. Coulliette, professor of physics, Birmingham-Southern College, re-elected for one year. The treasurer, John Xan, head of the chemistry department, Howard College, has two more years to serve, and the secretary, Septima C. Smith, associate professor of zoology, University, has one more year.

An executive council meeting and a morning and afternoon business session, which disposed of routine business, were held on Friday. Three important new committees were approved for appointment by the president for expanding the personnel, influence and value of the academy to the members and to the state. These are: The Committee on the Promoting of Membership and the Activities of the Academy; the Committee on Research and the Publications Committee, an editorial board which is to assist the editor in furthering the quality of publications in the journal.

SEPTIMA C. SMITH

UNIVERSITY OF ALABAMA

# SPECIAL ARTICLES

## ISOLATION FROM BEEF PANCREAS OF A CRYSTALLINE PROTEIN POSSESSING RIBONUCLEASE ACTIVITY

A CRYSTALLINE protein which acts as a powerful digestive enzyme for yeast nucleic acid has been isolated from fresh beef pancreas. The digestion of the acid is accompanied by little, if any, release of inorganic phosphorus. The split products, unlike the undigested yeast nucleic acid, are not precipitable with glacial acetic acid or in 0.5 M hydrochloric acid. The products of digestion readily diffuse through collodion or Cellophane membranes that are impermeable for the undigested yeast nucleic acid. The nuclease activity of the crystalline protein is only very slowly diminished when boiled at pH 2.0. Boiling at pH 5.0 or higher brings about a gradual denaturation of the protein with a corresponding percentage loss of nuclease activity.

The nuclease activity of the new crystalline protein appears to correspond to the thermostable pancreatic nuclease activity described first by Jones[1] and later confirmed by Dubos,[2] Dubos and Thompson[3]

[1] W. Jones, *Am. Jour. Physiol.*, 52: 203, 1920.

[2] R. J. Dubos, SCIENCE, 85: 549, 1937. Dr. Dubos kindly tested the effect of the new crystalline material on the staining characteristic of two strains of Pneumococcus (heat killed). He found "that their staining characteristics are altered after a few hours incubation"; like the material which he described,[3] the new crystalline protein "decreases the affinity of the bacterial cells for basic dyes" (personal communication from Dr. Dubos).

[3] R. J. Dubos and R. H. S. Thompson, *Jour. Biol. Chem.*, 124: 501, 1938.

and Schmidt and Levene.[4] The latter authors considered the thermostable pancreatic nuclease to have only a depolymerizing effect on nucleic acid without the production of Cellophane dialyzable products such as mononucleotides. Hence they named the enzyme "ribonucleodepolymerase." However, as mentioned before, the split products formed from yeast nucleic acid by the new crystalline protein were found to diffuse readily through collodion and Cellophane membranes; hence the more general term "ribonuclease" has been provisionally retained for this crystalline protein until more definite information becomes available about the chemical nature of the process.

The procedure for the isolation of the crystalline protein follows: Fresh beef pancreas is extracted with cold 0.25 N sulfuric acid, as described in the publications on the isolation of chymotrypsinogen and trypsinogen.[5] The acid extract is brought to 0.7 saturation with solid ammonium sulfate and filtered. The filtrate is then brought to 0.8 saturation with more ammonium sulfate and is refiltered with suction.

*Crystallization:* 10 gm of the semi-dry precipitate is dissolved in about 10 ml of water. The solution is filtered with the aid of about 0.5 gm of Standard Super-Cel (Celite Corporation) through soft filter paper on a small Büchner funnel; the residue on the paper is washed with water. The combined filtrate and washings are brought to a final volume of 20 ml. Saturated ammonium sulfate is then added slowly with stirring until a very faint turbidity appears. The pH of the solution is adjusted first to about pH 5.0 (brick red color with 0.01 per cent. methyl red solution on test plate) with the aid of a few drops of 1.0 N sodium hydroxide and then to pH 4.2 (orange color with 0.01 per cent. methyl orange) by means of 1.0 N sulfuric acid. The solution is allowed to stand at about 20° C. An amorphous precipitate rapidly forms. This changes within one or two days into a mass of fine needles or aggregates of long thin plates. The crystals are filtered after 2 or 3 days. The filtrate on further addition of saturated ammonium sulfate yields more crystals. The recrystallization is performed by adding saturated ammonium sulfate to an aqueous solution of the crystals until a very faint turbidity appears.

The crystalline material contains about 16 per cent. total nitrogen; 7 per cent. of the total nitrogen is free amino nitrogen. It does not diffuse through ordinary collodion membranes to any significant amount.

A solution of the crystalline material is precipitated completely in 10 per cent. trichloracetic acid and incompletely in 2.5 per cent. trichloracetic acid. It gives the usual protein color tests. The tyrosine-tryptophane content is about 15 per cent. of the total dry weight. The ribonuclease activity of the material becomes constant after the second crystallization.

Further investigation of the physical and chemical properties of the new crystalline protein and of the chemical changes brought about by its nuclease activity is in progress.

M. KUNITZ

THE ROCKEFELLER INSTITUTE FOR
MEDICAL RESEARCH,
PRINCETON, N. J.

[4] G. Schmidt and P. A. Levene, *Jour. Biol. Chem.*, 126: 423, 1938.

[5] M. Kunitz and J. H. Northrop, SCIENCE, 78: 558, 1933; 80: 505, 1934; *Jour. Gen. Physiol.*, 18: 433, 1935; 19: 991, 1936.

## ISOSTERISM IN THE VITAMIN B COMPLEX

THE physiological effect of both nicotinic acid and thiamine is characterized by exceptional specificity. Numerous investigations in the recent literature show that even small changes in the loading of these two heterocycles greatly affect their physiological activity. It seemed of special interest, therefore, to investigate some isosters of these two vitamins.

The concept of isosterism as proposed by Grimm[1] and investigated by Erlenmeyer[2] and others has been applied with particular success to nuclear derivatives where ring sulfur and an aromatic –CH=CH– group are mutually replaceable. According to them a 3-substituted pyridine compound is isosteric with a 5-substituted thiazole compound. This permits consideration of a relation between nicotinic acid and thiamin which has hitherto been unsuspected.

We have found that thiazole-5-carboxylic acid, isosteric with nicotinic acid,[3] stimulates the growth of dysentery bacilli on Koser's synthetic medium.[4] Its activity is of the order of .1 per cent. of that of nicotinic acid. Its activity in curing black tongue in dogs has been investigated to some extent, but the results have been inconclusive.

2-methyl-3-β-hydroxyethyl-N-[(2-methyl-6-amino-pyrimidyl-(5))-methyl]-pyridinium bromide hydrobromide isosteric with Vitamin $B_1$ hydrobromide has been synthesized by condensation of 2-methyl-3-β-hydroxyethyl pyridine with 2-methyl-5-bromomethyl-6-amino pyrimidine hydrobromide. 2-methyl-3-acetyl pyridine was obtained from 2-methyl-3-cyanopyridine by a Grignard reaction. Bromination of the ketone followed by hydrolysis and Clemmensen reduction yielded the new 2-methyl-3-hydroxyethyl pyridine (picrate M.P. 129° uncorr.). Fed to a series of rats with medium or acute polyneuritic symptoms the new condensation product shows Vitamin $B_1$ activity. The experimental data do not as yet permit exact quantita-

[1] *Naturw.*, 17: 535–40, 557–64, 1929.

[2] *Helv. Chim. Acta.*, 16: 733–8, 1933.

[3] Erlenmeyer, *Helv. Chim. Acta.*, 20: 204, 1937.

[4] *Jour. Infectious Diseases*, 62: 212, 1938.

tive evaluation and suggest possibilities of modified action.

Further experiments are in progress.

F. C. SCHMELKES

RESEARCH LABORATORY,
WALLACE AND TIERNAN PRODUCTS, INC.,
BELLEVILLE, N. J.

## A REVERSED ALDOL CONDENSATION

DURING the past years many steps in the mechanism of glycolysis in muscle as well as in yeast have been cleared up. One of the remaining questions is: What causes the disruption of the easily fermentable hexose diphosphate ("primaeres Veresterungsproduct" of Meyerhof, etc.), to form two triose phosphates? Another open question is the position of the phosphoric acid rests in this hexose diphosphate. I would like to record an observation made a few years ago which may throw some light on these questions. Further work (which I am unable to undertake) is necessary to test whether this is a true or a false light.

The splitting of the hexose carbon chain to form two trioses is, chemically speaking, the reversal of an aldol condensation (I). I could observe a similar breakdown of a carbon chain in the case of α-keto γ-acetoxy acids. When incubating α-keto γ-acetoxy valeric acid [(II: R-H)] at 37° with water, the thick oil slowly dissolved within a few days and pyruvic acid, acetic acid and acetaldehyde could be isolated and identified in form of derivatives. The next higher homologue [(II: R-$CH_3$)] gave the same decomposition, while aldol, acetaldol, β-acetoxybutyric

I II

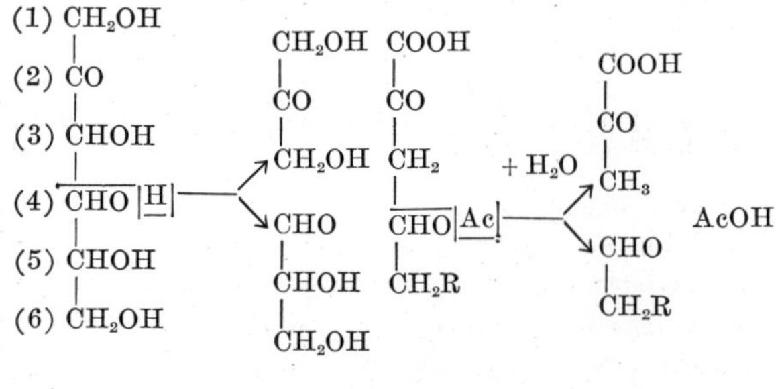


acid and β-acetoxy δ-keto-pentane were quite stable under these conditions. It appears that an acid pH of the solution or an acid group in the molecule is an essential condition for this breakdown, as well as an oxo-group in β-position to an esterified alcoholic one; this latter alcoholic group forms the new aldehyde group after the rupture of the chain. In analogy one is tempted to suppose that the readily fermentable hexose diphosphate ("primaeres Veresterungsproduct") is a ketose, carrying one phosphoric acid group in position 4. This might weaken the C-C-link between carbon atoms 3 and 4 sufficiently to cause a spontaneous formation of two trioses under our experimental conditions and the zymohexase might only be needed to catalyze this reaction to proceed with the necessary speed.

HEINZ FRAENKEL-CONRAT

## THE PRODUCTS OF THE CYCLIZING DEHYDRATION OF 1-BETA-PHENYLETHYLCYCLOHEXANOL-1 AND THE SYNTHESIS OF SPIROCYCLOHEXANE-1,1-INDANONE-3

BY a cyclizing dehydration of 1-*beta*-phenylethylcyclohexanol-1 with 85 per cent. sulfuric acid, Perlman, Davidson and Bogert[1] observed the simultaneous formation of octahydrophenanthrene and spirocyclohexane-1,1-indane.

Recently, Cook, Hewett and Lawrence,[2] and Cook, Hewett and Robinson,[3] by cold oxidation with chromic acid of a glacial acetic acid solution of the mixture of hydrocarbons resulting from the cyclization of *beta*-phenylethylcyclohexene-1, obtained a mixture of ketones, which they converted into the corresponding oximes, and then separated the latter by fractional crystallization. They thus isolated three oximes, which melted, respectively, at 187.5°, 175–177° and 124°. The first of these, they believed to be the oxime of spirocyclohexane-1,1-indanone, the second that of the *trans*-ketoöctahydrophenanthrene, and the third (m.p. 124°) that of its *cis*-isomer.

We have been occupied lately in the synthesis and study of the pure spirocyclohexane-1,1-indane, to learn more about its behavior when subjected to dehydrogenation reactions, and how its monacetyl derivative compares with those of the *cis*- and *trans*-octahydrophenanthrenes reported by Van de Kamp and Mosettig.[4]

In the course of this investigation, we synthesized the spirocyclohexane-1,1-indanone (VI), and found that its oxime melted at 137–137.8° (corr.). This wide divergence from the melting-point of 187.5° recorded by Cook *et al.* for their oxime, led us to reinvestigate the aforementioned hydrocarbon mixture, by a procedure essentially identical with that of our English colleagues with the result that we isolated the following oximes:

(1) An oxime, m.p. 187–188° (corr.).

(2) An oxime, m.p. 136.5–137° (corr.), which m.p. was not depressed when the compound was mixed with the oxime (m.p. 137–137.8°, corr.) of our synthetic spiroketone (VI). Each oxime was nitrated separately in cold concentrated sulfuric acid with powdered potas-

[1] Perlman, Davidson and Bogert, *Jour. Org. Chem.*, 1: 288, 300, 1936. See also Perlman and Bogert, *Jour. Am. Chem. Soc.*, 59: 2534, 1937.

[2] Cook, Hewett and Lawrence, *Jour. Chem. Soc.*, 1936, 71.

[3] Cook, Hewett and Robinson, *ibid.*, 1939, 168.

[4] Van de Kamp and Mosettig, *Jour. Am. Chem. Soc.*, 58: 1062, 1936.

sium nitrate, and the nitro oximes were then hydrolyzed with dilute sulfuric acid. The nitro ketones so obtained were identical and both melted at 192° (corr.). Further, direct nitration of our synthetic spiroketone (VI) gave the same nitro ketone (m.p. 192°, corr.).

(3) An oxime, m.p. 123–124° (corr.), which yielded a nitro ketone, m.p. 149–150° (corr.). This is evidently the same as the oxime, m.p. 124°, whose nitro ketone melted at 150–150.5°, and which Cook *et al.* suggested was probably the oxime of the *cis*-ketoöctahydrophenanthrene.

The only difference between our operations and those of Cook *et al.* was that our mixture of hydrocarbons was obtained by the action of 85 per cent. sulfuric acid upon the phenylethylcyclohexanol, while theirs was the result either of the action of phosphorus pentoxide upon the cyclohexanol, or of aluminum trichloride upon the corresponding cyclohexene.

The spirocyclohexane-1,1-indanone (VI) was synthesized by the following steps, in which "R" represents the group

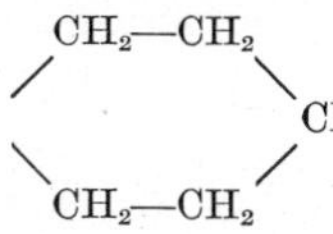

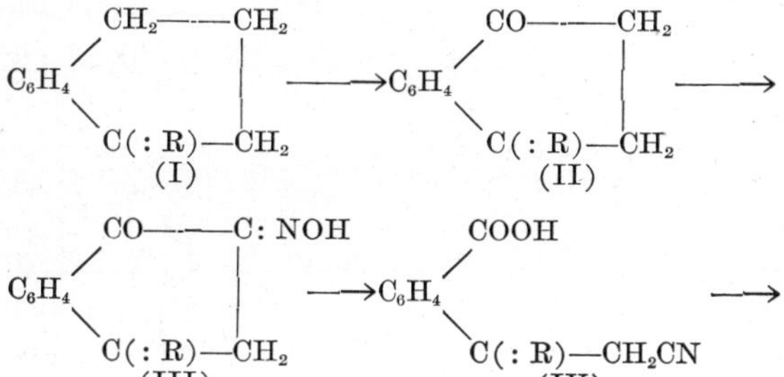

(I) (II) (III) (IV)

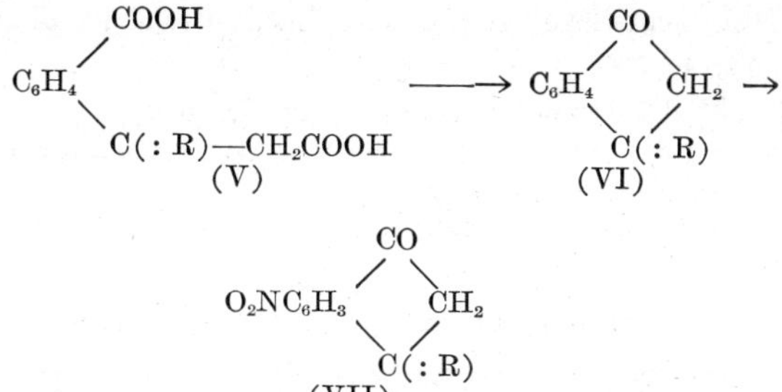

(V) (VI) (VII)

The pure spirocyclohexane-1,1-indanone (VI) was obtained as a white crystalline solid, m.p. 58–59° (corr.); oxime, m.p. 137–137.8° (corr.).

All products described in the foregoing gave on analysis figures substantiating the formulas assumed.

SUMMARY

(1) Spirocyclohexane-1,1-indanone (VI) has been found among the oxidation products of the hydrocarbon mixture which results when 1-*beta*-phenylethylcyclohexanol-1 is dehydrated, or when 1-*beta*-phenylethylcyclohexene is cyclized by aluminum trichloride, and its constitution has been proved by synthesis.

(2) Its oxime melts at 137–137.8° (corr.). The oxime of m.p. 187.5°, reported by Cook *et al.* therefore must be derived from some other ketone, perhaps the trans-ketoöctahydrophenanthrene, since we were unable to isolate any oxime of m.p. 177°, the figure which they reported for this compound.

MEYER LEVITZ
DAVID PERLMAN
MARSTON T. BOGERT
LABORATORIES OF ORGANIC CHEMISTRY,
COLUMBIA UNIVERSITY

# SCIENTIFIC APPARATUS AND LABORATORY METHODS

## AN X-RAY DENSITOMETER FOR MEASURING RELATIVE DENSITIES OF MUSCLE, BONE AND OTHER TISSUES

IN the studies of child growth and development undertaken by the Developmental Health Inquiry of the Associated Foundations it became evident that an objective method for measuring muscle, bone and other tissue densities would be a valuable aid. An x-ray densitometer has been designed and constructed for that purpose and is now in use.

Two other x-ray densitometers have recently been reported, one by P. B. Mack,[1] which is being used at Pennsylvania State College to determine the degree of mineralization of bone in a nutritional study and one by R. G. Bloch,[2] at Chicago University, designed for a study of tuberculous calcifications. Although the apparatus described here is similar in principle to these, its differences are the result of an attempt to obtain an optimum degree of accuracy combined with rapidity of operation and simplicity in interpretation of readings in a unified portable instrument.

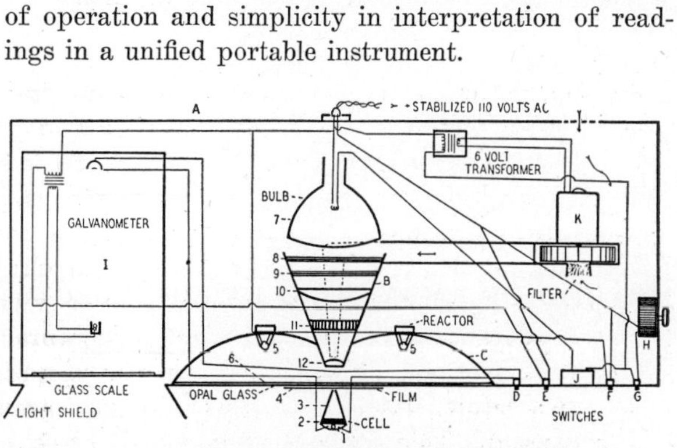


FIG. 1. Top view and circuit diagram.

As shown in Fig. 1, the various components of the

[1] P. B. Mack *et al.*, SCIENCE, 89: 467, 1939.

[2] R. G. Bloch *et al.*, *Am. Jour. of Roentgenol. and Rad. Therapy*, 41: 642–647, 1939.

instrument have been mounted in a special metal case (A) and only 110-volt alternating current is required.

The light source (7) for density measurement is centered in a new type vertical x-ray illuminator (C). Controls (D, E, F, G and H) are grouped on the right-hand panel, and the galvanometer (I) is in the same case to the left. A vertical arm (1) mounting a photo-E.M.F. cell (2) for measuring the light transmitted by any square mm area of film is hinged to turn out of the way while the illuminator is used for other purposes. A brass cone (3) with its interior surface chromium-plated and a 1 mm circular opening at the apex is fitted over the cell. The film (4) is held in place by hinged rubber-tipped arms and can be moved freely to place any desired portion under the cone aperture for density measurement. In the new x-ray illuminator mentioned above, two 18-inch tubular fluorescent bulbs (5) in the special reflector (C) provide a cold blue light for the flashed opal glass (6).

A 150-watt floodlight bulb (7) in the optical system is directed toward the large end of an aluminum cone (B) which contains two glass filters (8, 9), two condensing lenses (10, 12) and a disc of lucite (11), to project an intense spot of cool monochromatic light on the opal glass. A rheostat (H) and voltmeter (J) in the bulb circuit provide a control for intensity of the spot, and a voltage regulator is employed to reduce line voltage variations to $\pm 1$ per cent. at all values. Heat generated by the bulb in the optical system is dissipated by well-directed streams of filtered air from a rotary fan (K), thus keeping the temperature rise at the film to 9° C. above room temperature under the most intense light. Cell output current is registered on the sensitive portable galvanometer (I) of reflected-beam, enclosed-spotlite type.

A calibration table has been made which permits relative tissue density values, based on absolute film densities, to be noted at a glance for each millimeter of galvanometer deflection. Effects of variations in exposure time, developing and emulsion are suppressed by subtracting the reading for a standard film area from each other reading on that film. The total range of the instrument in units of film density is from 0.3 to 3.0, which includes all the x-ray films in our files.

HUGH E. WEBBER

LABORATORY OF ANATOMY AND
ASSOCIATED FOUNDATIONS,
WESTERN RESERVE UNIVERSITY

## METHOD OF EMBALMING LARGE INSECTS[1]

ANY one who has mounted numbers of grasshoppers or other large insects appreciates the difficulties encountered in drying the specimens without deterioration, discoloration or destruction by the larvae of flies.

[1] Contribution No. 205 from the Department of Zoology, University of Oklahoma, Norman.

The following technique was devised by the writer to improve the quality of dried insect specimens by eliminating the difficulties mentioned above. Although the method is original as far as the writer is concerned, others may have suggested similar procedures.

An embalming fluid is prepared as follows:

60 ccs of toluene (or xylene)
25 ccs of tertiary butyl alcohol
15 ccs of ethyl alcohol
5 grams phenol
20 grams paradichlorbenzene
10 drops of balsam in xylene as used in microtechnique

Mix the ingredients in the order named.

The fresh specimen is injected by inserting the needle of a hypodermic syringe in a posterior abdominal segment and running it forward to or into the head, then slowly withdrawing the needle while injecting the fluid. Care should be taken not to force too much fluid into the body cavity at once, as the abdominal segments may be ruptured. After injection, lay the specimen aside a few moments, then pin it in position on a drying board and place in an open place for twenty-four or more hours.

The writer has found that the largest grasshoppers will ordinarily dry in less than forty-eight hours following this treatment. No color changes occur in the injected specimens.

The fluid may also be used as a preservative without injection by merely dropping the specimens into a jar and covering with the liquid. Green-colored grasshoppers bleach somewhat if stored in the fluid. I have other specimens which were stored in the fluid for over a year, then dried, which show very little color change.

Museum pests, mice and flies are effectively repelled by this treatment.

CHARLES CLINTON SMITH

UNIVERSITY OF OKLAHOMA

## BOOKS RECEIVED

ANDERSON, ARTHUR K. *Essentials of Physiological Chemistry.* Second edition. Pp. ix + 323. 36 figures. Wiley. $2.75.

CLEMENTS, F. E. and V. E. SHELFORD. *Bio-ecology; A Correlation of the Fields of Plant and Animal Ecology.* Pp. vi + 425. 85 figures. Wiley. $4.50.

EGGELING, W. J. and C. M. HARRIS. *Forest Trees and Timbers of the British Empire; Vol. IV, Fifteen Uganda Timbers.* Pp. 120. 15 figures. 16 plates. Oxford University Press. $2.50.

HUXLEY, JULIAN. *The Living Thoughts of Darwin.* Pp. 151. Longmans, Green. $1.00.

KROGH, AUGUST. *Osmotic Regulation in Aquatic Animals.* Pp. 242. 54 figures. Cambridge University Press, Macmillan. $4.00.

LEMON, HARVEY B. and FITZ-HUGH MARSHALL. *The Demonstration Laboratory of Physics at the University of Chicago.* Pp. 127. 10 figures. 26 plates. University of Chicago Press. $1.50.

PRESSEY, SIDNEY L., J. ELLIOTT JANNEY and RAYMOND G. KUHLEN. *Life; A Psychological Survey.* Pp. xxxiii + 654. 105 figures. Harper. $2.50.

SCIENCE

VOL. 90 FRIDAY, AUGUST 11, 1939 No. 2328

*The American Association for the Advancement of Science:*
*Darwinian Ethics and Its Practical Applications:* DR. S. J. HOLMES 117
*The Stanford University Meeting of the Pacific Division:* PROFESSOR J. MURRAY LUCK 123
*Scientific Events:*
*Exhibits at the British Natural History Museum; The Byrd Antarctic Expedition; Preliminary Program of the Dundee Meeting of the British Association; The Boston Meeting of the American Chemical Society. Recent Deaths and Memorials* 131
*Scientific Notes and News* 134
*Discussion:*
*The Correlation between Ionization in the Ionosphere and Sun-Spot Numbers:* DR. FRED L. MOHLER. *A Whale Shark in the Hawaiian Islands:* DR. E. W. GUDGER. *Toxicity of the Sodium Salt of Dinitro-o-Cresol to Venturia inaequalis:* PROFESSOR G. W. KEITT. *Seeds for the Study of Root and Root-hair Structure in Botanical Laboratories:* DR. JOSEPH KRAMER 137
*Special Articles:*
*Action of Ketene on the Pituitary Lactogenic Hormone:* DR. CHOH HAO LI, DR. MIRIAM E. SIMPSON and DR. HERBERT M. EVANS. *The Effect of Cocarboxylase upon Metabolism and Neuro-psychiatric Phenomena in Pellagrins with Beriberi:* DR. T. D. SPIES and OTHERS. *Evidence for the Existence of a Respiratory Neurohormone:* PROFESSOR THEODORE KOPPANYI and CHARLES R. LINEGAR. *The Reducing Groups of Egg Albumin:* DR. M. L. ANSON 140
*Scientific Apparatus and Laboratory Methods:*
*An Improved Type of Ketene Generator:* DR. CHOH HAO LI. *A Simple and Efficient Precipitate Dryer:* ARNOLD LOWMAN. *Turntable for Exercising Rats:* DR. EDMOND J. FARRIS and GUSTAV ENGVALL 143
*Science News* 6

SCIENCE: A Weekly Journal devoted to the Advancement of Science, edited by J. MCKEEN CATTELL and published every Friday by

THE SCIENCE PRESS
New York City: Grand Central Terminal
Lancaster, Pa. Garrison, N. Y.
Annual Subscription, $6.00 Single Copies, 15 Cts.

SCIENCE is the official organ of the American Association for the Advancement of Science. Information regarding membership in the Association may be secured from the office of the permanent secretary in the Smithsonian Institution Building, Washington, D. C.

# THE AMERICAN ASSOCIATION FOR THE ADVANCEMENT OF SCIENCE

## DARWINIAN ETHICS AND ITS PRACTICAL APPLICATIONS[1]

By Dr. S. J. HOLMES
PROFESSOR OF ZOOLOGY AT THE UNIVERSITY OF CALIFORNIA

IT not infrequently happens that when one is called upon to deliver a presidential address he chooses a subject quite outside his own field of competence. This procedure has its dangers, of course, especially for the naive and unwary. In extenuation of my own intrepidity in venturing to discuss Darwinian ethics I may explain that in spite of the extensive literature which this subject has called forth it has rarely received adequate treatment and is not infrequently grossly misrepresented. Few people who accept the Darwinian theory of evolution realize its far-reaching import, especially in the social sciences. Sir Arthur Keith has remarked that "even our leading biologists and masters of history are evolutionists only from the lips outwards." The same statement is even more applicable to writers on ethics. Although there has been a number of relatively scholarly discussions of Darwin's views, in most books on morals the Darwinian standpoint is presented, if at all, in a few words, followed by a more elaborate criticism of the ethics of Spencer, which has commonly been treated as typifying the ethics of evolution. The subject has now lost its novelty. Ethics is still closely affiliated with metaphysics and theology, and Darwin,

[1] Presidential address before the Western Division of the American Association for the Advancement of Science, Stanford University, June 27, 1939.

having been assigned to his proper little niche, is passed by with little appreciation of the real extent of his contribution.

Darwin's views on ethics are a logical outgrowth of his theory of the causes of evolution. Although this theory has encountered no dearth of adverse criticism, I think I am justified in saying that its essential features are now more widely accepted than at any previous stage of its history. Certainly no other theory has succeeded in approaching the status of a formidable rival. If we assume that this theory is correct and carry it out consistently in all its implications, where will it lead us in the field of ethics? On this assumption we, like the lower animals, owe our native endowments of mind and body to the preservation of favorable variations in the struggle for existence. Our explanation of how we came to be constituted as we are falls into the same general formula as our explanation of the origin of a tough hide or sharp teeth. These latter characteristics are obviously very useful adjuncts to survival in this world of strife, and natural selection would seem to be peculiarly suited to afford a naturalistic explanation of their origin. But the attempts to explain man, with his superior intelligence, his high sense of duty and his capacity for esthetic appreciation and religious feeling as the outcome of the same process of selective survival naturally aroused strenuous opposition. The co-discoverer of the principle of natural selection, Alfred Russell Wallace, who was more of a natural selectionist than Darwin in relation to most evolutionary problems, stopped short of applying the theory of natural selection to explain the distinctive endowments of man. A similar position is held by many philosophers and liberal-minded theologians and by the more enlightened leaders of Catholic thought who accept the doctrine of evolution. But Darwin, who had become pretty much emancipated from all theological prepossessions when he wrote the "Descent of Man," was of a different cast of mind. In the "Origin of Species" he said almost nothing in regard to the application of evolution to the human species, beyond the remark that "light will be thrown upon the origin of man and his history." But it was this very aspect of Darwin's theory that made the strongest impression upon people in general, who were much more concerned with their own origin and what this might imply than they were with speculations on the origin of species.

The "Descent of Man" formed an original and very apposite sequel to the "Origin of Species" because it afforded the opportunity to round out the general doctrine and to show its important bearing on human psychology and the social sciences. Aside from that part of the work dealing with sexual selection, the "Descent of Man" is devoted to setting forth the evidence from morphology, embryology, etc., indicating the descent of man from animals resembling the apes, to showing that the human intelligence differs from animal intelligence only in degree instead of in kind, and that morality, and even religion do not imply the possession of unique endowments but are outgrowths of man's superior intellectual development and the social instincts and emotions which man shares to a certain extent with the higher mammals. In the "Descent of Man" Darwin ventured upon relatively unfamiliar territory when he discussed the moral sense and the standard of ethical conduct. Traditionally, the field of ethics had been appropriated almost exclusively by theologians and philosophers. Darwin, who never concerned himself with the subtleties of metaphysics, approached the subject apologetically, with the remark that the moral sense "has been discussed by many writers of consummate ability and my sole excuse for touching on it is the impossibility of here passing it over; and because, so far as I know, no one has approached it exclusively from the side of natural history." Only as a naturalist, therefore, did Darwin presume to touch upon the great problems of morals, and he did so for the simple reason that it lay across his path. If man is, as Spencer states, organically moral, Darwin's theory must be able to explain how he came to be so. A thoroughgoing Darwinian can hardly afford to admit the existence of entirely unique endowments that do not have at least their roots in more primitive forms of life.

Social life in animals is possible only on the basis of a certain degree of altruism. As Zell has shown in his work on "Morale in die Tierwelt," animals have a sort of moral life which in its fundamental features is much like our own. Man is a social animal, and because of this fact he is a moral animal.

> Any animal whatever [says Darwin] endowed with well-marked social instincts, the parental and filial affections being here included, would inevitably acquire a moral sense or conscience as soon as his intellectual powers had become as well or nearly as well developed as in man . . . the moral sense follows, firstly, from the enduring and ever-present nature of the social instincts; secondly, from man's appreciation of the approbation and disapprobation of his fellows; and thirdly, from the high activity of his mental faculties, with past impressions extremely vivid. . . . Owing to this condition of mind, man can not avoid looking both backwards and forwards, and comparing past impressions. Hence after some temporary desire or passion has mastered his social instincts, he reflects and compares the now weakened impression of such past impulses with the ever-present social instincts; and he then feels that sense of dissatisfaction which all unsatisfied instincts leave behind them, he therefore resolves to act differently for the future—and this is conscience.

This view of the origin and nature of conscience, here sketched in merest outline, was utterly at variance with the prevailing notions of the time. Conscience has always proven to be a very troublesome faculty for the moralists anyway. The recent searching analysis by T. V. Smith in his volume "Beyond Conscience" has effectually disposed of most of the attempts to justify conscience as a dependable guide to good conduct. If we grant that conscience always means well, we must remark that it has often approved the burning of witches and heretics, and countless other foolish and wicked actions. Apparently there is no atrocity or baseness that it will not condone if it is subjected to the right sort of preliminary education. No one, except perhaps Nietzsche and his followers, would deny that conscience, despite its obvious shortcomings, is a very valuable if not indispensable aid to decent living in an organized society.

That conscience is not infallible when it might be expected to be according to many theories of its nature and origin has sorely perplexed moral philosophers for ages. But the annoying imperfections and inconsistencies of this unreasonable faculty are not at all disturbing to one who considers it purely from the standpoint of natural history. When the Darwinian looks on the organic world he expects to find adaptation, at least in a broad and general way, but not perfection. He is as much pleased with a vestigial eye or a useless ear muscle as he is with a remarkable case of protective coloration. They are all grist for his mill, provided that their origin may plausibly be interpreted according to the principle of natural selection. A conscience that is always right would fill the Darwinian with dismay.

It is evident that conscience is no single discrete faculty or organ of the mind, but a general term for a class of intellectual and emotional reactions. Its emotional components impel us to follow what we judge to be right, and our judgments on this score are usually determined by the mores of our associates. Its voice is the voice of the group or, as Clifford has called it, the tribal self. We are social animals endowed with social instincts which make us sensitive to the esteem or disregard of our fellows, and with sufficient intelligence to reflect upon our acts and to judge them in accordance with prevailing standards. Hence, according to Darwin, we are moral animals and have a conscience which is on the whole a fair though far from perfect guide to the kind of conduct which meets with moral approval.

Unquestionably, one of the greatest contributions of Darwinism to the social sciences is the light which it throws on the constitution of human nature. The traditional explanation prevailing in Darwin's time was that man is as he is because he was so created, although his original divine image was sadly marred as a result of the fall and the continued machinations of Satan and his cohorts of evil spirits. From the moral standpoint man is an exceedingly variable animal. He is at once courageous and cowardly, kindly and cruel, honorable and deceitful, proud and humble, generous and grasping, just and partial. He is capable of attaining sublime heights of moral excellence, and, on the other hand, there is no depth of infamy and degradation to which he will not descend. We need not concern ourselves with the theological interpretations of these remarkable diversities of character. Devils, evil spirits, principles of evil and doctrines of total depravity, notwithstanding the high ability and profound learning of many of their apologists, we may dismiss without further comment. The efforts of the various proponents of the experience philosophy to explain the development of mind and character have proceeded along much more scientific lines, but their failure is now commonly recognized. It is a noteworthy fact that up to the time of Darwin we had no scientific explanation of human nature that was worth a rap. The history of human thought is strewn with interpretations of human nature of the most artificial and wooden description. Man has never understood man, and the worst feature of this failure is that his misunderstandings have been fraught with incalculable evils throughout the course of human history. Flogging the insane and keeping them chained in filthy dungeons, the barbarous treatment of criminals and the petty cruelties inflicted in the discipline of children are among the many evils growing out of mistaken views of the nature of man which are gradually giving way to a more rational understanding. With a more scientific interpretation of man the cruelties of witchcraft, the horrors of religious persecution and the multitudinous barbarous practices that have been the outgrowth of superstition would not have occurred. Human history has emphasized the tremendous importance of the maxim, "Know thyself." For ages man has occupied the unfortunate position of a sort of meeting ground between the natural and the supernatural. Through sorcery and other magic powers he might influence others for good or for ill, and demoniacal possession accounted for disease. The demons are not yet all exorcized by the growing light of science, but our progress toward a rational understanding of the human animal has been among the most potent influences in humanizing man's treatment of his fellow man.

In organized society a large part of our activities consists in dealing with other people. Obviously, the better we understand our fellow creatures the better we should be able to deal with them effectively. It is only within the past two or three generations that educators have discovered that it is necessary to understand children in order to educate them in the proper way. The natural aptitudes, instincts and interests of the child were largely disregarded and he was put through a regimen which was prescribed on *a priori* grounds, and frequent flogging was resorted to in order to supply an adequate motive for serious application. In dealing with criminals, delinquents and the insane, as well as with normal human beings, we need not merely good intentions but insight and understanding. Hence, any theory that throws a flood of light upon the nature of man and the whys and wherefores of human behavior can not fail to have a salutary influence on all our efforts at moral reform.

The Darwinian theory, I believe, does just this. One who accepts the Darwinian theory of natural selection and applies it consistently has, so to speak, his interpretation of human nature cut out for him. Man's traits, in so far as these are a part of his inheritance, owe their origin and biological meaning to their survival value. In fact, the Darwinian theory could not well account for the evolution of any other kind of creature. All the natural traits and impulses of human beings must therefore be fundamentally good if we consider the good as the biologically useful. Cruelty, selfishness, lust, cowardice and deceit are normal ingredients of human nature which have their useful role in the struggle for existence. Intrinsically they are all virtues. It is only their excess or their exercise under the wrong conditions that justly incurs our moral disapproval. For the Darwinian the categorical distinctions between good and bad take on a new meaning. His standpoint is, in Nietzschean phraseology, "beyond good and evil." The old distinctions between sins, venial or otherwise, and ordinary wrong acts melt away. Immutable principles of good and evil go by the board. They are the inventions of philosophers and have no place in reality. What we call bad conduct is usually the result of maladjusted egoistic impulses that are not properly subordinated to the needs of social life. Our good conduct, on the other hand, commonly springs from social impulses which the Darwinian would explain as the result of group selection. As expressed by a thoroughgoing Darwinian, Professor Karl Pearson:

> The struggle among primitive men of tribe against tribe evolved the social instinct. The tribe with the greater social feeling survived; we have to thank the struggle for existence for first making man gregarious and then intensifying, stage by stage, the social feeling. Such is the scientific account of the origin of our social instincts; and if you come to analyze it, such is the origin of what we term morality; morality is only the developed form of the tribal habit, the custom of acting in a certain way toward our fellow beings, upon which the very safety of the tribe originally depended.

If this gives us a true natural history of our moral sense, we should not be perplexed by the great diversity of character exhibited by different men. Man, as we should expect in the light of his origin, is no angel; neither can he be accused of total depravity in the absence of divine grace. He is loyal and sympathetic toward his own, hostile to the stranger, amenable to leadership and subordination and willing on occasion to sacrifice his own welfare in the interest of his group. At times he is cruel, revengeful, cowardly or otherwise a pliant creature of his purely self-regarding impulses. In the eternal conflict between egoism and altruism he obeys now the one and now the other kind of urge. Human nature bears the imprint of having been molded in the stern school of strife. On the whole it is just about what we would expect it to be in the light of its method of evolution.

If we wish to gain a proper insight into the native and uncamouflaged impulses of human beings there is perhaps no more instructive procedure than to study the group behavior of chimpanzees. There you will find the mutual sympathy, the group pugnacity, the egoism and the altruism which are so curiously blended in man. They are more crudely exhibited, to be sure, but they have a more adequate adjustment to the needs of the group.

"Nature," says William James, "implants contrary impulses to act in many classes of things and leaves it to slight alterations of the conditions of the individual case to decide which impulses shall carry the day." It is this endowment of varied and seemingly contradictory traits that accounts largely for the remarkable diversity of human character to which I have alluded. Basically, most of us have the same natural impulses. Our differences of character, like our differences of bodily structure, are mainly matters of emphasis. If the purely egoistic impulses are grossly hypertrophied we may become highly undesirable members of society. On the other hand, normally virtuous tendencies may become vices if carried to excess. After all, there is much wisdom in Aristotle's doctrine of the Golden Mean.

We sublimated simians have no reason to be ashamed of our origin. We owe to our more primitively moral ancestors our good as well as our bad traits. Our nature is much less closely adapted to the environment in which we live, for reasons very easy to understand. We owe much more than any lower animal to the influences of our environment. This environment has changed greatly in the last few thousand years. Human nature seems to have been developed for life in small, quarrelsome clans which afford ample opportunity for the exercise of the complementary traits of mutual aid and group pugnacity. The complex civilization which has appeared in recent times has developed so rapidly that the innate endowments of man have not kept pace with environmental changes. We shall probably be more and more concerned with problems arising out of the maladaptiveness of human nature to its conditions of life. For the proper solution of these problems, therefore, a really scientific understanding of human nature will become more and more imperative.

The influence of Darwin upon ethics consisted not only in giving us a new standpoint in relation to human nature, including man's moral sense, but in affording a standard of right and wrong which, if not necessarily associated with the doctrine of natural selection, is a perfectly logical and consistent conclusion from Darwinian principles. The proper standard of conduct is a subject upon which moralists have furnished us with a most varied assortment of theories. Throughout the recorded history of mankind most peoples have lived under moral codes which were assumed to owe their origin and binding force to supernatural authority. A perfectly typical example of such a system is furnished by the ancient Hebrews, who were instructed concerning right and wrong by special revelations from Jehovah, who not only furnished them with the Ten Commandments, but, through the inspired authors of Leviticus and Deuteronomy, with meticulous instructions as to what they should and should not eat and the fine points of conducting sacrifices. For the Hebrew being good consisted in acting according to the revealed code, and sin was disobedience. When our original parents ate the forbidden fruit, when all the inhabitants of the earth, with the exception of Noah and his immediate family, departed from ways of righteousness, when the inhabitants of Sodom and Gomorrah were given over to their scandalous ways and when the unfortunate Onan ventured on the first recorded experiment in contraception, an outraged Jehovah visited upon them the full measure of his wrath. It behooved the faithful Hebrew to walk in the ways of the Lord. That was morality.

The ethical teachings of Jesus, though greatly refined and humanized as compared with those of the Jews in their semi-barbaric period, were still authoritarian in character. Amid the various modifications of ethical doctrine that had grown up during the history of Christianity, the authoritarian basis of morals, in one form or another, has remained one of its most stable features. In the Roman Catholic church this doctrine has come to be more deeply intrenched, inasmuch as this body has definitely claimed to be the final court of appeal on all questions of morals as well as religion. Here we have perhaps the sharpest and most vital issue that remains between science and theology. Catholicism purports to speak on matters of morals with a voice from which there is no appeal. Questions of astronomy have long since been passed over to the astronomers. The healing art, once held to be the peculiar province of the priest, is now generally, but by no means exclusively, conceded to be the legitimate occupation of the physician. But in the opinion of a large part of even the educated public the field of morals belongs not to the scientist but to the man of God. Supernaturalism in morals is still very much alive. Not only does it continue to enjoin many observances of no intrinsic moral significance, but it is very influential in determining attitudes on many questions of real importance. There is, of course, a broad basis of agreement in practically all moral codes. Murder, lying, stealing and adultery are all condemned in almost every list of forbidden acts, but of course no code can cover all the varied situations in which questions of right and wrong may arise. There are many problems of morals upon which people differ sharply. Among these we may mention the justification of divorce, birth control and euthanasia. When we look into the alignment of opinion on these controverted questions we find that it is determined largely by whether or not the individual forms his moral judgments on the basis of authority or upon considerations of human welfare. There is no gainsaying the fact that whether our moral judgments are determined by authority, the greatest happiness principle, the categorical imperative, some form of self-realization or the Darwinian criterion of rightness may determine our attitude on many important moral problems.

Where differences of opinion as to the morality of an act arise from differences in criteria by which the act is judged, discussion comes to an *impasse*. If agreement is reached it is only when both parties come to view the act from a common standpoint, such as the promotion of human welfare, which they both adopt in principle, whether consciously or not. In our present age notions about the basis of morals vary greatly. The rank and file of people still base their conduct on some form of authoritarian ethics, and the authority is coming to have less and less hold upon them. Many drift along with no clearly defined moral standpoint, being guided by their natural impulses under the restraining influence of law and custom. For the most part they get along fairly well. After all, social instinct and social traditions are much more effective than moral philosophy in keeping people in the straight and narrow path.

The common criticism directed against standards of conduct is that their practical application would lead to very undesirable consequences. Evolutionary ethics, especially Darwinian ethics, has been denounced as subversive of everything that humanity has considered most worthy. Darwinism consistently applied would measure goodness in terms of survival value. Darwin never developed this phase of his doctrine fully, but his view is indicated by the following remark made in discussing general happiness as a standard of conduct: "The term general good may be defined as the rearing of the greatest number of individuals in full vigor and health, with all their faculties perfect, under the conditions to which they are subjected. As the social instincts, both of man and the lower animals, have no doubt been developed by nearly the same steps, it would be advisable, if found practicable, to use the same definition in both cases, and to take as the standard the general good or welfare of the community rather than the general happiness." According to this viewpoint, the end of the moral life, speaking teleologically, is the same as the biological life of the organism. Morality becomes just one phase of the adjustment of the organism to its conditions of existence. As a good body is one which runs smoothly and efficiently in the maintenance of its vital functions, so a good man is one whose conduct not only maintains his own life on an efficient plane, but conduces to the enhancement of the life of his social group. In making the preservation and perpetuation of life the true function of morals, as it is a function of life itself, Darwinism affiliates ethics more closely with the biological sciences. Moral life is the expression in human conduct of true and effective living. Through being moral we have life, and have it more abundantly.

Of course, human beings are free to choose any criterion of conduct they please and to order their lives accordingly. There may be a number of perfectly justifiable ends of moral endeavor. The Darwinian, however, would maintain that, wittingly or not, people have been led to approve of conduct that makes for survival and to condemn conduct that is socially destructive. As Walter Bagehot remarks in his "Physics and Politics," "the moral groups cohere and therefore prevail." Tribes having the most effective codes have continually been selected in the competition of opposing groups. Peoples may believe that their moral customs derive from a supernatural source, but one potent reason for their adoption is their conduciveness to survival. The Darwinian standard may be said, therefore, to be in a sense nature's own. If peoples depart too widely from the kind of conduct it prescribes, they are courting the fate of all ill-adjusted variations in the struggle for life.

The Darwinian would maintain that his standard makes explicit what is implicit in all codes in so far as their prescriptions are morally valid. Although peoples may ascribe the origin of their codes to the commands of their gods, or whatever else, the true cause for their development is their survival value. Whether or not we agree with Ritchie that "natural selection . . . is a perfectly adequate cause to account for the rise of morality," we must concede that it affords a plausible interpretation of the differences in the moral codes of peoples living under different conditions. Although there is a good deal of maladjustment in the moral customs of peoples, as there is elsewhere in organic nature, differences in moralities, as Westermarck has shown in his "History of Moral Ideas," are to a large extent explicable as an outgrowth of the varied environments to which a people must adjust itself.

In speaking of applying the concept of natural selection in the field of ethics I must here guard against a possible misinterpretation. The application of the principle of selection to interpret the adaptive modifications of moral codes does not compel one to assume that moral sentiments and, still less, the particular acts which are approved or condemned, are matters of biological inheritance. In social evolution tradition plays a role very similar to that of heredity. Complex sentiments as such are not transmitted through the germ-plasm, although they may rest upon a basis of instinctive components. Tribes with the best codes will tend to prevail, whatever be the method by which the more useful moral customs are handed on. Natural selection has made man a social animal as a result of his heredity. Selection, experience and social tradition have led him to adopt moral practices which favor survival.

There are many people who are very suspicious of Darwinian ethics and are disturbed over what might happen if we proceeded to order our conduct in accordance with its dictates. I think that we can assure ourselves that nothing very dire would happen, because to a large extent people order their lives according to its dictates now. They really approve honesty, courage, loyalty and benevolence because these qualities have led to greater fulness of life. Fundamentally, therefore, our ethics is Darwinian, whether we like it or not. It is only imperfectly so, however, and I venture to suggest that current moral practice might be considerably improved if it became more consciously and definitely regulated in terms of the Darwinian standard.

There are several ways in which the practical application of Darwinian principles would affect our conduct and our ideals. One can not imagine a Darwinian finding anything particularly heinous about eating meat on Friday or playing cards on Sunday. Neither, if smitten, would he be likely to turn the other cheek. On occasion he would feel quite justified in going to war. He would doubtless contend that conflict has played an important role in shaping the evolution of man, although if he followed Darwin and many of his adherents, he would point to the highly dysgenic effects of modern warfare. He would emphasize the importance of eugenics, both positive and negative, and all measures that make for healthful and wholesome life and the improvement of its adjustment to its environing conditions, material and social. For every ethics that seeks its sanctions in the welfare of mankind every moral problem is a scientific problem to be solved like other problems by the employment of scientific methods. For such a view-point ethics is not a field that can be sharply demarcated from other disciplines and made the province of priestly authority. As John Dewey remarks, "ethics is ineradicably empirical, not theological, nor metaphysical, nor mathematical. Since it directly concerns human nature everything that can be known of the human mind and body in physiology, medicine, anthropology, and psychology is pertinent to moral inquiry."

A scientific ethics would insist, as the Greeks did, upon the moral obligation of wisdom. One unfortunate influence of Christian ethics has been its tendency to divorce wisdom from morality. The good will alone is a very inadequate guide to good conduct. It is impossible to be really effectively good without being wise. There are circumstances under which practically all rules must be broken in order to lead the good life. Where different codes are followed in a community there is bound to be more or less conflict of moral aims. The people of Christian nations profess allegiance to a code which the exigencies of their life compel them to continually violate. The result is confusion and conflict and a constant incentive to hypocrisy.

In many ways the attempt to follow authoritarian ethics leads to conduct at variance with that which is dictated by considerations of human welfare. One of the most serious obstacles to several moral reforms is the blind adherence to moral codes that command unquestioning obedience. Were all questions of morality frankly recognized as scientific problems, much of the conflict I have mentioned would disappear. Many unsettled problems would of course remain, but by the applications of scientific methods they might finally be settled. It is only through becoming a true science that ethics can perform its greatest service. In this respect ethics is on precisely the same footing as medicine and other fields of applied science. Darwin, the great naturalist, in approaching ethics purely from the standpoint of natural history in the two famous chapters in his "Descent of Man," has contributed greatly toward making ethics scientific, and hence of greater value to mankind.

# THE STANFORD UNIVERSITY MEETING OF THE PACIFIC DIVISION

**Edited by Professor J. MURRAY LUCK**
SECRETARY

The twenty-third annual meeting of the Pacific Division, American Association for the Advancement of Science, and of seventeen associated societies was held at Stanford University, California, during the week of June 26, 1939.

The meetings may be considered noteworthy in several respects. They were characterized by a number of symposia of outstanding quality and were followed by a five-day symposium of fascinating interest on "The Cell and Protoplasm." Following upon this, in turn, was the sixteenth National Colloid Symposium, which brought to the university a third contingent of distinguished visitors. The results of such meetings can never be properly evaluated. The stimulus to scientific research is admittedly great, and the interest awakened within the layman in the contributions of science to the social order is, we suspect, more than transitory. The only index available for measuring the "success" of the meeting is to be found in the registration figures—a total of 882 for the divisional meetings alone. This is much greater than that of any previous meeting and may be compared with the registration total of 377 at the last Stanford University meeting (1924).

All the general sessions were held in the Memorial Theater and in Cubberley Hall—two new buildings provided with excellent auditoria and other facilities necessary for large meetings of this character. Guests were housed in Lagunita Court—a splendidly equipped dormitory which was placed in commission by the university only a few years ago. In every respect the material facilities were all that could be desired.

Local arrangements for the meeting were in the care of a committee consisting of S. B. Morris (*chairman*), Ernest R. Hilgard (*secretary*), Norris E. Bradbury, Eliot Blackwelder, Paul H. Kirkpatrick, Eliot Mears, George S. Parks, Templeton Peck, Gilbert M. Smith, Victor C. Twitty.

The first general session, which was held on the morning of June 27th, took the form of a symposium on "Radiation and Life." Four invited speakers participated. Since it is manifestly impossible to describe in detail the papers presented, it may be sufficient to list the titles and speakers: "Radiation," W. V. Houston, California Institute of Technology; "Radioactive Elements as Tracers in Metabolic Studies," John H. Lawrence, University of California; "Radiation and the Hereditary Mechanism," M. Delbruck, California Institute of Technology; "Medical Applications," Robert R. Newell, Stanford University Hospitals.

The afternoon of the same day was devoted to surveys of current research—a program which has been repeated annually by the division for many years. J. W. McBain, of Stanford University, reviewed a number of the recent advances in colloid chemistry. A. R. Davis, of the University of California, dealt with mineral metabolism in plants, and H. Borsook, of the California Institute of Technology, surveyed some of the recent contributions to knowledge in that lively field of research, biological oxidations and reductions. A paper in the field of psychology was contributed by J. W. Macfarlane, of the University of California, who discussed research on personality development.

The evenings of Tuesday, Wednesday and Thursday were given over to addresses of general interest to the visiting members as well as to the lay public. That of Tuesday evening by Professor S. J. Holmes, president of the Pacific Division, on "Darwinian Ethics and its Practical Applications" evoked a great deal of interest and much comment in the press because of its challenge to authoritarian concepts of right and wrong. On Wednesday evening Professor V. Gordon Childe, of the University of Edinburgh, presented an address on the neolithic economy in northwestern Europe—a subject in which he is a recognized authority. The concluding address of the series, delivered by Professor J. D. Bernal, of the University of London, consisted of a graphic description of the structure of protein molecules.

Several events of a social character were arranged for the entertainment of visiting members and guests. Mention should be made of the reception tendered by the university on Tuesday afternoon, a visit to several private gardens in the Palo Alto—Atherton region and a special concert by the Roth Quartette on Friday afternoon.

In addition to organized visits to the Ryan High-Voltage Laboratory and the Laboratory of Plant Biology, Carnegie Institution of Washington, attractive excursions were made to Lick Observatory on Mount Hamilton, the Radiation Laboratory of the University of California and the Hopkins Marine Station at Pacific Grove.

Meetings of the executive committee and of the council were held in the course of the week. Dr. Lewis M. Terman, professor of psychology at Stanford University, was elected to the presidency of the division for the ensuing year, and R. E. Clausen and J. Murray Luck were reelected vice-president and secretary-treasurer, respectively. Ian Campbell, of the California Institute of Technology, was elected to the executive committee in succession to W. V. Houston, who retires on completion of his term of office. E. O. Essig, of the University of California, and C. V. Taylor, of Stanford University, were elected to the council as members-at-large for the customary four-year term.

Announcement was made that the next meeting, national in character, will be at the University of Washington, Seattle, during the week of June 17, 1940.

## SESSIONS OF AFFILIATED SOCIETIES

Seventeen of the affiliated and associated societies participated in the meeting, and over 440 papers were presented. The reports of the various sessions follow.

### American Physical Society

(*Report by Paul Kirkpatrick*)

Sessions for the presentation of brief contributed research reports were held on Thursday, Friday and Saturday forenoons. These reports, fifty-seven in number, touched upon theoretical and experimental investigations in varied fields, with nuclear researches in the place of prominence.

Three symposia, concerned with applications of physics in the adjacent fields of astronomy, electrical engineering and biology, were presented at the afternoon sessions. On Wednesday afternoon the society met in joint symposium with the Astronomical Society of the Pacific to consider the phenomenon of limb darkening. Papers by C. D. Shane, Edison Pettit and A. B. Wyse on aspects of this problem were followed by a paper on the design and construction of the 60-inch cyclotron by E. M. McMillan. The symposium of Thursday afternoon presented aspects of the ultra-high frequency radio investigations in progress in the Stanford Physics Department. Papers by W. W. Hansen, D. L. Webster and S. F. Varian were accompanied by demonstrations of new devices (Rhumbatrons, Klystrons) applicable to communication. A symposium on methods and results of x-ray structure determination, held on Friday afternoon, was addressed by M. L. Huggins, J. D. Bernal and O. L. Sponsler, the first speaker defending the hypothesis of the existence of hydrogen bridges in crystals, and the succeeding ones discussing respectively the structures of plant virus particles and of the super-molecules of protein and cellulose existing in living organisms.

A dinner on Thursday evening, organized jointly by the American Physical Society and the Astronomical Society of the Pacific, was addressed by J. D. Bernal, who spoke of the social and human responsibilities of science.

### American Meteorological Society

(*Report by John A. Riley*)

The American Meteorological Society held five sessions, with twenty-eight papers on the program. About one hundred persons were present.

The first session on Wednesday morning was concerned primarily with the meteorological problems of the Pacific Ocean as related to the weather in the western United States and Alaska and to transpacific aviation. In the absence of Dr. Reichelderfer, chief of the Weather Bureau, Major E. H. Bowie gave a brief report on pending developments in meteorology, stressing the need for expansion and improvement of the vessel weather reporting service in the Pacific, with four complete reports daily. W. H. Clover spoke on the relation of meteorology to the operation of Pan American clippers across the Pacific; T. R. Reed discussed the relations between the general pressure field and the weather in California. "Occlusions on the Alaska Coast"' was the subject of A. B. Carpenter's paper.

The afternoon session was devoted to upper-air investigations and their application to forecasting and to aviation. A new field of observation and research has been opened by the use of the radiosonde, which now penetrates the stratosphere daily and transmits by radio data on the atmospheric conditions aloft for current use. A résumé of the first year of these observations at Oakland was presented by J. W. Smith and C. R. Elford. E. M. Vernon discussed a constant level synoptic chart based on free air data. John A. Day spoke on aviation wind forecasts for long hops over the Pacific, and C. L. Smalley demonstrated an instrument for rapid calculation of winds at flying levels from pressure and temperature fields and adaptable for use on charts of various size. Results of an investigation of cloud heights over the Plateau Region, referred to sea level, were reported by H. Dean Parry, of Salt Lake City.

A symposium on atmospheric radiation on Thursday morning consisted in the demonstration of instrumental equipment, theoretical studies and practical applications. L. W. K. Boelter, of the University of California, discussed the construction and operation of a sensitive yet inexpensive radiometer for use in measuring nocturnal and terrestrial radiation. C. Lorenzen, Jr., gave a report on some results obtained with the instrument in citrus orchards during the frost season. Walter M. Elsasser, of the California Institute of Technology, reviewed the theoretical considerations leading to a graphical method for the determination of radiative transfer. Edward M. Ashburn discussed the application of these results in computing the transfer of heat in the lower layers of the atmosphere in connection with summer stratus clouds on the California coast.

In the afternoon, N. E. Bradbury, of Stanford University, described the theory and practice of a continuously recording apparatus for the measurement of the density of atmospheric condensation nuclei; a report on the diurnal variation and vertical distribution of these nuclei was given by E. A. Yunker. The results of measurements of atmospheric charges with electric field recorders were presented by R. E. Holser, of the University of New Mexico. "Statistical Relationships of Seasonal Rainfall Records," by Charles P. Conroy, was followed by a report on varves and rock strata as recorders of cycles by Halpert P. Gillette.

During the last session, in "Melting Snow as a Flood Factor in the Sierra Nevada," E. H. Fletcher pointed out that, contrary to popular belief, the melting of snow by rain alone is a slow process and the presence of considerable snow on the ground acts as a damper in retarding a rapid run-off. C. P. Smith pointed out the need of accurate temperature forecasts for natural gas dispatching in California. Dean Blake spoke on the origin of tropical Pacific air in the Southwest, R. C. Counts on storm effects on tides in the Golden Gate and A. Breese on meteorological aspects of a historic disaster in Moscow. E. E. Eklund explained administration of the San Francisco Weather Bureau. The sessions closed with an illustrated talk on Alaskan and western mountains as climatic factors by L. H. Daingerfield.

### ASTRONOMICAL SOCIETY OF THE PACIFIC

*(Report by Gerard F. W. Mulders)*

A joint session was held with the American Physical Society on Wednesday afternoon, June 28, with an attendance of about eighty. C. D. Shane, University of California, gave an outline of the theory of limb-darkening for a star and discussed the importance of limb-darkening measurements as a means of determining the wave-length dependence of the continuous absorption coefficient. Edison Pettit, of the Mount Wilson Observatory, described measurements of the limb-darkening in the sun and in the stars, respectively.

E. M. McMillan, of the University of California, described the design and construction of the recently completed 60-inch cyclotron at Berkeley. This instrument, the largest of its kind in the world, is capable of producing deuterons with an energy of 16.5 million volts.

Sessions for papers were held on Thursday, June 29, with an attendance of about forty-five. Twenty papers from five different institutions were presented and several points of special interest were noted. J. H. Moore reported on a spectroscopic determination of the rotation period of Saturn, showing that this planet rotates more slowly at higher latitudes than it does near the equator, which is similar to the rotation of the sun. R. M. Petrie described three spectroscopic investigations at the Dominion Astrophysical Observatory, Victoria, B. C., by W. E. Harper, C. S. Beals and himself. A. H. Joy gave a summary of the behavior of variable stars of intermediate periods, which he divided into two distinct groups with periods of 88 and 111 days. The members of the first group usually have a G-type spectrum which changes considerably between minimum and maximum brightness, while the second group has a spectrum of class M which shows little change.

The absorption lines of neon, usually rather faint in stellar spectra, are very strong in Upsilon Sagitarii, as Paul W. Merrill showed, which must be due to a high neon content of this star. N. U. Mayall described the occurrence of emission lines of ionized oxygen in the spectra of a great number of extragalactic nebulae. Roscoe F. Sanford reported on observation of interstellar lines of sodium and calcium in the spectra of various stars. G. E. Kron reported on an extremely accurate photoelectric determination of the color of an eclipsing variable star.

Modifications of the Schmidt camera were discussed by W. H. Christie and Franklin B. Wright, an amateur astronomer. Sophia H. Levy described a determination of mean elements and perturbations by the Berkeley Tables for four minor planets, while Damon M. Beard gave a new orbit method, which he had applied to the recently discovered eleventh satellite of Jupiter.

W. F. Meyer, A. H. Joy and Gerard F. W. Mulders presided at the various sessions. Astronomers and physicists met informally at a joint dinner on Thursday evening, June 29, while an excursion to the Lick Observatory took place on Friday, June 30.

### Association of Pacific Coast Geographers

(*Report by H. F. Raup*)

The fifth annual meeting of the Association of Pacific Coast Geographers was held on Thursday and Friday, June 29 and 30. The first speaker to be introduced was John E. Kesseli, with a paper entitled, "The Origin of the Valley of June and Silver Lakes, Mono County, California." In his paper, Mr. Kesseli evaluated the several factors which have been responsible for the formation of the valley and the lakes. The second speaker, Walter A. Hackler, also dealt with physical aspects of the landscape. He showed many views of the widely publicized landslip near Sargent, California, and discussed the conditions under which the landslide occurred. J. O. M. Broek then gave a presentation of the demography of the California counties, with special emphasis placed upon the reasons for the decline of population and changes in economy of residents of the northern Coast Range counties. The present and past use of the North Branch of the Susquehanna River as a trans-Appalachian route of travel was discussed by H. F. Raup.

The afternoon session of June 28 began with an historical study of eighteenth and nineteenth century American geographers and their publications, by James F. Chamberlain. This was followed by a paper by Eliot G. Mears, "Some Locational Problems in British Industry," in which he treated of recent changes responsible for the location of British industry, in comparison with the traditional location factors such as fuel supply, markets, etc. Helen M. Strong, speaking as a guest of the association, gave an informal talk on the relationship between land use and geographical conditions in widely separated parts of the United States. She was followed by Willis H. Miller, who spoke on "Geography and State Planning," with special emphasis on California planning. The final paper of the session was presented by George C. Kimber, in which he advocated a wider use of geography in determining the political wishes and views of the people under a democratic form of government.

The annual dinner was held on June 29 with members present from many parts of the Pacific Coast, and one introduced guest, Dr. Pakstas, from Lithuania. The 1939–1940 officers, recently elected, were announced: *President,* Peveril Meigs, 3rd, of Chico State College; *Vice-President,* Forrest Shreve, of the Carnegie Institution Desert Laboratory, Tucson; *Secretary-Treasurer,* Frances M. Earle, University of Washington; *Editor,* Otis Freeman, Eastern Washington School of Education, Cheney. The address of the evening was given by the retiring president, John B. Leighly, of the University of California. His topic, "The Historical Background of Carl Ritter's Geographic Theory," was in part concerned with the relationship between the ideas of Ritter and Pestalozzi.

The concluding meeting on Friday, June 30, was addressed by J. W. Hoover, who showed many views of the terraced hills of southern Arizona, the "Trincheras de Cerros." Howard H. Martin followed with an illustrated talk on the Kabyles of Algeria, a people living under conditions of isolation in a mountain environment. Frances M. Earle described conditions of health among the white residents of tropical Queensland, where she found disease no longer a deterrent to occupation of this tropical region by white men. Margaret Carstairs gave the concluding paper, "The Intensification of Agriculture in Subtropical Japan," in which she described the unusually intensive cropping of fields on the southern islands of the archipelago. The meetings concluded with the annual business session of the association.

### American Society of Ichthyologists and Herpetologists, Western Division

(*Report by Margaret Storey*)

Two regular sessions were held on Wednesday, June 28, at which twelve papers were presented: "Problems in the Classification of Some California Fresh-Water Fishes," Leo Shapovalov; "Preliminary Studies of the Denning of the Desert Tortoise, *Gopherus agassizii,*" A. M. Woodbury and Ross Hardy; "Darwinism in Contemporary Social Evolution," Paul D. R. Rüthling; "Specimen Species and Real Species," G. F. Ferris; "The Species of *Triturus* in British Columbia," Gertrude Smith Watney; "Observations on the Philippine Sea Snakes," A. W. Herre; "Notes on Metabolic

Levels of *Dipsosaurus dorsalis* (Crested Lizard) and *Sceloporus occidentalis* (Western Blue-Bellied Lizard) over a Period of Five Months under Temperature Control," F. M. Baldwin and P. W. Eberle; "Some Notes on the Physiology of Warm-Spring Fishes," F. B. Sumner; "Reproductive Cycles in the Sagebrush Lizard, *Sceloporus g. graciosus,*" A. M. Woodbury and Marian Woodbury; "Observations on the Rate of Development of the Pacific Dogfish, *Squalus suckleyi,*" L. E. Griffin; "Remarks on the Systematics of California Skinks," T. L. Rodgers and H. S. Fitch; and "The Herpetological Collections of the Stanford Natural History Museum," G. S. Myers. A collection of live herpetological specimens was on display at the Natural History Museum on Thursday afternoon. At the business meeting on Wednesday the following were elected to office for the coming year: *President,* Wilbert McLeod Chapman, Seattle, Washington; *Vice-President,* Tracy I. Storer, Davis, California; *Secretary-Treasurer,* Margaret Storey, Stanford University. Attendance at the various sessions ranged from 45 to 150.

The symposium "Dams and the Problem of Migratory Fishes" was presented on Thursday morning jointly with the Western Society of Naturalists. For this first authoritative summary of a timely and important problem in conservation the invited speakers included the men directly responsible for the fish-ways and fish-conservation measures at the great new dams on the West Coast. Dr. F. B. Sumner, president, introduced the following speakers: Willis H. Rich, of Stanford University and director of research, Fish Commission of Oregon, Portland, "Fishery Problems Raised by the Development of Water Resources"; Harlan B. Holmes, U. S. Engineers Corps, Portland, "The Passage of Fish at Bonneville Dam"; Wilbert M. Chapman, of the Washington State Department of Fisheries, Seattle, "Fish Problems Connected with the Grand Coulee Dam"; Harry A. Hanson, U. S. Bureau of Reclamation, Stanford University, "The Sacramento River Salmon-Salvage Problem"; and Alan C. Taft, chief of the Bureau of Fish Conservation, California State Division of Fish and Game, "Summary of the Present Status of Dams versus Migratory Fishes on the Pacific Coast, with Especial Reference to Problems in California." An interesting discussion followed, which was recorded, and a resolution was unanimously passed that before starting construction, surveys of the fisheries resources be made by qualified experts, to parallel engineering surveys, over a minimum period of five years, or sufficient to cover the life cycles of all economically important fishes concerned. Publication is planned for the entire symposium, including the discussion and resolution. Those desiring further information may write to Professor George S. Myers, Natural History Museum, Stanford University, California.

### American Association of Economic Entomologists, Pacific Slope Branch

(*Report by Roy E. Campbell*)

The twenty-fourth annual meeting of the Pacific Slope Branch was undoubtedly the best one held so far, not only in attendance, which exceeded 200, but in the program. Almost every phase of entomology was covered, including experimental, taxonomy, teaching and demonstration. Tuesday morning included papers on new fumigants, hop insects, tomato worms, the pea aphid and the honey bee. Tuesday afternoon topics were fumigation and citrus scales, the addition of toxicants to oil sprays and recent progress in the control of other citrus pests. A motion picture was shown depicting the development and progress in fog spraying.

What was probably the outstanding feature of the meeting was the demonstration of spraying and dusting equipment Wednesday morning. At least a dozen commercial companies exhibited equipment, from small hand dusters and sprayers for backyard use to large high-powered machines mounted on trucks capable of reaching the tops of trees 150 feet high and covering orchards at the rate of 10 acres per hour. Fog and dust sprayers were also demonstrated as well as fumigating apparatus. The demonstration was attended by members of several other societies as well as the entomologists. The demonstration was followed by several technical papers on spraying, taxonomy and thrips.

On Wednesday afternoon papers on attrahents and repellents were given, together with several on forest insect problems. A sound picture on the production and use of sulfur was followed by one on the control of live-stock parasites. Thursday morning's session was devoted to papers on a variety of topics, including filbert and walnut insects, design of field plots, dried fruit insects, grasshoppers, insects for classroom use and a new alfalfa weevil. The final session was held in Golden Gate Park, San Francisco, jointly with the Pacific Coast Entomological Society.

Another notable feature of the meeting was the extensive exhibits of chemicals used as insecticides, mounts of injurious insects; insects, manuals and apparatus for classroom use; models of cages, dusters and field and laboratory apparatus used in insect studies. Officers elected were: *Chairman,* B. G. Thompson, Oregon State College; *Secretary-Treasurer,* Roy E. Campbell, Alhambra, California.

### Botanical Society of America, Pacific Section

(*Report by Ira L. Wiggins*)

The Botanical Society of America, Pacific Section, held three general sessions, with an average attendance of fifty-five, at which thirty papers were presented. The standard of the papers was high, with particularly good ones on anatomy and morphology, cytogenetics, marine algology, mycology and experimental taxonomy. D. M. Crooks described a "Translongitome" with which it is possible to cut transections and longisections, alternately, from the same block of material, both types of sections appearing in the same ribbon. G. L. Stebbins, Jr., and Lotti Steinitz reported that mitosis in *Hordeum* seedlings is inhibited under anaerobic conditions; H. S. Reed described the cytological effects of the little leaf disease; Eubanks Carsner reported that flowering of sugar beets is increased by shading of the soil or by early planting; and J. V. Harvey reported the discovery of several new watermolds.

Three symposia were held. One, a joint session with the Ecological Society of America, Western Section, dealt with "Recent Contributions of Botany and Ecology to Society" and was ably presented by E. B. Babcock, Tracy I. Storer, E. P. Meinecke and H. L. Shantz. At a joint symposium with the Western Section of the American Society of Plant Physiologists the views of two schools of thought on "Translocation of Solutes in Plants" were presented and excited brisk discussion. The third symposium centered about the opportunities for botanical research in western North America. Papers by five speakers indicated that many such opportunities still exist.

On Friday, June 30, a luncheon of the American Society of Plant Taxonomists was followed by the final session, during which ten taxonomic papers were read. D. D. Keck and J. Clausen described recent results obtained in experimental taxonomy. H. F. Copeland discussed some communications opposing and others supporting his recent proposal to make four distinct kingdoms of the old animal and plant kingdoms. Opinion was about equally divided between support and opposition.

A joint field trip to Año Nuevo Point was made by twenty-four ecologists and botanists on Saturday, July 1. Much interest was shown in the partially consolidated, unpetrified plant material exposed along the beach and in the vegetation occurring on and among the dunes.

At a brief business meeting George B. Rigg and C. Leo Hitchcock, of the University of Washington, Seattle, were elected to serve as president and councilor, respectively, during the ensuing year.

### American Chemical Society, Pacific Intersectional Division

(*Report by F. O. Koenig*)

The session on Wednesday morning, June 28, opened with a series of four papers, chiefly by collaborators of Dr. Pauling, on molecular structure as determined by the diffraction of x-rays and of electrons. Of particular interest because of its bearing on the exact theory of protein structure at present being striven for on many fronts, was the conclusion of Dr. R. B. Corey regarding interatomic distances in proteins: from the complete crystal structure analysis of glycine and of diketo-piperazine it is probable that these distances are: C–C, 154° A; αC–N, 1.40° A; keto C–N, 1.33° A; C–O, 1.25° A. The four further papers of Wednesday morning dealt respectively with complex formation by hemoglobin derivatives (2 papers), the reduction of nitrobenzene by metals and the valence states of osmium.

The Wednesday afternoon session was devoted to two photochemical papers by Dr. Leighton and collaborators, four thermochemical papers by Dr. Parks and collaborators, a paper on liver proteins and a paper on the theory of diffusion.

On Thursday morning there were read first six papers by collaborators of Dr. McBain, dealing with the adsorption, the phase rule diagrams and the hydrolysis of various soaps. These were followed by a paper on the theory of strong electrolytes and one on the theory of cells with liquid-liquid junctions.

The session of Thursday afternoon began with a historical paper on Alexander Butlerov. This was followed by seven papers dealing respectively with the introduction of substituted amino groups into the aromatic nucleus, the quantitative determination of bismuth in certain antisyphilitic agents, the flotation of galena in the presence of xanthates, the oxidation of pigments in freshly killed leaves, the rate of salt infiltration into chilled fish, allylic rearrangements and the bioassay of riboflavin.

### American Society of Plant Physiologists, Western Section

(*Report by A. S. Crafts*)

The program of the Western Section this year consisted of three symposia, three half-day sessions for submitted papers and the annual dinner.

A joint symposium with the Western Society of Soil Science on Wednesday morning, June 28, considered problems of nutrient availability in soils. Professor Burd's discussion of the mechanics of phosphate retention by soils and the description of the process of contact exchange between plant roots and soil colloids by Hans Jenny were outstanding contributions.

While the symposium with the Botanical Society on "Translocation of Solutes in Plants" was marred by the absence of T. G. Mason and O. F. Curtis, an interesting presentation of the anatomy of vascular tissues by Dr. Esau and descriptions of virus, auxin and radioactive isotope movement in plants provided an interesting program. A discussion of the mechanics of organic solute movement concluded the session.

The symposium on "Growth," which started with a description of growth in meristems by Dr. A. S. Foster and considered the nutritional factors involved and the role of vitamin B and auxin, was of broad interest and attracted a good audience.

The Wednesday afternoon program of submitted papers concerned soil-plant relations as affected by water and nutrients. The physiology of yeasts, problems of plant biochemistry and the response of plants to x-rays and radioactive elements were topics considered on Thursday morning. Studies on phloem exudate from grape were also described. The Friday afternoon session presented some papers of outstanding interest on mineral nutrition, salt flux and accumulation and growth factor requirements of roots.

Officers for the coming year, as announced at the dinner on Friday evening, are: *Chairman,* W. M. Atwood; *Vice-Chairman,* A. S. Crafts; and *Secretary,* J. van Overbeek.

An extremely interesting trip through the greenhouses and laboratories of the Division of Plant Nutrition at Berkeley, personally conducted by Professor D. R. Hoagland and members of his staff, was enjoyed by a number of visiting plant physiologists on Saturday morning.

### AMERICAN PHYTOPATHOLOGICAL SOCIETY, PACIFIC DIVISION

*(Report by L. D. Leach)*

The meetings of the Pacific Division of the American Phytopathological Society were featured by a larger attendance and greater diversity of program than for several years. Thirty-two papers reporting research projects were presented during four half-day sessions. Of the eight papers on virus diseases, the presentation of evidence of the production of curly-top virus antibodies or antibody-like substances in Turkish tobacco by J. M. Wallace created the most discussion. Other papers of general interest were those of C. E. Yarwood on attempts at the *in vitro* culture of certain powdery and downy mildews and of J. T. Barrett on the occurrence of overwintering mycelium of downy mildew in the California wild grape. A group of papers on control of *Armillaria* by soil fumigants was presented by H. E. Thomas, L. O. Lawyer and P. D. Caldis. Prevention of apothecial formation of *Sclerotinia fructicola* by soil treatments was reported by G. A. Huber.

Thursday morning was devoted to a symposium on teaching of plant pathology. Certain phases of the problem were discussed by W. W. Robbins, J. T. Barrett, W. B. Hewitt, H. R. Stanford and T. E. Rawlins.

A field trip of unusual interest, consisting of visits to several greenhouses and commercial plantings of ornamentals between Palo Alto and San Francisco and a tour through one of the large estates occupied all of Friday.

Officers of the society for the ensuing year are as follows: *President,* B. F. Dana, U. S. Department of Agriculture, Corvallis, Oregon; *Vice-President,* T. E. Rawlins, University of California; *Secretary-Treasurer,* L. D. Leach, University of California, Davis; *Councilor,* E. Carsner, U. S. Department of Agriculture, Riverside.

### WESTERN SOCIETY OF NATURALISTS

*No Report Received*

### ECOLOGICAL SOCIETY OF AMERICA, WESTERN SECTION

*(Report by H. de Forest)*

The society cooperated with the Botanical Society of America in organizing a symposium on "Recent Contributions of Botany and Ecology to Society," held on Wednesday, June 28. T. I. Storer and H. L. Shantz spoke for the Ecological Society on animal and plant ecology, respectively.

On Thursday, June 29, a session for the presentation of papers occurred. Eight papers were given, two of these being invitational, by R. W. Chaney on Tertiary forests and by A. H. Hutchinson on a method of polygonal graphing of ecological data containing several variables. H. P. Hansen read a paper on ring-growth and dominance in a spruce-fir forest, and G. A. Pearson one on growth in southwestern pine forests. E. Fritz gave an interesting account of anomalous growth rings in redwood. L. C. Cole described an electrical apparatus for measuring several environmental factors. The Hutchinson and Cole work held as much of interest for zoologists as for botanists. The more distinctively zoological papers, which were placed in the latter half of the program because of an unexpected A. A. A. S. botanical excursion to the Carnegie Institution Laboratory of Plant Biology in the later afternoon, were by W. H. Rich on the influence of environment on salmon migration and by C. T. Vorhies on the habitat and shelter preferences of *Neotoma albigula.* Both of these called forth interesting discussion.

The society participated in the Biologists' Dinner of Wednesday evening, June 28. On Saturday, July 1, an enjoyable joint field excursion took place with the Botanical Society of America. During the day redwood forests, streamsides, chaparral and other scrubs and the coastal sand dunes of Año Nuevo Point were visited. The plant life was commented on by L. R. Abrams and I. L. Wiggins, of Stanford University.

### SOCIETY FOR EXPERIMENTAL BIOLOGY AND MEDICINE

*(Report by Charles Weiss)*

The Pacific Coast and the Southern California branches of the Society for Experimental Biology and Medicine met jointly on June 30, 1939. A total of 19 papers was presented and also an invited address on vitamin K by H. J. Almquist, of the University of California, Berkeley.

P. J. Hanzlik, W. C. Cutting and G. B. Robson reported on the gastro-intestinal absorption of insulin in animals. Astringents, simple alcohols, poly-alcohols, detergents, antiseptic dyes, local anesthetics and agents which increase permeability favor absorption in animals. Results in man are unsatisfactory.

James B. McNaught, R. R. Beard and F. DeEds reported on the efficacy of phenothiazine in experimental trichinosis. R. H. Wilson and F. DeEds concluded that the continued feeding of cadmium-containing diets produces cardiac hypertrophy traceable to the anemia produced.

E. F. Cannon, S. P. Lucia and E. H. Benson, of the University of California Medical School, conclude that the difference induced in the circulation time after exercise is not significant as a test for cardiac efficiency.

N. S. West and R. H. Vaughn, of the University of California, reported that coliform organisms of the genus *Citrobacter* might be responsible for gassy deterioration of olives.

Ira A. Manville, of the University of Oregon, Portland, reported that sorbitol is well tolerated by diabetic patients and provides a good source of energy; it also favors the deposition of glycogen in the liver. F. J. Reithel, of the University of Oregon, Portland, reported that the presence of food in the stomach decreases the concentrtaion of alcohol after the ingestion of intoxicating liquors. Effective foods are sugar, apple juice, milk, bread, egg albumen, butter, cream and amino acids.

H. S. Reed, Department of Botany, University of California, read a report sent by Dr. J. Dufrenoy, of Bordeaux, France. Certain springs which had been used since Roman times to cure sick people were found to favor the proliferation of willow cuttings. These are the springs of St. Roche and Tambour in the Pyrenees Mountains.

### WESTERN SOCIETY OF SOIL SCIENCE

(*Report by L. T. Kardos*)

The Western Society of Soil Science held five half-day sessions at which were submitted 33 papers. The attendance ranged from fifty to seventy persons.

The papers on Monday and Tuesday were devoted largely to problems of land classification, land utilization, evaluation of soils, soil conservation, drainage, erosion, soil permeability, soil moisture, bound water in soils, flocculation of soil, fixation of arsenic by soils, organic matter in soils, base exchange capacity and bacterial activity in soils.

On Wednesday morning a session was held jointly with the American Society of Plant Physiologists in which four papers were presented in a symposium on the "Availability of Nutrients in Soils to Plants." The speakers were W. T. McGeorge, of the University of Arizona; John S. Burd, of the University of California in Berkeley; H. D. Chapman, of the Citrus Experiment Station in Riverside, and Hans Jenny, of the University of California in Berkeley.

The following officers were elected for the ensuing year: *President,* W. T. McGeorge, University of Arizona, Tucson; *Vice-president,* G. B. Bodman, University of California, Berkeley; *Secretary-Treasurer,* L. T. Kardos, State College of Washington, Pullman; *Council Representative,* O. C. Magistad, Regional Salinity Laboratory, Riverside.

## CONCURRENT MEETINGS OF OTHER ORGANIZATIONS

### AMERICAN ASSOCIATION OF PHYSICS TEACHERS

(*Report by Paul Kirkpatrick*)

The Wednesday morning session was devoted to the presentation of brief contributed reports, relative chiefly to apparatus useful in the teaching of physics but containing also reports of historical and theoretical interest. At the luncheon which followed, Vice-President A. A. Knowlton spoke briefly of the general affairs of the association. During Wednesday afternoon apparatus used in elementary and upper-division physics courses in Stanford was on display in the laboratories. This equipment is mainly of local design and construction.

The evening meeting of the same day consisted of three invited papers. V. F. Lenzen discussed "The Operational Theory in Elementary Physics," criticizing constructively a number of the concepts and definitions regularly presented in the teaching of general physics. "Historical View-Point and Allusion in Physics Teaching" was the subject of a paper by E. C. Watson, which the author illustrated by slides made from materials in his private collection of historical matter related to physics and technology. R. D. Richtmyer showed a series of related absolute experiments for the electrical-measurements laboratory, performing the manipulations and carrying out numerical results in the course of his presentation.

### AMERICAN SOCIETY FOR HORTICULTURAL SCIENCE, WESTERN SECTION

(*Report by W. W. Aldrich*)

In the case of previously nitrogen-deficient grapefruit trees near Yuma, Arizona, the maintenance of a high nitrogen level (as indicated by nitrogen content of leaves) during the spring and summer resulted in fruit of a coarser texture and greener color that fall.—W. E. Martin, University of Arizona.

The sugar prune, which normally sets a heavy crop one year and then fails to blossom the next year, blossomed heavily the following year when entire trees or limbs two inches or more in diameter were completely deflorated or defruited within 14 to 30 days after full bloom. Strangely, either the upper or lower half, if completely deflorated, would differentiate with large numbers of blossom buds, while the undeflorated half was apparently not affected.—L. D. Davis, University of California.

As a means of covering emasculated blossoms, to keep out insects and windblown pollen, a web of rubber cement can be spun by a small electric fan, with attachment for feeding cement at constant pressure. Web has thus far shown no deleterious effects to pollen or to pistil.—J. R. King, University of California.

In a ten-year study of rootstocks for the Satsuma orange, the Morton citrange showed promise of permitting as good tree growth and yield as the sweet orange. Trifoliate stock was definitely inferior.—H. J. Webber and L. D. Batchelor, University of California.

# SCIENTIFIC EVENTS

## EXHIBITS AT THE BRITISH NATURAL HISTORY MUSEUM

RECENT additions to the Natural History Museum, South Kensington, include a number of mounted heads and skulls of hoofed mammals from Northern Rhodesia, an area from which the museum has hitherto not possessed much material of this kind. They were collected, chiefly at Mpika, by the late F. H. Medland, and have been given by Mrs. Medland. Among them are some very fine sable and roan antelope heads which are of special interest as representing transition stages from the types found in South Africa to the more northerly forms of Tanganyika Territory and Kenya Colony.

Two large collections of South American mammals, one from Dutch Guiana and the other from Ecuador, have been purchased. The latter contains a series of specimens representing a remarkable genus of Diprotodont marsupials (*i.e.,* marsupials having the kangaroo type of dentition), *Caenolestes,* one of the genera of opossum mice.

A series of specimens of "Darwin Glass" from Mount Darwin, Tasmania, collected by the late Hartwell Conder, has been given by his widow. This is a silica glass of a pale olive color, thousands of tons of which are found, in the form of small rounded or rod-like pieces, over an area of 60 square miles. It is thought to have been formed by the heat caused by the impact of a large meteorite.

A British mineral of which good crystals are very rare is withamite, a pink variety of epidote, an iron aluminium silicate which is usually green. The type-locality is Glencoe, and some excellent specimens from there have now been presented to the museum by Mr. W. G. Myers, a local A.A. scout, who found them when the new road was cut through the lava in which they occur. The Mineral Department has also acquired a large rough crystal of microcline feldspar from Norway, measuring 14 inches by 12 inches by 10 inches and weighing about 100 pounds.

Two new exhibits have been put on view in the central hall. One is devoted to the Coelacanth fish, lately discovered off the South African coast, and belonging to a type which was supposed to have been extinct for 50,000,000 years. The fish has been named *Latimeria Chalumnæ* by Dr. J. L. B. Smith, of Grahamstown, who first recognized its nature and importance. A life-size photograph is shown, together with models illustrating the close similarity of *Latimeria* to its fossil relatives.

The second exhibit illustrates the method used by the museum to reconstruct extinct animals (the particular beast chosen is the large amphibian *Cyclotosaurus* from the Triassic ironstone of New South Wales) from the impressions of their skeletons in rock.

## THE BYRD ANTARCTIC EXPEDITION

A CONFERENCE was held in Washington on July 24 under the auspices of the National Academy of Sciences and the National Research Council concerning scientific arrangements for the coming Antarctic Expedition.

According to press reports, thirty-two scientific men from twenty government agencies and representatives of institutions of learning and research discussed the scientific program of the expedition with Rear Admiral Byrd, commander. Dr. Isaiah Bowman, president of the Johns Hopkins University, presided. He was assisted by Dr. Henry B. Bigelow, director of the Oceanographic Institution at Woods Hole, Mass.

Plans for meteorological observations and for the mapping of a region some 5,000,000 miles in extent, 3,000,000 miles of which is still to be explored, were discussed at length. The desirability of making arrangements to insure the continuation of these observations over a series of years was also taken up.

It is planned to establish for the expedition three bases, one at Little America, another about 1,400 miles to the eastward, and a third between the two, with twenty-two men at each base, though not continuously. They will come and go as specialists replacing each other to engage in their respective activities.

Members of the expedition, which it is expected will start in October, will include: Dr. F. Alton Wade, geologist, Miami University; Dr. Thomas Poulter, physicist, director of the Research Foundation of the Armour Institute of Technology; Richard Black, engineer surveyor, who is attached to the Division of Territories and Island Possessions of the Department of the Interior, and Paul Sipel, who was the Boy Scout member of the last Byrd Expedition and who since has taken his Ph.D. at Clark University.

## PRELIMINARY PROGRAM OF THE DUNDEE MEETING OF THE BRITISH ASSOCIATION

ACCORDING to the preliminary program of the meeting of the British Association for the Advancement of Science to be held at Dundee, under the presidency of Sir Albert Seward, from August 30 to September 6, the following are among the principal subjects announced for presentation:

WEDNESDAY, AUGUST 30

Presidential Address by Sir Albert Seward, on "The Western Isles through the Mists of Ages."

THURSDAY, AUGUST 31

Presidential Addresses in the Sections:
A—R. S. Whipple, on "Instruments in Science and Industry."
B—Professor E. K. Rideal, on "Film Reactions as a New Approach to Biology."
D—Professor J. Ritchie, on "Perspectives in Evolution."
G—H. E. Wimperis, on "The Future of Flight."
L—Dr. A. P. M. Fleming, on "Education for Industry."
M—Sir Thomas Middleton, on "Practice with Science. The Farmer's Position and the Scientific Worker's Program."

Discussions, etc., in the Sections:
A—"Television."
B, I—"Tissue Respiration."
C—"Local Geology."
E—"A National Atlas" (with speakers from Sections C, D, F, H, K, M).
G—"Problems of Transatlantic Aviation."
L—"Education as a Preparation for Industry."

Division for the Social and International Relations of Science—Papers and discussion on coordination of scientific research, on population and other topics.

FRIDAY, SEPTEMBER 1

Presidential Addresses in the Sections:
E—A. Stevens, on a subject to be announced.
H—Professor W. E. Le Gros Clark, on "The Scope and Limitations of Physical Anthropology."
J—R. J. Bartlett, on "Measurement in Psychology."
K—Professor D. Thoday, on "The Interpretation of Plant Structure."

Discussions, etc., in the Sections:
A, B—"Applications of Artificial Radio-Elements."
C—"Raised Beaches of Forth and Tay."
D—"The Natural History of Salmon and Trout: Exhibition of Biological Films."
F—"Scottish Problems."
G—"Air Conditioning."
I—"The Problem of Pain" (whole-day session, at St. Andrews).
L—"Educational Facilities in Industry."
M—"Agricultural Education."

Discussion on Jute (under the auspices of appropriate Sections).

Conference of Delegates of Corresponding Societies.—Presidential Address by Professor H. L. Hawkins, on "Local Scientific Societies and the Community"; papers and discussion.

SUNDAY, SEPTEMBER 3

Division for the Social and International Relations of Science.—Address by Sir Richard Gregory, on "Science and Social Ethics."

MONDAY, SEPTEMBER 4

Sectional Presidential Address:
C—Professor H. H. Read, on "Metamorphism and Igneous Activity."

Discussions, etc., in the Sections:
A—"Problems of High-speed Flight."
A—"Surface Temperature of Stars."
B—"Light Alloys."
D—"Problems of Freshwater Biology."
H, I—"Nutrition and Physique."
L—"Educational Research in Scotland."
M—"Grass Conservation."

Conference of Delegates of Corresponding Societies.—Papers and discussion.

TUESDAY, SEPTEMBER 5

Presidential Addresses in the Sections:
F—Professor H. O. Meredith, on a subject to be announced.
I—Professor D. Burns, on "The Assessment of Physical Fitness."

Discussions, etc., in the Sections:
A—"High Temperature Problems."
A—"Solar and Terrestrial Relationships."
B—"Intra-molecular Changes."
C—"Old Red Sandstone-Carboniferous Boundary."
H—"Teaching of Anthropology."
I—"The Assessment of Physical Fitness."
L—"Discussion on Spens Report."
M—"Seed Potato Growing."

Discussion on Jute (continued from Friday).

Evening Address by Dr. Isaiah Bowman.

WEDNESDAY, SEPTEMBER 6

Division for the Social and International Relations of Science. Discussion on Nutrition.

## THE BOSTON MEETING OF THE AMERICAN CHEMICAL SOCIETY

ALL the eighteen professional divisions of the American Chemical Society will meet in Boston from September 11 to 15 in connection with its ninety-eighth convention. Numerous symposia will supplement the regular sessions.

The divisions and their chairmen are: Agricultural and Food, Dr. Roy C. Newton, of Swift and Company, Chicago; Biological, Dr. Joseph J. Pfiffner, of Parke, Davis and Company, Detroit; Cellulose, Professor George L. Clark, of the University of Illinois; Chemical Education, Martin V. McGill, of Lorain High School, Lorain, Ohio; Colloid, Professor Lloyd H. Reyerson, of the University of Minnesota; Fertilizer, Egbert W. Magruder, of the F. S. Royster Guano Company, Norfolk, Va.; Gas and Fuel, Dr. Frank H. Reed, of the Illinois Geological Survey; History of Chemistry, Professor Tenney L. Davis, of Massachusetts Institute of Technology; Industrial and Engineering, Dr. Walter L. Badger, of the Dow Chemical Company, Ann Arbor, Mich.; Medicinal, Professor Walter H. Hartung, of the University of Maryland; Microchemistry, Lawrence T. Hallett, Eastman Kodak Company, Rochester, N. Y.; Organic, Professor Werner E. Bachmann, of the University of Michigan; Paint and Varnish, Professor William H. Gardner, of the Polytechnic Institute, Brooklyn, N. Y.; Petroleum, Dr. Per K. Frolich, of the Standard Oil Development Company, Elizabeth, N. J.; Physical and Inorganic Chemistry, Professor George Scatchard, of Massachusetts Institute of Technology; Rubber, Dr. G. K. Hinshaw, of the Goodyear Tire and Rubber Company, Akron, Ohio; Sugar Chemistry and Technology, A. R. Nees, of the Great Western Sugar Company, Denver, Colo.; Water, Sewage and Sanitation, Professor Alvin P. Black, of the University of Florida.

The divisions will hold symposia as follows:

The Division of Agricultural and Food Chemistry is sponsoring a symposium on Nitrogen-Free Extracts, with Dr. C. A. Browne, of the U. S. Bureau of Chemistry and Soils, Washington, D. C., in charge, and another on Plant Hormones. Together with the Division of Medicinal Chemistry, the food chemists will cooperate with the Biological Division in a program on Vitamins and Nutrition. Papers on other agricultural and food topics will also be heard.

The Division of Biological Chemistry will devote a day to a symposium on Methods in Protein Chemistry. It will also join the Medicinal Division in a symposium on Sterols and Related Compounds. General papers in the field of biological chemistry will be given at other sessions. The Cellulose Division will hear a variety of general papers.

Dr. Mary L. Sherrill, of Mount Holyoke College, will be chairman of a symposium on the Training and Opportunities for Women in Chemistry to be held by the Division of Chemical Education. The Colloid Division will participate in a symposium on X-Ray Studies of Substances of High Molecular Weight, with Dr. Maurice L. Huggins, of the Eastman Kodak Company, presiding. The Fertilizer Division will have a program of general papers in three sessions.

A symposium on the Combustion of Solid Fuels under the chairmanship of Martin A. Mayers, of the Coal Research Laboratory of the Carnegie Institute of Technology, will be sponsored by the Gas and Fuel Division. A comprehensive session on Industrial Wastes is planned by the Division of Industrial and Engineering Chemistry and Water, Sewage and Sanitation Chemistry. Dr. Walter A. Schmidt, president of the Western Precipitation Company, will be chairman.

A third Unit-Process Symposium will be held by the Industrial and Engineering Division, with Professor R. Norris Shreve, of Purdue University, presiding. A symposium on Resins and Plastics from Hydrocarbons is planned by the Petroleum, Paint and Varnish, and Rubber Divisions.

The Division of Physical and Inorganic Chemistry, of which Professor Harold C. Urey, of Columbia University, is secretary, will have a program of a hundred and thirteen papers. Professor F. G. Keyes, of the Massachusetts Institute of Technology, will preside at a symposium on Low Temperature Research, and Professor W. C. Fernelius, of the Ohio State University, at a symposium on Compounds with Elements in Unusual States of Valence. Dr. Scatchard, Professor Charles P. Smyth, of Princeton University, and Professor Urey will be chairmen of the sessions on physical chemistry, while Professor G. Frederick Smith, of the University of Illinois, will preside at the sessions on inorganic and analytical chemistry.

A symposium on Vulcanization in addition to a special celebration of the centenary of the discovery of the vulcanization of rubber by Charles Goodyear will be sponsored by the Rubber Division. Numerous general papers on rubber chemistry are also scheduled.

## RECENT DEATHS AND MEMORIALS

Dr. Wendell Clay Mansfield, geologist of the U. S. Geological Survey, died suddenly on July 24 at the age of sixty-five years. His principal line of research was the late-Tertiary mollusks of the southeastern states, particularly of Florida.

Dr. Burtis Burr Breese, who retired two years ago as head of the department of psychology at the University of Cincinnati with the title of professor emeritus, died on July 31 at the age of seventy-two years.

John Ritchie, of Malden, Mass., died on July 22 at the age of eighty-eight years. Mr. Ritchie was interested in astronomy and for many years was in charge of the collection and distribution of astronomical news from the Harvard Observatory. He also was active in conchology and in other scientific subjects.

John Harvey Lovell, known for his work with bees, biological editor of "Cyclopedia of Bee Culture" died on August 2 at the age of seventy-eight years.

Professor Archibald Young, Regius professor of

surgery in the University of Glasgow, died on July 23 at the age of sixty-five years.

THE Agricultural Experiment Station at New Haven, Conn., will include brief addresses in memory of the late station botanist, Dr. G. P. Clinton, and the state entomologist, Dr. W. E. Britton, in the Field Day exercises to be held at the station farm at Mount Carmel on August 16. Dr. Clinton died two years ago after thirty-five years of state service, and Dr. Britton, who had served the state since 1893, died last February. Immediately after luncheon Director W. L. Slate, of the station, will open a short program which will include an address by Dr. Henry G. Knight, chief of the Bureau of Chemistry and Soils, Washington, D. C. Mr. David Clarke, of Milford, will say a few words about the work of the late Dr. Clinton, and Mr. Fred S. Baker, of Cheshire, will speak about Dr. Britton. Later the new state entomologist, Dr. Roger B. Friend, and the station botanist, Dr. J. G. Horsfall, appointed early this summer, will be introduced.

To mark the two hundredth anniversary of the founding of the Swedish Royal Academy of Science, the Swedish Post Office issued a set of commemorative stamps on June 2. The designs are: 15 öre brown and 50 öre grey, with a portrait of the naturalist Linnaeus; 10 öre violet and 30 öre blue, with a portrait of the chemist Berzelius.

# SCIENTIFIC NOTES AND NEWS

DR. W. L. BRAGG, Cavendish professor of experimental physics in the University of Cambridge, has been elected a corresponding member in the section of mineralogy of the Paris Academy of Sciences.

THE Royal Academy of Sciences at Rome has awarded the Cannizzaro prize for chemistry to Professor Otto Hahn, of the University of Berlin.

THE gold medal of the Society of the Medical and Natural Sciences at Jena has been awarded to Dr. Werner Heisenberg, professor of theoretical physics at the University of Leipzig.

MEDALS of the Royal Scottish Geographical Society for 1939 have been awarded as follows: the Livingstone Gold Medal to the Right Hon. Lord Hailey, for his direction of the African Research Survey under the auspices of the Royal Institute of International Affairs; the Mungo Park Medal to Dr. E. B. Worthington, for his share in the work of the African Research Survey; the Research Medal to Dr. Herbert John Fleure, professor of geography and anthropology in the University of Manchester, "for his many original contributions to geography and anthropology and his furtherance of these sciences in the British Isles."

*Nature* states that the Royal African Society has awarded a silver medal to the late C. F. Massy Swynnerton, formerly director of tsetse research in Tanganyika Territory.

DAVID G. THOMPSON, senior geologist, and Albert G. Fiedler, senior engineer, of the U. S. Geological Survey, were awarded at the annual convention of the American Water Works Association at Atlantic City the John M. Goodell Prize for their paper entitled "Some Problems Relating to Legal Control of Use of Ground Water." This prize was established by *The Engineering News Record* as a memorial to John M. Goodell, one-time editor of the journal and a former editor of the *Journal* of the American Water Works Association. It is awarded annually for "a notable contribution to the science or practice of water works development."

ESTELLE LACASE, a member of the Junior Academy of Science of New Orleans, has been awarded a prize consisting of a subscription to SCIENCE for one year in a recent contest based upon a written review of the contents of Volume 88 of SCIENCE.

DR. HOWARD I. YOUNG, president of the American Zinc, Lead and Smelting Company and of the American Mining Congress, was awarded the honorary degree of doctor of engineering at the commencement exercises of the School of Mines and Metallurgy of the University of Missouri.

ON commemoration day at the University of Glasgow the doctorate of laws was conferred on Sir Andrew Rae Duncan, chairman of the executive committee of the British Iron and Steel Federation; W. J. Goudie, emeritus professor of the theory and practice of heat engines, University of Glasgow; I. M. Heilbron, professor of organic chemistry, University of London; H. J. Paton, White's professor of moral philosophy, University of Oxford; F. J. M. Stratton, professor of astrophysics, University of Cambridge, and G. G. Turner, professor of surgery, University of London.

DR. GUSTAVUS AUGUSTUS EISEN, from 1893 to 1900 curator of the California Academy of Sciences, later for five years connected with the U. S. Department of Agriculture, known for his work in biology, anthropology and archeology, celebrated his ninety-second birthday on August 2.

DR. CLYDE E. KEELER, instructor in the Bussey Institution of Harvard University, has been elected a fellow of the Wistar Institute of Anatomy and Biology, Philadelphia.

DR. R. RUGGLES GATES, professor of botany at King's College, the University of London, has been appointed president of the section of cytology of the seventh International Botanical Congress for the meeting to be held at Stockholm from July 17 to 25, 1940.

HARRY W. CAVE, of the Kansas State College, has been appointed head of the department of dairy husbandry at the Oklahoma Agricultural and Mechanical College. He succeeds Earl Weaver, who resigned some time ago to accept a similar position at the Michigan State College.

DR. IVER JOHNSON, of the University of Minnesota, has been appointed professor of farm crops at the Iowa State College. He will specialize in plant breeding.

DR. ROY S. HANSLICK, of New Haven, Conn., has been appointed assistant professor of chemical engineering at Vanderbilt University.

DR. CARL L. STOTZ, visiting lecturer in geography for the last three years in the summer sessions of the University of Pittsburgh, has been elected assistant professor of geography at the university.

DR. T. V. I. STARKEY, lecturer in physics and mathematics at Rotherham College of Technology, has been appointed head of the physics department of the Technical College, Swansea, in place of Dr. E. Thomas, who has been appointed director of education for Caernarvonshire.

DR. DEAN BURK, associate professor of biochemistry at Cornell University Medical College, New York City, has been appointed senior chemist in the National Cancer Institute of the U. S. Public Health Service. He will be engaged in a study of tissue metabolism fundamental to cancer, under the auspices of a grant from the National Advisory Cancer Council made to the department of biochemistry. Collaborating in the investigations will be Dr. Fritz Lipmann, formerly fellow at the Rockefeller Institute with Dr. P. A. Levene and recently research associate with Dr. Albert Fischer and Dr. Herbert Sprince on a Parker fellowship from Harvard University.

IN the statement in regard to the reorganization of the work in zoology at Cornell University, printed in the issue of SCIENCE for July 28, those doing work in vertebrate taxonomy, ecology and anatomy should have been given as: Professor A. H. Wright, Assistant Professor W. J. Hamilton, Jr., Dr. W. C. Senning and Dr. E. C. Raney, instructors.

DR. VLADIMIR KARAPETOFF, for thirty-five years professor of electrical engineering at Cornell University, who has been made professor emeritus, will reside in Leonia, N. J., where he will engage in research and consulting work. He will next year give a course of lectures on electromagnetic waves in the new evening post-graduate school for metropolitan engineers at the Stevens Institute of Technology, Hoboken, N. J.

THE second International Congress for the Investigation of Biological Rhythm will be held at Utrecht on August 25 and 26.

THE third International Congress of Agricultural Engineering, according to *The Experiment Station Record,* will be held in Rome from September 20 to 23 at the International Institute of Agriculture. The program of the congress has been drawn up by the International Commission on Agricultural Engineering. Irrigation, drainage and land reclamation works, provisions for hygiene and buildings in rural areas, production of motive power by means of new combustible materials, standardization of tests of agricultural machinery, applications of electricity in agriculture, agricultural engineering and its social implications and scientific management in agriculture are the main subjects in the agenda. Additional information may be obtained from the Secretariat, Via Regina Elena, 86, Rome, Italy.

BEFORE the formal conferences of the fifth International Congress of Genetics at Edinburgh, there will be a gathering in London and organized visits to the plant-breeding work at Wisley and to the Galton Laboratory and various parts of the University of London. The next move will be to Cambridge, where the delegates will visit the leading research centers engaged in animal and crop-breeding work. The arrangements have been worked out in such a way as to bring scientific and practical breeders together for discussion and interchange of views. The formal congress will open at the University of Edinburgh on Wednesday, August 23, when the Russian scientist, Professor Vavilov, will deliver his presidential address. He will be followed by well-known American, Dutch and other foreign research workers. Receptions have been arranged for delegates by the City of Edinburgh, by his Majesty's Government and various organizations. The general secretary of the congress is Professor F. E. Crew, of the Institute of Animal Genetics, West Main Road, Edinburgh.

AT the ninth annual meeting of the American Malacological Union, held in the Royal Ontario Museum of Zoology in Toronto from June 20 to 23, the following executive council was elected: *Honorary Presidents:* Mrs. Ida S. Oldroyd, Stanford University; Dr. Henry A. Pilsbry, Academy of Natural Sciences, Philadelphia; and Mrs. Harold R. Robertson, Buffalo Museum of Science; *President,* Dr. H. B. Baker, Zoological Laboratory, University of Pennsylvania; *Vice-president,* Dr. Harald A. Rehder, U. S. National Museum; *Corresponding Secretary,* Norman W. Lermond, Knox

Academy of Arts and Sciences, Thomaston, Me.; *Financial Secretary,* Mrs. Harold R. Robertson, Buffalo Museum of Science; *Councillors at Large,* Dr. Myra Keen, Stanford University; Dr. Henry van der Schalie, University of Michigan Museum; Dr. H. E. Wheeler, Birmingham, Ala.; Aurela LaRocque, Canadian National Museum; *Past Presidents,* Dr. Joshua L. Baily, Jr., San Diego, Cal.; Dr. Paul Bartsch, U. S. National Museum, Washington, D. C.; William J. Clench, Museum of Comparative Zoology, Cambridge; Calvin Goodrich, University of Michigan Museum; Dr. Henry A. Pilsbry, Academy of Natural Sciences, Philadelphia; Maxwell Smith, Lantana, Fla.; Dr. Carlos de la Torre, Museo Poey, Havana. The 1940 meeting will be held in Philadelphia.

THE Museums Association of Great Britain celebrated its jubilee at the annual conference which was held at Cheltenham during the week beginning on July 2. In addition to Lord Bledisloe, who delivered the presidential address, speakers from related organizations included Lord Balniel, representing the Standing Commission on Museums and Galleries, Lord Amulree, president of the Royal Society of Arts, Dr. Arundell Esdaile, president of the Library Association, and Sir Robert Witt, chairman of the National Art-Collections Fund. Papers read during the conference included those of Lord De La Warr on "Museums and Education," and of Don Salvador de Madariaga, chairman of the International Museums Office, Paris, on "Museums and World Peace."

THE John Burroughs Association desires to get in touch with all organizations in the United States and elsewhere that have been established in honor of John Burroughs, to learn whether such groups would be interested in a yearly publication containing reports from these various units, as well as articles about John Burroughs. Communications should be addressed to Dr. Clyde Fisher, president of the association, at the American Museum of Natural History, New York City.

IT is announced by the London *Times* that the general council of the Trades Union Congress has appointed J. Hallsworth, the chairman, H. H. Elvin, E. Bevin and Sir Walter Citrine to meet representatives of the British Association to discuss the procedure of the Scientific Advisory Council which is to be jointly established. J. Marchbank has been appointed a deputy representative. The *Times* states that it is more than eighteen months since the first steps were taken to bring together members of the British Association and the Trades Union Congress. There have been informal talks, but the work of the advisory council has not yet taken shape.

THE William R. Warner and Company, Inc., New York City, announces the establishment of the following research fellowships under the Warner Institute for Therapeutic Research, for the year beginning July 1, 1939: At Columbia University, College of Physicians and Surgeons; under Professor James W. Jobling, department of pathology: a post-doctorate fellowship to Dr. Henry S. Simms, for the continuation of his work on arteriosclerosis; at the University of Maryland, School of Pharmacy; under Professor Walter H. Hartung, department of pharmaceutical chemistry: (1) a post-doctorate fellowship to Dr. Melvin F. W. Dunker, for work in organic synthesis; (2) a post-graduate fellowship to George P. Hager, for work in organic synthesis; (4) a post-graduate fellowship to Kenneth E. Hamlin, for work in organic synthesis; at the Warner Institute for Therapeutic Research, under Dr. Marvin R. Thompson, director: (1) a post-doctorate fellowship to Dr. P. P. Zapponi, for studies in physical chemistry.

A COLLECTION of 8,257 herbarium sheets, consisting of plants from England, Western Continental Europe, northeastern United States and adjacent sections of Canada, has been presented to the New York Botanical Garden by Mrs. T. W. Edmondson. They are the collections made by her husband during vacations over many years. Dr. Edmondson was professor of mathematics and physics and, before his death last autumn, professor emeritus at New York University. The garden has also acquired about a hundred volumes of botanical books from Dr. Edmondson's library.

L. J. BRASS, botanist of the Archbold Expedition to Dutch New Guinea, returned to Brisbane by the flying boat *Coogee* on June 28. The expedition was led and sponsored by Richard Archbold in the scientific interests of the American Museum of Natural History. The principal method of transport was by the flying boat *Guba.* The personnel, equipment and stores of the expedition were flown from sea level to Lake Habbema at 11,000 feet in the mountains. The botanical collections made by Mr. Brass include over 5,000 numbers. These were mostly obtained from regions above 3,000 feet. It is understood that these specimens will be allocated for determination to various American and European specialists by Professor E. D. Merrill, administrator of the botanical collections of Harvard University. Another result of the work is a collection of a hundred and fifty $10 \times 8$-inch negatives of landscapes typical of the regions worked over by the expedition. Mr. Brass is leaving Brisbane this month for New York, where he will complete his work upon some of the collections.

THE first International Exhibition for Polar Exploration will be held at Bergen in 1940. Dr. Grau Bögh has been appointed Commissioner-General by the Norwegian Government. In connection with the exhibition an international conference of Polar explorers is being arranged.

A LARGE new exhibition hall, devoted to comprehensive archeological and ethnological collections from the lands of Budda and other Oriental countries, has been opened at the Field Museum of Natural History. The museum already had important collections of Chinese and Tibetan material. The opening of the new hall, which is devoted to Korea, Siam, Siberia, India, Burma, Ceylon, the Ainu of Yezo, and the Andaman and Nicobar groups of islands in the Pacific, rounds out the representation of life in the Far East. The hall contains hundreds of objects, large and small, varied in character, including pieces remarkable for their beauty, for their ingenuity and for their extreme oddity. They have been gathered over a period of many years and come from various sources. One of the most striking features in the hall represents the ancient Siamese ancestors of the modern motion pictures—that is, the figures used in shadow plays. Mounted on glass and illuminated from behind, these are displayed much as they would appear in performances given in their place of origin.

ACCORDING to the Paris correspondent of the *Journal* of the American Medical Association, the drop in the birth rate in France as compared with the increase in the number of deaths is causing much anxiety. A committee was appointed several months ago by the Académie de médecine of Paris to study methods of checking the drop in birth rate. At the April 26, 1938, meeting Professor Lereboullet submitted the report of the committee. The chief causes of the decline in the birth rate were found to be contraceptive methods and the wide-spread use of abortifacients or induced abortion. There were only 630,000 births in 1937 as compared to a little over a million in 1876. From 1935 to 1937, inclusive, there were 57,117 more deaths than births in France, as compared to an excess of 950,000 births over deaths in Germany and of 775,000 in Italy during 1936 and 1937. The committee believed that the causes of the denatality in France were chiefly moral and economic. It made the following recommendations: (1) That the gravity of the denatality question be made known to the public by every possible method. (2) That an appeal be made to the moral and spiritual forces of the country to encourage the raising of large families by granting large subsidies which increase proportionately to the number of children. (3) That the danger of induced abortions be impressed on the women of the country and that the laws already in existence which entail imprisonment and heavy fines for abortionists be rigorously applied.

# DISCUSSION

## THE CORRELATION BETWEEN IONIZATION IN THE IONOSPHERE AND SUN-SPOT NUMBERS

STUDIES of the ionosphere over a period of years have indicated a close correlation between the ionization in the ionosphere and the Wolf sun-spot numbers. A detailed analysis of the National Bureau of Standards data by Smith, Gilliland and Kirby[1] shows that the relation is particularly striking when 12-month running averages of critical frequencies and sun-spot numbers are compared. In the period of 1934 to 1937, the average sun-spot number increased from 5 to 110, while the average $f^{\circ}_{F2}$ critical frequency at noon increased from 6.3 Mc/sec to 11.5 Mc/sec, corresponding to a range of electron concentrations from $0.38 \times 10^6/cm^3$ to $1.42 \times 10^6/cm^3$. Since noon values of electron concentration are nearly equilibrium values, the intensity of the ionizing radiation is proportional to the square of the electron concentration. Hence the intensity has increased about 14-fold, with an increase of 22-fold in the sun-spot number. In the same period the radiation producing ionization in the E layer and $F_1$ layer has increased by factors of 2.4 and 3, respectively. The correlation between sun-spot numbers and monthly averages of $F_2$ values is not so close, and Goodall[2] has shown that the solar characteristic giving the best correlation is the character figure for central zone calcium flocculi given in bulletins of the International Astronomical Union.

It is the purpose of this note to point out a possible reason for this correlation in the case of $F_2$ ionization. This ionization is variously ascribed to atomic oxygen, atomic nitrogen and molecular nitrogen,[3] but in all these cases the threshold wave-length for ionization is equal to or less than 910A. This is the Lyman series limit of hydrogen, and because the solar atmosphere is largely hydrogen in the normal state, its atmosphere will be extremely opaque for wave-lengths less than 910A. The light of a given wave-length comes from a depth in the solar atmosphere which varies inversely as the opacity at that wave-length, the average depth being such that the radiation is reduced to 1/e. Taking the atomic absorption coefficient as $0.6 \times 10^{-17}$ it follows that the radiation occurs at a level where the hydrogen pressure is $3 \times 10^{-3}$ dynes. The pressure at the photosphere[4] for visible radiation is roughly 300 dynes/cm² so the ionizing radiation comes from a level of the chromosphere several thousand kilometers above the photosphere.

[1] *Jour. Research,* NBS 21: 835, RP-1159, 1938.

[2] "The Solar Cycle and the $F_2$ Region of the Ionosphere." In press.

[3] Hulburt, *Phys. Rev.,* 53: 344, 1938; Wulf and Deming, *Terr. Mag. and Atmos. Elec.,* 43: 283, 1938.

[4] Unsöld, "Physik der Sternatumosphären," Julius Springer, 1938.

The opacity at 910A is comparable with the opacity in the strongest solar absorption lines. The atomic absorption coefficient of H$\alpha$ is roughly $10^4$ times that at the Lyman limit, but since less than $10^{-8}$ atoms per $cm^3$ are in a state to absorb H$\alpha$ the opacity at H$\alpha$ is much less than at 910A. The opacity in the K line of $Ca^+$ is estimated[4] to be roughly 4,000 times the opacity near the center of H$\alpha$ and is comparable in order of magnitude with the opacity at the Lyman limit.

A spectroheliogram made with the K line of $Ca^+$ gives a photograph of the solar atmosphere near the pressure level for emission of radiation beyond the Lyman limit. The picture is complicated by Doppler effect and by variations in chemical composition of the atmosphere, but primarily it gives a picture of the temperature distribution over the sun at the given pressure level. The spectroheliogram is characterized by bright flocculi in the region of sun-spots, while most of the disk is relatively dark. This contrast would be enormously enhanced in the far ultra-violet for a spot 4 times as bright as the solar disk at 3,900A would be 400 times as bright at 910A.

Roughly quantitative considerations show that nearly all the ionizing radiation must come from bright spots rather than the disk as a whole. It has been shown[5] that if the disk radiated as a black body at 6,000°, the quanta of wave-length less than 910A could account for the $F_2$ ionization, but there is no reason to assume that the solar atmosphere at these low pressures is at 6,000°. The temperature as measured by the brightness at the center of a strong absorption line is less than 5,000° and the radiation at 5,000° can not account for 1 per cent. of the observed effect. However, if less than 1 per cent. of the solar disk is at a temperature of 7,500° or more, these bright spots could account for the observed ionization. The hypothesis that nearly all the ionizing radiation comes from the flocculi normally associated with sun-spots can well account for the type of correlation found between $F_2$ ionization and sun-spot numbers. The average intensity over long periods of time will be nearly proportional to the number of spots, simply because flocculi are associated with spots; but because of variation in brightness of flocculi, the day-to-day values will vary in a random way. A similar correlation is found between the "character figures" giving the number and brightness of K flocculi and the sun-spot numbers.

Ionization of the E layer probably comes from molecular oxygen[6] with a threshold near 1,000A, and bright line emission of Lyman lines in the flocculi may be an effective source of ionization. There is no basis for predicting the relative effectiveness of the radiation of the solar disk and the flocculi in this spectrum range, but the variation of E-layer ionization with sun-spot number indicates that at sun-spot maximum more than half the effect comes from flocculi, while at minimum most of the effect comes from the disk as a whole. The origin of $F_1$ ionization is quite uncertain, but the rate of variation with sun-spot number suggests that the threshold is at a wave-length greater than 910A.

It is well recognized that bright chromospheric eruptions produce radio fade-out,[7] but the disturbance seems to come from ionization below the E layer with little or no change in the F layer.[8] The radiation from normal flocculi rather than from these transient eruptions must be invoked to explain $F_2$ ionization.

The above considerations indicate that $F_2$ ionization can not be maintained by the temperature radiation from the solar disk as a whole. The hypothesis that the ionizing radiation comes from bright flocculi accounts for the observed correlation between ionization and sun-spot numbers, but it will be a difficult problem to show whether or not the continuous radiation from these bright spots can quantitatively account for the ionization.

FRED L. MOHLER
NATIONAL BUREAU OF STANDARDS

[5] Hulbert, *Phys. Rev.*, 53: 344, 1938.
[6] Wulf and Deming, *loc. cit.*

[7] Dellinger, *Jour. Research* NBS, 19: 111, 1937.
[8] Dellinger, *Phys. Rev.*, 50: 189, 1936.

## A WHALE SHARK IN THE HAWAIIAN ISLANDS

IT is interesting to note that the whale shark, *Rhineodon typus,* can be said almost to abound in both the western and the eastern waters of the Pacific Ocean. But it has been so sparingly reported from the Central Pacific, that it might be thought almost absent from those vast reaches. Hence definite information of its occurrence in the Hawaiian Islands seems worthy of record.

Of its relative abundance in the western Pacific from the eastern coast of Japan to that of New South Wales in Australia, I have brought together all the evidence as of December 31, 1934, in an article on the geographical distribution of this greatest of the sharks.[1] As of that date 26 specimens were listed from the Western Pacific, and 15 of these were from Philippine waters. This abundance and the fact that it had been known (but not described) in these waters since 1800 (first record, 1816) lead me to believe that *Rhineodon* originated in the Philippine-Sulu Sea region and was distributed thence by ocean currents to all parts of the three great central oceans. This article was illustrated with maps showing all recorded occurrences.

Interestingly enough, *Rhineodon* seems almost as abundant in eastern Pacific waters—along the shores of the Americas from Lower California to Callao in Peru. I produced records for 23 specimens, of which 14 are listed from the lower part of the Gulf of California—

[1] E. W. Gudger, *Proc. Zool. Soc., London,* pt. 2, 863–893, pl. and 2 charts, 1934.

mainly around Cape San Lucas. Since that date, Dr. William Beebe has found them almost abundant and almost tame in those same waters. And more recently (1938), I have recorded that whale sharks are so abundant on the outer coast of Lower California from Hippolito Point to Cape San Lucas and so entirely unafraid as to be almost a nuisance to the tuna fishermen.[2]

From the Central Pacific but two whale sharks have ever been reported so far as I know—and these interestingly enough from the same group of islands. In 1929, Rougier[3] described a *Rhineodon* skin in the little museum in Papeete, Tahiti. This had come from a 17.3-foot specimen taken at Takaroa, Tuamotu Archipelago, in 1928. The second record is one I made in 1937 of a whale shark about 40 feet long impaled on the bow of a steamer near Tikehau Atoll in the Tuamotus.[4]

To these two records, I am now fortunate in being able to add a specimen of the whale shark, found in Hawaiian waters. These data came to me through the courtesy of Captain G. S. Bryan, hydrographer, U. S. Navy Department. This is but the last of many accounts of the wide-spread occurrence of this great fish communicated by the Hydrographic Office—to which my debt is heavy. This excellent account, sent in by Second Officer R. C. Willson, of the S. S. *Mapele* of the Matson Navigation Company, San Francisco, has been forwarded to me, and from it the following data on coloration and behavior are put on record.

On September 4, 1938, the *Mapele* was moored off Kukuihaele Landing on the north coast of Hawaii in Lat. 20° 08′ N. and Long. 155° 33.5 E. At 2:30 P.M. local time, a whale shark was seen slowly and fearlessly swimming around the ship among the sweepings and larger debris thrown overboard. The shark, seen by all hands, was about 25 feet long and about 4 feet wide across the broad blunt head. The description of the markings indubitably identify this fish as a whale shark. The head was covered with many white spots varying from one to two inches in diameter. These were scattered in random fashion over head and neck region. On the other hand, the body was covered with white spots in vertical rows separated by vertical white stripes. These extended from the back down the sides as far as the curve of the belly permitted sight. The rows of spots were about 6 inches apart, and the white stripes were about 2 inches wide. Spots and stripes both decreased in size from above downward and from the neck region toward the tail. The dorsal fin was about 18 inches high and had on it 7 distinct spots.

At about 3:30 the shark disappeared, but at 6:00 P.M. it was again seen swimming about under the stern amid slops and scraps thrown overboard from the ship's galley. "It swam leisurely around for about 20 minutes, bumping into the mooring lines a number of times. Once as it was swimming over one of the lines to a buoy the ship lifted, throwing the shark partly out of the water. Then it swam slowly off toward the west and was seen no more."

This behavior tallies almost exactly with the actions of another whale shark in swimming around a steamer in the harbor of St. Marc, Haiti, in 1937.[5] It is also very like that described of various specimens off the outer coast of Lower California. This great fish has no enemies and seems entirely unafraid of vessels and of men.

E. W. GUDGER

THE AMERICAN MUSEUM OF NATURAL HISTORY, NEW YORK

## TOXICITY OF THE SODIUM SALT OF DINITRO-o-CRESOL TO VENTURIA INAEQUALIS

POSSIBILITIES of direct chemical attack on fungi that cause certain types of plant disease now combated chiefly by repeated applications of protectant fungicides have been studied by the writer and associates.[1] It is sought by an eradicant fungicidal treatment at a vulnerable stage in the life-history of the pathogen to reduce the primary inoculum to a level at which the disease may be more surely and economically controlled. A preliminary report on further experiments with the apple scab pathogen, *Venturia inaequalis* (Cke.) Wint., follows.

In small-scale experiments in the spring of 1938, overwintered apple leaves bearing abundant mature ascocarps of *V. inaequalis* were sprayed with Elgetol, a proprietary preparation containing 12 per cent. by weight of the sodium salt of dinitro-o-cresol with a supplement to aid its penetration. Similar leaves sprayed with water served as controls. Studies of treated and untreated leaves indicated that Elgetol in water at 1 per cent. by volume reduced ascospore discharge by 99.7 per cent. (average of 3 trials).

Toximetric studies with agar plate cultures by a method reported by Palmiter and Keitt[2] indicate that the lethal concentration of Elgetol to the 2 isolates of *V. inaequalis* tested was near .05 per cent. by volume.

These small-scale experiments show that Elgetol has a high degree of eradicant effectiveness against *V. inaequalis*. Conclusions regarding its practical adap-

[2] E. W. Gudger, *Calif. Fish and Game*, 24: 420–421, 1938.

[3] Emm. Rougier, *Bull. Soc. Etudes Oceanogr.*, Papeete, 3: 318–319.

[4] E. W. Gudger, SCIENCE, 85: 2204, 314, 1937.

[5] E. W. Gudger, *Copeia*, 1: 60, 1937.

[1] G. W. Keitt and D. H. Palmiter, *Jour. Agr. Res.*, 55: 397–438, 1937.

[2] D. H. Palmiter and G. W. Keitt, *Jour. Agr. Res.*, 55: 439–452, 1937.

tation for apple scab control must await the results of further experiments, which are in progress.

G. W. KEITT
UNIVERSITY OF WISCONSIN

## SEEDS FOR THE STUDY OF ROOT AND ROOT-HAIR STRUCTURE IN BOTANICAL LABORATORIES

IN connection with studies made of the invasion of the bunch grass prairies by weeds, extensive germinations were made with *Bromus tectorum* L., one of the most common and abundant weeds invading deteriorated prairies in western Montana.

Under ordinary laboratory conditions, *B. tectorum* germinates easily in two days, giving usually from 90 to 98 per cent. germination. Its very fine single seminal root appears to me a most excellent material for the study of root-hair structure in undergraduate laboratories. All zones of the young primary root can be easily seen under both low and high powers of the microscope. The root-hairs stand out very clearly and prominently, giving a full series from the youngest epidermal cell just bulging out to the fully developed hair, in which streaming of protoplasm is usually evident.

A very convenient way, without the use of blotters, is to scatter the seed in the moist chamber, in which water has been poured to a depth of say one half to one mm. The chamber may be placed either in a lighted or in a darkened place; in two or three days the roots will be of the proper length. The seeds will also germinate if dropped in a tumbler-full of water.

I'll be glad to send on the receipt of a mailed and stamped envelope enough seed for any size class.

JOSEPH KRAMER
MONTANA STATE UNIVERSITY

# SPECIAL ARTICLES

## ACTION OF KETENE ON THE PITUITARY LACTOGENIC HORMONE

IN their study of the acetylation of pepsin, Herriott and Northrop[1] found that the primary amino groups play no significant role in the activity of the pepsin molecule. Later, White[2, 3] reached the same conclusion in a study of insulin and emphasized the importance of the tyrosine molecule in all hormones of protein nature. In contrast with their conclusions we have found that the primary amino groups in the lactogenic hormone appear to be important for its biological activity.

The lactogenic hormone contains 0.53 per cent. amino nitrogen, as determined by Van Slyke gasometric apparatus. Herriott and Northrop have shown that amino groups are acetylated by ketene at room temperature in not more than five minutes, whereas the phenolic hydroxyl groups remain unchanged.[4] We have also found that ketene treatment for five minutes at room temperature was sufficient to block all amino groups in the lactogenic hormone. If the reaction is carried out at 0° C, for five minutes, only 30 per cent. of the amino groups is acetylated. The acetylation is achieved by passing a constant stream of ketene into a suspension which contains 10 mg protein per cc in pH 5.6 M acetate buffer. Ketene is obtained by the improved type of generator designed by one of us.[5]

[1] R. M. Herriott and J. H. Northrop, *Jour. Gen. Physiol.*, 18: 35, 1934–35.

[2] K. G. Stern and A. White, *Jour. Biol. Chem.*, 122: 371, 1938.

[3] A. White, Cold Spring Harbor Symposia on Quantitative Biology, 6: 262, 1938.

[4] There is as yet no experimental evidence to show that the phenolic hydroxyl of tyrosine in the lactogenic hormone is also important for its biological activity.

All ketene experiments were done with a preparation of lactogenic hormone (Li-P)[6] which, as Table I shows, gives a pronounced reaction when a total dose of 1 mg is injected intramuscularly into one-month-old squabs.

It will be seen from the results in Table I that the free amino groups in lactogenic hormone are essential for its activity. The results of the present work are in contrast with those secured by Stern and White[7]

TABLE I

| Lactogenic preparation (Li-P) | Amino groups acetylated per cent. | Dose/Squab mg | Number of squabs | Crop sac reactions |
|---|---|---|---|---|
| Untreated ........ | 0 | 1.0 | 3 | pronounced |
| Acetylated at 0° for 5 minutes ..... | 30 | 1.0 | 3 | 2 minimal<br>1 negative |
| Acetylated at 20° for 5 minutes ... | 100 | 1.0 | 6 | negative |
| | 100 | 4.0 | 6 | negative |

in the acetylation of insulin, and are especially interesting because of several striking similarities in the two hormones. Stern and White treated insulin with the same reagent—ketene—under conditions similar to those here employed, and found that the free amino groups of insulin played no significant role in its phar-

[5] C. H. Li, SCIENCE, this issue, page 143.

[6] The authors are most grateful to Dr. W. R. Lyons for the potent preparation of lactogenic hormone employed. The minimal effective dose was 0.2 mg when divided into four daily doses and administered intramuscularly. We have had the opportunity of studying a similarly potent preparation of adrenotropic hormone, due to the kindness of W. R. Lyons and H. D. Moon. The activity of adrenotropic hormone is not destroyed by ketene by five minutes of treatment. This method may conveniently eliminate the lactogenic activity in adrenotropic fractions.

[7] *Loc. cit.*

macodynamic action. These groups are essential for the activity of the lactogenic hormone.

CHOH HAO LI
MIRIAM E. SIMPSON
HERBERT M. EVANS
INSTITUTE OF EXPERIMENTAL BIOLOGY,
UNIVERSITY OF CALIFORNIA,
BERKELEY

## THE EFFECT OF COCARBOXYLASE UPON METABOLISM AND NEURO-PSYCHIATRIC PHENOMENA IN PELLAGRINS WITH BERIBERI[1]

THE present communication is a report of observations on eight selected cases of pellagra with beriberi which were studied from chemical, neurological and psychiatric standpoints. Preceding and following the administration of cocarboxylase, each patient was studied repeatedly by the following methods: (1) Analysis of blood samples for metabolites, including sulfite combining substances. (2) Neurological examination, including chronaximetric measurement. (3) Estimation of the psychiatric status.

The intravenous administration of 50 milligrams of cocarboxylase (Merck) to persons who exhibited signs of an "active process" was followed, in every instance, by dramatic and rapid improvement. The bisulfite-binding substances decreased in quantity. The pathological signs of peripheral and cranial nerves, which had become increased in patients who were being treated with nicotinic acid and riboflavin, became less conspicuous or disappeared. The irritability of a number of muscles, measured in terms of their strength-duration curves, returned from underexcitability before treatment to normal values and in some cases even progressed to overexcitability. Correspondingly, the increased threshold of sensibility to touch and prick in arms and legs was reduced to normal, and the depressed pupillary and corneal reflexes improved quantitatively, often becoming normal.

Following the administration of cocarboxylase, some beneficial effect occurred, in some persons within an hour and in all persons within four hours. Improvement continued for from one to four days thereafter. Since the unbalanced diets of these persons remained essentially unchanged, in the absence of further therapy the patients tended to regress rapidly to their condition preceding treatment. A psychoneurotic syndrome which was recognized in these persons and which responded promptly to the administration of cocarboxylase will be described separately. In contrast, in the persons selected for control, there was no decrease of bisulfite-binding substances in the blood and no improvement in the neurological and psychoneurotic symptoms following cocarboxylase therapy.

The present study shows that the neuropathy accompanying pellagra represents a clinical entity (beriberi), distinct from a deficiency of nicotinic acid or of riboflavin. It shows also that cocarboxylase (pyrophosphate of thiamin) has a striking effect upon certain intermediate products of carbohydrate metabolism and induces improvement in the affected peripheral and cranial nerves. Furthermore, the decrease of bisulphite-binding substances in the blood is accompanied by a decrease or disappearance of certain neurological signs and of psychoneurotic symptoms.

F. H. LEWY
MEDICAL COLLEGE OF THE UNIVERSITY
OF PENNSYLVANIA
H. E. HIMWICH
ALBANY MEDICAL COLLEGE
J. P. FROSTIG
UNIVERSITY OF CALIFORNIA
T. D. SPIES
UNIVERSITY OF CINCINNATI COLLEGE
OF MEDICINE

[1] From the Department of Neurosurgery, Hospital of the University of Pennsylvania, Philadelphia, Pennsylvania; Department of Physiology and Pharmacology, Albany Medical College, Albany, New York; Department of Psychiatry, University of California, Berkeley, California; and Department of Internal Medicine, University of Cincinnati General Hospital, Cincinnati, Ohio. This study was aided by grants from the Child Neurology Research (Friedsam Foundation) and from the Rockefeller Foundation.

## EVIDENCE FOR THE EXISTENCE OF A RESPIRATORY NEUROHORMONE

IN the course of studies on the pressor effects of acetylcholine, it was observed that amounts of acetylcholine which produce pressor effects and contraction of the nictitating membrane also increase the rate and depth of respiration for brief intervals. It was also observed that the larger the dose of acetylcholine the longer the duration of respiratory stimulation and the greater the depth of respirations. The pressor effect always outlasts the respiratory stimulation.

The minimum amounts of acetylcholine producing respiratory stimulation in atropinized dogs and cats are 0.15 to 0.2 mgm or more per kilogram, but in the presence of optimum amounts of eserine (about 1.5 mgm per kilogram) as little as 0.005 mgm of acetylcholine may produce respiratory stimulation. If 0.05 mgm of acetylcholine is used throughout in atropinized animals, the smallest dose of eserine which is required to produce respiratory stimulation from this amount of acetylcholine is 0.04 to 0.05 mgm per kilogram. In the same animals doses of epinephrine which produced blood pressure elevation and withdrawal of the nictitating membrane also caused a decrease but never an increase in the rate of respiration.

In five cats and eight dogs the carotid sinuses were removed and in some of these animals the vagi above the ganglia nodosa as well as the sympathetics above the superior cervical ganglia were sectioned. In these animals, which were treated with atropine and eserine,

0.05 to 0.1 mgm of acetylcholine did not produce respiratory stimulation.

In another group of animals treated with atropine and eserine, 3 to 6 mgm of nicotine per kilogram abolished not only the pressor effects of acetylcholine but also diminished or abolished its respiratory stimulant action.

The respiratory effect of intravenously administered acetylcholine appears after a delay of seven to twenty seconds, and slow or rapid injection of comparable doses into the common carotid artery does not accelerate the onset of the respiratory effect. In several dogs acetylcholine in doses effective as respiratory stimulants when administered by the femoral vein produced no or feeble respiratory stimulation when given by the carotid artery.

It is concluded that the respiratory stimulation following acetylcholine injections depends upon the presence of the carotid body and that the active principle is not acetylcholine but a sympathin liberated at the nerve terminations following stimulation of sympathetic ganglia by acetylcholine. Nicotine prevents this stimulation by producing ganglionic paralysis or depression. Examination of the tracings published by Magoun, Ranson and Hetherington[1] and by Harrison, Wang and Berry[2] reveals that sympathins liberated following hypothalamic stimulation in adrenalectomized animals produce not only pressor effects and withdrawal of the nictitating membrane but also marked and brief stimulation of respiration.

It is tentatively suggested that a sympathin, not identical with epinephrine, possesses (via the carotid bodies) properties of a respiratory stimulant.

THEODORE KOPPANYI
CHARLES R. LINEGAR
GEORGETOWN UNIVERSITY

[1] Magoun, Ranson and Hetherington, *Amer. Jour. Physiol.*, 119: 615, 1937.

[2] Harrison, Wang and Berry, *Amer. Jour. Physiol.*, 125: 449, 1939.

## THE REDUCING GROUPS OF EGG ALBUMIN

IT has long been known that SH reducing groups can be detected by the nitroprusside test in denatured but not in native egg albumin. In some other proteins SH groups can be detected with nitroprusside even when the protein is native.[1] Various methods have been developed for the quantitative study of protein-reducing groups.[2, 3, 4]

In the present experiments measurements are made of the amount of ferricyanide reduced by denatured egg albumin in the presence of the synthetic detergent Duponol PC and of the effects on the amount of ferricyanide reduced of previous reactions of the protein with iodine and iodoaceticacidamide. These experiments show the kinds of complications which may be involved in the study of protein groups generally. They also illustrate some of the remarkable effects of synthetic detergents on proteins, which I shall describe more completely elsewhere.

At pH 9 ferricyanide oxidizes not only the SH groups of denatured egg albumin but weaker reducing groups as well. The amount of ferrocyanide formed is greater the longer the time of reaction and the higher the concentration of ferricyanide.[5] This also is true at pH 6.8. In addition, the results at pH 6.8 are variable because they depend on the physical state of the denatured protein. Other things being equal, the more the denatured protein is aggregated,[6] the less ferrocyanide is formed.

If, however, denatured egg albumin is oxidized by ferricyanide at pH 6.8 in the presence of Duponol PC, the oxidation takes place at a much lower concentration of ferricyanide than in the absence of Duponol, and the amount of ferrocyanide formed is independent, within wide limits, of the time and temperature of the reaction and of the concentrations of ferricyanide and Duponol. No reduction of ferricyanide takes place if the SH groups of denatured egg albumin are first abolished with formaldehyde or iodoaceticacidamide.

The proper conditions for the reaction between ferricyanide and denatured protein vary from protein to protein. In the case of egg albumin, the reaction is carried out for 10 minutes at 37° C. in 3 cc of a pH 6.8 solution containing 0.002 mM of ferricyanide and 10 mg of Duponol PC (du Pont), a mixture of the $C_{10}$—$C_{18}$ compounds of $CH_3(CH_2)_nCH_2OSO_3Na$. 0.001 mM of ferrocyanide are formed from 10 mg of denatured egg albumin. There is no increase in the amount of ferrocyanide formed if the reaction is carried out for 100 minutes instead of for 10 minutes or if the rate of reaction is increased by increasing the amount of ferricyanide 25 times and the amount of Duponol 10 times or by raising the temperature from 37° to 100° C.

Urea[7] and guanidine,[8] like Duponol, promote the

[1] M. L. Anson, "The Chemistry of Amino Acids and Proteins," Chapter IX. Edited by C. L. A. Schmidt, Springfield, 1938.

[2] A. E. Mirsky and M. L. Anson, *Jour. Gen. Physiol.*, 18: 307, 1935.

[3] R. Kuhn and P. Desnuelle, *Zeits. Physiol. Chem.*, 251: 14, 1938.

[4] J. P. Greenstein, *Jour. Biol. Chem.*, 125: 501, 1938.

[5] A. E. Mirsky and M. L. Anson, *Jour. Gen. Physiol.*, 19: 451, 1936.

[6] M. L. Anson and A. E. Mirsky, *Jour. Gen. Physiol.*, 15: 341, 1932.

[7] I have used urea for many years to promote the reaction between protein-reducing groups and the uric acid reagent.

[8] Greenstein (see note 4) has studied the effect of guanidine on the oxidation of denatured egg albumin by porphyrindin. I shall discuss his results elsewhere.

ferricyanide reaction. They are much less effective reagents than Duponol.

Ferricyanide, iodine and iodoaceticacidamide all react with the SH groups of simple SH compounds like cysteine, which is a constituent of egg albumin. Ferricyanide, although it reacts with denatured egg albumin, does not react with native egg albumin.[5] Iodine and iodoaceticacidamide, nevertheless, do react with native egg albumin. 10 mg of native egg albumin treated with 1 cc of 0.0015 N iodine at pH 3.2 and then neutralized and denatured by Duponol, no longer reduces dilute ferricyanide. 10 mg of native albumin treated with 0.01 mM of iodoaceticacidamide at pH 9 and then denatured reduces only half as much ferricyanide as untreated albumin.

In connection with the observation that native egg albumin reacts with iodoaceticacidamide but not with ferricyanide, it is interesting to note that urease is inactivated by iodoaceticacidamide[9] but not by ferricyanide.[10] The effect of iodoaceticacidamide on viruses is now being tested.

The fact that ferricyanide does not react with native egg albumin does not prove that the SH groups of native egg albumin are linked or inaccessible. On the other hand, it can not be assumed, without independent evidence, that in the present experiments ferricyanide, iodine and iodoaceticacidamide are reacting only with SH groups. All three of these reagents can, under suitable conditions, react with protein groups other than SH groups. It is possible, furthermore, that there are reducing groups in denatured egg albumin which are not SH groups but which are oxidized by dilute ferricyanide only in the presence of SH groups.

M. L. ANSON

THE ROCKEFELLER INSTITUTE FOR MEDICAL RESEARCH

[5] M. L. Anson, Jour. Gen. Physiol. (footnote not on this page)

# SCIENTIFIC APPARATUS AND LABORATORY METHODS

## AN IMPROVED TYPE OF KETENE GENERATOR

RECENTLY Herriott[1] described a ketene generator which was improvised from that previously suggested by Ott, Schroter and Packendorf.[2] In our studies of the acetylation of pituitary hormones we have developed a new design of generator, giving a more efficient and workable apparatus. A diagram is given in Fig. 1.

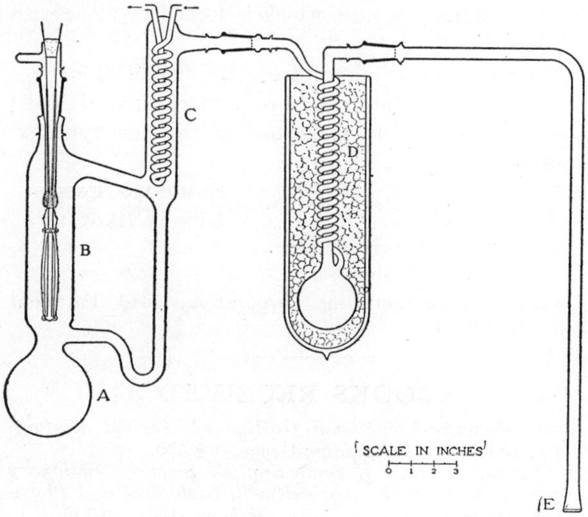


FIG. 1

Vaporized acetone from flask A is decomposed by the heating filament B, which is kept at a bright-red heat. The mixed vapors pass through the condenser C in order to remove the unchanged acetone vapor and most of the ketene polymers. More complete removal of these two substances is then effected by the trap D, which is immersed in a freezing mixture of salt and ice. Ketene then passes into the solution through a sintered glass plate E. The sintered glass plate is particularly useful for bubbling gas; it gives more effective contact between the solution and the gas, and it stirs the solution sufficiently to make unnecessary a mechanical stirrer as generally suggested.

The removable filament-support is the same as described by Herriott. The 40 mill tungsten leads are sealed permanently into the glass and the replaceable tungsten filament (15 mill) may be attached to them in the manner illustrated in the figure. The rate at which ketene is generated can be controlled by varying the current which passes through the heating filament.

CHOH HAO LI

INSTITUTE OF EXPERIMENTAL BIOLOGY, UNIVERSITY OF CALIFORNIA, BERKELEY

## A SIMPLE AND EFFICIENT PRECIPITATE DRYER

IN the course of preparing enzymes, protein was precipitated with ammonium sulfate at 70 per cent. saturation. The filtered, wet precipitate contained a large amount of mother liquor. If the precipitate was allowed to dry on the filter paper more than half its dry weight would be salt and not the active material desired. Drying first on blotting paper and then on a porous plate was tried. By this method all the water was absorbed; but as it began to evaporate,

[1] R. M. Herriott, *Jour. Gen. Physiol.*, 18: 69, 1934.

[2] E. Ott, R. Schroter and K. Packendorf, *Jour. Prakt. Chem.*, 130, N.S.: 177, 1931.

[9] C. V. Smythe, *Jour. Biol. Chem.*, 114: 601, 1936.

[10] L. Hellerman and M. E. Perkins, *Jour. Biol. Chem.*, 107: 241, 1934.

ammonium sulfate was redeposited as an efflorescence on the surface of the protein precipitate.

A method was devised which reduces efflorescence to a minimum, purifies the protein precipitate and shortens drying time. An apparatus was constructed which consisted of a galvanized iron box open on one side. Inside the box, on the bottom, an electric socket is fastened and the wires pass through a hole in one side. In the top, over the lamp and also along the lower edge of each side of the box, holes are bored to allow circulation of air. A drying plate, made of plaster of Paris, about five eighths of an inch thick, fits vertically into the open side, closing the box. This face plate is pushed into the open side of the box until flush with the outer edges. It should fit snugly. In order to be able to remove the plate easily, thumb holes are made by cutting out a small "V" from the middle of each edge against which the plate rests.

Before use the plate should always be oven dried. A 60- or 75-watt lamp is then placed in the socket, the plate adjusted, and the lamp turned on for 5 or 10 minutes to allow the box to warm up. The precipitate is removed from the filter paper, roughly dried on blotting paper and spread in a thin layer on the surface of the plaster plate. The plaster absorbs the mother liquor. As the inside surface is at a higher temperature than the outside, most of the evaporation takes place there, and ammonium sulfate deposits on the inside face. The protein meanwhile dries readily on the outside. When dried to the point of cracking into small pieces it can be scraped off and ground to a powder in a mortar.

The plaster plate is reconditioned for further work by completely scraping off the last traces of any remaining precipitate with a knife or spatula. If the apparatus remains unused for some time the plate should be dried in an oven before use, as it will have become saturated with moisture from the air.

Arnold Lowman

University of California Medical School,
San Francisco

## TURNTABLE FOR EXERCISING RATS

The turntable herewith described is very satisfactory for exercising rats. It is permanent, inexpensive and easily removed from the cage for cleaning. This new exerciser has been tested thoroughly in the dormer cage[1] used in the animal colony of The Wistar Institute.

It consists of an aluminum disc[2] (Fig. 1) 12½ inches in diameter of 3S18 gage sheet aluminum of 20-minute alumilite finish, with a ¼ inch outer edge flange for

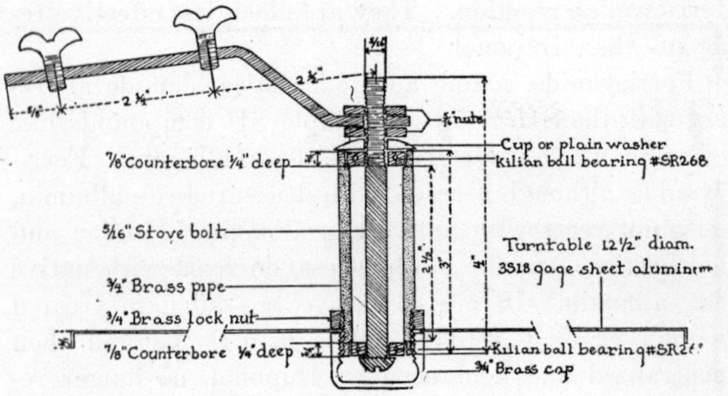


Fig. 1

strength, and a center hole of 1–1/16 inches. This new disc replaces the monel metal and stainless steel discs used formerly, preventing pitting caused by animal excretions and the brittleness in the metal with consequent cracking around the hole.

The housing is made from a piece of standard ¾ inch brass pipe, 3 inches in length, threaded on one outer end, with a ⅞ inch counterbore on each end ¼ inch deep. Inserted in each counterbore is ⅞ inch × ¼ inch Kilian ball bearing[3] SR 268, 5/16 inch bore. A 5/16 round head stove bolt, 4 inches in length, serves as a shaft. The stove bolt is inserted in the thread end of the housing, through the ball bearings, covered with a brass washer and locked with a 5/16 inch standard hexagonal nut. On one end of bolt is placed a 1 inch × ⅛ inch × 6 inch hanger of galvanized steel for fastening to the ceiling of the cage with two ¼ inch thumb screws. On threaded end of housing is placed a ¾ inch lock nut, then the aluminum disc, which is locked in place with a ¾ inch brass cap.

The new brass hub replaces the modified bicycle[1] front wheel hub and axle, to prevent rusting. It costs about two dollars to make one of the new type exercisers.

Edmond J. Farris
Gustav Engvall

The Wistar Institute of
Anatomy and Biology

[1] M. J. Greenman and F. L. Duhring, "Breeding and Care of the Albino Rat for Research Purposes," 2nd ed., The Wistar Institute, Philadelphia, Pa., 1931.

[2] The Aluminum Cooking Utensil Company, New Kensington, Pa.

[3] Kilian Manufacturing Corporation, 1640 Fairmont Avenue, Philadelphia, Pa.

## BOOKS RECEIVED

Bone, Robert G. *Visual Outline of Ancient History.* Pp. iv + 124. Longmans, Green. $0.75.

De Vries, Louis. *German-English Science Dictionary for Students in the Agricultural, Biological and Physical Sciences.* Pp. x + 473. McGraw-Hill. $3.00.

Heffron, Roderick. *Pneumonia; with Special Reference to Pneumococcus Lobar Pneumonia.* Pp. xvii + 1086. Commonwealth Fund, New York. $4.50.

Legget, Robert F. *Geology and Engineering.* Pp. xviii + 650. Illustrated. McGraw-Hill. $4.50.

Oppenheimer, Carl and Kurt G. Stern. *Biological Oxidation.* Pp. ix + 317. 17 figures. Nordemann. $8.25.

Reihlen, Hans. *Remsen's Einleitung das Studium der Chemie; Neu Bearbeitet und Neu Herausgegeben.* Pp. xv + 324. 59 figures. Steinkopff, Dresden.

# SCIENCE

Vol. 90 | Friday, August 18, 1939 | No. 2329

*Food, Drink and Evolution:* Professor Charles T. Brues ... 145
*Scientific Events:*
*The First Hundred Years of Photography; Foreign Markets for Medicinal Products of the United States; The Rochester Athenaeum and Mechanics Institute; Biochemical Research at the University of Pittsburgh; The Third International Cancer Congress; The Bicentenary of the Royal Swedish Academy of Sciences; The Hundredth Anniversary of the Birth of Robert Henry Thurston; Recent Deaths and Memorials* ... 150
*Scientific Notes and News* ... 153
*Discussion:*
*Compound Words:* Professor Sterling B. Talmage; R. H. Baugh; Dr. Oran Raber; Marjorie Fuller and Jane McMasters. *Value of Characters of the Undeveloped Shoot in Identifying Plants:* Professor H. D. Harrington. *Cystine and Methionine Requirements for Growth and Lactation:* Dr. J. R. Haag and L. D. Wright ... 155
*Scientific Books:*
*The Theory of Numbers:* Professor George D. Birkhoff. *Principles of Insect Physiology:* R. E. Snodgrass ... 158
*Societies and Meetings:*
*The Royal Society of Canada* ... 159
*Special Articles:*
*Copper and Vitamin C Effects upon the Excised Frog Heart:* Dr. Hubert B. Peugnet. *Prolonged Therapeutic Effect of Subcutaneously Implanted Crystals of Ovarian Hormone in Women:* Dr. Udall J. Salmon, Robert I. Walter and Samuel H. Geist. *The Influence of 3-Indole-Acetic Acid on Pollen Germination:* Paul F. Smith. *The Vitamin C Content of Spring Greens:* Professor R. C. Burrell and Helena A. Miller ... 162
*Scientific Apparatus and Laboratory Methods:*
*A Thermal Method for the Separation of Gases and Isotopes:* Dr. Arthur Bramley and Dr. A. Keith Brewer ... 165
*Science News* ... 8

SCIENCE: A Weekly Journal devoted to the Advancement of Science, edited by J. McKeen Cattell and published every Friday by

THE SCIENCE PRESS
New York City: Grand Central Terminal
Lancaster, Pa. Garrison, N. Y.
Annual Subscription, $6.00 Single Copies, 15 Cts.

SCIENCE is the official organ of the American Association for the Advancement of Science. Information regarding membership in the Association may be secured from the office of the permanent secretary in the Smithsonian Institution Building, Washington, D. C.

# FOOD, DRINK AND EVOLUTION[1]

By Professor CHARLES T. BRUES
HARVARD UNIVERSITY

The three primary animal instincts, to secure sustenance, to gain protection and to enjoy the opportunity of reproducing their kind, are related either individually or collectively to every biological problem, however narrow its scope. Although the impress of each of these necessities is to be found in the behavior and structure of every species, it is by no means evident to the same extent, nor alike at all periods of ontogeny. Reproduction is confined to a limited part of the life span even in the most primitive types of animals, and the period of reproductive activity is still more obviously restricted in the insects, where it becomes an attribute of only the final, unchanging imaginal stage. This stage must thus suddenly disclose all the adaptations of the sexually mature animal.

Protection from destructive agencies is on the other hand a constant necessity, common to all periods of the life span. It is, however, in part passive, as it may depend to a great extent upon bodily characteristics, not necessarily associated with specialized behavior.

The instinct to secure food is equally a constant necessity during post-embryonic growth, for only by its gratification can growth and development take place. Even more than reproductive activity the taking of food by animals is rhythmic, cyclical or interrupted by periods of varying length. Furthermore, food requirements in insects are proportionally much greater during the preparatory stages, when large reserves of fat are produced and stored within the body. Feeding is thus by no means a uniform or continuous process, but its association with the several stages is far more extended than is reproduction. Also, it is a purely active, never a passive, process, and in consequence we find that it has modified struc-

[1] Annual public address of the Entomological Society of America at its meeting in Richmond, Va., December 29, 1938.

ture and behavior even more profoundly than have the needs for protection.

The relations of insects to their food supply are very diverse and complex and taken together are unparalleled in any other group of living organisms. We have as yet made slow progress in unraveling the details and have been tempted to make many assumptions and generalizations which it must be admitted rest upon a rather flimsy basis. For this reason I feel that it behooves us as entomologists to take brief stock of our present knowledge concerning the food and feeding habits of insects as they appear to have influenced the course of insect evolution.

With reference to their choice of foods we may roughly group the insects into two categories, one of which includes herbivorous species, feeding directly on plants, and the other represented by those that are carnivorous, preying on other living animals or consuming those dead from other causes. The number of species in each group is approximately equal, but it is a striking fact that the great majority of the carnivorous forms depend upon other insects on which they are either predatory or parasitic. In this respect the insects are almost human, for the most important predatory and parasitic enemies of civilized man are other groups of men. Some of them accept and thrive upon the foliage and other tissues of numerous, often unrelated plants without evincing a pronounced preference for any particular kind. The number of such polyphagous species is large, but not so great as we once thought. Even some of our common grasshoppers restrict their feeding to one or at most to a very few species of plants. They may, however, under stress of hunger partake of many plants they would otherwise avoid, while other Orthoptera and even lepidopterous caterpillars may occasionally become cannibals. Such transgressions again are "almost human" and recall the behavior of mobs. They are of definite biological significance, for they show conclusively that the normally restricted diet of these insects is not a physiological necessity, since the unaccustomed substances cause neither digestive disturbances nor other metabolic derangement sufficient to interfere with normal growth and development.

Viewed in the light of our own appetites such a restricted dietary is utterly incomprehensible. We, as entomologists, are so accustomed to this peculiarity among many insect pests that we take it for granted and have shown little inclination to inquire into its evolutionary history.

Carnivorous insects exhibit many of the fundamental characteristics of their vegetarian relatives with reference to food, despite their more spectacular behavior. They are almost equally fastidious in confining themselves to diets as circumscribed as those affected by vegetarian species. Thus, certain ground beetles of several related genera restrict their food to snails. Lady-beetles consume great numbers of aphids and scale insects either generally or with great specificity. The solitary wasps store their nests with spiders and insects of all kinds, but we find, generally, that each species limits its provisioning to members of a single family or still more closely restricts its choice, sometimes, to a single species of prey. Such behavior is again difficult to reconcile with our own human appetites.

Parasitic insects present undoubtedly the most striking series of highly specialized food habits to be found in the whole animal kingdom, and their behavior is modified for several reasons. The vast majority, known as entomophagous or insect-eating, parasites, present a picture that is fundamentally different from the more conventional types of parasitism among other organisms. They are members of the holometabolous orders of insects in which it is almost invariably only the preparatory stages that dispense with a free-living existence. One result of this dual mode of life is the acquisition of totally different food-habits by the larval and imaginal stages of the insects concerned. This is paralleled, but to a far lesser degree, by the nectar-loving butterfly that suddenly discards the carrots or cabbage that nurtured it as a caterpillar. Such vagaries should not surprise us, as they are quite in keeping with our own personal habits when we feed our offspring on milk and spinach and deny them the liqueurs and lobster that we smugly reserve for the age of discretion. Nevertheless, this proved to be an innovation for insects as it initiated the development of the many remarkable modifications which now follow independent lines of evolution in the larval and imaginal stages. This condition reaches its highest development among parasitic insects. The free-living imagines are morphologically of quite ordinary structure, but the female is endowed with very highly adaptive and complex instincts associated with host-selection and oviposition. The larvae on the other hand commonly show unusual physiological, morphological and behavioristic peculiarities that enable them to develop successfully within the eggs or bodies of the many diverse insects on which they are parasitic. Individual species are narrowly restricted in the selection of host insects, even more regularly so than the free-living vegetarian and predatory types.

We have already mentioned the fact that one of the most extraordinary features of this horde of entomophagous parasites is their selection almost exclusively of other insects as hosts and that the same is true of predatory insects. For this reason the insects are a much more self-contained series of organisms than any other group of animals. That is to say, the balance of nature which determines the fluctuations of organic populations is among the insects dependent to a large extent upon the abundance and activities of other insects.

It is perfectly obvious from the foregoing very inadequate summary that food and food-selection play a very important part in the present economy of the insects as a whole. Thus we may readily surmise *a priori* that their evolution and diversification through the ages have been determined in great measure by the changes and specializations that have established the complex picture just presented.

We may now inquire to what extent the evolution of insects has been directed or modified by the persistence of stabilized food habits and by the acquisition of new methods of securing sustenance in a living world that has itself undergone vast changes.

Since vegetarian insects are at the present time the mainstay of the entire series it is natural to suppose that this type was the first to appear on the earth, but this appears dubious when we examine it critically. The present vegetarian insects depend mainly on the seed plants, and these were not in existence till long after insects had become highly differentiated. Moreover, specialized predators, like the dragon-flies and mantids, are included among the early arrivals, quite contemporaneous with the precursors of vegetarian types.

The obvious conclusion to be drawn from these facts is that the several types of food habits have persisted without change for very long geological periods. This may be most naturally attributed to physiological or anatomical necessity. That is to say, to assume that animal foods are the only ones suitable for the proper nutrition, growth and reproduction of carnivorous insects and that plant foods are similarly required by vegetarian insects. Two plausible reasons for such an assumption readily come to mind. The restriction may be functional or physiological, depending upon the ability of the animals to utilize the materials which they eat. Or it may, on the other hand, depend upon the morphology of the mouthparts and digestive system or upon structures accessory to the feeding process such as prehensile legs or unusually delicate sense organs. Such mechanistic explanations do not suffice, so as a third alternative we may blame it on the pure cussedness of the "critters" and call it blind instinct. We shall have to leave this question in abeyance till we have considered some other aspects of the problem.

It is quite axiomatic that there is usually a high correlation between form and function in animals, meaning form in a wide sense. An extension of this idea to behavior, habits or bionomics as an integral part of "function" is justified, partly because of the necessarily loose way that these terms must be applied to the activities of animals. Also, it is impossible to find any discontinuity as we pass gradually from a purely physico-chemical type of functional activity to the complex train of events involved in the search, capture, mastication, digestion and final utilization of food by a predatory insect. Such associations are the essence of the division of labor between the parts of the animal body, and they lose their true significance once we attempt to deal with them as independent or even separable units. Nevertheless, we shall proceed to do this very thing, as there seems to be no other approach. We perceive everywhere niceties of structure that are obviously suited to the food-habits of their possessors. The asymmetrical grinding mandibles of a grasshopper are better fitted for chewing foliage than for tearing flesh, although they may draw blood from our finger if it is offered to them. The composite sucking jaws of an ant-lion suit their purpose admirably, but they would make little headway if their owner elected to eat a tasty bit of spinach. The scissor-like mandibles of the worker amazon ant are fine for a formicine pogrom, but render the ants useless in their own nursery as they can not even pick up their babies without danger of inflicting mortal injury.

Without prolonging this familiar inventory, we will agree that such profound modifications are important factors in limiting the choice of food.

Nevertheless, if we should continue to enumerate further such similar structural adaptations of mouthparts we would reach the point where the correlation was far less patent. Then we could not honestly say that a transition, for example, from predatism to vegetarianism would entail any mechanical difficulties.

Indeed, some of the most interesting and instructive evidence bearing on the evolution of food habits is furnished by the sporadic appearance of aberrant diets in insects belonging to groups that are otherwise homogeneous in this respect. The acquisition of carnivorous habits by butterflies or moths and the occurrence of a few vegetarian members among the enormous series of parasitic chalcid flies are examples of this phenomenon.

Clear-cut examples are to be found which show that there have occurred occasionally shifts in food habits whereby changes comparable to structural mutations have resulted in the appearance of vegetarian habits in a purely carnivorous group or *vice versa*. Likewise between the four types, phytophagy, predatism, parasitism and saprophagy, similar shifts may be noted. One of these relates to the very obnoxious Mexican bean beetle.

It is well known that the lady-birds or coccinellid beetles form an almost uniformly predatory group. They spend their entire developmental and adult life gobbling up helpless aphids or scale insects and hence represent the acme of virtue to the economic entomologist. To him the bean beetle is *persona non grata* for the subfamily Epilachninae into which she was born gave up the murderous habits of their ancestors and became gentle vegetarians many millions of years before it became a fad in America to visit Battle Creek for this purpose.

Together with a number of similarly degraded relatives the bean beetle forms the cosmopolitan genus Epilachna, so named because it has a fuzzy back in the place of the hairy chest that adorns the real meat-eating he-beetles. For this reason the term lady-bird is particularly appropriate. A few distant cousins forming two other genera are equally disreputable vegetarians with specific food plants. A second species, *Epilachna borealis,* is common in eastern North America, feeding on the foliage of our native wild cucumber and also mutilating cultivated squash and pumpkin vines. We have thus in our region two species, each with sharply restricted food plants. In Europe two species feed on cucurbits, usually on native palearctic species, and one of these may on occasion attack potato foliage when its preferred food plants are absent, but no European species are known to feed on legumes. Further eastward, from India to Japan, Malaya and Australia a common oriental species is often a pest of potatoes and may be frequently found feeding on other solanums and related genera, while a Japanese species feeds on both Cucurbitaceae and Solanaceae. In South America two species eat cucurbits, but none are known to eat solanums. Finally in Africa no less than five species attack cotton, a malvaceous plant that is never known to harbor the beetles on other continents except in one or two isolated cases that have been reported.

From this complicated situation we may draw several inferences. The integration of food plants and Epilachnas throughout their entire range demonstrates quite conclusively a genetic relationship in their diets traceable to a common origin of their vegetarian habits. Since that time, which was probably at least well back in the Tertiary, the genus has attained its present cosmopolitan distribution, has undergone differentiation into numerous species and split off two minor vegetarian genera. On the basis of related food-plants in adjacent areas we might even trace its migrations in space and time just as paleontologists have done for certain mammals on the basis of their fossil remains. From the foregoing it is evident that phytophagy appeared full-blown, like a structural mutation, and that the insects became addicted to particular plants which they were loath to leave even during the long period required for speciation to the present level. Other coccinellids are known to feed occasionally on foliage, pollen or fungi although retaining their primary predatory habits. The fixation of such an aberration would produce the kind of sudden change that we have just described.

Changes from parasitic to vegetarian habits are well illustrated by a number of chalcid flies of the order Hymenoptera. The members of this enormous group of minute insects are entirely parasitic, except for scattered genera or species that have turned to plants for food. In such cases this involves changed instincts in the adult wasps and an utterly strange environment for the larva, which becomes an internal feeder within the seeds or other plant tissues, sometimes with the production of galls or malformations in the host plant. Contrary to the condition in the lady-beetles, the food of the adult chalcid-fly undergoes no change. Phytophagous habits have appeared in at least six of the fifteen families that compose this group, and they are so scattered that no one can question their independent origin. A quite recent inception is indicated in some cases where the vegetarian forms are not even generically distinct from the parasitic ones.

Here again we encounter fundamental changes in larval food and imaginal instinct, but no correlated structural modifications. As a matter of fact the changes are occasionally not so great as they appear at first sight when we come to examine them closely. For example, in the Eurytomidae, the primitive members of the family are parasites of gall-making insects, so that the mother wasp must lay her eggs within the galls in order to reach the host larva that is enclosed therein. Some of the derived forms, like the abundant and destructive species of Harmolita, still lay their eggs within the tissues of grains and other grasses, but the larva is a vegetable feeder and, what is most remarkable, its larva also produces gall-like swellings of the grass-culms within which it feeds. It is thus in the same sort of immediate environment as its parasitic forbears, but is eating the plant directly.

We have mentioned the great age of the derived vegetarian habits of the bean-beetle and we could readily present evidence to show the antiquity of other similar shifts from one method of feeding to another that have taken place.

We have already referred to the development of quite independent lines of evolution in the larvae of insects without correlated modifications in the reproductive stage. This condition is involved to some extent in shifts from one type of food habits to another, but we have seen that these do not necessarily involve a high correlation between form and function, but that rather the reverse is true.

However, slow-moving, non-aggressive larvae tend to be vegetarian and the opposite holds for predatory forms. Glaring exceptions come to mind, such as the highly degenerate apodous, blind and almost jawless larvae of syrphid Diptera and certain predatory gall-midges that suck the juices of aphids for a living.

If we turn from these poor moronic maggots to the trim aphis-lion, enjoying the same diet, we are confronted with the very quintessence of adaptation: good vision, strong active legs, jaws of marvelously complicated and appropriate form and all in all a creature that looks and acts the part. "Ain't Nature wonderful" when we contemplate the inscrutable tenacity of purpose that enables all these creatures to keep "off relief" and successfully cope with their environment?

This leads us to another phase of the food problem among insects that has had a profound influence on the evolution of many vegetarian groups, especially among the social insects. I now refer to those that have established symbiotic relations with, and cultivated certain fungi and micro-organisms of several types. In this way they have been able to exploit their environment by fostering the growth of plants for food just as civilized man has done through the development of a farmer class. But we must not apply this comparison too closely, for the similarity is quite superficial. They have not bartered away their own products, wishing to acquire others in their place, but have lived the self-contained life that is characteristically theirs as insects. Consequently, they have been able to maintain themselves in a biocoenosis that excludes many undesirable meddlers and parasites.

The mycetophagous food-habits of the ambrosia beetles and the fungus-growing ants and termites are familiar to all of us. Their origin is obscure, but we may be reasonably certain that they arose through chance associations with fungi growing in the wood or other vegetable material where the ancestors of these insects fed. During the course of time, at least some of the fungi have undergone marked evolutionary changes which set them off from their non-symbiotic relatives. At the same time various structures have been developed by the insects like the bristly heads of the ambrosia beetles and instincts like the leaf-cutter ant-queen, who takes a neat little packet of the fungus spawn along when she goes in search of a new home. The precious treasure is stuck in her cheek like a quid of tobacco to be later erupted as the nucleus for the garden that is destined to nourish her future household. Here we see that in spite of the fundamental changes in food habits only slight structural or instinctive modifications are required to render the new system at once self-perpetuating.

Concerning the symbiotic relations of termites to the fauna of highly specialized flagellate Protozoa that inhabit the alimentary tract of these insects we have quite a complete picture. The ability of these symbionts to digest cellulose renders them at once absolutely necessary in the economy of the wood-consuming termites, by a direct trophic relationship. This is perpetuated by the unhygienic habit prevalent among socially minded insects of transferring food from one to another just as the communal lolly-pop insures the propagation of mumps and measles. The great age of this association is shown by the large number of termite protozoans and their differentiation into many taxonomic groups.

Concerning the intracellular symbionts that occur in many insects, we have as yet insufficient knowledge to do much more than speculate about their probable origin and present importance to the insects that harbor them.

From their irregular distribution among insects and the occasional occurrence of more than one species of symbiont in a single insect we are safe in assuming that symbionticism is of multiple origin. That they have played a part in guiding the evolution of food-habits in insects seems quite certain.

Another interesting corollary which greatly strengthens the conclusions we have reached concerning the great age of the numerous sorts of food habits may be derived from an entirely independent source. Over the course of many years I have devoted some time to purely taxonomic studies of certain Tertiary insects, especially those in Baltic amber of Oligocene age. Gradually the impression has developed that the insect fauna at that remote period, at least so far as certain groups are concerned, was not only as extensive and varied as the living one, but that many of the complex associations like myrmecophily and parasitism existed in the form that we encounter them to-day.

What in brief are the general conclusions that may be drawn from the material I have endeavored to parcel out in more or less independent categories? Has the evolution of insects been influenced and guided to an exceptional extent by their highly specialized food-habits? If so, can we point out any obvious reasons why they should differ from any other group of animals in this respect?

Many lines of structural evolution (if you will pardon the term) owe their origin and direction to the several types of food-habits. You may say this is putting the cart before the horse, but I think not, for it is the persistence of instinctive feeding habits over long periods that has provided a long, straight course for natural selection to act in the good old-fashioned way. Lest you throw me out as a nineteenth century biologist I hasten to repeat an earlier statement, that at least many of the shifts in food habits so conspicuous among insects have arisen as mutations in instinct that appear *de novo* and unexpectedly in perfectly serene ecological associations.

This is, I believe, the crux of the matter in that instinctive behavior, particularly with reference to food, is in insects of such paramount importance that its influence has transcended the cruder characteristics on which we can put our fingers and resolve into smaller particles under the microscope.

# SCIENTIFIC EVENTS

## THE FIRST HUNDRED YEARS OF PHOTOGRAPHY

An exhibition illustrating the first hundred years of photography is on view at the Science Museum, South Kensington. The exhibition, according to the London *Times,* has been arranged by the museum in collaboration with the Royal Photographic Society. It is in three sections—the first consisting of early photographs and apparatus; the second of photographs, drawn from the society's collection, illustrating the history and development of pictorial photography down to the present; and the third of the commercial and scientific applications of photography.

In the third section are exhibits illustrating photo-engraving; various methods of color photography; the making of aerial surveys; and the use of photography in astronomy, mineralogy and electrical research. One case shows the improvement which has taken place in the sending of press photographs by cable across the Atlantic between the primitive results of 1927 (when a crude outline effect was achieved) and those of 1934, 1936 and 1939. Radiography also figures largely in this section, with a life-size human skeleton in one corner, a number of medical x-ray photographs and a miscellaneous and amusing collection of others, among which the head and spine of a fish—a species of ray—appear as most astonishing gnome-like monsters.

The *Times* states that exhibits in the early historical section illustrate the massive character of some of the early photographic apparatus. In particular there are a dark-room tent of about 1853 which had to be trundled around on a little two-wheeled pushcart, and a wet-plate outfit of 1855, standing on a tripod and large enough to have served, at need, as a quite sizable dovecote. The display also includes relics of the two men whose work made 1839 so greatly notable as the starting-point of modern photography, Daguerre and Fox Talbot. The Fox Talbot exhibits are drawn from the collection of his apparatus and photographs presented to the museum by his granddaughter, Miss M. T. Talbot, who was present at the opening of the exhibition. Some of the Fox Talbot prints, in spite of the publicity his work has had, are quite unfamiliar. D. O. Hill, Mrs. Cameron and Roger Fenton are other early photographers who are well represented.

## FOREIGN MARKETS FOR MEDICINAL PRODUCTS OF THE UNITED STATES

According to a world survey entitled "Foreign Markets for American Medicinal Products," made available by the Chemical Division of the Department of Commerce, the United States is one of the world's largest exporters of medicinal products, with shipments going forward regularly to more than a hundred foreign countries and trading areas.

Ten years ago when a similar survey was conducted, the United States was the largest exporter of medicinals and accounted for twenty per cent. of the import demand for such products. The present survey shows that although the United States exports approximately the same amount of medicinal products as ten years ago, it is now in the fourth place, following closely behind the United Kingdom and France. Germany is the principal exporter with sales almost double those of its nearest competitor.

The study deals at considerable length with the market for such products abroad, detailing the extent of the demand, local production, methods of distribution, advertising, branch factories, local packaging of imported bulk products, regulations, local preferences and other data.

An important point brought out is the changed character of the export trade of the United States. A decade ago practically all the medicinal and pharmaceutical products entering into foreign trade channels were packaged and ready for the ultimate consumer. Now many of these products are exported in bulk or in concentrated form, and are elaborated or packaged in the country of destination. Medicinal chemicals, for example, are elaborated and pressed into tablets or pills, and liquid products arriving in the country of destination in concentrated form are diluted with syrup, alcohol, water or other bulky ingredients before being packaged. These elaborating and packaging operations are carried out either in branch plants of the parent American companies or in local laboratories by license or other arrangements with the American brand or patent owners. This situation has been brought about by legislation enacted in various foreign countries, designed to stimulate the domestic medicinal and pharmaceutical industries.

A number of branch factories have been established abroad during the last ten years by American medicinal and pharmaceutical manufacturers, but the aggregate value of medicinal exports from the United States has been well maintained. Beginning with 1928 the value of exports of such products moved up somewhat, reaching a peak of $21,322,500 in 1929. Following that year foreign demand declined sharply and exports reached the low of $9,816,000 in 1933. From this low point, however, the total advanced steadily to approximate $18,000,000 in the years 1937 and 1938.

## THE ROCHESTER ATHENAEUM AND MECHANICS INSTITUTE

The Rochester Athenaeum and Mechanics Institute has been offered an anonymous gift of $400,000 provided that $600,000 additional can be raised for endowment purposes. The donor pointed out the long record of meritorious service of the institute to the community as reason for the offer. The need for additional endowment is said to be one of the most pressing needs of the institute, the present endowment and trust funds amounting to $1,500,000 being entirely inadequate.

The following members of the Board of Directors have been appointed to a committee to make plans to raise the $600,000: James E. Gleason, *chairman;* Herbert W. Bromley, Dr. Albert K. Chapman, George H. Clark, M. Herbert Eisenhart, Dr. Mark Ellingson, Charles K. Flint, Edward A. Halbleib, Sol Heumann, P. Richard Jameson, Frank W. Moffett, Oscar H. Pieper, Herman Russell and Albert F. Sulzer.

Mr. Gleason in discussing the matter said that by the addition of a million dollars to the endowment funds a long step would be taken toward financial independence. Income from endowment has been steadily declining, and as tuition at the institute covers only about fifty per cent. of the cost of operation, the extension of its services makes additional support imperative.

The offer provides that the $600,000 to be raised must be secured by pledges on or before December 31, 1940. This does not necessarily mean that contributions must be made at once; pledges payable over periods as long as five years will be acceptable under the terms of the offer.

The institute was founded in 1829. It is Rochester's oldest educational institution, and during the past year has had a student body of nearly 3,400 day and evening school students. In the day school, instruction is offered to high-school and college graduates in the applied arts, publishing and printing, general home economics, food administration, retailing, photographic technology, construction, chemistry, electricity and mechanics. Over a hundred and forty courses are offered in the evening division for employed men and women. It has pioneered in the individualization of education, in the cooperative plan and in its counseling program.

## BIOCHEMICAL RESEARCH AT THE UNIVERSITY OF PITTSBURGH

DR. ALEXANDER SILVERMAN, head of the department of chemistry in the University of Pittsburgh, announces the continuation of the biochemistry research project which has been subsidized by the Buhl Foundation of Pittsburgh. The personnel for 1939–40 follows: Max O. Schultze (Ph.D., University of Wisconsin), senior fellow; Herbert E. Longenecker (Ph.D., Pennsylvania State College), senior fellow; Theodore H. Clarke (Ph.D., University of Pittsburgh), senior fellow; Rade R. Musulin (Ph.D., University of Pittsburgh), senior fellow to September 1; Carl V. Smythe (Ph.D., University of California), senior fellow reporting September 1; Carter J. Harrer (B.S., University of Pittsburgh), research assistant; George W. Jack (B.S., Grove City College), research assistant; Mary L. Dodds (M.S., University of Pittsburgh), research assistant.

The grant covers researches on animal nutrition, tissue respiration and molecular structure. Dr. C. G. King, professor of biochemistry at the university, is director, and Dr. Gebhard Stegeman, professor of physical chemistry, is associate director.

To broaden the investigation which has been in progress for several years in the department of chemistry, additional funds have been provided by the Buhl Foundation, so that cooperative studies will be made with the departments of physics and biology and with the School of Medicine. The total available for the entire project is $60,000.

## THE THIRD INTERNATIONAL CANCER CONGRESS

THE third International Cancer Congress will meet at Atlantic City, N. J., from September 11 to 15. The program, which has now been issued, includes papers on both the research and clinical phases of cancer, by authors from the United States, Canada, Mexico, South America and Europe. The following grouping has been adopted; Biophysics, Chairman Dr. Gioacchino Failla; Genetics, Chairman Dr. Clarence C. Little; Experimental Pathology, Chairman Dr. William H. Woglom; General Pathology, Chairman Dr. Milton C. Winternitz; Surgery, Chairman Frank H. Lahey; Diagnostic Roentgenology, Chairman Dr. John D. Camp; Therapeutic Radiology, Chairman Dr. Ursus V. Portmann; Statistics and Education, Chairman Dr. Burton T. Simpson, and finally a General Section which will be conducted by the president of the congress, Dr. Francis Carter Wood, for papers which arrive too late for classification under the different specialties.

A number of innovations have been made in planning the sessions of the congress. One of these is the appointment of a number of vice-chairmen, so that when a chairman must be absent from his section there will be available an assistant who is familiar with the program and the speakers. It has been ruled that all papers must be read at the time printed in the program.

The facilities for projection and demonstration will be unusually complete. Through the generosity of two large foreign instrument houses projection apparatus will be available for full-size radiographic films. There will be also, in a special room, a high-power projection apparatus for microscopic preparations, which will make it possible for groups interested in the finer details of a paper to study at leisure the microscopic lesions while the writer demonstrates his points. The usual lanterns and projectors for films also will be continuously available.

Each evening there will be lectures surveying special fields. The lecturers include the U. S. Surgeon-General, Dr. Thomas Parran, Jr., who will speak on "Cancer and the Public Health" on Wednesday evening after the president's dinner, and Professor James Ewing, who will close the meeting on Friday with an address on "Cancer, Present and Future," in which he will survey the accomplishments of the congress and express his opinions on methods for attacking the cancer situation in the next decade.

## THE BICENTENARY OF THE ROYAL SWEDISH ACADEMY OF SCIENCES

THE preliminary program of general events for the Bicentenary Jubilee of the Royal Swedish Academy of Sciences, which meets in Stockholm from September 23 to 25, has been issued. The principal events are as follows:

*Saturday, September 23*

At 2:30. Delegates and specially invited guests gather in the academy building at Frescati, where there will be arranged, in the assembly rooms, an exhibition of pictures, manuscripts and books, which will be demonstrated by the librarian of the academy.

After about an hour's stay in the academy building an opportunity will be given to visit the near-by Institute for Experimental Physical Research, the various sections of the Museum of Natural History, the Geological Survey of Sweden and the Bergius Botanical Garden.

At 6:30. An informal dinner will take place at the restaurant Hasselbacken to welcome the delegates and specially invited guests.

*Sunday, September 24*

At 2:00. Bicentenary festival in the Concert Hall of Stockholm in the presence of the King of Sweden and other members of the royal family. Further details will be given in a special program.

*Monday, September 25*

At 10:00. Departure by steamer to Saltsjöbaden (alternatively by motor coaches at 11:00).

At 12:00. Demonstration of the Stockholm Observatory at Saltsjöbaden.

At 1:00. Lunch at the Saltsjöbaden Grand Hotel or at some restaurant in Stockholm.

About 5:00. The guests of the academy are invited to tea at the Royal Palace in Stockholm.

At 8:00. The guests of the academy are invited to a gala performance at the Royal Opera House.

Those wishing to attend are advised to order in time hotel rooms for their stay in Stockholm from September 23 to 25. According to an agreement with the Organization Committee of the Academy the travel bureau "RESO," Stockholm, will undertake to provide hotel accommodation.

## THE HUNDREDTH ANNIVERSARY OF THE BIRTH OF ROBERT HENRY THURSTON

THE hundredth anniversary of the birth of Robert Henry Thurston will be celebrated by Cornell University with the cooperation of the American Society of Mechanical Engineers on October 25.

The preliminary program follows:

Convocation in Bailey Hall, 10:00 A.M.

Dr. Edmund Ezra Day, president of Cornell University, presiding.

*Speakers*

Dr. William Frederick Durand, professor of marine engineering, Cornell University, 1891–1904; emeritus professor of mechanical engineering, Stanford University; past president, American Society of Mechanical Engineers, and author of "Robert Henry Thurston: a Biography."

Dr. James Pickwell Adams, vice-president of Brown University.

Admiral Wilson Brown, superintendent of the United States Naval Academy.

Dr. Harvey N. Davis, president of the Stevens Institute of Technology and past president of the American Society of Mechanical Engineers.

Dean S. C. Hollister, College of Engineering, Cornell University.

During the afternoon, guests will have the opportunity to inspect the College of Engineering and meet informally with members of the faculty. There will be exhibits of Dr. Thurston's publications and of apparatus he designed.

The program gives the following sketch of Professor Thurston's life and work:

ROBERT HENRY THURSTON
October 25, 1839–October 25, 1903

Robert H. Thurston has been recognized as the leading mechanical engineer of his time and as the most influential educator in this field. While teaching at Annapolis, where the U. S. Navy transferred him after his period of active service in the Civil War, Thurston began to develop a plan for training engineers that would supplant the current vocational courses in mechanic arts. He put his plan into operation at Stevens Institute between 1871 and 1885, founding the first mechanical laboratory for purposes of instruction, assembling and at times inventing the necessary apparatus, and writing a pioneer manual, "The Materials of Engineering," for his students. In 1885 President Andrew D. White called Dr. Thurston to Cornell, where for 18 years he directed instruction in mechanical engineering, setting up a more comprehensive laboratory, writing additional textbooks, surrounding himself with able teachers and establishing educational standards and programs that set the pattern for modern engineering education. His biographer and former colleague at Cornell, Dr. W. F. Durand, has stated that his work at this university gave "to the College prestige and standing in the very front rank of the engineering schools of the country and of the world."

Throughout his career as a teacher and administrator, Dr. Thurston continued the practice of engineering and wrote voluminously for technical publications. He was one of the organizers and the first president of the American Society of Mechanical Engineers, serving for two terms; three times a vice-president of the American Association for the Advancement of Science, and a member of the American Society of Civil Engineers and of numerous other technical and academic organizations in this country and abroad. He also served on several important state and federal commissions.

Dr. Thurston was considered an authority on materials of construction, steam engines and boilers, and the history of engineering, as well as on the philosophy of education. His most widely known work, "A History of the Growth of the Steam Engine," published originally in 1878, is scheduled for republication this year as part of the celebration of the centennial of his birth.

Training engineers to meet the problems of the future was a subject of perennial interest to Dr. Thurston and will be the theme of the Anniversary Convocation. Thurston, the pioneer, proclaimed values and enunciated principles that have a bearing to-day, and the spirit of Thurston counsels boldness in grasping the immense opportunities of to-morrow.

### RECENT DEATHS AND MEMORIALS

Dr. Lewis D. Roberts, professor of physical chemistry at the University of Southern California, died by suicide on August 3. He was in his fifty-sixth year.

Dr. Clyde Mason Shaw, professor emeritus of the College of Pharmacy at the University of Illinois, Chicago, died on August 5, at the age of seventy-one years.

Dr. Cooper Curtice, who retired as veternarian at the Bureau of Animal Industry of the U. S. Department of Agriculture in 1930, known for his work in the eradication of cattle ticks and cattle-tick fever, died on August 8, at the age of eighty-three years.

*Nature* reports the death on July 28 of Professor R. W. Reid, emeritus regius professor of anatomy in the University of Aberdeen; and of Scoresby Routledge, known for his investigations among the Akikuyu of East Africa and of the archeology and ethnology of Easter Island, on July 31, in his eightieth year.

According to *Nature* a teak memorial seat to the late Sir William Perkin, the chemist, is to be unveiled and dedicated to the public at Sudbury, Middlesex, on August 12. The memorial will be outside a recreation ground, and opposite the site where Sir William's house and laboratory stood. The cost of the memorial has been met by public subscription.

## SCIENTIFIC NOTES AND NEWS

Dr. Robert A. Millikan, of the California Institute of Technology, accompanied by Dr. H. Victor Neher and Dr. W. H. Pickering, sailed for Australia on August 16. They will engage in cosmic ray research in Australia, Tasmania, the East Indies, India and Egypt, returning in February, 1940.

The Royal College of Physicians has made the following awards: the Baly Gold Medal to Dr. C. H. Best, professor of physiology in the University of Toronto, for his physiological researches; the Moxon Gold Medal to Sir Arthur Hurst, senior physician to Guy's Hospital, for his researches and observations in clinical medicine; the Weber-Parkes Medal and Prize to Sir Pendrill Varrier-Jones, founder and medical director of the Papworth Village Settlement, for his work on tuberculosis.

The gold medal of the Royal Agricultural Society of England has been awarded to Sir George Stapledon, professor of agricultural botany at the University College of Wales at Aberystwyth and director of the Welsh Plant Breeding Station, "for his distinguished services to agriculture."

The prize of the Senckenberg Foundation of the value of about 4,000 marks, which was established a hundred and seventy-five years ago, was awarded on the occasion of the twenty-fifth anniversary of the university at Frankfurt-a/M, to Dr. Ernst Ruska for his work with the electron microscope. The prize is awarded every three years to a German investigator for contributions to the advancement of medicine or science.

The *Journal* of the American Medical Association reports that at the annual meeting of the Minnesota State Medical Association it was voted to present the distinguished service medal and scroll, awarded to members for special contributions to the work of the association, to the late Drs. William J. Mayo and Charles H. Mayo. Their photographs will be hung in the Medical School of the University of Minnesota.

Dr. George H. Fancher, professor of petroleum engineering at the University of Texas, has been elected a fellow of the International Institute of Petroleum, which has its headquarters in London.

The University of Edinburgh has conferred the doctorate of laws on Dr. Francis H. A. Marshall, fellow of Christ's College, Cambridge, and reader in agricultural physiology in the University of Cambridge, in recognition of his work in the physiology of reproduction.

Professor Luigo D'Amato, director of the Medical Clinic of the University of Naples, has been made a senator of Italy.

Dr. Laignel-Lavastine, professor of the history of medicine at the University of Paris, has been elected president of the International Society of the History of Medicine.

THE *Experiment Station Record* states that Dr. E. C. Van Dyke, professor of entomology at the University of California, retired with the title emeritus on July 1 after twenty-six years of service. He will be succeeded by Dr. E. O. Essig, whose work will be taken by Dr. Guy F. MacLeod, professor of economic entomology at Cornell University. Drs. E. Gordon Linsley and Robert L. Usinger have been added to the staff as instructors in entomology, the former to be stationed at Berkeley and the latter at Davis.

DR. RICHARD W. JACKSON has been promoted to an associate professorship of biochemistry at the Cornell University Medical College, New York City.

DR. ALFRED L. ANDERSON, acting head of the department of geology at the University of Idaho, has been appointed assistant professor of geology at Cornell University. He will give lectures on economic geology.

DR. CHARLES H. NORRIS has been appointed instructor in biology at the University of Colorado.

DR. NOËL FIESSINGER, professor of experimental pathology at the University of Paris and co-editor with his father, Dr. Charles Fiessinger, of the *Journal des Praticiens,* has been nominated professor of clinical medicine in succession to Professor Carnot, who is retiring on reaching the age limit.

DR. W. G. BARNARD, consultant histologist of the Public Health Department of the London County Council, has been appointed from October 1 to the chair of pathology of the University of London, tenable at St. Thomas's Hospital Medical School.

THE John Lucas Walker Studentship of the University of London for original research in pathology, of the value of £300 a year for three years, has been awarded to J. C. Colbeck.

DR. F. WOOD JONES, professor of anatomy at the University of Manchester, will retire at the end of the Michaelmas term.

BRAYTON EDDY, lecturer on entomology, was recently appointed administrator of the Office of Entomology and Plant Industry for the State of Rhode Island.

ROBERT J. CHEATHAM, now in charge of cotton utilization research in the Bureau of Agricultural Economics of the U. S. Department of Agriculture, has been made head of the Cotton Processing Division of the Southern Regional Research Laboratory at New Orleans. He will direct investigations involving the processing and utilization of cotton lint, including work on developing new and improved manufacturing processes, yarns, fabrics and other products composed wholly or in part of cotton.

DR. RAYMOND C. PARKER, until recently an associate in experimental surgery at the Rockefeller Institute for Medical Research, New York, has accepted a position with E. R. Squibb and Sons, at New Brunswick, N. J., where he will be in charge of the Virus Division of the Biological Laboratories.

THE Committee on Scientific Research of the American Medical Association has made a grant to Dr. Fritz Schiff, of the department of bacteriology and serology of Beth Israel Hospital, New York City, to be applied toward his work on the serological classification of Salmonella, and a grant in support of work on the physiology of the peripheral blood vessels by Dr. Roy H. Turner, of the department of medicine of Tulane University.

DR. MARGARET E. LEWIS, of the Johns Hopkins University, will join the staff of the new Crocker Radiation Laboratory of the University of California. She plans to undertake an investigation of the effect of neutrons on tissue cultures.

AT Lehigh University Dr. Lawrence Whitcomb is in charge of the summer school of geology. Dr. R. D. Butler is with the London Mines and Milling Company, Alma, Colo. Dr. D. M. Fraser is engaged in prospecting for petroleum for the Atlantic Refining Company in Cuba. Dr. B. L. Miller has continued his investigations of the geology of Lehigh County, Pennsylvania. Dr. Bradford Willard is engaged in studies of the Ordovician shales of Berks and Lehigh Counties. Drs. Fraser, Miller and Willard have recently received *per diem* appointments with the Pennsylvania Topographic and Geologic Survey.

VICTOR E. LEVINE, professor of biological chemistry and nutrition at the School of Medicine of Creighton University, is on his fifth trip to the Arctic, continuing medical and biological studies of the Eskimo under the auspices of the U. S. Public Health Service. His base this year is Kotzebue, north of the Arctic Circle.

THE eighteenth International Geological Congress will be held in London from July 31 to August 8, 1940. Titles of papers to be presented must be in the hands of the General Secretaries, Dr. W. F. P. McLintock and Professor W. B. R. King, Geological Survey and Museum, Exhibition Road, South Kensington, London, S.W. 7, not later than June 1 and the manuscripts by July 1, in a typewritten form, with illustrations, etc., ready for publication. A large number of excursions under the guidance of leading specialists both before and after the congress have been arranged. These include practically all places of geological interest in Great Britain.

AN Institute for the Consideration of the Blood and Blood-forming Organs will be held by the Medical School of the University of Wisconsin on September

4, 5 and 6. The Wisconsin Alumni Research Foundation has made available the necessary funds to finance this institute. Among those who will take part are Dr. L. J. Witts, professor of chemical medicine at the University of Oxford, and Dr. E. Meulengracht, professor of chemical medicine at Copenhagen. The subjects to be discussed include various forms of anemia and the therapy of anemia; the etiology and therapy of granulocytopenia; the formation of hemoglobin; hemorrhagic diseases; leukemia; diseases affecting lymph nodes.

THE name of the Eugenics Record Office, at Cold Spring Harbor, Long Island, N. Y., has been changed to Genetics Record Office. This office is associated with the Department of Genetics of the Carnegie Institution of Washington.

THE chairman of the Board of Agriculture of Bermuda, Sir Stanley Spruling, has outlined the results of an emergency survey recently completed by the Department of Agriculture. Cultivated and uncultivated lands of Bermuda have been surveyed as to crop potentialities and employment in the event of war. The whole plan would not go into operation immediately on the outbreak of war unless the tourist trade, the mainstay of business in the island, had declined seriously. It was stated that an agricultural survey by experts from Cornell University might be undertaken.

MANY bird-watchers in the British Isles, according to the London *Times,* have collaborated in field work under the British Trust for Ornithology, of which the fourth report has been issued. More than one hundred observers recorded day by day the exact song-periods of the misselthrush, songthrush, blackbird, chaffinch, yellowhammer and skylark. This inquiry was continued until recently, because of the abnormal weather of last winter and spring, which caused a scarcity of winter song. More than 150 heronries in 64 counties of the British Isles were visited last year by trust observers, who found that the breeding stock of herons is about at the level of ten years ago, although one Kent heronry had reached a size never before recorded since a systematic census work on this species began in Great Britain. For the little owl inquiry 73 helpers sent material from 34 counties, apart from a large number who sent notes but no material. The national bird-marking scheme was taken over by the trust last year, when more than 45,000 wild birds were marked with rings in the British Isles. Among interesting results of this work were the finding of a rook aged twelve and a blue tit aged at least eight which is still flourishing.

SIR BUCKSTON BROWNE, retired surgeon, donor and honorary curator of Down House, Kent, which was for forty years the home of Darwin, has written the following letter to the London *Times:* "Sir Charles Lyell's second edition of his 'Elements of Geology' appeared in 1841. He annotated a copy in view of another edition, and on the fly-leaf, under 'Addenda,' in his own hand, the following entry appears—'Darwin recommends a short chap. on metallic veins, giving the present state of our knowledge. He denies seeing a beginning to each crop of species. Jan. 26, 1842.' Mrs. Lyell, Sir Charles' sister-in-law, afterwards gave the book to the late Mr. Benjamin Harrison, the celebrated, self-taught, village geologist. It is now in the possession of Mr. Sidney Spokes, M.R.C.S., of Lewes, and will be presented to Darwin's old home, Down House, Downe, Kent, now preserved as a national memorial. This precious little bit of manuscript shows that in 1842 Darwin had fully realized his 'Origin of Species.' He was, however, so patient, so conscientious, in his search for truth that 17 years were to pass before, in 1859, the immortal book appeared."

# DISCUSSION

## COMPOUND WORDS

IN the current issue of SCIENCE, just received, Dr. H. J. Conn presents an interesting discussion[1] of the confusion occasioned by the orthodox use (and non-use) of hyphens in the making of multiple compound words. The examples are well chosen from biological terms; but the biologists have no monopoly on such hyphenated chaos. The current issue of *Economic Geology* presents a very instructive example.

An article by E. C. Dapples[2] is entitled: "Coal Metamorphism in the Anthracite-Crested Butte Quadrangles, Colorado." To any one familiar with the region, it is quite obvious that the territory under discussion comprises two adjacent areas, designated respectively as the Anthracite Quadrangle, and the Crested Butte Quadrangle; to others, the connective implication of the hyphen, as used, suggests a butte crested with anthracite. Evidently the "others" include the headline writer for the journal in question; for, in compressing the title to a page heading, he eliminates the pseudo-adjective "anthracite-crested," and has, as a condensed title at the top of fourteen pages, the amazing and amusing contraction: "Coal Metamorphism in Butte Quadrangles." Any geologist will at once connect the term "Butte Quadrangles" with an area in Montana, in which no coal occurs.

In the closing paragraph of his discussion, Dr.

1 H. J. Conn, SCIENCE, 89: 582–3, 1939.

2 *Economic Geology,* 34: 4, 369–398, June–July, 1939.

Conn expresses the hope that some system may be devised "to show which elements belong most closely together and which are related to the others more indirectly." His wording here is excellent, and clearly expresses the crux of the problem. It appears that originally the hyphen was used rather freely as a connective; later practise has tended to eliminate the hyphen in compound nouns, except in connecting words of strictly coordinate import. This rule works well for simple or singly compounded words; but with multiple compounds, we need a connective factor for the units of the simple compounds and a separative factor for the compound units of the larger and more complex terms.

In the examples that Dr. Conn cites, it appears that the omission of the hyphen (according to standard practise) suggests a separation of the words in the unit-compounds, while the use of the hyphen between the unit-compound elements appears to tie together those factors that should be separated. Perhaps this seems as pedantic as the question whether the primary function of the mortar in a wall is to hold the bricks together or to hold the bricks apart (I once saw two tipsy brick-masons stage a fight to settle that problem!); but I think it contains the key to the solution of our difficulty.

If the connective implication of the hyphen is so strong as to be confusing, what might we use as a separative factor? May I suggest the disused colon? The colon has gone almost out of fashion in present-day writing; but the mathematicians still use it in their formulas to express a definite comparative relationship. Why may we not do the same in technical writing?

The suggested use of the colon as a separator and the hyphen as a connector is as simple as it is unorthodox. It includes only two rules, which are: (1) In multiple compound words, the single terms of each compound unit are to be connected by a hyphen (whether or not the hyphen would be so used if the unit term stood alone). (2) The compound units are to be separated by colons.

Using Dr. Conn's terrifying examples, they would be expressed as "safranin: orange-G: crystal-violet technic," and as "iron-alum: hematoxylin-phenol: Bismarck-brown Y schedule" (or perhaps "Bismarck: brown-Y schedule"; I am afraid that I shall have to ask Dr. Conn to interpret that one).

The sole merit of such a system is that it makes the meaning of a multiple compound term entirely clear. I have used it repeatedly in class discussions, and it has proved quite adequate, at least in blackboard work.

STERLING B. TALMAGE
NEW MEXICO SCHOOL OF MINES

THE recent discussion on compound words by Weatherby[1] and Conn[2] presented two interestingly different points of view. The former treated the question without even mentioning that admirable if ancient device, the hyphen, although the heading of his communication, "Compound Words in *Present-day* English," embodied the principle that he failed to invoke. One wonders whether the "mental epidemic" of compounding which he foretells (giving as a sample, "Costanalysis of Scholarlyperiodicalprinting") will not have been started, not by the Greeks and the Germans, but by the author of "Ulysses" and "Finnegan's Wake"? (On the first page of the latter occurs the curious portmanteau "upturnpikepointandplace"—just for example.)

Conn's entertaining picture of the endless editorial battle of the hyphen added details that had seemingly been overlooked by Weatherby. Single-word compounds (*e.g.*, blackbird) are likely to have hyphened compounds (black-bird) as their forerunners; and as Fowler[3] says, "The conversion of a hyphened word into an unhyphened single one is desirable as soon as the novelty of the combination has worn off, if there are no obstacles in the way of awkward spelling, obscurity, or the like." But often there are such obstacles. And that same indispensable mentor, *ibidem*, offers something like the "rules," for hyphening "double-barrelled adjectives," that Conn (and perhaps all of us) cannot find in our grammar-books:

> Mr. Lloyd George (without a hyphen) forms the Lloyd-George Government (with one); the need [for hyphens] is still greater when further complications come, but the result is then unsatisfactory—the Lloyd-George-Winston-Churchill Government. Obviously connexions of a different power are needed; a short & a long hyphen (-, –), or a single & a double one (–, =), would do (the Lloyd-George—Winston-Churchill Government, the Lloyd-George=Winston-Churchill G.); but this is an innovation that would hardly find acceptance; *&* is better than — or = (the Lloyd-George & Winston-Churchill G.); better than either is some evasion, the George-Churchill G., or the G. of Messrs. Lloyd George & Churchill.

Their unfamiliarity aside, there might still be some (rather remote) possibility of confusing the "long" hyphen with the dash, the "double" hyphen with the "equals" sign. (These objections could be disposed of—except perhaps among the typographical profession—by setting the new symbol slightly above or slightly below the center of the line of type.) Is it not more likely that the "real" reason why such devices would not be generally acceptable is merely that it will always

[1] C. A. Weatherby, SCIENCE, 89: 413, 1939.
[2] H. J. Conn, SCIENCE, 89: 582, 1939.
[3] H. W. Fowler, "A Dictionary of Modern English Usage," Clarendon Press, p. 244.

be easier not to seek precision—not to "bother," even about "short" and "single" hyphens? And yet, as any reader of these musings who knows the work of Korzybski[4] will already have reminded himself, "Hyphens allow us in principle to make compound words structurally similar to the non-elementalistic world we happen to live in."

R. H. BAUGH

COLLEGE OF PHYSICIANS,
PHILADELPHIA

WEATHERBY in a recent note[1] says that "The English language is rapidly acquiring a facility in forming compound words comparable to that possessed by ancient Greek and contemporary German." It should not be difficult to convince writers who wish to be understood that they might follow better models than classical Greek, which has now become a "dead" language, or modern German, which has never been known especially favorably either for clarity or ease of reading. Moreover, I question whether the language really *is* changing. *Unit modifiers* always have been used, especially by scientists who were poorer writers than researchers. What is now happening is that we are losing our critical faculties in writing English; the result is that technical writing is full of errors that any one well grounded in the proper use of English would notice immediately. Weatherby cites a few examples of "present-day" English to prove that the language is changing; he is merely proving that it is possible to write poorly and "get away" with it. For instance, he says that thirty years ago no one would have put forth such a title as 'Cost Analysis of Scholarly Periodical Printing." It is still true that no one would write such a title if he hoped to be understood perfectly. Does that title mean, as Weatherby suggests, "An Analysis of the Cost of Printing Scholarly Periodicals?" Perhaps so, but rather it seems to mean "An Analysis of the Cost of Printing Periodicals Scholarly" —a cost (one feels sure after reading much of the current scientific balderdash) that would be much more than that of printing scholarly periodicals. Maybe Mr. Weatherby is right, and in the somedaydistant-future we shall all be compoundedlyunitmodifying, but if this mentalepidemicurge he speaks of ever truly possesses us, Heaven help our desiringtounderstandus-readers.

ORAN RABER

SOUTHERN FOREST EXPERIMENT STATION,
NEW ORLEANS

[4] A. Korzybski, "Science and Sanity," Science Press Printing Company, pp. 31, 243; "General Semantics," Arrow Editions, p. 34.

[1] SCIENCE, May 5, 1939, p. 413.

GRANTED that at best hyphenation is a bothersome subject, your correspondent, H. J. Conn, editor of *Stain Technology,* does not seem to be aware of two common rules which simplify the matter somewhat. One is the rule followed by the Chicago University Press and many other people: "Hyphenate adjectival phrases formed of two or more words when preceding the nouns modified, where ambiguity might result." Mr. Conn's phrase "safranin-orange G-crystal violet technic" would become "safranin orange-G crystal-violet technic." The other rule from the same source: "Where one of the components of a compound adjective contains more than one word, an en dash should be used in place of a hyphen." This would make "the Great Northern–Northern Pacific railway system" a manageable term and could be applied also to the "safranin" phrase if preferred.

Mr. Conn has further complicated his problem by not having discovered that the current unabridged Webster (1935) omits the hyphen after non- as a prefix and has made one word of "sporeformer." "Nonsporeformer" is a good example of the very trend Mr. Conn has been desiring.

MARJORIE FULLER
JANE MCMASTERS

THE TECHNOLOGY REVIEW

## VALUE OF CHARACTERS OF THE UNDEVELOPED SHOOT IN IDENTIFYING PLANTS

IN many cases foresters and range workers find they must identify woody plants such as forest trees or shrubs in winter condition. In range surveys or quadrat studies it often becomes necessary to ascertain the name of a grass in the early season before the appearance of the inflorescence. Various keys and description are available for this purpose, but very often a positive specific identification can not be made, due to the very nature of the material. Where the plant can be studied again later in the season, this difficulty is not serious. Often this later check can not be carried out. It is the purpose of this article to call attention to the characters of the undeveloped shoot as an aid to the immediate identification of such material.

The leaves and flowers inside the winter buds of woody plants can be so studied. In grasses information gained by dissecting out the small inflorescence which lies in the sheath tube about at ground level may allow for a more definite determination.

The technique of this dissection is not intricate. In woody plants the bud scales can be removed and the shoot exposed for study. In order to have both hands free the writer uses a dissecting microscope equipped with a foot-focussing device. This machine was described in SCIENCE[1] and is now for sale by the Spencer Lens Company of Buffalo, N. Y. However, even with a good hand lens leaf characters, such as vernation, general shape, type of base and apex, kind of margin and venation, can usually be made out. In addition, the buds may inclose flowers far enough along so that floral characters such as number and type of sepals, petals, stamens and pistils can be ascertained. In many cases unknown species can actually be run through the keys of manuals based on floral and leaf characters.

In grasses the sheath tube of a large vigorous culm can be split longitudinally and the incipient inflorescence exposed. The type of inflorescence can be determined, in most cases the florets of a spikelet can be counted and many of their characters can be made out.

In many instances these undeveloped, concealed characters in woody plants and grasses are definite enough to actually allow for identifying the plant in ordinary manuals. However, in most cases their greatest value will probably be in helping decide between several possibilities or in allowing for a positive check on what otherwise might be an uncertain identification.

H. D. Harrington
Colorado State College

## CYSTINE AND METHIONINE REQUIREMENTS FOR GROWTH AND LACTATION

Recent studies have shown that the sulfur-containing amino acids promote lactation in rats when fed with rations in which the protein is derived from casein or alfalfa leaf meal. Since these proteins are deficient for growth in their combined contents of cystine and methionine, it does not necessarily follow that cystine and methionine should be regarded as lactation stimulants merely because they promote lactation when fed with these proteins.

We have recently determined the growth and lactation responses in rats fed alfalfa leaf meal proteins supplemented with various levels of cystine. We have also determined the growth and lactation responses to cystine and methionine when fed with peanut meal protein. Cystine does not significantly improve the growth- and lactation-promoting properties of peanut meal protein. Methionine improves both properties. Our results indicate that the combined requirements for cystine and methionine and the conditions governing the interchangeability of cystine and methionine are of essentially similar orders for growth and lactation.

J. R. Haag
L. D. Wright
Oregon State Agricultural College

# SCIENTIFIC BOOKS

## THE THEORY OF NUMBERS

*An Introduction to the Theory of Numbers.* By G. H. Hardy and E. M. Wright. The Oxford University Press. Octavo: xvi + 403 pp. $8.00.

Mathematics undergoes continuous revitalization through two main currents of thought: the one flowing from the inexhaustible supply of simple conundrums concerning the positive integers; the other flowing out of new conceptual ideas necessary for the comprehension of natural laws. For example, to quote Cajori,[1] "in the study of the right triangle there arose questions of puzzling subtlety. Thus, given a number equal to the side of an isosceles right triangle, to find the number the hypotenuse is equal to. . . . The problem may have been attacked again and again. . . . In some such manner arose the theory of irrational quantities"—as a byproduct of the attempt to solve an arithmetic problem without rational solution. Similarly the imposing edifice of Euclidean geometry grew out of the physical concepts based on exact spatial measurement.

In the fascinating volume by G. H. Hardy and E. M. Wright under review here we find a remarkably happy and varied selection of important arithmetic problems treated with consummate clarity and distinction. The book will appeal to the many non-professional devotees of number theory and to professional mathematicians generally. As a basis for an attractive and profitable first course on the theory of numbers one could not find a better text. The title is the same as that of a well-known volume by our great American number-theorist, L. E. Dickson. But there is little overlapping, and no real confusion will be caused.

It will enhance the value of the work to mathematicians that one of the two distinguished authors (Hardy) has not only contributed greatly to the advancement of the subject on the side of the so-called "analytic theory of numbers" but also has long been one of the most inspiring mathematical figures in the world. We recall too his close association with the short-lived genius, Ramanujan of India, with the lamented Landau of Göttingen and with his remarkably gifted colleague Littlewood at Cambridge, all of whom have done so much for number theory.

Although the pages of the book treat a large variety

[1] H. D. Harrington and R. W. Poulter, Science, 79: 368–369, April 20, 1934.

[1] "History of Mathematics," second edition, pp. 56–57.

of topics, nevertheless it is truly stated by the authors in the preface that "in the first eighteen chapters we assume nothing that is not commonly taught in schools, and any intelligent university student should find them comparatively easy reading. The last six are more difficult, and in them we presuppose a little more, but nothing beyond the content of the simpler university courses." The authors have discussed the distribution of primes, Farey series, the geometry of numbers of Minkowski, irrational numbers, the theory of congruences, Fermat's theorem and related topics, decimal representation of numbers, continued fractions, approximation of irrationals by rationals, algebraic integers, Diophantine equations, the familiar arithmetical functions, partitions, representation of numbers by two or four squares, Kronecker's theorem in one or more dimensions. In every case the discussion given is on an elementary level so far as technical knowledge is presupposed, but on a genuinely professional level as far as insight and thoroughness are concerned.

A valuable feature of the book is the bibliographic material in small print at the end of each chapter, which furnishes an excellent orientation in the relevant literature.

It is much to be hoped that other mathematical works having the appeal of the book by Hardy and Wright will soon be written; and that a much wider public than at present will come to realize how through such works the highest artistic and intellectual enjoyment may be obtained, only to be compared with that to be derived from literature, art and music.

George D. Birkhoff

### THE PRINCIPLES OF INSECT PHYSIOLOGY

*The Principles of Insect Physiology.* By V. B. Wigglesworth, London School of Hygiene and Tropical Medicine. 434 pp., 316 illustrations. London, Methuen and Company, Ltd. 1939. 30 shillings net. New York, E. P. Dutton and Company.

With the appearance of "The Principles of Insect Physiology" the subject of entomology acquires a new dignity and the right to claim a place in the higher ranks of biological science. Too long we have been fed with mere "wonders" and "marvels" of insect life. The numerous citations given in the present work show, however, that during the last few decades many serious workers, unproclaimed to the general public, have been diligently searching for the underlying causes and principles of the much-heralded wonders and marvels, with the result that we now have a full-fledged text on insect physiology. The author of the book, himself a leading investigator in this field, has brought together in admirable form the gist of what may now be regarded as a sound basis for the scientific study of insect functions and behavior. The book should be welcomed particularly by all teachers and students of entomology, since it is well recognized that further advance in economic entomology must depend largely on an understanding of insect physiology.

Unfortunately it is not possible for most entomologists to be trained physiologists, but the style of "The Principles of Insect Physiology" is such that the text can be read and understood by any entomologist whether or not he has been schooled in physiological technique and terminology. The treatment is informative rather than discussional, and the book is not a manual of laboratory practice. The subject-matter is divided into 15 chapters under the following headings: Development in the Egg; Integument; Growth, Muscular System and Locomotion; Nervous System; Vision; Mechanical and Chemical Senses; Behaviour; Respiration; Circulatory System and Associated Tissues; Digestion and Nutrition; Excretion; Metabolism; Water and Temperature; Reproductive System. Each chapter is accompanied by a list of references, cited by numbers in the text, varying from 48 to 265 for single chapters, a total of over 2,000 with a few repetitions. The 316 illustrations are entirely line drawings, and thus give a pleasing uniformity to the general appearance of the pages. Anatomy and histology are given briefly wherever necessary for the elucidation of the subject-matter, and in many cases the up-to-date information on these subjects contributes much to the value of the book.

R. E. Snodgrass

## SOCIETIES AND MEETINGS

### THE ROYAL SOCIETY OF CANADA

The annual meeting of the Royal Society of Canada was held at the invitation of the University of Montreal in the new Botanical Building from May 22 to 24. A large attendance of fellows from all parts of Canada had an opportunity of seeing this splendid new development of a Botanical Garden in Montreal with its research laboratories, greenhouses and large park still in the process of completion as a works project financed by civic and government authorities and under the direction of Frère Marie-Victorin, of the University of Montreal.

The presidential address was delivered by Dr. Victor Morin, who spoke on "La Chanson Française a travers les siecles," with interpretations of songs by the *Quatuor des Alouettes.* This address was preceded by the introduction of new fellows and by the presentation of medals awarded by the society. The Flavelle Medal was awarded posthumously to the late Professor J. Playfair McMurrich in recognition of his distinguished work in anatomy. Dr. Wilfred Bovey received the Lorne Pierce medal, and the Tyrrell medal was presented to Dr. E. Z. Massicotte. A unique social feature of the meeting was the operetta-dinner held in the ballroom of the Mount Royal Hotel, at which the fellows and their wives were the guests of the City of Montreal. This fanciful dinner-play was written by the president of the society, Dr. Morin, as a reconstitution of the feasts given by the "seigneurs" of olden times. Parodical rhymes on gastronomical subjects adapted to the music of well-known operas of the French repertory were sung by artists in cook's and maid's costumes, as the several dishes of the dinner were served. At the concluding general meeting, Dr. H. M. Tory was elected the new president of the society.

Section III (Chemical, Mathematical and Physical Sciences) was held under the presidency of Professor S. Beatty, who delivered the presidential address on "Generalization as a Principle of Mathematics." Three new members were elected to this section, Professor H. N. Brocklesby, Professor M. F. Crawford and Professor G. Herzberg. In all, 120 papers were presented and the section divided into the three subdivisions to facilitate the giving of the papers during the time of the meeting. Space permits reference to only a few papers read. Professor E. F. Burton spoke on a number of papers contributed by his co-workers, among which special mention should be made of the recent results obtained by Johns, Wilhelm and Grayson Smith on the flow and viscosity of liquid helium, in which it was proved by using glass capillaries ranging from 0.025 cm to 010036 cm in diameter and with lengths varying from 2 cm to 26 cm that normal laminar flow was obtained for He I with a viscosity of the order of $10^{-5}$ c.g.s. units, while for He II, the flow could be expressed as the sum of a laminar flow plus an additional pressure-independent flow. The laminar portion obeyed Poiseuille's law and gave a viscosity of the order of $10^{-5}$ c.g.s. units. The new electron microscope constructed by A. Prebus and J. Hillier and photographs obtained with it indicating high resolving power were described by Dr. Burton. Among the papers presented by Professor J. A. Gray, one in collaboration with J. S. Marshall and A. G. Wood contained results on the scattering of $\beta$ rays using metallic foils, which were in contradictions to those obtained by other observers using expansion chamber methods. Dr. D. C. Rose described an electromagnetic pick-up device used with a cathode ray oscillograph for investigating vibrations in aeroplanes during flight. A new method of observing the Raman effect in small amounts of liquid with short exposure times was presented by Professor M. F. Crawford and H. L. Walsh. A description of the methods now being used to determine the upper earth structure from data obtained by registering the seismic waves from rock bursts occurring in mines was given by Dr. E. A. Hodgson. Other papers on field results of geophysical investigations were given by Dr. A. A. Brant, Professor L. Gilchrist and Professor D. A. Keys. The results of an analysis of meteorological data by A. Thomson showed that the average winter temperature was 4° F. warmer in Manitoba and Saskatchewan for the period of 1919–38 than for the period 1884–1903, which was explained by the increase in the temperature of the air masses moving in from the Arctic circle.

Among the fifteen papers presented by Professor O. Maass and his associates, particular interest was taken in those dealing with the measurements of viscosity, opalescence, specific heat, density and solubility relations of various liquids and vapors in the critical temperature region. The influence of intense mechanical stirring on the temperature at which the disappearance of the meniscus takes place shows that a wide range of overall density gives identical critical temperatures. Professor E. W. Steacie presented eight papers dealing with various aspects of photosensitized decomposition. Professor R. H. Clark and his collaborators contributed fourteen papers, among which special mention may be made of the results obtained on activators of zymase. The plant hormones activate live yeast but have little accelerating effect on zymin. Another paper of interest was on the mechanism of the flotation of galena in the presence of xanthate which is applied in the mining industry in Canada. Professor H. Hibbert spoke on the results obtained in his laboratory carried out with various collaborators in lignin and other wood products.

In the mathematical and astronomical section, M. S. McPhail and Professor R. J. Jeffery spoke on "Stieltjes Integrals," with applications to fractional integrals. The profiles of hydrogen line in the spectrum of H. D. 190073 by C. S. Beals and an investigation into the hydrogen line contours in the spectra of solar type stars by K. O. Wright were given by Dr. W. E. Harper. Dr. A. V. Douglas, D. C. West and D. E. Guignard described an investigation on the profiles of hydrogen lines in two class B stars.

Professor J. A. Gray was elected president of the section and Professor J. K. Robertson secretary.

In Section IV (Geological Sciences) the presidential address by Dr. M. E. Wilson outlined the development of ideas about the Canadian Precambrian and discussed certain Precambrian problems. Eighteen papers were presented. Two papers dealt with Sudbury, one by Dr. H. C. Cooke, in which some new ideas about the general geology of the district were given, and the other by Dr. A. B. Yates, concerned with the ore deposition. Dr. H. C. Gunning and J. W. Ambrose outlined the results of five years detailed investigation of the so-called Timiskaming-Keewatin contact in Rouyn-

Harricanaw Area, Quebec. The whole succession of volcanic and sedimentary rocks is apparently conformable, and the investigations show the need for complete revision of our conceptions of Archean stratigraphy and structure in this part of the Canadian shield.

The paleontological papers included descriptions of a Helderber fauna from the eastern townships of Quebec by Dr. T. H. Clark, some species of Neo-Triassic ammonites by Dr. L. H. McLearn. Dr. J. T. Wilson presented an interesting paper on the eskers northeast of Great Slave Lake, N.W.T. The information was gained chiefly from the study of aerial photographs.

Dr. H. W. Fairbairn presented a paper on the fracture hypothesis of quartz orientation in tectonites. Dr. M. B. Baker discussed the floor of the Paleozoic rocks in Canada.

The presidential address of Section V (Biological Sciences) was delivered by Dr. J. M. Swaine, of Ottawa, on "Scientific Research as the Key to Progress in Agriculture."

The program comprised seventy-two papers, of which nineteen came before the medical subsection and twenty-nine were botanical.

Dr. N. H. Grace reported upon the relative physiological activity of the members of a series of naphthyl acids when applied to plant cuttings, showing that those with an even number of carbon atoms in the side chain are the more active. Drs. E. Gordon Young and R. W. Begg found certain small proportions of copper, calcium, magnesium and iron to be required in bacterial culture media. Factors affecting stomatal movement in the dark were described by J. H. Whyte. That increased permeability of the host accompanies increased susceptibility to parasites and diseases in plants was shown by F. S. Thatcher. The importance of boron for normal cell division, enlargement and maturation in plants was described by J. G. Coulson and R. O. Lachance, while studies related to hardiness of plants were reported by Messrs. J. Levitt and D. Siminovitch. R. B. Thomson discussed the structure of the pollen cone of Austrotaxus and its phylogenetic significance, showing it to be a highly specialized derivative of the usual conifer type, and C. N. Haldenby described the distribution and origin of horizontal resin canals in Coniferae. A series of papers by Frère Marie-Victorin was devoted to various taxonomic and distributional studies of the plants of Quebec and of Cuba, interesting contributions to the problem of relic floras being made, particularly in papers by Mm. Roussear and Gauthier.

In the field of genetics, a definite relationship between sterility and chromosome segregation with translocations was demonstrated in wheat crosses by W. P. Thompson and the actual causes of failure of seed-setting in certain intergeneric cereal crosses were described in another paper by the same investigator. F. H. Peto gave an account of the production of fertile amphibolypoid plants from sterile hybrids of Triticum species and *A. glaucum* by temperature and colchicine treatments, with cytological studies of the processes involved. Certain chromosome mutations in oats were shown by H. G. F. Sander to involve loss of all or parts of one chromosome and studies on the chromosomes of Trillium by G. B. Wilson and H. B. Newcombe gave data which can not readily be fitted to any existing theory of crossing over but suggest a new partial hypothesis.

Features of the morphology of the circulatory system of Amia, particularly in relation to an air-breathing mechanism, were described by V. C. Wynne-Edwards, and the presence of a vessel of portal nature connecting the hypothalamus in the frog was reported by E. Horne Craigie. The latter also demonstrated wide and important differences in the vascular richness of hypothalamic centers in the rat. Various studies on the white whale were reported by V. D. Vladykov, who also discussed sexual dimorphism in the trout populations. An account of differential growth rates and of regeneration in the hind limb of the frog was offered by A. Emerson Warren. A study of temperature relations of the numerous species of midges (Chironomidae) occurring in a lake was described by R. B. Miller.

B. P. Babkin and associates showed that ergosterol and parathyroid hormone effect gastric secretion in the dog chiefly by depressing its nervous phase. Early cessation of growth in rats on a rich fat diet was found by R. G. Sinclair and traced to the masking or suppression of synthesis of essential fatty acids. The effect of guaiacols on the respiratory passages was described by E. M. Boyd. Authentic notochordal tissue in a dermoid cyst of the ovary was reported by J. L. Riopelle. The structure and development of certain renal tumors led P. Masson to believe that the metanephros is not mesodermal but is derived from the neural crest; while his associate, P. Simard, found a constant neuro-insular complex in the mammalian apparatus. Drs. A. Scott and A. M. Fisher gave an account of the effects of certain chemicals in activating insulin and showed by moving picture film that each insulin crystal has two parallel square surfaces relatively close together, connected by four oblique quadrilateral surfaces. James Craigie showed that the Guarinieri inclusion bodies are probably not intracellular colonies of a virus. The chemotactic attraction of staphylococci for leucocytes from mouse spleen was found by J. W. Stevenson and G. B. Reed to vary inversely with their pathogenicity, while Alma Howard reported an inverse relationship between chiasma frequency in chromosomes and susceptibility to mammary gland carcinoma in mice.

# SPECIAL ARTICLES

## COPPER AND VITAMIN C EFFECTS UPON THE EXCISED FROG HEART[1]

In a preliminary report, Urban and Peugnet[2] showed that vitamin C exerts a powerful beat-strengthening action upon the perfused frog heart. Since that time, Peugnet and Urban[3] have shown that: (1) Vitamin C also accelerates the beat frequency of the abnormally slow pacemaker, with little or no effect upon the normal rate—in which it differs from adrenalin; (2) vitamin C frequently increases the diastolic "tonus," though not as yet reproducibly; (3) inotropic effects are obtainable in concentrations as low as .05 mg per cent.; (4) vitamin C action is independent of and additive with that of perfusate glucose; (5) vitamin C action is not due to atropine-like vagus paralysis, nor to removal of inhibitory action of perfusate potassium, nor to calcium contamination of the vitamin C; (6) oxidized (iodine) vitamin C is inactive.

In the present communication, the author wishes to present experiments proving that the action of vitamin C on the frog heart requires the presence of copper.

The method is that of Straub, described in detail by McLean and Hastings.[4] Ringer (glucose-free) solutions are made with Kahlbaum (analytical) chemicals and Pyrex-distilled water, and contain $NaHCO_3$ (0.2 per cent.), being continuously bubbled, both in reservoir vessels and in cannula, with 95 per cent. $O_2$–5 per cent. $CO_2$. Vitamin C is the synthetic crystalline material.[5]

The experimental evidence for the necessity of copper in the action of vitamin C is briefly as follows:

(1) The inotropic action is always present (about 40 experiments) with ordinary "reagent quality" chemicals and metal-distilled water.

(2) The effect is absent (14 out of 16 experiments) with Kahlbaum chemicals and Pyrex-distilled water.

(3) The heart which fails to respond to vitamin C alone does respond when copper is added to the perfusate (0.1–4.0 micro-mols per liter copper ion, as chloride).

(4) In the same heart, copper alone is ineffective until the addition of vitamin C.

(5) Vitamin C alone can not maintain the inotropic increase, but requires the continued presence of copper in the perfusate.

(6) The heart which does respond to vitamin C alone gives a greater response with copper in addition.

It is particularly to be noted that the response to the addition of copper (vitamin C already present) occurs only after a latent period, or "induction" period, whereas the response to vitamin C addition (copper already present) begins immediately. (The technique in the two cases is as nearly identical as possible; the copper and the vitamin C are freshly mixed with Ringer a few seconds before each application.) This induction period is never seen with vitamin C, and appears to be a constant phenomenon with copper. The duration of the latency varies roughly inversely with the copper concentration (see Table I).

TABLE I

| Frog Date | Copper Ion. micro-mol./L | Induction per. (sec.) |
|---|---|---|
| 5–25–39 | 0.4 | 240. |
| 6–4 | 2.0 | 90. |
| 5–10 | 2.5 | 110. |
| 5–24, A | 4.0 | 30. |
| 5–24, B | 4.0 | 35. |

As to the nature of the induction period, it appears certain that this delay is not due to any *in vitro* reaction or "activation" time, since the time during which the two are in contact *in vitro* is the same whether or not the tissue has been previously exposed to the copper alone; and, as already mentioned, the previous "conditioning" of the tissue with copper abolishes the delay. Apparently, then, the copper is necessary in some part of the tissue system which utilizes vitamin C. Further experiments on this question will be presented at a later date.

Hubert B. Peugnet
Washington University,
St. Louis

[1] Aided by grant of the Ella Sachs Plotz Foundation.

[2] F. Urban and H. B. Peugnet, *Am. Jour. Physiol.*, 123: 207, 1938.

[3] Exhibited with F. Urban at the American Medical Association Convention, May, 1939.

[4] F. C. McLean and A. B. Hastings, *Jour. Biol. Chem.*, 107: 337, 1934.

[5] Donated by Merck and Company.

## PROLONGED THERAPEUTIC EFFECT OF SUBCUTANEOUSLY IMPLANTED CRYSTALS OF OVARIAN HORMONE IN WOMEN

The investigation reported here was undertaken to determine whether it is possible to prolong the physiologic effects of a given dose of estrogenic hormone in humans by implanting crystals of the hormone, subcutaneously. It appears from the results of various investigations that the high dosage of estrogens required to relieve symptoms caused by ovarian failure and to maintain the endometrial and vaginal mucosa in a normal physiologic state is in a great part attributable to the rapid absorption and excretion of the hormone. To achieve a satisfactory therapeutic effect at present it is necessary to administer intramuscular injections of a solution of the hormone in oil at frequent intervals for periods of many weeks. Aside from the inconvenience caused the patient by the necessity for frequent injections, there is the additional factor of expense which places this form of therapy beyond the means of the majority of patients. In the interests of economy and the patient's comfort, it would appear to be highly advantageous to have an estrogenic preparation which would be absorbed slowly so that the patient may derive a fuller measure of benefit from a given amount of the hormone and obviate the necessity for frequent injections. An attempt was made to achieve this objective by the implantation of crystalline a-estradiol benzoate, subcutaneously.

### Technique

Crystals of the hormone were placed in small glass tubes measuring 3 mm in diameter and 1½ cm in length and sterilized by autoclaving. The amounts varied from 4 to 7 mgm. The implantation was performed in the gluteal region. The skin was prepared with tincture of iodine and alcohol. An area of skin measuring approximately 1½ inches in diameter was infiltrated with 2 per cent. novocaine. An incision measuring 1 inch in length was made and the capillary oozing controlled with a dry packing. The estradiol benzoate crystals were then implanted into the wound and the skin edges approximated with 2 silk sutures. The sutures were removed 5 days later.

A total of 10 menopause cases were so treated, including patients with surgical as well as natural menopause. All the patients had typical menopause symptoms and morphologic evidence of estrogen deficiency. The vaginal smear was used as an indicator of estrogen deficiency and estrogenic effect. Vaginal smears were taken twice weekly after the implantation.

### Results

The majority of the patients reported improvement in their symptoms as early as 6 days after the implantation. Complete relief of symptoms usually occurred within 2 weeks and has persisted to date (periods varying from 60 to 98 days after the implantation). Objective evidence of the biologic effect of the implanted crystals was noted in the vaginal smear changes as early as 4 days after the implantation. The "atrophy" cells and leucocytes began to diminish in number, being replaced by large squamous epithelial cells. At the end of 7 to 10 days, the smears consisted entirely of large squamous epithelial cells exhibiting the characteristics of the smear of the normally menstruating woman. This evidence of continued activity has persisted to date (periods varying from 60 to 98 days).

Inasmuch as 1 mgm of a-estradiol benzoate is equivalent to 6,000 R.U., these patients were given doses varying from 24,000 to 42,000 R.U. of estrogenic hormone. This amount, when administered in solution in oil, in a single dose, intramuscularly, will, in the average menopause case with a well-developed menopause syndrome, produce only an incomplete effect both on the symptoms and vaginal smears. Unless repeated injections are administered the symptoms recur in their original intensity and the smears show evidence of regression to the pre-treatment state within 7 to 14 days after the injection.

It appears that crystalline a-estradiol benzoate, when implanted subcutaneously in women who have clinical and morphologic evidence of ovarian deficiency, exerts an effect which is strikingly more pronounced and more prolonged than is obtained with comparable doses of the hormone administered intramuscularly in solution in oil. This prolonged effect is attributed to the slow rate of absorption and excretion of the hormone.

Judging from the prolonged effect exerted by the small amounts of hormone used here, it is logical to expect that by implanting larger amounts of hormone (25 to 50 mgm) it will be possible to keep a patient symptom-free for periods of many months. This method of administering estrogens, it seems to us, has great therapeutic potentialities. In addition to being applicable to various types of cases of ovarian failure (natural menopause, functional amenorrhea, x-ray and radium castrates, etc.), it is suggested that it can be employed prophylactically at the time of surgical removal of the ovaries to prevent the development of the artificial menopause.

Further studies are being carried on in a larger series of cases to determine the duration of the effect in relationship to different amounts of the hormone implanted in order to ascertain the optimal amount of hormone for various clinical conditions.[1]

Udall J. Salmon
Robert I. Walter
Samuel H. Geist
Mt. Sinai Hospital, New York

## THE INFLUENCE OF 3-INDOLE-ACETIC ACID ON POLLEN GERMINATION

The presence of auxin in various kinds of pollen has been shown by several investigators.[1] Although several hundred papers have been published on growth substances, apparently no work has been done on the influence of auxin on the germination and growth of pollen tubes. The present writer is studying the effects

[1] We are indebted to Dr. Erwin Schwenk of the Schering Corporation, Bloomfield, N. J., for the crystalline a-estradiol benzoate used in this investigation.

[1] F. W. Went and K. V. Thimann, "Phytohormones." New York, 1937.

of heteroauxin on the rate of germination, the percentage of germination and the rate of elongation of the pollen tubes of several different species. The results obtained from five species seem worthy of a preliminary report.

Pollen grains of *Tradescantia canaliculata, T. occidentalis, Polygonatum commutatum, Lathyrus odoratus* and *Pinus Austriaca* Höss were cultured in solutions of sucrose (C.P.) in twice-distilled water. A 3 per cent. sugar solution was used for *Polygonatum* and the two species of *Tradescantia*; a 10 per cent. solution was used for *Lathyrus* and *Pinus*. These concentrations were chosen because preliminary trials had shown that they caused no plasmolysis or plasmoptysis. For each experiment two solutions were prepared with exactly the same concentration of sucrose, and to one of them enough 3-indole-acetic acid was added to be of a concentration of one part per million parts solution. The other solution was used as a control. The solutions were made up each time a group of cultures were started in order to prevent bacteria and mold from bringing about changes. The pH of the solutions was $6.4 \pm 0.1$ as determined by the calomel electrode potentiometer. Brink's[2] hanging drop technique was employed. Although no attempt to control the temperature was made, it varied only within the range of 25°–27° C. A large number of slides were carried through for each species in both the sugar series and the sugar-heteroauxin series. Representative fields were counted from each slide by means of the compound microscope (100X). To determine the rate of germination, the elapsed time between inoculation and the first protuberance of the intine was noted on each slide. Extensive four-hour counts were made on all species except *Pinus* (in which case twelve-hour cultures were counted) to determine the percentage of germination. Measurements of the pollen tubes were made also on these four- and twelve-hour cultures using an ocular micrometer.

These data indicate that 3-indole-acetic acid in concentrations of 1:1,000,000 produces the following effects: (1) germination is stimulated in such a way that the pollen tube appears in considerably less time than in the control, (2) the rate of elongation of the tube is increased, (3) a much higher percentage of germination is achieved, (4) greater tube lengths are found at the end of four hours, and (5) the pollen of *Pinus Austriaca* is stimulated to germinate, whereas no germination occurred in the control.

TABLE I

MEASUREMENTS ON POLLEN GERMINATION AND TUBE GROWTH WITH AND WITHOUT 3-INDOLE-ACETIC ACID

| Pollen | Rate of germination in minutes | | No grains counted | | Percentage germination | | Average four-hour tube length in microns* | |
|---|---|---|---|---|---|---|---|---|
| | Test | Control | Test | Control | Test | Control | Test | Control |
| *T. occidentalis* .... | 2–3 | 4–6 | 1453 | 1274 | 84% | 61 % | 920 | 590 |
| *T. canaliculata* .... | 2–3 | 4–6 | 1240 | 1042 | 80 " | 62.5 " | 350 | 208 |
| *Polygonatum* ...... | 15–18 | 25–28 | 1272 | 1240 | 58 " | 37 " | 450 | 220 |
| *Lathyrus odoratus* . | 25–30 | 90–100 | 1475 | 1535 | 76 " | 40 " | 163 | 86 |
| *Pinus Austriaca* ... | 6 hrs. | No ger. | 1200 | 1500 | 51 " | 00 " | 75 | 00 |

* The tube measurements on *Pinus* were made in twelve hours.

PAUL F. SMITH

UNIVERSITY OF OKLAHOMA

## THE VITAMIN C CONTENT OF SPRING GREENS

IN connection with a course in local flora, determinations were made of the ascorbic acid (vitamin C) content of certain wild plants which have been reported as being used for spring "greens" in southern Ohio. Young leaves, collected during the spring as soon as good growth had started, were analyzed in duplicate by the 2,6 dichlorophenolindophenol indicator method as described by Bessey.[1] The results are reported as milligrams of ascorbic acid per gram of fresh weight.

TABLE 1

ASCORBIC ACID CONTENT OF CERTAIN WILD PLANTS USED AS SPRING GREENS

| Common name | Botanical name | Mg ascorbic acid per gram of fresh weight |
|---|---|---|
| Burdock | *Arctium minus* | 0.696 |
| Chickweed | *Stellaria media* | 0.377 |
| Curly dock | *Rumex crispus* | 1.349 |
| Dandelion | *Taraxacum officinale* | 1.546 |
| Milkweed | *Asclepias syriaca* | 6.556 |
| Pokeweed | *Phytolacca americana* | 2.735 |
| *Shepherd's purse | *Bursa bursa-pastoris* | 1.296 |
| Skunk cabbage | *Spathyema foetida* | 3.150 |
| *Slender nettle | *Urtica gracilis* | 1.007 |
| Smaller leaved milkweed | *Asclepias incarnata* | 2.537 |
| Sorrel | *Oxalis stricta* | 1.765 |
| Sow thistle | *Sonchus oleraceaus* | 0.633 |
| *Water cress | *Sisymbrium nasturtium-aquaticum* | 1.875 |
| *Wild carrot | *Daucus carota* | 0.748 |
| Wild lettuce | *Lactuca canadensis* | 0.636 |

[2] R. A. Brink, *Am. Jour. Bot.*, 12: 149–162, 1925.

[1] Otto A. Bessey, *Jour. Am. Med. Asn.*, 111: 1290–98, 1938.

Plants which are starred in Table 1 gave extracts colored by anthocyanins. These were removed by treating with a small quantity of Lloyd's reagent (hydrated aluminum silicate) and centrifuging. This also removes a little of the ascorbic acid but was the most satisfactory reagent for the decolorization that could be found out of a great many that were tested. It is also realized that certain other substances besides ascorbic acid can reduce the dye and that in cooking, particularly when the liquid is discarded, there may be large losses of vitamin C. The values as determined for the fresh samples are given in Table 1.

For comparison, the average of several samples of fresh spinach by the same method was 0.812 milligrams of ascorbic acid per gram of fresh weight.

R. C. BURRELL
HELENA A. MILLER
THE OHIO STATE UNIVERSITY

# SCIENTIFIC APPARATUS AND LABORATORY METHODS

## A THERMAL METHOD FOR THE SEPARATION OF GASES AND ISOTOPES

Two methods are available for the separation of isotopes in quantity; one is the chemical, the other the physical. The chemical method, which will not be discussed in this paper, has been developed to a high degree of perfection by Professor Urey, of Columbia University. The physical method depends for its operation on the difference in the thermal behavior of the isotopes. As early as 1917 Chapman and Dootson[1] observed that when a gas consisting of two isotopes is placed in a tube heated at one end a slight concentration of the light component is induced in the heated portion of the tube by thermal diffusion. The effect in itself, however, is too small to serve as an efficient device for separating gases or isotopes. Within the last year processes have been developed which put the physical method on a practical basis. Clusius and Dickel[2] observed that, in an apparatus consisting of a cooled vertical tube with a heated wire down the center, an appreciable concentration of the heavy component of the gas is obtained at the bottom, while the light component rises to the top. The details given of the apparatus are so meager that an accurate description is impossible; it is stated, however, that the tubes vary in height from one to thirty meters and that the temperatures of the central wire range from 300 to 600° C. With the thirty-meter tube several liters of $HCl^{37}$, 99.4 per cent. pure, have been separated. These investigators describe the mechanism of operation as one arising from the combined action of thermal diffusion (the Chapman effect) which concentrates the light component at the heated wire, and to an overall convection current action which causes the gas to move upward along the heated wire and down along the cold wall. In this process the light gas is transported to the top of the tube and the heavy to the bottom.

Another modification of the thermal method has been developed in this laboratory.[3] The mechanism of separation depends on the combined action of the Chapman effect and an internal diffusion which results from the fact that molecules of different mass have different velocities when in thermal equilibrium. The basic principles involved in internal diffusion have been described in detail by Mulliken and Harkins.[4] The most effective design of apparatus so far constructed here consists of two vertical concentric glass tubes, the outer one water-cooled, while the inner one is heated electrically. In a device of this type the heat is transferred from the hot wall to the cold by a series of swirls in the intervening gas and not by an overall convection current up the hot wall and down the cold. Direct transference of heat by conduction occurs only in a thin layer adjacent to the walls. It is a well-known fact that if two molecules, one light, the other heavy, impinge on a heated plate they receive the same amount of energy, except for a slight difference due to their accommodation coefficients. In the case of isotopes the accommodation coefficients are obviously the same. In consequence, the lighter molecules, on coming in contact with the heated inner tube, rebound with the greater average velocity and hence go ahead to enrich the front rank of the expanding gas. The reverse process occurs at the cold wall. This effect is still further enhanced by thermal diffusion, which tends to concentrate the light gas at the hot surface. As a consequence of this enrichment more light than heavy molecules are trapped by the overlying gas swirl, the net result being that the light gas moves upward and the heavy downward.

The operation of the apparatus is illustrated by the following experimental results. The object of these experiments was to determine the most efficient design of instrument and not the separation of large quantities of material. The tubes were all one meter in length and the outside diameter of the inner cylinder was 1 cm. A 50–50 mixture of methane and ammonia was used, because analysis could be made quickly by freezing out the ammonia with liquid air. The effect of wall

1 Chapman and Dootson, *Phil. Mag.*, 34: 248, 1917.
2 Clusius and Dickel, *Naturwiss.*, 26: 546, 1938.
3 Brewer and Bramley, *Phys. Rev.*, 55: 590 (A), 1939; Bramley and Brewer, *Am. Chem. Soc. Abs.*, Baltimore meeting, April, 1939.
4 Mulliken and Harkins, *Jour. Am. Chem. Soc.*, 44: 37, 1922.

clearance was studied in a series of tubes in which the distance between the walls was varied from 1.3 mm to 22.0 mm. The gas separation (ratio of ammonia to methane) rose sharply with increasing wall clearance to a rather broad maximum at 7 mm. The effect of gas pressure was investigated from 11 to 60 cm of Hg for the different tubes. The 7 mm tube gave a maximum gas separation of 27 per cent. at 20 cm pressure. The pressure however is not critical nor is the optimum pressure the same for all gas mixtures. In these tests the temperature difference between the walls was 350° and the average temperature of the gas close to 150°. By varying the power input it was found that the final gas separation increased with the temperature difference between the walls. The rate of separation was investigated for a wall clearance of 7 mm and a temperature difference of 350°. The separation rose to 90 per cent. of its final value in 15 minutes. The absolute rate at which gas could be removed without decreasing the separation factor was not determined with accuracy; it was observed, however, that 1 cc of gas (N. T. P.) could be removed every 15 minutes without influencing the percentage separation. This speed suggests that a continuous flow method of operation should be feasible.

A number of gas mixtures have been studied in addition to the one mentioned above. The operation of the tube can be shown in a striking manner with a uniform 50–50 mixture of helium and bromine. In the course of a few minutes the bromine completely disappears from the top of the tube and becomes concentrated at the bottom. The separation of isotopes is easily demonstrated with HCl, in which gas the ratio of $Cl^{35}$ to $Cl^{37}$ was changed at a pressure of 20 cm from 3.2, its normal value, to 2.8 in a few minutes. The optimum conditions of operation depend, of course, on the nature of the gas. The results obtained with different gas mixtures lead to the conclusion that the separation depends primarily on the difference in mass of the two components divided by their sum.

Experiments have been performed which throw additional light on the mechanism of operation. When the entire tube was inclined 13° from the vertical the separation was decreased from 27 per cent. to 5 per cent. In another apparatus a series of corrugations was placed every 3 cm along the inner tube in such a manner that any gas moving along the heated wall would be deflected into the intervening space. In a 50–50 methane-ammonia mixture the average temperature of the gas was reduced about 15° and the final separation enhanced about 4 per cent. The design of the tube also appears to have a marked effect on the gas separation. A tube was built along the lines described by Clusius and Dickel with a heated tungsten wire extending down the center and a 7 mm clearance. After a run of several hours a smaller final separation of the chlorine isotope was observed with an 800° difference in temperature than was obtained in 15 minutes with the concentric glass tubes for a 350° difference in temperature. A 350° difference in temperature gave only a negligible separation. A similar tube with a 4 mm platinum ribbon down the center failed to show an appreciable separation. It is evident that separation is augmented by symmetry of the two surfaces. An all-glass apparatus in which the outer wall was heated and the inner cooled gave a separation value only slightly lower than when the inner wall was heated; the average temperature of the gas, however, was materially higher.

The rate of mixing of the separated gases has been investigated for various tubes. The results show that the rate of back diffusion increases with wall clearance and becomes very rapid for outside tubes of larger diameter.

Reviewing the above results as a whole, it is evident that conditions involving both wall symmetry and corrugations enhance swirl definition and thereby enhance separation. On the other hand, separation is materially lower in straight wire or ribbon-centered tubes as well as in tubes having small wall clearances in which swirls are either poorly defined or impossible. It appears that the mechanism of separation is different in the two cases. Under conditions where swirls are well defined the separation results from the combined action of initial and thermal diffusion within the swirls. In wire-centered tubes or glass tubes with small wall clearances where the swirls are poorly defined, the mechanism may involve thermal diffusion and an overall convection current.

We wish to thank Mr. Leonardo Testa, the glassblower, for constructing the large number of tubes used in these experiments.

ARTHUR BRAMLEY
A. KEITH BREWER
BUREAU OF CHEMISTRY AND SOILS,
U. S. DEPARTMENT OF AGRICULTURE

## BOOKS RECEIVED

CONWAY, EDWARD J. *Micro-diffusion Analysis and Volumetric Error.* Pp. xiii + 306. 49 figures. Crosby, Lockwood, London. 25/–.

CUMMINGS, ALEX., CHARLES, and SNYDER A. KAY. *A Text-book of Quantitative Chemical Analysis.* Pp. xv + 496. 85 figures. Van Nostrand. $5.00.

*Meeting the Needs of the Mentally Retarded.* Bulletin No. 420 of the Department of Public Instruction, Commonwealth of Pennsylvania. Pp. 158. Illustrated. The Department, Harrisburg.

MILLS, CLARENCE A. *Medical Climatology.* Pp. vii + 296. Illustrated. Charles C Thomas. $4.50.

POPE, CLIFFORD H. *Turtles of the United States and Canada.* Pp. xviii + 342 + v. 99 plates. Knopf. $3.75.

WOLF, RALPH F. *India Rubber Man; The Story of Charles Goodyear.* Pp. 291. Illustrated. Caxton Printers, Caldwell, Idaho. $3.00.

# SCIENCE

VOL. 90 | FRIDAY, AUGUST 25, 1939 | NO. 2330

*The American Association for the Advancement of Science:*
*Standards of Living as Functions of Science and of Social Organization:* DR. STUART A. RICE ... 167
*Obituary:*
*Heinrich William Poll:* PROFESSOR HAROLD CUMMINS. *Recent Deaths* ... 172
*Scientific Events:*
*The New British Non-Ferrous Metal Research Laboratories; Expedition to the Pacific Islands; Courses in Public Health at Harvard University and the Massachusetts Institute of Technology; Establishment by the American Mathematical Society of a New Periodical; Award of the Chandler Medal* ... 173
*Scientific Notes and News* ... 176
*Discussion:*
*The New Nomenclator Zoologicus:* PROFESSOR T. D. A. COCKERELL. *A New Color Reaction of Vitamin* $B_1$*:* DR. GILBERTO G. VILLELA and ALUISIO M. LEAL. *On the Nature of Friction:* PROFESSOR G. W. HAMMAR and GORDON MARTIN. *The Conscience of the Past and the Practise of the Present:* PROFESSOR M. F. ASHLEY-MONTAGU ... 178
*Scientific Books:*
*Science in Africa:* HAROLD J. COOLIDGE, JR. *The Advance of Medicine:* PROFESSOR CHAUNCEY D. LEAKE ... 180
*Societies and Meetings:*
*The Seismological Society of America—Eastern Section:* A. J. WESTLAND, S.J. ... 183
*Special Articles:*
*Studies in the Physical Chemistry of Insulin:* PROFESSOR EDWIN J. COHN and OTHERS. *Type-Specific Antibody Production with Living Pneumococci in the Rabbit:* PROFESSOR JULES FREUND and MARTHA A. BEHAN. *The Significance of the Amino Acids in Canine Nutrition:* PROFESSOR WILLIAM C. ROSE and ELDON E. RICE ... 183
*Scientific Apparatus and Laboratory Methods:*
*Deep-Sea Photography:* PROFESSOR E. NEWTON HARVEY. *A Glass Electrode Vessel for the Determination of Blood pH:* DR. VIVIAN G. BEHRMANN and PROFESSOR MARION FAY ... 187
*Science News* ... 6

SCIENCE: A Weekly Journal devoted to the Advancement of Science, edited by J. MCKEEN CATTELL and published every Friday by

THE SCIENCE PRESS
New York City: Grand Central Terminal
Lancaster, Pa. Garrison, N. Y.
Annual Subscription, $6.00 Single Copies, 15 Cts.

SCIENCE is the official organ of the American Association for the Advancement of Science. Information regarding membership in the Association may be secured from the office of the permanent secretary in the Smithsonian Institution Building, Washington, D. C.

# STANDARDS OF LIVING AS FUNCTIONS OF SCIENCE AND OF SOCIAL ORGANIZATION[1]

By Dr. STUART A. RICE

CHAIRMAN, U. S. CENTRAL STATISTICAL BOARD

THE purposes of my paper as first projected for inclusion in the symposium on "Science and Society" were: "(1) to take stock of the extent to which the standards of living of the people in the world have been raised in recent times; (2) to examine the extent to which production must still be expanded in order to provide satisfactory standards of living." It was hoped thus to "provide a factual basis on which to consider the needs for further applications of science to productive enterprise."

The phrasing of these intended specifications implies an attempt at statistical precision. "Take stock," "extent," "raised," "factual basis," "further applications," are expressions appropriately used in discussing measurable and measured or enumerated phenomena. Alas! Quantitative evidences of changes in the world's standards of living are not to be here presented. The concept "standard of living" is a will-o'-the-wisp. Its incarnate shapes and dimensions at different times in different climes have not been calibrated.

Alfred Marshall avoids the term "standard of living"[2] and distinguishes between the *standard of life,* meaning "the standard of activities adjusted to wants," and the *standard of comfort,* "a term that may suggest a mere increase of artificial wants, among which perhaps the grosser wants may predominate." "A rise in the standard of life implies an increase in intelli-

1 Condensed from the address on "World Standards of Living" of the retiring vice-president and chairman of Section K, of the American Association for the Advancement of Science, at the Ottawa session, June 28, 1938.

2 "Principles of Economics," 8th ed., Chapter XIII, on "Progress in Relation to Standards of Life."

gence and energy and self-respect; leading to more care and judgment in expenditure, and to an avoidance of food and drink that gratify the appetite but afford no strength, and of ways of living that are unwholesome physically and morally. . . . It is true that every broad improvement in the standard of comfort is likely to bring with it a better manner of living, and to open the way to new and higher activities; while people who have hitherto had neither the necessities nor the decencies of life can hardly fail to get some increase of vitality and energy from an increase of comfort, however gross and material the view which they may take of it."

The concepts underlying factual studies of standards of living probably include now one and now the other of Marshall's standards. In "The Encyclopaedia of the Social Sciences,"[3] Carl Brinckmann asserts that "the concept . . has yet to be worked into definitive form." Brinckmann himself comes closer than Marshall to precise definition when he says: "The underlying idea of a standard of living would seem to be that of a particular system of wants as connected with a specific system of productive services designed to transform these wants into efficient demand in the market." This concept must be distinguished not only from Marshall's standard of life and standard of comfort but also from what are sometimes called the "plane of living" and the "cost of living," although all these to a certain extent approach each other.

The standard of living, to expand Brinckmann's definition, is a composite. On one side it is a "system" or complex of wants. This complex, in turn, is composed in part of certain natural or physical requirements for existence and in part, and more significantly, of material and immaterial elements related to the customs, attitudes and valuations peculiar to the group. These latter are not subject, as Marshall implies in describing the standard of life, to judgments outside of the group itself as to what is wholesome or "unwholesome . . . morally," conducive to a "better manner of living" or promotive of "higher activities." There is room for many differences of evaluation and of reference when such terms are used. The Florida kidnapper and murderer of little Jimmy Cash "claimed he wanted the better things of life for his wife and himself."[4]

From the side of human wants, then, a standard of living is a mixture of physical or natural *and cultural* elements. In its second, or complementary aspect, a standard of living involves the possibility of satisfying wants. The wants must not be merely conceptual, fantastic or utopian. They must exclude the moon, even though the baby cries for it. Ownership of a motor car may be part of the standard of living of a well-paid American workman, even though he does not have one in his possession; while the standard of living of a Mexican peon may exclude this item because the possibilities and expectations available to his status make such ownership fantastic. Brinckmann says: "Standards of living, besides representing the natural or physical conditions of certain minima of existence, derive their greatest economic and social significance, first, from the ways these conditions are reacted upon and developed, so that they result in cultural instead of natural minima, and, second, and even more important, from the productive contributions that societies or groups are able and willing to make in order to attain such minima."

All this bears upon the task initially undertaken for this paper because it indicates that the supplementary concepts of "raising the standard of living" and "measuring improvements in standards of living" are mixtures of definite and realistic and of indefinite or unreal elements.

If the standard of living includes the "natural or physical conditions of certain minima of existence," these conditions, taken together, will comprise, as it were, a *minimum* minimum standard of living. This will include certain ranges of altitude, of heat and cold, of access to food, of means, in general, for the survival and prolongation of life. These things are capable of examination by quantitative methods. While some of them may be related to human existence as constants or discrete phenomena rather than as variables, their combined effects produce variation in the possibilities of living or not living. The transition of desert to fertile land through irrigation would represent a gain in the *minimum* minimum standard of living, as would also the recession of the frontier for wheat production in western Canada—both of them triumphs of applied science. So, too, would medical discoveries. Indexes of change in the *minimum* minimum standard of living could be found in periodic data showing the numbers of the world's population, or in comparisons, at intervals, of the average expectation of life.

When we pass from the natural or physical conditions of existence and examine the cultural components of a standard of living, we immediately encounter individual and social values, improvements in which can not be assumed or measured except in relation to artificially fixed points of reference. Universal agreement upon these points of reference will be rendered difficult if not impossible for all time to come because of the great diversity of human cultures.[5]

[3] "Standards of Living," Vol. 14, p. 322.

[4] Statement of the Chief of the Federal Bureau of Investigation, *The New York Times*, June 11, 1938, p. 1.

[5] Cultural anthropologists distinguish between material culture and immaterial culture. The latter would include such items as beliefs, speech habits, ethical ideas or scientific knowledge. Material culture would include dwellings, machines, incendiary bombs, microscopes and frying

The assumption which is general in Euro-American culture that standards of living are continuously improving as a result of scientific development appears to be a thinly disguised version of the belief in social progress. The concept of social progress has been somewhat discredited and confused by events since the outbreak of the World War. The development of communism and of fascism are cited by Russians and Germans, respectively, as evidences of social progress, while the success of both doctrines is responsible for dimming the belief in progress in the United States and Canada.

If standards of living are functions of cultural standards of value which are highly diverse, no means seem available for accurate comparisons of the standard of living among races and nations, or among groups and classes within the same racial or national structure or within the same nation or group at differing periods of time. Even individuals of the same group and social status may have widely differing standards at the same moment of time.

May I illustrate by describing an afternoon which I spent some years ago at the English country home of one of the world's leading social scientists. I sat with him in a small, frugal study, chilled to the bone by the raw drizzle through which we had walked from the station. It contained tiers of books, a simple oak table, two dilapidated chairs and a tiny grate containing a single, partially burned but unlit coal. That was all.

Outside in the garden he proudly exhibited neat rows of vegetables and—a rock-garden. The younger and middle-aged generations, he said sadly, are rushing around in motor cars and losing their capacity to construct and enjoy rock-gardens. This he regarded as a definite loss to living standards—a decline in one of the recognized norms of the English home, important in itself no less than as a symbol of that quiet contentment and domestic stability that makes every Englishman's home his castle.

Figures are no doubt available showing the production and use of motor vehicles in Great Britain, with estimates of passenger miles driven. These doubtless would show upward trends since the World War. But I am sure that no indexes have yet been devised to determine the relationships of such figures to the essential values in his nation's standard of living that alone seemed worth preserving to this distinguished scholar.

How, then, may we determine "the extent to which the standards of living of the people of the world have been raised in recent times?" I believe that there is no satisfactory quantitative answer to this problem. The question is on a par with such others as: To what extent have men gained wisdom in and satisfaction from the spending of their incomes? What improvements can be shown in the world's choices of occupations? In how far have human customs and manners been improved? Such questions are unreal, first, because of the absence of norms from which to measure deviations; second, because they assume the existence of criteria external to the productive system of which, in actuality, such criteria must be a part. One is reminded of the question allegedly asked of Abraham Lincoln, "How long should a man's legs be?" And his alleged reply, "Long enough to reach the ground."

The only practical means which I can discern by which to approach such questions have already been disclosed. First, we may agree to accept as a norm some pattern of standards which is held for the moment by a given group, presumably our own. This solution is implicit in all missionary activity, political, economic or religious. It is especially congenial to a nation which finds its motion pictures, its manners and its forms of industrial organization increasingly demanded or imitated throughout the world. As other peoples seek to become more like ourselves it is easy to agree that their standards of living are improving, and it would probably be possible to devise some indexes of the process.

For example, we might reduce to an annual index the world total, broken down by countries, of exhibitions of motion picture films or even of theater attendance. (The data required are not, I believe, available; but they could become so.) The areas of higher and lower living standards, as gauged by the index, would be clearly disclosed. If the land of Ghandi, who, I believe, spurns Hollywood art no less than our mechanical gadgets, should appear as one of the darker areas on the map, this would substantiate the vast superiority of American standards. Those who do not admire our gods show themselves to be heathen; and being heathen, what would you expect? However, the darker areas would be a challenge to the evangels of higher standards. Experience has shown that sales resistance can be overcome, and intensification of marketing efforts would be indicated. It is largely by such efforts that living standards, in the sense that I now employ the term, have actually been raised throughout the world.

A second approach to the problem of gauging im-

pans. Theoretically, it might be possible to obtain periodic quantitative measures of material culture, by weight, by number of units, by monetary value, by variety or otherwise. Thus it has been estimated that one million distinguishable types and varieties of commodities enter into trade in the United States, and this might be taken as a measure of our material culture. The relation of the material culture to standards of living depends upon its relationship to the *minimum* minimum standard or, more often, to the values contained in the immaterial culture. Thus increases in the quantity of opium in the United States would be increases in its material culture but probably not in its standards of living. A new aqueduct to supply pure water to a city, on the other hand, would be an unquestioned addition to the standard of living because it would be favorable to human life itself.

provements in world standards of living is to limit the examination to the *minimum* minimum standard. This has incidental statistical advantages, since it tends to avoid many questions of qualitative differences, of national or group averages, of deviations within the group, of the valuation to be placed on the consumption of leisure and the disvaluation to attach to forms of discontent arising from constraints upon individuals. Thus human life may be postulated as a good in itself. The development during several centuries past of the medical, hygienic, nutritional, political, sociological, productive and distributive sciences, technologies and arts, has brought about increases in the expectation of life and possibly also in opportunities to be born. The net result, in any event, has been an increase in the world's population. To science may be attributed the primary credit for the fact that there is undoubtedly more human life on our planet to-day than at any time before in its known history.[6] This brings me to the second of my initial undertakings: "to examine the extent to which production must still be expanded in order to provide satisfactory standards of living" and thus to "provide a factual basis on which to consider the needs for further applications of science to productive enterprise."

As already indicated, specifications for a "satisfactory" standard of living of world-wide application are unrealistic. At the same time, I believe that living standards in my own country are far from satisfactory, and that in most of the remaining countries of the world they are probably even less so. One third of the nation, according to our President, is "ill-fed, ill-clad and ill-housed." But such negative statements are easier to make than are their complementary positives. I could not say when, if all individual real incomes were to be raised at the same constant rate, "one third" would have been reduced to zero. Once the nation had attained a "satisfactory" level for every one, we should in the process have developed new opinions as to what is "satisfactory."

Two assumptions in my initial project caused me the most difficulty; first, that satisfactory standards of living are to be achieved by the expansion of production; second, that such an expansion depends upon "further applications of science." Both of these are partially true but omit a major consideration. In the case of the second, I can resolve the difficulty by placing my own interpretation upon the term "science."

The overlooked consideration is that natural science alone, without social organization to sustain it and put its achievements to work, would be a modern form of monasticism. By "social organization" I do not refer to the organization of scientific laboratories, faculties, staffs and associations merely; but rather to the entire structure and organized processes by means of which men live, produce and consume together. I mean in combination what the economist means by "the economy," the sociologist by "the society" and the political scientist by "the state," in so far as these differ. As an economy the system may be capitalistic or communistic or something between; as a society it may veer toward individual freedom or toward autocracy; as a state it may be democratic or totalitarian. Social organization of some kind there must be if the masses of men are to receive benefits from the laboratories and cloisters of the men of science.

A recent Associated Press dispatch from Shanghai will illustrate the way in which natural science, when implemented by social organization, may extend the lives of persons who are utterly lacking in knowledge of its aims and methods; "In this war-shocked, disease-ridden city any resistance on the part of a Chinese war refugee against vaccination is efficiently countered by health workers with strong-arm methods. While a sock on the jaw or the application of a half-Nelson may seem a bit drastic, such measures are often the only means of overcoming the Oriental fear of a bit of arm-scraping and a dose of vaccine." In its essentials, this mode of applying science through social organization is familiar to all of us.

But while social organization in cooperation with natural science is saving lives, social *disorganization,* especially on an international level, is destroying the lives and the cultural achievements of millions and reducing the standards of living of hundreds of millions. Science has been unable to prevent and in some respects has actually furthered social disorganization. How long will social organization, in forms competent to translate natural science into living standards, be able to endure as against the forces throughout the world making for war and other forms of social disintegration?

In the United States, we find: One third of the nation ill-fed, ill-clad and ill-housed; tremendous surpluses of food products and cotton; the producers of lumber, steel, glass, cement and other building materials operating well below capacity. Are the greater possibilities of improving standards of living in the United States to be found in expansions of production or in improvements in distribution? In further applications of science to productive enterprise or in perfecting the social organization?

In the *long run,* in my opinion, further applications of science to the increase of production will be required. From both the short-run and the long-run standpoints improvements in the mechanism of distribution and a recasting of present forms of social organization are essential. What shapes the recasting

[6] *Cf.* "Science," F. R. Moulton, SCIENCE, June 18, 1937, Vol. 85, No. 2216.

will produce I do not know. *Laissez-faire* in my opinion, and that of the publication *Fortune*,[7] is dead. The forms of departure from *laissez-faire* known as fascism, communism and national socialism all seem to me highly objectionable. I believe that ways can be found to reconcile social and political democracy with social efficiency in a system which will permit the untrammeled development of science and the distribution of its benefits to all the people. Hence, it would appear that *just now*, in accordance with the economic principles of *increasing* and *diminishing returns*, additional increments of scientific development would be most profitable in the fields of distribution and in respect to the perfection or recasting of social organization. These are tasks for social science rather than natural science.

These are questions of deadly seriousness for our present industrial civilization. Since the beginning of the industrial revolution in Europe, there has been a general upward trend in the possibilities of life—the *minimum* minimum standard of living. There has also been a great increase in material culture, though whether this has contributed more to the "standard of life" or to the "standard of comfort," using Marshall's distinction, is not certain.

Prior to the World War there seemed to be progress in the development of certain elements of immaterial culture which most people like ourselves deemed "desirable." These included "democracy," "civic consciousness," personal liberty, liberalism, universal education, cultural leveling, the free development of individuality, scholarship, research, tolerance, sophistication, urbanity, cosmopolitanism, pacification and perhaps pacifism, world-wide economic and intellectual interdependence, international justice, international law, humane sentiment, attention to personal cleanliness and appearance, esthetic sensitivity and appreciation, "sincerity" in architectural standards and more frequent and more rapid intercommunication over wider areas. Most of these are still regarded as desirable by people such as we. Others are being widely challenged and some have an interest mainly historical. The war brought subtle and often imperceptible changes in our valuations. Even in 1918, John Maurice Clark, Walton H. Hamilton and Harold G. Moulton pointed to "the establishment of new industrial standards, the enlarged domain of control, *the changes in personal habits and the newer conceptions of what is worth while in national and individual life*"[8] that would affect the transition from war to peace.

Before the war, the social mechanism, both internationally and within each nation, was becoming more subject to failure of parts to intermesh. The sacrifices of war were made endurable to democratic peoples by the faith that it would recast the worn-out parts and reset the ill-fitting gears. It was a war to make the world safe. These faiths have been very largely dissipated. World tensions have been growing more rapidly than before the war to end war. What meanings can be obtained from these experiences? What are the near-term prospects for human life and civilization on this planet? The world confronts two types of hazards, in my opinion: first, a catastrophic breakdown in its social organization; second, a slow disintegration and decay of social organization.

I have referred above to "war and other forms of social disorganization." This really begs an important question. Warfare has served at many historical junctures as a force making for social unification, organization and cultural diffusion; just as slavery, also, has had its periods of usefulness as an instrument of progress. But warfare, with the World War marking a turning point, has radically changed its character.

Traditionally, war has been a conflict between armies. The morale of the civilian populations behind the lines was usually strengthened by it, and nations could emerge from war with the social fabric more firmly inter-knit than before. To-day there are no lines to stay behind. The destruction of the morale and social organization, not to speak of the civilian lives, of the enemy nation have become major military objectives. Technological progress has facilitated the prosecution of these objectives, as by the development of aerial warfare. Technology has also increased the vulnerability to attack of social organization; first, by contributing to social complexity; second, by increasing social dependence upon material structures open to physical attack, such as central power stations, transportation and communication systems, and concentrated centers of manufacturing production.

For these reasons, a catastrophic breakdown in social organization, as a result of another world war involving unparalleled destructive efficiency, seems a distinct possibility. This is the forecast of H. G. Wells in his "Things to Come."

The possibility of slow decay in social organization arises from more subtle forces of disintegration at work within the social structure itself. The retardation of the birth rate; the prospective stabilization or decline of national populations; the weakening or disappearance of traditional sanctions for individual behavior; and the failure, in western liberal, capitalistic countries, to devise efficient means for the distribution of the products of technology, seem to be among these forces.

The existence of both of these hazards is an evidence of the seeming limitations upon man's capacity to

[7] "Business and Government," *Fortune Magazine*—February, March, April, May, 1938.

[8] Clark, Hamilton and Moulton, "Readings in the Economics of War," University of Chicago Press, p. 6, 7. Italics are mine.

direct a mechanism so complex as his own social organization.

A characteristic of periods of social stress and strain seems to be the tendency of peoples to seek escape into phantasy or *other-worldliness* from the over-difficult perplexities of real life. A leading economist said to me during the trough of the depression that we were headed in the United States for the "——est religious revival that this country has ever seen." His expectations were not realized, perhaps, because of the economic recovery that rapidly ensued thereafter. However, we see many evidences to-day of the same basic phenomenon to which he alluded. With a certain attitude of desperation the world is sacrificing its hopes of higher living standards on behalf of towering, non-productive armaments; meanwhile seeking psychological compensation in phantasy. The unprecedented "success" of Walt Disney's "Snow White and the Seven Dwarfs" and the wide appeal of James Hilton's "Lost Horizon" illustrate the point.

I think it significant that the present-day pessimism in the nations which are striving to preserve simultaneously liberalism, capitalism and democracy, is not engendered by fear that natural science and technology, of themselves, may fail to provide foundations for further expansions of production. It arises from fear of universal warfare and the general breakdown of existing social institutions. Science itself, in the latter event, might perforce be compelled to retreat again into the cells to which it was once confined by medieval theology. Even now, in large and important nations, science has been commandeered by the priests of force and intolerance. Without understanding that science can prosper only when abundantly supplied with the air of freedom, they would drive it to serfdom and prostitution on behalf of bastard political and anthropological doctrines.

We whistle and believe that "it can't happen here." This keeps up our courage. I believe that we must do more. Natural science and social science must join their efforts in undertaking the realistic task of constructing social organization, national and international, that can function and produce for the well-being and improvement of mankind. Only then can we believe with confidence that improvements in world standards of living are a reality.

# OBITUARY

## HEINRICH WILLIAM POLL

DR. HEINRICH POLL, anatomist and biologist, died suddenly on June 12, 1939, in his sixty-second year. Long denied common decencies of human living in the home country which he loved even to the end, he had found refuge in Lund, Sweden. It was here that he died after but a few days of freedom, tragically burdened by concern over the welfare of Mrs. Poll (Dr. Clara Poll Cords), who remained in Germany.

Poll was born on August 5, 1877, in Berlin. In 1900 he received the degree of doctor of medicine from the University of Berlin, where during 1899 he served as assistant to Oscar Hertwig. Appointed privatdocent in the Berlin Institute of Anatomy and Biology in 1904, he was elevated to professorship in 1907 and to extraordinary professorship in 1922. In 1924 he removed to the University of Hamburg, to occupy the ordinary professorship and to serve as director of the Institute of Anatomy and Human Genetics. Displaced from this position in 1934, he remained thereafter without institutional connection.

In 1928–29 Poll presented the first series of Flexner Lectures at Vanderbilt University, and on the occasion of this visit in the United States lectures were given also at the University of Chicago, Columbia, Harvard, Washington University and Yale.

Poll's first publications appeared in 1896; as a youth in the late teens he was already driven by the urge which made of him a scholar in all that the true sense of the word implies. That urge never deserted him. Even through the dark years which followed 1934 Poll did not cease his studies, hampered though he was by material obstacles and stresses, which for another might have stultified productive work. His bibliography, numbering over one hundred titles, closes with two papers in press, and other investigations were left unfinished.

His studies for the most part lie in three fields: physical anthropology, the endocrines and genetics. It is significant to note that his two first publications are concerned respectively with physical anthropology and endocrinology. Both these interests endured through a working career of over four decades, and for a large part of this period genetical investigations claimed a share of his attention. To each of the three fields Poll contributed distinct advances, not only directly but through his students as well. His most important work in physical anthropology is perhaps that concerned with finger prints, a subject which commanded first place in his interests during the later years. He developed a novel and revealing methodology, with the use of which he investigated racial variation, geographic variation within single races, constitution and symmetry. In endocrinology, his early demonstration (1896) of survival of transplanted adrenal tissue, the discovery of adrenal-like elements in invertebrates and a series of studies on the interrelation of the sex glands and adrenal are noteworthy. His genetical studies chiefly relate to hybridization of birds. Poll (1914) was among the first to appreciate the promise of the twin-method and to utilize it in genetical research.

Poll's stimulating discussions of scientific matters would alone hold him close in the memories of those who knew him. But his friends have gained much more from the man, the warmth and fullness of his understanding, be it in sharing a sunrise or in united attack on some entangled problem.

HAROLD CUMMINS

DEPARTMENT OF ANATOMY,
TULANE UNIVERSITY

## RECENT DEATHS

DR. ALGERNON COOLIDGE, since 1911 professor emeritus of laryngology at the Harvard Medical School, died on August 16 at the age of seventy-nine years.

DR. CLEMENT ROSS JONES, since 1932 dean emeritus of the College of Engineering of the West Virginia University, died on August 16 at the age of sixty-eight years.

DR. ALBERT COULSON BUCKLEY, professor of psychiatry at the Graduate School of Medicine of the University of Pennsylvania and honorary consulting psychiatrist at Philadelphia General Hospital, died on August 17 at the age of sixty-six years.

# SCIENTIFIC EVENTS

## THE NEW BRITISH NON-FERROUS METAL RESEARCH LABORATORIES

OLIVER STANLEY, president of the British Board of Trade, opened on June 29 the new laboratories of the British Non-Ferrous Metals Research Association in London. According to an article in the London *Times,* in the entrance hall he unveiled a bronze portrait plaque, erected as a memorial to Thomas Bolton, who from 1920 to his death in 1937 was chairman of the association.

The new premises provide a center for the research necessary in the metallurgical industries. Non-ferrous metals have been extensively used to show their advantages in modern building. The heating installation, electrical conduit, certain water supplies, plumbing and principal rain pipes are in copper; other water supplies are in BNF ternary lead alloy No. 2; water fittings in nickel silver and bronze; the principal stair balustrade has a nickel silver handrail, with anodized aluminium tubular standards, and door furniture is of nickel silver, anodized aluminium and bronze.

At semi-basement level there is a melting shop, with furnaces of many kinds, and nearby is a galvanizing and welding shop. The mechanical testing laboratory includes a constant temperature room, maintained at 68 deg. F., with a control to within plus or minus half a degree, so that no two points in the room differ by more than one degree. The machine shop includes a guillotine capable of cutting sheet steel up to 18 gauge. The physics laboratory is equipped with highly sensitive instruments for spectrographic analysis, general physical testing, thermal conductivity, specific-gravity determinations and reflectivity measurement.

In one of the two rooms reserved for metallography, photographic work is carried out on a large projection microscope with which magnifications from three to 2,500 diameters can be obtained. There are also chemistry laboratories, a pyrometry and heat treatment laboratory, laboratories for investigating corrosion, a general laboratory, a development department which interprets and demonstrates the result of the association's researches, offices, a library containing 4,000 books and 20,000 pamphlets and a store room.

The building is steel framed, with brick panel walls. Easy access to the flat roof makes it convenient to expose specimens to atmospheric corrosion.

The British Non-Ferrous Metals Research Association is a national organization of producers, manufacturers and users of non-ferrous metals, established in 1920 for the promotion and use of scientific knowledge in industry. It has grown to a large organization with nearly 300 subscribing members and a total income exceeding £30,000 a year, a proportion of which is received from the Department of Scientific and Industrial Research on a basis which provides for increased government grant as the industrial income increases. The association conducts researches on technical problems of common interest to groups of members and assists in the application to industrial practice of its own research results and of other advances in science.

## EXPEDITION TO THE PACIFIC ISLANDS

AN expedition to the Pacific Islands, under the auspices of the National Geographic Society and the University of Virginia with the cooperation of the U. S. Coast Guard, will sail from San Francisco shortly after the middle of September on board the U. S. Coast Guard cutter *Hamilton,* a 328-foot vessel.

Professor Wilbur A. Nelson, of the University of Virginia, will be the leader of the expedition and in charge of its geological work. Dr. C. S. Piggot, geophysicist, of the Carnegie Institution of Washington, will make studies from cores of mud taken from the ocean bottom. Professor Maurice Ewing, geophysicist of Lehigh University, will carry on gravity investigations at sea and will make special studies by means of artificial "earthquakes" produced by explosions on the ocean floor. Lieutenant A. J. Hoskinson, geophysicist of the U. S. Coast and Geodetic Survey, will measure gravity on land. Dr. J. W. Green, geophysicist of the Department of Terrestrial Magnetism of the Carnegie Institution of Washington, will conduct magnetic investigations, and Dr. Waldo L. Schmitt, marine biologist of the Smithsonian Institution, will make studies of sea life.

Other members of the expedition are F. Barrows Colton, science writer of the National Geographic Society, and R. H. Stewart, staff photographer, both of Washington; Jon M. Larson, of Princeton, N. J., radio engineer of the National Broadcasting Company; and the following assistants: R. M. Maddex and George T. Nelson, of Charlottesville, Va.; Leslie Manning, of Baltimore; Charles R. Smoot, of Washington, D. C.; A. C. Vine, of Garrettsville, Ohio; E. G. Uhl, of Elizabeth, N. J.; J. L. Worzel, of Staten Island, N. Y.; and O. Roy McClunin, of Washington, D. C. Leon J. Canova, 2nd, of Washington, is the secretary of the expedition.

In addition to the eighteen members of the expedition, the *Hamilton,* under the command of Captain Stephen Safford Yeandle, will be manned by a crew of 110. The ship will cover the island-studded area of the central and south Pacific extending 5,000 miles in an east-west direction and 2,500 miles north-and-south. Landings will be made on many of the islands in order to establish bases for instrumental observations.

## COURSES IN PUBLIC HEALTH AT HARVARD UNIVERSITY AND THE MASSACHUSETTS INSTITUTE OF TECHNOLOGY

A NEW course, designed to train school supervisors, and especially supervisors of education in health, in the technique of educating the public concerning the protection and promotion of health, will be offered at the Harvard School of Public Health beginning this September.

The course, open to college graduates and extending one or two years, has been planned in recognition of the growing realization that those who are engaged in health education work must not only understand individual health measures, but they must also know what public health is, what its aims are, and what administrative measures are used in the fulfillment of its aims. Because it is equally essential that the student understand educational techniques, the Harvard Graduate School of Education will cooperate with the Harvard School of Public Health in giving this new course.

There will be no prescribed curriculum; each student will be assigned a personal program after an individual conference to determine his or her needs, in the light of prior training and experience. Credit may be granted for previous academic work in public health and in educational methods, and for experience in the field.

The training offered in this course is based on the principle that the person going into the field of health education needs first of all a basic knowledge of anatomy, physiology and the fundamental medical sciences. He will need to know the diverse functions of health departments and how such departments are organized. The student will, therefore, according to his individual needs, be assigned to work in the Harvard School of Public Health, in the Harvard Graduate School of Education, in the Harvard Faculty of Arts and Sciences, in Radcliffe College and in the Harvard Medical School.

A graduate course in public health engineering has been established at the Massachusetts Institute of Technology in the department of biology and public health, of which Dr. Samuel C. Prescott is head. This new course will consider such subjects as water supplies, water purification, sewerage, industrial waste disposal, stream pollution and purification and the sanitation of shellfish grounds. In addition, consideration will be given to the most advanced practice in the collection and disposal of refuse, sanitation of swimming pools, rural communities and camps, as well as the sanitation of food supplies, stores and restaurants. Students will also receive instruction in the relationship of insects and rodents to disease; the atmosphere in relation to health and comfort, housing and health, school sanitation and industrial hygiene. There will be training in the organization and activities of health departments, the collection, analysis and interpretation of vital statistics, epidemiological methods, the value and conduct of public health surveys, and the use of standard health appraisal forms.

The course will lead to the degree of master of science in one year, and will be open to qualified men of outstanding scholastic attainment and professional promise who are graduates in engineering of a recognized school or college. Candidates must have had at least one year of experience with a city, county or state department of health, the United States Public Health Service or some other recognized health agency.

Professor Murray P. Horwood, of the department of biology and public health, will direct the courses in public health engineering and vital statistics. Professor T. R. Camp, of the department of civil engineering, will give the course in hydraulic and sanitary engineering and sanitary design. The courses in health department practice and industrial hygiene will be given by Professor Clair E. Turner and the course in sanitary biology by Professor Marshall W. Jennison. Students will be required to present a satisfactory thesis dealing with some original investigations.

## ESTABLISHMENT BY THE AMERICAN MATHEMATICAL SOCIETY OF A NEW PERIODICAL

THE American Mathematical Society has received grants from two foundations to found a new international mathematical abstracting journal to be known as *Mathematical Reviews.* During the past quarter of a century while the United States and Canada have been gradually assuming a more prominent part in mathematical research, there has been sentiment expressed from time to time among mathematicians that there should be a review journal sponsored by American organizations. But doubts as to whether the scientific and financial resources could be spared caused the postponement of the undertaking. However, the rapid growth of American mathematical resources and the availability of funds have resolved these doubts, and it has been decided to proceed immediately.

The first number of *Mathematical Reviews* is to appear late in 1939 or early in 1940; the material to be reviewed begins with the latter half of 1939. It is proposed to review all fields of pure mathematics and also those of applied mathematics and mathematical physics which are of pronounced interest to mathematicians. The new journal, which will be issued approximately once a month, will contain several thousand reviews annually and will run to approximately eight hundred large double-column pages. Professors J. D. Tamarkin and Otto Neugebauer will be the first editors. A strong group of collaborators for the initial period is assured.

The Carnegie Corporation has appropriated $60,000 for the new journal. The Rockefeller Foundation has made a gift of $12,000 to cover some of the initial costs. Brown University is housing the project and aiding in the editorial work. The American Mathematical Society and the Mathematical Association of America are each starting off with a subsidy of $1,000 for the first year. Annual subsidies are being sought from other organizations, and plans for the permanent financing of the project are being considered. On account of the subventions, the subscription price will be set below actual cost.

Partly with a view to aiding indirectly in the support of this journal, the Rockefeller Foundation has made a gift to Brown University for an experiment in the dissemination of mathematical publications through the distribution of microfilm. This money is to be used to augment the mathematical library at that university, a collection which is already internationally known as outstanding. Out-of-print journals will be put on film and made available to mathematicians; rare books of general use will be filmed; on request from a subscriber to the new journal, any article reviewed will be sent on film or as film-print. This service will be extended to all parts of the world at a price not exceeding cost.

## AWARD OF THE CHANDLER MEDAL

THE seventeenth Charles Frederick Chandler Medal of Columbia University has been awarded to Thomas H. Chilton, director of the technical division of the engineering department of E. I. du Pont de Nemours and Company, Wilmington, Del.

Mr. Chilton was chosen "for his outstanding achievements in the discovery and formulation of principles underlying the unit operations of chemical engineering, and in the application of these principles to process development, equipment design and chemical plant construction and operation," according to the citation of the award committee. The medal will be presented to him on November 16, when he will deliver the annual Chandler Lecture on "Engineering in the Service of Chemistry."

The committee has issued the following statement in which it gives grounds for the award:

> Mr. Chilton's studies have brought to light unknown facts concerning distillation, heat transfer, fluid flow and absorption—factors which are present in nearly every manufacturing process.
>
> His published works are to the chemical engineer what the classics are to the student of literature. Principles discovered by his researches are used in the design and operation of chemical plants. There are few industrial processes involving chemical reactions in which his researches can not be applied.
>
> In addition to conducting these researches, Mr. Chilton has developed a method of producing formaldehyde, of prime importance in the manufacture of synthetic resins, from methane, the chief constituent of natural gas. Because of the wide use of formaldehyde, this development has made many chemical processes more economical to operate.
>
> The efficiency of the process by which nitric acid is manufactured from the oxidation of ammonia has been increased through Mr. Chilton's work. With the introduction of the nitrogen-fixation process into industry, ammonia became a relatively cheap and plentiful product. Its use as raw material for the production of nitric acid has greatly lowered the cost of the latter.
>
> Heat and fluids are associated with nearly all chemical apparatus. In attacking the problem of how heat flows through various substances and determining the characteristics of fluid flow under different circumstances, he has clarified these fundamental subjects.

# SCIENTIFIC NOTES AND NEWS

DR. E. D. MERRILL, administrator of botanical collections at Harvard University and director of the Arnold Arboretum, has been elected a corresponding member of the Institut national Genevois.

A FELLOWSHIP in the Rochester, N. Y., Museum of Arts and Sciences has been conferred on Dr. Carl E. Guthe, director of the University Museums and the Museum of Anthropology of the University of Michigan. Dr. Guthe's certificate of fellowship carried a citation which said, in part: "It is a recognition of your eminence in the field of museum administration and your leadership in the coordination of anthropological and archeological organizations resulting in the founding of the Society for American Archeology and to numerous important convocations of anthropologists and students interested in the study of early man in America."

T. E. WALLIS, reader in pharmacognosy in the University of London, has been awarded the Hanbury Medal of the Pharmaceutical Society of Great Britain.

DR. W. A. WESLEY, assistant director of the Research Laboratory, International Nickel Company, Bayonne, N. J., was awarded the annual gold medal of the American Electro-Platers' Society at its twenty-seventh annual convention in Asbury Park, N. J., in recognition of his paper on "Physical Properties and Uses of Heavy Nickel Deposits."

AT the fourth annual conference of the British Speleological Association, which opened at Swansea on August 5, a silver key was presented to Sir Cyril Fox, director of the National Museum of Wales, by Dr. R. R. Marett, president of the association.

PROFESSOR THEODOR VAHLEN, president of the Prussian Academy of Sciences, has been awarded the Goethe Medal for Art and Science by the German Chancellor.

PROFESSOR JAROSLAV PERNER, professor of paleontology in the Charles University, Prague, recently celebrated his seventieth birthday.

DR. R. E. COKER, head of the department of zoology and chairman of the division of natural sciences of the University of North Carolina, has been made Kenan professor of zoology in the place of Professor H. V. Wilson, who died on January 4.

DR. C. A. MCCUE, dean and director since 1920 of the Agricultural Experiment Station of the University of Delaware, who has been connected with the institution since 1907, has retired. George L. Schuster, professor of agronomy and research agronomist, has been appointed director.

DR. W. E. SHULL, associate professor of entomology at the University of Idaho, has been appointed head of the department. He succeeds Dr. Claude Wakeland, who has resigned.

DR. RICHARD O. SUTHERLAND, formerly of the University of Wisconsin and of Carleton College, has been appointed assistant professor of chemistry at Hamilton College, Clinton, N. Y. Dr. Asa Emanuel McKinney has been advanced to a professorship in that department, to take the place of Dr. Arthur Percy Saunders, who has been connected with the college since 1900.

DR. NATHAN SCHWID, of Montana State College, Bozeman, has been named assistant professor of mathematics at the College of Mines and Metallurgy, a branch of the University of Texas at El Paso. He succeeds Dr. Hugh L. Turrittin, who has resigned to join the faculty of the University of Minnesota.

DR. JULIA SOUTHERD LEE, formerly of Purdue University, has been appointed assistant professor of textiles and clothing at the Iowa State College.

DR. FRANCES L. HAVEN, associate professor at the University of Rochester School of Medicine and Dentistry, has been awarded a research fellowship by the National Cancer Institute at Washington.

DR. HUGH NICOL, of the Rothamsted Experimental Station, has been appointed scientific assistant to Sir John Russell, director of the station.

PROFESSOR ERNST FREUND has resumed his work as director of the Pearson Research Laboratory, which has been removed from Vienna to London. The laboratory, which has specialized in work on food chemistry and nutrition in its relation to cancer, was founded by Frederick Pearson, an American now living in England. Dr. Freund's assistant, Dr. Gisa Kaminer, who was for many years surgeon at the Rudolf Hospital in Vienna, is also working in the laboratory at London.

DR. JAMES R. WITHROW, of the Ohio State University, is one of a group of American chemical engineers who have been invited by the Swiss Government to visit the chemical and other industries of Switzerland in connection with the International Exposition of Swiss Industries at Zurich.

DR. JOHN A. KOLMER, professor of medicine at Temple University, Philadelphia, has been invited by the Health Section of the League of Nations to represent the United States at the fourth International Conference on the Serologic Diagnosis of Syphilis, to be held in Copenhagen from September 25 to October 6.

ACCORDING to *Industrial and Engineering Chemistry*, Charles M. A. Stine, vice-president in charge of research at the E. I. du Pont de Nemours and Company, Inc., has accepted an invitation to address the Second International Chemical Engineering Congress, convening in Berlin during the week of June 23, 1940. Dr. Stine will represent the American Institute of Chemical Engineers, of which he is a director. His address, "Chemical Engineering and Industry," will be one of the four papers to be delivered during the general session. The other speakers will be Sir Harold Hartley, representing England; Georges Claude, France, and Richard Kuhn, Germany.

PROFESSOR FRANCESCO PENTIMALLI, professor of pathology at the University of Naples and a member of the Italian Parliament, arrived in New York on August 17. He plans to attend the International Congress of Microbiology in New York and the Cancer Research Congress in Atlantic City.

DR. RHEINHARDT DOHRN, director of the Naples Zoological Station, reports an active spring session at the laboratory this year. He states that an important result was the isolation of fertilizin (F. R. Lillie) from sea urchin eggs by Dr. Max Hartmann and his collaborators. Dr. Dohrn expresses regret that there were no American applicants this year. The American table is supported by the National Research Council under the direction of Professor R. E. Coker, chairman of the division of biology.

THE Advisory Council on Human Relations, authorized at the Richmond meeting by the executive committee of the American Association for the Advancement of Science, has organized with Dr. Horace B. English, of the Ohio State University, as *chairman,* and Dr. C. E. Lively, University of Missouri, as *secretary.* Other members of the council are: Dr. J. L. Hypes, University of Connecticut; Dr. C. C. Zimmerman, Harvard University; Dr. W. M. Krogman, University of Chicago; Dr. R. E. Coker, University of North Carolina; Dr. Douglas Fryer, New York University, and Fred C. Pederson, state forester, Charlottesville, Va. The council was appointed at the suggestion of the U. S. Forest Service to act as a central advisory and coordinating body for research into the human-relations problems of reforestation and soil conservation and such other problems as may arise.

THE twenty-ninth National Conference on Weights and Measures was held in Washington from June 6 to 9. The following officers were elected for the ensuing year: *President,* Dr. Lyman J. Briggs, director, National Bureau of Standards. *Vice-presidents,* Charles C. Read, state superintendent of weights and measures of New Jersey; C. E. Tucker, chief, State Division of Weights and Measures of California; H. N. Davis, supervisor, State Department of Weights and Measures of Vermont; A. J. Jenson, state inspector of weights and measures of North Dakota; Alex Pisciotta, director, Bureau of Weights and Measures of New York City; James O'Keefe, inspector of weights and measures, of Chicago, Ill. *Secretary,* F. S. Holbrook, National Bureau of Standards, Washington, D. C. *Treasurer,* George F. Austin, Jr., supervising inspector of weights and measures of Detroit, Mich.

THE British American Engineering Congress, dedicated to the subject, "Engineering Aids World Progress," will be held in New York City from September 4 to 8. It meets with the American Society of Mechanical Engineers, the Institution of Mechanical Engineers of Great Britain, the American Society of Civil Engineers, the Institution of Civil Engineers of Great Britain and the Engineering Institute of Canada and other participating engineering organizations. These include the American Engineering Council, United Engineering Trustees, the Engineering Foundation, the Engineers' Council for Professional Development, Engineering Societies Library, the American Institute of Mining and Metallurgical Engineers, the American Institute of Electrical Engineers, the Society of Automotive Engineers, the Society of Naval Architects and Marine Engineers, the Society of American Military Engineers and the Institute of the Aeronautical Sciences.

THE seventh congress of the Association pour la Documentation photographique et cinématographique dans les sciences will be held in Paris on October 12 and 13. Members will meet on the first day at the Palais de la Découverte and on the second day at the Musée Pedagogique de l'État. Further information may be obtained from Dr. Charles Claoué, 39, rue Scheffer, Paris, 16.

THE twenty-seventh International Congress of Americanists was opened on August 5 in Mexico City, under the patronage of President Cardenas, with an attendance of over three hundred students of archeology, anthropology and history. Dr. Alfonso Caso, director of the National Institute of Archeology and History, Mexico City, was elected president, and General Cardenas honorary president. The honorary vice-presidents include T. A. Joyce, lately of the British Museum, and M. Paul Rivet, of the Museum of Man in Paris. An excursion was made to the pyramids and the museum at San Juan de Teotihuacan.

THE twelfth International Congress of the History of Medicine will be held in Berlin from September 22 to 28, 1940, when the chief subjects for discussion will be the evolution of medicine in different countries from Harvey to Haller, the epoch of medical philosophers, introduced by Dr. Laignel-Lavastine, professor of the history of medicine in the faculty of medicine of the University of Paris, and the history of typhus, introduced by Professor Zeiss, director of the Institute of Hygiene of the University of Berlin.

The hundredth anniversary of the presentation of the daguerreotype process of photography to the French Academy by Louis Jacques Daguerre, father of photography, was commemorated on August 17 at the Eastman Kodak Building at the World's Fair with the opening of an exhibition of daguerreotype equipment, including a camera operated by Charles H. Tremaine, the only daguerreotypist in the United States. The exhibition includes an original daguerreotype by Daguerre, an 1837 photograph, which is the earliest existing still-life; an 1845 daguerreotype panorama of Niagara Falls, and many early photographs.

The regular summer meeting of the Pennsylvania Academy of Science was called at Laporte, county seat of Sullivan County, on August 11, 12 and 13 by President R. W. Stone. Ninety-eight members and guests were present. Laporte is on the Allegheny Plateau at an elevation of almost 2,000 feet and is ideally situated for field trips, particularly in botany, as many rare plants occur in the neighborhood, including a number of unusual northern species. Field trips were held to the Haystacks, Lincoln Falls, Whirls End, High Knob and other points. On the evening of the eleventh, an out-of-door meeting open to the public was held. Talks, partly illustrated by lantern slides, were given on the local forestry, botany and geology. A correspondent writes that an unusually fine display of the aurora was visible that evening, adding materially to the interest of the meeting.

The Rockefeller Foundation has recently granted Stanford University the sum of $200,000, for the continued maintenance, during a ten-year period, of a program of biological research supported since 1934 by previous grants from the same foundation. The project is under the general supervision of Professor C. V. Taylor, and has included individual investigations on biochemical factors in eye-color control in Drosophila, by G. W. Beadle; bioelectric phenomena in plant cells, by L. R. Blinks; the reorganization processes in induced encystment and excystment of ciliates, by C. V. Taylor; hybridization and embryonic transplantation experiments with Amphibia, by V. C. Twitty; the determination of polarity in developing ova, by D. M. Whitaker, and biochemical studies of bacterial synthesis, by C. B. van Niel.

Additional facilities for the scientific study of problems confronting the fishing industry on the Atlantic Coast will be provided by the Bureau of Fisheries through the construction of a new laboratory building at the University of Maryland, College Park, to be built at a cost of $100,000. Preliminary plans call for the erection of a building to permit consolidated housing of the technological laboratory units now in operation at College Park and at Washington. A laboratory for research into West Coast fishing problems is maintained by the bureau at Seattle. The College Park building will provide for the first time similar unified facilities for the benefit of Atlantic Coast fishermen.

# DISCUSSION

## THE NEW NOMENCLATOR ZOOLOGICUS

Scientific workers can not avoid a considerable amount of bibliographic drudgery, but in the nature of things some of this most necessary work can not be undertaken by single individuals. This is especially true in regard to generic and subgeneric names, which, according to the rules, may not be duplicated in the whole realm of zoology. Sherborn's "Index Animalium," listing, with bibliographical references, the generic names proposed up to 1850, has been invaluable; and particulars concerning later names may be found in the annual volumes of the *Zoological Record.* The various nomenclators, that of Scudder being the most important, listed the generic names, with dates. Yet with all these aids, there was clearly urgent need for a new nomenclator, bringing the subject up to date, and including some five thousand names which had been omitted from earlier lists. Such a work was projected by Dr. S. A. Neave, assistant director of the Imperial Institute of Entomology, in 1934. As a result of incessant labor by many workers, it has been completed, and is published by the Zoological Society of London. The first volume (A–C) is now published; three others (with over 900 pages each) will appear at intervals of about six months. The whole work is sold for eight guineas, post free, "a price which bears no relation to the initial cost, but which, it is hoped, will enable many individual zoologists, as well as institutions and libraries, to purchase copies." There are more than 225,000 entries, each occupying one or more lines of print. The generic names are in bold face and thus much easier to read than those in Scudder's work, which is in any case almost impossible to obtain, being long out of print. Looking up numerous names which are familiar to me, I have failed to detect any errors. The cost of preparation was borne by the Zoological Society of London, which publishes the work at its office in Regent's Park, London, N.W.8. Contributions towards the cost of printing were made by the Carnegie Corporation of New York, the Royal Society and a generous anonymous donor. Recorders were paid, but surely not in proportion to their labors.

J. R. le B. Tomlin unreservedly turned over for the use of the editor his great manuscript list of the generic names used for mollusca, on which he has been working for many years.

Such a work as this serves to emphasize the international and cooperative features of scientific work, and to show that it is possible to maintain a great republic of workers, without regard for race and without any external coercion. In the field of science we have a working League of Peoples, which may well serve as a model for other efforts to unite humanity for the common good.

T. D. A. Cockerell
University of Colorado

## A NEW COLOR REACTION OF VITAMIN $B_1$ (THIAMIN, ANEURIN)

Studying the influence of pure synthetic vitamin $B_1$ (thiamin, aneurin) on blood phosphate fractions[1] by Fiske and Subbarow's technic we were surprised by the great increase of the values when thiamin was added. More accurate investigations showed that pure thiamin produced alone an intense blue color by the use of ammonium molybdate in sulfuric acid solution and aminonaphthosulfonic acid solution. This reaction being nevertheless non-specific permits, however, the determination of the vitamin when the concentration is above 100γ in pure aqueous solution. Since the color reaction follows the Beer's law it was possible to determine the optimal spectral zone for photometric readings. A Pulfrich spectrophotometer was employed, using filter S 72. The absorption index, $\frac{\text{concentration}}{\text{extinction coeff.}}$ was calculated and found to be 0.375. The technic for the determination is easy and rapid. To a 25 ml flask the thiamin solution (more than 100γ) is added together with 5 ml of a 2.5 per cent. ammonium molybdate solution in 3N sulfuric acid and then 1 ml of a 0.25 per cent. aminonaphthosulfonic acid containing sodium bisulfite and sodium sulfite (as prepared for blood phosphorus determination by Fiske and Subbarow).[2] The flask is filled to the mark with distilled water and the color read after 10 minutes using a 3 ml cup and filter S 72 in a Zeiss photometer. The extinction value is multiplied by 0.375 to obtain the thiamin in the sample.

When phosphorus is also present in the solution the color intensity represents the vitamin plus phosphorus content. By destroying organic matter with sulfuric-nitric mixture in another sample and neutralizing, then proceeding as above, the color developed represents only the phosphorus content. The difference between the first and the second determinations gives the thiamin content.

[1] G. G. Villela and A. M. Leal, *Compt. Rend. Soc. Biol. Paris,* in press.

[2] C. H. Fiske and Y. Subbarow, *Jour. Biol. Chem.,* 66: 375–400, 1925.

A more detailed study of this reaction will be published elsewhere.

Gilberto G. Villela
Aluisio M. Leal
Oswaldo Cruz Institute,
Rio de Janeiro, Brazil

## ON THE NATURE OF FRICTION

Friction between solid surfaces is ordinarily thought of as due to the interlocking of surface irregularities. That static friction also depends on the molecular attractions between the surfaces has recently been shown in a series of experiments on the tangential force between two smooth, clean glass surfaces in contact.

We placed a short piece of fire-polished glass tubing inside of a longer straight glass tube. This tube had a sufficiently large bore so that the smaller piece could slide freely within it. This assemblage was thoroughly heated and carefully evacuated by means of an efficient mechanical vacuum pump after which the outer tube was sealed off in the evacuated state. The assemblage was then enclosed in a water jacket for temperature control and clamped on a tilt table. This arrangement permitted us to determine accurately the angle at which the small glass tube started to slide under gravity within the larger tube.

During the course of the experiments it was discovered that the static friction, as computed from the angle of slip, was much larger for surfaces baked in a vacuum than for surfaces which were exposed to the air in the laboratory. The lower friction of the exposed surfaces undoubtedly was due to a moisture and gas film between them.

Several assemblages were constructed, baked out and sealed under vacuum. In each the coefficient of static friction decreased almost rectilinearly with the number of passes of the slider. In one case, where both slider and enclosing tube were made of soft soda glass, the coefficient of static friction decreased to one half its original value in 44 passes of the slider.

The appearance of the sliding surfaces was much modified during the experiment. The fresh surfaces looked perfectly smooth under a microscope, but after a few passes of the slider the surfaces became pitted. The pits were approximately round and not elongated in the direction of the motion, showing that parts of the surfaces had been torn out as if welded junctions had been broken.

In all our experiments, using baked and evacuated apparatus, the coefficient of static friction decreased with wear. How far this decrease in friction continues is not known as yet, but it is not likely to go much below one half of its virgin value. Certain difficulties with the breaking of the outer tube due to the impacts of the slider have prevented us from extending the experiment indefinitely with a given tube.

Our interpretation of these results is that a large

fraction of the static friction between two clean, smooth glass surfaces in contact is due to molecular attraction between those parts of the surfaces which are so close to one another that their molecular adhesions come into play. This assumption would explain both the formation of the observed microscopic pits and the decrease in friction with decreased smoothness of the surfaces. If this interpretation applies to all friction between smooth, solid surfaces it would indicate that the friction is largely determined by the molecular attractions between the two surfaces in contact and by their mean distance apart.

G. W. HAMMAR
GORDON MARTIN
THE UNIVERSITY OF IDAHO

## THE CONSCIENCE OF THE PAST AND THE PRACTISE OF THE PRESENT

INCREASING awareness among scientists of the barbaric uses to which their discoveries and inventions have so frequently been put—and in many cases are at the present time threatening the destruction of millions of human beings—has caused many scientists somewhat belatedly to take thought how best they can in future prevent such misuse of their labors. In our own day one of the greatest mechanical inventions of this or any other century, the aeroplane, has been turned into an instrument which power-crazed governments use to threaten not only the peace but the civilization of the world. It is therefore of peculiar interest for us to-day to hear what the inventor of the first airship, Father Francesco Lana (1631–1687), considered to be the strongest objection to his invention.

After enumerating the six technical objections which he foresaw to his invention (actually in his poverty he was unable to construct the ship), he goes on to say:

> Other Difficulties I see not, which may be objected against this Invention, besides one which to me seems greater than all the rest, and that is, That it may be thought, that God will never suffer this Invention to take effect, because of the many consequencies which may disturb the Civil Government of men. For who sees not, that no City can be secure against attack, since our Ship may at any time be placed directly over it, and descending down may discharge Souldiers; the same would happen to private Houses, and Ships on the Sea: for our Ship descending out of the Air to the sails of Sea-Ships, it may cut their Ropes, yea without descending by casting Grapples it may over-set them, kill their men, burn their Ships by artificial Fire works and Fire-balls. And this they may do not only to Ships but to great Buildings, Castles, Cities, with such security that they which cast these things down from a height out of Gun-shot, cannot on the other side be offended by those below.

This passage occurs in the author's "Prodromo," which was published in 1670. The first account and criticism of this work in English (probably by Robert Hooke) appeared in the *Philosophical Collections,* No. 1, 1680, pp. 18–29, and it is from this account that the translation given above is reproduced.[1]

M. F. ASHLEY-MONTAGU
HAHNEMANN MEDICAL COLLEGE,
PHILADELPHIA

[1] A contemporary English translation of the relevant fifth and sixth chapters from the "Prodromo" is "The Aerial Ship, by Francesco Lana." The Aeronautical Society of Great Britain, London, 1910, 12°, pp. vi–7–27. The following are the studies which I have thus far been able to discover relating to Francesco Lana's invention: Wilhelm Balthasar, "An der Wiege der Luftschiffart. Francesco Lana und Barthol. Laurenço de Gusmao." *Frankfurter Zeitgemässe Brorchüren,* Hamm, Vol. 28, pp. 137–198, 1909; Anton von Brandis, "Studien über die Verfassungs-Geschichte der Gemeinde Lana," *Zeitschrift des Ferdinandeums für Tirol und Vorarlberg,* 3 Folge, Heft. 18, pp. 159–196, (Geschichtliche Abtheilung), Innsbruck, 1873; Angelo Ferretti-Torricelli, "Padre Francesco Lana nel terzo centanario dalla nascita," Ateneo di Brescia. Commentari, Brescio, 1931/32, pp. 331–390. See also Francesco Lana Terzi, *Magisterium Naturae, et Artis,* Brixiae, Libri 3, (1) 1684, (2) 1686 and (3) 1692.

# SCIENTIFIC BOOKS

## SCIENCE IN AFRICA

*Science in Africa.* By E. B. WORTHINGTON. New York: Oxford University Press, 1939. Pp. xv + 746. Illustrated. Maps. $4.00.

LORD HAILEY, the director of the African Research Survey, writes in the Foreword:

> This book is one of a series of reports prepared in connection with the African Research Survey. The problems of Africa, as they present themselves to those whose concern is with the development of the continent, are discussed in "An African Survey." The purpose of this volume is to summarize the present position of studies in the various sciences which have a bearing on African conditions.

Mr. Worthington starts in by pointing out the interrelations between branches of science, and then as an aid to the appreciation of the interdependence of scientific studies in Africa he mentions important points about the changing environment. For example, he says, "The picture really presented by Africa is one of movement, all branches of physical, biological and human activity reacting on each other, to produce what biologists would refer to as an ecological complex."

Mr. Worthington's first chapter deals with some problems of research in which he makes many practical suggestions arising from his investigations; for example, he points out the practical advantages of separating research organization from the executive work of the technical departments and placing it under a separate director of research, as in the system applied in the Anglo-Egyptian Sudan. He then shows how such an organization might be set up, taking the three subjects of Agriculture, Veterinary Service and Forestry.

He emphasizes the value of financing research, especially that of the long-range type such as land survey work, from special funds raised by loan rather than from current revenue, which fluctuates so much with economic conditions.

He points out, under the "Waste of Research," that great quantities of material are published mainly in official documents, such as several department reports, bulletins, pamphlets, etc. Information in this form is not readily available to the scientific expert. He suggests adopting a common format for the separation of scientific fact from administrative detail, a standardization of form for statistical tables and some means of referring to the contents.

In recent years organizations for the promotion of scientific studies in the colonies have been formed in Paris, Brussels, Portugal and Rome as well as in South Africa and England, but in spite of all this, which is mostly recent, this continent, which has been developed almost wholly in the twentieth century, has been led by economic development.

The rest of the book is divided into 17 chapters dealing with the following subjects: Surveys and Maps, Geology, Meteorology, Soil Science, Botany, Forestry, Zoology, Fisheries, Entomology, Agriculture, Crop-plants, Plant Industry, Animal Industry, General Health and Medicine, Human Diseases, Health and Population, Anthropology.

There follows an alphabetical list of 192 authorities who have assisted by providing information or commenting on the drafts, also 73 governmental departments in British Africa which were helpful.

There is a 64-page bibliography, arranged alphabetically by chapters, an index and a physical map of Africa.

In various chapters of the book, the author refers to the important work being carried on by the Royal Botanic Gardens at Kew in botanical investigations, the Imperial Forestry Institute at Oxford in forestry, the forest organization of the Union of South Africa, the British Museum (South Kensington) in Zoology and Entomology, the Zoological Society with its largest collection of living African mammals, the Society for the Preservation of the Fauna of the Empire stressing conservation, the four National and Provincial Museums in South Africa in Zoology, the Bureau of Animal Population at Oxford in ecology, the Imperial Institute of Entomology in the identification of insects, the East African Agricultural Research Station at Amani—one of the projected control research stations in the Tropical Empire—the London and Liverpool Schools of Tropical Medicine, and the Bureau of Hygiene and Tropical Diseases that abstracts articles of interest to Empire workers.

In this book Mr. Worthington has most effectively set forth the interrelation between sciences in Africa, the part they can play in its further development and the importance of scientific knowledge in coping with such problems as erosion, locust plagues and sleeping sickness.

One is impressed by the enormous job there is to be done and what a good start has been made on several fronts.

If we grant that the author has attempted to cover too wide a field within the covers of a single volume, nevertheless the title is misleading. Applied science in British or South African controlled territories, south of but not including the Anglo-Egyptian Sudan, would more nearly apply to the areas and subjects treated in the book. In most sections French, Belgian and Portuguese territories have been sketchily dealt with if they are mentioned at all.

The author in his own preface states that a shortage of time has resulted in the omission of much interesting work and that there is consequently a lack of proportion in the treatment of some subjects. This is unfortunately true. For example, such sections as the ones dealing with soil science, applied entomology, crop-plants or the plant industry are competently dealt with, whereas his chapter on anthropology or his treatment of the preservation of flora and fauna seem by the same standard to be extremely inadequate.

It is extraordinary that in a survey of this kind significant scientific reports on African research by American and other foreign investigators should have been completely overlooked and not even find a place in the bibliography; for example, Dr. Richard P. Strong's two-volume report on "The African Republic of Liberia and the Belgian Congo," published in 1930, covering a wide range of scientific subjects reported on by competent investigators in the fields of medicine, botany, entomology and zoology, and Dr. Wilfred D. Hambly's two-volume "Source Book for African Anthropology," published in 1937 by the Field Museum of Chicago.

In "Science in Africa" mollusks and invertebrates outside of insects are hardly mentioned at all.

Mr. Worthington has succeeded in producing a readable book covering a wide range of interest written in a uniform style, and at the same time valuable for reference on account of its splendid double index, helpful maps and bibliography as well as the thoroughly sound recommendations which he makes in his opening (not concluding) chapter. It is most fortunate that such a competent zoologist was selected for this task and that he was a man of such wide vision with a sound critical judgment. Let us hope that many of his excellent recommendations may be favorably acted upon in the years to come.

HAROLD J. COOLIDGE, JR.
MUSEUM OF COMPARATIVE ZOOLOGY,
CAMBRIDGE, MASS.

## THE ADVANCE OF MEDICINE

*Thus We Are Men.* By SIR WALTER LANGDON-BROWN, emeritus professor of physic and fellow of Corpus Christi College in the University of Cambridge. xii + 344 pp. Kegan Paul, Trench, Trubner and Co., Ltd., London, 1939. 10s. 6d.

*The March of Medicine. Selected Addresses and Articles on Medical Topics, 1913–1937.* By RAY LYMAN WILBUR, president of Stanford University, California. x + 280 pp. 1938. $2.75.

*Milestones in Medicine: Laity Lectures of the New York Academy of Medicine.* Introduction by JAMES A. MILL, president of the New York Academy of Medicine. vii + 276 pp. D. Appleton-Century Company, New York, 1938. $2.00.

THESE three volumes have a certain similarity in that they illustrate the manner in which various and diverse individual essays may be integrated about a single theme. This is an increasingly popular way by which busy intellectual leaders may coordinate a series of brief efforts about a more general philosophy.

Sir Walter's volume is deliberately planned in this spirit. Its general theme is stated in the first essay, the 1936 Maudsley Lecture, "The Biology of Social Life," in which it is pointed out that the demands of human evolution for a functioning social unit combining full cooperation with individual freedom are currently causing great stress as we bumble along in trial and error toward a surviving fitness. Psychological factors impose the greatest obstacles in this evolutionary process. To proceed we should learn more about our minds and the way they work. As Sir Thomas Browne phrased it three centuries ago, "Thus we are men and we know not how." Sir Walter's next essay has the provocative title, "We Have Reason to Think." He deals with the perplexing phenomenon of the "retreat from reason" in literature and politics on the basis of individual failure to evolve smoothly from infancy to manhood.

About this theme Sir Walter now plays many variations. A set of six essays deal with psychological states as illustrated from literature and science. The fascinating character of these studies is indicated by the titles: "Myth, Phantasy, and Mary Rose," "Robert Bridges—the Poet of Evolution," "Sir William Osler," "The Psychology of Authorship," "Dr. Jekyll Diagnoses Mr. Hyde" and "The Background to Harvey." In the latter it is recalled that Sir Thomas Browne (1606–1682) first used the word "electricity" and that he was an experimental scientist of considerable merit, especially in chemical embryology.

Another set of six studies deals with applications of this social and psychological evolutionary idea to art and religion. The discussion on "The Evolution of Death" brings the volume to a notable climax. Sir Walter's great scientific and literary ability make these essays stimulating and delightful reading.

President Wilbur's volume includes twenty-nine addresses delivered at various important functions since 1913 and dealing generally with current non-technical problems of biology, medicine and public health. Many of the earlier ones contain much wisdom resulting from years of experience on methods of teaching in medicine. The later ones are more concerned with the economic consequences of medical advance, and with the social significance of public health. As chairman of the Committee on the Costs of Medical Care, Dr. Wilbur summarized his views on these matters in his address before the National Conference on the Costs of Medical Care, at the New York Academy of Medicine, November 29, 1932.

For several years the New York Academy of Medicine has sponsored a series of "Laity Lectures" in which distinguished leaders in various medical fields have summarized recent significant developments in lay terms, or have dealt historically with interesting or practically important lines of progress. In 1936 the lectures were collected in a volume entitled "Medicine and Mankind," and included surveys of anatomy and physiology, an account of the medicine of the Amerinds, constitutional make-up in relation to disease, vitamins and a Carrel mystification on death. The 1937 lectures have now been published under the title "Milestones in Medicine." These titles are not quite appropriate. The books might better be titled "Laity Lectures in Medicine," giving then the year so that the series might be kept distinct.

The current volume includes an historical survey of psychiatry by Smith Ely Jelliffe, a discussion of the mechanisms of heredity by Charles R. Stockard, a diverting discussion of medicine at sea in the days of sail by Karl Vogel, a description of the evolution of the human brain by Frederick Tilney, a stimulating and documented "history of medical history" by Henry E. Sigerist, a historic account of leprosy by Newton E. Wayson and a survey of current knowledge of the glands of internal secretion by Walter Timme. Non-medical scientists will find that these essays afford a pleasant way to follow the historical development of medical ideas. Judicious documentation might add to their value for this purpose without detracting from their readability.

CHAUNCEY D. LEAKE
MEDICAL SCHOOL, UNIVERSITY OF CALIFORNIA,
SAN FRANCISCO, CALIF.

# SOCIETIES AND MEETINGS

## THE SEISMOLOGICAL SOCIETY OF AMERICA—EASTERN SECTION

THE Eastern Section of the Seismological Society of America held its fourteenth annual meeting in Freeman Hall on the campus of Fordham University, New York City, June 9 and 10, 1939. The Reverend Joseph Lynch, S.J., well-known seismologist and head of the department of physics, welcomed the guests and members of the section.

The sessions were officially opened on Friday morning at 9:15 by the chairman, H. E. McComb, of the U. S. Coast and Geodetic Survey. To allow time for more informal discussion and a tour of some of the scientific exhibits of the World's Fair, a departure was made from the usual procedure. Two days are customarily devoted to the presentation of committee reports, election of officers and the reading of papers. This year the seismologists continued in session until 7:15 in the evening, completing the scheduled program and stopping only long enough at 1:30 to enjoy a buffet luncheon as guests of the university. Because of the warm weather the lunch was served in one of the basement laboratories, where suction flasks and pyrex beakers provided the necessary "scientific" atmosphere.

Reassembled again at 2:30 P.M., the delegates resumed with presentation of papers and reports. Animated discussion attended the reading of the report of the committees on microseisms and amateur seismology and the paper of A. C. Chick, Providence, R. I., on "Trends in Earthquake Insurance since 1933." Other papers of special interest should be mentioned: "The Nature and Origin of Microseisms," by J. Emilio Ramirez, S.J., of Bogotá, Colombia; "The Problem of Earth Deformation," by M. King Hubbert, Columbia University, and a report by A. G. Ingalls, of the editorial staff of the *Scientific American*, on "Amateur Seismology." The formal meeting was terminated by the reports of the resolutions and nominating committees and the election of officers for the ensuing year. The unanimous choice was as follows: *Chairman*, A. C. Ruge, of the Department of Civil Engineering, Massachusetts Institute of Technology; *Vice-Chairman*, A. J. Westland, S.J., Department of Physics, Spring Hill College; *Secretary*, W. A. Lynch, Department of Physics, Fordham University; *Treasurer*, H. Landsberg, Geophysical Laboratory, Pennsylvania State College; *Fifth Member of the Executive Committee*, H. E. McComb, of the U. S. Coast and Geodetic Survey.

At 10 o'clock Saturday, June 10, practically the entire group assembled again for a three-hour informal discussion of current seismological problems. Topics of timely import were, a new speed control for seismograph drums, demonstrated by A. C. Ruge; the necessity of putting all our seismographs to work; the new instruments and equipment at cooperative stations of the U. S. Coast and Geodetic Survey; the need for more sensitive instruments in the Gulf Coast States.

A. J. WESTLAND, S.J.

SPRING HILL COLLEGE,
SPRING HILL, ALA.

# SPECIAL ARTICLES

## STUDIES IN THE PHYSICAL CHEMISTRY OF INSULIN[1]

### I. THE SOLUBILITY AND DIELECTRIC PROPERTIES OF INSULIN AND ITS CRYSTALLIZATION WITH RADIOACTIVE ZINC

INSULIN, which can be crystallized in a state of high purity, and possesses unusual chemical stability, as well as specific physiological properties, is a very suitable protein for quantitative physical chemical studies. This paper gives preliminary results of a series of investigations in progress in these laboratories upon the physical chemical properties of insulin and its interaction with ions and dipolar ions.

Crystalline zinc insulin[2] was dissolved in sufficient N/10 hydrochloric acid to bring the final pH to 2.5, electrodialyzed against N/300 hydrochloric acid in a Brintzinger type electrodialyzer for four hours, and then freed from acid by continuing the electrodialysis against distilled water for twenty hours. The protein precipitated in amorphous form; the supernatant solution had a conductivity of about $3 \times 10^{-6}$ ohm$^{-1}$ cm$^{-1}$ and was chloride-free. The insulin was washed with conductivity water.

Measurements of solubility in water and glycine solutions were carried out at 5° by rotating portions of amorphous insulin prepared in the above manner with successive aliquots of solvent. After each equilibration, lasting from two to eight days, the suspension was allowed to settle, and the supernatant solution filtered through sintered glass. Analysis was performed by precipitating the insulin with trichloracetic acid, washing free of solvent with dilute trichloracetic acid solution, digesting the protein and determining the nitrogen colorimetrically with Nessler's reagent.

[1] From the Department of Physical Chemistry, Harvard Medical School, and the Jefferson Physical Laboratory, Harvard University.

[2] Furnished through the kindness of Eli Lilly and Company.

The solubility in water of insulin thus prepared never exceeded 0.027 grams per liter, but diminished to approximately a third of this value upon repeated equilibration with water. Although denaturation of the insulin with prolonged washing is not precluded, pharmacological activity[3] had not diminished in a sample which had been washed fifteen days, the solubility of which had decreased to 0.014 grams per liter. The average solubilities, when a constant level had been reached, are designated by the hollow circles in Fig. 1, initial solubilities by circles with crosses.

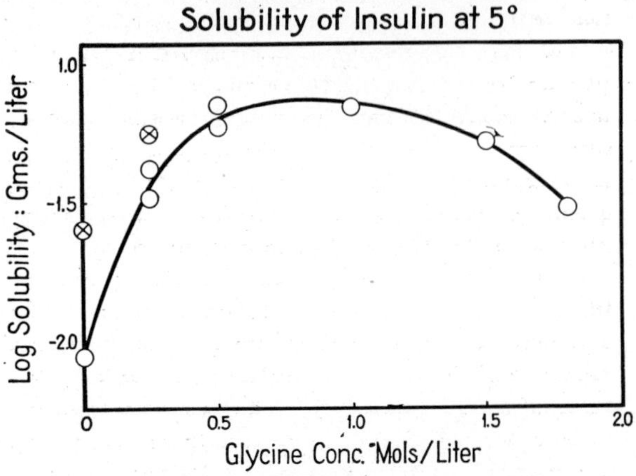


FIG. 1

Solubility of insulin in solutions containing 0.5 M glycine or more did not diminish upon re-equilibration with solvent, but remained constant for as many as nine equilibrations over a period of thirty days. These solutions saturated with insulin always had a pH close to 6.1, characteristic of pure glycine, rather than of the isoelectric point of the insulin. The average solubility was 0.065 grams per liter in 0.5 M glycine, 0.069 grams per liter in 1.0 M, 0.052 grams per liter in 1.5 M and 0.030 grams per liter in 1.8 M glycine. The occurrence of maximum solubility at a glycine concentration not greater than 1.0 M indicates a large "salting-out" effect. Indeed, the solubility in 1.8 M glycine is smaller than in 0.5 M glycine, whereas for hemoglobin[4] the "salting-out" effect reduces solubility at this concentration only to approximately that in 1.0 M glycine. The observed solvent action of glycine upon insulin, if corrected for the "salting-out" effect by an equation comparable to that previously employed for hemoglobin ([5], equation 5), would suggest interaction between these two dipolar ions somewhat greater than observed for hemoglobin. Lactoglobin has thus far been studied[6] only at glycine concentrations lower than half molal, where no "salting-out" effect could be detected and the observed interaction was far greater than with insulin or hemoglobin.

The rôle of the dipole moments in the interactions of dipolar ions has previously been stressed.[5] Taking the dipole moment of glycine as 15, that of hemoglobin[7] has been estimated as 500 and of lactoglobulin[6] as 700, on the basis of measurements of dielectric constant increments of 0.33 and 1.4, respectively, per gram per liter.

The concentration of insulin prepared as above, even in 1.0 M glycine, is too low to contribute appreciably to the dielectric constant of the solution. Accordingly electrolyte-free solutions of insulin in quantities sufficient to study its dielectric properties were prepared in other solvents. Solutions of 1.9 grams per liter in propylene glycol, 3.2 grams per liter in propylene glycol containing 10.2 per cent. and 3.6 grams per liter in propylene glycol containing 20 per cent. of water were studied. The total dielectric increments from high to low frequencies, $\Delta\varepsilon_t$, were 0.26, 0.29 and 0.38 per gram per liter, respectively, in these three solvents. The dispersion curves are given in Fig. 2, where the relative increase in dielectric constant is plotted against the logarithm of the frequency. The mean relaxation times in the three solvents, when divided by the viscosities relative to water, agreed within 10 per cent., the average value being $1.7 \times 10^{-8}$ seconds.

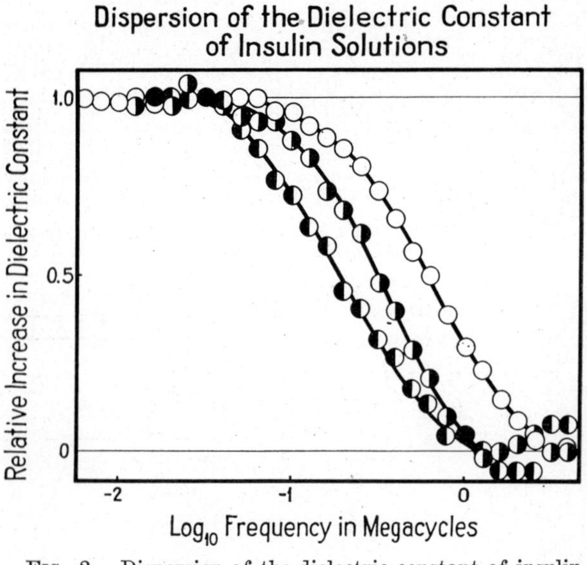


FIG. 2. Dispersion of the dielectric constant of insulin at 25° C. in ◐ propylene glycol (viscosity relative to water, $\eta_r = 47.5$), ◑ propylene glycol with 10.2% water ($\eta_r = 28$), ○ propylene glycol with 20% water ($\eta_r = 17$).

The viscosities and dielectric constants of these solu-

[3] As judged by mouse test, for which we are indebted to Dr. W. T. Salter, of the Department of Medicine, Harvard University.

[4] M. M. Richards, *Jour. Biol. Chem.*, 122: 727, 1938.

[5] Cohn, McMeekin, Ferry and Blanchard, *Jour. Phys. Chem.*, 43: 1, 1939.

[6] Ferry, Cohn, Oncley and Blanchard, *Jour. Biol. Chem.*, Proceedings (1939).

[7] J. L. Oncley, *Jour. Amer. Chem. Soc.*, 60: 1115, 1938.

tions differ so greatly from those of water that insulin is also being studied in other solvents, such as aqueous solutions of serum proteins in which it is appreciably soluble. The far lower solubility of insulin in water than in propylene glycol, a type of behavior characteristic also of zein, indicates that insulin may be considered a crystalline animal prolamine.

After repeatedly electrodialyzing crystalline zinc insulin in the preparation of the amorphous material used in the above experiments, it occurred to us to recrystallize the amorphous insulin with radioactive zinc. For this purpose a sample of zinc containing the radioactive $Zn^{65}$ isotope, of half-life 250 days, was employed.[8] The electrodialyzed insulin was crystallized with radioactive zinc from acetate buffers, and amorphous commercial insulin was crystallized from phosphate and recrystallized from acetate buffers, following the method of Scott.[9] The radioactivity of the dried crystals was determined with a Lauritsen type quartz fiber electroscope. The radiation was filtered through 2.35 mm of aluminum in order to record only the gamma rays, which are much less affected than beta particles by self-absorption in samples of varying bulk. Comparison was made in each case with a standard sample of zinc sulfide or zinc ammonium phosphate prepared from the same sample of zinc. Under the conditions of electrodialysis given above, no more than 0.31 per cent. radioactive zinc was detected in our final products of crystalline insulin. Scott reports that crystalline zinc insulin contains 0.52 per cent. zinc. In order to determine whether our lower content of radioactive zinc depended upon incomplete removal of zinc by electrodialysis under the conditions employed, a commercial amorphous preparation[10] believed to contain not more than 0.03 per cent. Zn was crystallized with radioactive zinc. These crystals were estimated to contain 0.36 per cent. radioactive zinc.

Further experiments with radioactive zinc will be undertaken in order to determine the maximum content of radioactive zinc that can be introduced into crystalline insulin, and the conditions under which the zinc can be removed from insulin by dialysis or electrodialysis in acid or neutral solutions, or by interchange with blood and tissue proteins. Our experiments thus far indicate that none of the radioactive zinc introduced into insulin is removed at neutral reactions by electrodialysis or prolonged dialysis, but that at the isoelectric point of insulin the radioactive zinc is quantitatively lost to normal horse serum. When, however, insulin containing two atoms of radioactive zinc per mole was separated from serum at neutral reaction, by precipitation with the protamine, salmin,[2] the resulting precipitate retained 0.14 per cent. radioactive zinc, corresponding approximately to a mono-radioactive zinc insulin protaminate.

EDWIN J. COHN
JOHN D. FERRY[11]
J. J. LIVINGOOD
MURIEL H. BLANCHARD

[8] Livingood and Seaborg, *Phys. Rev.*, 55: 457, 1939.

[9] Scott, *Biochem. Jour.*, 28: 1592, 1934; Scott and Fisher, *Biochem. Jour.*, 29: 1048, 1935.

[10] We are indebted to Dr. George B. Walden, of Eli Lilly and Company, for this material.

[11] Society of Fellows, Harvard University.

## TYPE-SPECIFIC ANTIBODY PRODUCTION WITH LIVING PNEUMOCOCCI IN THE RABBIT

IT is generally held that only virulent strains are satisfactory as antigens for preparing antipneumococcus sera and that it is at least doubtful that immunization with living pneumococci is of value.[1] Griffith[2] writes that "living attenuated culture is useless for preparation of protective serum, and, as is known, this is due to the absence of type-specific antigen in such strains. This essential complex is liable to disintegration in living cultures, both prior to and subsequent to inoculation, with the result that non-type-specific antibodies are produced in the serum."

It was found recently[3] that a strain of attenuated tubercle bacilli, *Bacillus* Calmette-Guerin, induces antibody formation against virulent bovine tubercle bacilli more readily than heat-killed suspension of virulent micro-organisms. This observation stimulated us to determine whether living attenuated pneumococci are more effective immunizing agents than killed suspensions of virulent strains. Pneumococci of low virulence agglutinable by the type-specific antibody can be procured by repeated subcultures on blood bouillon and omission of the customary passage through mice. The first series of experiments were carried out with a Type III strain because sera against this type are of low potency and mouse-virulent strains are of relatively low virulence for rabbits. The lethal dose of the strain used is more than 20 cc for adult rabbits.

The centrifugalized sediment of five hours pepton bouillon cultures was suspended in 1 cc of bouillon per dose of "vaccine" and inoculated intravenously into rabbits weighing from two to three and one-half kilograms. Most of the rabbits received the sediment of 5 cc of culture on three successive days of the week for four weeks; later the doses were increased to 5, 5 and 10 cc. Agglutinin and precipitin titers of the sera of rabbits so immunized are considerably higher than those of animals immunized with killed suspension of cultures passed through mice frequently. Type-specific antibody nitrogen determination made by Dr. Kenneth

[1] B. White, E. S. Robinson and L. A. Barnes, "The Biology of Pneumococcus," The Commonwealth Fund, New York, 1938; H. Zinsser, J. F. Enders and L. D. Fothergill, "Immunity Principles and Application in Medicine and Public Health," The Macmillan Company, New York, 1939.

[2] F. Griffith, "A System of Bacteriology," Vol. II, His Majesty's Stationery Office, London, 1929.

[3] J. Freund, J. Casals and E. P. Hosmer, *Proc. Soc. Sxp. Biol. and Med.*, 37: 509, 1937; J. Freund and E. L. Opie, *Jour. Exp. Med.*, 68: 273, 1938.

Goodner of the Rockefeller Institute have shown in a small group of rabbits that the majority of the sera contained from one to two mg antibody nitrogen per cc, and one exceptional serum contained approximately 6.4 mg.

Similar experiments are being carried out with pneumococci of Type I. The results indicate that the method described above is applicable to production of Type I antipneumococcic serum.

JULES FREUND
MARTHA A. BEHAN

DEPARTMENT OF HEALTH
OF THE CITY OF NEW YORK
BUREAU OF LABORATORIES,
ANTITOXIN LABORATORY,
OTISVILLE, N. Y.

## THE SIGNIFICANCE OF THE AMINO ACIDS IN CANINE NUTRITION[1]

IN previous publications from this laboratory[2,3] it has been shown that only ten of the twenty-two amino acids known to exist in proteins are *indispensable* dietary components. These are tryptophane, lysine, histidine, phenylalanine, leucine, isoleucine, threonine, methionine, valine and arginine. With the exception of arginine, the removal of any one of these compounds from the food leads to a profound nutritive failure, accompanied by a rapid decline in weight, loss of appetite and eventual death. On the other hand, the exclusion of arginine from the ration is followed by much less pronounced effects. The subjects continue to gain, but at a suboptimal rate. This is accounted for by the fact that arginine, in contrast to the other members of the indispensable group, can be manufactured by the cells,[4] but at a speed which does not quite keep pace with the demands of *normal* growth. The twelve remaining amino acids are dispensable in the sense that they can be synthesized in adequate amounts out of materials ordinarily available in the organism.

In arriving at the above conclusions young rats served as the experimental animals. Consequently, it does not follow necessarily that the findings are applicable to other species. Indeed, a *quantitative* difference in the arginine requirement has already been recorded in the literature. The growth of chicks is said to be accelerated by the addition of this amino acid to the ration, even when the latter contains 18 per cent. of casein[5] (equivalent to a dietary arginine content of approximately 0.68 per cent.). This amount of casein furnishes more than three times the quantity of arginine necessary for the growing rat.[2] It becomes of importance, therefore, to ascertain whether the rat is singularly proficient in the synthesis of amino acids, or whether other mammals also manifest the ability to thrive on relatively simple mixtures.

The nutritive rôle of the individual amino acids has now been established for the adult dog. This was undertaken as a preliminary to extensive investigations on the maintenance of nitrogen equilibrium in various species by oral and intravenous alimentation. The program has advanced sufficiently to warrant a brief report at this time. The experimental findings and the details of the technique will be presented elsewhere.

Adult females were used throughout. As a rule, they were first brought into nitrogen equilibrium upon a casein diet, and were then transferred to a similar ration in which mixtures of highly purified amino acids served as the sole sources of nitrogen, except for traces introduced unavoidably as contaminants of the vitamin B concentrates. The urine samples were collected by catheterization at intervals of twenty-four hours, and the feces were divided into periods of seven days by the administration of carmine capsules.

The first dog received a ration containing the ten amino acids found previously to be indispensable for the growing rat. She promptly manifested a slight positive nitrogen balance, and continued to do so, with a moderate gain in weight, for the duration of the test (4 weeks). Obviously, *the amino acids which are dispensable for the growing rat are also dispensable for the adult dog.* At the beginning of the fifth week, arginine was dropped from the diet. The change was without influence upon either the body weight or the nitrogen balance of the subject. Thus, *for the adult dog arginine is not a necessary dietary component.* This finding was not unexpected. Nearly two years ago we[3] predicted that arginine would prove to be dispensable for full-grown animals. The experiment was discontinued at the end of the eighth week, at which time the dog was in perfect nutritive condition.

Three dogs were employed in determining the physiological importance of the other amino acids of the indispensable group. Invariably, the removal from the food of any one of these compounds was followed by a pronounced negative nitrogen balance. Furthermore, the restoration of the missing amino acid to the diet uniformly resulted in a positive nitrogen balance. These data demonstrate that *the qualitative amino acid needs of the dog are identical with those of the rat.* The fact that two widely different species require for their well-being the same components of the protein molecule, increases the probability that other mammals, including man, may manifest like responses.

In the experiments herein described the amino acid

1 The researches upon which this report is based were supported in large measure by a grant from the Rockefeller Foundation.

2 W. C. Rose, SCIENCE, 86: 298, 1937.

3 W. C. Rose, *Physiol. Rev.*, 18: 109, 1938.

4 C. W. Scull and W. C. Rose, *Jour. Biol. Chem.*, 89: 109, 1930.

5 A. Arnold, O. L. Kline, C. A. Elvehjem and E. B. Hart, *Jour. Biol. Chem.*, 116: 699, 1936; A. A. Klose, E. L. R. Stokstad and H. J. Almquist, *Jour. Biol. Chem.*, 123: 691, 1938.

intakes, though low, were not reduced to the minima. Repeatedly we[2, 6, 7] have pointed out that mixtures of purified amino acids, compounded in accordance with the quantitative needs of the cells for each component, may prove to be the most efficient type of nitrogen ever devised for the uses of the animal organism. For some time investigations have been in progress[7] to establish the lowest intakes of such preparations which are capable of maintaining nitrogen equilibrium in the rat and in the dog. The results will be reported later. Inasmuch as the successful use of synthetic mixtures of amino acids in nutrition studies was made possible by the discovery of threonine in this laboratory, it seems not inappropriate to expect that a reasonable period of time will be allowed for the consummation of the program outlined above before similar studies are undertaken by others.

Wm. C. Rose
Eldon E. Rice

University of Illinois, Urbana

# SCIENTIFIC APPARATUS AND LABORATORY METHODS

## DEEP-SEA PHOTOGRAPHY

Interest in deep-sea animals had led me to assemble an automatic camera mechanism in a pressure chamber[1] capable of withstanding two miles of depth in the sea, two tons per square inch, with a considerable safety factor. In this self-contained device, two six-volt storage batteries supply the current to run the motor (12 volts) for a 16 mm moving picture camera, a 50 candle power headlight with reflector (8 volts), and a timing motor (4 volts). The light shines through one "herculite" glass window, while the camera takes pictures through another. A pressure gage with electric contacts, which can be set for any depth, activates the mechanism by means of a lock relay. This starts the timing motor whose contacts turn on the movie camera and light (each through a separate relay) for 1.2 second and then turn them off for 11.1 seconds, when the process is repeated. The camera is set to take 16 pictures a second, and the films when developed show 20 light frames between 3 dark ones, since the filament takes some time to reach incandescence and the motor some time to stop. In 100 feet of film, there are about 170 chances of photographing something. Since the pictures are taken in the zone of perpetual darkness, a lure is hung 4 feet in front of the pressure chamber and the camera with stop f 1.5 focused on it. This lure is a wooden fish resembling a deep-sea fish, with rows of photophores painted on it with self-luminous zinc sulfide paint.

In June, through the kindness of Dr. J. F. G. Wheeler, of the Bermuda Biological Station for Research, I had the opportunity of testing the camera, which was let down from the ketch, *Culver*, permanently stationed in Bermuda for oceanographic work under the auspices of the Royal Society of London. Five descents were successfully accomplished in the region 5 to 10 miles southeast of Bermuda, where Beebe[2] has made over 1,500 hauls with nets and many descents with the bathysphere. Three 100-ft rolls of super XX panchromatic film were taken at 500 fathoms, one at 800 fathoms, and one at 1,320 fathoms ($1\frac{1}{2}$ miles). In the latter, the chamber touched bottom (although the chart indicated plenty of depth), knocking off a support and turning the camera out of position so that nothing appeared on this film. The other four films showed the lure clearly but no fish or large organisms. However, 17 small creatures, the largest about one centimeter in diameter, too small to be identified, moved across the beam of light in the 300 feet of film taken at 500 fathoms, the depth where Beebe obtained most material in his hauls with the nets. The film at 700 fathoms only showed two small creatures.

Since the lens angle of the camera subtended a rectangle $8 \times 11$ inches at 2.5 feet and $20.5 \times 26$ inches at 6 feet, the depth of focus for f 1.5 stop, we can think of the camera as sampling a frustum of about 7 cubic feet or one fifth of a cubic meter. Because of the drift of the boat, 510 samples were made in the three films exposed at 500 fathoms and 17 organisms photographed. This is one medium-sized organism per 30 samples or 210 cubic feet (6 cubic meters) of sea.

While no striking photos were obtained of deep-sea fish attacking the lure or one another, the experiments show that deep-sea photography is quite feasible and might be developed into a method of estimating the density of organisms at different depths.

E. Newton Harvey

Princeton University

## A GLASS ELECTRODE VESSEL FOR THE DETERMINATION OF BLOOD pH

The Beckman pH meter may be employed effectively in estimating the pH of whole blood under anaerobic conditions through the use of a special glass electrode assembly. The determination can be made directly on

6 W. C. Rose, *The Harvey Lectures*, 30: 49, 1934–35.

7 W. C. Rose, *Proc. Inst. Med. of Chicago*, 12: 98, 1938.

1 It gives me great pleasure to acknowledge the advice of Dean Greene and Dr. Moody, of the Engineering Department of Princeton University, in the design of the pressure chamber, which was a most acceptable gift of Mr. Owsley Brown, president of the Springfield Boiler Company, manufacturers of the chamber. To Mr. Charles Butt, research assistant in physiology, I am grateful for skilful arrangement of the wiring mechanism.

2 Wm. Beebe, "Half Mile Down," Harcourt, Brace and Company, New York, 1934.

the blood within 40 to 50 seconds after collection. In a series of determinations made upon dogs, we have obtained consistent and readily reproducible results.

A small glass vessel, illustrated in the figure, was made, having two side arms. This vessel may be attached to the standard Beckman glass electrode by winding firmly with thin rubber dam and fastening with rubber cement. After a little practice an air-tight connection can readily be made. If the Beckman electrode with the ground glass collar is available, the

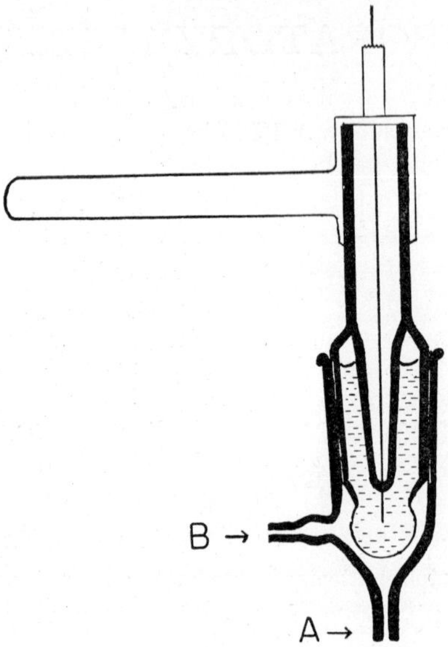


FIG. 1

vessel may be ground to fit this collar. The ground glass connection permits of more rapid adjustment and is more convenient for washing, but we have found the rubber connection to be perfectly satisfactory. The side arm, A, is attached by the shortest possible length of rubber tubing to a syringe adapter. If desired, this side arm may be made of a syringe tip, sealed into the cup, thus making a direct connection for the needle.[1] A ten-inch length of 3 mm rubber tubing attached to a mouthpiece is fastened to side arm, B, to be used in filling the vessel. The total capacity of such a chamber is 0.3–0.4 cc.

The procedure for performing a blood pH determination is as follows: Saturated KCl solution is warmed to 40° C. and placed in a small wide-mouthed vessel of about 50 cc capacity. This is supported so that the calomel half-cell dips into it and a thermometer is immersed in the solution, which serves as a bath and a salt bridge. Sufficient 1 per cent. neutral oxalate (pH 7.0) at 38° C. is drawn through A into the electrode vessel and a small clamp placed on the rubber tubing near the mouthpiece. A venipuncture is made with a hypodermic needle and when a constant flow of blood is obtained, the chamber is attached to the needle and the blood drawn into the vessel by opening the clamp and exerting suction on the mouthpiece. From 0.5–0.7 cc of blood is drawn into the vessel and tubing to insure complete replacement of the oxalate. It is essential that the chamber remain free from air bubbles. The electrode is disengaged from the needle, plunged immediately into the bath and the connection made rapidly. The temperature of the bath will usually have fallen to 38° C. and can be checked with the thermometer and adjusted, if necessary, by adding warmer or colder KCl solution. A steady E. M. F. is obtainable within 30 to 40 seconds after the electrode is attached to the pH meter.

As soon as the reading is obtained the electrode is removed and the vessel washed free of blood by drawing in warm distilled water. It is then rinsed and refilled with oxalate in preparation for the duplicate determination. During the interval necessary for the pH reading and the washing of the vessel a syringe may be attached to the needle and a blood sample taken for analysis. This total procedure can be done in from 2 to 4 minutes. When stasis is avoided, duplicate determinations check within the error of the instrument (± 0.01 pH). If this agreement is not obtained, a third determination should be done. Before each determination, we find it advisable to calibrate the electrode with standard buffers in the pH range of blood at 38° C., using the procedure as outlined for blood.

VIVIAN G. BEHRMANN
MARION FAY
WOMAN'S MEDICAL COLLEGE OF PENNSYLVANIA

[1] Both types of vessel were made for us by Mr. J. D. Graham, at the University of Pennsylvania.

## BOOKS RECEIVED

BRODE, WALLACE R. *Chemical Spectroscopy.* Pp xi + 494. Illustrated. Wiley. $5.00; professional edition, $6.00.

CAMPBELL, NEIL. *Qualitative Organic Chemistry.* Pp. ix + 213. 13 figures. Van Nostrand. $2.60.

*Contributions from the Biological Laboratory of the Science Society of China; Vol. X, Botanical Series, No. 3, April, 1938.* Pp. 207–308. 7 figures. The Society, Nanking.

DA ROCHA-LIMA, HENRIQUE, JOSÉ REIS, KARL SILBERSCHMIDT. *Methoden der Virusforschung.* Pp. viii + 384. 54 figures. Urban and Schwarzenberg, Berlin.

MOY-THOMAS, J. A. *Palaeozoic Fishes.* Pp. ix + 149 + 8. 33 figures. Chemical Publishing Co. $2.00.

OPPENHEIMER, CARL and KURT G. STERN. *Biological Oxidation.* Pp. ix + 317. 16 figures. W. Junk, The Hague. 15 fl.

VICKERY, HUBERT B., GEORGE W. PUCHER, ALFRED J. WAKEMAN and CHARLES S. LEAVENWORTH. *Chemical Investigation of the Rhubarb Plant; Bulletin 424, May, 1939.* Pp. 157. 38 figures. Connecticut Agricultural Experiment Station, New Haven.

WILSON, A. H. *Semi-conductors and Metals.* Pp. viii + 120. 39 figures. Cambridge University Press, Macmillan. $2.00.

# SCIENCE

VOL. 90 FRIDAY, SEPTEMBER 1, 1939 No. 2331

*The British Association for the Advancement of Science:*
*The Western Isles through the Mists of Ages:* SIR ALBERT SEWARD ... 189

*Scientific Events:*
*The Forests of Great Britain; The Australian Meteorite in the Collection of the Smithsonian Institution; The Proposed Inter-American University in Puerto Rico; The New York Meeting of the Electrochemical Society; Lectures at the Dundee Meeting of the British Association. Recent Deaths and Memorials* ... 200

*Scientific Notes and News* ... 203

*Discussion:*
*Conditions and Opportunities at the Naples Zoological Station:* DR. R. E. COKER. *One-Man Authority Citations:* DR. CORNELIUS H. MULLER. *Spraying with Plant Growth Substances to Prevent Apple Fruit Dropping:* DR. F. E. GARDNER, P. C. MARTH and DR. L. P. BATJER. *"Distinction" in "Science":* DR. C. STUART GAGER ... 206

*Special Correspondence:*
*Research in Venezuela:* DR. GEORGE GAYLORD SIMPSON ... 210

*Scientific Books:*
*Malaria in Panama:* PROFESSOR W. H. TALIAFERRO 211

*Societies and Meetings:*
*The North Carolina Academy of Science:* PROFESSOR H. L. BLOMQUIST ... 212

*Special Articles:*
*Chemical Composition of the Tumor-producing Fraction of Chicken Tumor I:* DR. ALBERT CLAUDE. *Vitamin K Activity of Synthetic Phthiocol:* DR. ERHARD FERNHOLZ and DR. S. ANSBACHER. *Human Vaccination against Equine Encephalomyelitis Virus with Formolized Chick Embryo Vaccine:* DR. J. W. BEARD, DOROTHY BEARD and HAROLD FINKELSTEIN ... 213

*Science News* ... 10

SCIENCE: A Weekly Journal devoted to the Advancement of Science, edited by J. MCKEEN CATTELL and published every Friday by

THE SCIENCE PRESS
New York City: Grand Central Terminal
Lancaster, Pa. Garrison, N. Y.
Annual Subscription, $6.00 Single Copies, 15 Cts.

SCIENCE is the official organ of the American Association for the Advancement of Science. Information regarding membership in the Association may be secured from the office of the permanent secretary in the Smithsonian Institution Building, Washington, D. C.

# THE WESTERN ISLES THROUGH THE MISTS OF AGES[1]

By Sir ALBERT SEWARD
PROFESSOR OF BOTANY EMERITUS OF THE UNIVERSITY OF CAMBRIDGE

## INTRODUCTORY

TWENTY-SEVEN years ago, when the British Association met for the second time in Dundee, Sir Edward Schäfer chose as the subject of his presidential address "The Nature, Origin and Maintenance of Life"; he discussed problems that will long continue to exercise the ingenuity and stimulate the imagination of biologists and chemists. A theme such as his is far beyond my reach. Seventy-two years ago the association met for the first time in this city. The Duke of Buccleuch occupied the presidential chair, and the opening words of his address are applicable to one who now finds himself in this privileged position; the Duke said: "No man has a title to state that he is unworthy of the post he is called on to fill, whatever may be his private feelings as to his fitness for the post. To state that he is unworthy to be there placed is not only a disparagement to himself, but is no great compliment to those who thought him worthy of being so placed."

This, in my opinion, is not an occasion on which it is desirable to follow the easier course and address oneself in technical language to fellow workers in the pursuit of natural knowledge. The position which it is my great privilege to occupy affords a rare opportunity of talking to a large and, I venture to hope, a sympathetic audience, including some at least who are repelled by the jargon of specialists. My intention is to speak in ordinary language on a subject of which I know enough to realize how little that knowledge is, and briefly to describe an example of the way in which, within one small patch of an illimitable field, a student asks questions of nature and does his best to interpret the answers.

[1] Address of the president of the British Association for the Advancement of Science, Dundee meeting, August 30, 1939.

### AN EXCURSION INTO THE PAST

I invite my audience to accompany me on an excursion of a kind which has substantially contributed to the enjoyment and enrichment of my own life, an excursion into a world that knew not man, with the object of deciphering from such records as we find in the rocks a few pages of the story-book of the earth. Each one of us can say with Shakespeare's soothsayer:

In Nature's infinite book of secrecy
A little I can read.

As that great Scotsman, Hugh Miller, wrote nearly a century ago: "We find the present incomplete without the past—the recent without the extinct." To reinforce his own opinion he quoted Samuel Johnson: "Whatever makes the past, the distant, or the future predominate over the present, advances us in the dignity of thinking beings." We shall try to reconstruct a small part of an ancient land, a remnant of which is now called Scotland, and envisage a scene at a stage in the history of the earth separated from the present by at least sixty million years, a stretch of time difficult for us who have been called "the afterthoughts of creation" fully to appreciate. When we substitute geological standards for the modest time-scale of the human period and remember that the earliest chapters of the world's history are recorded in rocks at least two thousand million years old, sixty million years dwindle to comparative insignificance. All that it is possible to do is to lift a corner of the veil separating us from the world as it was and view through dimly illuminated vistas the forests and undergrowth on an ancient continent that is now represented by a few widely scattered, dismembered pieces.

### THE HISTORY OF PLANT LIFE

The history of plant life in the sea and on land is a branch of natural knowledge not unworthy of consideration by us human beings who owe our existence to the vegetable kingdom. Green plants in one vital sense are our superiors: from air and water they build up the complex organic substances necessary to our life, a feat beyond man's power. As members of a subject race we should be interested in endeavoring to unravel the history of the plant kingdom—in trying to trace the origin and relations of the several classes and groups as defined by botanists. The documents that are the sources of the botanical historian are contained in the earth's crust: as a preliminary it is worth while to ask ourselves of what these documents consist; how they came to be preserved in the rocks. In order to bring to life the past we must take the present for our guide. "Speak to the earth, and it shall teach thee." There is no reason to think of nature's methods as other than continuous. If we stand by the bank of a river flowing past tree-covered slopes we see on the sand and mud by the edge of the channel or floating on the stream leaves, twigs and seeds that are random samples of vegetation scattered by wind or shed from overhanging boughs, debris swept along with offscourings from the rocks to be carried eventually to a delta or an estuary where the water-borne material comes to rest. Beds of old sands and mud, with included fragments of contemporary trees and other plants, exposed on the faces of cliffs and ravines, are layers of sediment that have been raised to a higher level. In addition to leaves, twigs and other scraps easy to see on the split surface of sandstone or shale, sediments of former ages, especially such as are peaty, occasionally furnish another valuable source of information invisible to the unaided eye. Minute grains of pollen may be carried by wind to places where conditions are favorable for their preservation: fortunately the grains or at least most of them, are protected by highly resistant coats and retain almost for all time their characteristic form and surface sculpturing. With hardly any exception it is possible for a specialist, by comparative microscopical examination of fresh material, to assign fossil pollen-grains to their generic and occasionally their specific position in the plant kingdom.

There is another natural agency to which students of extinct plants are not infrequently indebted: the formation of rocks by volcanic action. From time to time volcanoes that have long been dormant eject clouds of ash; these with streams of lava poured over the rim of a crater spread havoc among trees and shrubs that had colonized precarious sites during a peaceful interlude. Vulcanicity is not only destructive: paradoxical as it may seem, forces inimical to life have contributed to the reconstruction of life which they destroyed. Scotland is exceptionally rich in botanical treasures that are legacies from ages of fire, and indeed the fossil plants with which we are concerned this evening owe their preservation to volcanic forces.

The following botanical retrospect is based mainly on results obtained during the last two or three years, but not yet published, by the joint efforts of Mr. W. N. Edwards, keeper of geology in the British Museum; Dr. J. B. Simpson, of the Geological Survey, and myself.

### RECONSTRUCTION OF A FOREST SCENE

#### A. *The geological background*

(1) *Prolonged and intermittent volcanic activity.* In order to present in true perspective the scene which it is my aim to bring to life, it will be helpful to visualize the physical features of northwestern Europe some thousands of years antecedent to the phase of geological history chosen for closer examination. The chalk downs of England and part of the cliffs on the Antrim coast of Ireland are made of upraised calcareous material that was once a soft white ooze on the

floor of a clear sea, a sea which had swept slowly and irresistibly over an enormous stretch of land, embracing the greater part of England, northern Ireland and part of the region that is now western Scotland. With the uplifting of the chalky ooze from the ocean bed and the gradual recession of the waters a new land was born; a new chapter was inaugurated in the history of the earth. Following the great upheaval, as a consequential phenomenon, subterranean forces that had long been quiescent gained the upper hand: floods of semi-molten rock from deeply hidden reservoirs surged as a fiery deluge over the chalk downs, and over other and older rocks, converting thousands of square miles into barren lava-fields, extending over an area, not less than 2,000 miles from south to north, which reached far beyond the Arctic Circle. This unprecedented manifestation of volcanic energy, by no means confined to Europe and the arctic regions, but recorded on an equally titanic scale in the peninsula of India and elsewhere, is one of the wonders of geology; it is convincing evidence that the earth after the lapse of many hundred million years had not lost her youth; there was no sign of senescence. During the period we are considering most of Britain was land: we know that at a slightly later date a broad sea lay over the whole of what is now southern England. Travelers in the tube-railway in the London district may perhaps derive pleasure from the knowledge that they are being conveyed through a stiff clay upraised from the floor of that ancient sea. As an appropriate designation for the great northern land an American geologist suggested the name Thulean continent or province (see accompanying map). In the early days of the period called by geologists the Tertiary era, the greater part of the Thulean province was covered with sheets of sombre-colored lava in nearly horizontal layers, products of a series of outbursts from deep fissures rent in the earth's crust under the compelling strain of subterranean forces and from localized volcanic centers of eruption. The columnar basalts of the Giant's Causeway, the columns of the "cathedral of the sea" at Fingal's Cave, the basalts of Mull, Skye, Canna, Eigg and other western isles, weathered into step-like terraces, which form a characteristic feature of Hebridean cliffs, the flat-topped McLeod's Tables of Skye (1,600 feet), precisely similar basaltic platforms on the hills of Disko Island and the mainland of western and eastern Greenland—all these are parts of one stupendous whole, a plateau covering half a million square miles, that was once the Thulean continent. The wide-spread lava-flows represent one phase of volcanic activity in an age of exceptional unrest. Another phase is illustrated by more coarsely crystalline rocks, such as those of the dark Cuillin hills of Skye. They were not poured out as lava-streams over the land, but were forced upwards as great dome-like masses from a deeply seated subterranean source and, as their coarser texture proves, slowly cooled under the pressure of a thick superincumbent load: the comparatively large size of the crystals indicates gradual solidification from a molten mass. These two phases of prolonged rock-building help us to appreciate the immensity of geological time. Describing the lava-flows of Mull, Sir Archibald Geikie wrote: "On Ben More we can walk over each bed of basalt from the sea-level to the mountain top, a height of 3,169 feet." The basaltic lavas we see in the cliffs of Mull and many other islands are but a part of the original pile. Those that remain furnish an impressive example of rock construction which must have extended over an enormous period of time. The second phase, on the other hand, is an equally impressive example of rock destruction as a measure of geological time. We see the jagged peaks of mountains rising to a height of 3,000 feet above sea-level which, at no distant date as earth history is reckoned, were buried under a considerable thickness of younger rocks that have been utterly destroyed by the ceaseless operation of denuding agents.

The world to our limited vision appears to be almost static; the mountains we have been accustomed to think of as symbols of eternity, seen through geological spectacles, take their place as episodes in a series of events which have moulded the changing features of the earth's face. The rocky covering of the world viewed by geologists, "foreshortened in the tract of time," reveals itself as a dynamic, mobile crust responding from age to age to constructive and destructive forces which have operated since the earth's early youth following a still earlier stage when, in the imagery of the poet,

> This world was once a fluid haze of light.

(2) *Plant-bearing sediments indicative of quiescent intervals.* So far the events chronicled in rocks of igneous origin have been spoken of as though there had been continuous outpourings of lava with occasional showers of ash and, in some districts, upwelling of molten material that remained hidden below the surface until in the course of time the covering rocks were removed by erosion. There is, however, clear proof that the extrusion of lava and other rocks was intermittent: intercalated among the lava-beds are layers of sedimentary material, hardened sand and mud, layers of coal and beds of fine-grained limestone containing beautifully preserved leaves, a few fruits and other plant fragments, also rare examples of insect wings and shells. The richest plant-containing layers occur near the base of the pile of basaltic lavas on Ardtun Head, the low "headland of the waves" near the southwestern corner of Mull, the island on which from his home on Iona—which has been aptly named "the light of the western world"—Saint Columba must often have gazed. Trees, shrubs and other plants were

able to colonize portions of the lava-field during the long pauses between recurrent outbursts of volcanic fires.

The association of sedimentary material with the basalts at Ardtun Head was noticed by Abraham Mills as long ago as 1790; but it was not until the middle of the nineteenth century that Mr. McQuarrie, of Bunessan, discovered the fossil plants, which were very briefly described by Professor Edward Forbes in an appendix to an important paper by the Duke of Argyll published by the Geological Society of London in 1851. The Duke spoke of the leaves as having been shed "autumn after autumn into the smooth still waters of some shallow lake, on whose muddy bottom they were accumulated, one above the other, fully expanded and at perfect rest." By far the richest collection of

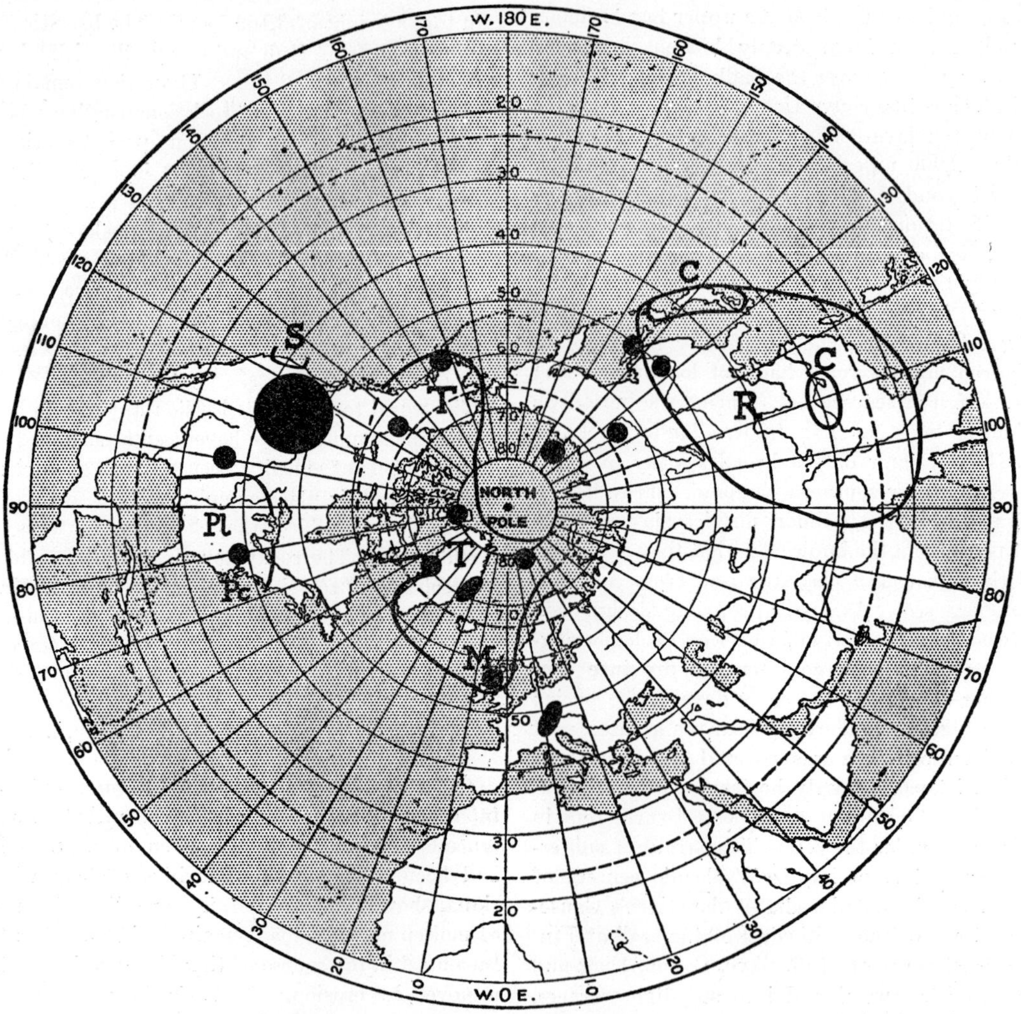


MAP OF THE NORTHERN HEMISPHERE ILLUSTRATING SOME OF THE SUBJECTS DEALT WITH IN THE ADDRESS

C, C. The present geographical distribution of *Cercidiphyllum,* a Japanese and Chinese tree. *Black patches* mark localities and districts where fossil specimens of *Cercidiphyllum* have been found. Arctic and sub-Arctic regions: Alaska, Mackenzie River, Grinnell Land and Ellesmere Land, West and East Greenland, Spitsbergen, New Siberian Islands, Lena River. Canada and the United States of America: several localities from British Columbia and California, and east of the Rocky Mountains in Montana, Wyoming, Oklahoma, etc. The oldest examples of *Cercidiphyllum* leaves are from early Cretaceous rocks in Maryland—the Potomac formation (Pc). Others are recorded from Europe—Mull, Switzerland, Bohemia, Silesia; Eastern Asia; Sakhalin Island and the Bureja River. M. Mull and neighboring islands. Pl. The geographical distribution of the occidental plane. R. Approximate boundary of the area within which are the present homes of the majority of trees and shrubs most closely related to extinct species of the Hebridean flora. S. The present distribution of *Sequoia sempervirens* (Redwood) and *Sequoia gigantea* (Mammoth tree). T. Hypothetical boundaries of the Thulean province.

fossils was made by Mr. Starkie Gardner rather more than fifty years ago and partially described by him in a paper read to the Geological Society of London in 1887. Descriptions of several fossil plants from the Mull beds have also been published by Dr. T. Johnson. The main collection is now in the British Museum. Additional specimens have been obtained by other collectors in more recent years. The work of deciphering the botanical records from Mull, Skye and a few of the other islands is rendered mildly exciting by the danger of misinterpretation. Fossil leaves, we are often reminded, are very uncertain guides—records left by nature in a mischievous mood to mislead the unwary and over-confident student. Sir Joseph Hooker, in an address to the British Association at Norwich in 1868, spoke of fossil botany as "this most unreliable of sciences"; but he added by way of consolation—"the science has of late made sure and steady progress, and developed really grand results." One may cheerfully take the risk of being called an unscientific optimist by colleagues whose chief concern is with living plants. Botanists who confine their attention to recent plants have ample sources of information, not merely detached leaves but twigs bearing leaves, flowers and fruits. It is natural, therefore, that they should tend to underestimate the value of leaf-form and venation, characters that are often the only criteria available to the paleobotanist.

B. *The ancient flora of the Inner Hebrides*

What, then, is it possible to say about the ancient flora of the Inner Hebrides without transgressing the limits of probability? We know very little of the smaller and simpler plants which lived under the shade of the forest trees or clung to the surface of stems where they were washed by trickling rills of rain-water. The three smallest plants which have left recognizable fragments are a fungus and two liverworts or, as they are often called, hepatics, a group allied to the mosses but of simpler construction. The fungus was found by Mr. Edwards several years ago on some detached leaves of a conifer from the Mull plant-beds; the manner of its discovery illustrates an interesting technique often employed with success by students of fossil plants. In many instances leaves preserved on shale are covered with a very thin, black coaly film produced as the result of chemical change in the plant tissues after death. It is often possible, by detaching a piece of the film and treating it with certain clearing agents, to remove the carbonaceous matter and obtain a sample of the surface skin of the leaf that is brown in color, transparent and suitable for microscopical examination. After treatment the Mull leaves showed some minute dark spots on the surface film, and these on magnification were found to be circular discs made of rows of radially disposed cells. The discs were identified as organs of a fungus closely resembling reproductive structures of a living genus *Phragmothyrium,* a fungus now mainly tropical: the occurrence in Mull of a nearly allied form is, however, probably indicative of a moist rather than a tropical climate. One of the liverworts bears a close resemblance to a living species, *Pellia epiphylla,* which has a wide geographical distribution and is very common on damp earth in Britain; it has a flat green, forked body barely an inch in length. The other hepatic is a member of a different family, characterized by a slender thread-like stem bearing two rows of minute leaves; it bears a striking resemblance to some living species included in the order Jungermanniales. These two fragmentary remains of liverworts are worth mentioning because fossil examples of such plants are comparatively rare; also for another and a more important reason. A few years ago Professor J. Walton, of Glasgow, published a description of some liverworts discovered for the first time in rocks containing remains of plants which grew in the forests of the Coal Age about 200 million years ago. The interesting fact is this: the Paleozoic liverworts differ hardly at all in the construction of the delicate plant-body from the much later forms from the Thulean continent; both are essentially modern and yet both are surprisingly ancient. We do not know much about the history of these plants, but it is clear that some liverworts persisted through a succession of geological periods with practically no modification of their simple design.

The only fern so far discovered is very nearly related to the sensitive fern, *Onoclea sensibilis,* a familiar species in North America, ranging from Florida to Newfoundland and as far west as Saskatchewan; it occurs also in northern China, Manchuria, Japan and Corea; it has what is called a discontinuous geographical distribution. *Onoclea,* no longer a native of Europe, is often cultivated. The fossil fronds from Mull, both sterile and fertile, differ hardly at all from those of the living fern. Records of the rocks show that *Onoclea* formerly grew in northwestern Europe and in Greenland, regions where, through the vicissitudes of climate, it long ago failed to survive. Evidence furnished by fossils and the facts of geological history affords a clue to the present discontinuous range; in all probability *Onoclea* originated on the Thulean continent, perhaps north of the Arctic Circle, whence it spread radially into America, Europe and the Far East; in the European region it became extinct, sharing the fate of many other plants that were unable to survive the rigors of the Ice Age. Its territory was originally continuous; now it is restricted to North America and eastern Asia. Another member of the class to which the ferns belong is the familiar *Equisetum,* the horsetails: one species, closely comparable with the living *Equisetum limosum* —widely distributed in north temperate and arctic lands—has been found in the sediments of Ardtun

Head. *Equisetum* may be described as an emblem of changelessness: nearly related forms grew in Paleozoic forests at least 150 or 200 million years ago: less closely related plants in the same forests—the calamites—were comparable in size with trees. The slender horsetails of the Coal Age and their much more robust and woody allies remind us that in the course of evolution some of nature's early experiments survived unaffected by the production of new competitors, while others, less successful, left no direct descendants. As we follow the march of plant-life through the ages evidence of progress accompanied by retrogression becomes recurrently apparent: in the varying green mantle of the earth there can be traced threads running through the whole, changing very slightly as we follow them onwards and upwards, preserving all the time a remarkable uniformity in essential characters.

By far the greater number of fossils from Ardtun are leaves of trees or shrubs, which belong to one or other of the two great classes of seed-bearing plants. In Gymnosperms, including conifers and some other less familiar plants, the seeds are naked. In members of the other class, the highest, the most various and most abundant in the vegetable kingdom, the seeds are more efficiently protected and are contained in a closed case; hence the name Angiosperms. Conifers played a prominent part in the Hebridean forests, but their representatives were not such as we find in modern Europe. A single and well-preserved seed attached to a relatively large wing affords evidence of the occurrence of a conifer allied to the silver fir (*Abies pectinata*) and some other species commonly cultivated in Britain. Firs, using the term for trees belonging to the genus *Abies* and excluding the spruce fir (*Picea*), now occur in Europe, northern Africa, northern Asia and America; there is no British species of *Abies*. The Mull seed, it is important to note, agrees most closely with seeds of firs now living in China and Japan. Among other conifers discovered in the plant-beds of Mull and Skye are *Cephalotaxus, Cryptomeria* and *Sequoia*. Recent species of *Cephalotaxus* are comparatively small trees confined to the Far East; some kinds are cultivated in our gardens. The foliage of the Mull species bears a striking resemblance to that of *Cephalotaxus fortunei,* a small tree widely distributed in China. Another genus which we believe to have been a member of the Hebridean flora is *Cryptomeria;* the fossils from northern Ireland and the Isle of Skye include foliage shoots, cones and pollen-grains. The solitary living species is the Japanese *Cryptomeria japonica,* which occurs also in China—this is the tree of the famous avenue of Nikko in Japan, a notable memorial of a peasant who was too poor in worldly goods to contribute the usual building stone or a bronze lamp to the mortuary temple of an emperor, and instead offered to plant trees to protect visitors against the heat of the sun.

One of the most interesting of all living conifers is the genus *Sequoia,* of which there are two species confined within the narrow strip of hill ranges bordering Oregon and California on the Pacific coast—the Redwoods (*Sequoia sempervirens*) of the Coast Range, watered in the dry season by mists from the western ocean, and the Mammoth trees (*Sequoia gigantea,* often called *Wellingtonia*) of the Sierra Nevada (see map, S). *Sequoia* is an impressive example of the light thrown by fossil plants on the past history and wanderings over broad regions of the earth's surface of trees that, without man's protection, would be in danger of extinction. In earlier periods *Sequoia* was almost cosmopolitan; it ranged over wide spaces in the old and the new world and overstepped the limits of the northern hemisphere. Foliage shoots preserved in the sediments of Mull were in all probability borne by trees closely related to the living Redwoods, trees which are well worthy of inclusion among the wonders of the world; they attain a height of over 300 feet and the rings on cross-sections of giant trunks that have been felled bear witness to an age of 3,000 years and more. They were growing where they stand to-day 1,000 years before the Christian era. Trees next of kin to the Redwoods once lived within a short distance from the Polar Sea several hundred miles farther north than the present tree-limit. Another species of *Sequoia,* more nearly allied to the Mammoth tree, lingered on in Britain long after the disappearance of the Thulean forests: this we know from the discovery of fossil twigs and cones in the sediments of an old lake on the edge of Dartmoor in Devonshire. The two surviving species live in splendid isolation, dreaming of a greater glory that was theirs, their memories stored with secrets man can never know.

There was another naked-seeded tree in the forests into which we have intruded, a species of *Ginkgo,* the Maidenhair tree. The barbarous name *Ginkgo,* invented in 1712 by the German naturalist Kaempfer, is in the opinion of the Reverend Dr. Moule, formerly professor of Chinese at Cambridge, a false transcription of Sankyo, which probably means hill-apricot. Leaves perfect in form and venation were found in the chalky sediment of a lake that filled a hollow in the Hebridean lava-field; they differ from the foliage of the living tree only in a few minor features detected by the practiced eyes of Dr. Florin of Stockholm in the microscopical structure of the superficial cells. Dr. Simpson discovered *Ginkgo* pollen-grains at another locality. The story of the Maidenhair tree has recently been told[2] and the temptation to linger over it this evening must be resisted. *Ginkgo* of all trees furnishes

[2] *Science Progress,* January, 1938.

the most thrilling of a link with the past; its history, compiled from fossils of many geological ages and in many parts of the world, is an enthralling romance. This is but one of many histories recorded in nature's storybook which makes us share the thought of Edward Fitzgerald: "Yes, as I often think, it is not the poetical imagination but bare science that every day more and more unrolls a greater epic than the Iliad." It would be rash definitely to assert that the Maidenhair tree still exists under strictly natural conditions as a wild tree of the forest. Botanists who have searched for it in China, the country believed to be its last home, failed to discover convincing evidence of the occurrence of specimens which could not be ascribed to man's agency. On the other hand, a few years ago a Chinese botanist expressed the opinion that *Ginkgo* still grows wild in the province of Chekiang in eastern China. The oldest living examples occur in China and Japan, often in places where, as is fitting, they are venerated as trees endowed with healing properties. The history of *Ginkgo* has been traced to periods antedating by millions of years the Thulean forests. We do not know of what sort its progenitors were; but we know that it is a survival from an age too remote for us to measure in terms which we can fully appreciate. We also know that *Ginkgo,* now a lonely relic in the present world, is a primitive and isolated type, the sole representative of a large family, including many different members, all of which save the Maidenhair tree long ago fell by the way in the struggle for existence. When the tree lived in the Hebridean forests it was common in other parts of the Thulean continent from northern Canada to Greenland and Spitsbergen, in North America, Europe and Asia. It was as widely distributed geographically as oaks, pines and firs in the modern world. The history of *Ginkgo* is a record of endurance, of persistence with apparently little change in an unstable world. When we recall the amazing life-story of the tree and its forbears the autumnal color acquires a deeper significance—we see in the pale yellow of the leaves a reflection of the golden age of a family that left a precious legacy. Would that the Maidenhair tree were endowed with the oracular power of the oaks of Dodona and, in the trembling accents of its fluttering leaves, could tell us not of the future but of the varying fortunes of the family as age succeeded age.

The *Ginkgo* of Mull was not the last of its race in Europe. Well-preserved remains have been found in younger rocks in France and Germany proving that it survived in the western world, though probably only in a few places, to an age preceding by a comparatively short period the invasion of temperate Europe and North America by arctic ice-sheets and glaciers, which had a far-reaching effect upon the vegetation in the western world.

Leaving the naked-seeded plants, we pass to the flowering plants or Angiosperms. This class is more recent in origin than the Gymnosperms, at least so it would seem, and as in present-day floras so also in the Thulean forests, flowering plants contributed the greatest number of genera and species. We shall take first a few trees and shrubs which have descendants still living in Europe, and afterwards mention others that have no near relations in European floras. There were, we think, three or four kinds of oak, all different from those now living in Europe and America. The largest leaves from Mull assigned to the genus *Quercus* are oval, with a broadly rounded base and relatively small teeth; they resemble the foliage of a few Indian species, but the oak with leaves most closely resembling the fossil form is *Quercus serrata,* a native of China, the rain-forests of Assam, Japan, Corea and the Himalayas. A second species from Mull is closely comparable with other Indian and Far Eastern oaks; and a third form of leaf is very similar in shape and venation to a species that now has its home in China, Assam and the island of Formosa. It is noteworthy that none of the oaks of the Thulean forests conformed in pattern of the foliage to our familiar British trees.

One of the most conspicuous trees in the Hebridean woodland was a plane (*Platanus*) with large handsome leaves almost, but not quite, identical with those of the existing occidental plane of North America. The fossil evidence in this instance is supplied by male flowers and fruit-balls as well as leaves. As in all living planes the expanded base of the leaf-stalk enclosed and protected a bud. There is, however, one interesting feature in which the leaves of the Mull tree differ from those of any living plane: there were two fairly large leaflets attached to the long leaf-stalk between the main part of the leaf and the base of the stalk. The significance of this peculiarity need not be discussed; it is one of those botanical problems of academic interest which excite the specialist. A more important fact for us is that plane trees in the period we are considering occupied a territory which extended very much farther north than the present area of distribution. Remains of plane trees have been found as far north as Spitsbergen in rocks approximately equivalent in age to those of Mull. There are in the world to-day six or possibly eight different kinds of plane: the oriental plane (*Platanus orientalis*), the only species native in Europe, is one of the noblest living trees; it recalls the groves of the Academy in the golden age of Greece. One of the oldest specimens is the venerable stump bearing enormous arms in the market place on the island of Cos, where, legend would have us believe, Hippocrates, more than two thousand years ago, gave advice to his patients under the shade of the youthful tree. The oriental plane extends from Greece and the Aegean islands eastward to Asia Minor and the Caspian Sea; it is sometimes said to be wild in Persia and northern India, but more probably this eastward spread should be attributed to man. The most widely distributed species in the New World is *Platanus occidentalis,* growing usually in river valleys from Lake Ontario to Florida and west to Texas and Nebraska (see map, Pl.). On the western side of North America there are other species, in Mexico and along the Coast Range hills of California. The most familiar cultivated species in Britain is *Platanus acerifolia,* the so-called London plane: this favorite urban tree is regarded by some botanists as a hybrid between the oriental and the occidental plane; the time and place of its origin are not known with any certainty. The geological record of *Platanus* affords a striking example of contrasts between past and present areas of distribution. Some of the oldest known fossil leaves and fruits are from early Cretaceous beds in Greenland, at least 300 miles north of the Arctic Circle. The occurrence of these remains in sediments that were deposited in a remote northern estuary before the chalk of the British Isles had been upraised from the sea-floor affords definite proof that plane trees lived in arctic forests millions of years before they spread to the southern part of the Thulean continent. The birthplace of *Platanus* may have been in the far north, whence in course of time it spread to Iceland and Spitsbergen, from arctic to temperate North America and Europe, and wandered as far east as Sakhalin Island on the eastern confines of Asia.

One of the comparatively few trees in the Hebridean forests related to recent British species was a *Corylus* with leaves similar to those of our hazel but still more like the foliage of species now living in India and the Far East. Hazels were associated with planes not only in the ancient flora of Mull but in circumpolar forests from which they traveled, in response to the urge of climatic change, to fresh and more genial homes farther south. Another tree in the Thulean forests was a cornel, a species of the genus *Cornus,* which has a far-flung distribution, in arctic and sub-arctic countries, in North America, Europe and Asia. While fully conscious of the danger of placing excessive trust in leaves as evidence of affinity, we believe that a Chinese cornel (*Cornus chinensis*) agrees most closely in foliage with the Mull species. The cornels are members of an old stock represented in northern forests as long ago as the Cretaceous period.

Among the larger fossils from Ardtun Head are a few almost perfectly preserved leaves of a vine, which we believe to be specifically identical with specimens previously discovered in Alaskan rocks of approximately the same geological age as those associated with the lava-flows of Mull. Similar leaves have been described from Greenland, Iceland, Spitsbergen and more southern localities in America and Europe. Vines were widely distributed even as far back as the Cretaceous period. There is now only one European species, the wine-producing *Vitis vinifera,* but its leaves are unlike the fossils from Ardtun. The striking contrast between the present distribution of the vine in Europe and its former, much more extended distribution, which included arctic and north temperate regions, raises the difficult problem of changes in climate from one age to another. Vine scrolls are a fairly common ornament on early Northumbrian Anglo-Saxon crosses, a motif adopted in still earlier ages by Greek and Roman sculptors, which, after the lapse of centuries, reached the highest expression of naturalistic treatment in England in the last two decades of the thirteenth century. Millions of years before vine leaves and fruit were fashioned in stone, one kind lived in prehuman days on the Thulean continent; and it is noteworthy that its nearest counterpart in the modern world occurs in the Far East.

We turn now to trees and shrubs belonging to genera which are no longer living in Europe. The first tree to be considered furnishes a striking contrast, in the narrow limits of its present geographical area, to the widely spread cornels and oaks. *Cercidiphyllum* is now confined to Japan and mountain valleys in some parts of China (see map, C). The name *Cercidiphyllum* was chosen because of a superficial resemblance of the leaves to those of the Judas tree, *Cercis siliquastrum.* Only a single species, with a few varieties, has survived, *Cercidiphyllum japonicum,* familiar to many tree lovers who cultivate it for the sake of the exceptionally beautiful gold, pink and red parti-colored autumnal foliage. In common with some other trees of ancient lineage, *Cercidiphyllum* lacks any near relations in the present age; it is one of a select company of nature's anachronisms. Like the Maidenhair tree, it is an aberrant type, a relic living within a comparatively small area in the Far East; formerly it was one of the most widely distributed forest trees on both sides of the Atlantic Ocean. Several beautifully preserved leaves have been found in the plant-beds of Ardtun Head, leaves and occasionally fruits of *Cercidiphyllum* have been found in Grinnell Land and Ellesmere Land on the northeastern corner of the Canadian Archipelago, in Alaska and at several localities on the Pacific and Atlantic coasts of North America, in Greenland, Iceland and Spitsbergen, as well as in Switzerland and other parts of Europe (see map). Leaves, superficially at least indistinguishable from those of the existing species, are recorded from sedimentary beds in the valley of the Potomac River in Maryland assigned to the early days of the Cretaceous period when flowering plants were comparatively few in number and had not yet come into their own as the dominant class in the plant kingdom. When we remember the remote antiquity of *Cercidiphyllum* and its wanderings over the earth's surface during the passing of millennia, the autumnal glory of its foliage is enhanced a hundredfold and acquires a symbolic meaning.

The plant-beds on the headland of Ardtun have yielded very few recognizable fruits and seeds. Among the rare examples of fruits are some, about half an inch long, consisting of a slightly elongated seed-vessel surmounted usually by five leaflets, the enlarged and persistent covering of the young flowers, which served as efficient aids to dispersal by wind. The fossil winged fruits and associated leaves present a remarkably close resemblance to those of some living species of *Abelia,* a genus named after Mr. Clarke Abel, who discovered the shrub in China about one hundred and twenty years ago. *Abelia* is a member of the honeysuckle family (*Caprifoliaceae*); most of the existing species have their home in central China and are cultivated as flowering shrubs in European gardens. There are a few species in Japan, the Himalayas and Mexico. Fruits of a Chinese *Abelia* agree most closely with the fossil specimens. Similar though not specifically identical fruits were discovered thirteen years ago by Mrs. Clement Reid and Miss Chandler in a collection of fossil plants from Bembridge in the Isle of Wight. The Bembridge flora is younger geologically than the flora of Mull and indicates a warmer climate. Other examples were recorded long ago from southeastern France. It is therefore clear that shrubs next of kin to Abelias now living in China were once native in western and northern Europe. The introduction to British and continental gardens in our time of *Abelia, Cercidiphyllum* and other trees and flowering shrubs may be described as the reinstatement, through man's desire for horticultural novelties, of plants that had long been exiles from western woodlands where as natives they were never seen by human eyes.

So far attention has been confined to a selection of plants identified from leaves and a few fruits. If time permitted, the list could be substantially enlarged by inclusion of the interesting results of Dr. Simpson's intensive study of pollen-grains, which he found by microscopical examination of broken-up pieces of lignite and coal, associated with sandy beds in Mull and on the adjacent peninsula of Morven. The pollen-bearing layers of rock are below the basaltic lavas and therefore slightly older than the leaf-beds of Ardtun Head. Dr. Simpson discovered several conifers and flowering plants confirmatory of identifications based on leaves; he also made many additions to the list compiled from leaves, fruits and seeds. Three of his discoveries are selected for brief reference. He found pollen-grains of two kinds of alder (*Alnus*). The pollen of alders has a very characteristic structure and can easily be recognized. The occurrence of alders in the Hebridean flora supplies one of the few links between the extinct and the present European vegetation. The second genus chosen from Dr. Simpson's list is *Magnolia;* it is now represented by many species, both trees and shrubs, and is widely distributed on two sides of the Pacific Ocean—in Asia along the Himalayas and in parts of Tibet, over a large area in China, Japan and Corea, the Malay Archipelago and Indo-China; in America from southern Ontario as far south as Central America and Cuba. It was shown many years ago that *Magnolia* formerly lived in Europe and flourished as far north as latitude 70° N. in Greenland; we now know that it played a part in the adornment of the Thulean forests.

Finally a few words on the discovery of pollen-grains believed to belong to a species of *Nelumbium;* this genus is one of the most attractive water plants, a plant held sacred in ancient Egypt and venerated in the Far East. One of the living species is the sacred lotus, native in China and Japan and established as far west as the Caspian Sea; the other species has an extended range in North America, spreading as far south as the West Indies and Brazil. *Nelumbium* no longer grows in the Nile: long years ago it had a wide distribution in Europe, both in the Cretaceous period and in later ages. Looking backwards we see its great circular leaves spread over the still waters of a Thulean lake.

It is important to note that Dr. Simpson's comparative investigation of fossil and recent pollen shows a preponderance of eastern Asiatic species in the Hebridean flora.

### FANCY WITH FACT

We have attempted to recreate a scene in the past, and it is natural to ask—how does our reconstruction compare with reality? As it is impossible to satisfy curiosity by an actual flight to the Thulean continent, we can at least imagine ourselves miraculously transported to a destination where the past has become the present. At a very early stage of the backward journey we should see the greater part of the land being gradually obliterated by a covering of snow and ice; glacial conditions would be succeeded by a climate becoming more and more genial. Human beings would be missed before one fiftieth of the flight had been completed. At last, after observing the moving panorama of land and sea, fluctuations in climate and changes in the character of the vegetation, let us imagine ourselves at the journey's end. Combining fact with fancy, we find ourselves, where in day-dreams we have often been, among the plants on the lava plateau. Thanks to the artistic cooperation of Mrs. Gwendy Caröe, it has been possible to give substance to our mental picture based on geological and botanical facts. It requires a special effort for us, who think of ourselves as overlords in nature's realm, to visualize a world in which man has no place. Alone in a world which for millions of years to come would be uninhabited by the human race, we could hardly fail to look upon the beauty of nature's pageantry with a strange and more penetrating vision:

> Beauty, the eternal Spouse of the Wisdom of God
> and Angel of his Presence thru' all creation.

We should realize as never before man's insignificance: on the other hand, our estimate of spiritual values would be raised to a higher level and we should experience a deeper sense of union with the infinite. Our tendency is to think of the past, as we think of the present—in relation to man; we forget his very recent participation as an actor in life's drama. As we look at nature as into a mirror our own image obtrudes itself into the foreground. Had man been a dweller on the Thulean continent he would have seen, as we see, the sun by day setting in motion the living machinery of trees and herbs; the splendor of the evening sky; he would hear the wind in the trees, the music of running water and the songs of birds. The beauty of nature is eternal. To the east and north beyond the lava-fields the Caledonian mountain ranges would be seen rising to greater heights than any of their peaks reach to-day; they were still to be exposed for millions of years to the destructive operation of nature's sculpturing tools. Making a fresh demand upon our imagination, let us take a longer view over the curve of the earth towards the heart of Europe and far to the east to northern India. We should look in vain for the Pyrenees, the Alps, the Carpathians and the Himalayas: these and other mountain ranges had not yet been lifted up; the time of their birth was not far off. We should see in their place a broad belt of water stretching from the Atlantic to the Indian Ocean, linking West and East. On the bed of this ancient sea—the Tethys Sea of geologists—sediments had long been accumulating, and these, with other rocks of igneous origin, would be involved at no distant date in a complete transformation of the earth's features and the crumpling of the crust into the "everlasting hills."

Returning to the Thulean continent at a place near the present geographical position of the Inner Hebrides, let us take a survey of the vegetation. We should be impressed by its luxuriance: at first sight the general aspect would seem familiar, but on closer examination of the trees and shrubs we should find only a few recalling modern European species; many would remind us of exotic plants of eastern origin. Despite the immensity of the time interval separating us from the world we had left, we should not be aware of any such marked contrast in the general character of the vegetation as we might have expected. The plants had already put on their familiar dress and would seem to us surprisingly modern. But—and this would be the deepest impression—we should feel that we were among trees and shrubs that were reminiscent of remote eastern forests. We should be conscious of the dynamic character of the plant-world; we should be driven to the conclusion that the forests were mainly composed of wanderers resting for a time in a temporary home whence, as conditions changed, they would pass to other stages in the long journey to their present refuges in Asia.

### EVOLUTION

There remains another question which is always asked by those who attempt to reconstruct the vegetation of past ages: What contributions do the records of plant-life make towards a better understanding of evolution? The riddle of evolution remains a challenge and, as knowledge increases, we make fresh guesses. As a Cambridge friend writes in a recent volume of "Provocative Verse":

> That life evolves was guessed of yore,
> Darwinians prove it true;
> Of how and why we know but little more
> Than old Lucretius knew.

The little more we know urges us to continue in hopeful expectancy the long and endless prying into nature's methods. What then do we learn from the ancient flora of the Western Isles? The facts do not substantially help us to trace the unfolding of life in the long interval separating the older part of the Tertiary era from the present time. There is little difference between the past and the present vegetation of the world as a whole in the nature of trees, shrubs and ferns; our knowledge of the earlier history of herbaceous plants is very meager. The fossil flora of Mull represents an early phase of what may be called the modern type of vegetation, which overspread the world in the later stages of the Cretaceous period and has persisted with few major modifications until now. Evolution seems to have been characterized by bursts of production when new and successful types exercised a transforming influence; and these periods of exceptional creative activity were separated by periods of relative stability. The early Tertiary floras belong to a stage when a new order had become well established and an older order had passed its prime. The one great difference that emerges from comparison of the Mull flora and the existing European floras is not a difference in the components of the world forests, but a contrast in the geographical positions occupied by the various genera in the northern hemisphere: for the most part a western home has been exchanged for a home in the Far East.

### DRIFTING CONTINENTS

If we followed the vegetation on the southern part of the Thulean land farther to the north, we should be impressed by its apparent indifference to changing physical conditions as we traveled beyond the Arctic Circle; we should fail to notice any zonal distinguishing characters in the floras such as in our day reflect the passage from temperate to arctic regions. The evidence of fossil plants forces us to the conclusion that the vegetation on the Thulean continent, its northern boundary within a short distance of the polar sea, its southern border on the latitude of northern Ireland and western Scotland, was astonishingly uniform. How, we ask, can we explain this surprising and well-attested fact? There must, it is generally agreed, always have been climatic belts; high arctic and much lower temperate regions can not have supported closely comparable floras possessing several species in common. Some of us are convinced that changes in geography from one period to another, land connections where there are now arms of the sea, interference with paths of ocean currents and consequential changes in temperature are inadequate as explanatory causes. What then remains? Were it possible for us to make a survey of the Thulean continent as it was, we might find that the geographical relation of the northern part of the forest-clad land to the North Pole was by no means the same as it is now. It is difficult, it is probably impossible, to explain the facts without calling to our aid the hypothesis of drifting continents usually associated with the late Professor Wegener and recently discussed in an able book by Professor Du Toit, of South Africa. This is a controversial subject beyond the scope of my address. I can do little more than reaffirm adherence to the view that plant records from rocks of many ages raise problems which seem to be insoluble unless we postulate movement and sliding of the earth's crust. As icebergs are slowly drifted by ocean currents, as masses of cumulus clouds rapidly changing shape pass across a blue sky; so, the rate of travel enormously reduced, large slabs of the outermost rocky shell of the world may have shifted their position in the course of geological time. It must, however, be admitted that as yet refined methods of measurement have not furnished any evidence of crustal movement. Dr. Nörlund, of Copenhagen, has stated that longitudinal determinations, carried out by the Danish Geodetic Institute in 1927 and 1936 with a modern transit instrument, both times on the same pillar at a locality on the west coast of Greenland, gave practically the same result. In his presidential address at the Norwich meeting of the association in 1935 Professor W. W. Watts made an interesting and judicial reference to the Wegener hypothesis: he spoke of it as having been hailed by many classes of investigators as almost a panacea, and quoted one of several critics who called it a beautiful dream, the dream of a great poet.

Proof or disproof of the Wegener hypothesis will be forthcoming in the more distant future when the precision of modern methods of measurement has been available long enough to provide trustworthy data. Meanwhile we must be content to wait in sanguine expectation that an interpretation of the overwhelming evidence furnished by fossil plants will be provided by research workers in the geophysical field.

One of the most impressive examples of the bearing of fossil plants upon the fascinating problem of climatic conditions in the past has been furnished by Professor Harris, of Reading. The facts are briefly these: Several years ago Professor Nathorst, of Stockholm, described a large collection of fossil plants from rocks in Scania, the southernmost province of Sweden, demonstrating the existence of a flora many million years older than the one we have been considering. It was a very rich flora composed of numerous ferns, conifers and other plants; it probably lacked flowering plants. More recently Professor Harris made a still larger collection of fossils during a long visit to eastern Greenland in the ice-bound district of Scoresby Sound, where, under extreme arctic conditions, only a few stunted plants are able to exist. Nothing could be more striking than the present contrast between the floras of eastern Greenland and southern Sweden. The arctic fossil plants of the same age as those from Scania demonstrate the former existence of a flora even richer than that from southern Sweden; comparison of the two floras affords no indication of any difference in the size of individual plants and no difference in the vegetation as a whole. A luxuriant and uniform vegetation occupied an area stretching from central Germany to southern Sweden and a thousand miles farther north beyond latitude 70° N. The fossils preserved in rocks at localities within this far-flung geographical area from south to north give no indication of any such change in the plant communities as we should expect and as we find when we contrast arctic and temperate floras in the present world. This uniformity, I venture to think, is inexplicable unless we assume a very considerable movement and reshuffling of the earth's crust. The geological historian needs the cooperation of astronomers and physicists in his endeavor to reconstruct the world at the successive stages of its development; he looks to them to prevent him from making assumptions inconsistent with conclusions reached by workers in other fields. On the other hand, geologists and paleontologists contribute facts that are incontrovertible, however much they seem to be in opposition to the views of students whose primary interest is in geophysical problems.

### NEGLECT OF EARTH HISTORY IN EDUCATION

There are still some people who ask, What is the use of the kind of information given in this address? My reply is that knowledge gained from a first-hand study of nature, both animate and inanimate, has a value beyond price. Enjoyment of the romance of creation as recorded in the life of the past and of the present is within the reach of all who have the desire to read the open pages of nature's book. In the rocks we find the soul of history: the whole world throbs with life, and the joy of it all is ours to share:

> I said it in the meadow path,
> I said it on the mountain stairs—
> The best things any mortal hath
> Are those which every mortal shares.

This evening we have caught through the mists a glimpse of a scene on earth's stage separated from the present by a small fraction of time in relation to the whole span of geological history. The Thulean forests which we have visited included trees, shrubs and other plants of surprisingly modern aspect, though it is not to be supposed that they were absolutely identical specifically with their living descendants; from the material available it is impossible to define or assess the difference. What we have seen throws little light on the evolution of the plant-world; it is equally true that the main conclusion forced upon us by our retrospect can not fail to convince us that it is impossible to understand the present distribution of plants over the earth's surface unless we extend our survey into the past. Darwin spoke of geographical distribution as a noble science, "almost the keystone of the laws of creation." The living world can not be fully appreciated as an expression of creative energy unless we free ourselves from the cramping influence of the environment in which we live.

As a botanist whose first love was geology, may I make a plea for wider recognition of physical geography and geology as branches of knowledge possessing an inestimable value as a means of bringing young people into close companionship with nature and as a source of refreshment, a stimulus and an inspiration. Most of us would probably agree with the spirit of a remark made a good many years ago by the late A. C. Benson: "I find it hard to resist the conviction that, from the educational point of view, stimulus is more important than exactness." Arguments in favor of introducing geology into schools were put forward in a "Report on Scientific Education" presented at the Dundee meeting seventy-two years ago, and in 1936 and 1937 the association published two reports on the same subject. Let me add another argument of no little value: Hugh Miller wrote in a letter to a friend, "geology is, I find, a science in which the best authorities are sometimes content to unlearn a good deal." That is worth much; geology helps us to cultivate the not too common virtue of admitting that it is possible to make a mistake. In conclusion, I can not do better than quote with whole-hearted agreement words spoken by Sir William Bragg in his presidential address to this association eleven years ago: "Some speak of modern science as tending to destroy reverence and faith. I do not know how that can be said of the student who stands daily in the presence of what seems to him to be infinite." These words apply with equal force to searchers after truth whose main interest is in the living world no less than to those whose objective is the elucidation of the structure of matter that is called by contrast dead and yet vibrates with life. The earth was once lifeless; when and how living protoplasm had its birth we do not know, nor do we know whereupon were the foundations of the earth laid. We can only echo in our hearts the voice out of the whirlwind:

> Whereupon were the foundations thereof fastened?
> Or who laid the corner stone thereof;
> When the morning stars sang together,
> And all the sons of God shouted for joy?

# SCIENTIFIC EVENTS

## THE FORESTS OF GREAT BRITAIN

ACCORDING to the report of the British Forestry Commission for the year ending September, 1938, approximately 54,000,000 trees were planted during the year. Forty-seven per cent. of these trees were Norway and Sitka spruces, 24 per cent. Scots and Corsican pines, 9 per cent. European and Japanese larches, 1 per cent. Douglas fir and 16 per cent. broad-leaved species. The total addition to the woodland area of Great Britain as a result of the commission's operations during the year was 20,300 acres. Including reafforestation in the former Crown woods and replanting areas damaged by fire, 24,100 acres were planted, of which 21,600 acres were planted with conifers and 2,500 acres with hardwoods.

By the end of the forest year the commissioners had 125 forests in England and Wales and 107 forests in Scotland. The total area afforested is now 365,000 acres, and is being increased by some 30,000 acres a year. During the year 92,000 acres of land were acquired, including 64,100 acres of plantable land. The commission now controls 1,100,000 acres in Great Britain. The commission mainly plants conifers, principally because the demand for coniferous timber, called softwood, is about nine times the demand for hardwood, and the commission's policy is to afforest land of little agricultural value, which is generally unsuitable for hardwoods.

The year under review was one of the worst for forest fires, which burnt 2,100 acres of planted land and cost £39,900. The worst year on record was 1929, when the damage from fire amounted to £46,000.

Railways and the general public were mainly responsible.

The number of forest workers directly employed by the commission varied between 4,555 in the summer of 1938 and 5,395 in the following winter. Further forest workers' holdings, which have an average of 11 acres each, were established, and increased the total number of holdings to nearly 1,400.

Seven eighths of the woodland in Great Britain is privately owned. A census of all those woodlands of not less than five acres was started early in 1938, and will provide reliable information on the condition and contents of the woods in view of the importance of the reserves of standing timber for national defense.

The commissioners have continued to assist planting and direct sowing by local authorities and private owners by means of grants up to £2 an acre for conifers and up to £4 an acre for hardwoods, and by a proceeds sharing scheme. So far 120,000 acres have been planted privately with the aid of grants.

Enthusiastic use has been made of the camping grounds in the Argyll National Forest Park, opened to the public by the commissioners in 1936. The number of visitors who made use of the facilities provided there was 29,500, compared with 20,400 in the previous year. Progress has been made with plans for establishing the Snowdonia and Forest of Dean National Forest Parks. The Dean National Forest Park will be opened shortly.

## THE AUSTRALIAN METEORITE IN THE COLLECTION OF THE SMITHSONIAN INSTITUTION

A 2,000-POUND meteorite, probably a fragment of one of the largest to have struck the earth, has been added to the meteorite collection of the Smithsonian Institution. This specimen was found in 1903 near the town of Pearcedale, not far from Melbourne, Australia—the general area of the Cranbourne meteorite which was discovered in 1854.

The largest piece of the Cranbourne meteorite, weighing over three tons, is now in the British Museum; the second largest piece, weighing about one and a half tons, is in the Melbourne Museum. Smaller fragments are displayed in museums all over the world.

It is not known definitely whether this meteorite is actually a part of the Cranbourne fall, but according to E. P. Henderson, of the institution, it will probably prove to be so. That two separate meteoric falls of such large size would occur within such a limited area is quite improbable. The meteorite probably exploded in midair and fragments may be found some distance apart. It will shortly be placed on exhibition at the U. S. National Museum. A study will be made to determine its composition and relationships to the Cranbourne meteorite, which must be considered as one of the major collisions between the earth and a body from space. It is, however, said to be by no means the largest known meteorite.

Stony meteorites are more numerous than the iron variety, but all the largest falls, both as to size and weight, are iron meteorites. There are many scars upon the surface of the earth where meteorites have struck, notable among which is the great Meteor Crater in Arizona. The fall of 1908 which struck in northern Siberia produced a shock observed on seismographs far distant from the point of impact.

The Smithsonian has added thirty different falls to its collection so far this year. Most of these have been found in the United States. The Australian iron is by far the largest received this year, but several good-sized ones have come in from Chile and Mexico.

## THE PROPOSED INTER-AMERICAN UNIVERSITY IN PUERTO RICO

SECRETARY ICKES has made public the report of the commission appointed by President Roosevelt to make recommendations for the proposed establishment of an Inter-American University consisting of six graduate schools and research units grouped about the University of Puerto Rico, of which they would be an expansion but not an integral part.

The chairman of the commission was Dr. Isaiah Bowman, president of the Johns Hopkins University. Other members were Senator Elbert D. Thomas; Frank P. Graham, president of the University of North Carolina; David L. Crawford, president of the University of Hawaii; Dean Thomas E. Benner, of the University of Illinois; Alvin Johnson, director of the New School for Social Research, New York; Victor S. Clark, economic consultant, Library of Congress; Richard Pattee, of the Division of Cultural Relations of the State Department, and Max Radin, professor of law, University of California.

Of the six special service units recommended for inclusion in the program, one already is in existence. This is a School of Tropical Medicine, the increased support and enlargement of which is recommended, as well as its merger with the proposed organization.

The other units would be a Graduate School of Tropical Agriculture, a Graduate School of Economics and Business, an Institute of Languages, Literature and History of the Americas, an Institute of Law and a Tropical Fishery Research Laboratory.

These units would form the Inter-American Institution of the University of Puerto Rico. Their control as a group by a single board independent of the university is recommended, although an interlocking relationship between this board and the board of trustees of the university is suggested.

Virtually the entire burden of building and supporting the proposed institution must be borne outside of Puerto Rico, which already is contributing as much as it can toward maintenance of the present university.

Operating costs are estimated at about $1,250,000 a year after the institution "gets well under way," and during the first few years there would be in addition capital expenditures for erecting and equipping essential buildings.

Responsibility for the undertaking must be assumed chiefly by the United States Government, with as much assistance as possible from private foundations and individuals and from universities throughout the Americas.

## THE NEW YORK MEETING OF THE ELECTROCHEMICAL SOCIETY

THE seventy-sixth meeting of the Electrochemical Society, an international organization, will open at the Hotel Commodore, New York City, on Monday morning, September 11, and will continue through Wednesday evening, September 13.

The session on Monday morning, which is in charge of Professor Hiram S. Lukens, of the University of Pennsylvania, will be devoted to "Modern Methods in Electro Analysis." Experts in the field will describe how, with the aid of the electric current, accurate analyses can be carried out in a few minutes, as against hours consumed in ordinary chemical analysis. The Tuesday morning session on "Corrosion" is in charge of Dr. Robert B. Mears, of the Aluminum Company of America. No other subject is of more general and vital interest to both scientific men and engineers. Twelve papers will be presented covering the latest findings of research laboratories, including those of the National Bureau of Standards, the University of Cambridge, the Separator Laboratories of Stockholm, of Vienna, Berlin, Prague, Princeton, Pittsburgh and Philadelphia. The Wednesday morning session will cover electrochemical subjects of a general nature, including the electrometallurgy of lead, silver, nickel, manganese and arsenic and a paper on the cadmium-nickel storage battery.

Monday, September 11, has been set aside by the New York World's Fair as Electrochemical Day. In the afternoon Professor Bradley Stoughton, of Lehigh University, will give a popular illustrated address on "Modern Marvels of Electrometallurgy." The meeting will be held in the Science and Education Building at the World's Fair Grounds and will be open to the public. On Tuesday evening the Edward Goodrich Acheson Medal dinner will be given at the Hotel Commodore, when the Acheson Medal and $1,000 Prize will be presented to Dr. Francis Cowles Frary, director of the Research Laboratories of the Aluminum Company of America. Following the dinner and medal ceremonies there will be dancing.

## LECTURES AT THE DUNDEE MEETING OF THE BRITISH ASSOCIATION

AN extensive program of lectures was arranged for the Dundee meeting of the British Association for the Advancement of Science, the inaugural general meeting of which was held on the evening of August 30, when Sir Albert Seward delivered his presidential address. This is printed in the present issue of SCIENCE.

The evening lectures, several of which already have been announced, include:

*Saturday, September 2*

Public lecture by Dr. M. A. H. Tincker on "Science in Gardening—Making More Plants."

*Sunday, September 3*

Division for the Social and International Relations of Science. Address by Sir Richard Gregory, Bt., F.R.S., chairman of the division, on "Science and Social Ethics."

*Tuesday, September 5*

The British and American Association Lecture, being the first lecture under the arrangement concluded in 1938, between the British and the American Associations for the Advancement of Science, by which, in alternate years, an American speaker will address the British Association and a British speaker the American Association: Dr. Isaiah Bowman, president of the Johns Hopkins University, on "Science and Social Pioneering." A public lecture, at University College, by Dr. D. A. Spencer on "Some Aspects of Color Photography," is announced for the same evening.

In addition to lectures to be given before the association in Dundee public lectures have been arranged in neighboring places. These are:

*Arbreath*, September 1. Professor Allan Ferguson on "Splashes and What They Teach."

*Brechin*, September 5. Dr. G. B. Harrison on "Color Photography."

*Carnoustie*, September 5. Sir Gilbert Walker, F.R.S., on "The Dynamics of Sport."

*Cupar*, September 1. Professor J. L. Myres on "Nomadism."

*Dunfermline*, September 5. Professor W. T. Gordon on "Gem Stones."

*Forfar*, September 5. Sir John Russell, F.R.S., on "The Comparative Value of Organic as against Inorganic Manures."

*Montrose*, C. W. N. Lock on "The Work of the Aerodynamics Department of the National Physical Laboratory."

*Perth*, September 1. Dr. C. G. Darwin, F.R.S., on "Cold Temperatures."

*St. Andrews*, September 1. Dr. W. T. Calman, F.R.S., on "The British Museum (Natural History)."

A lecture for school children, illustrated by zoological films, will be given by Donald Alexander on September 5.

## RECENT DEATHS AND MEMORIALS

DR. ERNEST C. DICKSON, professor of public health and preventive medicine at the School of Medicine of Stanford University, San Francisco, died on August 23 at the age of fifty-eight years.

DR. MILTON A. BRIDGES, assistant professor of medicine in the New York Post-Graduate Medical School and Hospital, with which he had been associated since 1922, died on August 19 at the age of forty-five years.

DR. OTTO WOLFGANG WICHELHAUSEN, research bacteriologist in the Hospital of the Johns Hopkins University, died on August 14, at the age of thirty-five years.

PROFESSOR CHARLES PEABODY, formerly curator of European archeology at the Peabody Museum of Harvard University, died on August 17. He was in his seventy-second year.

DR. JAMES A. SHAW, director of the minerals division of the Conservation Department of Louisiana, died by suicide on August 20. Dr. Shaw was to have been a witness in the federal trial of former Governor Richard W. Leche and Seymour Weiss.

HENRY PARK HOLLIS, assistant at the Royal Observatory at Greenwich from 1881 to 1912, died on August 8 at the age of eighty-one years.

A CORRESPONDENT writes: "D. LeRoy Topping died on July 20 in Honolulu, after a long illness. He was born in North Harpersfield, N. Y., on November 2, 1861. Mr. Topping was interested in botanical field work, particularly in ferns, assembling large and important collections not only from various parts of the United States, but also in the Philippines, where he served for many years; in Siberia, where he served with the American Red Cross following the World War; in British North Borneo, particularly on Mount Kinabalu, and in the Hawaiian Islands, where he has lived since his retirement in 1922."

THE fiftieth anniversary of the death of Henry Shaw, who gave the Missouri Botanical (Shaw's) Garden and Tower Grove Park to the City of St. Louis, was commemorated on August 25, when a wreath was placed in the mausoleum at the garden where Shaw is buried. The ceremonies were conducted by Dr. George T. Moore, director. Henry Shaw was born in England and went to St. Louis in 1819. He established a hardware business from which he amassed a fortune. He died in 1889 at the age of eighty years. Mr. Shaw, after his retirement from business, established Shaw's Garden and provided for its maintenance in his will.

ACCORDING to *The New York Times,* the villa at Pontecchio, a small village near Bologna, where Marconi made his first experiments in radio transmission, has been presented by his heirs to the Guglielmo Marconi Foundation, created by Il Duce at the Royal Academy of Italy to perpetuate his memory. On the front of the house a monument will be erected. Inside relics will be preserved with documents concerning his inventions and of the technical and scientific progress derived from them. The memorial will be completed by next Marconi Day, April 25.

# SCIENTIFIC NOTES AND NEWS

DR. GERALD B. WEBB, research director of the Foundation for Research in Tuberculosis at Colorado Springs, received the Trudeau Medal of the National Tuberculosis Association during the annual meeting of the society in Boston, in recognition of his attempts "to produce specific immunity against tuberculosis by the inoculation of animals with very minute numbers of tubercle bacilli."

THE Ebert Prize for pharmaceutical research of the American Pharmaceutical Association has been awarded to Dr. B. V. Christensen, director of the University of Florida School of Pharmacy, in recognition of his paper on "biological assaying" presented at the 1938 convention of the association. Dr. Christensen will become director of the Ohio State School of Pharmacy at the opening of the academic year.

DR. GUSTAV EGLOFF has been elected a fellow of the Institute of Petroleum of London.

DR. LUDWIG JOST, professor of botany in the University of Heidelberg, has been awarded the Charles R. Barnes honorary life membership of the American Society of Plant Physiology.

DR. FRIEDRICH-KARL KLEINE, honorary professor of hygiene in the University of Berlin, known for his work on tropical diseases, has been awarded the shield of nobility of the German Reich.

THE University of Edinburgh has conferred the degree of doctor of laws on Dr. G. N. Watson, professor of mathematics at the University of Birmingham.

A DINNER in honor of Dr. Roy W. Wright, professor of surgery at the Medical School of the Louisiana State University, who has been elected director of the Charity Hospital, New Orleans, was given on August 24 by his colleagues and by leaders in business and education. A desk set was presented to him by Dr. Spencer B. McNair, chairman of the dinner committee, in behalf of the hospital staff. The speakers included Dr. C. C. Bass, retiring dean of the Medical School of Tulane University, and Dr. Maxwell Lapham, dean-elect; Dr.

Paul Hebert, acting president of Louisiana State University, and Governor Long.

DR. JAMES E. RICE, professor emeritus of poultry husbandry at Cornell University, was elected president of the World's Poultry Congress, which met in Cleveland, Ohio, from July 28 to August 7. He succeeds Karl Vetter, of Berlin.

SIR HAROLD BECKWITH WHITEHOUSE, Birmingham, was chosen president of the British Medical Association at the annual meeting in Aberdeen, and Dr. Thomas Fraser was installed as president. Sir Ernest Kaye Le Fleming, Wimborne, chairman of the council for several years, was elected a vice-president. Next year's meeting will be in Birmingham.

DR. DUNCAN GRAHAM, of Toronto, was made president-elect of the Canadian Medical Association at the recent Montreal meeting; Dr. Frank S. Patch, of Montreal, was installed as president. The next meeting will be in Toronto.

AT the eighteenth annual meeting of the Jesuit Science Association of the Eastern States, held at Fordham University on August 17 and 18, the following officers were elected: *President,* the Rev. John A. Tobin, S.J., head of the department of physics at Boston College; *Secretary,* the Rev. John J. Blandin, S.J., of Loyola College, Baltimore; *Treasurer,* the Rev. Francis W. Power, S.J., associate professor of chemistry at Fordham University.

LORD BERTRAND RUSSELL, philosopher and mathematician, who lectured last year at the University of Chicago, will be a member of the faculty of the University of California at Los Angeles during the present academic year.

DR. J. W. BUTLER, of the University of Edinburgh, has arrived in the United States. He will join the department of chemistry at Princeton University at the opening of the university this month.

DR. BRUNO ROSSI has been appointed research associate in the department of physics of the University of Chicago, where he will work with Professor Arthur H. Compton. The appointment has been made possible by a grant from the Emergency Committee in Aid of Displaced Foreign Scholars. Dr. Rossi was deprived of his professorship at the new Physical Institute of Padua by the government's decrees of September, 1938. For three years he had been in charge of planning and building the new institute and equipping it for research in atomic and nuclear physics.

DR. MARGARET HESS, head of the department of biology at Judson College, Marion, Ala., has been made head of the department of biology at Winthrop College, Rock Hill, S. C.

DR. GEORGE H. REED, of the University of Illinois, has been appointed associate professor of chemistry at Knox College.

DR. J. RIGNEY D'AUNOY has presented his resignation as dean of the Medical Center of the Louisiana State University. He will remain as professor of pathology and bacteriology, but will relinquish his position as chief pathologist and medical consultant at the Charity Hospital. In accepting the resignation Dr. Paul M. Hebert, acting president of the university, wrote in part, "I wish to express the appreciation of the university for the constructive accomplishments of your administration of the medical school."

DR. WILLIAM C. BAGLEY, professor of education at Teachers College, Columbia University, became on September 1 editor of SCHOOL AND SOCIETY, a weekly journal of education. He succeeds Dr. J. McKeen Cattell, who founded the journal in 1915 and has since edited it.

DR. THEODORE T. ZUCK, a member of the staff of the Brush Foundation, Cleveland, since its establishment in 1929, has been appointed director to succeed the late Dr. T. Wingate Todd.

AT the Armour Institute of Technology, Philip Conrad Huntley, professor of mechanical engineering and head of the department, has been appointed director of the civil engineering curriculum, and James Clinton Peebles, professor of experimental engineering and director of the insulation laboratory of the Research Foundation, has been appointed acting head of the department of mechanical engineering.

DR. ROBERT STUART TIPSON, research associate of the Rockefeller Institute for Medical Research, and Warner Carlson, who held a research fellowship during the past year in the Industrial Research Foundation at the Ohio State University, have been appointed fellows of the Mellon Institute in the department of research in pure chemistry.

DR. CHARLES V. AKIN, chief quarantine officer of the Port of New York since 1936, has been detailed as assistant surgeon general of the U. S. Public Health Service in charge of the division of sanitary reports and statistics.

DR. WILLIAM MALAMUD, professor of psychiatry at the College of Medicine of the State University of Iowa, has resigned to become clinical director and director of research at the Worcester State Hospital, Massachusetts.

DR. EMIL OTT, formerly assistant professor of chemistry at the Johns Hopkins University, has been appointed director of research of the Hercules Powder Company, with headquarters in Wilmington, Del. Since 1937 he has been at the head of the research department of the experiment station of the company.

DR. BERNARD L. OSER, who directs the work of the Food Research Laboratories, Inc., of New York City, in the field of biological assaying of vitamins, has been appointed vice-president of the laboratories.

BY an order of the Committee of the British Privy Council, made after consultation with the Medical Research Council and with the president of the Royal Society, Dr. A. J. Clark, professor of materia medica in the University of Edinburgh, and Dr. T. R. Elliott, emeritus professor of medicine in the University of London and consulting physician to University College Hospital, have been appointed members of the Medical Research Council in succession to Professor H. S. Raper and Professor J. A. Ryle, who retire in rotation on September 30.

DR. ROBERT S. LIVINGSTON, associate professor of physical chemistry at the University of Minnesota, who has been working for the past year with Dr. Frank at the University of Chicago under a fellowship awarded from the Lalor Foundation, has returned from an extended European trip, during which he visited the chief centers of research in physical chemistry in England and on the continent.

DR. CHRISTOPHER H. ANDREWES, a member of the British Medical Research Council, gave a series of lectures at the Medical School of the University of Wisconsin from July 25 to 28, under the auspices of the Wisconsin Alumni Research Foundation. His subjects were: "The Nature and Properties of Viruses," "Viruses in Relation to New Growths," "Recent Work in Influenza" and "Immunity in Influenza and Other Virus Infections."

THE fifth annual meeting of the Canadian Physiological Society will be held at Queen's University, Kingston, Ontario, on Friday and Saturday, November 3 and 4.

AUSTIN WRIGHT, the general secretary of the British-American Engineering Congress, which was to have met from September 4 to 8 in New York City, reports that a cable has been received from England, announcing that British delegates have cancelled reservations to sail and that the congress will not be held. A hundred and eighty delegates from England and two hundred and fifty from Canada were expected to attend.

APPLICATIONS must be on file with the United States Civil Service Commission at Washington, D. C., for the position of associate physical oceanographer, Treasury Department, at $3,200 a year, not later than September 18. An open competitive examination to fill an existing vacancy at Woods Hole, Mass., and future vacancies that may occur in positions requiring similar qualifications will be filled from this examination, unless it is found in the interest of the service to fill any vacancy by reinstatement, transfer or promotion. Applications must also be on file on September 18 for positions with the Children's Bureau, U. S. Department of Labor, and the U. S. Public Health Service, Federal Security Agency, of psychologist with a salary of $3,800 a year; of associate psychologist, $3,200 a year, and of assistant psychologist, $2,600 a year.

THE firm of Messrs. P. Blakiston's Son and Company, Inc., specializing in scientific and medical books, has been purchased from the estate of Kenneth M. Blakiston by Horace G. White, executive vice-president of the firm. The business was established in 1843 by Presley Blakiston and was continuously in the Blakiston family until the death of Kenneth M. Blakiston in 1937. It will now be carried on under the name The Blakiston Company. Mr. White will be president of the company; Charles C. Norris, Jr., and Robert F. Bowman, vice-presidents; Edmund J. Glaser, treasurer, and Edward B. Barnes, secretary.

GROUND was broken recently for a new building for the Institute of Therapeutic Research of Merck and Company, Rahway, N. J. It is reported in *Industrial and Engineering Chemistry* that the building will be constructed of brick and concrete in a colonial design to harmonize with the research laboratory and administration buildings. It will have three stories and basement and will be 47 feet wide and 100 feet long. The entire second floor will be air-conditioned. The building will contain equipment for studies of the circulatory, nervous and respiratory systems by means of electrocardiograph, x-ray, cathode ray oscillograph, etc.; facilities for housing and feeding several thousand small animals for nutrition studies and investigation of the action of vitamins, synthetic drugs, etc.; and offices and laboratories for the staff of about twenty-eight workers.

To prevent unnecessary duplication of research and to coordinate work in the future, the paper industry has undertaken a cooperative program which will contribute to better control of sanitation in the manufacture of paper, the establishment of sanitation standards, the development of methods of analysis to accompany such standards and cooperation with health agencies. This coordinated program, to be administered through the American Paper and Pulp Association, will relate, it is hoped, investigations now in progress and suggest the trend of new experiments. The association has enlisted the Institute of Paper Chemistry to carry on the fundamental work prerequisite to the establishment of standard technics and to expand through the use of these technics the understanding of sanitary problems involved in the manufacture and conversion of paper to be used in the packaging of foods. Acting with the institute in an advisory capacity will be Dr. Fred W. Tanner, professor of bacteriology at the University of Illinois. Dr. Tanner and the institute will work closely with a special committee of experts from the paper industry.

A CORRESPONDENT from Cannes of the London *Times* writes that at St. Michel de Provence, on the plateau of Aurifeuille, five miles from Forcalquier, a new observatory has been built which is not only the largest but the most favorably placed climatically in Europe. The site, which is at an altitude of over 2,000 feet, was decided upon after ten years of research. The 80-inch telescope at present in service at the Paris Observatory will be transported there. The observatory and the buildings attached have been designed in the Provençal style of architecture. They owe their existence to the initiative of M. Jean Perrin, who secured the financial backing while he was Under-Secretary of State for Scientific Research.

# DISCUSSION

## CONDITIONS AND OPPORTUNITIES AT THE NAPLES ZOOLOGICAL STATION

JUST a few years ago there were a number of American subscriptions to tables in the Stazione Zoologica di Napoli, but at the present time apparently there is only one—that of the National Research Council to which subscription was first made for the year beginning July 1, 1938. The fact that up to this time no applications for this table have been received may perhaps be attributed to distrust of conditions in Europe at the present time, or it may be that merely by chance the year has been one in which the need of American biologists for the facilities and materials of foreign stations has been at a temporary minimum. It has been thought, too, that with some persons there might be uncertainty as to the normality of operation of the laboratory. In reply to an inquiry addressed to Dr. Dohrn, director of the station, he has written, giving information that may be of interest to American biologists in general. He says:

It is quite natural that there should be some apprehension over things as they stand at present. However, during the past and the current year biologists have come to work in Naples from all parts of Europe, and, what is more, they have been able to work in an atmosphere of almost unruffled calm, and certainly one of happiness and contentment. It is therefore a great pity that this apprehension should not have been overridden. The presence here of American biologists is always a welcome addition to the body of workers with us and a most effective means for securing continued cooperative relations between biologists of our two countries.

However, it seems to me quite as possible that the fundamental trouble is lack of knowledge of the Stazione Zoologica in America, and of the facilities that it offers. Probably, too, some knowledge of the present activities of the Station would serve as a stimulus to American biologists, and to this end I am enclosing a list of the more important figures of the scientific world who have worked here during the past year, with a note appended to each of the subjects under investigation.

As to facilities it is, I suppose, natural to stress the quantity and variety of living material obtainable at Naples. Then there is the excellence of the conditions under which organisms can be kept in captivity in the Station and, no less important, the conditions under which the biologist himself may work. I am enclosing two leaflets which will perhaps do something to illustrate the extent of the apparatus and supply of reagents which are available to all. Finally we have here at Naples one of the richest biological libraries in the world for scientific periodicals, journals and abstracts; this is of eminent value to the research worker who has constantly to refer to literature relevant to his work.

I would also like to emphasize the value of foreign experience for the young American biologist, especially in reference to the contact which he can thus make with techniques and scientific ideas of European biologists, with the human element of the contact by no means the least important. As a sideline, too, I might perhaps mention the excellent opportunity for picking up a working knowledge of Italian and German, while working at Naples. Lastly, what perhaps requires no words of mine to stress is the beauty of Naples and of its environs.

You suggested very kindly in your letter to me that you could perhaps do something to give publicity to a few of the things I have mentioned about work at the Stazione Zoologica. I hope and think that this would improve the possibility of our seeing Americans working here next year, and for this reason I trust most sincerely that you can do so. If there should be any further details which you would like me to let you have, I shall be only too glad to forward them.

I cannot close this letter without thanking you once more for the special kindness and thought that you have shown to the Station, and I do most sincerely hope that we may soon return to the conditions of fruitful cooperation so valuable in the past. I shall be very thankful for anything that you can do to help bring about such a situation.

Sincerely yours,

/s/ PROF. R. DOHRN

The lists to which Dr. Dohrn refers, an extended inventory of more recently acquired biological and physical apparatus and rolls of leading investigators from many countries, predominantly British and German, engaged in work at the station in 1938 and the early part of 1939 are, of course, available for consultation in the office of the Council in Washington.

R. E. COKER

NATIONAL RESEARCH COUNCIL,
WASHINGTON, D. C.

## ONE-MAN AUTHORITY CITATIONS

THE recent agitation on the subject of citation of authorities in botanical nomenclature[1] is being so prolonged that it seems advisable to review the various attacks on the existing system along the line of a comparison of the present degree of efficiency with that which might be expected from the various proposals.

Clausen's very clear reply[2] to Peattie's argument indicates that the principle of authority omission is not attractive to the practicing taxonomist. The subsequent papers by Jacot and by Baily, though agreeing with Peattie in the proposal to dispense, totally or in part, with authority citation, do not agree on the method or system to be substituted. Apparently no one is able to suggest a system sufficiently attractive to win agreement from his fellow critics of the existing method.

Dr. Samuel Johnson's oft-quoted remark is called to mind: "Every other author may aspire to praise, the lexicographer can only hope to escape reproach." The same is true of taxonomists working in any field of biology. If they are too conservative and too ready to allow variations to creep into their concept of this species or that, they are speedily made aware of the fact by the non-systematic biologist for whom they are engaged in making identifications. If, on the other hand, their species concepts are narrow and result in more numerous and less readily recognized species (no matter how sound taxonomically), they are again assailed. In short, the work of taxonomists is a service rendered to the general field of biology and as such is subject to attack from all sides, and the taxonomists must regard their productions as tools in the hands of other workers and fashion them accordingly.

On the other hand, the general field seems not to realize the urgent need in the field of taxonomy for an unfailing system of bibliographic citation, nor to appreciate the difficulties of setting in order an exceedingly complex group which has been dabbled in by a dozen taxonomists in the past two centuries and subjected to as many species concepts. (Though perhaps not in the case of this controversy, the objections to authority citation on any ground whatsoever usually have come from biologists other than taxonomists.)

Peattie (*loc. cit.*, p. 128) cited some very excellent arguments *against* his own proposal of omission of authorities, and his rebuttal of these arguments can hardly be regarded as complete. They need further examination:

(1) "The original author is deprived of credit." Of this Peattie says the purpose of authorities is not to give credit but to lead the reader to the original description. With that statement every botanist would agree; it constitutes strong argument in favor of retaining authority citations. It makes little difference to any of us if, a hundred years from now, our names remain attached to our new species and combinations, but for some reason it matters greatly whether or not those species are recognizable to the next several generations.

(2) "The one-man citation might encourage name-jugglers to attach their names to everything." Peattie points out the "remarkable activities" in this field of Kuntze and Greene in spite of two-man citation. The fact that two-man citation allows as much juggling as one-man citation is hardly an argument for the superiority of one-man citation. It is unbelievable that any botanist would fail to transfer a species from one genus to another if it obviously fit better by being changed. So long as there remain species in the wrong genera, they need to be changed, no matter whose name is attached. Actually, taxonomists are highly appreciative of the drudgery which Kuntze and Greene performed in making new combinations for the sake of accuracy.

(3) One-man citations "conceal the history of the species." Peattie wants to know "why, except in elaborate taxonomic work, should it be revealed?" It is doubtful that any biologist would admit that his work need be less accurate than that of taxonomists. If it is objectionable to a worker to reveal the history of the species he cites, he can not care much if his species names are recognizable in the next century. The history of a species often shows clearly whether one or another interpretation of the name is meant. In any study, such as host-parasite relations, ecology, physiology and genetics, in which exact identity of species and varieties is of extreme importance, complete citation of authorities facilitates subsequent identification.

The efforts of taxonomists to meet the demands of biology with a workable classification of the thousands of existing species have resulted in the building up amongst most workers of the type concept for reference purposes. That this practice is not only practical but essential is readily demonstrated in the genus *Quercus*. Even by means of modern lengthy and detailed descriptions it is in many cases quite impossible so to characterize a species that it can be recognized by subsequent workers. Linnaeus described *Quercus rubra* in the eastern United States. Du Roi misunderstood the description and applied the name to what is now known as *Q. maxima* (Marshall) Ashe. He was followed in that by numerous authors. When subsequently it was discovered that Linnaeus' name had been meant to apply to what had been known as *Q. falcata* Michaux, an attempt was made to apply the name correctly. However, so many authors were using the name to designate the more northern *Q. maxima* that

[1] SCIENCE, 88: 128, August 5, 1938; 240, September 9, 1938; 474, November 18, 1938.

[2] SCIENCE, 88: 299, September 30, 1938.

complete misunderstanding resulted, so that Professor Rehder has recently moved to abandon the name *rubra* and allow both species to carry the names subsequently proposed for them. How much difficulty and misunderstanding might have been eliminated, had there been a type specimen to help du Roi avoid his initial error, one can only guess.

No one, it is hoped, would suggest that taxonomists abandon the type system. Yet, the system would be greatly hampered by the suggested omission of one or the other of the authority citations. Full citation tells a taxonomist at a glance that at least two treatments are available, and he invariably needs to study both, unless he wishes to run the risk of perpetuating the many errors which have not yet been weeded out of botanical nomenclature. The first citation in most cases aids to fix the type. The second reveals a critical study of the species, which may or may not be accurate. To omit either would be as serious an error as the omission of a citation from the card catalogue of the Congressional Library.

Jacot (*loc. cit.*, p. 240) places undue faith in existing monographs. His suggestion that the name of the monographer giving the fullest description be cited would result in the greatest confusion. With the adoption of such a rule one could imagine every describer of a new species writing descriptions so ample that each one would cover several pages. There still remain thousands of species which have not been fully described in any monograph but were recognized beyond doubt from their original descriptions and subsequently have been changed from one genus to another. Which authority would one cite under Jacot's proposal in such a case? Jacot's notion that the old original descriptions and the authorities for them are of no practical value but only of historic value is dangerous in extreme. Ecologists, morphologists, geneticists, etc., perhaps do not realize that each of the species with which they deal is painstakingly run through the mill of "ancient" descriptions by some modern taxonomist before he dares drop it into the lap of his biological public. Only so can he be sure that he is contributing to a reasonably sound nomenclature. It is not for nothing that each succeeding International Botanical Congress has carefully revised the code of nomenclature in an effort to guide its constituent membership to greater stability.

Baily (*loc. cit.*, p. 474) charges that authority citation "augments the confusion instead of diminishing it." He cites the example of Solander's species which were published in Dillwyn's catalogue. It is easy to add numerous other examples, such as Duval's species in A. De Candolle's Prodromus. The accepted method of citation under those circumstances is "Solander in Dillwyn," "Duval in A. De Candolle" or the proper abbreviations of those names. Either method permits ready reference to the original description, particularly with the aid of Index Kewensis.

Baily recognizes the prime importance of determining the original identity of a plant name and proposes setting up a periodical to function as a receptacle for the authority citations, synonyms, etc., which so many workers wish to omit from their writings. He does not state why the Index Kewensis and the Gray Herbarium Index do not amply fill our needs, and it is not at all apparent how any other form of index could be more helpful.

It would be interesting, however, to learn how the exponents of authority omission would propose to locate in any index some of the names they might encounter. For instance, *Quercus hypoleuca* might conceivably be recommended to our nurserymen as a desirable ornamental. Without further information the nurserymen would refer to Baily's proposed periodical, where they would find *Q. hypoleuca* Engelmann credited to the American Southwest. But there is also the earlier published and quite different *Q. hypoleuca* Miquel in southern Asia. The American species is known under the present system as *Q. hypoleucoides* A. Camus. Its synonym is cited as *Q. hypoleuca* Engelmann, not Miquel. How could this information be furnished without the use of authors' names?

Even under the present system too many errors and misunderstandings arise. These certainly can not be diminished by the adoption by taxonomists of a more lax system. In fact, in the interest of an ideal of accuracy, complete authority citation (and the citation of any other information which might be helpful in subsequent identification) should be practiced by non-taxonomic botanists as well. Unfortunately, an appalling proportion of these do not even bother to collect or preserve specimens for identification.

CORNELIUS H. MULLER

BUREAU OF PLANT INDUSTRY

## SPRAYING WITH PLANT GROWTH SUBSTANCES TO PREVENT APPLE FRUIT DROPPING

ORCHARDISTS need no introduction to the subject of late fruit dropping, a trouble which occurs with many apple varieties and other fruits just prior to and during harvest time and which annually results in substantial losses. For those less familiar with the problems of apple growing, for instance, it may be stated that this tendency of the fruit to drop is, in general, a characteristic of early ripening varieties, but is also of frequent occurrence with a number of important midseason and late apples. As the fruit approaches the proper maturity and color for harvesting, the danger of loss from dropping becomes more and more acute. With varieties susceptible to this trouble, each day that the fruit is allowed to remain on the tree to attain these desirable market qualities becomes a gamble with fate. With some varieties, Stayman Winesap, for example, a disastrous drop may, without warning, occur almost overnight. On the other hand, McIntosh, a notorious dropper in many fruit sections, may fall steadily for several weeks prior to harvest time.

It is well known that climate and weather influence fruit dropping and are therefore important factors determining the feasibility of growing certain varieties in a given region. It is conceivable that elimination of the danger of dropping, in addition to safeguarding those varieties which consistently show this characteristic, may also widen the growing range of certain others, which drop badly only in the more southern regions.

Most of the commercial so-called plant growth substances have the propensity, in varying degrees, of delaying the normal abscission of various plant organs. Among a number of these substances tested naphthalene acetic acid and naphthalene acetamide have been reported[1, 2, 3] as being particularly effective in delaying the abscission of flowers of the date and holly, in the latter case, resulting in parthenocarpy. The frequent observance of the effect of these compounds in delaying the abscission of floral structures, stems and also of petioles on treated cuttings led to the attempt to apply them in a practical way to the problem of apple fruit dropping by spraying the trees. The results to date have been more than gratifying.

Thus far, trees of seven varieties, including Yellow Transparent, Williams Early Red, Oldenburg, Early McIntosh, Wealthy and three new early varieties, as yet unnamed, have been sprayed with various concentrations of the growth substances and a record obtained of the percentage of the total crop dropping from the trees over a period of time in comparison with the drop from untreated trees. Naphthalene acetic acid and naphthalene acetamide applied just prior to fruit maturity have proved to be particularly effective with all the varieties thus far treated. In addition to these two substances, indole acetic and indole butyric acids have been used, although the indications are that these indole compounds are much less effective in preventing abscission than either of the two naphthalene compounds.[4]

In the first experiments much stronger concentrations were used than are now proving to be necessary. Williams Early Red, as an outstanding example, was sprayed with .001 percentage of naphthalene acetic acid on July 13. By July 25 the unsprayed control trees had dropped from 64.2 to 90.8 per cent. of their total crop on actual fruit count, whereas the sprayed trees had dropped only from 1.3 to 1.5 per cent. of their fruit. Concentrations of .00025 per cent. on other varieties have since been found to bring about very marked inhibition of dropping. The effectiveness of some of these compounds in such dilute concentrations would definitely recommend their usage as a practical orchard procedure. Their practicability becomes enhanced if the present indications, that they can be added to the regular spray schedule, are borne out by additional experiments.

It is anticipated that a detailed account of the experiments will be issued in the near future when the results are compiled on additional experiments, now underway, related to various practical phases of application. This brief report, it is hoped, may serve to call to the attention of other investigators the possibility of using these compounds to advantage in the numerous problems involving the abscission of various other fruits and plant organs.

F. E. GARDNER
P. C. MARTH
L. P. BATJER
U. S. HORTICULTURAL STATION,
BUREAU OF PLANT INDUSTRY,
BELTSVILLE, MD.

[1] *Bot. Gaz.*, 99: 184–195, 1937.
[2] *Ibid.*, 100: 868–871, 1939.
[3] F. E. Gardner and P. C. Marth, *Bot. Gaz.*, 101: No. 1, 1939.
[4] Acknowledgment is made to Franklin D. Jones, of the American Chemical Paint Company, Ambler, Pa., for supplying in generous quantities all the compounds used in this work.

## "DISTINCTION" IN "SCIENCE"

ACCORDING to a news item in the *Herald-Tribune* for July 19, 1939, the Postmaster General, James A. Farley, has authorized the issuance of a special series of postage stamps in honor of Americans who have "achieved fame" in the arts and sciences. The list of scientists chosen for this honor is as follows: Luther Burbank, Dr. Crawford W. Long, Dr. Walter Reed, John James Audubon and Jane Addams.

The official news release of the Postoffice Department stated that the stamps are to honor "famous Americans who have achieved outstanding distinction in the arts and sciences." "Outstanding distinction" from what source? Without intending the least disparagement of the services rendered by the Postoffice "scientists," Heaven help us if this list of names is a true index of the public's understanding and evaluation of what science is and of scientific accomplishment in the United States.

One can not help wondering who the committee was, if any, that made the selection of "scientists." Certainly it could not have been referred to either the American Association for the Advancement of Science, or the National Academy of Sciences, which is the official adviser to the Government in such matters.

C. STUART GAGER
BROOKLYN BOTANIC GARDEN,
JULY 24, 1939.

# SPECIAL CORRESPONDENCE

## RESEARCH IN VENEZUELA

THE activities of three previous Scarritt Expeditions of the American Museum of Natural History have previously been reported in this journal.[1] The general program of these expeditions and of the related office and laboratory work has been to contribute to knowledge of fossil mammals of North and South America and of the relationships between them. This program has been continued and broadened by recent work in Venezuela, under the direction of the writer, as were the three earlier expeditions. The Venezuelan work has been a cooperative undertaking between the American Museum of Natural History and the Venezuelan Government, through the Ministry of Fomento (development and exploitation), under the Minister, Dr. Manuel R. Egaña, that ministry defraying all field expenses and the museum paying costs of transportation and of preparation and study of materials. The museum's participation was made possible by continued sponsorship of Mr. H. S. Scarritt, of New York.

Field work in Venezuela developed into two distinct major expeditions and two reconnaissance trips. The first objective, reached in September, 1938, was the vicinity of Barquisimeto, in the State of Lara, in western Venezuela. Here Brother Nectario María, a teacher in the local Salesian school, had made several important and interesting discoveries of Pleistocene mammals. With his cooperation a camp was established about thirty miles southwest of Barquisimeto, near the village of San Miguel, and numerous fossil prospects were examined. These proved disappointing at first, but a new locality was soon found which turned out to be by far the richest deposit of fossil mammals yet known between Argentina and the United States. With the help of numerous local workmen, who proved to be unexpectedly intelligent and energetic, a large quarry was opened and this has been worked almost continuously, except for an interval of heavy rains, from October to the present time. Modern methods of extracting fragile and broken bones were employed for the first time in Venezuela, and native workmen were trained in these methods, a result which may mean even more for the future of vertebrate paleontology in Venezuela than do the collections already made.

This quarry has yielded almost innumerable bones of fossil mammals, with many jaws and at least two skulls. It is anticipated that the materials already in hand will permit the assembling and mounting of several essentially complete large skeletons. Most of the material belongs to still unidentified and probably new species of megatheres and toxodonts, with more fragmentary remains of several other groups.

[1] SCIENCE, 80: 2070, 207–208, August 31, 1934; 83: 2140, 13–14, January 3, 1936.

When the work here was well advanced and the men had become skilled in the collection of bones under these conditions, the San Miguel Quarry was left in charge of Brother Nectario, and a reconnaissance trip was made into the great llanos (plains) region south of Caracas, broad areas of which are underlain by middle and later Tertiary sediments. North of Zaraza, at a locality where the well-known geologist, Dr. Peter Christ, had already collected an important astrapothere jaw, the nearly complete carapace of a new fossil turtle was collected. With the cooperation of geologists working for the Standard Oil Company, two other promising prospects in the Miocene were located in this general region. There is every reason to hope that quarrying of these localities and more intensive search of the scattered and generally poor exposures will yield important fossil mammals, turtles and crocodiles.

A second reconnaissance, in April, 1939, was made into the higher Venezuelan Andes, as far as Mérida. In the vicinity of Valera deposits of fossil mammals, probably of late Tertiary age, were exactly located for future work. Even aside from strictly paleontological aspects, these promise to be exceptionally valuable because they are in the youngest beds definitely folded in the Andine orogeny and hence will serve to date the end of this activity.

Between these two reconnaissance trips, the writer and his wife accompanied a large Venezuelan expedition to the southern part of the country. This expedition, the Comisión Exploradora de la Gran Sabana, was one of two organized this year by the Ministry of Fomento to explore and map parts of the enormous and very poorly known Venezuelan Guayana, the great area south and east of the Orinoco, mainly inhabited by uncivilized Indians. At various times the expedition included three geologists and topographers, a mining engineer, a medical doctor, two astronomers, a soil expert, a colonization expert, an airplane pilot and a mechanic, and numerous assistants and native workmen. The writer and his wife worked with the expedition for about six weeks as naturalists. The general results of the extensive and excellent work done by this party will later be made public by its organizers and experts in other fields, and in the present note only brief mention will be made of our own results.

The first and principal base camp was established by airplane transport in Camarata, the broad open valley south of Auyantepuy, a large mountain about 300 kilometers south—southeast of Cuidad Bolívar on the Orinoco. Here, as was anticipated, no fossils of any sort were found, but during the month spent there we made collections of recent mammals and plants as well as very detailed study of the Kamarakoto Indians, a poorly known and hitherto unstudied Carib group which preserves most of its aboriginal culture intact. From here we flew to Santa Elena, a mission station near the Brazilian border in the region of Mount Roroimá.[2] Since the Indians of this region are very, and the flora and fauna fairly well-known, we spent only about ten days here, obtaining comparative observations for the study of our Camarata materials.

During all the work in Venezuela the writer was accompanied by his wife, Dr. Anne Roe Simpson, who collected mainly recent mammals for the museum and ran our camp when we were working independently.

Except for the botanical collections, which will remain in Caracas for study and preservation, all the material collected, paleontological, mammalogical and ethnological, will be sent to New York for preparation and study, which has already begun as regards part of it. When this is completed, the collections will be divided between New York and Caracas, where they will form the nucleus of a national collection of fossil vertebrates. The results already obtained show that Venezuela is a very promising and still almost untouched field for such studies.

GEORGE GAYLORD SIMPSON
THE AMERICAN MUSEUM OF NATURAL HISTORY

# SCIENTIFIC BOOKS

## MALARIA IN PANAMA

*Malaria in Panama.* By Lieutenant Colonel J. S. SIMMONS, Medical Corps, U. S. Army with the collaboration of Lieutenant Colonel G. R. Callender, Medical Corps, U. S. Army; Major D. P. Curry, Medical Reserve Corps, U. S. Army; Lieutenant Colonel S. C. Schwartz, Medical Corps, U. S. Army, and Lieutenant Colonel R. Randall, Veterinary Corps, U. S. Army. *The American Journal of Hygiene,* Monographic Series No. 13. The Johns Hopkins Press, Baltimore, 1939. $1.10 net, postpaid.

WORKERS in public health, tropical medicine and parasitology, in general, and in malariology, in particular, welcome source books regarding malaria in any region. The present volume is particularly important because it deals with Panama, a region of outstanding importance in the development of methods of malaria control and yet one which is often misunderstood.

The book is divided into three main sections. Part 1, which deals with malaria on the Isthmus from 1501 to 1938, gives in one chapter a most interesting series of notes on the history of the disease and in another an account of the present distribution of malaria in the Republic of Panama. Part 2 is a more detailed consideration of malaria in the Canal Zone from 1904 to 1938. Its seven chapters give information of the utmost importance on various geographic features, meteorology, Health Department and vital statistics of the Zone; malaria among the canal employees; malaria carriers in the Zone, Anopheline mosquitoes, and sanitary methods used for the control of malaria in the Zone. Part 3 is concerned with malaria in the military forces on the Zone and in four chapters considers malaria among U. S. troops; distribution among the various military posts; factors concerned in the relatively high incidence of the disease among the troops, and an evaluation of methods used to control the disease among the troops.

Each chapter is a compendium of material taken from a wide variety of sources, including many official records and results of the authors' own research. Much of this material is stated in synoptic form, but at the end of most chapters a concise, readable comment is given. Finally, there is a terminal résumé in which the authors give their main conclusions in five pages. With such a mass of detail it is possible to select only a few conclusions of general interest.

According to the available data, malaria seems to have been common on the Isthmus for several centuries, and recent surveys show conclusively that the disease is widely spread in all the provinces of the Republic of Panama. This wide-spread distribution serves as a reservoir of potential infection for the sanitated regions. At the present time the sanitated areas are situated chiefly around the terminals of the Canal (including the cities of Colon and Panama in the Republic) and the locks. In these locations most of the Canal employees, military forces and their families are concentrated. Elsewhere on the Zone, where there is no anti-mosquito work or general sanitation, the employees are furnished with thoroughly screened quarters. Within the sanitated areas, the records are conclusive in showing that control measures have been effective in reducing the incidence of the disease among the employees since 1904, when Gorgas, Carter, LePrince and their associates arrived on the Zone. At the same time they also show why, even with the extensive resources at hand, it has been impossible to control the breeding of *Anopheles* in many bodies of water and why it has proved possible to sanitate only relatively small areas near the principal towns occupied by employees and around military posts. For example, Gatun Lake presents a tremendous problem, since from it mosquitoes can apparently fly into the sanitated areas at certain times of the year. This 165-square-mile lake, built as a necessary part of the high level lockage system of the Panama Canal, is relatively shallow, and vast areas of it harbor aquatic plants. These plants, especially in the dry season, are exposed in surface mats level with the water's surface and appear to be ideal breeding places for *Anopheles albimanus* and *A. albitarsis.* The former appears to be the chief malarial vector. No satisfactory means of controlling the growth of

[2] Widely, but incorrectly, publicized as Roraima.

these plants and of the mosquitoes breeding among them have, as yet, been devised. The detailed descriptions of the sanitary methods used for the control of malaria in the Zone will be of particular interest to students of malaria. Chief reliance has been placed on screening and on reducing mosquitoes by larvicides, by drainage and by filling. The situation among the troops stationed on the Canal Zone is noteworthy. Although malaria has declined among them since 1911, when they were first stationed on the Zone, the morbidity rates are higher than among the civilian employees of the Canal or among U. S. troops stationed elsewhere. Inasmuch as the barracks are located in well-sanitated areas, the authors believe the higher rate to be due to infection at night during official and unofficial visits in the Republic of Panama, in unsanitated areas of the Zone and, even to a certain extent, in sanitated areas of the Zone.

The entire book is written from the standpoint of the most up-to-date conception of malarial control and leaves little room for criticism. One disappointing feature is the untrustworthy nature of the older records—which is obviously no fault of the authors. The book, besides supplying a much needed source book on Panama, is another demonstration of the difficulty of controlling malaria in the tropics at a reasonable cost and the imperative need of further research. It is to be hoped that the various agencies carrying on research in the Republic of Panama and the Canal Zone will continue their excellent work.

W. H. TALIAFERRO

UNIVERSITY OF CHICAGO

# SOCIETIES AND MEETINGS

## THE NORTH CAROLINA ACADEMY OF SCIENCE

THE thirty-eighth annual meeting of the North Carolina Academy of Science was held at Wake Forest College, N. C., on May 5 and 6. About 250 members and visitors attended the meeting. Seventy-three papers and several exhibits made up the program.

The general section met the first day with the president, John W. Lasley, Jr., presiding. This meeting consisted mostly of the reading of papers of general interest and continued, except for the luncheon hour, till 4:30 P.M., when the annual business meeting was held.

At the business meeting reports of the various committees were called for. The executive committee reported the election of 33 new members and the reinstatement of 6 former members. The losses in membership were reported as follows: from non-payment of dues, 12 members; from resignation, 2 members; from death, 1 member. The committee announced the acceptance of the invitation from Davidson College to hold the thirty-ninth annual meeting at Davidson, N. C., in 1940. The committee also recommended that H. B. Arbuckle, department of chemistry, Davidson College, and W. C. Coker, department of botany, the University of North Carolina, be made life members.

The committee on high-school science reported that in the essay contest sponsored by the academy, first prize for 1939 had been awarded to Alfred Gallant, of the Central High School, Charlotte, N. C., for his essay entitled "Quartz Crystals for Radio Transmitters." The committee also reported the nomination of Ralph Kiser, Central High School, Charlotte, and Miss Eugenia Cox, Old Town High School, Winston-Salem, for junior membership in the American Association for the Advancement of Science.

In the report of the conservation committee resolutions were presented as follows: (1) that the Conservation Committee of the North Carolina Academy cooperate with the Virginia Academy "to arrange and carry out such cooperation as may be of mutual benefit to the two academies in the proposed study of the Dismal Swamp Area"; (2) that the two areas which make up the "Primeval Forest" at Highlands, N. C., be preserved and that, therefore, the U. S. Forest Service and the National Forest Reservation Commission be urged to acquire this tract immediately and add it to the Nantahala National Forest.

The committee of the American Association for the Advancement of Science research grant reported that the grant for 1939 had been awarded to F. H. McCutcheon, department of zoology, North Carolina State College, for use in his "investigation of possible experimentally induced seasonal variations in the oxygen affinity of hemoglobin in mammals."

The committee on the academy medal reported that the 1939 medal had been awarded to F. H. McCutcheon, department of zoology, North Carolina State College, for his paper entitled "The Respiratory Mechanism of the Grasshopper."

The following officers of the academy were elected for 1940: *President,* H. L. Blomquist, Duke University; *Vice-president,* John N. Couch, the University of North Carolina; *Secretary-Treasurer* (three years), Bert Cunningham, Duke University; *Member of the Executive Committee,* Earl H. Hall, Woman's College of the University of North Carolina; *Representative to the Academy Conference and the Council of the A. A. A S.,* Bert Cunningham, Duke University.

After the reading of a memorial report honoring

the late Henry van Peters Wilson, the business meeting adjourned.

At 8:30 P.M. the evening meeting was held with the vice-president, Donald B. Anderson, presiding. After a brief address of welcome by Dean Bryan, of Wake Forest College, President John W. Lasley, Jr., gave his retiring address entitled "The Relation between Mathematics and the Sciences."

On Saturday afternoon the academy met in the following sections: General, Botany, Mathematics, Physics, Zoology, The North Carolina Section of the American Chemical Society and the High School Science Teachers.

The following officers were elected by the various sections:

ZOOLOGY SECTION

*Chairman:* J. P. Givler, Woman's College, University of North Carolina.
*Secretary:* Z. P. Metcalf, North Carolina State College.

MATHEMATICS SECTION

*Chairman:* T. F. Hickerson, University of North Carolina.
*Secretary:* J. A. Greenwood, Duke University.

PHYSICS SECTION

*Chairman:* H. E. Fulcher, Davidson College.
*Secretary:* F. W. Lancaster, North Carolina State College.

NORTH CAROLINA SECTION OF THE AMERICAN CHEMICAL SOCIETY

*Chairman:* E. C. Markham, University of North Carolina.
*Vice-Chairman:* W. E. Jordan, North Carolina State College.
*Secretary-Treasurer:* Ivan D. Jones, North Carolina State College.

HIGH SCHOOL SCIENCE TEACHERS

*Chairman:* Clifford Beck, Salisbury, N. C.
*Secretary:* Harry MacDonald, New Bern, N. C.

H. L. BLOMQUIST,
*Secretary*

# SPECIAL ARTICLES

## CHEMICAL COMPOSITION OF THE TUMOR-PRODUCING FRACTION OF CHICKEN TUMOR I

THE agent transmitting chicken tumor I can be separated from tumor extracts quantitatively, and partially purified, by a method of centrifugation at high speed.[1] The material prepared in this manner is found to be composed of small granules, visible in the dark-field microscope, approximately 70 mμ in diameter,[2] with a corresponding particle weight of about $2.3 \times 10^{-16}$ grams and a molecular weight of *ca.* 140 millions.[3] The tumor-producing power of ordinary tumor extracts varies a great deal, and only preparations exhibiting high activity were retained for this study. Tests were made by injecting the freshly prepared material intracutaneously in adult hens. Tumors were usually present after 8 days and the final results were recorded not later than 18 days after injection. In these experiments, the smallest dose to produce actively growing tumors was about $4 \times 10^{-13}$ grams, in terms of dry weight, of the purified substance. The relation between this weight and the weight of the individual particles indicates that the minimal active dose contained approximately 2,000 of the elementary granules.

The purified tumor fraction contains 8.5 to 9.0 per cent. nitrogen, a confirmation of previous analysis, and 1.5 per cent. phosphorus. Tests for proteins are positive. A typical Feulgen reaction, characteristic of thymonucleic acid, is absent. However, an intense reaction is obtained with the Schiff reagent, which suggests the presence of aldehyde groups in the material. Tests for pentoses are strongly positive.

Previous work has shown that the purified tumor fraction could be decomposed into two chief components, namely, a lipoid fraction and a protein fraction.[4] The chemical and physical properties of these fractions have been investigated further, and the results of this study is the matter of the present note.

The lipoid material associated with the tumor-producing fraction of chicken tumor I, and extracted by ether, had been found to represent about 24 to 26 per cent. of the whole substance.[4] The results of a somewhat more vigorous extraction by treating the dry substance with ether-alcohol and chloroform, at room temperature, indicates that at least 35 per cent. of the total dry weight of the purified material is lipoid in nature. This complex lipoid material contains about 2.4 per cent. phosphorus and 1.6 per cent. nitrogen.

Two main fractions can be separated from it. (*a*) One fraction is soluble in cold acetone. At room temperature it is a soft, yellow-colored mass which crystallizes in narrow plates arranged in rosettes. This fraction contains about 1.8 per cent. phosphorus and 0.9 per cent. nitrogen, figures which suggest that about half of the material may be in the form of phospholipids. The test with the Schiff reagent is negative or weakly positive. (*b*) The second fraction, which is the most abundant, has the general composition and

[1] J. C. G. Ledingham and W. E. Gye, *Lancet*, 1: 376, 1935; C. R. Amies, *Jour. Path. Bact.*, 44: 141, 1937; A. Claude, *Jour. Exp. Med.*, 66: 59, 1937, *Am. Jour. Cancer*, 30: 742, 1937, and SCIENCE, 87: 467, 1938.

[2] W. J. Elford and C. H. Andrewes, *Brit. Jour. Exp. Path.*, 17: 422, 1936.

[3] A. Claude, *Jour. Exp. Med.*, 66: 59, 1937; K. G. Stern and F. Duran-Reynals, SCIENCE, 89: 609, 1939.

[4] A. Claude, *Jour. Exp. Med.*, 61: 41, 1935; SCIENCE, 87: 467, 1938.

physical properties of phosphatides. It is precipitated by cold acetone and contains 3.8 per cent. phosphorus and 1.8 per cent. nitrogen, 0.3 per cent. of which is in the form of amino-nitrogen. A characteristic property of this lipoid component is that it gives a strongly positive reaction for aldehydes, when tested with the fuchsin-sulfurous acid solution of Schiff. The reaction is accelerated by acid, by heat and acid, by mercury bichloride and by trichloracetic acid. This aldehyde component of the tumor material resembles closely the substance demonstrated in the cytoplasm of certain cells, under the name of plasmalogen, by Feulgen and Voit.[5] The plasmal reaction of Feulgen, carried out on frozen sections, showed the cytoplasm of chicken tumor cells to be loaded with this lipoid.

The occurrence, in the purified chicken tumor material, of relatively large quantities of a substance which may exhibit the properties of an aldehyde is of interest, as regards tumor production, but this point is still undetermined. It is also possible that this chemically active group, which can be uncovered easily, plays a part in the so-called spontaneous inactivation of the tumor agent.

The complete lipoid fraction can be taken up in water or in salt solution, making a stable and homogeneous colloidal suspension. This is accomplished more easily under moderate heat or when traces of alcohol, which can be removed later, are present. Under the dark-field microscope this suspension appears to be composed of small particles which, as regards size and shape, are indistinguishable from those making up the original, unfractionated material. This observation suggests that the lipoid components of the purified tumor fraction may play an important role in the morphology of the active granules.

The portion of the tumor material, which is left after lipoid extraction, contains 12.6 to 13.2 per cent. nitrogen and about 1 per cent. phosphorus. Tests for protein are positive. In contrast to the complete fraction, the test with the Schiff reagent is negative, in agreement with the fact that the substances giving the reaction are removed by organic solvents. Thymonucleic acid is absent, or is not present in appreciable quantities, as shown by negative Feulgen and Dische tests. Tests for pentoses are positive. These observations support the view, stated previously, that the nucleoprotein which forms a large portion of the purified chicken tumor fraction is of the ribose type.[6]

A nucleic acid has been prepared from this material, by alkaline hydrolysis.[7] The separation is readily accomplished by leaving the freshly prepared tumor suspension in 0.1 N NaOH for 6 to 12 hours at 4° C. The alkaline mixture is then brought to pH 4.7 with 0.1 N acetic acid. The flocculent precipitate which settles at this point is removed by the centrifuge. The supernatant liquid is clear and colorless, and gives a negative biuret reaction. The Feulgen test for thymonucleic acid is negative, but tests for pentoses are strongly positive. The solution absorbs ultra-violet light in the manner of nucleic acid, with the position of the maximum at λ2575 and the minimum near λ2400.[8] The intensity of absorption of ultra-violet light and the phosphorus content suggests that 10 to 15 per cent. of the protein may be nucleic acid.

From the above nucleic acid fraction, guanylic acid was isolated by further alkaline hydrolysis. The substance gave positive tests for pentoses and the characteristic absorption spectrum of guanine.[9]

Previous studies have shown that active fractions of chicken tumor I, prepared by various methods, present a characteristic ultra-violet absorption spectrum, with a broad maximum in the region of λ2550–2575.[10] The present work is in agreement with these findings, as both the complete tumor fraction and the "nucleic acid" derived from it also show the typical maximum of absorption at $\lambda \simeq 2575$.[8] These observations indicate, either that the substance responsible for the absorption in that region is not yeast nucleic acid, which has its maximum at λ2600,[10] or that the material contains an absorbing element which causes the maximum to be consistently displaced toward the shorter wave-lengths. The separation of a guanine nucleotide which has a broad absorption band in the region of $\lambda = 2500$, and evidence from unpublished experiments,[11] suggests that this effect might be caused by guanine as a predominating element in the molecule. A quantitative study of the various nucleotides must await the preparation of suitable quantities of material.

By the same method of differential centrifugation at high speed, it is possible to separate from normal chick embryo a fraction which, in many respects, resembles the active fraction of chicken tumor I.[12] Further analysis of this chick embryo material has emphasized the similarities between the two substances. The chick embryo material, like the tumor fraction, is found to consist essentially of a phospholipid-aldehyde portion, associated with a nucleoprotein of the ribose type.[13, 14]

ALBERT CLAUDE

ROCKEFELLER INSTITUTE,
NEW YORK, N. Y.

[5] R. Feulgen and K. Voit, *Arch. Ges. Physiol.* (*Pflügers*) 206: 389, 1924.

[6] A. Claude, SCIENCE, 87: 467, 1938.

[7] P. A. Levene and L. W. Bass, "Nucleic Acids," The Chemical Catalog Co., Inc., New York, 1931.

[8] The ultra-violet absorbing power of the solutions was determined by Dr. A. Rothen.

[9] F. F. Heyroth and J. R. Loufbourow, *Jour. Am. Chem. Soc.*, 56: 1728, 1934; T. Caspersson, *Scand. Arch. Physiol.*, 73: Supplement No. 8, 1936.

[10] A. Claude and A. Rothen, *Am. Jour. Cancer*, 26: 344, 1936; A. Claude, *Am. Jour. Cancer*, 30: 742, 1937, and SCIENCE, 87: 467, 1938.

[11] In collaboration with Dr. G. I. Lavin.

[12] A. Claude, *Proc. Soc. Exp. Biol. Med.*, 39: 398, 1938.

## VITAMIN K ACTIVITY OF SYNTHETIC PHTHIOCOL

ALMQUIST and Klose[1] recently announced that pure synthetic phthiocol (2-methyl-3-hydroxy-1,4-naphthoquinone) has antihemorrhagic activity. With a sample of phthiocol, synthesized according to Anderson and Newman,[2] we were able to confirm the fact that phthiocol has some vitamin K activity.[3] Thayer *et al.*[4] have also published a confirmatory report. It is now fairly well established that a variety of naphthoquinones cure the vitamin K deficiency of chicks in a single dose of an order of magnitude of a milligram. The sample of phthiocol reported in our first communication had an activity of one unit[5] in 0.5 mg. We have since found that the vitamin K activity of phthiocol prepared according to Anderson and Newman is to a large extent due to traces of an impurity, presumably 2-methyl-1,4-naphthoquinone, which can be removed by washing its solution in alkali with ether. A sample so purified was found to have one unit in 2 mg, and is therefore only one fourth as active as the original sample. The melting point is not changed by this special purification procedure.

This is understandable in view of the unusually high potency of 2-methyl-1,4-naphthoquinone and the diacetate of the corresponding hydroquinone which serve as a starting material for the preparation of phthiocol. Since our original publication,[6] we have investigated the potency of these two compounds more extensively. The minimum effective dose is even lower than that of vitamin $K_1$.[7] While 2 $\gamma$ of vitamin $K_1$ are required for a unit as used in our laboratory, the diacetate of 2-methyl-1,4-naphthohydroquinone requires 1 $\gamma$ and 2-methyl-1,4-naphthoquinone only 0.5 $\gamma$. The duration of the curative effect of a single dose of 0.5 $\gamma$ of the methyl-naphthoquinone dissolved in 0.1 cc of cod liver oil given to severely deficient chicks with a blood clotting time of over 90 minutes is illustrated by Table 1.

TABLE 1

DURATION OF THE CURATIVE EFFECT OF 0.5 $\gamma$ OF 2–METHYL–1,4–NAPHTHOQUINONE

| Chick No. | Weight gr. | Clotting time (minutes) after 6 | 18 | 48 | 72 | 96 hours |
|---|---|---|---|---|---|---|
| 7316 | 60 | 2 | 1 | 2 | 5 | 7 |
| 7350 | 75 | 5 | 2 | 2 | 6 | 6 |
| 7366 | 70 | 3 | 1 | 2 | >30 | >30 |
| 7393 | 60 | 3 | <½ | 2 | 4 | 8 |
| 7403 | 65 | 3 | 1 | 2 | 3 | 7 |
| 7414 | 70 | 6 | 2 | 2 | 5 | >30 |
| 7430 | 65 | 3 | 1 | 2 | 8 | >30 |
| 7449 | 70 | 2 | 2 | 2 | 5 | >30 |

The activity of 2-methyl-1,4-naphthoquinone is so high that a contamination of the repurified phthiocol with 0.025 per cent. of the substance would account for the vitamin K activity. We have, therefore, submitted our phthiocol to chromatographic adsorption, using a benzene solution and calcium sulfate for adsorbent. The substance was readily adsorbed and drawn out to a homogeneous orange column on continued washing. The column was then divided into two equal parts and both parts separately eluted with ether. The activity of both fractions was equal and the same as before adsorption, showing that no fractionation had occurred. This degree of activity is probably a genuine property of phthiocol, although a biological assay of natural phthiocol would still be of interest.

A report of a successful application of phthiocol to a patient with low prothrombin time has already appeared in the literature.[8] Also 2-methyl-1,4-naphthoquinone is now being studied for its effect in raising the prothrombin content of the blood of such patients. In all of a considerable number of cases it has been found effective in a daily dosage of one milligram.

ERHARD FERNHOLZ
S. ANSBACHER
THE SQUIBB INSTITUTE FOR MEDICAL RESEARCH,
NEW BRUNSWICK, N. J.

[13] In another paper (footnote 12), a positive reaction with the Schiff reagent was erroneously referred to as a positive Feulgen test. On closer examination it was found that, as in the case of the tumor fraction, the intense reaction obtained with the fuchsin-sulfurous solution was given by the lipoid components of the chick embryo material, whereas a typical reaction for thymonucleic acid was apparently absent.

[14] The work has now been extended to a variety of other avian and mammalian tissues, especially mouse embryo and mouse tumors. By the use of the same procedure it has been possible to isolate from these tissues a fraction, likewise composed of small granules, which presents physical and chemical properties similar to those already described for chicken tumors and chick embryo fractions. The material separated and purified in the centrifuge may represent as much as 2 to 8 per cent. of the whole cellular body. These observations indicate that a phospholipid-ribose nucleoprotein complex is probably a general constituent of normal and tumor cells.

[1] H. J. Almquist and A. A. Klose, *Jour. Am. Chem. Soc.*, 61: 1611, 1939.

[2] R. J. Anderson and M. S. Newman, *Jour. Biol. Chem.*, 103: 405, 1933.

[3] S. Ansbacher and E. Fernholz, *Jour. Am. Chem. Soc.*, 61: 1924, 1939.

[4] S. A. Thayer, L. C. Cheney, S. B. Binkley, D. W. MacCorquadale and E. A. Doisy, *ibid.*, 1932.

[5] S. Ansbacher, *Jour. Nutrition*, 17: 303, 1939.

[6] S. Ansbacher and E. Fernholz, *loc. cit.*

[7] S. A. Thayer, L. C. Cheney, S. B. Binkley, D. W. MacCorquadale and E. A. Doisy, *loc. cit.*

[8] H. P. Smith, S. E. Ziffren, C. A. Owen and G. R. Hoffman, *Jour. Am. Med. Assoc.*, 113: 383, 1939.

## HUMAN VACCINATION AGAINST EQUINE ENCEPHALOMYELITIS VIRUS WITH FORMOLIZED CHICK EMBRYO VACCINE[1]

THE pathogenicity of equine encephalomyelitis virus for man[2] has been proved by recognition of infections

[1] This work was supported by a grant from Lederle Laboratories, Pearl River, N. Y.

[2] K. F. Meyer, *Ann. Int. Med.*, 6: 645, 1932.

with the virus under natural conditions[3] and following laboratory contact with virus-diseased chick embryo tissues.[4,5] The occurrence of unrecognized infection in man has been demonstrated,[5] and in a recent study[6] of the incidence of such subclinical infections we have examined 184 human sera,[7] 69 of which were from individuals exposed to the Eastern strain virus. In 23 of these 69 sera antibodies sufficient to neutralize 100 to 1,000 infective doses of virus were found, and in one instance the serum fixed complement in the presence of Eastern strain virus purified by ultracentrifugation. Similar though less definite results were obtained in parallel studies with the Western strain. These findings have introduced the problem of protective vaccination, especially in workers frequently exposed to virus-diseased tissues and animals. We have vaccinated a group of men and women with formolized chick embryo vaccine[8] and have studied the probable effectiveness of the procedure by the examination of their sera for the presence of neutralizing antibodies.

Injections were made with a "bivalent" vaccine, prepared in the routine way for the immunization of horses. Vaccines consisting of 40 per cent. suspensions of diseased chick embryo tissue formolized to 0.4 per cent. were prepared separately for the Eastern strain and Western strain viruses. These were centrifuged at low speed, mixed in equal parts and used without further treatment. Two injections were made with an interval of 7 days. In some instances 1.0 cc was given as the first dose and 2.0 cc for the second. The majority, however, received two doses of 2.0 cc each. Routine injections were made deep in the gluteal muscles in two areas to lessen reactions to the formalin. Injections into the deltoid muscles of three individuals caused painful local reactions. Blood was drawn prior to the first vaccination and after 7, 14 and 21 days.

Slight general reactions were observed in a few of 89 volunteers vaccinated. Sharp transient pain was experienced locally in most instances, followed occasionally by low-grade dull pain for from one to three days.

Sera from 23 of those vaccinated have been tested[9] for neutralizing antibodies against the Eastern strain virus, and a typical protocol is shown in Table 1. In 9 of the 23, serum taken 7 days after the first injection seemed to protect mice. In every case after 14 days, antibodies nearly as effective as those after 21 days were observed. After the latter interval the antibody content was sufficiently great to neutralize completely 100 to 1,000 infectious units of virus, except in one individual, whose serum neutralized only 10 units. In one instance, the serum drawn 21 days after a single injection of 1.0 cc vaccine protected against 1,000 infectious units.

TABLE 1

MOUSE PROTECTION TESTS AGAINST EQUINE ENCEPHALOMYELITIS VIRUS (EASTERN STRAIN) WITH SERUM OF WOMAN VACCINATED WITH FORMOLIZED CHICK EMBRYO VACCINE

| Case | Serum | Date bled | Date vaccinated | Amount vaccine | Number of deaths in 4 injected mice — Virus dilution $10^{-4}$ | $10^{-5}$ | $10^{-6}$ | $10^{-7}$ | $10^{-8}$ |
|---|---|---|---|---|---|---|---|---|---|
| | a (control) | May 2 | May 2 | 1.0 cc | 4 | 3 | 2 | 2 | 0 |
| L. H. | b | May 9 | May 9 | 2.0 cc | 4 | 4 | 3 | 1 | 0 |
| | c | May 16 | | | 1 | 1 | 0 | 0 | 0 |
| | d | May 23 | | | 0 | 0 | 0 | 0 | 0 |

The crude bivalent vaccine was thus found to be effective in the induction of antibodies against the Eastern strain virus, and to cause little discomfort. Vaccines containing less formalin and chick tissue debris may prove as effective and more useful for human vaccination.[10]

J. W. BEARD
DOROTHY BEARD
HAROLD FINKELSTEIN
DUKE UNIVERSITY SCHOOL OF MEDICINE

[3] L. D. Fothergill, J. H. Dingle, S. Farber and M. L. Connerley, *New England Jour. Med.*, 219: 411, 1938.
[4] R. R. Case, personal communication, Dr. R. W. G. Wyckoff.
[5] P. K. Olitsky and I. M. Morgan, *Proc. Soc. Exp. Biol. and Med.*, 41: 212, 1939.
[6] H. Finkelstein, D. Beard and J. W. Beard. Unpublished work.
[7] Obtained through the generous cooperation of members of the staff of Lederle Laboratories, Pearl River, N. Y., and Sharp and Dohme Company, Philadelphia, Pa.
[8] J. W. Beard, H. Finkelstein, W. C. Sealy and R. W. G. Wyckoff, SCIENCE, 87: 490, 1938.
[9] P. K. Olitsky and I. M. Morgan, *loc. cit.*
[10] R. W. G. Wyckoff, SCIENCE, 89: 542, 1939.

## BOOKS RECEIVED

BIGGER, JOSEPH W. *Man Against Microbe.* Pp. 304. 17 figures. 18 plates. Macmillan. $2.50.

HARRISON, GEORGE R. *Massachusetts Institute of Technology Wavelength Tables, with Intensities in Arc, Spark, or Discharge Tube.* Pp. xxviii + 429. Wiley. $15.00.

SCHEINFELD, AMRAM and MORTON D. SCHWEITZER. *You and Heredity.* Pp. xvii + 434. Ilustrated. Stokes. $3.00.

TINKLE, WILLIAM J. *Fundamentals of Zoology.* Pp. xvi + 492. 278 figures. Zondervan, Grand Rapids, Mich. $3.00.

TRELOAR, ALAN E. *Elements of Statistical Reasoning.* Pp. xi + 261. 47 figures. Wiley. $3.25.

WEEKS, MARY E. *Discovery of the Elements.* Pp. v + 470. Illustrated. Journal of Chemical Education, Easton, Pa. $3.00.

# SCIENCE

VOL. 90 FRIDAY, SEPTEMBER 8, 1939 No. 2332

*The British Association for the Advancement of Science:*
*Film Reactions as a New Approach to Biology:* DR. ERIC K. RIDEAL ... 217

*Obituary:*
*The Mayo Brothers and Their Clinic:* PROFESSOR HARVEY CUSHING. *Recent Deaths and Memorials* ... 225

*Scientific Events:*
*Marine Engineering at the Massachusetts Institute of Technology; The New Research Vessel of the Bureau of Fisheries; The Association for the Study of Systematics in Relation to General Biology; The International Congress of Genetics; Opening of the International Congress for Microbiology* ... 226

*Scientific Notes and News* ... 229

*Discussion:*
*The Mode of Action of Sulfanilamide:* DR. ARTHUR LOCKE and DR. R. R. MELLON. *Red Color in Apples:* DR. R. B. DUSTMAN and DR. I. J. DUNCAN. *A Fire-Fly "Spinthariscope":* PROFESSOR R. W. WOOD. *The First Articles on Group Theory Published in America:* PROFESSOR G. A. MILLER ... 231

*Scientific Books:*
*An Anecdotal History of Electricity:* DR. F. C. BROWN ... 234

*Special Articles:*
*An Analysis of Skin Pigment Changes after Exposure to Sunlight:* EDWARD A. EDWARDS and S. QUIMBY DUNTLEY. *Presence of a Leukocytosis-Promoting Factor in Inflammatory Exudates:* DR. VALY MENKIN. *Glycogen in Sweet Corn:* DR. DANIEL LUZON MORRIS and CAROL TILDEN MORRIS ... 235

*Scientific Apparatus and Laboratory Methods:*
*A Method for the Continuous Recording of Gastric pH in Situ:* DR. JAMES FLEXNER, MICHAEL KNIAZUK and JAN NYBOER. *Chromosomes from Leaves:* PROFESSOR J. T. BALDWIN, JR. ... 239

*Science News* ... 6

SCIENCE: A Weekly Journal devoted to the Advancement of Science, edited by J. MCKEEN CATTELL and published every Friday by

THE SCIENCE PRESS
New York City: Grand Central Terminal
Lancaster, Pa. Garrison, N. Y.
Annual Subscription, $6.00 Single Copies, 15 Cts.

SCIENCE is the official organ of the American Association for the Advancement of Science. Information regarding membership in the Association may be secured from the office of the permanent secretary in the Smithsonian Institution Building, Washington, D. C.

# FILM REACTIONS AS A NEW APPROACH TO BIOLOGY[1]

By Dr. ERIC K. RIDEAL, M.B.E., F.R.S.

PROFESSOR OF COLLOID SCIENCE, UNIVERSITY OF CAMBRIDGE

TOWARDS the end of the last century the biologist and physiologist were agreed that the biological entity was the whole living unit. This century has seen an attack on biological problems by the physical and organic chemist. The study of the living unit has been dropped and in its place we find investigations on specialized processes such as oxidation and reduction or catalytic reactions. It is an unfortunate fact, as the late Sir William Hardy clearly pointed out, that in this method of approach the mechanism of the coordination or the integration of the activities of an assemblage of cells must remain insoluble. It is this very point which I think deserves some consideration. We know for example that at death the catalysts escape from control since the molecular structure of the moving parts gets disorganized. Again, Loeb showed that unfertilized sea urchin's eggs could be made to develop by immersion in salt solutions of sufficient concentration. In development a whole series of complicated chemical reactions are set in operation and it is clear that in the quiescent unfertilized egg all the chemical ingredients for the reactions are present but await some change in organization before reaction sets in. We must conclude that the mechanism of integration is at any rate dependent on a pre-existing organization of at least the major operative portions of the assemblage of cells. This raises a number of important problems such as, what types of organization are to be found in living material; how far control over chemical reactions can be effected by modification of the type or extent of such organization and finally how far different types of organization can modify such important factors as the chemical or physical state of

[1] Address of the president of the Section of Chemistry, British Association for the Advancement of Science, Dundee, August 31, 1939.

a material or chemical equilibria in reacting systems, and lastly what new properties or reactions make their appearance as a direct result of organization.

Whilst it has been frequently stated that one of the chief characteristics of living matter is that it contains a relatively large proportion of matter in what we designate the colloidal state, a closer analysis indicates that in fact the colloidal properties of living matter are due to the fact that an exceptionally large fraction both of material and of energy is present in films, membranes, fibers, fine capillaries and the like. It thus seems pertinent to inquire a little into the properties of surfaces of separation between bulk phases or of matter in the boundary state. These surfaces of separation can be considered as a new phase—the interphase—and for our discussion we must examine this phase and find in what respect it differs from the enclosing bulk phases.

Whilst we must pay attention to the static properties such as composition, form and orientation we must not forget that it is the dynamic properties of ingress and egress, of flow and chemical action in and with the two-dimensional contents of the phase that we are particularly interested in, but any integrating features of the former are of great importance if it can be shown that they produce effects in the dynamics of the system which are not to be found in non-structural liquid or vaporous phases.

We already know that the composition of the interphase differs from that of either of the bulk phases in contact with it and the general principles governing relationship between its composition and its three dimensional partners were clearly enumerated by Willard Gibbs and Sir J. J. Thomson. Equally important are the considerations of Sir William Hardy and Irving Langmuir, who showed that in many cases when dealing with an interphase we were actually examining a monolayer—a hypothesis suggested by Lord Rayleigh. Finally we know the molecules contained in the monolayer are orientated with respect to one another and to the plane of the interphase. I need not enlarge at this point on the structure and different physical states as well as the effects of variation of the external variables on the equilibria of the phases of monolayers of simple molecules such as derivatives of both paraffinic and cyclic hydrocarbon, since these have been exhaustively examined during the last twenty years, but monolayers both of macromolecules as well as those composed of binary and components of a higher order posseses a number of interesting and somewhat unexpected properties.

We find, for example, that macromolecules such as the methylated or acetylated starches and celluloses or the native proteins can be spread as monolayers. The chains are extended at the interface and in general the non-polar side chains penetrate into one (the non-polar) and the polar side chains into the other (the aqueous) phase. This separation of the side chains by the solvent action of the homogeneous phases can only be effected by suitable partial rotation along the chain involving the usual cis-trans motion. Thus no single protein chain can acquire along its entire length either the $\alpha$ or $\beta$ keratin configuration unless the side chains alternate in polarity in suitable fashion. Monolayers of both the proteins and of the derivatives of starches and celluloses when suitably compressed acquire rigidity and interesting elastic properties; we are forming in fact a two-dimensional gel, the prototype of a membrane. We shall return to some of the reactions which are observed with such monolayers, but may observe in passing that these macromolecules in a monolayer are in part crossing one another by the accident of distribution, in part associate with one another through three separate factors: (*a*) the non-polar side chains forming a hydrophobic surface to a triplex sheet; (*b*) association through the –CO–NH linkages in the chains; (*c*) association between some of the polar heads in the substrate. It appears that at extremely great surface dilutions of many proteins actual molecular separation occurs, and we are thus presented with a simple method of determining the molecular weight from the relation $FA = RT$ of these complex bodies.

We have referred to the fact that molecules in a monolayer are orientated relative to one another and to the substrate and that this orientation can be altered by extension or compression. If the molecules in the monolayer undergo reaction with a reactant dissolved in the substrate the rate of reaction may be modified by the charge in molecular orientation of the former. This is equivalent to a control of the steric factor and determining the path of approach of a reacting molecule or ion to the reactive portion of the other reactant. In this way both the reaction velocity and the height of the energy barrier or apparent energy of activation may be altered.

In Tables 1 and 2 and Fig. 1 are given three different examples of such a variation in reaction effected by change in compression of a monolayer.

It is interesting to observe that these film reactions can be carried out with minute concentrations of strongly adsorbed reactants. Thus in the case of the attack of lecithin by snake venom to form lysolecithin a half life of about one hour is obtained with a concentration of venom as low as $2 \cdot 5 \times 10^{-6}$ per cent. When cobra venom is examined by this method it is found that only in extreme dilutions does any reaction occur. This inhibition at higher concentrations is due to proteins present in the cobra venom which are absorbed in preference to the enzyme by the lecithin monolayer. Egg albumin, although not so effective when added to black tiger venom, will produce a similar result. In addition to lecithinase present in snake venoms, other enzymes have been studied and amongst them crystalline trypsin and crystalline pepsin which rapidly digest monolayers of caseinogen, the former at pH 8 and the latter at pH 2. When the purified and crystalline enzyme preparations are employed, these enzyme actions on the protein monolayers behave exactly as

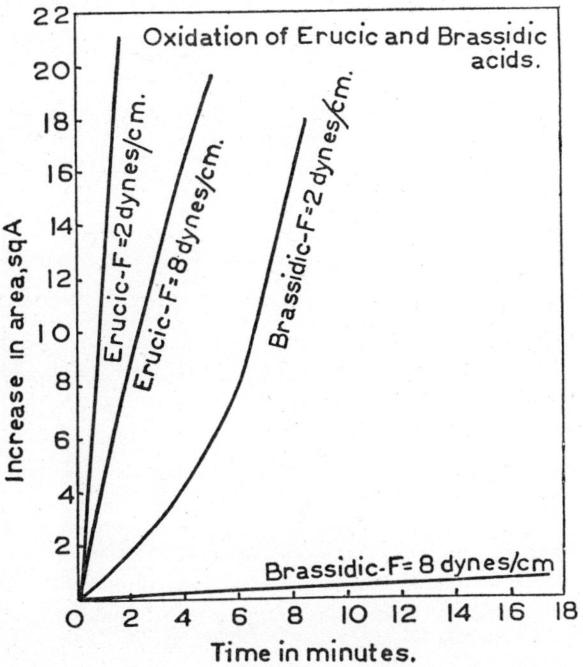


FIG. 1. Oxidation of Erucic and Brassidic acids by 0.005 per cent. $KMnO_4$ and N/100 $H_2SO_4$.

in bulk phase, although the protein has undergone a process akin to denaturation. With unpurified proteolytic ferments, on the other hand, fatty acid protein complexes are invariably present which give rise to other phenomena.

TABLE 1

HYDROLYSIS OF TRILAURIN ON N/5 NAOH. T = 20°

| F dynes/cm | E cals./gm mol. |
|---|---|
| 5·4 | 10,000 |
| 10·8 | 13,200 |
| 16·2 | 16,100 |

In the reactions which we have discussed the chemical processes involved do not differ from those which would occur in similar systems in the disorganized state, and the only effects of molecular organization into oriented monolayers are noted in the alterations produced in accessibility of the groups as revealed by the rapidity of the reactions and in the apparent energies of activation.

TABLE 2

ATTACK ON LECITHIN MONOLAYERS BY 0·001 PER CENT. BLACK TIGER SNAKE VENOM AT 20° AND pH 7·2

| No. of lecithin molecules per sq. cm × $10^{-14}$ | Half life in minutes |
|---|---|
| 1·04 | 0·5 |
| 1·27 | 4 |
| 1·57 | 32 |
| 2·11 | 90 |

A further consequence of molecular orientation at interphases is found in those cases where radiation incident on the surface produces photochemical action after absorption of quanta by chromophoric groups in the monolayer. If, as is the case in ring compounds, the extinction coefficients are different along the three molecular or group axes, the photochemical reaction rate can be varied by alteration of the orientation by compression. Thus the rate of photochemcial hydrolytic fission followed by oxidation in protein monolayers at those points along the chain where the chromophoric groups are situate can be varied within wide limits by simple expansion or contraction.

There are several processes in which an alteration in the properties of an interphase bring about a number of varied biological processes of great importance. I may mention the phenomena of lysis, agglutination, sensitization and the lethal activities of certain substances on various types of cells and micro-organisms. It is true that we are not yet certain in any one case as to the exact composition, structure or thickness of the cell membrane, but we are certain that the surface structure must be organized in the sense that forces of molecular orientation must be operative in the membrane. Whilst, as we have seen, a monolayer membrane of a protein may be destroyed by suitable enzymes, yet the phenomena which I am now referring to do not appear to be the result of chemical action in the usual sense of the word. The reactions themselves do not appear to possess large temperature coefficients indicative of sensible energies of activation, although it must be admitted this fact is frequently obscured by other processes operative at the same time. We may mention in passing the thermal denaturation of proteins is a reaction in which the apparent and true energies of activation are markedly different, a fact emphasized by the investigations of Steinhardt and La Mer. A second criterion is to be found in the fact that these processes are nearly all catastrophic in character, *i.e.*, the process under investigation being recorded as a hit or miss. As far as quantitative results are possible in such systems it appears that a definite quantity of reactant related naturally to the extent of all surface is required to bring about the reaction, and further that this quantity is removed from the environment on to or into the cell wall. One further point of interest is that the relation between the quantity on or in the cell wall and the concentration in the environment can be expressed in terms of an adsorption isotherm. Not too much stress may be laid on this last point, because the adsorption isotherm may equally well be replaced for existing experimental data by a partition function between two phases or by the mass law operative between easily dissociable salts.

Whilst the extent of mutual miscibility of two liquid phases is usually interpreted in terms of the relative internal pressures of the two liquids, we note from the molecular point of view, especially in the case of the large complex and the biologically important material, that we are really concerned with specific molecular interactions which may be identified as being due to those forces operative between the non-polar and the polar portions of the molecules respectively. In two component monolayers the two molecular species are adlineated in respect to one another, and we should thus anticipate that it might be possible to form relatively stable two-component complexes which in three dimensions would only be detectable in terms of mutual solubility and when a mutual solvent was present as a third component might not be observable at all. These conclusions are indeed fully borne out by investigations on two component monolayers. It is found, for example, that strong complexes are formed in mixed monolayers of a variety of substances such as saponin with cholesterol or digitonin or cetyl amine or sulfate with cholesterol.

Examination of a great variety of these systems has demonstrated that the free energy of formation of the complex is constitutive in the sense that its magnitude is dependent on the extent of interaction between the polar reactive groups and also that of the Van der Waals interaction between the non-polar portions of the reacting species. The difference in properties of mixed films containing cholesterol on the one hand and those containing, for example, epi-cholesterol is most marked, but when models are made of the two molecular systems, it becomes quite evident that the ease of adlineation of the hydrophobic portions of the molecule and the relative orientation of the polar group with respect to the axis of the molecule are the determining factors. The free energy changes involved in formation of these two-dimensional complexes is of the order of some 10,000 cals. per gm. mol. Complexes containing the constituents in ratios other than one to one can be prepared; thus cetyl alcohol and cetyl sulfate can form both a 1:1 and a somewhat unstable complex in the ratio of 1:3, whereas elaidyl alcohol produces an unstable 1:2 but no 1:3 complex. It is probable that with a more extended investigation of these interesting systems the basis for the most elementary form, *i.e.*, a two-dimensional crystallography of the type envisaged by Patterson may be laid down.

I might mention in passing that the effects of cis-transisomerism on the free energies of the complexes are very characteristic and fully confirm the hypothesis we have advanced as to the importance of molecular adlineation; thus saturated aliphatic hydrocarbon chains with different reacting polar groups will form stable systems, likewise trans-olefinic chains can penetrate and pack both with one another and with saturated chains, but the cis form is not capable of such adlineation. From the biological point of view I think that the most interesting property of these systems lies in the mechanism of their formation, for on injection of one of the reactants beneath a monolayer of the other it is found that penetration of the latter by the former will take place to form the complex monolayer. This penetration, if carried out at constant area, naturally involves a rise in the two-dimensional pressure, or if at constant pressure a rise in area is involved. We have indeed examined the formation of complexes under both these conditions, and the changes involved are frequently remarkable, thus the injection of a few mgm of saponin under a film of cholesterol compressed to a pressure of 10 dynes/cm will cause an increase of pressure of over 50 dynes/cm. Whilst a film of cetyl alcohol at 20 $A^2$ per molecule expands to no less than 78 $A^2$, even when the pressure is maintained at 23 dynes/cm on the injection of only 1 mgm in 300 cc of cetyl sulfate.

If sodium cetyl sulfate be injected beneath a monolayer of cholesterol this substance will penetrate to form, as we have seen, a complex. By suitable adjustment of the pressure this complex can be maintained at the definite composition of one to one, excess of the sodium salt being ejected as the pressure is raised. It is found that the pressure on the film has to be raised as the concentration of sodium salt in the substrate is raised; some of the values obtained are given in Table 3.

TABLE 3

| Conc. sodium cetyl sulfate gms/cc × $10^{-7}$ | Equilibrium pressure in dynes/cm for the 1·1 complex formation |
|---|---|
| 1·0 | 17 |
| 2·0 | 32 |
| 3·0 | 38 |
| 4·0 | 45 |
| 5·0 | 47 |
| 6·0 | 48 |

We conclude that there must be a more or less complete layer of the sodium sulfate adsorbed beneath the surface of the complex. We are thus led to the view that in many oil-in-water emulsions as well as in the micellar aggregates found in soap solutions the gegen ion atmosphere around the emulsion particle or micelle must contain a number of molecules of the emulsifying soap, a somewhat novel conclusion as to their structure. Further, that emulsions formed from such complexes should be remarkably stable with a low interfacial energy. In some cases a small alteration in the pH of the substrate may affect the ease of penetration of a reactant to a marked extent. In the diagram is shown the effect of such a variation on the rate and extent of penetration of bilirubin into cholesterol as a function of the pH. It is possible to examine the reactivity of various substances in respect to penetration of monolayers. I have referred to the penetration of monolayers of cholesterol and we note that some substances such as digitonin or cetyl sulfate or amine possess this property to a remarkable extent. Of the other important cell wall constituents we include phospholipins and the proteins. Little information as yet is available on phospholipins, but our knowledge of the reactions of this type in the case of the proteins,

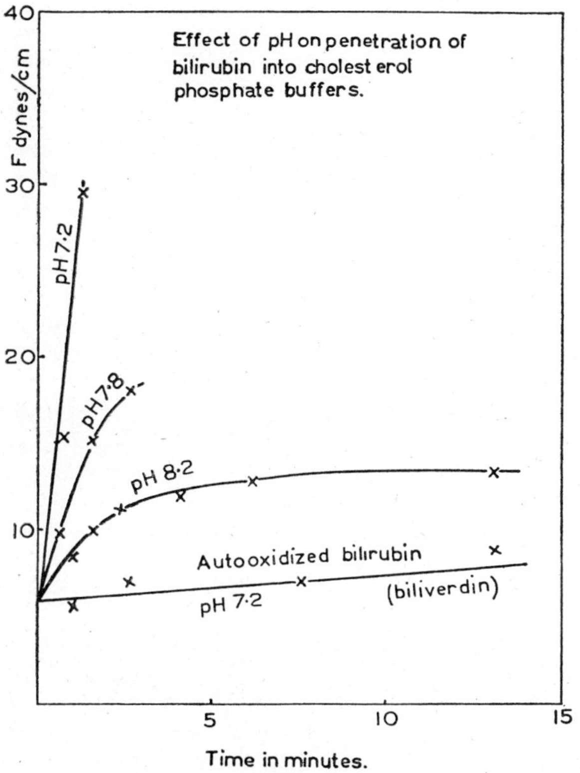

FIG. 2

especially the alcohol soluble and thus readily dispersible protein gliadin, has been greatly extended in recent years.

The stability of the protein monolayer is, as we have seen, due partly to their mutual association; if these are broken down by stronger associating reactants we might anticipate a dispersion of the monolayer resulting in a solution of the protein in the form of a protein-reactant complex. This phenomenon is readily observed on injection of even minute quantities of such substances as sodium oleate, cetyl sulfate or psychosin beneath a protein monolayer.

Other substances may react by penetration into the protein layer but not effect dispersion. By spreading monolayers with various head groups and examining the reactions caused on injection it is possible to identify the reacting group in the protein monolayer. A characteristic group of protein complexes formed in monolayers are the lipo proteins; thus gliadin forms a remarkable complex with cholesterol in the ratio 4:1 by weight. Here the cholesterol is anchored to specific groups in the gliadin, in particular the amino and carboxylic groups. At high pressures (20 dynes) the cholesterol is forced up above the protein monolayer, and the surface becomes one essentially of cholesterol. Nevertheless the cholesterol is still anchored to specific portions of the protein, for on release of the pressure the lipo-protein film is re-formed. This extrusion and re-forming process can be repeated several times before the complex structure breaks down. It is interesting to note that saponin, which penetrates cholesterol with extreme ease, but proteins only slightly, will penetrate these lipo-protein films except at those pressures where the cholesterol is separated from the substrate by the protein monolayer to which the cholesterol is anchored.

It thus appears not unlikely that the materials such as cytoplasm, and especially in the more stratified chloroplasts, must be regarded as a protein gel framework to which is attached the enzymes, the phosphatides and lipoids and the means of attachment is as we have seen due to the interaction both of the non-polar as well as of the polar portions of the molecules concerned. Another important conclusion to be drawn from monolayer experiments is that these penetrative reactions involve not only a new head group interaction, but in many cases also the breaking of such a head group interaction already existing in the monolayer prior to penetration. Several biological analogies may be mentioned—thus since lysis of blood cells can be brought about both by protein and cholesterol penetrants we must conclude that it has lipo-protein surface. Several micro-organisms can be sensitized for lysis by cholesterol penetrants by a prior treatment with cholesterol. Again, cilia of mytilus appear to be mainly lipoidal, those of paramoecia chiefly protein, as judged by the criterion of penetration.

The carrier action of desoxycholic acid on fatty acids can readily be demonstrated in monolayers, as desoxycholic acid does not interact with other lipoids nor to any great extent with proteins. We find also that the hemolytic activity of a long chain alcohol is negligibly small, owing to the fact that it is practically insoluble in water, but it readily forms a soluble complex with a long chain sulfate and can be transported to the cell wall in this form. There both the sulfate and the alcohol can penetrate separately, the former acting both on the protein and on the lipoid, the latter only on the protein, and produce lysis.

Yet another reaction of this type has been described by Peters and Wakelin, who found that the complex ovoverdin containing protein and astacin could be split to form a lipo-protein containing soap by the addition of small amounts of saturated long chain fatty acids setting free the astacin. On the addition of calcium ions the process is reversed. They likewise draw attention to the fact that it seems probable that the co-enzyme in an oxidase system may be separated from the enzyme by the formation of such a lipo-protein complex.

Somewhat more complex in behavior are the blood coagulants heparin and the synthetic sulfate celluloses. It is found that their biological activities run parallel to the ease with which they penetrate films of cholesterol. It is not unlikely that they operate by breaking down a cholesterol cephalin complex, setting the latter free.

We have referred to the fact that for the penetration of a monolayer by a substance injected into the substrate primary interaction between the reactive head groups occurs, followed by solution, *i.e.*, penetration and adlineation, of the tail. In the case of reactants containing two or more reactive head groups it is found that these can associate with head groups in the monolayer and thus form a series of links. Here another important factor is found operative. If the injected bipolar molecule possess a hydrophobic portion of such a structure that it can pack or adlineate with its neighbors beneath the monolayer, the resultant composite film is remarkably stable. Thus the long chain dibasic acids are adsorbed on to, but do not penetrate monolayers of amines, whilst the diamidines are adsorbed by, but do not penetrate monolayers of cholesterol. Substances containing the phenolic group are of particular interest in this respect as they include a number of biologically important substances. They react with amine groups quite readily and to a less extent with the imido group in a polypeptide chain. Gallic and tannic acids react with great ease with monolayers both of amines and with proteins. It is interesting to note that the reactivity of tannic acid with the spaced amine groups of the protein is high and that subsequent injection of fatty acids beneath such treated monolayers in the dispersion of the galloyl-amine or galloyl-protein complex film, but not in the tanned one—an indication of the effectiveness of the interlinkage produced in the non-dispersible network

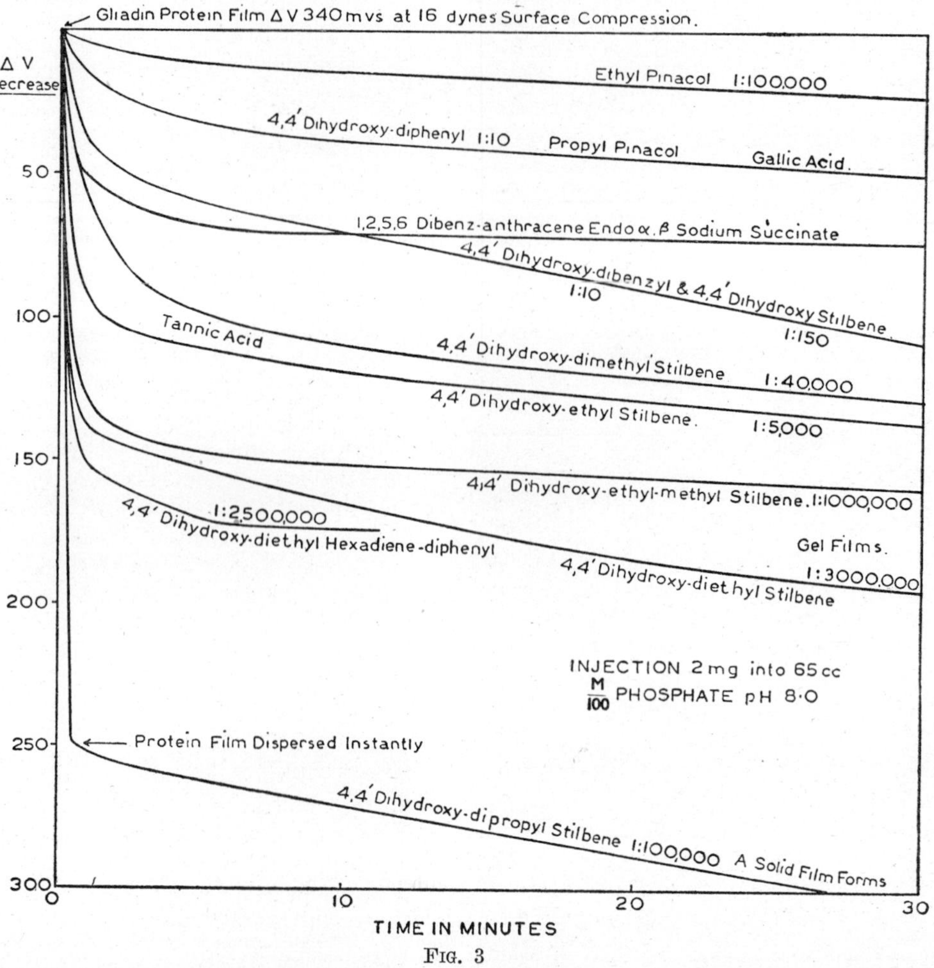

FIG. 3

by the multiple point contact of the large tannic acid molecules.

The extremely reactive oestrogenic compounds of Dodds and Lawson, of which the *pp'* dihydroxy diphenyl hexadiene and stilbene derivatives form a definite series in which the ratio of hydrophobic to hydrophilic portion can be varied, present an interesting series, the results of injection of which under a protein monolayer are shown in the attached curve.

It will be noted that reaction sets in rapidly, but equilibrium is only finally attained after some 15 to 20 minutes, and that there is a parallelism between the estrogenic activity and the protein adsorption except in the first and the last members, points we shall refer to later.

In apparent conformity with Traube's view, there is a marked increase in adsorption with increase in the number of $CH_2$ groups in the molecule, and this adsorption is cut down by the insertion of polar groups. This effect is clearly exemplified in comparing the diethyl stilbene or dibenzyl compounds with the corresponding pinacols. If, however, reactive polar groups, *e.g.*, the phenolic hydroxyl, had been inserted instead of the primary alcoholic groups in the pinacols, a marked increase rather than a decrease in adsorption would have been observed, for the following compounds react in order of increasing adsorption on both amine and protein monolayers—cresol, gallic acid, digallic acid, purpurogallin and tannic acid. This order is, however, reversed to give a normal Traube series when these substances are injected under a relatively non-reactive monolayer such as a long chain acid.

A wide variety of substances have been examined from this point of view, namely, their extent of interaction with protein monolayers, and it has been found that there is a direct parallelism between their extent of interaction and their lethal action on paramecia. Another significant biological similarity has been noted when we measure the extent of penetration of a series of substances containing identical hydrophobic "tails," *e.g.*, a $C_{12}$ chain but with different head groups, into a monolayer of a typical lipoid such as cholesterol. In all cases the extent of interaction as measured by the increase in surface pressure caused by the injection of 0.33 mgm/100 cc under a film of cholesterol originally extended to 40 $A^2$ per molecule is found to be closely parallel to the hemolytic activities and lethal activities on paramecia of these substances.

These latter can be placed in order both of monolayer penetration and biological activity as follows:

$$RNH^+_3 > RSO'_4 > RSO'_3 > RCOO' > RN(CH^+_3)_3 > RNH(C^+H_3)_2 > \text{Bile acids.}$$

We may conclude that the most reactive group in the protein macromolecule is the amino group, since the –NH–CO– group is poorly reactive, a point of some interest when we examine the reactions of lecithin and of cephalin. This order of head group reactivity receives confirmation when penetration into monolayers containing these head groups is examined, *i.e.*, on inverting the system. When we compare the reactivities of a series of long chain compounds with identical head groups it is found that biological activity and film penetration commences with $C_9$ when attached to a very reactive head group, with $C_{12}$ when attached to a poorly reactive group, and reaches a maximum value at *ca.* $C_{18}$. It is interesting to note that it is not necessary for all the carbon atoms to be in the form of a chain but may be enclosed in ring systems; thus activity commences with diphenyl derivatives and increases with addition of carbon atoms to an optimum as in the bile acids, stearic acid, diethyl stilbene and benzpyrene. By examining the reactivity of substances containing two reactive groups at various spacings underneath protein monolayers, it is possible to obtain some idea as to the statistical distribution of the reactive groups in the monolayer. It would appear that some 12·5 A is the mean distribution of the amine groups beneath a gliadin film. In the native protein such spacings are naturally different, and thus reactions involving two-point contact will not take place in bulk phase unless the spacing is unaffected by two-dimensional unrolling of the protein.

We have referred to the modification which must be introduced into either the Overton Meyer or Traube concepts of biological activity, *i.e.*, lipoid solubility or capillary activity necessitated by the concept of specific head group interaction. We see that a definite limit is also set to the hydrophobic portion of the molecule, not only on account of the decreasing solubility in the aqueous phase causing difficulty in transport and on account of the ease of adlineation or packing having an optimum of $C_{18}$ for association with sterols or fats, but also because a new phenomenon, as exemplified in the figure, sets in with long chains, *viz.*, dispersion of the monolayer, most marked in the case of 4 4' dihydroxy dipropyl stilbene. It is possible that this phenomenon of film collapse and dispersion may be a generally important factor in setting the upper limit to the chain length or more generally the capillary activity of homogeneous series of biologically important substances, *e.g.*, anesthetics. This dispersion of protein films may have biological counterparts in adsorption on specific portions of the cell surface similar to the hemolytic activity of long chain compounds such as oleic acid, which readily disperses protein films. Another interesting parallelism has been observed in the surface reactivities and estrogenic powers of two isomeric compounds (*pp'* dihydroxy diethyl dibenzyl), one being markedly differentiated from the other in both protein adsorption and in estrogenic activity. Here models indicate that the trans arranged rings can pack laterally with one another in sheet form much more readily and with a greater degree of adlineation than the cis structure, imparting stability to the adsorption complex formed with the former substance.

In advancing these somewhat novel principles based upon the hypothesis of a parallelism of film reactions and biological activity, it is desirable to point out exceptions. It is found, for example, that 4 4′ dihydroxy diethyl pinacol is a much more effective estrogenic agent than either its paramecicidal activity or adsorption on protein monolayers would suggest. The view might be advanced that on certain living tissues it can be partly converted by enzymitic dehydration to the extremely active 4 4′ dihydroxy diphenyl hexadiene. Another interesting exception is to be found in desoxycholic acid, which is the only hemolytic agent in the bile acid (*ca.* 1:550) series and is likewise lethal on paramecia. It is as we have seen unreactive to films of protein, cholesterol and glycerides, and in fact a specific interaction with fatty acids is involved.

This method of attack permits us to investigate the nature of the coatings of cells or unicellular animals and plants by examining the effects of lipoid or protein penetrating substances on them.

Thus both red cells and paramecia are affected by both lipoid and protein monolayer penetrating (cytolyzing) or adsorbing (agglutinating) agents, and we deduce that their surface structures must contain lipoproteins or consist of a lipoid protein mosaic; whereas certain other unicellular animals frequently found associated with paramecia and in addition the cilia of mytilus are not affected by protein dispersants but are readily influenced by lipoid penetrating agents, and their coatings in consequence must be chiefly lipoidal in nature.

Examination of the carcinogenic hydrocarbons by the monolayer technique reveals the interesting fact that whilst they themselves are unreactive they are readily converted into extremely reactive water-soluble photo-oxides. These substances are not only reactive to protein monolayers like the water-soluble dibenzanthracene endosuccinnate, but also are paramecicidal, the parallelism between the biological activity and monolayer reaction being maintained.

Many attempts have been made to construct model systems to yield potential differences analogous to the bioelectric potentials observed in tissues. The work of Beutner, Bauer, Cremer and others suggests that potential differences of magnitude corresponding to those found in living systems can be obtained by interposing suitable oil phases between electrolytes of different composition, and the fact that the penetration of large molecules into living cells frequently follows their lipoid solubility has given support to the theory that the seat of the bioelectric potential lies in the lipoid-like cell wall. The order of thickness of such cell walls can not exceed a few molecular layers, and we must take this fact into consideration. We have noted that at the lipoid-water interface there will exist an orientated layer of dipoles, and on placing a monolayer at the interface, the original array of solvent dipoles will be replaced by one consisting of the material of the monolayer. If an electrolyte be brought to equilibrium in both the homogeneous phases, it is clear that opposite the monolayer in both the aqueous phase and in the lipoid phase adsorption and electrokinetic potentials[2] will be built up of such magnitudes that the total potential fall across the interface, which may be written $\xi_{oil} + \Delta V + \xi_{water}$, must be zero. If the lipoid phase be replaced by air no diffuse double layer can be built up, since the gaseous ions produced by the usual radioactive source are continually drawn into the liquid phase; there is in consequence a permanent potential fall equal to $\Delta V + \xi_{water}$, which is the one customarily measured.

It is evidence that a bioelectric potential difference may be caused by a sudden alteration in $\Delta V$, for the compensating potential differences $\xi_{oil}$ and $\xi_{water}$ must take time to readjust themselves by diffusion to the new equilibrium values. Since in general the electrolyte concentration in the aqueous phase is high, it seems probable that $\xi_{water}$ will adjust itself to the new value acquired by $\Delta V$ as rapidly as $\Delta V$ can be caused to change either by mechanical, electrical or chemical means. Thus surges in potential difference across the interface due to a periodic alteration in $\Delta V$ may be caused by the slow readjustment of $\xi_{oil}$, for it is in this phase that the ionic concentration is low.

Another source of biological potentials is to be found in the case where the chemical potential of the electrolyte is not the same in the two phases, bringing into existence a diffusion potential across the interface from source to sink. It is clear that a monolayer can only affect the diffusion potential provided that its permeability to the ions is not only comparable to that of the homogeneous phases on each side, but that it also is not equally permeable to both ions. Experiments have shown that monolayers and even built-up multilayers of considerable thickness of proteins are surprisingly permeable to ions and we must presume that the bioelectric potentials do not involve only a protein membrane between the ionic source and sink.

[2] Whether adsorption or electrokinetic potentials will be built up in any specific case will depend on whether short or long range forces are involved *i.e.*, on the magnitude and spacing of the dipoles. If the dipole system occurs across a relatively thick multilayer the potentials will be purely electrokinetic.

It thus appears that there is some justification for the assumption that it must be a lipoid or a lipo-protein membrane.

It has been the purpose of this address to re-emphasize the importance of the fundamental concepts introduced by Sir W. Hardy and Dr. I. Langmuir as to the structure of matter in the boundary state. I have attempted to show that there is implicitly contained in the concept of molecular orientation a whole series of properties and events for which there are no analogies in homogeneous bulk phase systems. We note that many of the modes and types of the reactions which can be effected in monolayers, and which can be defined with precision and their mechanism established with a considerable degree of assurance, are unique for such interphases, but are again observed in living and organized material. It is with this object of ultimate correlation with biological behavior that we have taken up the detailed study of interfacial reactions at Cambridge, and I should like to express my deep indebtedness to my colleague, Dr. J. Schulman, who has been associated with me in this object.

Many "vitalistic" models have been proposed in the past, and whilst it might be correct, although unscientific, to suggest that the ultimate level of integration in living matter is incapable of examination and definition, yet I believe that one is justified in asserting that at least one of the important levels to which due attention must be given for a proper understanding of biological activities is that of the ordered interface.

# OBITUARY

## THE MAYO BROTHERS AND THEIR CLINIC

There was nothing mysterious or supernatural about this twentieth century Lourdes at whose doors incredible numbers of the lame, halt and blind have for years been daily delivered from the ends of the earth. Nothing supernatural—unless possibly the flawless, life-long devotion of two brothers for one another be so regarded. Not since the somewhat mythical attachment of those fifth-century physicians, Cosmos and Damian, both of whom in due time came to be sanctified, has there been anything quite like it.

Rochester, Minnesota, fifty years ago, then scarcely on the map, was a prairie town near the headwaters of the Mississippi where in a humble way, at St. Mary's Hospital, the Clinic had its beginning. It was, to be sure, a Catholic foundation in which Sisters of Mercy doubtless prayed for the recovery of their patients. But it was not primarily for prayer, however efficacious, that the afflicted as by a magnet came to be drawn to that particular shrine.

It was rather the world-wide reputation of two forward-looking men whom I like to remember as they were thirty years and more ago, young and vigorous; each blessed with rare surgical judgment, each with hands which seemed possessed, in an emergency, with an uncanny ability to do, unflustered, just the right thing at the right moment.

At this shrine there was plenty of ritual, to be sure, but it was the ritual of the well-drilled, silent, operating room where for every movement there is a reason; where the incense in the air is not to conceal corruption but to produce painless sleep; where the water in which gloved fingers are dipped is holy only because it is sterile.

Their father, the senior Dr. Mayo, pioneer and Indian fighter, was still alive when I first came to know the place in its early simplicity. There were then but two operating tables, at one of which "Dr. Will" officiated, at the other in an adjoining room "Dr. Charlie." They were thus affectionately differentiated by every one—staff, patients, employees and fellow townspeople—not to mention the countless visiting doctors who even then were wearing a path to their door.

For these also soon came from all parts of the world, often by special trains, to see for themselves what modern miracles were being performed daily in this once obscure country town. To what they could learn and carry away for their own use they were more than welcome, for our profession has no trade secrets. The more widely knowledge can be disseminated, the better for every one.

And so, as the years slipped rapidly by, a great tower of healing, known everywhere as the Mayo Clinic, was finally erected—a living memorial to a great idea, not a mere place of worship for tradition dead and gone, like the Basilica of SS. Cosmos and Damian built some fifteen centuries ago in Rome by Pope Felix IV.

Another contemporary pair of no less self-effacing brothers—Wilbur and Orville Wright of Dayton, Ohio—were also at about the same time dreaming dreams of a different sort that in no less spectacular fashion came likewise to be fulfilled. Like the Mayos, they seem to have imbibed in their youth the flavor of the old Northwest Territory where the offspring of the early settlers were reared to think more highly of serving mankind than of helping themselves.

One is led to wonder whether imaginative visions of such kind are not more likely to occur and be more possible of realization for those who live where horizons are broad than for those cooped up in metropolitan centers where, even could the rising or the setting sun ever be seen, there would be no time to stop and commune with it.

Different as W. J. and C. H. Mayo were from each other, I have always felt that there was something Lincolnesque about them both. It was shown not only by their modesty and self-effacement, but in their shrewd appraisal of other people in whatever walk of life and in their quiet dry sense of humor. About this there was nothing boisterous, but I have known them to save with Lincoln-like readiness many an awkward situation by an appropriate story more often turned on themselves than otherwise.

Lincoln of course was pitchforked out of his native environment in the old Northwest into a position of responsibility he could not refuse. So the Mayos were ready to serve when called, as they did during the war; but they very much preferred their own countryside with its comparatively simple life despite the ever-increasing responsibilities and laborious routine of their professional work. They felt only an amused pity for those who thought they were wasting their talents in a small town and who ventured to offer them positions elsewhere of supposedly wider influence.

W. J. once said to me, "When Charlie gets so busy on his farm he forgets to have his shoes cleaned, he takes a night sleeper to Chicago knowing that he will find them well polished under his berth in the morning." Had he been encountered by some traveler on the train who with Mid-West informality asked his occupation, he would have replied, "A Minnesota farmer." Had Dr. Will been similarly asked who he was by some chance companion, he probably would have replied: "I'm C. H. Mayo's elder brother."

After Charlie's death, their friends knew the separation could not be for long. There is a tradition among surgeons that they are likely to meet their end by the same malady in the treatment of which they have themselves specialized. So it was entirely consistent that "Dr. Will" when nearly eighty should calmly submit to an operation whose difficult technique he had not only perfected but countless times had successfully carried out on persons of younger age who still survive to bless him.

The modern world is all too accustomed to gauge success in terms of net income, and thus measured the returns from the Mayo Clinic exceeded the dreams of avarice; but when in 1915 the Mayo Foundation was established Dr. Will simply stated: "We never regarded the money as ours; it came from the people and we believe, my brother and myself, that it should go back to the people."

HARVEY CUSHING

THE SCHOOL OF MEDICINE,
YALE UNIVERSITY

## RECENT DEATHS AND MEMORIALS

DR. HENRY SMITH PRITCHETT, president emeritus of the Carnegie Foundation for the Advancement of Teaching, died on August 28 at the age of eighty-two years. Before becoming president of the foundation in 1906, Dr. Pritchett had been professor of astronomy at Washington University, St. Louis; superintendent of the U. S. Coast and Geodetic Survey, and president of the Massachusetts Institute of Technology.

THE death is announced of Professor L. Lévy-Bruhl, professor of philosophy in the Sorbonne from 1899 to 1927, president of the Institut française d'Anthropologie during 1927–30, aged eighty-two years.

*The British Medical Journal* reports the death of Professor M. B. Krol, director of the clinic for nervous disorders at the All-Union Institute of Experimental Medicine. Born in 1879, Professor Krol was chief physician at the Kremlin Hospital from 1934 to 1938, and in 1935 he was chairman of the Soviet delegation to the second International Neurological Congress in London.

ON the eleventh anniversary of the death of Dr. Hideyo Noguchi, of the Rockefeller Institute for Medical Research, in Accra, West Africa, where he had gone for work with yellow fever, a memorial hall was dedicated at his birthplace in Okinajima, Japan.

# SCIENTIFIC EVENTS

## MARINE ENGINEERING AT THE MASSACHUSETTS INSTITUTE OF TECHNOLOGY

THE prospect of expansion in naval and merchant ship-building during the next ten years and a demand for naval engineers of exceptional qualifications has led to the establishment at the Massachusetts Institute of Technology of an advanced course in marine engineering. The course will last for one year and will lead to the degree of master of science. While it is designed primarily for graduates of Annapolis, and arranged with the cooperation of the Navy Department, it will be offered also to a group of selected civilian graduate students. It is expected that ten experienced officers of the United States Navy will be detailed to the institute for this course and that five civilians will be admitted.

The naval building plans call for replacement of a large part of the present fleet, including battleships, cruisers, destroyers, submarines and various service ships, while the Maritime Commission is planning construction of 500 ships for the merchant marine. This program requires engineers with special training in the design and construction of marine propulsion machinery, for the major ships involved in both the Navy and merchant marine programs must be designed to give the utmost in economy of operation and reliable service. The training is designed to prepare engineers for solution of essential problems of marine engineering, including the use of marine power plants operating at high pressures and temperatures. There is also the problem of the application of Diesel engines with hydraulic, electrical or gear drive, the solution of which involves familiarity with its thermal, metallurgical and mechanical limitations.

The basic objective of the course is to give the student a unified and scientific approach to engineering problems within this field, with special emphasis on investigation of fundamental methods of analysis applied to new problems in marine engineering. Cooperating in the course, in addition to the department of naval architecture and marine engineering, will be the departments of mechanical and electrical engineering. The entire resources of the institute will be available for various aspects of the training.

Professors Evers Burtner, Lawrence B. Chapman, Frank M. Lewis, all members of the staff of the Pratt School of Naval Architecture, will give instruction in advanced marine engineering and mechanical vibration in ships, and Professor Lewis will give special attention to instruction in propeller theory and experimental research in this field. Professor Harold L. Hazen, head of the department of electrical engineering, will have charge of advanced problems in his subject; Professor C. Richard Soderberg, of the department of mechanical engineering, a designer of heavy power machinery, will devote his attention to advanced problems in mechanical engineering; the subject of internal combustion engines, particularly Diesel power plants, will be covered by Professor C. Fayette Taylor, one of the leading authorities in engine design; instruction in heat transfer will be given by Professor William H. McAdams, of the department of chemical engineering.

## THE NEW RESEARCH VESSEL OF THE BUREAU OF FISHERIES

AIDED by the commercial fishing industry, the Bureau of Fisheries is about to place in service a first-class research vessel for offshore work in the North Atlantic. Through the cooperative interest of the General Seafoods Corporation of Boston, arrangements are being made for the transfer of the *Harvard,* a 152½-foot trawler, to the Bureau of Fisheries. As soon as the transfer of the vessel has been completed, Public Works Administration funds to the amount of $125,000, allotted late in June, will be made available for the reconditioning and outfitting of the vessel.

Repairs and alterations to the hull and superstructure and installation of equipment for oceanographic studies and experimental fishing are expected to be completed in time to put the vessel into operation on the fishing grounds next summer. Since the *Albatross II* was taken out of service because of lack of operating funds in 1932, the Bureau of Fisheries has possessed no ship suitable for use on the fishing banks of the Atlantic.

One of the most important problems to be studied with the aid of the new research facilities will be that of maintaining stocks of fish on the nearer banks, a day's run from the New England ports. Under intensive fishing, supplies of haddock in the Georges Bank area have been so reduced in recent years that it has been necessary for much of the fleet to operate on the distant Nova Scotian banks.

As a result of several years' investigation of the haddock fishery, William C. Herrington, in charge of the biological fishery investigations in the North Atlantic area, last fall announced a theoretical basis for operating the haddock fishery of Georges Bank at a level that would maintain a stable yield and guard against reduction of the basic stock. With the aid of a seagoing research vessel, Mr. Herrington and his staff now expect to determine the actual poundage that represents the optimum yield for the haddock fishery.

The program of investigations to be carried out includes an annual survey of the fishing grounds from Nantucket Shoals to the Laurentian Channel to discover the localities in which the greatest numbers of fish are concentrated.

With gear to be installed in the new vessel, biologists will be able to make a census of young haddock too small to be caught in commercial nets. Experiments will be undertaken with commercial fishing gear to develop and encourage the use of nets of a type that will release undersized fish without loss of marketable sizes.

Fluctuations in the catch of mackerel, which may vary more than 50 per cent. from year to year, have been shown by past investigations of the Bureau of Fisheries to be closely linked with the fate of young mackerel during the first months of their lives. It is now planned to make definite measurements of the effects of oceanic conditions on the survival of the young; and to make annual censuses of the newly hatched and one-year-old mackerel so that it may advise the industry whether to expect good or poor fishing. Cruises are also contemplated to discover the location of schools of adult mackerel in years when they do not congregate in the usual areas, as happened in 1937. Tagging of mackerel will be done at sea to further explore the movements of the fish.

## THE ASSOCIATION FOR THE STUDY OF SYSTEMATICS IN RELATION TO GENERAL BIOLOGY

THE Association for the Study of Systematics in Relation to General Biology has issued, according to the London *Times,* a statement in regard to its aims and constitution. Hitherto its constitution has been as loose as possible, and there has been no subscription. In spite of this, useful work has been done, discussions have been organized in connection with the Zoological Society, the Linnean Society and the British Association, and "The New Systematics," a book of essays on recent progress in taxonomy in relation to other branches of biology, edited by Dr. Julian Huxley, will be published soon by the Oxford University Press.

It has now, however, been decided that, in order that the association may function still more effectively, a regular income is necessary, and a subscription of 5s. a year has been fixed for the first three years. An agreement has been made with the Linnean Society, whereby the association may use the society's rooms for meetings, joint discussions are to be held, and the annual report will appear in the *Proceedings* of the Linnean Society.

The general aim of the association is to remedy the isolation which modern specialization has inevitably created in the various branches of biology. Its objects include the study of the bases and practical aims of taxonomy; the examination of the criteria employed in defining species and other systematic categories; the consideration of modifications of the existing categories in the light of various branches of specialized research; the promotion of research; the investigation of methods of teaching systematics; and the promotion of cooperation between workers in different branches of biology and taxonomic problems. The association plans eventually to produce a uniform series of handbooks on the British fauna and flora.

The chairman of the association is Dr. Julian Huxley; J. S. L. Gilmour is botanical secretary; H. W. Parker, zoological secretary, and Dr. J. Smart, treasurer. The address of the treasurer is care of the British Museum (Natural History), London, S.W. 7.

## THE INTERNATIONAL CONGRESS OF GENETICS

BEFORE the opening of the International Congress of Genetics at Edinburgh a special cable to *The New York Times,* signed by Ritchie Calder, reported that Professor N. I. Vavilov, president of the congress, together with fifty of his colleagues had withdrawn from the congress and that Soviet science would not be represented either by a delegation or by individuals. The official explanation, contained in a letter to Professor F. A. E. Crew, secretary-general of the congress, is that the Russians could not participate because the congress should have been held in Moscow instead of Edinburgh.

Mr. Calder wrote that this announcement, which was received on the eve of the congress, came as a complete surprise. Two years ago plans to hold the congress in Moscow were abandoned because of differences and restrictions that foreign geneticists could not accept. By a decision of the international committee that organizes the congress, the meeting was transferred to Edinburgh, but it was also decided that the president should be Professor Vavilov as arranged and that the Russians should have a dominant part in the proceedings.

Three weeks before the opening, Professor Vavilov, who for eighteen months had been actively participating in the arrangements, discovered that the project for meeting in Moscow had not been "abandoned" but only "postponed" and that the Edinburgh proceedings were therefore out of order.

Russian papers, including the presidential address, had been received and printed. They had to be suppressed and all the program had to be readjusted and reissued to close the fifty gaps caused by this wholesale retreat.

No one, according to the *Times,* seriously accepted the official explanation. It is known that there have been growing differences of opinion among Russian geneticists, and one section is demanding "Marxist genetics." Thus Soviet biology has become involved with ideology.

It is also thought that the turn of international events has had some bearing on the fact that the Russians had not received their passports.

About a quarter of the German geneticists had also withdrawn. Six out of twelve members in the field of human genetics were "unable to attend," but thirty-two were expected to be present at the opening of the Congress. One of the principal papers planned for that day was a study of heredity and environment through identical twins by Professor Fritz Lenz, of Berlin. About twenty Italians were expected to take part. The American contingent numbered 120, and there were large delegations from France, the Netherlands and Scandinavia.

## OPENING OF THE INTERNATIONAL CONGRESS FOR MICROBIOLOGY

THE third International Congress for Microbiology opened at the Waldorf-Astoria Hotel, New York City, on September 2. According to the *New York Herald Tribune* many scientific men from abroad who expected to be present were unable to attend and others must return as soon as transportation can be arranged.

Nearly all the forty-two official delegates designated by the German government actually sailed on the Hamburg-American liner *Hansa,* but the boat was recalled to Hamburg. Several official delegates designated by the Italian Government were to have sailed on the Italian liner *Conte di Savoia,* but the sailing was cancelled, and the ship is still in Naples.

Some of those who were unable to attend were already in the service of their governments. Among these is Dr. G. Ramon, director of the Pasteur Institute in Paris, who was to have headed the French delegation. He is engaged in preparing vaccines and anti-toxins for the French Government. Dr. Pierre Lepine, head of the rabies and virus diseases department of the Pasteur Institute, took his place.

The first general session of the congress on Monday was to have been devoted to addresses by Professor Dr. A. J. Kluyver, of Delft, the Netherlands; Dr. Paul Fildes, of London, and Dr. C. Levaditi, of Paris, and Wednesday's general session to addresses by Professor Dr. Eduard Reichenow, of Hamburg, Germany; Professor A. Missiroli, of Rome, and Dr. B. O. Dodge, of New York. Of these speakers only Dr. Dodge was able to be present. Mayor F. H. La Guardia and Dr. John L. Rice, commissioner of health, welcomed the delegates at the opening ceremonies at the Waldorf-Astoria. Other speakers included Dr. Thomas M. Rivers, director of the Hospital of the Rockefeller Institute and president of the congress; Sir John C. G. Ledingham, director of the Lister Institute, London, and Dr. Lewis R. Jones, of the University of Wisconsin.

# SCIENTIFIC NOTES AND NEWS

THE British Association for the Advancement of Science adjourned on September 1 after meeting for only three days. Before adjournment Sir Richard Gregory, formerly editor of *Nature,* was elected president in succession to Sir Albert Seward.

COLUMBUS ISELIN, 2nd, assistant professor of oceanography at Harvard University, was appointed director of the Woods Hole Oceanographic Institution at the recent annual meeting of the Board of Trustees. He succeeds Dr. Henry B. Bigelow, who was elected president of the corporation in succession to Dr. Frank R. Lillie.

P. H. BATES, chief of the Clay and Silicate Products Division of the National Bureau of Standards, has been awarded the Turner Gold Medal of the American Concrete Institute. The award was made for "contributions to science, direction of research and outstanding leadership in advancing the intelligent utilization of cement and concrete."

AT the San Antonio meeting of the American Home Economics Association, Dr. Icie G. Macy-Hoobler, director of the research laboratory of the Children's Fund of Michigan, Detroit, was presented with the 1939 gold medal and the $1,000 prize of the Borden Company for research achievement in applied nutrition.

PROFESSOR JOSEPH RIGNEY D'AUNOY, who recently resigned as dean of the Medical Center of the Louisiana State University, remaining as professor of pathology and bacteriology, has been decorated with the Order of Commendatore of the Crown of Italy "in recognition of his achievements in the fields of medical research and education."

THE honorary doctorate of the medical faculty of the University of Freiburg/Br. has been conferred on Dr. Eugen Fischer, professor of anthropology at Berlin. He has also been awarded the Goethe prize for art and science.

THE following corresponding members of the Prussian Academy of Sciences have been elected: Dr. Heinrich Vogt, professor of astronomy at Heidelberg; Dr. Peter Adolf Thiessen, professor of physical chemistry at Berlin, and Dr. Siegmund Shumacher, professor of histology and embryology at Innsbruck.

DR. A. FRANKE, of Arnstadt, Germany, has recently received the honorary doctorate of the University of Jena for his contributions to geology, especially in the field of micropaleontology.

AT Teachers College, Columbia University, Dr. Jean Broadhurst, professor of bacteriology, and Dr. M. A. Bigelow, professor of biology, have been appointed emeritus professors. Successors have not been appointed because the Division of Practical Science and the Institute of Practical Science Research have been discontinued.

DR. EDGAR HULL, for the past eight years a member of the Medical Center, New Orleans, has been made acting head of the department of medicine of the Louisiana State University. He succeeds the late George S. Bel.

DR. KARL BRANDT, professor of agricultural economics in the Food Research Institute of Stanford University, has joined the staff of the Giannini Foundation of Agricultural Economics of the University of California.

DR. RALPH W. BOST has been made head of the department of chemistry of the University of North Carolina. He takes the place of Dr. Edward Mack, Jr., who resigned to become a member of the staff of the Battelle Memorial Institute, Columbus, Ohio.

DR. NELSON F. MURPHY, of the chemical engineering staff of the General Chemical Company, New York City, has been appointed assistant professor in chemical engineering in the College of Applied Science, Syracuse University.

DR. LLOYD H. DONNELL, of the Goodyear Zeppelin Corporation, has become associate professor of mechanical engineering at the Armour Institute, Chicago.

IT is reported in *The Collecting Net* that Dr. William C. Young, assistant professor of biology at Brown University, has been appointed associate professor of primate biology at the Yale University School of Medicine. He will work at the Laboratories of Primate Biology, Orange Park, Fla., and at New Haven, Conn.

DR. HARVEY DIEHL, assistant professor of analytical chemistry at Purdue University, has been appointed to a similar position at the Iowa State College.

THE Anderson Clayton Company of Texas is continuing the support of industrial research fellowships, for the study of industrial utilization of hemi-cellulosic constituents of plants, at the Iowa State College. Professor E. I. Fulmer is director of the research. Dr. John A. Dunning will hold a fellowship for the coming year.

THE *Journal* of the American Medical Association reports that Dr. James R. Martin, chief surgeon at the State Hospital for Crippled Children, Elizabethtown, Pa., and director of the state program for crippled children under the Social Security Act, has been appointed James Edwards professor of orthopedic surgery at Jefferson Medical College, Philadelphia. He succeeds Dr. J. Torrance Rugh, who has resigned after holding the chair since 1918 and who will become professor emeritus.

DR. KENNETH M. SODERSTROM, of Seattle, has been appointed a member of the staff of the division of epidemiology in the Washington State Department of Health in charge of tuberculosis control.

DR. WESLEY COCKER, assistant lecturer in organic chemistry at University College, Exeter, has been appointed lecturer in chemistry at King's College, Newcastle, Durham, in place of Dr. R. D. Haworth, who has been appointed to the chair of chemistry in the University of Sheffield. J. A. Lyddiard, of the Standard Telephones and Cables, Limited, New Southgate, has been appointed to a new lectureship in electrical engineering.

CHANGES in the department of hygiene at the University of California have been announced as follows: Lecturers appointed include Dr. Jacques P. Gray, who has resigned his position as director of public welfare in San Francisco, and Dr. A. Stampar, professor of public health at the State University of Zagreb, formerly director of public health in Yugoslavia and expert in rural health matters for the League of Nations. Dr. Eschscholtzia L. Lucia, associate professor of biometry, has been promoted to a professorship. Dr. Frank L. Kelly, for several years assistant professor of public health administration and now city health officer of Berkeley, will serve as lecturer in public health in the second semester.

O. C. DURHAM, chief botanist of the Abbott Laboratories, Chicago, will make a study of pollen grains in the upper air. The trip by commercial airplanes will extend from the Gulf of Mexico to Alaska, across the Atlantic to England and across the Pacific to China. Mr. Durham is continuing the work of Dr. Fred C. Meier, of the Department of Agriculture, and Dr. Earl B. McKinley, dean of the George Washington Medical School, who died in the crash of an airplane in the South Pacific while making aerial studies of the distribution of pollen, spores and disease germs.

THE Swiss Society of Naturalists has announced that the one hundred and twentieth annual meeting will be held at Locarno from September 23 to 25 in conjunction with the Swiss Medico-Biological Society.

THE eighth annual convention of the Biological Photographic Association will be held at the Mellon Institute for Industrial Research, Pittsburgh, from September 14 to 16, under the presidency of Louis Schmidt, of the Rockefeller Institute for Medical Research. There will be a session on the uses of scientific photography at which the speakers will include Robert Cook, Washington, D. C., editor of the *Journal of Heredity;* Watson Davis, director of Science Service, Washington, and David Dietz, science editor of the Scripps-Howard newspapers, Cleveland.

THE department of industrial medicine of the medical school of Northwestern University will hold its third annual symposium on Industrial Disease and Hygiene on September 25 and 26. There will be four sessions presided over by Drs. Merritt Paul Starr and M. Herbert Barker, assistant professors of medicine at the university; Wilber E. Post, clinical professor of medicine, and Edward A. Oliver, associate clinical professor of dermatology, both of Rush Medical College.

AT a meeting held on August 29, the board of directors of the Union Carbide and Carbon Corporation approved an agreement for the acquisition by the corporation of all the assets of the Bakelite Corporation, founded by Dr. L. H. Baekeland over twenty-five years ago. The Carbide Corporation is a producer of chemical raw materials and the Bakelite Corporation a user of chemicals. According to the announcement it is expected that "the coordination of technical knowledge, research, production methods and distribution facilities of these two organizations will result in the improvement of existing products, the development of new plastics and other chemical compounds, and the discovery of new uses for such materials."

IT is stated in the *Journal* of the American Medical Association that the Utah State Board of Health with the collaboration of the U. S. Public Health Service and the Utah Industrial Commission has begun a study of occupational disease under the direction of State Health Commissioner John L. Jones, of Salt Lake City, who has leave of absence for two years. The state legislature has appropriated $25,000, which will be used for the conduct of the study with a view to developing a permanent occupational disease service. The federal public health service will participate in the first six months of the investigation, the major problems of which will be exposure to silicious dusts and dusts in bituminous coal mines, lead and other metallic dusts and fumes and certain gases. Later, health hazards in other industries will be investigated.

A NEW siderite, or iron meteorite, to be called the Mapleton meteorite, has been acquired by Field Museum of Natural History from Mr. Harvey Meevers, Mapleton, Iowa. This is the first iron meteorite to be reported from that state. Previous to the discovery of this iron, four other meteorites were known from Iowa, three of which were aerolites or stone meteorites, and one a meso-siderite or variety of iron-stone meteorite. No conclusive evidence is at hand regarding the date and time of the fall of the meteorite, which probably does not represent much more than half of the original mass. It weighs 49 kilograms (108 pounds). Its greatest length, breadth and height are 17½ inches, 9⅞ inches and 6 5/16 inches, respectively.

THE Committee on Sedimentation of the Division of Geology and Geography of the National Research Council has prepared a symposium on recent marine sediments. This consists of thirty-four papers by specialists in different fields of this subject. Emphasis has been placed upon the processes affecting the deposition of sediments. Because of the bearing of this subject on petroleum geology, the symposium has been published by the American Association of Petroleum Geologists. Dr. Parker D. Trask, associate geologist of the U. S. Geological Survey, became chairman of the committee four years ago. At that time he proposed the assembling in a single volume of the large amount of information that had been obtained in the previous ten or fifteen years by investigators of conditions in the oceanographical, geological, biological and other publications in many parts of the world. This idea received favorable reception, and a book of 740 pages, which is now about ready for distribution, is the result.

*The E. W. Scripps,* the research vessel of the Scripps Institution of Oceanography of the University of California, sailed from San Diego early in August for a study of ocean currents and undersea strata from San Diego to Santa Barbara. Samples of undersea strata will be taken about thirty miles off shore. Dr. Roger Revelle, member of the institution, is in charge of the cruise. Dr. R. T. Young, physicist of the Worcester Polytechnic Institute, will make a special study of the transmission of light in sea water. *The E. W. Scripps* returned recently after a cruise of 1,200 miles of the Pacific from the Oregon border to Cedros Islands in Mexico. The cruise, which lasted two months, was made in cooperation with the Federal Bureau of Fisheries, which was interested in studying the distribution of sardine eggs off the California coast. General hydrographic conditions were observed at a number of stations from just off shore to as far as 360 miles at sea.

# DISCUSSION

## THE MODE OF ACTION OF SULFANILAMIDE

DR. PHILIP SHAFFER'S communication on this subject in the issue of SCIENCE[1] for June 16 suggests that both the therapeutic and toxic actions of sulfanilamide may be exerted through a "mechanism by which the sterilizing oxidation intensity of molecular oxygen is applied nearly at its maximum to bacteria and unavoidably also to some extent to host cells."

The undersigned are in agreement with this conception to the extent that it indicates a source of sulfanilamide toxicity. They do not find the available evidence compatible with a concept of identity between the mechanisms producing the known toxic and therapeutic effects nor with an explanation of the therapeutic usefulness of sulfanilamide in terms of capacity to act as a reservoir for an intermediate substance of high oxidizing intensity.

[1] P. 547.

*The Shaffer premises:* Ingested sulfanilamide is assumed to become (1) converted by a process of biologically mediated oxidation into derivatives which act, in turn, as oxidizing agents; (2) producing injuries to the cellular reducing systems; (3) less easily tolerated by the invading pathogen than by the resisting host.

The acting derivatives are assumed to form a reversible electrode couple (as do ferrous and ferric iron) composed of p-hydroxylamino and p-nitroso benzene sulfonamide "or the corresponding semiquinone free radicals."

The cell components mentioned as especially susceptible to injury by this oxidizing combination are: catalase, hemoglobin, glutathione and ascorbic acid. The injuries are presumed to be more readily tolerated by the host than by the invader because of "the relative immunity of host tissues to toxic effects . . . due to their lower oxygen tension, their higher metabolism and to higher catalase content."

*Association of the oxidizing potentialities of the postulated intermediate with the nitroso and not with the hydroxylamine component:* Nitrous acid, in the orientation present in p-nitroso benzene sulfonamide, is an effective oxidizing agent, producing damage to the capacity of hemoglobin to transport oxygen and to the capacity of the body to maintain circulation. Hydroxylamine is not an oxidizing agent at the pH of the blood, excepting toward substances of unusually powerful reducing capacity or under conditions of catalytic mediation. *In vitro,* it reduces Fehling's solution much as glucose does. *In vivo,* it becomes converted into nitrite[2,3]—again acting as a reducing, not an oxidizing agent. The point is emphasized because hydroxylamine is known to block catalase action in concentrations as small as M/100,000.[4]

*Insusceptibility of catalase to oxidative injury of the type postulated:* The oxidizing potentialities of p-nitroso benzene sulfonamide would be a source of injury to hemoglobin, glutathione and ascorbic acid, but not to catalase. Keilin and Hartree[5] and K. G. Stern,[6] authorities on the properties of catalase, report it to be so extraordinarily resistant to oxidation as to suggest that the iron content of that enzyme may be in the ferric condition, passing fleetingly into the ferrous condition only after *reduction* by hydrogen peroxide.

*Successful chemotherapeutic action is directed against a type of vulnerability, in the pathogen, not shared by the host:* Oxidizing actions against hemoglobin, glutathione and ascorbic acid are directed against oxygen-carrying power and against capacity to sustain circulation. They are highly toxic because they strike at the host where he is most vulnerable in his defense against oxygen want. The pathogens responsive to sulfanilamide are less vulnerable to oxygen want[7] and more vulnerable to peroxide.[8] The maximum chemotherapeutic possibilities are obviously not to be sought in an action striking at the defenses against oxygen want but in an action striking at the defenses against peroxide, namely, against catalase.[9,11] For this action, the reducing, hydroxylamine derivative of sulfanilamide is definitely available[9,11] *not* the oxidizing nitroso derivative, which is a source of toxicity.

*Alternative suggestion:* There can be no question but that p-hydroxylamino and p-nitroso benzene sulfonamide are obtainable from sulfanilamide by biologically feasible types of oxidation. They may not, however, be produced together but, rather, stepwise: the hydroxylamine derivative being formed within the locus of infection[9,11] by the metabolic process which *yields* peroxide, and the nitroso derivative being formed following diffusion of the hydroxylamine from the areas vicinal to the cell substance of the pathogen, into the blood.

This stepwise production, first of the therapeutically active derivative and, secondly, of the toxic derivative, is possible in the manner outlined. It would not be possible as a result of the peroxide-mediated type of oxidation postulated by Shaffer. The latter type of oxidation is, however, not indicated: (1) because the pathogens most responsive to sulfanilamide are not those producing the most peroxide and permitting accumulation of peroxide to highest levels—as is demanded by a hypothesis of conversion mediated by peroxide—and (2) because such a type of oxidation contains no factor of self-limitation. (Production of active intermediate as a function of available peroxide concentration would increase progressively with increasing peroxide concentration until the pathogen was destroyed. Sulfanilamide does not act, *in vivo,* in any such drastic fashion. It produces only a degree of growth retardation, in infections responsive to its action, sufficient to hold down the *numbers* of the pathogen to be disposed of, by the host, to levels within possibility of control.[10,11]

An assumption of stepwise production of the therapeutically active and toxic agents opens up the possibility of using, in place of sulfanilamide, an agent making hydroxylamine available, within the locus of infection, in a form not so readily oxidized to a nitrous acid derivative as is p-hydroxylamino benzene sulfonamide. The comparative anti-catalase and anti-hemoglobin potentialities of hydroxylamine linked to the sulfon group, following blockade of the p-amino group against oxidation, should be explored in this connection.

Adjuvant measures should be taken, during sulfanilamide therapy, to counteract toxic actions on hemoglobin and on circulatory capacity so as to permit full realization of therapeutic effect.[10,11]

ARTHUR LOCKE
R. R. MELLON
THE WESTERN PENNSYLVANIA HOSPITAL,
PITTSBURGH

2 J. W. Mellor, "A Comprehensive Treatise on Inorganic and Theoretical Chemistry," Vol. 8. Longmans-Green, New York, 1928.

3 T. Sollmann, "A Manual of Pharmacology," W. B. Saunders, Philadelphia, 1936, p. 479.

4 M. G. Sevag and L. Maiweg, *Biochem. Zeitschr.*, 288: 41, 1936.

5 *Proc. Roy. Soc. (London)*, B124: 397, 1938.

6 *Jour. Gen. Physiol.*, 20: 631, 1937.

7 A. Locke and E. R. Main, *Jour. Infect. Dis.*, 46: 393, 1930.

8 J. W. McLeod and J. Gordon, *Jour. Path. Bact.*, 26: 326, 1923.

9 A. Locke, E. R. Main and R. R. Mellon, SCIENCE, 88: 620, 1938.

10 A. Locke, R. B. Locke, R. J. Bragdon and R. R. Mellon, SCIENCE, 86: 228, 1937.

11 A. Locke, E. R. Main and R. R. Mellon, *Jour. Immunol.*, 36: 183, 1939.

## RED COLOR IN APPLES[1]

In 1936 the authors[2] published a paper identifying and describing the chemical nature of the red pigment of the Winesap apple, and a few months later Sando[3] confirmed these findings with the Stayman and Jonathan varieties. The red pigment of three varieties thus has been shown to be idaein, a glycoside which yields cyanidin and galactose on hydrolysis.

At the time the pigment was identified the work was carried out of the laboratory into the orchard in an effort to study the various factors involved in its formation and, if possible, to influence the color produced in certain varieties of moderate or low color. In the summer of 1936 we were fortunate in finding a substance which seemed to enhance the red color of the Stayman, and subsequent work in each succeeding summer has confirmed this result and developed a method of treatment which has been more or less effective in improving the red color of several varieties, including Stayman, Rome, Delicious, McIntosh, Jonathan and others. Under certain conditions even such varieties as Golden Delicious and Grimes Golden, which normally carry little or no blush, were affected by the treatment in such a manner as to increase *slightly* the amount of blush present on the fruit.

We are now conducting trials for the fourth consecutive season and believe that the tests have gone sufficiently far to indicate the general trend involved and to justify announcement of the method employed. The effective agent appears to be the thiocyanate ion applied in combination with any one of a number of substances representing the positive group. The materials are applied in relatively low concentration, as a spray, to the foliage and fruit on the tree during the growing season. Up to this year all treatments have been applied with a hand-sprayer, but at present the university power-spray outfit is being employed on somewhat larger-scale operations than have been tried heretofore. Many important questions remain unanswered and final evaluation of the procedure including practical application, if any, must await future work. This notice is being written to invite the attention of any or all interested in the improvement of color in fruits.

R. B. Dustman
I. J. Duncan

West Virginia Agricultural Experiment Station,
Morgantown

## A FIRE-FLY "SPINTHARISCOPE"

It must be well known that the lantern of a fire-fly, teased by being held with the fingers, emits irregular flashes from minute point-sources in the lantern which follow the normal flash, the light of which fills the entire lantern. I am wondering, however, if the very astonishing spectacle presented by a fly which has been bitten by a spider has been described. Within a few minutes after a few "nips" have been made by the spider, if the fly is removed from the web, the lantern will be observed to glow with a faint green light which shows the same "shimmering" quality as the radium paint on the dial of a watch. Examination with an ordinary hand magnifying glass, of moderate power, shows the lantern filled with bright points of light, which at first sight appear to be in rapid vibratory motion, and at the end of half an hour we have a seething cauldron of hundreds of bright points, dancing and flashing, and giving an almost perfect picture of a screen of zinc sulphide under a terrific bombardment of "Alpha" particles (spinthariscope). The phenomenon persists with undiminished intensity for 48 hours but finally dies out, the fly apparently having returned to normal. The spinthariscope effect is frequently accompanied by an occasional normal flash, which ceases if the fly is decapitated, though the other effect continues.

The normal flash of the lantern is obviously due to the simultaneous excitation of all the luminous centers by nerve impulses from the brain, but the scintillations persist even after the lantern has been severed from the body. Both types of illumination cease if the fly is placed in a narrow glass tube through which a stream of carbon dioxide is flowing. I have produced the spinthariscope effect by inoculations with 1 : 1000 solution of snake venom, but in this case the fly did not recover.

Under a microscope, with a low power objective, the individual flashes of green light are seen against a black background and the strong vibratory movement, seen with a hand magnifier, appears to be due chiefly to the quenching of a flash at one point accompanied by the successive flash of a luminous center in its immediate vicinity. My impression is, however, that I have seen single flashes quiver, though in this case it may be merely the spreading of the chemical reaction which produces the light, from one part of a cell to another. The phenomenon, seen with the microscope, is really an amazing sight.

The spiders were, in most cases, small ones found in window webs, with bodies not much larger than a grape-seed, and they usually made their first bites on the leg joints of the fly. The sparkling green flashes appeared first along the upper edge of one or both of the two lanterns, sometimes on one side only. The phenomenon then spread rapidly throughout the entire volume of the lantern. It seems possible that some

[1] Published with the approval of the director of the West Virginia Agricultural Experiment Station as Scientific Paper No. 224.

[2] *Jour. Amer. Chem. Soc.*, 58: 1511–14, 1936.

[3] *Jour. Biol. Chem.*, 117: 45–56, 1937.

information about the nervous system of the fly might be gained by recording the position of points inoculated by the spider and the point or points in the lantern at which the scintillations first appear, but the problem is one for a biologist rather than a physicist.

R. W. WOOD

EAST HAMPTON,
LONG ISLAND, N. Y.

## THE FIRST ARTICLES ON GROUP THEORY PUBLISHED IN AMERICA

IN 1878 the first volume of the *American Journal of Mathematics* was published under the auspices of the Johns Hopkins University. This volume was edited by J. J. Sylvester (1814–1897) and contains two very short articles written by A. Cayley (1821–1895), who was then professor of mathematics at Cambridge University, England, and one of the most eminent mathematicians in the world. Each of these two articles covers less than three pages, and the former was largely embodied verbatim by its author in a longer article which appeared during the same year in the *Proceedings of the London Mathematical Society.* It contains the absurd statement that there are three groups of order 6, notwithstanding the fact that about twenty-four years earlier A. Cayley stated correctly that there are only two such groups, in the *Philosophical Magazine,* Volume 7, page 40 (1854).

The two articles by A. Cayley to which we called attention in the preceding paragraph seem to be the earliest articles on group theory published on the American Continent, but it is not true that the *American Journal of Mathematics* was the first mathematical journal founded on this continent, as stated by H. Weyl in his "The Classical Groups," page 27 (1939). The most conspicuous exception is *The Analyst,* founded at Des Moines, Iowa, in 1874, which appeared in ten volumes and was noted in the "Jahrbuch über die Fortschritte der Mathematik" for 1875 and later. It contains articles by G. W. Hill, S. Newcomb and other well-known mathematicians of that time and was the forerunner of the *Annals of Mathematics,* which is now published by the Princeton University Press.

The fact that no article on group theory was published in America before 1878 throws much light on the early history of mathematics in our country, since articles on this subject began to appear in Europe about one hundred years earlier and soon attracted considerable attention on the part of various European mathematicians living in different countries. This interest was greatly stimulated by the work of N. H. Abel (1802–1829) and E. Galois (1811–1832), both of whom died early but attracted much attention by their tragic lives and fundamental discoveries at an early age. The work of these men was published in Europe about fifty years before work along similar lines was published in America and the latter work had actually been done by a European mathematician and was only published in our country. It took about ten years more until such work was both accomplished and published in this country.

At present important advances made in Europe soon attract attention in America so that the slowness with which American mathematicians entered upon the study of group theory is in striking contrast with present conditions and throws light on the isolation of early American mathematicians. Their interests were for a long time practically confined to the writing of elementary text-books which were frequently based largely on the European text-books which had been in great favor but confined themselves to the treatment of elementary mathematical subjects. About half a dozen mathematical periodicals were published in America before the *American Journal of Mathematics* was established, and some of them had contributors who resided abroad, but the *American Journal of Mathematics* was the first to publish articles by eminent mathematicians residing abroad.

Just as in the case of the first article on group theory published in America the first text-book on this subject to be thus published was written by a mathematician residing in Europe. This text-book appeared in 1892 under the title "Theory of Substitutions" and was a translation of a work by E. Netto. This was about twenty-two years after a similar work had appeared in Europe under the title "Traité des substitutions," by C. Jordan. Enough may have been said to show how the backwardness of the early mathematics in America is reflected in the history of one advanced subject and to emphasize once more the rapid forward strides made by American mathematicians in recent years. The developments in group theory represent some of the most conspicuous advances, especially in the central and the western parts of our country.

G. A. MILLER

UNIVERSITY OF ILLINOIS

# SCIENTIFIC BOOKS

## AN ANECDOTAL HISTORY OF ELECTRICITY

*Sparks, Lightning, Cosmic Rays.* By DAYTON C. MILLER. ix + 192 pp., 183 illustrations. The Macmillan Company, 1939, $2.50.

THE author describes his book as an anecdotal history of electricity. It is based on the Christmas Week Lectures for young people by the Franklin Institute in December, 1937. Both the book and the lectures form a natural tribute to the honor of Benjamin Franklin.

The material in the book in the main is objective and is chosen from the highlights of history. The settled accomplishments of the human race form easy stepping-stones for the lay reader to reach a fascinating picture of electricity as a part of the world. A museum of electricity outlined from this book would be a grand institution. Not only are abstruse and difficult mathematical derivations omitted, but there are also a minimum of mathematical relationships. Likewise worthy attempts to correlate electrical forces with gravitational forces are not considered.

The first part of the book is designated as "Sparks" or the "Beginnings of Electricity." The illustrations are numerous and in keeping with the writing. Particularly the illustration of "Queen Elizabeth watching Gilbert's Experiments" is appropriate to an anecdotal account. Perhaps the explanation of the electrophorus would have been improved if attention had been given to the fact that Volta devised it as a voltage multiplier which enabled him to establish the relative values of the different metals in the Volta series. Also the reproduction of the scene where Volta was showing the Voltaic Pile to Napoleon Bonaparte would fit. An artist's conception of Madame Galvani discovering the twitching of frog legs when an electrical discharge took place in her kitchen would dramatically mark the advent of the first galvanometer. In the reference to the "attracted disk electrometer" of William Snow Harris and later by Lord Kelvin one may make the valuable implication that the advance in the knowledge of electricity is contingent upon instruments of measurement.

The second part of the book is under the caption, "Lightning," in which simple experiments by Franklin and others lay solid foundation for the science of electricity. Franklin's inspiration for this science was incited at the age of forty when he saw some experiments by Dr. Spence. Within a year he had well stated the theory of positive and negative electricity. Within a few years he experimented in every practicable manner. His procedure was simple and direct, and his interpretation has stood well. He showed that lightning was an electric discharge, and he gave the world an electrostatic motor, the lightning rod, the electric chime and the basis for the "inverse square law" from the "ice pail experiment" as interpreted by Joseph Priestley. Besides the author presents the versatile Franklin as making contributions to book-printing, flying machines, optics, eye-glasses, chemistry, geology, submarine boats, whirlwinds, stoves, street cleaning, musical instruments, aerial warfare, etc. In reading of Franklin's discussion of science before royalty and the greatest characters of the time, it would seem that as a salesman for science he is a model.

The author quotes Franklin's philosophic attitude, "nor is it of much importance to us to know the manner in which nature executes her laws. It is enough if we know the laws themselves. It is of real use to know that china (ware) left in the air unsupported will fall and break; but how it falls and why it breaks are matters of speculation. It is a pleasure indeed to know them, but we can preserve our china without it. Thus in the present case, to know this power of points (to discharge electricity) may possibly be of use to mankind, though we should never be able to explain it."

The reviewer would like to have seen reproductions of the early precursors of the Vande Graaff electrostatic generator such as were made by Sir William Thomson, Righi or Gray.

The third part of the book treats of modern electrical science up to and including cosmic rays. Maxwell's work is stated necessarily briefly, but the lay reader would hardly suspect him as the greatest intellect of all, whose work guided perhaps more research than any other man. Perhaps if Maxwell's electromagnetic model had been illustrated and explained, the reader might glimpse the great man's plight and vision. Nevertheless, this last part is an excellent short survey and should encourage many to learn more.

A commanding pageant, "Electricity," could be enacted in a three-hour period by selecting characters, apparatus and wording from Dr. Miller's book. Perhaps it would be bold for an ordinary reviewer to suggest that Dr. Miller could direct the staging of a film encompassing the outline and spirit of this book. By such works as these, other men may become inspired by science as Franklin was at forty.

F. C. BROWN

MUSEUM OF SCIENCE AND INDUSTRY,
CHICAGO

# SPECIAL ARTICLES

## AN ANALYSIS OF SKIN PIGMENT CHANGES AFTER EXPOSURE TO SUNLIGHT

WITH the use of the Hardy recording spectrophotometer and the methods set forth in an earlier paper,[1] we have been able to determine objectively the pigmentary changes in the skin after irradiation by sunlight. Here we demonstrate the events following a single one-hour exposure to the mid-day sun (in August, 1938).

[1] E. A. Edwards and S. Q. Duntley, *Am. Jour. Anat.*, 65: 1, 1939.

A normal male adult served as the subject, and the sacral region was used for the analysis. This area had not previously been exposed to direct sunlight for two years, and it was kept from further exposure after the start of the experiment. Readings were made with diminishing frequency for a total of nine and a half months. The changes following exposure are illustrated by the selected spectrophotometric curves here reproduced (Fig. 1).

The curve made before the exposure (upper curve, Fig. 1) is typical of the sacral region. The blood here is quite venous, as shown by the bluntness of the curve between 500 and 600 millimicrons. Carotene is evidenced by the extremely shallow depression or absorption band at 482 millimicrons, and melanin is moderate in amount as shown by the general upward slope from 400 (violet end) to 700 millimicrons (red end).

Hyperemia was the first effect of the radiation. It was marked in two hours, and maximum in eleven hours. The curve at this time (Fig. 1, lower curve) shows a great lowering in reflectance with pronounced oxyhemoglobin absorption bands, characteristic of an active arterial blood flow (hyperemia). The regression of the hyperemia was rapid in the next few days, and the local blood volume diminished, although it remained distinctly higher than normal. Moreover, there was a shift from oxyhemoglobin to reduced hemoglobin, indicating blood stagnation. This shift could be detected at four days, and is striking in the nineteen-day curve shown in Fig. 1. This curve indicates the gradually decreasing blood volume by the increased reflectance in the region of the twin bands of oxyhemoglobin, while the reduced arterialization is evidenced by the marked blunting of these bands. The venous trend is even more strikingly shown by the fact that despite a diminished blood volume, the nineteen-day curve passes below the eleven-hour curve in the red region of the spectrum (600 to 700 millimicrons). Reference to published curves of reduced and oxyhemoglobin[1] shows that this crossing indicates an increased venous blood content.

During the succeeding months the blood volume slowly receded but did not reach the pre-irradiation level. The shift to a more venous blood continued for four and a half months, after which the blood became fairly constant in its proportions of oxy- to reduced hemoglobin. Thus, while the hyperemia was an acute reaction, the blood stagnation persisted and was still detectable at nine and a half months. This illustrates that solar radiation exerts a long-lasting effect on the blood vessels, a fact previously mentioned by Finsen.[2]

Since melanin gives no sharply demarcated bands in the visible spectrum, but rather imparts a general slope to the curve, an increase in this material will be indicated by a depression of the violet end of the spectrum (400 millimicrons). The concomitant effect of the changes in the other pigments must, however, be kept in mind in drawing deductions as to the amount of melanin present. An increase in melanin was apparent in two days, increasing to a maximum on the nineteenth day. The rate of formation of melanin was slowed after this time, and at one month its total quantity also began to diminish. The nine and a half month curve shows the melanin to have returned to approximately the same level as before exposure.

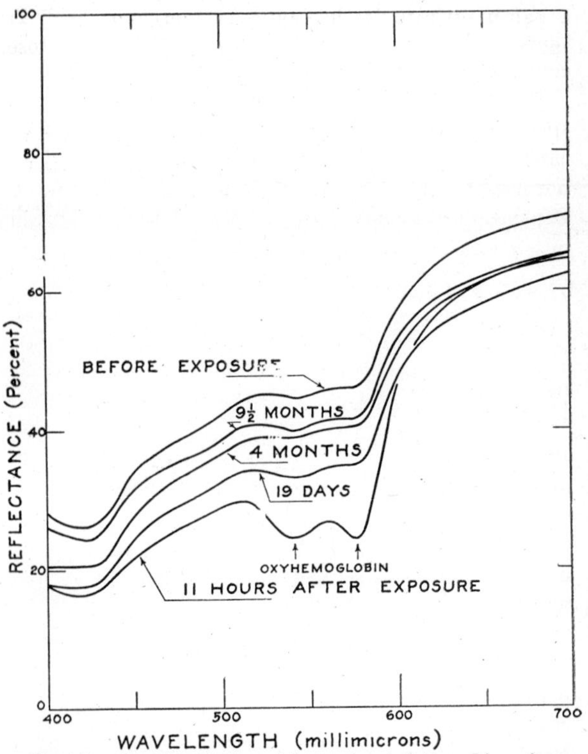


FIG. 1. Spectrophotometric curves of the skin after a single exposure to sunlight. Hyperemia (oxyhemoglobin) is maximal at 11 hours, melanin at 19 days, and melanoid at four months. Blood stagnation, as registered by reduced hemoglobin, persists from the time of the early disappearance of hyperemia for over nine months.

We have previously pointed out that the degeneration of melanin produces an allied pigment which we have named melanoid.[1] The presence of this pigment is shown by a flattening of the spectrophotometric curve near 400 millimicrons. This flattening can be seen in the curve at nineteen days and is maximum at four months, but one fails to find it at nine and a half months. Thus it is seen that the initial appearance of melanoid depends on the formation of considerable melanin. Melanoid increases for some time after the production of new melanin diminishes. Finally, with the disappearance of most of its mother substance, the melanoid ultimately fails to be recognizable.

[2] N. R. Finsen, *Meddelelser fra Finsens Medicinske Lysinstitut*, 1: 6, 1899.

While carotene showed some fluctuation from time to time, there were no changes in this pigment which could be definitely related to the irradiation.

From the purely physical data represented by spectrophotometric curves, the psychophysical specification of the color stimulus received by the eye of a normal observer was computed[3] for I. C. I. Illuminant C using data standardized by the International Commission on Illumination in 1931.

| | Relative brightness | Dominant wave-length | Excitation purity |
|---|---|---|---|
| | Per cent. | mμ | Per cent. |
| Before exposure ....... | 48.6 | 580 | 20.2 |
| 11 hours after exposure | 31.8 | 590 | 20.5 |
| 48 hours after exposure | 31.8 | 592 | 20.9 |
| 4 days after exposure | 36.9 | 587 | 20.7 |
| 19 days after exposure | 37.4 | 585 | 20.7 |
| 4 months after exposure | 42.6 | 580 | 20.5 |
| 9½ months after exposure | 43.6 | 583 | 20.1 |

In this color language "relative brightness" is a measure of the quantity of light reflected by the skin, while "dominant wave-length" and "purity" describe the quality of this light. Thus, hyperemia caused the skin to be much darker and noticeably more red, but it produced only a very slightly more pure or saturated color. At the end of four days the skin was less red but still much darker than normal. This is ascribable not so much to melanin as to the venous stagnation previously referred to. After four months the color of the skin had returned to its original quality, but its brightness was reduced by melanin. The gradual recession of this substance is shown by the increased brightness of the nine and a half months' data. Even at this time the skin was darker than before exposure.

EDWARD A. EDWARDS
DEPARTMENT OF ANATOMY,
HARVARD MEDICAL SCHOOL

S. QUIMBY DUNTLEY
DEPARTMENT OF PHYSICS,
MASSACHUSETTS INSTITUTE OF TECHNOLOGY

## PRESENCE OF A LEUKOCYTOSIS-PROMOTING FACTOR IN INFLAMMATORY EXUDATES[1]

THE recent studies of the writer have indicated the presence of a crystalline nitrogeneous substance liberated in areas of acute inflammation, capable *per se* of increasing capillary permeability and of inducing prompt leukocytic migration at the site of injury.[2, 3, 4] This substance has been termed leukotaxine. Its liberation and recovery from injured tissue offer a reasonable explanation for two of the basic initial sequences in the development of the acute inflammatory reaction. Leukotaxine has been shown to have no manifest physiological property in common with histamine.[2, 4, 5]

Leukotaxine, injected either subcutaneously or intravenously, fails to induce an increase in the leukocytic level of the circulation in both the dog and the rabbit. Repeated injections of 30 to 50 milligrams of the material over an interval of several days leave the number of circulating leukocytes essentially unaltered. The independence of the chemotactic factor (leukotaxine) from that concerned with leukocytosis is not wholly surprising when it is recalled that certain inflammatory processes characterized by marked leukocytic infiltration can even be accompanied by distinct leukopenia.

Having apparently eliminated leukotaxine as the factor responsible for the state of leukocytosis accompanying inflammation, studies were undertaken in an endeavor to determine whether the active principle might not be liberated in the exudate as a result of tissue injury. Ponder and MacLeod[6] recently expressed the opinion that in the blood stream of rabbits with peritonitis the shift to the left of polymorphonuclear counts is probably referable to the absorption of breakdown products of the cells appearing first in the exudate.

Inflammatory exudates were obtained by a variety of methods. In the majority of instances the exudative material resulted from an intrapleural injection of 1.5 cc of turpentine in dogs. Several of the exudates studied, however, were derived either after the intrapleural injection of 0.1 cc 10 per cent. croton oil in olive oil, the combined irritating action of several substances (*e.g.*, magnesium carbonate, staphylococcus *aureus* toxin and a mixture of aleuronat and colibactragen), or finally by physical injury. The latter consisted in recovering exudative material from a severe burn induced under nembutal anesthesia by scalding the limb of a dog in water heated to about 90° C. The exudate was obtained by removing the edematous subcutaneous tissue, and gently expressing the oozing and abundant exudative fluid content.

From 15 to about 25 cc of whole or cell-free exudate was injected by intracardiac puncture into the circulating blood stream of a normal dog. The results of eighteen such experiments indicate that there is a conspicuous rise in the leukocytic counts several hours after the introduction of an exudate into the blood. The increase in the number of circulating leukocytes averages 70 per cent.

[3] A. C. Hardy, "Handbook of Colorimetry," Technology Press, Cambridge, 1936.

[1] Aided by grants from the Milton Fund of Harvard University, from the International Cancer Foundation and from the Academy of Arts and Sciences.

[2] V. Menkin, *Jour. Exp. Med.*, 64: 485, 1936.

[3] *Ibid., Jour. Exp. Med.*, 67: 129, 1938.

[4] *Ibid., Physiol. Rev.*, 18: 366, 1938; *Proc. Soc. Exp. Biol. and Med.*, 40: 103, 1939.

[5] V. Menkin and M. A. Kadish, *Am. Jour. Physiol.*, 124: 524, 1938.

[6] E. Ponder and J. MacLeod, *Jour. Exp. Med.*, 67: 839, 1938.

The results of a considerable number of experiments clearly show that the products of injury liberated in an area of acute inflammation are *per se* capable of inducing in a normal dog a prompt leukocytosis to a degree reasonably comparable with that seen in the animal serving as source of the exudative material. Furthermore, some preliminary observations indicate that exudates from animals with marked leukopenia tend to contain a minimal amount of what might now be appropriately termed *leukocytosis-promoting factor*.

The effect on the leukocyte level of a dog manifested by the intravascular injection of an exudate transcends, as a rule, the maximum rise occurring during the rhythmical leukocytic variations. During the period of an experiment, *i.e.,* 6 to 8 hours, the maximum increase in leukocytes of several normal dogs averaged 23.8 per cent. This therefore roughly indicates that there is, as a result of a single injection of exudate, a threefold increase in the number of circulating leukocytes.

To extend the observations, dog serum, sterile broth, large doses of leukotaxine, a broth culture of an exudate and finally a culture of killed staphylococcus *aureus* were injected into the circulating blood of normal animals and of dogs which on other days had received exudates. A leukocytosis invariably failed to develop in these experiments.

For the following reasons it is improbable that the leukocytosis-promoting effect of exudates can be directly referred to the irritant *per se* or any of its derivatives:

(1) Exudates obtained by a variety of unrelated irritants produced in the blood stream an essentially similar effect on the level of circulating leukocytes. Turpentine incubated in serum for varying lengths of time failed to induce a leukocytosis when introduced into the blood stream. These observations, however, do not preclude the possibility that derivatives of turpentine formed in the exudate may still not be responsible for the cellular response. On the other hand, the variety of irritants employed, as well as the fact that a number of unrelated irritating substances fail when injected into the circulation to increase promptly the leukocytic level, suggest that the irritant *per se* bears no direct relation to the leukocytosis-promoting effect of exudates.

(2) The introduction into the circulating blood stream of exudative material obtained as a result of physical injury (*e.g.,* in the form of a severe burn) induces a state of leukocytosis. Such observations clearly indicate that it is unnecessary to refer the leukocytosis-promoting effect of exudate to either the presence of a chemical irritant or any of its derivatives.

The leukocytosis-promoting factor of exudate is thermolabile. Heating the exudate at 60° C. for several hours inactivates it. It is in large part indiffusible, failing to dialyze through a Cellophane membrane. The effect of the factor seems to be primarily on the bone marrow, producing an outpouring of granulocytes into the circulation. Histamine, adenosine, nucleic acid, all fail to reproduce the same pattern of reaction as does an exudate. The details of all these observations will form the subject of a separate communication to be published elsewhere. Further studies are now in progress in an endeavor to identify the nature of the leukocytosis-promoting factor which seems to offer an explanation for the mechanism of leukocytosis accompanying inflammation.

VALY MENKIN

DEPARTMENT OF PATHOLOGY,
HARVARD MEDICAL SCHOOL

## GLYCOGEN IN SWEET CORN

IT has previously been shown that certain tissue extracts exercise specific effects on the crystallization patterns of cupric chloride, and that the specific oat pattern is dependent on the presence of a polysaccharide in the extract.[1] It has since been found that there is a corresponding polysaccharide in sweet corn, which is essential for the production of the specific corn pattern. This polysaccharide is apparently glycogen.

Though glycogen has been found in a number of lower members of the plant kingdom—yeasts, bacteria, fungi, etc.—it has not previously been reported in any of the higher plants. The designation of a polysaccharide from a plant source as glycogen is rendered uncertain because certain dextrins have properties very similar to those of glycogen. The only striking difference between glycogen and some of the erythrodextrins is the fact that an aqueous solution of glycogen is opalescent, whereas dextrin solutions are usually clear. Hence it is insufficient to show that a polysaccharide exhibits all the usual characteristics of glycogen, but in addition it must be shown specifically that it is not a dextrin or a mixture of dextrins.

The corn polysaccharide has all the properties commonly associated with glycogen. Its aqueous solution is opalescent, it is resistant to the action of hot alkali, and with acids it is hydrolyzed quantitatively to glucose. Its specific optical rotation is +188° with sodium D light. When iodine is added to its aqueous solution a red-brown color is produced that fades when warmed and reappears when cooled. An erythrodextrin can be prepared whose properties differ essentially from these only in the lack of opalescence of its solution.

The glycogen and dextrin can be easily differentiated, however, by their effect on the cupric chloride crystal patterns. That of the corn glycogen is totally indis-

[1] Morris and Morris, *Jour. Phys. Chem.*, 43: 623, 1939.

tinguishable from those of the animal glycogens, whereas the dextrin pattern is entirely different.

The action of malt diastase on corn glycogen has been studied, since Glock[2] has shown that glycogen is hydrolyzed by the diastases at a much slower rate than are the starches. The corn glycogen has been compared with starches, with the erythrodextrin mentioned above and with glycogen from other sources. Table 1 shows the fraction of each polysaccharide hydrolyzed after one hour under identical conditions. The amount of hydrolysis was measured by determination of the reduction of the solution by Hanes method[3] calculated as maltose.

TABLE 1

| Polysaccharide | Source | Per cent. hydrolyzed |
|---|---|---|
| Glycogen | *Cysticercus fasciolaris*[4] | 10 |
| Glycogen | Oyster | 15 |
| Glycogen | Yeast | 31 |
| Glycogen | Sweet corn | 32 |
| Erythrodextrin | Corn starch | 50 |
| Starch | Rice | 60 |
| Starch | Corn | 65 |

It is evident that the corn glycogen is hydrolyzed at a rate much lower than that of the starches, higher than that of the animal glycogens, but nearly identical with that of yeast glycogen.

PREPARATION

The corn is soaked for a day or two, extracted with water, and the extract boiled and filtered. Two volumes of glacial acetic acid are added,[5] and the precipitated starch either centrifuged or allowed to settle. The acetic acid concentration of the supernatant solution is increased to 75 per cent.,[6] whereupon the glycogen precipitates. The starch should be redissolved and reprecipitated several times to increase the yield of glycogen, but the separations eventually become less efficient, since both starch and glycogen apparently combine with the acid to form more soluble compounds. Purification of the glycogen can be accomplished by the usual methods.

On one occasion 3.9 gm of glycogen were obtained from 30 gm of Golden Bantam sweet corn. The quantity in one or two kinds of field corn investigated was negligible.

SUMMARY

A polysaccharide apparently identical with glycogen has been extracted from sweet corn.

DANIEL LUZON MORRIS
CAROL TILDEN MORRIS

THE PUTNEY SCHOOL,
PUTNEY, VT.

# SCIENTIFIC APPARATUS AND LABORATORY METHODS

## A METHOD FOR THE CONTINUOUS RECORDING OF GASTRIC pH IN SITU

A METHOD has been developed for the determination and the continuous recording of gastric pH *in situ*. To obtain accurate results it was found necessary to keep the silver-silver chloride glass electrode isolated from the gastric mucosa. This was accomplished by a glass or bakelite guard or by a small balloon attached above the electrode. The wire from this electrode was shielded and encased in a Levine tube. In order to mix the gastric contents and to obtain samples another Levine tube was bound to that containing the electrode lead in such a way that the tip of this second tube extended a few centimeters beyond the electrode. With the exception of the opening adjacent to the electrode all other openings of this second tube were covered with balloon rubber. Contact with the saline silver-silver chloride reference electrode was made either on the skin or by means of a thread placed in the aspirating Levine tube. The electrode leads were connected through a Beckman pH meter to a recording potentiometer.

In order to insure accurate recording, certain precautions had to be observed. The exact position of the glass electrode in the stomach was determined by fluoroscopic observation. The gastric contents were constantly mixed by a continuous pump which alternately withdrew and reinjected 25–50 cc of gastric contents at 30-second intervals. By these technical refinements the wide variations reported by Eyerly and Breuhaus[1] between the values obtained by the use of the gastric electrode and those determined on the aspirated speci-

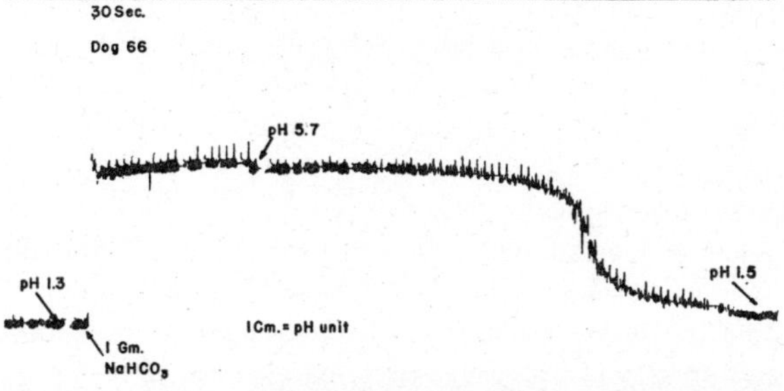


FIG. 1. Changes in gastric pH following administration of 1 gram of sodium bicarbonate in a dog of 17 kilograms, anesthetized with morphine and chloralose.

[2] G. E. Glock, *Biochem. Jour.*, 30: 1386, 1936.
[3] C. S. Hanes, *Biochem. Jour.*, 23: 99, 1929.
[4] The cysticercus glycogen was very kindly furnished by Dr. L. Frank Salisbury, of the Department of Chemistry, Yale University.

[5] *Cf.*, "Methods of Analysis of the Association of Official Agricultural Chemists," Washington, 1935, p. 357.
[6] *Cf.* Bell and Young, *Biochem. Jour.*, 28: 882, 1934.
[1] J. B. Eyerly and H. C. Breuhaus, *Am. Jour. Dig. Diseases*, 6: 187, May, 1939.

men were avoided, and the difference in the two types of pH determinations was maintained within 0.5 unit.

The accompanying Fig. 1 shows the accuracy of the method. The fasting contents of an anesthetized dog were diluted to 100 cc with distilled water and a control recording made. The introduction of 1 gram of sodium bicarbonate in 100 cc of distilled water followed by rinsing through the Levine tube with 50 cc of water caused a prompt increase in the pH value. The peak of this rise is conditioned by the pH of the alkaline solution, whereas the plateau level immediately following is the pH of the alkali and gastric content mixture. The duration of the plateau, shown by the gently sloping curve which is terminated by the sudden drop to a low level, is controlled by the amount of alkali added, the rate of acid secretion and the intermittent emptying of the stomach. The amount of emptying can be calculated if the gastric contents are measured after the pH has returned to the low level. By controlling the variables interesting data may be obtained on the efficacy of antacids and the rate of gastric secretion. Information pertaining to these experiments as well as further details concerning the method will be published elsewhere.

We are greatly indebted to Dr. N. R. Trenner for valuable suggestions as well as the construction of the glass electrodes and to Mr. L. Fernandez, who assisted during the earlier part of the experiments.

JAMES FLEXNER
MICHAEL KNIAZUK
THE MERCK ISTITUTE OF THERAPEUTIC RESEARCH,
RAHWAY, N. J.
JAN NYBOER
NEW YORK POST-GRADUATE MEDICAL SCHOOL AND HOSPITAL,
NEW YORK, N. Y.

## CHROMOSOMES FROM LEAVES

A MODIFICATION of Warmke's[1] method for making root-tip smears has been found by the writer to be effective for studying chromosomes in the leaves of certain plants: place young leaves in Carnoy's solution (3 parts chloroform, 2 parts absolute alcohol and 1 part glacial acetic acid) for five or more minutes; transfer momentarily to a solution of equal parts of 95 per cent. alcohol and concentrated hydrochloric acid; put the leaves back into Carnoy's, and, after several minutes, smear in iron aceto-carmine.

By this method the chromosomes of a number of genera have been investigated: *Smilax* L. (Liliaceae), *Sedum* L. (Crassulaceae), *Cercis* L. (Leguminosae), *Punica* L. (Punicaceae), *Sanicula* L. (Umbelliferae), *Pyxidanthera* Michx., *Diapensia* L., *Shortia* Torr. and Gray, *Schizocodon* Sieb. and Zucc., and *Galax* L. (Diapensiaceae), *Chimaphila* Pursh (Ericaceae), and *Plantago* L. (Plantaginaceae). Metaphase drawings of two species are shown here for purposes of illustration: Fig. 1, *Sedum pusillum* Michx., from Stone Mountain in Georgia, with 8 somatic chromosomes, the lowest number known for the extremely varied family; and Fig. 2, *Cercis canadensis* L., four trees on the grounds of the College of William and Mary, with 14 somatic chromosomes. Senn[2] reported a $2n$-number of 12, $n$-number of 6, for this species; his drawing of meiotic chromosomes suggests an interpretation of two bivalents in contact to be a single bivalent; his somatic number (not figured) was determined from an anther-wall division. The only other investigated species of *Cercis* has 14 and 7 chromosomes, respectively.[3]

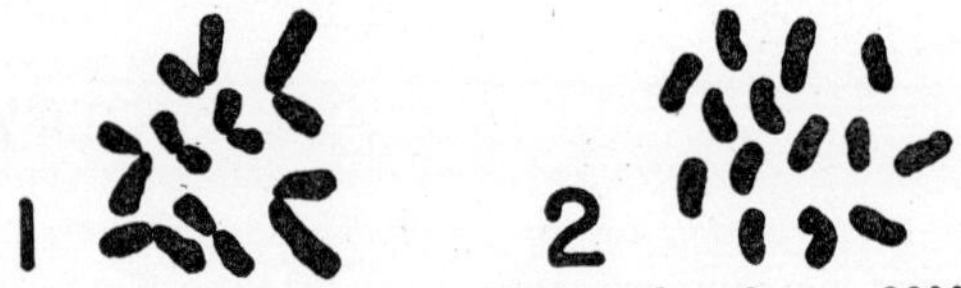


FIG. 1. *Sedum pusillum* Michx., $2n=8$, *ca.* 3800 ×.
FIG. 2. *Cercis canadensis* L., $2n=14$, *ca.* 4500 ×.

J. T. BALDWIN, JR.
COLLEGE OF WILLIAM AND MARY

[1] H. E. Warmke, *Stain Technology,* 10: 101–103, 1935.

[2] H. A. Senn, *Bibliogr. Genetica,* 12: 175–336, 1938.

[3] R. Corti, *Nuovo Giorn. Bot. Ital.,* N. S., 37: 679–680, 1930.

## BOOKS RECEIVED

DE BROGLIE, LOUIS. *Matter and Light; the New Physics.* Pp. 300. Norton. $3.50.

FLEMING, J. A., Editor. *Terrestrial Magnetism and Electricity.* Vol. VIII, *Physics of the Earth.* Pp. xii + 794. Illustrated. McGraw-Hill. $8.00.

FRASER, CHELSEA. *Heroes of the Air.* Pp. xl + 846. Illustrated. Crowell. $2.50.

FURNAS, C. C. *The Storehouse of Civilization.* Pp. xx + 562. Illustrated. Teachers College, Columbia University. $3.25.

GASSER, HERBERT S. and others. *Symposium on the Synapse.* (Reprinted from the *Journal of Neurophysiology.*) Pp. 361–474. 25 figures. Charles C Thomas.

GRAHAM, HARVEY. *The Story of Surgery.* Pp. xv + 425. 23 plates. Doubleday, Doran. $3.75.

HAUSMANN, ERICH. *Physics.* Second edition. Pp. vi + 756. 469 figures. Van Nostrand. $4.00.

HIBBEN, JAMES H. *The Raman Effect and its Chemical Applications.* Pp. 544. Reinhold. $11.00.

HUDDLESON, I. FOREST and others. *Brucellosis in Man and Animals.* Pp. xvii + 339. 40 figures. Commonwealth Fund, New York. $3.50.

MACDOUGALL, F. H. *Thermodynamics and Chemistry.* Third edition. Pp. ix + 491. Wiley. $5.00.

ROBBINS, WILLIAM J. and HAROLD W. RICKETT. *Botany; a Text-book for College and University Students.* Third edition. Pp. vii + 658. 440 figures. Van Nostrand. $3.75.

ROUSH, G. A. *Strategic Mineral Supplies.* Pp. xvii + 485. McGraw-Hill. $5.00.

SZEGÖ, GABOR. *Orthogonal Polynomials.* Vol. XXIII, American Mathematical Society Colloquium Publications. Pp. ix + 401. The Society, New York.

*Treatment in General Practice; the Management of Some Major Medical Disorders.* A symposium. Vol. I, pp. x + 259. Vol. II, pp. xii + 436. Little, Brown. $7.50.

# SCIENCE

Vol. 90 | Friday, September 15, 1939 | No. 2333

*The Species Complex in Biology and Education:* Dr. Albert Davis Mead ... 241

*Scientific Events:*
*The Cornell Ornithological Expedition; Balloon Flights into the Stratosphere; Courses in Modern Manufacturing and Research; Mouse Genetics; The American Association of Museums; The American Public Health Association* ... 246

*Scientific Notes and News* ... 248

*Discussion:*
*A Self-limiting Mechanism in Sympathetic Homeostatic Adjustment:* Dr. Amedeo S. Marrazzi. *Chlorazol Fast Pink BKS:* Dr. R. E. Rose. *"Stars" in American Men of Science:* J. H. G.; Professor Stephen S. Visher. *The Pacific Entomological Survey:* Professor G. D. Hale Carpenter ... 251

*Scientific Books:*
*Elementary Matrices:* Professor C. C. MacDuffee 253

*Societies and Meetings:*
*The French Association for the Advancement of Science. The Medical Library Association:* Anna C. Holt ... 254

*Special Articles:*
*Radioactive Ion Exchanges in Living Protoplasm:* Dr. Lorin J. Mullins and Professor S. C. Brooks. *The Denaturation of Proteins by Detergents and Bile Salts:* Dr. M. L. Anson. *The Configuration of the Glutamic Acid of Adenocarcinoma Protein:* Dr. L. Earle Arnow and Jeanette C. Opsahl. *Poliomyelitic Virus in Sewage:* Drs. John R. Paul, James D. Trask and C. S. Culotta ... 256

*Scientific Apparatus and Laboratory Methods:*
*Demonstration of the Shape of Cilia in Normal Motion:* A. M. Shanes. *A New Material for Mounting Nerve Tissue Sections in Paraffin for Silver Staining or Restaining:* Rosette Spoerri ... 259

*Science News* ... 10

SCIENCE: A Weekly Journal devoted to the Advancement of Science, edited by J. McKeen Cattell and published every Friday by

THE SCIENCE PRESS
New York City: Grand Central Terminal
Lancaster, Pa. Garrison, N. Y.

Annual Subscription, $6.00 Single Copies, 15 Cts.

SCIENCE is the official organ of the American Association for the Advancement of Science. Information regarding membership in the Association may be secured from the office of the permanent secretary in the Smithsonian Institution Building, Washington, D. C.

## THE SPECIES COMPLEX IN BIOLOGY AND EDUCATION[1]

By Dr. ALBERT DAVIS MEAD

PROFESSOR EMERITUS OF BIOLOGY AT BROWN UNIVERSITY

This afternoon I propose to discuss a certain mental trait which looms conspicuously in the background whenever I reflect upon the history of biology or upon academic procedures as I have observed them these many years. It is the innate propensity of active minds to form species, *i.e.,* successively to make distinctions, to point out similarities and then to assemble the things that are alike into their kinds. It applies to everything from chemical elements to college fraternities. Since the Latin word "species" is synonymous with the English word "kind" even to the point of being adequately indefinite I shall employ it in a wide and general sense which, indeed, accords with its earlier usage.

This mental trait is not a simple one. It is made up of a strong emotional factor, an inborn urge to put things in order and, alas, keep them there; of the intellectual faculty of discernment and discrimination which perceives distinctions and similarities; and of the constructive imagination which makes it possible to assemble in the mind things that are widely separated in space and time. For convenience I presume to call this trait the species-forming complex or, for short, the "species complex."

I shall first point to a few characteristic effects, good and bad, of the operation of the species complex in general; then to some of its accomplishments in the field of biology; and finally, shall venture to suggest that the recognition of the characteristics of this trait in human beings is desirable as we face the problems of the day inside and outside of the university.

The species complex often manifests itself in the

[1] Address at the Graduate Convocation of Brown University, June 17, 1939.

degree of importance assigned to nice distinctions and to exact definitions. It is, of course, to its credit that it does seek to make fine and clear-cut distinctions; but so highly is this function esteemed in academic circles that extraordinary powers of fine discrimination are sometimes mistaken, by the unwary, for scholarship itself. Again, instinctively we admire that which is definite, unequivocal and normal and we tend to ignore that which is vacillating, confused or abnormal, *i.e.*, mugwump, the mule and the freak. Is there not, however, a salutary moral to be found in the reflection that not long ago the political mugwump turned the tide of a major election in all but the two American states; that the hybrid established the science of genetics; and that the freak, under the polite name of mutation, largely restored the waning prestige of natural selection as a major factor in the modus operandi of evolution? Clear, sharp incisive definitions are admirable, but only when they do not throw out of proper consideration items which may be potentially important.

The most commonly recognized manifestation of the species complex is the blind adherence, or better the emotional adherence, to some particular definition of a species once it has been established, especially when the species in question is a doctrine of politics, economics, social organization, government or religion. Perhaps no other manifestation has greater possibilities for usefulness, and also for mischief. It engenders loyalty, it promotes solidarity, and it tends to satisfy the intuitive desire for a solid base or anchorage that is once and for all secure, immovable and permanent. But it tends also to favor dogmatism and to prevent or retard the candid, unprejudiced, fruitful study of relationships. It encourages debate and even war, and discourages deliberation as a method of deciding issues. This insistence upon permanence of species may sometimes have its explanation in proprietary interests or pride as the founder or beneficiary of the particular system, or in a long-time commitment to it as sponsor or adherent. But whatever the reason, and despite the useful service which it may perform in preserving the existing order, the sinister effects of this insistence are, as we all know, often very far-reaching. By way of contrast one of the significant contributions of science to humanity has been its attitude toward the permanence of its own hypotheses. For example, since many of us were studying science in college such fundamental tenets of classical physics as the indestructibility of matter, the conservation of energy and the integrity of the atom have been relinquished and superseded without serious emotional disturbance. We look forward toward the millennium when this attitude shall generally prevail, when deliberation shall everywhere be exalted above debate and missions shall give way to parliaments.

The greatest of all adventures in the study of species has been in biology; naturally so because of the characteristics of living material—the incomparable diversity of its forms and the paradox of their being at the same time persistent and changeable. Conversely, the greatest episode in biology has been the study of species plus the interpretation of its results. I refer to the stupendous enterprise which, in the eighteenth century, was inspired and for many years largely conducted by that extraordinary genius, the "immortal Swede," Linnaeus, and which was interpreted later in the Darwinian presentation of the hypothesis of evolution. This enterprise was a well-organized world-wide drive of which the objective was nothing less than to discover, describe, name and classify every living thing—as the housekeeper in Maine would say, to "neaten up" the living world and put it in "apple pie order." Literally the whole world was combed for new species by the agents and correspondents of the great impresario; and it should be remembered that the world was then a score of times larger than it is to-day.

As the work progressed it gained momentum, and in fact it has never ceased. At the present time the number of existing species of plants and animals recorded, described and named in accordance with the Linnaean system is considerably over a million, and new ones are being added continually. (Several have been announced this week.) It is evident, moreover, that the number of species existing to-day is only a fragment of the total number that have inhabited the earth.

Since this was by far the greatest, most systematic and most mature species study ever undertaken it should be profitable to review its consequences, immediate and latent. Directly from it two major generalizations were derived, both of them highly significant, and both utterly contrary to expectation and to immemorial tradition; first, that the number of species of plants and animals is of an entirely different order of magnitude than had ever before been imagined; second, that a specificity itself is an attribute equally of all living things, which means that every individual organism living or dead, animal or plant, the eagle or the earthworm, the rose or the mildew on its leaves, has an equally valid passport certifying its good standing as a regular member of some species; and that any individual amoeba, shellfish or insect, with respect to lineage and pedigree, stands, in the eye of nature, on equal footing with a Pharaoh.

So much for the direct consequences. The greater significance of this monumental labor was latent and potential. It became manifest and effective, not by the distinguishing of more species (although this work continued), but, on the contrary, by a half century of vigorous research into the relations between the very species that had been distinguished. Herein precisely is one of the practical lessons which this long and mature experience in biological species-study holds for the workers in other domains.

Several ingenious ways of getting at these relations were found out by the generations following Linnaeus. Let me recall very briefly three of them. First, the comparing of the whole internal and external structure of representatives of similar species established a new biological discipline, the science of morphology. With this work the name of Cuvier must always be associated, but it also held the distinguished attention of the poet Goethe and of a long list of savants of the early nineteenth century.

Another means of access to the relationships of species was paleontology, with which also the name of Cuvier must be associated. We commonly think of paleontology as relating to extinct species but, for purposes of this discussion, that which it reveals about living species is even more important. Through the study of fossils it became evident, not only that the kangaroo once lived a wild life in Paris, the mastodon (if not the elephant) was at home in Albany, the sabre-toothed tiger wrought havoc in Hollywood, and the superannuated giant-sloth retired to Pasadena, but also that man himself, and nearly all the kinds of animals and plants that are now living, have existed upon the earth only a few minutes of the geological day. Among all the creatures that have dwelt upon the earth since the beginning, they are comparatively recent arrivals.

A third means of access, geographic distribution, revealed a most significant relation among sciences; a relation which obtains also in human cultures and therefore directly concerns one of the paramount problems of our day and generation. The biologists have a name for it, but in plain English it is this: Species naturally occupy definite areas limited by barriers, geographic or physiologic, which, unaided, they can not cross but, once assisted across the barriers, they not only may continue to exist but may enjoy "the more abundant life," like rabbits in Australia and Buddhism in China and Japan. To this phenomenon in relation to human cultures, I shall revert later.

Now geographic distribution is not a subject to arouse the enthusiasm of the man on the street, yet it was the prolonged reflection upon this phenomenon, as he had observed it in the Galapagos Islands, that greatly stirred the imagination of the reputedly unemotional Darwin and first turned him toward the evolutionary interpretation of the nature of species. In 1844, seven years after returning from the voyage of the *Beagle,* he wrote to Hooker, the English botanist:

> . . . I have now been, ever since my return, engaged, in a very presumptuous work, and I know no one individual who would not say a very foolish one. I was so struck with the distribution of the Galapagos organisms, etc., and with the character of the American fossil mammifers, etc., that I determined to collect, blindly, every sort of fact, which could bear in any way on what are species. . . . At last, gleams of light have come, and I am almost convinced (quite contrary to the opinion that I started with) that species are not (it is like confessing a murder) immutable.

That all these general phenomena and others like them probably held the key to some great common mystery did not escape the notice and the comment of the savants of the nineteenth century. Questions about the significance of these constant relations were inevitable and insistent: Why the morphological resemblances? Why the short duration of a species? Why the apparently arbitrary restriction of a species to a single natural habitat?

The hypothesis of organic evolution as presented by Darwin in 1859 was formulated as an answer to these and similar irrepressible questions. A revised hypothesis of special creation as presented by Professor Louis Agassiz, also in 1859, was another and a very different answer.[2]

Great issues were at stake in these strictly alternative answers; nothing less in fact than the question of the place of man in the universe and of the operation of secondary causes in the living world.

The service which this gifted naturalist, Agassiz, performed in clarifying the evolution hypothesis by his adverse criticism, which was continued for fourteen years and up to the time of his death, is not always appreciated. Agassiz did not deny the validity of the relations between species as demonstrated in morphology, paleontology and geographic distribution—he emphasized them; but he gave to all of them severally and collectively an interpretation which showed what extraordinary postulates were required to adapt and adjust the time-honored doctrine of special creation to those newer findings.

In Agassiz's view, the human hand and the bat's wing have an identical plan of structure because the architect who designed both had the same plan in mind. He explained the fact that species live only a short period in geologic time by postulating an indefinite number of successive creative periods. To explain the

[2] Referring to the phenomena of morphology, paleontology and geographic distribution Agassiz wrote in 1863 in "Methods of Study in Natural History," pp. 100–102:

> What, then, does this correspondence teach us? . . . Surely not that the connection between animals is a material one. . . . If, then, this connection is not a material one, what is it?—for that such a connection does exist throughout the Animal Kingdom, as intimate, as continuous, as complex, as any series which the development theorists have ever contended for, is not to be denied. What can it be but an intellectual one? These correspondences are correspondences of thought . . . the same thought that spans the whole succession of geological ages controls the structural relations of all living beings as well as their distribution over the surface of the earth. . . .

enigma of geographic distribution, he postulated the special creation of each species in the region it now occupies.

The difference between the tenets of Darwin and Agassiz hinges on a cardinal difference in the definition of organic species or, as Darwin himself put it, on the question, "What are species?" To Darwin, species were abstract things, the temporary phases or manifestations of a continuous series, having separate entities only as infancy, childhood, youth, manhood and old age would have specific and separate entities if there were no knowledge of the transition from one to the other within a single individual lifetime. In fact, the child of five years has no direct knowledge of this transition, and so to him grandfather has always belonged to the distinct species "old man"; and father and mother too have always been grown-ups. In other words, were all facts known the exact lines separating species would be as elusive as lines separating the several stages of a man's life, and the search for them as futile as grappling for the equator. To Agassiz, on the other hand, a species was a concrete entity, in the sense that it was the sum total of all the individuals descended from an original pair. In summary, it might almost be said that Agassiz and his school sought to discover species; the evolutionists made them.

That, in biology, species turned out to be abstract entities and that species grade one into another does not mean that they have no legitimate status. It is legitimate and useful to distinguish infancy, youth and old age, although we know that somewhere in time one merges into another. For that matter, every biologist realizes that the term "individual," as applied to a particular animal or to a man as a physical organism, is also an abstract and indefinite one. The process of maturation, fertilization and early development of the egg are so perfectly continuous that, even when the whole span from one generation to the next is observed continuously under the microscope in concrete material form, the observer can not point to an exact moment when the egg becomes a new individual. To indicate that moment would be an utterly arbitrary act.

The profound, far-reaching consequences of the wide acceptance of the hypothesis of organic evolution is a matter of history. It directly involved mankind in new material relationships with the other animal species. It brought the living world wholly under the immediate operation of secondary causes, as the astronomical discoveries and interpretations had brought the inanimate world centuries earlier. It established a new kind of biological order. It created a new respect for things that lie in the indefinite zone between adjacent categories. It conduced to the general adoption of the genetic view-point in other domains of thought. Would that Linnaeus could behold how great a matter a little fire kindled!

As I reflect upon the considerable number of discussions which I have listened to or have read in the past four or five decades concerning the aims, purposes, organization, programs and procedures of collegiate education, the impression deepens that there is an increasingly abundant and diversified fauna and flora of educational propositions which would profit by the same kind of analysis and treatment; which invite and challenge the genius of a Linnaeus to distinguish the legitimate species, a Cuvier to compare them and to demonstrate their fundamental relationships, and eventually a Darwin to construct out of these relationships a new rational order and unity in a science of education.

However, this is the comprehensive task which confronts the generations to come. This afternoon I shall refer simply to one unfortunate characteristic of the species complex in the educational field, namely, the unconscious tendency to confuse convenient distinctions with incompatible alternatives—the tendency to set over against each other as more or less antithetical certain factors, in the methods of teaching and learning or in educational purposes, whose relationships to each other are really so very important that they ought not to be thus obscured; but, on the contrary, ought to be regarded as a subject of major concern.

For example: Humanities set over against the sciences as the substance of a liberal education; teaching against research as the function of the faculty and as a criterion of the usefulness of a professor; diversification against specialization as the way to comprehensive understanding; pedagogical training against knowledge of subject-matter as the best preparation for teaching; production of a continuous apostolic succession of "scholars" against the perfusion of the laity with the extract of scholarship, as the function of the university and the criterion in the selection and the training of students; classics against studies of modern thought and affairs as preparation for life; and many others.

The false antithesis between science and the so-called humanities is, perhaps, the most deplorable of all these examples. It is unwarranted and unnecessary, and is disastrous to the great interests of both. Philosophy, literature and art need constantly the substantial contributions of science. Science needs the penetrating criticism of philosophy to preserve its equilibrium and it needs the wings of literature and art to bear its conclusions to their destination.

Unhappily both the intellectual factor of the species complex and the emotional factor contribute to keeping science and the humanities apart. The chief role of science in college, that of aiding the student in building his own Weltanschauung, is not kept sufficiently in evidence. Again science is still defined occasionally as the study of the stage upon which man plays his part;

the humanities as the study of man himself. So to restrict science is, of course, to overlook that most pertinent corollary of organic evolution which admitted man into the association of animal species and conferred upon him all the rights and privileges thereunto appertaining. This made the manifestations of his mental and emotional life amenable to investigation by ordinary scientific methods. The findings of experimental and genetic biology and psychology are then common assets of science and the humanities.

Probably the instinctive or emotional component of the species complex must be held accountable for the notion that the sciences belong on McGuire's side of the railroad track; the nicer humanities on the other side in the older and better residential district. A former colleague at Brown used gleefully to relate the adventure of an ardent devotee of the humanities when on an exploring expedition through a biological laboratory; how her amazed delight over the exquisite beauty of color and texture of a section under a microscope suddenly turned to dismay when she learned that the object of her admiration was the kidney of a rat.

The idea that specialization necessarily conduces to narrowness of vision is a matter on which I speak with feeling and assurance, for I gave four years of merry youth to the intensive and extensive study of the egg of a worm under the impression, which has in no wise diminished through the years, that the polychaetous annelid in the ocean, as truly as "the flower in the crannied wall," is custodian of the eternal mystery. To change the figure abruptly; in delving below the surface in search of the underlying relations of things, one may start his tunnel from one point or from ten points or from fifty points. The number of entrances does not determine the extent of the ramifications.

To ask whether it is the obligation of the college to produce a succession of scholars or to educate the laity is like asking whether it is the business of the germ-plasm to produce more germ-plasm or to produce a corporeal body. It must do both, for if it fails in either the race perishes. In a democracy it is the prospective laity who will perpetually decide whether or not the college shall exist and, if existing, shall be bond or free. It is essential that the layman, even though himself not a scholar, shall have a sympathetic understanding of the content and aims of scholarship, and this is best learned in college. The prospective scholar, that is the academic germ-plasm, must then continue to produce still other scholars but also still other laymen.

Finally, a word concerning a general species problem of the future. If there are responsible institutions in the world, they are the colleges and universities situated in and supported by the democracies. These institutions must play the part of seers and prophets; they must lead and not follow in the thought of the times. Nevertheless, and because this is so, the conditions that obtain in the world in each generation are necessarily reflected in the total educational program of the college.

We have already observed that the biological phenomena attending geographic distribution of plants and animals, especially the effects of isolation, apply also to human cultures. Isolation, by means of more or less effective barriers, has been a primary condition both of the origin and the maintenance of these cultures; but it is abundantly evident that human cultures may thrive in regions other than those in which they originated. At the present time the confining barriers that have hitherto separated human cultures and have tended to maintain them as distinct are being broken down with unprecedented swiftness and unprecedented thoroughness.

The consequent complete, sudden, world-wide commingling of cultural species will be, I venture to say, the central problem of coming generations—even taking precedence over the problem of the vanishing frontiers.

It is true that the interpretation and mixing of cultures has been slowly going on for ages untold; that no human culture nor human race, for that matter, is pure, unmixed and homogeneous; but we have now entered upon a period of cultural diffusion that is something new under the sun. Hitherto cultures have spread from this or that center, sometimes very far indeed, but yet have had their territorial and ethnic limits. To-day they start from many centers at once and the earth is their limit. Hitherto the spread of a culture was determined by some governmental power which had a locus, Thebes, Athens, Rome, Agra, Peking. To-day it is spread by the instrumentality of science, which has no locus either territorial or political.

In the future, unless the existence of the science of physics and the technology of engineering are forgotten by civilized man, the airplane, telephone, radio, phonograph, cinema and their successors will continue to convey goods, persons and cultural ideas to and fro incessantly and almost or quite instantaneously over the whole world in defiance of every geographic and political obstacle. Not America, but the world is becoming the melting pot of cultural ideas.

What is to be the outcome of this, who can tell? It seems inevitable that the present cultural species, including systems of government, economics, ethics, morals, religions and philosophies, can not maintain themselves unmodified in the new conditions, but that from them new species will arise.

The species problem of the future is—how to direct the course of this inevitable cultural evolution so that the new species will include the finest elements that experience can contribute from all quarters of the world.

None should be better qualified to attack the problem than those prospective scholars, and laymen also, whose complex of impelling motives, powers of discernment and discrimination, and constructive imagination it is the privilege of the college and the university to educate.

# SCIENTIFIC EVENTS

## THE CORNELL ORNITHOLOGICAL EXPEDITION

THE Cornell Ornithological Expedition, under the leadership of Dr. Arthur A. Allen, head of the department of ornithology at the university, returned to Ithaca on September 3 after a four-months journey to the southwest and the west coast.

Color movies and sound records of the Attwater prairie chicken, the rare trumpeter swan and the almost extinct California condor were obtained.

Albert R. Brand, research associate in ornithology at Cornell, a retired stock broker who is an authority on the sound recording of bird-songs, provided funds for the expedition, which left Ithaca on May 2 in a sound truck and traveled over 12,000 miles. The truck was equipped not only for recording the songs and calls of birds and making color-films, but with camping facilities. Assistants to Dr. Allen were David Allen, his thirteen-year-old son and Charles Brand, son of the sponsor of the expedition.

The object of the trip was to secure recordings of the songs and calls of birds new to the Cornell collection; to make color-films of as many birds as possible; to inspect various wildlife refuges and conservation projects of the different states through which the expedition passed and of the Federal Government and to gather as much data as possible relative to the organization and management of these projects for course-work to be conducted at Cornell.

Describing the expedition, Dr. Allen said:

> We proceeded first to Texas and Louisiana, following the southernmost route, through Brownsville, El Paso and Tucson, to Pasadena and Berkeley, where I gave a course in ornithology at the University of California, between June 26 and August 4. On the return we took the northern route, through Oregon, Washington, Montana, North Dakota, Minnesota, Michigan and Ontario.
>
> We visited about two dozen of the state and federal wildlife projects, including seven of the national parks. We recorded the songs or calls of over a hundred kinds of birds not previously recorded; and we secured color-films of about 120 species, taking about 6,500 feet of color-film and 1,200 stills, which will greatly improve our classroom instruction, as well as being used to illustrate public lectures and general articles.

One of the accomplishments of the trip was the discovery of the nest of the coppery-tailed trogon, a tropical species which is found in the mountains of southern Arizona. The ornithologists of Arizona have been hunting for this nest unsuccessfully ever since the bird was first discovered in Arizona, about fifty years ago. The Cornell expedition was fortunate in being able to locate the nest and secure recordings of its voice and color-films of the bird, which has the reputation of being the most beautiful bird in North America. Other interesting or colorful birds recorded and filmed were the roseate spoonbills, on the Texas coast, the purple gallinules of Louisiana, wild turkeys, chachalacas, California, Gambel's and mountain quails, pelicans, vermillion flycatchers, cardinals, western tanagers and blue grosbeaks.

## BALLOON FLIGHTS INTO THE STRATOSPHERE

THREE recent flights into the stratosphere over Beltsville, Maryland, by means of groups of rubber sounding balloons reached heights of 14 to 16½ miles above the earth. The balloons, sent up as a joint project by the National Geographic Society and the National Bureau of Standards, carried on each flight with an "observer," an ingenious robot consisting of electric batteries, a tiny motor, photo-electric cells, moving screens and radio tubes.

The object of the flights was to gather additional information about the atmosphere's ozone layer—an important concentration of the gas which screens away from the earth's surface certain rays of sunlight injurious to vegetable and animal life. The metal and glass robot made "readings" of the varying concentrations of ozone at different altitudes and automatically radioed them to a receiving station on the ground. The results are being compared with other observations for a later report by the National Bureau of Standards.

On each of the three flights the lifting power was furnished by six rubber, hydrogen-filled balloons attached in tandem. Four-and-a-half feet in diameter when they were released, these balloons expanded to diameters of 14 feet or more in the rare upper air near the top of the ascents.

The string of balloons continued to rise until one of them burst as a result of expansion. The remaining balloons lowered the observing apparatus slowly to the ground and in every case it was recovered. The flights were made under the supervision of Dr. Lyman J. Briggs, director of the National Bureau of Standards, and Dr. W. W. Coblentz, chief of radiometry at the bureau.

In the hope of reaching greater altitudes for the cooperative study of ozone concentrations, the National

Geographic Society is now having large rubber balloons fabricated. In the meantime improved instruments for detecting ozone and for radioing information back to earth are under construction in the laboratories of the National Bureau of Standards.

## COURSES IN MODERN MANUFACTURING AND RESEARCH

New York University, the Polytechnic Institute of Brooklyn and the Stevens Institute of Technology, in cooperation with the Westinghouse Electric and Manufacturing Company, have announced a series of post-graduate courses in industry which will enable selected graduate engineers to study modern research and manufacturing methods and earn credit for masters' and doctors' degrees.

These courses are the first to be held in the New York metropolitan area in which an industrial concern has cooperated with a group of educational institutions to provide training for advanced degrees to graduate students. They will be similar to those held with the cooperation of Professor H. E. Dyche, head of the school of electrical engineering at the University of Pittsburgh. As a result of graduate study in these classes in the past twelve years, sixty-six students have been awarded masters' degrees and six students Ph.D. degrees.

Students chosen for enrolment in the New York classes will include graduate engineers now employed by the Westinghouse Company and graduate students in engineering from the three cooperating schools. A joint committee, including Dean Erich Hausmann, of the Polytechnic Institute of Brooklyn; Dr. H. J. Masson, of New York University; Dean F. C. Stockwell, of Stevens Institute of Technology, and J. H. Belknap, manager of technical employment and training for the Westinghouse Company, will examine students and supervise the courses.

Among the first courses authorized will be classes in advanced illumination and in symmetrical components. D. W. Atwater, manager of the commercial engineering department of the Westinghouse Lamp Division and past president of the Illuminating Engineering Society, has been appointed Westinghouse lecturer for the class in advanced illumination. The course, following advanced study procedure in technical schools, will consist of two-hour lectures each on Monday nights, for sixteen weeks at the Westinghouse offices in New York City. The course on symmetrical components, dealing with electrical distribution systems, will be taught by B. V. Hoard, engineer of the Westinghouse Meter Works at Newark, N. J., and S. H. Wright, of the engineering department at Pittsburgh. Instruction will include details of technical procedure in current laboratory research and commercial production. Engineers in the industry will present the latest developments in each field.

## MOUSE GENETICS

A circular letter signed by L. C. Dunn, W. H. Gates, G. D. Snell and W. L. Russell was recently forwarded to biologists interested in mouse genetics, asking for opinions with regard to the possible establishment of a Committee on Mouse Genetics Nomenclature and of a Mouse Genetics News Service. As a result, at the meeting of the International Congress of Genetics at Edinburgh Professors F. A. E. Crew and L. C. Dunn and Dr. G. D. Snell were appointed a Committee on Mouse Genetics Nomenclature.

A meeting with Dr. A. L. Hagedoorn (Holland) in the chair was called to consider a set of nomenclature rules drawn up by the committee and to discuss details of the News Service. Twenty-five members of the congress were present. The recommendations of the meeting as regards nomenclature were submitted to the committee.

The offer of the director and staff of the Roscoe B. Jackson Memorial Laboratory in Bar Harbor, Maine, for the publication in mimeographed form of the *Mouse Genetics News* was gratefully accepted. It was suggested that a register of stocks and the various Pure Lines should be drawn up in order to end the confusion in the naming of Pure Lines used in various laboratories which has arisen during the last few years. It was recommended that stock lists of all the laboratories concerned should be published from time to time. It was further suggested that notice should be given by a laboratory before any stocks are discontinued; it has happened several times in the past that valuable material has been irretrievably lost, because every laboratory has relied on other places for its maintenance. It is proposed that the News Service should also arrange for exchange of stocks, and it is hoped that its activities may be extended to rabbits and other rodents, and it is suggested that an appeal be made to all laboratories concerned to collaborate wholeheartedly by promptly answering correspondence and sending information.

The meeting discussed the establishment of centers, preferably in the United States for the maintenance and safe keeping of stocks, particularly of genes (pathological and otherwise). It was pointed out that the continuity of genetical work depends on keeping genes alive, as genes which have died out are as irrevocably lost as extinct animal or plant species. It was urged that this matter should receive the immediate consideration of the News Service and that an appeal should be made to the Carnegie and Rockefeller Foundations for financial assistance.

## THE AMERICAN ASSOCIATION OF MUSEUMS

The San Francisco meeting of the American Association of Museums, which met from June 26 to 28, drew, according to *Museum News*, an unexpectedly large attendance. More than 200 members were registered, of whom 150 were from out of town and 70 from east of the Mississippi. Three members came from Honolulu and two from Canada. It is reported in the *News* that the meeting was marked by especially successful entertainment features and by a generous spirit of hospitality on the part of the San Francisco museums and their friends and of officials of the Golden Gate International Exposition.

Dr. Clark Wissler, curator of anthropology and dean of the scientific staff of the American Museum of Natural History, was reelected president of the association, and Henry Butler Allen, director of the Franklin Institute, was elected a vice-president, succeeding Frank B. Jewett.

Section chairmen were elected as follows: Art Museums Section, George H. Edgell, director, Museum of Fine Arts, Boston; Art Technical Section, Francis Henry Taylor, director, Worcester Art Museum; Children's Museums Section, Mrs. Dean C. Osborne, president, the Auxiliary, Brooklyn Children's Museum; Education Section, Charles Russell, curator, Department of Education, American Museum of Natural History, New York; National and State Parks Section, Ned J. Burns, chief of the Museum Division, National Park Service, Washington, D. C.; Public Relations Section, Daisy Weld Warner, director of Publicity and Radio, Cleveland Museum of Art; Registrars Section, Imogene C. Robertson, registrar of the Buffalo Museum of Science; Science Museums Section, Carlos E. Cummings, director of the Buffalo Museum of Science; Science Technical Section, Ottmar F. von Fuehrer, staff artist, Carnegie Museum, Pittsburgh; Superintendents Section, Albert N. Henricksen, superintendent of the Brooklyn Museum, New York.

At the invitation of the museums of Detroit, Mich., that city was chosen as the meeting place for 1940.

### THE AMERICAN PUBLIC HEALTH ASSOCIATION

THE sixty-eighth annual meeting of the American Public Health Association and meetings of related organizations will open at Pittsburgh, Pa., on Sunday, October 15, closing on Friday, October 20. Thirty-five hundred health officers, nurses, engineers, school physicians, laboratory directors and other specialists are expected to attend. Every state in the Union, Canada, Cuba and Mexico, and many European countries will send delegates to participate in a scientific program that will cover the official public health activities of the North American continent.

The Sixth Institute on Public Health Education will open on Sunday, October 15. The meetings of the institute continue on Monday, October 16, at which time there will meet the International Society of Medical Health Officers, the American School Health Association, the Association of Women in Public Health and the National Organization for Public Health Nursing. The following conference groups also convene on Monday: the State Laboratory Directors, the State Sanitary Engineers, the Municipal Public Health Engineers, the Directors of Local Health Service and the State Directors of Public Health Nursing. Other organizations meeting during the week are the Pennsylvania Public Health Association, the Tri-State Food and Health Officials, the American Social Hygiene Association, Delta Omega and the American Association of State Registration Executors.

There will be six general sessions of the Public Health Association during the week at which "Medical Care," "Cancer," "Professional Education" and "The American Way as Seen from Abroad" are among the subjects to be discussed. The ten sections of the association have arranged an extensive series of joint and individual meetings covering topics of interest to health officers, laboratory workers, vital statisticians, industrial hygienists, public health engineers, food and nutritionists, child hygienists, public health education experts, epidemiologists and public health nurses. There will be a Health Exhibit with commercial and scientific displays. The headquarters will be at the William Penn Hotel. The preliminary program has been reprinted from the August issue of *The American Journal of Public Health* and may be obtained from the American Public Health Association, 50 West 50th Street, New York, N. Y.

## SCIENTIFIC NOTES AND NEWS

M. HENRI PIÉRON, professor at the Collège de France and director of the Institute of Psychology of the University of Paris, was elected at the Liège meeting president of the French Association for the Advancement of Science.

OWING to the early adjournment of the Dundee meeting of the British Association for the Advancement of Science Dr. Isaiah Bowman was presumably unable to give the first British and American Association lecture. The lecture, which is entitled "Science and Social Pioneering," will be printed in SCIENCE.

ON the occasion of the seventh assembly of the International Union of Geodesy and Geophysics, at a special convocation on September 11, Washington University conferred the honorary degree of doctor of science on Dr. Dan La Cour, director of the Danish Meteorological Institute, Copenhagen, who was president, and on Brigadier Harold St. John Loyd Winterbotham, British geologist and geophysicist, general secretary of the union. The degree conferred on Brigadier Winterbotham was *in absentia,* he having been recalled to England on account of the international situation.

THE American Congress of Physical Therapy meeting in New York City awarded on September 6 gold keys to four physicians in recognition of distinguished accomplishments in physical therapy. The presentation was made by Dr. William Schmidt, president of the congress. The awards were to Dr. Edward C. Titus, of New York, for his research in electrotherapy and light therapy; to Dr. A. Bern Hirsh, of New York, for his organization of physical therapy departments in hospitals and clinics; to Dr. Joseph Rivière, of Paris, for the introduction of electro-surgery into medical practice, and to Dr. James B. Mennell, of London, for contributions to physical medicine, particularly in massage.

THE American Amaryllis Society has awarded one of the William Herbert medals for 1939 to A. B. Stout, curator of education and laboratories at the New York Botanical Garden, for his work in breeding, cytology, genetics, introduction of new wild types and the production of fine horticultural varieties of Hemerocallis.

AT Syracuse University the establishment of three pioneer medals "in recognition of outstanding achievements" has been made possible by funds provided by George Arents, vice-president of the Board of Trustees. Dr. William Martin Smallwood, chairman of the department of zoology, was one of the first three recipients of the award. Dr. William P. Graham, chancellor of the university, made the following citation: William Martin Smallwood, distinguished educator; holder of degrees from Syracuse and Harvard; instructor and professor at Allegheny and Syracuse; eminent zoologist; member of various learned societies; author of widely used texts on biology; valued counselor on matters educational; pioneer investigator of the early teaching of science in the United States; donor of the Smallwood Library, an unmatched collection of books which have guided the development of science teaching in this country; for these and other reasons you are cited to receive a George Arents Medal for excellence in science.

F. T. LLEWELLYN, who retired on June 1 as research engineer of the United States Steel Corporation of Delaware after nearly fifty years' service, has been presented with an engrossed resolution of appreciation for his contribution to the structural steel fabricating industry by the American Institute of Steel Construction.

DR. LEONARD CARMICHAEL, since 1938 president of Tufts College, previously professor of psychology at Brown University and at the University of Rochester, was elected at the recent meeting at Berkeley, Calif., president of the American Psychological Association. He succeeds Dr. Gordon W. Allport, assistant professor of psychology at Harvard University.

DR. ROBERT P. FISCHELIS, secretary and chief chemist of the Board of Pharmacy of the State of New Jersey, was elected chairman of the Conference of Pharmaceutical Law Enforcement Officials, at the annual meeting held in Atlanta, Georgia, on August 24.

DR. WILLIAM HOPKINS CRAWFORD has been appointed dean of the School of Dentistry of Indiana University.

DR. ROBERT T. LEGGE, professor of hygiene at the University of California, who resigned as university physician a year ago and who has been on leave for the past twelve months, will return to the department of hygiene to continue his teaching and research on industrial hygiene.

MARGARET I. PINKERTON, superintendent of nurses at Barnes Hospital, St. Louis, has been made dean of the School of Nursing at Duke University, Durham, N. C.

DR. LEE T. SMITH, chemist in the research laboratories of the Bureau of Dairy Industry of the U. S. Department of Agriculture, has been selected to be head of the carbohydrate and derived products division of the Eastern Regional Research Laboratory of the Bureau of Agricultural Chemistry and Engineering. He will direct investigations concerned with the development of new uses of milk sugar and potato starch and products which can be prepared from these materials by fermentation and other means.

THE *Journal* of the American Medical Association reports that, pursuant to a law passed by the 1939 legislature, Governor Bushfield, of South Dakota, has appointed a basic science board. The members are: James D. Alway, Aberdeen; F. E. Burkholder, Sioux Falls; M. L. Severence, Aberdeen; Dr. William H. Waller, professor of anatomy of the School of Medicine at the University of South Dakota, and Dr. Gregg M. Evans, professor of chemistry and physics, Yankton College.

LIEUTENANT COLONEL L. T. POOLE, assistant professor of pathology at the Royal Army Medical College, England, has been promoted to the rank of colonel and has been appointed director and professor of pathology at the college in succession to Major-General H. M. J. Perry, who is retiring.

DR. EVARTS A. GRAHAM, Bixby professor of surgery at the School of Medicine of Washington University,

St. Louis, served this summer as head of the teaching surgical unit at St. Bartholomew's Hospital, London.

THE British Medical Research Council has appointed Dr. Donald Hunter, physician to the London Hospital, and Harold E. Clay, national secretary of the Passenger Services Group, Transport and General Workers' Union, to be members of the Industrial Health Research Board, in succession to Professor J. A. Nixon and R. Coppock.

THE status of director of the British Royal Air Force Medical Services has been advanced to that of director-general with the rank of air-marshal. Air Marshal Sir Albert Richardson, director of the medical services, thus becomes director-general.

DR. JOHN LAWRENCE, assistant professor of medicine at the University of California, a passenger on the British liner *Athenia,* is reported to have been rescued. Dr. Lawrence is a brother of Dr. Ernest O. Lawrence and a son of Dr. C. G. Lawrence, president emeritus of Northern State Teachers College, Aberdeen, S. D.

SIR FREDERICK BANTING, professor of medical research at the University of Toronto, has enlisted as captain in the fifteenth General Hospital of the Canadian Army Medical Corps.

DR. GEORGE S. AVERY, JR., professor of botany at Connecticut College and director of the Connecticut Arboretum, will return this month from the Carlsberg Laboratory in Copenhagen. He has been working with Professor K. Linderstrøm-Lang on enzyme micromethods and hormone-enzyme relationships.

DR. STACY R. METTIER, associate professor of medicine in the Medical School of the University of California, at San Francisco, has returned after spending six months in making a study of diseases of the blood in various clinics in London and elsewhere in Europe.

CHARLES B. HUNT, of the U. S. Geological Survey, has returned from his fourth field season in the Henry Mountains, Utah. Thomas A. Hendricks and Paul Averitt have returned from field work in the Ouachita Mountains, Okla. François E. Matthes has returned from a short field season devoted to the study of glacial deposits and physiography in the eastern Sierra Nevada. Mr. Matthes attended the meeting of the Geological Society of America at Berkeley from August 8 to 10 and, after the meeting, conducted an excursion in the Sierra Nevada.

THE eighth Congress of the Institut International d'Anthropologie was to have met at Istanbul from September 18 to 25 under the presidency of Professor E. Pittard of Geneva. Sections were planned covering paleontology and archeology, physical anthropology, heredity and blood groups, social anthropology, linguistics and the history of religions.

APPLICATIONS must be on file with the United States Civil Service Commission at Washington, D. C., not later than October 2 for the positions of senior aquatic physiologist at a salary of $4,600 a year and of associate aquatic physiologist at a salary of $3,200 in the Fisheries Service, Department of the Interior.

A STUDY of "The Place of Mathematics in Secondary Education" has been completed by the Joint Commission appointed in 1937 by the Mathematics Association of America and the National Council of Teachers of Mathematics, under the chairmanship of Dr. K. P. Williams, head of the department of mathematics of Indiana University. It has been carried on under a financial grant made by the General Education Board and will be published early in 1940 as the year-book of the National Council of Teachers of Mathematics. Members of the Joint Commission representing the Mathematics Association are: Professor Williams, A. A. Bennett, Brown University; H. F. MacNeish, Brooklyn College; H. E. Buchanan, Tulane University; U. G. Mitchell, University of Kansas; C. A. Hutchinson, University of Colorado, and F. L. Griffin, Reed College, and, representing the National Council, W. D. Reeve, Columbia University; William Betz, Rochester, N. Y., public schools; W. L. Hartung, University of Chicago; J. A. Nyberg, Hyde Park High School, Chicago; Mary A. Potter, Racine, Wis., public schools; G. H. Jamison, Northeast Missouri State Teachers College, and Ruth Lane, the State University of Iowa.

IN accordance with a resolution passed by the Board of Directors of the American Chemical Society at the Baltimore meeting, the chairman, Dr. Thomas Midgley, Jr., has appointed the following committee to formulate requirements for chemists in clinical laboratories and report to the directors: Frank C. Whitmore, *chairman,* Gustavus J. Esselen and Robert A. Keho. Any one interested in clinical laboratory work and in the proper qualifications for individuals directing or performing chemical work is asked to transmit his ideas to the chairman of the committee. *Industrial and Engineering Chemistry* states that the earlier notice on this subject is bringing in from the secretaries of the local sections and their members part of the information needed. While there is an interest in all clinical laboratories, special importance at this time is to be placed on any information regarding the quality of chemical work for which the public is paying the members of the medical profession in connection with the diagnosis of disease by the latter. It is stated that the preliminary results of the survey seem to indicate that most work of this kind is done by individuals having practically no chemical training. Those having pertinent information or knowing of others who may be able to give such information are requested to write to Dr. Frank C. Whitmore, State College, Pa.

The expedition led by Dr. Cecil Madigan across the Simpson Desert in Australia has returned to Adelaide after an absence of three months. Dr. Madigan said, according to the London *Times,* that he could not hold out much hope that the desert country was capable of development as pasture land or for any other purpose, though he did not think that there was danger that the desert would increase in area.

The Case School of Applied Science has received a grant from the National Advisory Committee for Aeronautics for a basic aerodynamic investigation of boundary layer control to study the effect of air upon the drag of airplane wings. Preliminary studies by Dr. John R. Weske have shown the possibility of reducing the wind resistance of airplanes through such a study.

Funds were appropriated in the third deficiency act for the investigation of strategic mineral deposits this year by the Geological Survey in accordance with the authorization, which had been previously passed by congress. These funds became available August 10, and the Geological Survey now has parties investigating strategic mineral deposits in several of the western states. These include manganese deposits in Montana, Washington, Oregon and New Mexico; chromite in Montana, Oregon and Wyoming; tungsten in Nevada; quicksilver in California, Oregon and Idaho; tin in Alaska, South Dakota and New Mexico; and nickel in Alaska. Investigation of certain tin and mica deposits in the southwestern states will begin shortly. Some of these investigations are essentially a continuation of those begun in the summer of 1938. The entire program is expected to continue for four years.

# DISCUSSION

## A SELF-LIMITING MECHANISM IN SYMPATHETIC HOMEOSTATIC ADJUSTMENT

It has been shown that adrenaline exercises a specific inhibitory action on sympathetic synapses.[1, 2] This has been demonstrated by recording the decrease in action potentials in the post-ganglionic nerves of the superior cervical ganglion of cats and rabbits when adrenaline was either liberated from the adrenals by splanchnic stimulation or was injected intravenously in amounts comparable to those known to be secreted under stress.[3] In each case as the adrenaline was destroyed recovery from inhibition took place.

It may appear paradoxical that adrenaline, which promotes sympathetic activity, also inhibits it, but I wish to suggest that a beneficial effect, important to the body economy, is served by the opposed actions. The ganglionic inhibitory action of adrenaline may constitute a self-limiting mechanism capable of checking the wide-spread activity produced by sympathico-adrenal discharge when this has reached a high level. The attempt to preserve maximum efficiency in the face of environmental change, *i.e.,* to maintain homeostasis, calls forth a marked, diffuse increase in sympathetic activity. This initiates the following sequence of events: Adrenaline liberated by the augmented splanchnic impulses prolongs and greatly enhances sympathetic activity. If this tends to become excessive, thereby partially defeating its purpose, the concentration of adrenaline in the blood rises to a level sufficient to produce ganglionic inhibition, and thus decreases the sympathetic discharge by obstructing the passage of impulses from the pre- to the post-ganglionic neurones. It may be supposed that a block is also interposed at the neuroadrenal junction, since it is structurally and pharmacologically of a ganglionic nature. The output of adrenaline is thus curtailed. With the lowered concentration of circulating adrenaline ganglionic inhibition is removed. Then, if the need for homeostasis still persists, sympathetic activity is once more allowed full play, until again restrained by the self-limiting influence of the rising blood adrenaline. This automatic safeguard adds another means of adjustment to the regulation exercised by other compensatory mechanisms, such as the carotid sinus.

Additional support for this view is found in the work of Tournade and Chabrol,[4] who observed a restrictive effect on sympathetically controlled functions in adrenalectomized recipient dogs when adrenaline is injected into the donors to which they are joined by adrenojugular anastomosis. Similar and more extensive effects are obtained in the same type of experiment when adrenaline is introduced into the donor by slow, continued infusion.[5] The inhibitory effects of adrenaline on the pressor action of nicotine and on reflexly induced sympathetic responses, described by Hoskins and Rowley[6] in 1915, are susceptible in part to a similar interpretation. So are the results of more recent workers,[7, 8] who have studied the depression of reflex sympathetic phenomena by adrenaline.

[1] A. S. Marrazzi, *Jour. Pharmacol. and Exp. Therap.,* 65: 395, 1939.

[2] *Ibid., Proc. Amer. Physiol. Soc.,* page 163, April, 1939.

[3] W. B. Cannon and D. Rapport, *Amer. Jour. Physiol.,* 58: 308, 1921.

[4] A. Tournade and M. Chabrol, *C.R. de la Soc. de biol.,* 94: 535, 1926.

[5] J. Malmejac, V. Donnet and E. Desanti, *C.R. de la Soc. de biol.,* 119: 1152, 1935.

[6] R. G. Hoskins and W. N. Rowley, *Amer. Jour. Physiol.,* 37: 471, 1915.

[7] L. W. Chu and F. Y. Hsu, *Quart. Jour. Exp. Physiol.,* 27: 307, 1938.

Were it not that the ganglionic nature of the neuro-adrenal junction prevents excitation of the adrenal by its own secretion,[9] adrenaline secretion once started might be self-perpetuating. Instead the nature of the junction introduces the possibility of self-limitation of adrenal discharge by the ganglionic inhibitory action of adrenaline. Work in progress is expected to yield data that will further test this view.

AMEDEO S. MARRAZZI
NEW YORK UNIVERSITY
COLLEGE OF MEDICINE

## CHLORAZOL FAST PINK BKS

IN the April 14 issue of SCIENCE there is a communication from Dr. Walter Modell drawing attention to the valuable characteristics of the azo dye known as Chlorazol Fast Pink BKS, Color Index No. 353, as an anti-coagulant.

This dye has been prepared in a pure form under my direction for quite a number of years in order to save the biological laboratory the necessity of purification, and has been supplied free of cost, in small quantities, to institutions of learning. Dr. Charles E. King, of Vanderbilt University, states that the material, as furnished, is so little toxic that he is able to give a full dose in one injection, although the slight shock, when this is done, can be avoided by dividing the amount and giving it in three portions.

This communication is made to inform those interested that, if they are in need of very small quantities, they can obtain these without the necessity of doing their own purification.

R. E. ROSE
E. I. DU PONT DE NEMOURS AND COMPANY,
WILMINGTON, DEL.

## "STARS" IN AMERICAN MEN OF SCIENCE

IN the "Distribution of the Younger Starred Scientists" by Professor S. S. Visher, which recently appeared in SCIENCE,[1] occurs the following statement: "Universities which had fewer starred men on their faculty in 1938 than in 1906 include Columbia, 60 in 1906, 39½ in 1938; Cornell 33, 25½; Dartmouth 6, 1; New York 9, 7; Clark 7, 1; Indiana 6, 3; Missouri 9, 1; Wesleyan 7, 4."

The casual reader would infer that these faculties had deteriorated or at least lost many of their most talented or creatively industrious members. A little further examination, however, reveals that the article contains no data as to actual numbers in 1938. In lieu of actual numbers for each institution, the article takes the total numbers of new names starred in 1921–1937 (third to sixth editions), mistakes them for totals on these faculties in 1938, and, comparing them with totals for 1906, finds in this particular group of institutions "fewer starred men" than in 1906.

As a simple and modest example, Dartmouth (which still prides itself on being a "liberal college" with no university aspirations) had in 1906 six starred members and actually six (rather than one as stated) in 1938. If an interested person should take the trouble to look up in the recent edition of American Men of Science the 1938 numbers for other institutions with diminishing returns, some of them, too, very likely would be removed from the black list.

A similar confusion appears in the two preceding paragraphs. The number of starred men included in the 1906 selection of 1,000 is compared with the total for each institution of selections in 1921, 1927, 1932 and 1937 (*ca.*, another 1,000). A list of institutions is given in which these total subsequent selections approximately equal the original selection for that institution: *e.g.*, Harvard 66 in 1906, compared with 69 (inadvertently identified with the unascertained number on the faculty in 1938).

Another list of institutions which have "gained notably" includes California, 27 in 1906 compared with 39, which is wrongly assumed to be the unascertained number on the faculty in 1938, but really is the total of the four selections made during the past 18 years.

If all the men and women starred in 1906 had died, or somehow become completely annihilated, before 1938, Professor Visher's statistical interpretation of the selections made during the last two decades would have been approximately correct.

J. H. G.
DARTMOUTH COLLEGE

THE portion of an article on this subject reprinted in the June 23 issue (89: 583–585) contains two inadequate statements. Although the study is concerned with the younger starred scientists, those starred in 1921–1937, and refers to the older group (those starred in 1903 or 1909) only for sake of comparison, a statement on the 1938 distribution of starred scientists does not make this limitation clear. What was meant was that certain institutions had in 1938 or earlier of the 1,101 scientists starred in 1921–1937 the numbers specified, which totals were greater or less than those institutions had of the 1,000 starred in 1903. A very few of these older men have not yet retired, whereas the quoted statements imply that they have all died or retired.

STEPHEN S. VISHER

## THE PACIFIC ENTOMOLOGICAL SURVEY

A NOTE under this heading in SCIENCE for June 16, 1939, over several signatures from Hawaii, has been

[8] C. W. Darrow and E. Gellhorn, *Proc. Amer. Jour. Physiol.*, page 58, April, 1939.

[9] P. Trendelenburg, *Ergebn. der Physiologie*, 21: 549, 1923.

[1] SCIENCE, 89: 583–585, June 23, 1939, reprinted (abridged) from *American Journal of Science*, 237 (1): 48–65, January, 1939.

brought to my notice by B. Ewart White, of 36 Bedford Row, London, W.C.1., in a letter to me dated July 12.

Exception is taken to the statement that E. P. Mumford, who has been completing the Marquesan work under my general supervision, has "no control over the collections made in the Marquesas" by himself and his assistants "nor over the publications resulting from their study," and that "All correspondence pertinent to the original survey" (which Mr. Mumford had been invited to direct, and towards the completion of which through the depression he and others outside of Hawaii had contributed financially) "should be addressed to Bernice P. Bishop Museum, Honolulu."

The facts are that the director of that museum had himself stated in official letters to Mr. White, "I understand perfectly that Mr. Mumford is responsible for checking the remaining taxonomic papers on the material collected by him and his assistants in the Marquesas and Society Islands." Mr. White continues: "the balance of funds on hand to the credit of the Pacific Entomological Survey in Hawaii in 1936 was transferred to me by order of the benefactors in Hawaii and elsewhere, and . . . I, as representative of these and subsequent subscribers, have here in safe keeping the original authorizations from Honolulu referring to the continued use of Pacific Entomological Survey Notes, correspondence, etc., and to the *continuation* of the 'work under the name of the Pacific Entomological Survey.'"

The statement in SCIENCE that the work now being carried on by Mr. Mumford under the auspices of Oxford University is a "new 'Survey' . . . distinct from the survey organized in Hawaii," is misleading. The authors of that statement make no reference to the account in the leading English scientific periodical *'Nature,'* January 29, 1938, of the means by which Mr. Mumford's work was continued at Oxford.

The reference to registration of a Pacific Entomological Survey "with headquarters at Oxford" is equally misleading. In 1936 a custodian of the abovementioned funds was necessary, and Mr. B. Ewart White consented to serve as a trustee. The name Pacific Entomological Survey was used for the time being to maintain the continuity of the work, as stated above, but the name Pacific Entomological Survey has not been, and will not be, employed in connection with the present phase of the work associated officially with Oxford.

It is to be deplored that attempts to interfere with the progress of this work should be made, even under a misapprehension. The only object in view should be to obtain, and make known, facts which will help in elucidating the problems of the Pacific Islands. It is appreciated by us that the Marquesan collections and certain other material now under the charge of Mr. Mumford will be deposited in the Bernice P. Bishop Museum, when the final results have been obtained. To further this end the Hope Department of Entomology of the University of Oxford, by means of grants from the University for five years from October, 1938, from the Royal Society and the British Association for the Advancement of Science and from benefactors through the trustee, Mr. B. Ewart White, is obtaining from sundry little known islands in the Pacific, new collections which it is hoped will aid in elucidating problems revealed by the Marquesan work that Mr. Mumford has been completing at Oxford.

G. D. HALE CARPENTER,
*Hope Professor of Zoology (Entomology) in the University of Oxford*

JULY, 1939

# SCIENTIFIC BOOKS

## ELEMENTARY MATRICES

*Elementary Matrices and Some Applications to Dynamics and Differential Equations.* By R. A. FRAZER, W. J. DUNCAN and A. R. COLLAR. xvi + 416 pp., 8vo. Cambridge: at the University Press. New York: The Macmillan Company.

Two of the authors of this beautifully printed volume are members of the Aerodynamics Department of the National Physical Laboratory of England, and the third is professor of aeronautics at Hull.

The book appears to have three main objectives. The first is the development of certain phases of elementary matric theory, the second is the practical solution of differential equations by means of the matric calculus, and the third is the application of these methods to mechanics, in particular to the dynamics of the airplane.

Clearly the book is intended primarily for students of applied mathematics who are not very familiar with modern algebra. Consequently, the elementary treatise on matrices which occupies the first 155 pages is quite lengthy and detailed. The usual theorems are given on quadratic and bilinear forms, latent (characteristic) roots, elementary operations and the elementary divisor theory. Infinite series of matrices are also treated and matrices of differential operators.

Throughout the text, computational methods are featured and many numerical problems are worked out in detail. Much attention is given to rapid methods of calculation by means of machines. For example, more than twenty pages are devoted to methods for calculating the reciprocal of a matrix, and one specimen calculation of the reciprocal of a sixth order matrix is given with some elements computed to the ninth decimal place. The solution of linear systems of algebraic equations is treated from the same standpoint, specimen solutions exhibiting methods which reduce labor to a minimum. Methods involving matrices are used to obtain dominant roots of algebraic equations of higher degree. Here the methods are interesting, but the results are not spectacular from the standpoint of the saving of labor.

After the four introductory chapters comes the treatment of differential equations and systems of differential equations by matric methods. While these methods are not essentially new, it is probably correct to say that this book takes more pains than any previous one to develop the theory in an elementary manner, and by means of many specimen problems to bring the methods within the range of the great number of workers who use differential equations in a practical way.

One interesting point in the matric method is its connection with the operational calculus of Heaviside. Some of the successful but unreasonable empirical methods which so delighted Heaviside appear quite reasonable and rigorous from the matric approach.

Next come chapters on kinematics and dynamics of systems, and systems with linear dynamical equations. The treatment is conventional, except that matric methods are used wherever possible, mainly in the solution of the differential equations involved, and that most of the problems relate to aerodynamics.

Chapter X is a collection of problems, each of considerable intrinsic interest, which are worked out in detail and with the expenditure of considerable labor. These problems are: (1) Oscillations of a triple pendulum. (2) Torsional oscillations of a uniform cantilever. (3) Torsional oscillations of a multi-cylinder engine. (4) Flexural oscillations of a tapered beam. (5) Symmetrical vibrations of an annular membrane. (6) A system with two equal frequencies. (7) The static twist of an aeroplane wing under aerodynamical load. (8) The oscillations of a wing in an airstream.

The remaining three chapters are devoted to the dynamics of the airplane, and in them some problems of considerable difficulty and practical importance are worked out by the techniques discussed earlier. The phenomena of ankylosis (or "sticking" of a degree of freedom), and flutter are treated at length with numerical problems and graphic interpretation of results. The last chapter is on pitching oscillations of a frictionally constrained aerofoil.

Judged by American and Continental standards, the book is verbose and somewhat nationalistic in referring to other authors. But clearly the book was written in the hope of converting many applied mathematicians to the use of more elegant and powerful mathematical tools, and it is so skilfully and attractively designed for this purpose that one should judge it from no other angle.

C. C. MACDUFFEE

UNIVERSITY OF WISCONSIN

# SOCIETIES AND MEETINGS

## THE FRENCH ASSOCIATION FOR THE ADVANCEMENT OF SCIENCE[1]

IN response to the kind invitation of the University of Liège, the French Association for the Advancement of Science met from July 17 to 22 for the third time in Belgium; the previous meetings were at Liège in 1924 and at Brussels in 1932.

The International Water Exhibition at Liège which marked the inauguration of the Albert Canal gave the meeting a special interest. Professor C. Fabry, president of the French Association, presided over the meeting, and Professor Dehalu, *administrateur-inspecteur* of the University of Liège, was president of the local committee.

The opening ceremony toook place on July 17 in the hall of the university. Professor Dehalu expressed his pleasure at receiving the Association at Liège for the second time, and Senator Buisseret, speaking on behalf of the burgomaster, welcomed the members of the congress. Professor C. D. Ellis, Wheatstone professor of physics at King's College, London, representing the British Association, and Dr. C. Romaña, representing the Argentine Association for the Advancement of Science, brought messages of good will for the success of the meeting. Professor Fabry, after having expressed the thanks of the association to the local committee at Liège, delivered his presidential address, on interstellar space.

Professor Fabry showed how a profound study of the light of the stars has enabled us to detect, in interstellar space, matter in a state of extreme rarefaction (1 kgm, nearly in a volume equal to that of the earth). In addition to matter, there exists also in interstellar space energy in the form of radiation emitted by the stars. These results have demonstrated the fruitfulness of collaboration of diverse scientific disciplines and of pure and applied science. Such collaboration is also the object of the French Association and of similar bodies.

The scientific meetings were held in the magnificent Institutes of Civil Engineering and Chemistry of the University of Liège at Val Benoît on July 17 and the following days. July 19 was devoted to an excursion on the Albert Canal and to a visit to a colliery at Beeringen. July 21, the day of the national fête of

[1] From *Nature*.

Belgium, was taken up with a visit to the Water Exhibition.

The several sections of the association showed great activity. The question of water occupied a prominent place in the program and was the subject of the following papers: M. Wyart, the states of solid and liquid water studied by x-rays; M. Cabannes, the Raman spectrum of liquid water; M. Kraft de la Saulx, history of the construction of hydraulic machines; M. Tongas, thermodynamic properties of steam; M. Trochon, microphysics of mists considered as aerosols; M. Roulleau, hygrometry; M. Rocard, kinetic theory of liquids; M. Hubault, pollution of waters, their industrial utilization and modifications of their fauna.

The Section of Civil and Military Engineering, under the presidency of M. Campus, was divided into three subsections: theoretical and applied hydraulics; navigable channels and ports; hydraulic works. One session was devoted to colonial hydrography.

The Section of Physics heard communications, among others, from Professors F. Joliot and F. Perrin. The work of the Section of Geology was completed by field excursions; the Section of Botany also had excursions in which the Royal Society of Botany of Belgium and the Liège Botanical Circle joined.

The Sections of Biogeography and of Zoology held several joint sessions with papers on the biology of equatorial lakes (M. Damas), the relations between the internal and external media in aquatic animals (M. Florkin) and the phreatic fauna (M. R. Leruth).

Mention should also be made of the communications presented to the Section of Geography (streams, their utilization and management, demographic and social aspects of water); and to the Sections of Medical Sciences (metabolism of water), of Psychology and Pedagogy, of Radiology and of Odontology.

Special subsections considered technical applications of water, applications of electricity, archeology and folklore.

The communications presented at the meeting will form a special volume published in connection with the Liège meeting.

## THE MEDICAL LIBRARY ASSOCIATION

THE Medical Library Association held its forty-first annual meeting from June 27 to 29, 1939, at the Academy of Medicine of Northern New Jersey, Newark. Officers for 1939–40 are: *President,* Colonel Harold W. Jones, Washington, D. C.; *Vice-president,* Dr. John M. Armstrong, St. Paul; *Secretary,* Miss Anna C. Holt, Boston; *Treasurer,* Miss Louise D. C. King, Baltimore; *Chairman of the Executive Committee,* Miss Mary Louise Marshall, New Orleans.

Miss Linda H. Morley described the varying services and requirements of three general types of medical libraries: those serving educational institutions; those serving organizations, and those affiliated and housed with a particular organization's staff.

Dr. George H. Lathrope answered the question, "Why Medical History for the Medical Librarian?" First, one's patrons are growing interested in this subject; second, it is a pleasant aid in developing acquaintance with medicine and its terminology; third, it has a distinct cultural value; and fourth, medical history is an almost untouched field for research.

"The Hospital Library and Its Administration" formed the subject of a most useful paper by Miss L. Margueriete Prime. She showed how the medical profession and friends of medical libraries have developed good hospital libraries. Standards have been established for them by the American Medical Association, the Canadian Medical Association and the American College of Surgeons. A general discussion of the organization and administration of the hospital library followed.

Another phase of the library connected with the hospital was portrayed by Miss Ethel Wigmore in her discussion of "The Responsibility of the Medical Library to the Nursing Profession." After sketching the development of libraries for nurses, with special reference to Bellevue, Miss Wigmore drew a picture of their present status in nursing education and of the growth of nursing literature.

Miss Margaret Bates showed in lantern slides a most interesting series of medical postage stamps.

Dr. Karl M. Scott gave a paper on "The Literature of Syphilis," in which he presented a broad picture of the whole subject and its application to the present-day campaign for control of the disease.

Real assistance in the association's endeavor to enlarge its supporting membership was rendered by Dr. Arthur H. Sanford, of the Mayo Clinic, who described the mutual benefits to be secured thereby. Dr. Joseph E. Raycroft's discourse on "Old Wine in New Bottles" quoted writings and archeological records to show that the ancients used certain treatments which are still valuable.

Dr. Max E. Soifer discussed "Dr. Horace Wells, the Discoverer of Anesthesia." "Problems of Microphotography," by Miss Dorothy Hale Litchfield and Dr. Mary A. Bennett, of the Film Library of Columbia University, dealt with the making, use and care of microfilms in libraries.

Dr. Charles H. Young made most interesting his account of the benefits and dangers of aviation to mankind. Aviation medicine is really preventive medicine.

The 1940 annual meeting of the association will be held in Portland, Oregon, at the invitation of the University of Oregon School of Medicine.

ANNA C. HOLT,
*Secretary*

# SPECIAL ARTICLES

## RADIOACTIVE ION EXCHANGES IN LIVING PROTOPLASM

PENETRATION curves for the entrance of radioactive ions into living cells of *Nitella coronata* have been described by Brooks,[1] who has also suggested that the initial increase in ion concentration in protoplasm during the first phase, which is at a maximum in about 15 minutes, is due to an exchange of a radioactive ion for some inactive ion. In the present study, the loss of radioactive ions from the protoplasm of *Nitella* by means of exchange was investigated. Ion exchange is here used to connote the replacement of an ion, possibly bound to an electrolyte by another ion. Ion exchange studies on barley roots have been described by Jenny and Overstreet[2] and on *Elodea* by Mazia.[3]

*Nitella* were taken from large outdoor ponds, separated into single cells and allowed to remain in pond water at 10° C. for a week. Only turgid cells with a length of 3.5 to 4.5 cm were used, in order to secure material which was as uniform as possible. Cells were immersed in 0.01 M solutions of K*Cl or Na*Cl dissolved in pond water at pH 8.2. After 15 minutes the cells were removed from the radioactive solutions, washed in triple distilled water, and the number of radioactive impacts measured with a Geiger-Müller counter. Cells were then placed in 0.01 M solutions of either LiCl, NaCl, KCl, RbCl or CsCl. Cells placed in either quartz-distilled $CO_2$-free water or in an ion-free 0.02 M sucrose solutions were used as controls. The temperature was 15 ± 0.1° C. After a 15-minute immersion, measurements of radioactive counts on each cell were made after 1, 2, 3, 5 and 10 minutes. Whole cells were used, the method of measuring consisting simply of placing each cell on a glass slide and putting this slide a known distance from the Geiger-Müller counting tube. The cell could then be returned to its solution and subsequent loss of radioactivity followed. There is no error because of the presence of sap, since there is no loss of Na* or K* to the sap as shown by separate analyses of the sap, protoplasm and wall in 15 minutes. The curves for the loss of radioactive ions from *Nitella* were exponential and followed equation (1)

$$C_p = C_o e^{-kt}, \quad (1)$$

where $C_p$ is the concentration of radioactive ion in the protoplasm, $C_o$ the initial concentration of ions in the protoplasm, $k$ a constant giving the slope of the logarithmic curve and $t$ the time of immersion of the cell in the solution of inactive ion. The values of $k$ which were found are given in Table I, and they represent the rate of loss of ions from the cell.

TABLE I

| Ion Exchanged | Value of k for Li | Na | K | Rb | Cs | HOH |
|---|---|---|---|---|---|---|
| Na* ...... | 0.33 | 0.26 | 0.23 | 0.20 | 0.19 | 0.05 |
| K* ....... | 0.12 | 0.16 | 0.83 | 2.00 | ... | 0.05 |

Some preliminary experiments with Rb*Cl and the alkali cation series indicate that in the exchange of Rb* for Li, Na, K, Rb or Cs, the results are similar to those in which K* was used, but the rate of loss is much greater.

Further preliminary experiments on the ion exchange properties of the vacuolar membrane of *Nitella* have been carried out by studying the changes in concentration of either K* or Rb* in both sap and protoplasm after the cell had been immersed in radioactive solutions for 24 hours, to allow for accumulation in the vacuole, and then placed in solutions of inactive alkali cations. The rate of loss of ions from the protoplasm was slower than when the cells had been immersed only 15 minutes. In the sap there was an initial rise after one minute and then a falling off in concentration. In the case of anions, where radioactive phosphorus (as $HPO_4^{=}$) was used and its exchange for the series F, Cl, Br, I, tested, there is a more rapid loss of P* in $F^-$ than in $I^-$ solutions.

In summary one may say that in the case of K*, the rate of loss followed the Hofmeister series, $Rb^+$ was the fastest and $Li^+$ the slowest in replacing K*. For Na* the Hofmeister series was reversed, $Li^+$ was the most rapid and $Cs^+$ the slowest in replacing Na*. In distilled water the rate of loss of ions was very low. It is suggested that there are at least two factors in operation, namely (1) a permeability effect which in the case of Na* reverses the lyotropic series because ions may not directly exchange, but, rather, be removed because of a decrease in the number of exchange positions on the membrane, and (2) the lyotropic series which governs the loss of ions from the cell in the case of K*.

LORIN J. MULLINS
S. C. BROOKS
UNIVERSITY OF CALIFORNIA

[1] S. C. Brooks, *Proc. Soc. Exp. Biol. Med.*, 38: 856–858, 1938.

[2] H. Jenny and R. Overstreet, *Proc. Nat. Acad. Sci.*, 24: 384–392, 1938.

[3] D. Mazia, *J. Cell. Comp. Physiol.*, 11: 193–203, 1938.

## THE DENATURATION OF PROTEINS BY DETERGENTS AND BILE SALTS

ALL the synthetic detergents and bile salts I have tried denature ordinary proteins such as hemoglobin and egg albumin at the isoelectric point and keep the denatured isoelectric protein in solution. Some detergents, such as Duponol PC,[1] in sufficiently high concentration, can prevent the precipitation of denatured protein by trichloracetic acid, tungstic acid and acid ferric sulfate.

Screenivasaya and Pirie[2] observed that the syn-

[1] Sodium dodecyl sulfate is the $C_{12}$ compound of the series $CH_3(CH_2)_nCH_2OSO_3Na$. Duponol Special WA Paste (du Pont) consists mainly of the $C_{12}$ compound. Duponol PC is a mixture of the $C_{10}$–$C_{18}$ compounds.

[2] M. Screenivasaya and N. W. Pirie, *Biochem. Jour.*, 32: 1707, 1938.

thetic detergent sodium dodecyl sulfate[1] in 0.5 per cent. solution slowly splits the large tobacco mosaic virus protein into smaller molecules and separates the nucleic acid from the protein, but does not denature the protein as shown by solubility and digestibility tests. Unfortunately the tests for denaturation were not carried out in an altogether satisfactory way. In any case, tobacco mosaic virus is much more resistant to sodium dodecyl sulfate than hemoglobin or egg albumin.

Hemoglobin is denatured by extraordinarily small amounts of Duponol PC. The addition of only 2 mg of Duponol PC to 10 mg of beef methemoglobin dissolved in 10 cc of pH 6.8 phosphate buffer solution suffices to denature the protein. This denaturation of methemoglobin in dilute solution can be followed optically. Native methemoglobin is a brown compound with a band in the red. Denatured methemoglobin in neutral Duponol solution is a red compound with no band in the red.

If 0.5 gm of Duponol PC is added to 10 cc of 2.5 per cent. hemoglobin and the excess Duponol is then removed by dialysis against water, the hemoglobin remains in solution after the dialysis and retains the color and spectrum of denatured methemoglobin. This result shows the great affinity of Duponol PC for denatured methemoglobin. The dialyzed hemoglobin is precipitated by 0.1 saturated ammonium sulfate, which does not precipitate native methemoglobin. It is digested by trypsin, which does not digest native methemoglobin. Duponol PC in sufficiently high concentration can prevent the precipitation by 0.1 saturated ammonium sulfate and can inactivate trypsin. This is why the excess Duponol is removed by dialysis before the solubility and digestibility tests.

It takes about 10 times as much of the bile salt, sodium glycholate, as of Duponol PC to denature hemoglobin.

0.2 N trichloracetic acid does not precipitate hemoglobin in 1 per cent. solution if 1.3 per cent. Duponol PC is present.

Hemoglobin can be estimated colorimetrically as denatured methemoglobin in 1 per cent. Duponol PC solution. This colorimetric procedure has two advantages over the usual acid hematin procedure. The amount of light adsorbed does not change with time and it is the same whether the Duponol is added to oxyhemoglobin or to methemoglobin.

Bacteria do not grow in the hemoglobin solution containing 1 per cent. Duponol, not even at 37° C.

The synthetic detergents and the bile salts all have the same type of hydrophobic-hydrophilic structure. Each synthetic detergent and bile salt consists of a large hydrophobic part with a small hydrophilic part attached to it. In actual chemical structure, the detergents and bile salts vary considerably. The hydrophilic group may be an acid group, such as $OSO_3^-$, or a basic nitrogen group. The hydrophobic part may consist of a long straight fatty acid chain, or it may contain a naphthalene or other ring structure.

The denaturation of protein and the solution of denatured protein by detergents and bile salts which differ widely in chemical composition must be attributed to the one property all the detergents and bile salts have in common, their general hydrophobic-hydrophilic character.

Bile salts have been used to extract the photosensitive protein pigment of the eye[3] and to extract a chlorophyll compound from the chloroplasts of spinach.[4] Chlorophyll, I have found, can be extracted from spinach by Duponol PC much more effectively than by bile salts. It is now clear, however, that a protein extracted by bile salts or detergents may no longer be in its original native undissociated form.

Physiologically, the bile salts emulsify fats, activate lipase and promote the absorption of various substances. The possibility must now be considered that the physiological reactions of the bile salts, like their reactions with proteins, depend not on their specific structures, but on their general hydrophobic-hydrophilic character, and that other substances with the same general hydrophobic-hydrophilic character can act as physiological substitutes for the bile salts.

M. L. ANSON

THE ROCKEFELLER INSTITUTE
FOR MEDICAL RESEARCH,
PRINCETON, N. J.

## THE CONFIGURATION OF THE GLUTAMIC ACID OF ADENOCARCINOMA PROTEIN

RECENTLY, Kögl and Erxleben[1] have reported that the glutamic acid of malignant tumor proteins is present in partly racemized form. Chibnall, Rees, Tristram, Williams and Boyland,[2] using the Foreman procedure, found only l(+) glutamic acid in Crocker mouse sarcoma and in bronchial carcinoma. Kögl and Erxleben[3] have offered evidence to show that the Foreman procedure is unsuited for the isolation of the unnatural glutamic acid isomer (d(–) glumatic acid). It is reported in a recent issue of *Science News Letter* (36:37, 1939) that the results of Kögl and Erxleben have been confirmed by Dr. E. Schroeder, of the Biochemical Research Foundation of the Franklin Institute.

[3] W. Kühne in L. Hermann, "Handbuch der Physiologie," Leipzig, 1879, 3: 264.

[4] E. L. Smith, SCIENCE, 88: 170, 1938.

[1] Kögl and H. Erxleben, *Zeit. f. physiol. Chem.*, 258: 57, 1939.

[2] A. C. Chibnall, M. W. Rees, G. R. Tristram, E. F. Williams and E. Boyland, *Nature*, 144: 71, 1939.

[3] F. Kögl and H. Erxleben, *Nature*, 144: 111, 1939.

Using the method employed by Kögl and Erxleben, we have isolated glumatic acid from two adenocarcinomas of the large intestine, and from a sample of normal intestinal tissue adjacent to one of the carcinomas. Our results indicate that approximately 41 per cent. of the glumatic acid in the first carcinoma, and approximately 26 per cent. of the glumatic acid in the second, were present as d(−) glutamic acid. These findings confirm the report of Kögl and Erxleben. Our experimental data are summarized below:

(1) *Adenocarcinoma of the sigmoid colon.* Initial weight, 97.5 g. Weight of dried combined protein, 14.0 g. Glutamic acid hydrochloride isolated, 97 mg. M. P., 205° C. $[\alpha]_D$, + 5.5°.

(2) *Adenocarcinoma of the cecum.* Initial weight, 108.5 g. Weight of dried combined protein, 15 g. Glutamic acid hydrochloride isolated, 140 mg. M. P., 201° C. $[\alpha]_D$, + 15.0°.

(3) *Normal tissue adjacent to adenocarcinoma of the cecum.* Initial weight, 150 g. Weight of dried combined protein, 19.1 g. Glutamic acid hydrochloride isolated, 19 mg. M. P., 205° C. $[\alpha]_D$,+ 31.0°.

It will be noticed that the yield of glumatic acid obtained from the adenocarcinoma of the cecum was considerably greater than that obtained from adjacent normal tissue. No conclusion can be drawn from this, however, since the insolation of the glumatic acid was not quantitative.

We are indebted to the departments of pathology and surgery of the University of Minnesota Medical School for giving us the tissues analyzed immediately after operation. Microscopic diagnoses of the tumors were made by Dr. Robert Hebbel.

L. EARLE ARNOW
JEANETTE C. OPSAHL

THE MEDICAL SCHOOL,
UNIVERSITY OF MINNESOTA

## POLIOMYELITIC VIRUS IN SEWAGE

WITHIN the past two years it has become increasingly apparent that poliomyelitic virus may be readily isolated from the stools of human patients during acute and convalescent stages of this disease. Many reports now testify to the ease with which this can be accomplished.[1] Consequently, whenever poliomyelitis occurs within a city, there is at least an opportunity for this virus to enter the local sewage system. But actually poliomyelitic virus has never been demonstrated in sewage, and there is no information as to the possible amounts which may be there, nor the length of time which this virus might survive in this medium.

An opportunity to test this situation has recently occurred in the City of Charleston, South Carolina, where poliomyelitis assumed epidemic proportions during the months of May, June and July of this year. From this same South Carolina epidemic a strain of virus was isolated from a specimen of feces received in our laboratory on July first. The stool was from a child (B.Cr.) three years old, who had contracted paralytic poliomyelitis in a small up-state town, but who had been hospitalized in Charleston. Part of the stool suspension was inoculated intraperitoneally into one rhesus monkey (No. 1213) on July fourth, and typical experimental poliomyelitis resulted after an incubation period of five days. This strain has been successfully carried to its third passage (monkeys No. 1230 and 1242) and is characteristic of poliomyelitic virus.

Subsequently, through the kindness of Dr. L. Banov, health officer of the City of Charleston, samples of sewage were collected by two of us (J. R. P. and J. D. T.) from a few sites throughout the city during the period of July 7 to 14, 1939. Particular attention was paid to one pumping station in which the sewage came not only from the hospital where poliomyelitis patients were isolated, but also from that part of the city where most of the cases had arisen. One sample (C) of this sewage, amounting to about 8 liters in volume, was collected on July 11 in a tall glass bottle and allowed to stand for a period of twenty-four hours. Ice was packed about the base of the bottle for part of this time. After the first two hours, a sample of sediment (C-1) amounting to 200 cc was removed and to it 24 cc of ether were added for bactericidal purposes. This sample was then taken to New Haven, where, on July 12 and 13, 75 and 45 cc, respectively, were inoculated intraperitoneally into one monkey (No. 1227). Another sample (C-2) amounting to 700 cc of the sediment, was removed from the original 8-liter specimen on July 12; 70 cc of ether were added to it, and the specimen was sent to New Haven, where one monkey (No. 1232) was inoculated intraperitoneally with 125 cc on July 14. Both of these animals developed experimental poliomyelitis. The incubation period in monkey 1227 was eight days from the last inoculation, and in monkey 1232 it was seven days. After a brief febrile period both animals developed quadriplegia, and both were prostrate on the third day of their disease. Monkey 1232 died on this day; no. 1227 was sacrificed. Spinal cord lesions, demonstrable histologically, were found to be very extensive in both animals. It is unusual in our experience to see rhesus

[1] (*a*) P. H. Harmon, *Jour. Am. Med. Asn.*, 109: 1061, 1937; (*b*) J. D. Trask, A. J. Vignec and J. R. Paul, *Jour. Am. Med. Asn.*, 111: 6–11, 1938; (*c*) P. Lépine and P. Sédallian, *Compt. rend, Acad. d. sci.*, 208: 129–130, 1939; (*d*) S. D. Kramer, B. Hoskwith and L. H. Grossman, *Jour. Exp. Med.*, 69: 49–67, 1939; (*e*) C. Kling, G. Olin, J. H. Magnusson and S. Gard, *Bull. Acad. méd.*, 121: 826–831, 1939; (*f*) J. R. Paul, A. J. Vignec and J. D. Trask, *Trans. Asn. Am. Phys.* (to be published). Also personal communications from: G. Y. McClure, Division of Laboratories and Research, N. Y. State Department of Health; and from C. Armstrong, National Institute of Health, Washington, D. C.

TABLE 1

TESTS FOR POLIOMYELITIC VIRUS IN SEWAGE SPECIMENS

| Sewage specimen | Original amount | Interim between collection and inoculation | Amount of inoculum | | Monkey No. | Result |
|---|---|---|---|---|---|---|
| | | | Intraperitoneal | Subcutaneous | | |
| (A) Pump | 3.5 liters | 6 and 7 days | 36 cc | 22 cc | 1229 | Abscess of abdominal wall; acute peritonitis. Killed on 4th day. |
| (B) Har. | 0.5 liter | 7 days | 24 " | | 1231 | Chronic and acute peritonitis. Died on 18th day. |
| (C) Pump (1) | 8 liters | 1 and 2 days | 120 " | | 1227 | Poliomyelitis. Killed on 10th day. Passage to monkey 1248 successful. |
| (2) | | 3 days | 125 " | | 1232 | Poliomyelitis. Died on 8th day. Passage not done. |
| (D) Hosp. (1) | 7 " | 5 " | 75 " | 125 " | 1239 | Infected abdominal wall. Died on 2nd day. |
| (2) | | 6 " | 25 " | 46 " | 1240 | Abscess of abdominal wall. Killed on 4th day. |

monkeys develop such a severe form of the experimental disease when inoculated with material from a human source, and so we have suspected that the amounts of virus in the inocula here were not small.

The results of our experiments to date on this type of material appear in Table I. Here it will also be seen that our other attempts to isolate virus from Charleston sewage were unsuccessful as a result of the premature death of the monkey from bacterial infection. Obviously, methods have not yet been perfected for handling or testing this type of material.

Our criteria for the diagnosis of poliomyelitis in these experiments have been practically the same as those we have used in previous work[2] on the isolation of poliomyelitic virus from extra-neural human sources, namely, that the inoculated animal developed signs and symptoms compatible with those of the experimental disease; that typical lesions were found in the spinal cord, and that the strain was successfully passed to another monkey. All these criteria were met in the case of monkey 1227; one of them is omitted in monkey 1232, for a passage of this strain was not attempted.

It is not evident from this work whether the presence of poliomyelitic virus in sewage is a direct or even an indirect link in the chain which leads this infectious agent from one patient to another in this disease. Our report merely calls attention to the fact that poliomyelitic virus may not only be present in urban sewage but also that it may possibly be present in appreciable quantities.[3]

JOHN R. PAUL

DEPARTMENT OF MEDICINE

JAMES D. TRASK

C. S. CULOTTA

DEPARTMENT OF PEDIATRICS,
YALE UNIVERSITY SCHOOL OF MEDICINE

# SCIENTIFIC APPARATUS AND LABORATORY METHODS

## DEMONSTRATION OF THE SHAPE OF CILIA IN NORMAL MOTION

IT is often desirable to demonstrate the shape and motion of cilia without the use of methods which may cause distortion or prevent an estimation of the rate of beating. An easily made stroboscope meets this need.

To make a periodically moving object like a cilium appear stationary, it must be made visible repeatedly at only one point in its path. This can be achieved by a light flashing on the object at exactly the same frequency as its motion. If the synchronization is not quite perfect, the cilium will appear to be moving very slowly because each flash of light will reveal it at a slightly different position. Should the synchronization be much poorer, the entire effect will be lost. These principles constitute the basis of the stroboscope.

An obvious means of producing a flashing light is to have a disk with a number of regularly spaced radial slits rotating in front of a fairly strong light source. Four slits have been found most suitable. In projection, it makes little difference where the disk is located; for convenience it may be placed between the ocular and the screen.

A satisfactory method for the adjustment of the disk's speed is an important element in the success of the stroboscope. A rheostat in series with the motor attached to the disk is adequate; however, finer adjustment is obtainable with two rheostats in series if the resistance per unit length of one is considerably larger than the other's. In the way of a motor, even those obtainable in metal construction kits are usable. A possible arrangement of the apparatus is shown in the diagram.

The rate of ciliary motion can easily be determined from the disk's speed when synchronization, as judged from the cessation of movement, is attained. In general, it will be found a simple matter to count the

[2] Criteria reviewed by A. J. Vignec, J. R. Paul and J. D. Trask, *Yale Jour. Biol. and Med.*, 11: 15–31, 1938.

[3] Aided by grants from the National Foundation for Infantile Paralysis.

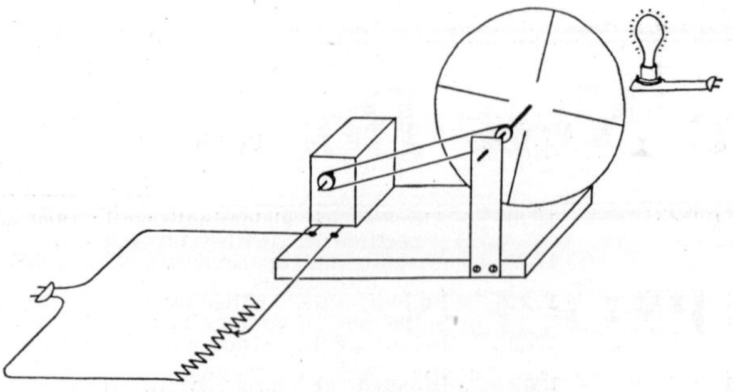

FIG. 1. A simple stroboscope.

number of rotations of the disk in a given period of time, which, when multiplied by the number of slits, will give the corresponding number of ciliary beats.

Organisms which will not move about much or side-view preparations of ciliated epithelium are best suited for demonstration purposes. Rotifers like Philodina and various attached Infusorians are excellent material, although with proper handling even an active form like Paramecium can be used.

A. M. SHANES

THE COLLEGE OF THE CITY OF NEW YORK

## A NEW MATERIAL FOR MOUNTING NERVE TISSUE SECTIONS IN PARAFFIN FOR SILVER STAINING OR RESTAINING

EGG albumin solution used to affix nerve tissue sectioned in paraffin to slides has not proven completely satisfactory. Sections so mounted are easily lost when the slides are passed through the various solutions. The histological picture obtained in those sections successfully carried through is not absolutely clear. While attempting to remove the haziness from such material, it soon became evident that the proteins of the albumin are responsible for the gray background. Some other mounting media were therefore considered. One which would have no reducing properties and which would, at the same time, hold the sections in place was desired. Because of the inertness of starch, a paste of this substance was tried. The following form of paste gave the most satisfactory results: 1 gm starch thoroughly mixed with 10 cc of cold water was added to 20 cc of boiling distilled water and constantly stirred until the suspension, which is opalescent, is uniform and free from lumps. Two drops of hydrochloric acid were then added, and the solution was boiled for an additional three to five minutes. After cooling, a small crystal of thymol was added as a preservative. The result is a clear thin paste which is used very much the same as the albumin fixative. The paraffin sections which are placed on the slide covered with the hydrolyzed starch suspension are allowed to dry for two to three days in an oven at 45° C.

This fixing material was used on sections from various sized blocks of tissue which had been impregnated with silver according to Bielschowsky's or Cajal's method. These blocks were sectioned and mounted serially. Out of 500 sections of one series, only one section was lost in the solutions. In all cases, the resulting pictures were clear. No precipitate was evident.

In another series of tests, fresh formalin fixed tissue was sectioned in paraffin and impregnated after being fixed to the slide. In this way a quite even staining reaction was obtained. The inevitable gradations which occur in mass staining were avoided. In addition, the time necessary for impregnation was reduced to less than half. These sections were mounted and dried, passed through xylol into water, through the graded alcohols, and washed for about fifteen minutes and then allowed to remain in pyridine over night. Next, the tissues were washed in distilled water for about ten minutes and put into a solution of 5 per cent. silver nitrate for three hours in the dark. They were then transferred into a solution of ammoniacal silver nitrate, *i.e.,* 200 cc of 5 per cent. silver nitrate solution plus 5 cc of 10 per cent. sodium hydroxide. Add ammonia, drop by drop, until the precipitate dissolves. The sections are allowed to remain in this solution for half an hour, then rapidly washed in distilled water, placed in a 10 per cent. formalin solution for about 5 minutes. After this, they are washed again and may be toned in gold and left in hypo for two minutes, then dehydrated, cleared and covered in the usual way.

This method stains the cells as well as neurofibrillae. Further work is being done in applying this method to other routine neurological techniques, such as Bodian's, modified Bielschowsky's and Ranson-pyridine methods.

ROSETTE SPOERRI

COLUMBIA UNIVERSITY AND
NEW YORK UNIVERSITY

## BOOKS RECEIVED

COLEMAN, LAURENCE V. *The Museum in America.* Vol. I, pp. viii + 218. Vol. II, pp. xiii + 221–428. Vol. III, pp. xviii + 431–730. Illustrated. American Association of Museums, Smithsonian Institution, Washington. Three volumes, $7.50.

HOLBROOK, STEWART H. *Iron Brew; a Century of American Ore and Steel.* Pp. viii + 352. Macmillan. $2.50.

KUDO, RICHARD R. *Protozoology.* Second edition. Pp. xi + 689. 291 figures. Charles C Thomas. $6.50.

NEURATH, OTTO. *Modern Man in the Making.* Pp. 159. Illustrated. Knopf. $2.95.

NORDENMARK, N. V. E. *Pehr Wilhelm Wargentin.* Pp. v + 464. Illustrated. Kungl. Svenska Vetenskapsakademien. Almqvist & Wiksells, Uppsala.

PORTER, ANNIE. *The Larval Trematoda Found in Certain South African Mollusca.* Publication No. XLII, Vol. VIII of the South African Institute for Medical Research. Pp. 492. 83 plates. 1 figure. The Institute, Johannesburg.

STEVENS, BLAMEY. *The Psychology of Physics.* Pp. xvi + 282. 59 figures. Sherratt & Hughes, Manchester, England. 7s. 6d.

# SCIENCE

Vol. 90 | Friday, September 22, 1939 | No. 2334

*The British Association for the Advancement of Science:*
*Local Scientific Societies and the Community:* Professor Herbert L. Hawkins ... 261

*Where Do Meteorites Come from?:* Professor C. C. Wylie ... 264

*Scientific Events:*
*The New Fishery Research Laboratory in Puerto Rico; The Expedition to Western Colorado of the Field Columbian Museum; Hurricane Warnings of the U. S. Weather Bureau; The Master of Science Degree in Engineering of Columbia University; Editors of the Publications of the American Chemical Society. Recent Deaths* ... 265

*Scientific Notes and News* ... 268

*Discussion:*
*Nutritional Physiology of the Adult Ruminant:* Dr. E. B. Forbes. *Heparin and Blood Clotting:* Dr. John H. Ferguson. *The Black Dye of the Navajos:* Professor Daniel T. O'Connell. *Appearance of a New Potato Disease in Northeastern Colorado:* Leslie B. Daniels ... 270

*Reports:*
*The Vulcanization of Rubber* ... 273

*Special Articles:*
*Androgens and Tumor Growth:* Professor J. R. Murlin and Others. *Ease of Body Heat Loss and Resistance to Infection:* Dr. Joseph W. Colvin and Dr. Clarence A. Mills. *The Muscle Hemoglobin of Seals as an Oxygen Store in Diving:* Douglas Robinson. *The Absorption of Radio Waves in Water:* Professor J. Barton Hoag ... 275

*Scientific Apparatus and Laboratory Methods:*
*A Spectrocolorimeter for Comparing the Spectra of Solutions of Different Depth:* Dr. Ely Perlman. *Periodic Discharging of Liquids and Intermittent Washing of Solids:* C. L. Graham and Dr. Raymond H. Lambert ... 279

*Science News* ... 6

SCIENCE: A Weekly Journal devoted to the Advancement of Science, edited by J. McKeen Cattell and published every Friday by

THE SCIENCE PRESS
New York City: Grand Central Terminal
Lancaster, Pa. Garrison, N. Y.

Annual Subscription, $6.00 Single Copies, 15 Cts.

SCIENCE is the official organ of the American Association for the Advancement of Science. Information regarding membership in the Association may be secured from the office of the permanent secretary in the Smithsonian Institution Building, Washington, D. C.

# LOCAL SCIENTIFIC SOCIETIES AND THE COMMUNITY[1]

By Dr. HERBERT L. HAWKINS
PROFESSOR OF GEOLOGY, UNIVERSITY OF READING

Through the whole range of nature, classification shows an underlying simplicity of principle expressed through various materials and in diverse grades. Gravitation controls galaxies and sand-grains, and evolution is the common destiny of genera and of individuals. Both of these fundamental principles tend inevitably to pile up aggregates of ever-increasing size and complexity. But such aggregates are collections of units, and, while appearing to acquire new properties, remain subject to the laws that govern units and dependent on the reaction of their components to those laws.

Human nature, despite the bombastic claims often urged by its exponents, illustrates the operation of the principle of evolution with painful fidelity, especially in its social reactions. From the lone hunter through the clan to the totalitarian state the process of aggregation goes on, with increasing complexity and decreasing flexibility, until Nemesis clears the stage for the next performance. Within the frame of natural or imperial unification are innumerable smaller aggregates, each so similar in type to the whole that one is reminded of a crystalline fabric, where each molecule has a shape consistent with that of the complete crystal.

A scientific society is but one example of this tendency towards congregation of kindred types. Whatever may be its peculiarities, its success or failure, each society has originated in much the same way as all the others. In most cases, its history can be traced back to the enthusiasm of an individual, who has attracted

[1] Address of the president of the Conference of Delegates of Corresponding Societies at the British Association for the Advancement of Science, Dundee, 1939.

and stimulated a small coterie of friends or disciples. Organization has followed; and, whether it was invented or adapted from previous models, it has produced a miniature copy of a democratic state, complete with cabinet and treasury.

The aims of these societies vary somewhat, some being devoted to research, others to instruction. The former type of society is in constant danger of decline, for it needs continuous stimulation by new enthusiasts in successive generations; the latter is fortunate if it avoids the comatose senility of a social club.

Sociability is, however, the key to the success, and almost a *raison d'être,* of a local society. Unless this is an association of friends, it belies its name and loses its efficiency. It is not in the academic eminence of its members, but in the spirit of cooperation and enjoyment, that the value of the society lies. For this reason a society that organizes field-excursions as an essential part of its program is a far more lively institution than one where the members meet only in the enforced silence of a lecture-hall. The element of friendly intercourse may, naturally, degenerate into a mere picnic; but even that is preferable to the priggish snobbery of a lion-hunt.

A society attracts to membership others besides those whose natural enthusiasm marks them as leaders in its enterprise. Although the danger of over-emphasis of the social side may be thus increased, such recruits are to be welcomed. Some may become interested and inspired, but all will contribute something, be it only a subscription, to help the society's work. No government can hope to carry out its schemes without the backing of a body of reasonably willing tax-payers.

The present is not altogether a propitious period for the advance of local societies. Although the proportion of the population capable of appreciating the aims of the societies is perhaps greater than formerly, the increase in the opportunities for recreation tends to reduce the personnel for any particular form of activity. Its local character is an essential aspect of a local society, and the metropolization of the provinces by transport and wireless telephony has obliterated much of the individuality of districts. Most societies deplore the lack of youthful recruits, and look forward with anxiety to decreasing membership.

In the great majority of cases, the members of local scientific societies are "amateurs" in the generally accepted sense of that term. Their scientific work is their hobby; and in the present pressure of business life few have time or energy to spare for a pastime that demands intellectual effort. The young prefer forms of recreation that involve strenuous and often exhausting physical exercise, while the middle-aged tend towards somnolent recreation. Not until retirement ensures leisure for following their own devices can most business men undertake the responsibilities or even enjoy the privileges of active membership. To such, a scientific society may offer hope of survival and of congenial activity, beyond the critical phase at which it used to be customary to receive an inscribed clock to mark the last few hours of life. Local societies can confer benefit on these and on themselves by attracting them to membership. Individually they may have poor actuarial prospects of permanence; but as a class they are available in ever-increasing numbers.

Probably the most fatal disease that can overtake a local society is that which gives it a reputation for erudition. If there is any truth in the fear of a prospective member that he or she would feel ignorant in a company of savants, membership should be avoided at all costs, for the society is not worth joining. Interest, not intellectual, should be the gauge of suitability; humble inquiry is more appropriate even to the specialist than declamation of a learning that is only ignorance in disguise. Mutual sympathy and encouragement must be the spirit of the society; all are there to learn, and no teacher needs to be reminded that he learns at least as much from contact with keen students as they are likely to learn from him.

So much of the useful work and maintenance of interest in scientific matters depends on casual everyday observation, that aspects of nature ready to hand for the majority of members are likely to receive and give most satisfaction. A society in a coastal town can obviously foster the study of marine conditions that would be outside the practical scope of one in a midland industrial city. While retaining an intelligent curiosity in respect of any and every thing in the universe, a healthy local scientific society will normally tend to focus its main efforts on locally appropriate topics. In this matter, the term "locally" may apply to some especially vigorous member, whose enthusiasm for his particular bent infects many of his colleagues, and, for his generation at least, overshadows the milder activities of those who have escaped contagion. Such waves of fashion are perhaps inevitable; but they are not altogether desirable. Hero worship falls very flat when the hero proves mortal.

Most local societies are devoted to "natural history"; very few take much cognizance of the physical sciences. When specialization is made, the two subjects of geology and archeology are those usually selected. Evidently the main function of a local society is its provision of relaxation for people who have no technical training in science. Outdoor interests offer far healthier spare-time hobbies than laboratory studies where elaborate calculations or stiff reading give no respite to jaded minds. An attractive feature of the natural sciences is the scope they afford for the making of collections. From early childhood the jackdaw-complex is deeply ingrained in most of us; and although specimen-collecting may become a vice, it shares that risk with all other virtues. So long as mere miserly acquisitiveness is avoided, the arrangement and study of collected material can revive memories of past thrills and prolong the joys of field-work. This matter of collections is so important that it may be discussed somewhat fully.

An important duty of every scientific society should be the control, by precept and example, of the mania for collecting. Especially in the case of living things, due regard for the preservation of rarities must check wholesale destruction. It is pleasing to be able to record a great improvement in this respect achieved in recent years, largely through the influence of local societies. The days when a rare plant or animal was ruthlessly slaughtered in the name of science are past—even game-keepers (who are rarely members of our societies) are less promiscuous in their attacks on any creatures worth preserving. We are even beginning, with the inspiration of the Council for the Preservation of Rural England and the National Trust, to frown upon, rather than to condone, vandalism done in the sacred name of Mammon.

But there yet remains ample scope for the training of collectors; and almost every society is likely to include some members who can guide and counsel the uninitiated. Collection involves dissociation of the specimen from its natural environment; in the majority of cases that environment is one of the most informative features of the specimen. It can not be brought away in substance, but it should always be recorded in writing with all possible detail. Paradoxical though it sounds, it is nevertheless true that a collection of specimens without adequate labels is less useful than a collection of labels without specimens. Every particular of the circumstances attending the collection of the specimen should be written down at the actual time and place—memories get blurred at the end of a day. Even details that seem irrelevant should be noted; wider experience may show that just such points had the greatest significance.

If all the material that clutters up our museums had been collected in accordance with that simple principle, its value for scientific research would have been enhanced a thousandfold; the charnel-house would have been a biographical library. One battered fragment with a history is worth a score of "plums" without a label; for there is more satisfaction in scientific circles over one poor specimen with particulars attached than over ninety-and-nine perfect examples that have no such accompaniment.

In the matter of collecting, the local society has no need to encourage an inborn instinct, but rather should guide and restrain. A collection made for a definite intellectual purpose is unlikely to lead to decimation of its materials. But the collecting of specimens is really a pandering to low instincts; a far more important and fruitful activity is the collecting of facts. Except when they are needed to substantiate a record or are required for intensive research, objects observed are often better left where they are. This policy of restraint does not apply to inanimate objects, which may be preserved by being taken under cover; but in the case of living things it is unusual, and surely unnecessary, to prove that one has met a friend by bringing his corpse home as a witness.

In the matter of research, the greatest contribution (other than encouragement) that can be made by scientific societies comes from their ability to keep, check and publish records of transient phenomena. Every recurrent seasonal event in nature invites, and often receives, accurate observation. Whether it be the first cuckoo or the last swallow, the flowering of the primrose or the ripening of the holly, it is apt for and deserves a permanent record. In such work the society, as distinct from the individual, has a special value; for records without independent confirmation are of uncertain use. Moreover, a record, however well authenticated, of a single phenomenon gains immeasurably in importance when taken in conjunction with other records of contemporary events. The dates of appearance and disappearance of living creatures are shorn of half their significance without statistics of the weather for the season. The arrival of a migratory bird in any district may prove to be controlled by the appearance of a particular insect, and this again may depend on the growth of the insect's food-plant, which may have been determined by the weather-conditions of the current or past season. The keeping of statistics thus becomes a matter of team-work; ideally every natural history society should include observers who keep accurate and unbroken records of data on every conceivable topic capable of such treatment.

Accurate prophecy is always based on knowledge of past history correlated with a perception of the laws of cause and effect. Statistical records such as those indicated would provide the raw material of prophecy; if such truly natural history of but a few decades were available, it would aid in forecasting just those tantalizing mysteries that every farmer, and so every consumer, wants to know. Just as a straw shows the way of the wind, so some obscure animal or plant might, if its significance were realized, provide an answer to problems of immense practical importance. The most sophisticated social order depends ultimately on nature, and common sense demands that the foundation of the social fabric should be studied. There is endless useful research awaiting the efforts of local observers in this indirect aspect of man's place in nature.

As regards geological and archeological studies, there can surely have been no period in the past more favorable than that in which we find ourselves to-day.

For one reason or another, excavation is a dominant feature of our present activities; and, however shallow it may be, every hole is likely to reveal something of interest. Modern methods of excavation are so speedy and mechanized that much of their revelations can be observed only by perpetual watching. Here the local society can find scope for important and urgent work. Every society should acquire a large-scale map of its area, and plot on it every site where a glimpse, however fleeting, of the subsoil has been possible. Pin-pricks on the map, with numbers written against them, to correspond with card-index entries giving all the particulars, would soon make the map a priceless record. Only accuracy and persistence are wanted to achieve results that could not fail to increase the knowledge that all local societies are nominally out to acquire. Probably most societies include one or more members with the business experience needed to keep the records in order, and every member could contribute to them directly or indirectly. The volume of local knowledge already stored in the minds of residents is impressive; if that knowledge were to be methodically recorded, it would outlive its original possessors and so contribute to something more permanently satisfying than reminiscent causeries.

The suggestions for activity outlined above may seem to be more concerned with the relation of scientific societies to science than with their reaction on the community at large. Such a view is not only narrow, but out of date. In the present critical times, statistics of the resources and character of the country are being feverishly compiled. There could surely be no better compilers than those residents in any district who have trained themselves to observe facts and to tabulate them methodically. Such problems as the yield of springs and wells, the availability of road-metal, sand and gravel, the quality of the soil, the incidence of blight and the usefulness or otherwise of our fellow inhabitants, are all of a nature that demand accurate observation on the spot. Many of them may involve elaborate technical study as well; but the first stage of all of them is within the capacity of any reliable observer. All who love their country (in both senses of the word) can find here congenial and valuable work that is needed urgently.

The proportion of the population likely to join, and participate in, a scientific society is inevitably small; but that is no reason why it should not serve as a leaven. The study of natural history produces a philosophic outlook that should supply a much-needed corrective to the world, and can mitigate the worst attacks of the flesh and the devil. The mere existence of a company of people declaring their interest in matters bigger than the squabbles of the political nursery, preferring to contemplate wider problems and vistas than those of the daily headline, should be enough to ensure a nucleus of stability in the quicksands of opportunism. Science is a search after the truth; its devotees should be sure of their gospel, and declare it in a world of falsehoods: *Magna est veritas, et prevalebit.*

# WHERE DO METEORITES COME FROM?[1]

**By Professor C. C. WYLIE**

STATE UNIVERSITY OF IOWA

SINCE the days of Schiaparelli and H. A. Newton, astronomers have considered three possible answers to the oft-repeated question, "Where do meteorites come from?" The three answers considered are: (1) that they come from the distances of the fixed stars; (2) that they come from the outer portions of the solar system, like most comets; and (3), that, like the closer asteroids, they have been traveling in orbits little larger than that of Mars.

Schiaparelli and others were impressed with the fact that the great majority of velocities as determined for the meteors dropping meteorites were high. They were so high that, if real, the meteors must have come from the distances of the stars. H. A. Newton, however, found that most meteors dropping meteorites came from the general direction of the anti-apex of the earth's motion. That is, before the meteors entered the earth's gravitational field, they had been traveling in the same general direction as the earth itself. This indicated that the meteors had been traveling in orbits little larger than the orbit of the earth, so Newton and others suspected that the high velocities found for bright meteors were fictitious.

When meteor work was instituted at Iowa some twelve years ago, it appeared that greater accuracy in the paths and velocities for spectacular detonating meteors was needed. To attain this greater accuracy, measurements of the angles and durations have been secured by personal interviews. The observer is asked to stand exactly where he was when the meteor was seen, and the angles are measured as he points them out. If there was definite action at the time of the fall of the meteor, he is asked to "reenact the scene," and the duration is determined with a stop-watch.

[1] Condensed from a paper presented before the American Astronomical Society at Berkeley, California, August 9, 1939.

This work has shown that the estimates received from the general public on spectacular meteors are subject to large systematic errors, which make the velocities much too high. If a sufficient amount of information is at hand, however, a person familiar with these psychological errors can eliminate most, and determine a path reasonably close to the truth, even from the information received by letter. Some of the more famous meteors of years ago have been studied in the light of this information.

Orbits have been calculated recently for a number of spectacular meteors; and six have been selected as representative. The first four are recent ones falling in the middle western United States, for which the paths and velocities are based on personal interviews, as explained above. The four meteors selected fell in the months of August, July, January and November, respectively. Numbers (2) and (3) fell in the evening hours, number (4) fell in the early morning hours just before dawn, and number (1) dropped meteorites in broad daylight.

The fifth meteor, which fell on February 9, 1913, in Canada, was selected because it is referred to as one whose path through the atmosphere was several thousand miles long. The information collected by Professor C. A. Chant, however, was sufficient to determine a reasonably accurate path, whose length was calculated as 116 miles.

The sixth meteor, which dropped meteors at Pultusk, in Poland, on January 30, 1868, was selected because it is referred to as coming in from the distance of the fixed stars. Dr. J. G. Galle, the discoverer of the planet Neptune, collected a great amount of material on this meteor. From this information we have calculated the elements of the orbit.

Table 1 gives for the orbits of the six representative bright meteors, the period in years, the mean distance from the sun in millions of miles, the inclination of the orbit to the orbit of the earth and the eccentricity.

TABLE 1

| | (1) | (2) | (3) | (4) | (5) | (6) |
|---|---|---|---|---|---|---|
| Period in years.. | 1.87 | 1.70 | 1.92 | 3.59 | 1.62 | 2.37 |
| Mean distance .. | 141 | 133 | 143 | 217 | 128 | 165 |
| Inclination .... | 7°.6 | 1°.9 | 7°.0 | 0°.9 | 17°.5 | 0°.8 |
| Eccentricity .... | 0.47 | 0.36 | 0.55 | 0.78 | 0.33 | 0.46 |

For comparison we give the same information in Table 2 for three of the closer asteroids.

TABLE 2

| | Adonis | Eros | 1932 HA |
|---|---|---|---|
| Period in years .... | 2.55 | 1.76 | 1.80 |
| Mean distance ..... | 173 | 135 | 137 |
| Inclination ........ | 1°.4 | 10°.8 | 6°.4 |
| Eccentricity ....... | 0.76 | 0.22 | 0.56 |

In Table 3 we give also this information for Encke's comet, which has the shortest period of any known comet, and for Halley's comet, which has the shortest period of any bright comet.

TABLE 3

| | Encke | Halley |
|---|---|---|
| Period in years ........... | 3.3 | 76.4 |
| Mean distance ............ | 205 | 1670 |
| Inclination ............ | 12°.9 | 162°.3 |
| Eccentricity ............ | 0.85 | 0.97 |

For an object coming from the distance of the fixed stars, the hypothesis favored by Schiaparelli and some later astronomers, the period would be millions of years (or infinity), and the eccentricity would be 1.00 or greater.

A comparison of the values shows that the orbits of these bright meteors resemble the orbits of the nearer asteroids much more closely than they resemble the orbits of the closer comets. Obviously, none came from the distance of the fixed stars or even from the distance of the average comet.

# SCIENTIFIC EVENTS

## THE NEW FISHERY RESEARCH LABORATORY IN PUERTO RICO

METHODS for the development of a modern fishing industry in Puerto Rico, which at present imports about 90 per cent. of the cured and canned fish used in local consumption, will be sought, according to *The Fishery Service Bulletin,* through scientific research by the U. S. Bureau of Fisheries.

With recent tabulations indicating that about 36,000,000 pounds of cured and canned fish are imported into Puerto Rico annually, it is obvious that many new avenues of employment would be provided if the fisheries industries of the island were expanded.

Preliminary plans call for the construction of a new $25,000 laboratory building on a site yet to be selected, where special studies may be made of fish preserving and marketing problems confronting not only Puerto Rico, but also the Virgin Islands and the Latin-American republics.

Situated at the "cross-roads" between North and South American waters and as the result of recent investigations by the President's Educational Commission on Puerto Rico, the new laboratory is designed to serve as the focal point for all fisheries research in the tropical areas.

Benefits from the research work of the laboratory

will be made available to Latin-American republics through a program of cooperation being worked out with the Puerto Rican Government's fisheries division and educational institutions. Under the plan, student assistants will be employed in the laboratory investigations, and, after two years of research work, should be in a position to aid their own governments in solving fisheries problems. As a result, the studies, covering the development of methods for preserving and marketing fishery products, as well as biological and fish cultural investigations, are expected to contribute to the economic welfare of all the Latin-American countries.

Construction of the new laboratory building in Puerto Rico was made possible by a recent grant of Public Works Administration funds.

## THE EXPEDITION TO WESTERN COLORADO OF THE FIELD COLUMBIAN MUSEUM

A NUMBER of important fossil finds of the Field Museum Paleontological Expedition to Western Colorado have been reported by Bryan Patterson, assistant curator of paleontology.

These include a skeleton of a prehistoric animal called Taeniodont, a representative of a small early group of hoofed mammals—a forerunner of a similar but larger creature excavated by Mr. Patterson in 1933 and known as Barylambda. The present specimen, according to Mr. Patterson, may constitute a new genus. He writes: "We have been on the track of this beast since 1932, but until now have never found more than a few fragments of it."

Other specimens collected by the present expedition include multituberculates (a group of small rodent-like animals characterized by many cone-like prominences on their teeth) and prehistoric turtles. Work has been begun on the excavation of a fossil crocodile, and a large collection of small fossil animals has been made.

Mr. Patterson is accompanied by James H. Quinn, a member of the staff, and by several volunteer collectors. The official announcement states that

> The field of operations lies in Mesa, Garfield and Gunnison counties, where an extensive series of formations belonging to various periods and eras in the earth's history is exposed. The work is mainly in late Paleocene and early Eocene deposits (the opening epochs of the Age of Mammals), with some attention also being paid to the late Cretaceous formations (the closing period of the Age of Reptiles). The main objective of the expedition is to collect fossil mammals from the Paleocene and Eocene. Specimens from these early horizons are of great interest to students of mammalian evolution. The dinosaurs and other reptiles that had previously dominated the earth were but a short time extinct (geologically speaking), and the mammals were just getting well under way. Many groups that no longer survive were flourishing, and several of the dominant mammalian types of the present time were represented by exceedingly primitive ancestors. Thus, for example, the horses of the early Eocene were small creatures no larger than foxes, and they possessed four toes in contrast to the modern horse's one.
>
> In addition to the work on vertebrates, attention is being given to geological observations and to the collecting of fossil plants. It is hoped that by means of the latter it will be possible to make somewhat more precise age determinations and correlations of the late Cretaceous formations than has hitherto been done.

## HURRICANE WARNINGS OF THE U. S. WEATHER BUREAU

THE U. S. Weather Bureau has issued a statement describing the methods used to chart storms during the hurricane season, which in the United States runs usually from July to October.

The hurricane warning service, according to F. W. Reichelderfer, chief of the bureau, is more efficient this year than ever before. Observations are taken twice daily from over eighty stations in the West Indies and the Caribbean, and two to four times daily from vessels in the Gulf of Mexico, Caribbean and West Indian waters. These observations are in addition to the reports from the regular system of stations in the United States and vessels in the North Atlantic.

Whenever there are indications that a tropical cyclone or hurricane is forming, special observations made at two to three hour intervals by ships and stations in the region of the hurricane are sent in so that the four forecast centers of the hurricane warning system—Washington, Jacksonville, New Orleans and San Juan—have information as to the location of the hurricane and its intensity long before it enters American waters or approaches the coast.

The effectiveness of this system was demonstrated recently in the case of the small hurricane which crossed the Florida Peninsula on August 11 and 12. This hurricane was first detected and warnings issued from the Jacksonville center on August 8 when it was located 175 miles northeast of San Juan. Subsequent advisory information was issued every six hours until the storm neared the Florida coast, after which the advices were increased to hourly broadcasts by radiophone until the storm passed across the Peninsula into the Gulf of Merico.

Mr. Reichelderfer points out that:

> These advices serve as examples of the remarkable accuracy with which the movement and intensity of violent storms can be foretold by means of the hurricane warning system. Many studies have been made of the formation and behavior of hurricanes which have moved toward our Atlantic and Gulf coasts during the past fifty years or more. Severe hurricanes do not often reach our coasts. But the Weather Bureau, through its system of hurricane

reporting stations and vessels which serve as outposts to detect and report the approach of a hurricane, is prepared to plot the position of these storms on the weather map long before they approach the coast and to give ample warning of the time of their arrival and their intensity.

As a further aid in insuring that the public will receive ample warning in the rare chance that a severe hurricane occurs this year, the bureau now has available a larger number of stations to make upper air soundings than ever before and is extending its dissemination of hurricane information and warnings by the installation of direct wire teletype connections at the larger population centers and is putting into effect special broadcast arrangements for weather warnings. Upper air observations are an important aid in calculating the direction and speed of movement of hurricanes from day to day.

## THE MASTER OF SCIENCE DEGREE IN ENGINEERING OF COLUMBIA UNIVERSITY

COLUMBIA UNIVERSITY has established a new master of science degree in engineering to enable candidates to obtain a broad background without specializing in one department. The degree was established chiefly for practicing engineers in the metropolitan district whose background and technical interests cross departmental lines. Before the introduction of the new general curriculum, it was necessary for graduate students to specialize in either chemical, civil, electrical, industrial or mechanical engineering.

Professor Joseph W. Barker, dean of the School of Engineering, announces that thirty-seven practicing engineers will supplement the instruction given by members of the faculty in fifty-seven courses, which will be given in the Extension Division of the university during the 1939–1940 academic year.

A course in physics, on "The Theory of Heat Conduction," has been added to the engineering curriculum, under the direction of Dr. Melvin Avrami, as part of a plan calling for an increase in scientific subjects dealt with from an engineering viewpoint. Other courses in heat transfer will be given under the direction of Professors C. E. Lucke and C. F. Kayan, of the department of mechanical engineering.

Four courses of an advanced nature have been designed particularly for engineers engaged in industrial activities who do not wish to work towards a degree. A sequence of three courses in electrical engineering has been arranged for students who have had a limited amount of training and who wish to obtain a background in the field. The application of chemical principles in the major chemical industries and the design of chemical equipment will be studied in two courses. Nine other courses will be given in the department of chemical engineering, two of which deal with the chemistry of textile processing. The department of civil engineering has planned fourteen courses, and the department of electrical engineering twelve courses covering every major sphere of electrical engineering.

The department of mechanical engineering will sponsor two courses in air conditioning, and will offer work in fluid dynamics, lubrication and power analysis. "Nomographic Charts and Empirical Equations" will be taught in a special course arranged for engineering students. Studies in engineering and architectural drafting will also be conducted.

Classes in the Extension Division will be held in the late afternoon, evening and on Saturday mornings in order that practicing engineers may enroll.

## EDITORS OF THE PUBLICATIONS OF THE AMERICAN CHEMICAL SOCIETY

AT the Boston meeting of the American Chemical Society Professor A. B. Lamb, of Harvard University, was reelected editor of the *Journal* of the American Chemical Society with associate editors as follows: Dr. C. S. Hudson, of the National Institute of Health, Washington, D. C.; Professor Lee Irvin Smith, of the University of Minnesota; Dr. Edward Mack, Jr., of Battelle Memorial Institute, Columbus, Ohio; Dr. R. H. F. Manake, of the National Research Council, Ottawa, Ontario, Canada; Professor Frederick G. Keyes, of the Massachusetts Institute of Technology.

Professor E. J. Crane, of the Ohio State University, was reelected editor of *Chemical Abstracts.* Dr. Harrison E. Howe, of Washington, D. C., was reelected editor of *Industrial and Engineering Chemistry.* Professor N. H. Furman, of Princeton University, and Professor I. M. Kolthoff, of the University of Minnesota, were reelected to the advisory board of the analytical edition of *Industrial and Engineering Chemistry.*

Professor W. Albert Noyes, Jr., of the University of Rochester, N. Y., was reelected editor of *Chemical Reviews.* Professors Robert C. Elderfield, of Columbia University, and E. R. Gilliland, of the Massachusetts Institute of Technology, were elected associate editors.

Professor Farrington Daniels, of the University of Wisconsin, and Professor Herbert Freundlich, of the University of Minnesota, were elected associate editors of the *Journal of Physical Chemistry.* Professor William T. Read, of Rutgers University; Dr. Charles A. Thomas, of Monsanto Chemical Company, Dayton, Ohio, and Dr. Bruce K. Brown, of the Standard Oil Company of Indiana, Chicago, were elected associate editors of the Technologie Monographs.

## RECENT DEATHS

PROFESSOR EMERITUS HENRY C. COWLES, for many years a member of the department of botany of the

University of Chicago, died on September 12. He was seventy years of age.

Dr. George Frederick Arps, professor of psychology and dean of the School of Education of the Ohio State University, died on September 16 at the age of sixty-five years.

Charles Ladd Norton, director of the Division of Industrial Cooperation and Research at the Massachusetts Institute of Technology, died on September 8 in his sixty-ninth year.

Dr. Hall Canter, professor of chemistry and geology and dean of the faculty at Randolph-Macon College, Ashland, Va., died on September 2 at the age of sixty-six years.

Dr. Horace J. Child, instructor in zoology and physiology at Sacramento Junior College, California, died suddenly on August 31 at the age of thirty-seven years.

George W. Tower, Jr., mining engineer on the staff of Guggenheim Brothers from 1918 to 1937, died on September 13 at the age of sixty-seven years.

Dr. Heinrich Karny, an entomologist specializing in orthoptera, formerly a member of the staff at the Botanical Garden at Buitenzorg, Java, died on August 7.

Sir Spencer Lister, director of the South African Institute for Medical Research at Johannesburg, died on September 6 at the age of sixty-three years.

# SCIENTIFIC NOTES AND NEWS

The National Academy of Sciences will hold its autumn meeting at Brown University, Providence, R. I., on October 23, 24 and 25. Dr. Henry Merritt Wriston, president of the university, will welcome the academy on Monday morning and there will be a response by the president of the academy, Dr. Frank B. Jewett. Scientific sessions will be held on Monday and Tuesday and on Wednesday morning. There will be luncheon daily in the Faunce House Art Gallery and dinners on the evenings of Monday and Tuesday.

Dr. M. R. Fenske, in charge of petroleum refining research and director of industrial research of the School of Chemistry and Physics at the Pennsylvania State College, has been elected a fellow of the Institute of Petroleum, London.

Sir David Milne-Watson has been elected president of the newly established British Gas Research Board of the gas industry.

Dr. Frank N. Freeman, professor of educational psychology at the University of Chicago, has been appointed to succeed Dr. W. W. Kemp as dean of the School of Education of the University of California.

Dr. Beryl I. Burns, director of the department of anatomy in the School of Medicine of the Louisiana State University, has been appointed dean of the school to succeed Dr. J. Rigney D'Aunoy, who retired on August 19.

Dugald C. Jackson, Jr., from 1935 to 1938 president of the Lewis Institute, Chicago, has been appointed dean of the College of Engineering at the University of Notre Dame. Professor Carl Wilcox, of the university, has become dean of the department of mechanical engineering, succeeding Professor William L. Benitz, who retired last spring.

Dr. P. Swings, associate professor of astrophysics and spectroscopy at the University of Liège, has been appointed a visiting member of the faculty of the University of Chicago. He plans to spend two months at McDonald Observatory and four months at the Yerkes Observatory. He will give lectures on astrophysics.

Dr. B. R. Teare, of the School of Engineering of Yale University, will direct the program of advanced study in electrical engineering at the Carnegie Institute of Technology, which has been made possible by a Buhl Foundation grant of $50,000. The project will be supported over a five-year period by the Buhl grant. The program has been planned so that engineers, already well trained in the electrical field, will pursue industrially useful research.

Dr. Parker Dooley, assistant professor of pediatrics at the Cornell University Medical College and associate attending pediatrician at the New York Hospital, has been appointed assistant professor of pediatrics at the University of Chicago.

Dr. Albert B. Sabin, associate of the Rockefeller Institute for Medical Research, New York, has been appointed assistant professor of pediatrics at the University of Cincinnati.

Dr. L. R. Kuhn, of Pitcairn, Pa., has been appointed assistant professor of bacteriology at the University of Georgia.

Dr. Krauch, authority on special problems of chemical production, has been appointed to an honorary professorship in the University of Berlin. He has directed the technical development of benzine production by hydrogenizing coal.

The following appointments at the Faculty of Medicine of Paris are recorded in the *Journal* of the American Medical Association: Dr. Aubertin, professor of therapeutics; Dr. Henri Bénard, professor of experimental pathology; Dr. Lévi Valensi, professor of the history of medicine, and Dr. Velter, professor of ophthalmology.

DR. CORNELIUS P. RHOADS, associate member of the Rockefeller Institute for Medical Research, has been elected director of the Memorial Hospital, New York City, in succession to Dr. James Ewing, professor of oncology at the Cornell University Medical College.

BARTLETT FROST has been appointed dioramist and Virginia S. Eifert, director of publicity, at the Illinois State Museum. Mr. Frost had been previously for four years dioramist with the National Park Service Museum Laboratories, and for one year with Joe Mora, the California sculptor, in preparing dioramas for the Golden Gate Exposition at San Francisco. At the Illinois State Museum he will continue a series of cultural dioramas begun last year by H. Brainerd Wright.

W. STEPHEN THOMAS, director of education at the Academy of Sciences of Philadelphia, has been appointed executive secretary of the Committee on Education and Participation in Science of the American Philosophical Society. This committee, under the chairmanship of Professor Edwin G. Conklin, executive vice-president of the society, will make a survey of adult education in science, using the Philadelphia region as an experimental area. The Franklin Institute, the Academy of Natural Sciences of Philadelphia, the Wagner Free Institute, the Museum of the University of Pennsylvania and other organizations will cooperate. Mr. Thomas has been granted a year's leave of absence by the Academy of Natural Sciences and during that time his place will be filled by Charles E. Mohr, of Reading.

DR. CARL L. HUBBS, curator of fishes at the University of Michigan, is making an investigation for the U. S. Fisheries Service of the fisheries, fur seals and other problems in Alaska. The work of the Bureau of Biological Survey is also being studied. Dr. Hubbs sailed from Seattle on July 4. He has traveled on the *Brant,* the vessel of the service, as well as by airplane and other means.

DR. W. C. MUENSCHER, professor of botany at Cornell University, who had leave of absence during the spring term, returned to Ithaca on September 8 from a trip of seven months through the southern and western states. The departments of botany in a number of colleges and universities were visited, and material for research and teaching was collected. More than 3,000 numbers of plant collections for the herbarium of Cornell University were obtained. Dr. Muenscher was one of the survivors of the party that was struck by an avalanche on July 22, on Mount Baker, Washington, in which six of the climbers lost their lives.

DR. HAROLD H. PLOUGH, Rufus Tyler Lincoln professor of biology at Amherst College, and Dr. Philip Ives and Dr. George Child, members of his department, who were passengers on the *Athenia,* are reported to have returned to the college.

THE first series of William Alanson White Memorial Lectures on "Modern Psychiatric Conceptions" will be given by Dr. Harry Stack Sullivan, president of the William Alanson White Psychiatric Foundation and president of the Washington School of Psychiatry, on Friday evenings in the auditorium of the Department of the Interior, Washington, D. C. The titles of the lectures are: October 27, "Conceptions of Modern Psychiatry"; November 3, "Organism and Environment"; November 10, "Diagnostic and Prognostic Syndromes"; November 17, "Explanatory and Therapeutic Conceptions"; November 24, "Prospective Developments and Research."

APPLICATIONS must be on file with the United States Civil Service Commission at Washington, D. C., not later than October 12 for the position of director of the Nautical Almanac at the Naval Observatory, Washington, D. C., at a salary of $6,500 a year. The qualifications of candidates will be passed upon by a special board of examiners composed of Dr. James Robertson, retired, formerly head of the Nautical Almanac Office; Dr. Dirk Brouwer, of Yale University; Dr. H. R. Morgan, principal astronomer, Naval Observatory, and A. W. Volkmer, examiner of the U. S. Civil Service Commission. The duties of the position will be to act as scientific and administrative head of the Nautical Almanac Office and professional consultant of the Navy Department in theoretical astronomy, calendarization and allied subjects; to have independent technical and administrative charge of the important, highly difficult work of producing the annual issue of the American Ephemeris and its supplementary volumes and to be responsible to the Navy Department for their scientific accuracy; to initiate, direct and report upon basic research problems in theoretical astronomy, performing developmental work in connection therewith and to be responsible for the difficult and highly technical mathematical deductions having to do with improving the tables forming the fundamental basis underlying the production of the annual volumes; to act as a member of the Astronomical Council of the Naval Observatory, advising as to the planning and execution of its work, and to take part in astronomical conferences of a national or international character, acting as the Navy Department's representative.

IN 1940 the spring meeting of the American Chemical Society, which now has 22,374 paid members, the largest number in its history, will be held in Cincinnati, Ohio; the autumn meeting in Detroit, Mich. In 1941 the spring meeting will be in St. Louis, and the autumn meeting in Atlantic City under the auspices of the Philadelphia section.

THE Bronx Health Unit, New York City, which is being erected at a cost of $400,000, was dedicated by Mayor Fiorello La Guardia on September 18. It is expected that the building will be completed by May, 1940. Health Commissioner John L. Rice presided. Invited speakers included Borough President James J. Lyons, Dr. George E. Milani, president of the Bronx County Medical Society, and Commissioner Irving V. A. Huie, of the Department of Public Works. The unit will include an auditorium, an exhibit room for health education, a staff lunchroom and kitchen and an air-conditioned storage vault in the basement. The first floor will contain the Bronx offices and child health, dental and maternal care quarters. Tuberculosis and venereal disease prevention activities will be housed on the second floor. Administrative headquarters for the health officer and his staff and health education and conference rooms will be on the third floor. The fourth floor will include borough offices for the sanitary superintendent, the Bureaus of Food and Drugs and Preventable Diseases and offices for visiting nurses and cooperating health agencies.

THE forty-fourth annual meeting of the American Academy of Ophthalmology and Otolaryngology will be held in Chicago from October 8 to 13 at the Palmer House. The academy will present courses of instruction to be given by more than a hundred specialists. There will be four afternoon programs of motion pictures and a scientific exhibit in addition to its formal scientific program. There will be one joint session at which Dr. George M. Coates, Philadelphia, will deliver his presidential address and Dr. Burt R. Shurly, Detroit, will be introduced as the guest of honor for the year and will deliver an address. At this session a symposium on essential hypertension will be presented by Drs. Albert C. Furstenberg, Ann Arbor, Mich., speaking from the standpoint of the otolaryngologist; Henry P. Wagener, Rochester, Minn., the ophthalmologist, and Roy W. Scott, Cleveland, the internist. Two foreign guests will address the section meetings, which will be held on alternate afternoons. Professor Josef Igersheimer, Istanbul, will discuss "The Optic Nerve and Diseases of Hypertension," and Arthur DeSa, Pernambuco, Brazil, will speak on "Ethmoiditis."

THE New York State Geographical Association will meet on September 23 at Syracuse University. In the morning there will be a series of papers on the teaching of geography. In the afternoon, Dr. Roy Price will lead a round table discussion on "The Relation of Geography to the Regents Investigation," and a similar discussion will be conducted by Dr. George B. Cressey on "The Place of Geography in the Secondary and High School." Dr. C. Grove Haines, of the department of history of Syracuse University, will speak at the banquet on "The Relationship of Geography and History in the Present European Crisis."

# DISCUSSION

## NUTRITIONAL PHYSIOLOGY OF THE ADULT RUMINANT[1]

IN this monograph Ritzman and Benedict set forth results of their own researches and also undertake to present a review "chiefly of the American literature" dealing with "the researches of the last few decades."

The authors' investigations are set forth *in extenso,* but the recognition of the work of others is highly inadequate.

The digestibility of the ash of feeding stuffs, as indicated by comparison of the constituents of feed and feces, is discussed (p. 13) as though significant, whereas it is thoroughly understood that the quantities of mineral substances in the feces signify nothing definite in relation to the digestibility of these components of the food.

[1] Comments on the monograph on this subject by E. G. Ritzman and F. G. Benedict, Carnegie Institution of Washington Publication No. 494.

The authors write uncritically as to certain practical matters; thus (p. 21) their statement that "at the larger stock yards of the country—fat steers are always bought subject to a 3 per cent. shrinkage in weight" is not true. Upon arrival at the central live-stock markets cattle are first given an opportunity to eat and drink. After they have been sold the packer-buyer pays for them at their actual weight, as they go over the scales, after eating and drinking.

In regard to methane production Ritzman and Benedict say (p. 26), "On the basis of seven "discordant results" in their calorimeter experiments Armsby and Fries concluded that 4 grams of methane result from every 100 grams of carbohydrate ingested, and this factor was later used largely by Forbes and by Mitchell to estimate the losses of energy by this path."

As a matter of fact the methane production has been experimentally determined in every calorimetric experiment conducted with cattle at this institute, and the writer has never used the above-mentioned factor for any purpose.

The authors present a graph (p. 75) in which the heat production is plotted against the insensible perspiration; and this graph is interpreted (p. 77) as showing that the insensible loss may be used as a basis of computation of the heat production; but the experiments involved were all conducted at about the same plane of nutrition. The results, therefore, do not establish a relationship of general significance. The authors should certainly have given careful consideration to Kriss's extensive studies of the relationship of the insensible loss to the heat production in cattle.

In regard to the "profound," "seriously challenging," "extraordinary" and "astounding" variability of the basal metabolism as observed with cows (p. 86)—the causes of the variability observed were not determined. Observations on the proximity of the period of oestrum to the time of determination of the basal metabolism would have been pertinent, as also a discussion of the normal body temperature of cattle, which is much more labile than is that of human beings.

One would prefer to maintain an open mind on this subject of lability of the basal metabolism of cows until the reasons therefor have been clarified, but we are told (p. 129) that "the overwhelming evidence presented here makes it obligatory on the part of every research worker to accept the demonstrated fact that the large domestic ruminant (particularly the genetically highly specialized dairy cow) has a very labile basal metabolism."

An attempt is made to support these findings in regard to cows by reference to determinations of so-called "standard metabolism" in steers (p. 130) by measurement of the heat production "in two or three successive half-hour periods while the animal was standing quietly, 24 hours after food."

According to the writer's understanding, measurements of the heat production of steers under the conditions stated would possess no standard significance, because of the brevity of the periods of observation and because the alimentary fill would be in no definite status.

Ritzman and Benedict imply (p. 178) that their observations on the lability of the basal metabolism of cows invalidates the four remarkably smooth and consistent curves of heat production in relation to the plane of nutrition, as determined, with steers as subjects, by Forbes and associates.[2] In our opinion the smoothness of these curves shows that the lability of the basal metabolism of cows, as observed by Ritzman and Benedict, is not characteristic of the metabolism of steers under successful experimental control.

[2] *Jour. Agr. Research,* 37: 253–300, 1928; 40: 37–78, 1930.

In discussing the energy expense of food utilization Ritzman and Benedict (p. 149) deplore the fact "that such a confusion of expressions to describe one and the same effect (the heat increment) exists," and then propose two more expressions for the same purpose. In this relation they state that "the Pennsylvania investigators" compute the heat increment to the basis of standing half the time and lying half the time. As a matter of fact the *heat production* has properly been so treated, but the heat increment, never.

Ritzman and Benedict conclude (p. 99) that the increase in heat production during standing exceeds that during lying to a greater extent during feeding than during fast, but the values they determined for percentage increase due to standing during fast all lie within the range of variation of such determinations during feeding, and there seems to be no statistical basis for the conclusion drawn.

As to the method of estimating the heat increment the authors say (p. 149): "Unfortunately the stimulating effect of food can at present only be determined by measuring the metabolism under this influence of food and without it, so that fasting becomes a necessary part of the technique of its determination."

The authors thus seem to ignore the fact (of which they are doubtless aware) that Kellner, Armsby and Forbes and associates have all measured heat increments for production by the differential method, above maintenance, without reference to fast; and they also ignore the conclusion of Forbes and associates (emphasized in several papers) that heat increments depending on measurements of heat production at planes of nutrition below the point of energy equilibrium are lower than the truth by the amount that the food diminishes the production of heat at the expense of body nutrients.

In the light of this conclusion Ritzman and Benedict's determination (pp. 169–176) of the dynamic effects of feeds with the basal metabolism as the base value is lacking in definite significance.

Ritzman and Benedict's idea (p. 186) that the high basal metabolism of lactating cows "suggests definitely that the stimulating effect of food is as much an essential to lactation as is the energy and other substance matter from which the milk is formed" seems to us to misinterpret a residual effect—a carrying over into the measurement of the basal metabolism—of the habit of high heat production resulting from the high food consumption of lactation.

Finally, the authors' assumption (pp. 187–8) "that the deposit value of metabolizable energy in amounts above maintenance is the same as for maintenance," based upon an opinion published by Armsby in 1919,[3] ignores extensive work on this subject which was

[3] *Jour. Agr. Sci.,* 9: 186, 1919.

planned and in the main conducted by Armsby, and, after Armsby's death, was completed by the writer and his associates, and published in 1926.[4]

In this work the energy outgo during fast was used as the base value of heat increments of food for maintenance, and the heat production of maintenance was used as the base value of heat increments of food for body increase and milk production. On this basis the relative efficiency of utilization of metabolizable energy for maintenance, milk production and body increase was found to be, on an average, as 79.1, 72.8 and 57.3 per cent., respectively.

During recent years, however, the writer and his associates have advocated another point of view in this relation, involving the conception of a new base value of heat production—that of fast minus the energy expense of utilization of the body nutrients katabolized during fast. The present indication, from investigations not yet completed, is that from this more fundamental point of view the utilization of metabolizable energy for maintenance and for moderate amounts of body increase may be indeed essentially the same.

E. B. FORBES

THE PENNSYLVANIA STATE COLLEGE

## HEPARIN AND BLOOD CLOTTING

IN a recent note[1] on this topic Astrup emphasizes the need for a plasma (or serum) factor necessary to the inhibitory action of heparin. It should be recognized that this was clearly enunciated by Howell and Holt[2] in the original work on heparin and, under the name of the *pro-antithrombic* (or *antithrombin-ogenic*) factor, has always held a prominent place in Howell's theory of blood coagulation. Quick[3] afforded evidence that the accessory factor was associated with the albumin rather than with the globulin fraction of the plasma proteins. Some recent investigations[4] confirm this point but stress a new interpretation which appears to clarify the "controversial statements" in the literature. It has been found that heparin readily *prevents* thrombin formation (the *antiprothrombic* action of Howell and Holt), provided that pure cephalin is used as the thromboplastic agent in forming thrombin from recalcified prothrombin. However, if tissue extracts (thrombokinase) or crystalline trypsin (thromboplastic enzyme[5]) are used instead of cephalin, the antiprothrombic action of heparin is overcome in all but the first minute or two of the process of thrombin formation.

The synergistic *antithrombic* (thrombin-*neutralizing*) effect of heparin-albumin mixtures is not dependent upon the mode of thrombin formation, in experiments which avoid thrombinolysis. Additional work is necessary to elucidate the true nature of "antithrombic" action, but there are clear indications that it shares with the process of thrombin formation a significant dependence upon the phospholipid-protein interrelationships in which a trypsin-like enzyme plays a leading rôle.

JOHN H. FERGUSON

UNIVERSITY OF MICHIGAN

## THE BLACK DYE OF THE NAVAJOS

CARNOTITE, a canary yellow mineral usually found as a powder in the sandstones and conglomerates of the Colorado Plateau, has been and still is used by the Navajo Indians to make a black dye to color the wool which they shear from their sheep to make the famous Navajo rugs.

Carnotite is known to-day to be an ore of radium, uranium and vanadium. It was not until 1898 that the chemical composition was determined by Fuedel and Cummenge, of Paris, from samples obtained from the Colorado Plateau by Kimball and Poulot. Long before that, the Navajo Indians had learned the art of preparing a rich black dye from the yellow mineral —"a uranium black." The yellow powder had formerly been reported as "yellow ochre," a form of limonite.

The writer is indebted to Mrs. Louisa Wade Wetherill, of Kayenta, Arizona, for the method used by the Navajo Indians in preparing the dye. The carnotite powder is roasted in a frying pan placed over an open fire until it changes in color from yellow to black. In a similar manner, the Navajos roast the pitch from the pinyon trees (stunted pines) that grow on the high mesas in the region. The pitch becomes brittle and breaks down to a black powder. These two black powders are then mixed and stirred into a solution prepared by boiling the entire plant of the squaw-berry bush (*Rhus trilobica*) in water until it assumes the color of tea. This makes a concentrated dye which is further diluted with water to the required strength.

In a rug which the writer obtained from the Western Navajo Indian Reservation, the uranium black dyed wool was used in combination with wools colored with natural vegetable dyes prepared from the root of the caniegra plant (wild pie plant or dock). Various colors may be obtained by varying the length of time the roots of the plant are boiled in water. The colors range from *old gold* through *greenish yellow* to a brown approximating the color of *burnt sienna*. The longer the period of boiling, the more brownish is the color obtained.

DANIEL T. O'CONNELL

THE COLLEGE OF THE CITY OF NEW YORK

4 *Jour. Agr. Research*, 33: 483–492, 1926.

1 T. Astrup, SCIENCE, 90: 36, 1939.

2 W. H. Howell and E. Holt, *Am. Jour. Physiol.*, 47: 328, 1918.

3 A. J. Quick, *Am. Jour. Physiol.*, 115: 317, 1936.

4 J. H. Ferguson, *Proc. Soc. Exp. Biol. and Med.* (in press).

5 J. H. Ferguson and B. N. Erickson, *Am. Jour. Physiol.*, 126: 661, 1939.

## APPEARANCE OF A NEW POTATO DISEASE IN NORTHEASTERN COLORADO

A new disease, apparently caused by the feeding of the pentatomid (*Chorochroa sayi* Stål), has appeared in the potato fields of northeastern Colorado.

On July 20 calls from farmers in Morgan County, Colorado, brought attention to what seems to be a general condition in the medium-early and late plantings of potatoes. The pentatomids were found associated with the disease in every case of the several hundred plants examined.

Cage experiments at the Greeley Potato Experiment Station begun on July 31 with plants known to be free of psyllids and disease, have demonstrated that the Say's pentatomid, feeding on the plants, is definitely responsible for the condition.

Medium-early plantings show 15 to 20 per cent. of diseased plants, while many late plantings in the Greeley area show 50 to 60 per cent. of pentatomid-affected plants.

The feeding may cause a complete wilting of the leaves or tips of the plants. Where the feeding is confined to the stems of the lower part of the plants, the symptoms become more general. Associated with the feeding is a basal curling of the terminal leaves, a yellowing followed by a reddish discoloration along the margin and an erect condition of the affected foliage. The tubers may be produced in chains or, in the more mature tubers, serious bumpiness and malformation may occur. The number of insects on each plant determines the severity of the disease. In the Morgan County area, an average of eleven adult insects was found on each plant. Plants attacked by three or four insects were only mildly affected, while those on which there were nineteen or twenty adult insects showed extreme symptoms.

The disease is very similar to "psyllid yellows," caused by the tomato psyllid, *Paratrioza cockerelli* (Sulc.).

Leslie B. Daniels

Experiment Station,
Colorado State College

# REPORTS

## THE VULCANIZATION OF RUBBER

The centenary of the discovery of the vulcanization of rubber by Charles Goodyear was celebrated on Wednesday, September 13, at the ninety-eighth annual meeting of the American Chemical Society. Numerous papers describing the progress of rubber research and manufacture in the United States were read at a general meeting in the afternoon.

At the banquet in the evening, Dr. Karl T. Compton, president of the Massachusetts Institute of Technology, spoke on "Looking Forward in Research"; Dr. James Bryant Conant, president of Harvard University, discussed "Lessons from the Past," and P. W. Litchfield, president of the Goodyear Tire and Rubber Company, Akron, Ohio, described "Rubber's Position in Modern Civilization."

In his address Dr. Compton said:

A good deal has been said about the ways in which science has been applied to make warfare more destructive, just as science has also been applied to bring about a certain compensating degree of protection against new weapons. But there is one possibility in science which seems to me to be far more significant than these, namely, the use of science to remove some of the major causes of war.

In so far as wars are caused by the natural ''cussedness'' of human nature, science can contribute if at all only very indirectly. It can probably not do much toward removing the desire which some men have for great domination. It can not remove ambition and envy from the human breast. But in so far as wars may be induced by economic considerations, science may do much to remove the causes.

One of the earliest incentives to war was the invasion of one country by another for the purpose of loot. Later, as we became more civilized, this took the form not so much of loot as of the control of population for the purposes of taxation and of exploitaton of labor and of natural resources. This is all part of the old primitive instinct of animals and men to secure the good things of life by taking them from someone else.

Science, however, has given mankind a method of gaining the good things of life without taking them from someone else and without working inordinately long and hard to produce them. Discovery and development of ''good things of life'' by science, engineering and invention are a far more certain and productive source than organized loot and robbery. To the extent therefore that great groups of people, such as nations, can be induced to support technological development directed toward these ends, to that extent can they satisfy their desires, without recourse to war.

More specifically, many nations have felt the urge to conquest in order to secure to themselves an assured supply of various materials which are necessary to the nation's economy. For example, Great Britain needs oil for her navy and food for her population, which can not be produced in the British Isles. Germany and Japan need rubber, food stuffs and mineral resources. Even the United States, richest of all nations in its mineral resources, is inadequately supplied with such important materials as rubber, tin and tungsten. Does national safety force these nations to conquest in order to assure themselves of these commodities?

The necessities of national economies could be taken care of by scientific research at a cost far less than that of a major war and within a time far less than that in which the effects of a major war could be recovered from. At the same time this could be done not only without hurting any one but with great indirect benefit to all concerned. Let me give a few examples.

The time will surely come in the not too distant future when a satisfactory motor fuel can be produced from coal at a cost which is not too far out of line with that of petroleum products. When this happens, Great Britain, for example, will no longer be critically dependent upon the Persian oil fields nor will we be so much worried about Japan's efforts to secure a foothold in Mexico.

When substitutes for rubber are produced which are satisfactory for automobile tires and which can be produced at a reasonably competitive price, then one of the great causes of anxiety and international haggling will have been removed. Perhaps the new development of "chemical agriculture" in which farm products are produced without soil by planting them so their roots are bathed in appropriately nutritive chemical solutions can be developed to remove the fear of food shortage which now causes so much anxiety in several nations, and will at the same time provide a diet which will be a distinct improvement on that which is now customary.

The development of suitable lacquers as substitutes for tin in the coating of containers for canned foods will make the United States less anxious about its access to the Bolivian tin supply. Or perhaps improved methods of extraction from our existing but rather poor tin deposits may accomplish the same result. To the extent that science can produce these materials or suitable substitutes, to that extent will be removed almost the only basis for war which can be intelligently argued for at the present time.

Dr. James B. Conant, president of Harvard University, holder of the William H. Nichols Medal of the New York Section of the American Chemical Society, said in an address on "Lessons from the Past":

One might claim that our scientific knowledge of large molecules and the chemical reactions which produce them is but a by-product of the ubiquitous motor car. Fifty years ago a celebration of Goodyear's discovery would have awakened almost no interest among chemists, for the science of rubber chemistry was hardly born. It would have awakened almost no interest among the general public, for the automobile was still unknown.

The total world's annual production of rubber was then less than 50,000 tons. It was not till the first years of this century that the production began to rise and not till the second decade that a phenomenal upswing commenced.

And why did the annual production reach 200,000 tons by 1916 and 500,000 tons by 1924? The answer is obvious. Tires for automobiles. From 1910 to 1930 the curves of rubber production and automobile registration rise together; during the last decade they rise and fall, somewhat, in almost parallel fashion. I venture to predict that if some industrious soul should count the number of articles published in scientific journals dealing with the chemistry of rubber and rubber-like compounds, he would find that the annual production from the laboratories followed the growth curve of the automobile industry.

One can have no adequate picture of scientific progress, I believe, without examining the social and economic conditions under which this progress took place. Admittedly, one can carry the economic interpretation of history, including the history of science, to absurd lengths. But one can also fail to understand the lessons of the past by reading the history of science solely as the story of scientific heroes who lived and moved in a vacuum.

Viewed in historical perspective, the contempt of the practical man for all scientific work, unless it has immediate utility, is seen to be shortsighted. Patience is needed by the scientist. It is no less needed by society in evaluating the work of our universities and research laboratories.

On the other hand, the scorn of some cloistered scientists and scholars for the inventor and the industrial worker is clearly equally shortsighted.

In science, as in other human activities, looking down one's nose at other people is worse than a ridiculous pastime. It is often equivalent intellectually to throwing a monkey wrench into the machinery. If my thesis is correct, that in the long run pure science and applied science are so closely interrelated as to be inseparable, then clearly when one lacks nourishment the other must eventually wither and inevitably die.

So industrialists and scientists may well join together in celebrating either a great discovery in pure science or a revolution in the industrial arts. For on close analysis both events are seen to be of equal significance for the attainment of these goals for which the two groups strive. And they may ask the other members of the community to join with them when they pay honor, as to-night, to a pioneer who opened doors to riches for mankind he little dreamed of. Treasures not measured in material terms alone, new weapons in man's intellectual armory—perhaps the only enduring wealth of modern times.

P. W. Litchfield, president of the Goodyear Tire and Rubber Company, Akron, Ohio, in an address on "Rubber's Position in Modern Civilization," said:

In fixing rubber's position in modern civilization it is possible to say that four million persons, the world over, are employed in the rubber business; it may also be pointed out that almost three billions of dollars are invested in facilities for the growing, manufacture and distribution of rubber; we may consider the fact that there are more than fifty thousand different and useful products made from rubber and that more than two billion pounds of pure rubber are consumed in a normal year.

But such measurements are inadequate. The influence and importance of rubber is so all-pervasive as to defy any rule of thumb. I believe we get closer to the real answer when we think of our social and economic structure as a living thing, the skeleton of which is composed of metal and stone, the arterial system of which carries a life stream of oil and the flexing muscles and sinews of which are of rubber.

I could go on indefinitely—into the building industry, into the modern conveniences of our homes and offices, into food packaging, into the operating rooms of the hospitals, into the mines and factories—and show to you the threads of vulcanized rubber which are woven back and forth through the fabric of modern living.

# SPECIAL ARTICLES

## ANDROGENS AND TUMOR GROWTH

THE observation of Murray[1] that male mice bearing ovarian grafts developed spontaneous mammary tumors, although normal males do not, and the observation of Lacassagne[2] that the same effect could be produced in males by means of injected estrogens suggested a possible antagonism between male and female sex hormones as regards their carcinogenic properties.[3] Accordingly, in the fall of 1935 experiments were begun on the effects of urinary androgens on the growth and metastasis of the Brown-Pearce epithelioma of the rabbit. Preliminary observations having proved encouraging the experiments have continued to the present, employing over 300 rabbits. In one paper[4] now in press the results with several chemically pure androgens, one estrogen and androgens extracted from human urine are presented in detail. In another[5] some further evidence is presented of the opposite effects on growth of the most active androgen and the most active estrogen available.

Urinary-extract androgens and chemically pure testosterone propionate, both in small doses, quite definitely inhibited the growth of the primary Brown-Pearce tumor implanted in the testicle. For a study of secondary growths (metastasis) four degrees of malignancy were recognized: (1) no secondary growths; (2) few, *i.e.,* less than four scattered small nodules; (3) several, *i.e.,* 3 to 6 sites with multiple nodules; and (4) extensive, *i.e.,* diffuse involvement of 6 or more sites. A summary of the longer-period experiments, running from 89 to 112 days, is given in Table 1. The androgens were injected daily in olive or sesame oil. Controls with and without oil alone showed no material difference in the spread of secondary growths. The average of these two control groups is taken as the unmolested incidence of such growths when the tumor is of average malignancy. Estradiol monobenzoate did not change the percentage of animals having any degree of metastasis or none. The urinary androgens, however, did very positively shift the incidence from the high side of the scale toward the low side. Still greater was the effect of testosterone propionate (10 to 50 I.U. daily) in the same direction. Instead of twenty-nine per cent. (average of the two control groups) having extensive metastases there were none in the group receiving this most potent androgen.

TABLE 1

LONG PERIOD EXPERIMENTS

| | | Degree of Metastases | | | | | | | |
|---|---|---|---|---|---|---|---|---|---|
| | | Extensive | | Several | | Few | | None | |
| | No. of rabbits | No. | Per cent. | No. | Per cent. | No. | Per cent. | No. | Per cent. |
| Control no oil. | 25 | 8 | 32 | 7 | 28 | 2 | 8 | 8 | 32 |
| Control oil only | 35 | 9 | 25.8 | 8 | 22.8 | 7 | 20 | 11 | 31.4 |
| Estradiol Monobenzoate | 18 | 5 | 27.8 | 5 | 27.8 | 3 | 16.6 | 5 | 27.8 |
| Urinary androgens 4.6 to 216 I.U. | 55 | 4 | 7.3 (– 21) | 14 | 25.4 (– 1) | 13 | 23.6 (+ 10) | 24 | 43.6 (+ 12) |
| Testosterone 37 & 39 I.U. | 22 | 9 | 40.9 (+ 12) | 7 | 31.8 (+ 5) | 2 | 9.1 (– 5) | 4 | 18.2 (– 14) |
| Testosterone Propionate 10 & 50 I.U. | 20 | 0 | 0.0 | 2 | 10.0 | 7 | 35.0 | 11 | 55 |
| Total | 175 | | (2– 29) | | (– 16) | | (+ 21) | | (+ 23) |

The figures in parentheses represent the changes in percentage from an average of the two control groups. The shift to the low side of the scale of metastases caused by urinary androgens and by testosterone propionate is impressive. The opposite effect of testosterone is not so great.

Conversely, instead of 32 per cent. having no metastases as in the controls there were 55 per cent. having none. Curiously enough, chemically pure testosterone had a moderate effect in the opposite direction.

In experiments which ran to only 60–62 days pure androsterone and dehydroandrosterone, in doses comparable to those used for most of the urinary androgen injections, had no material effect on either the rate of primary growth or the incidence of secondary growths. It is therefore probable that the urinary extracts contain one or more steroids, extractable by the same method as the known androgens, which are responsible for the inhibiting effects noted. Fractionation of such extracts has already been accomplished, and the chemically different groups will be tried soon for anti-carcinogenic properties.

In the short-period experiments also testosterone propionate in doses of 100 and 250 I.U. daily seemed to exacerbate the metastatic process. Dosage therefore is of great importance.

J. R. MURLIN
C. D. KOCHAKIAN
C. L. SPURR
R. A. HARVEY

UNIVERSITY OF ROCHESTER

[1] W. S. Murray, *Jour. Cancer Res.,* 12: 18, 1928.

[2] A. Lacassagne, *Compt. Rend. Acad. Sci.,* 195: 630, 1932.

[3] I. T. Nathanson and H. B. Andervont, *Proc. Soc. Exp. Biol. and Med.,* 40: 421, 1939.

[4] J. R. Murlin, C. D. Kochakian, C. L. Spurr and R. A. Harvey, *Arch. Path.,* in press.

[5] C. D. Kochakian, *Endocrinology,* in press.

## EASE OF BODY HEAT LOSS AND RESISTANCE TO INFECTION

WE wish here briefly to report a rather striking dominance exercised over resistance to infection by the ease with which body heat can be lost. White mice adapted to moist heat (90° F. and 65 per cent. relative humidity) exhibit a resistance to infection only one quarter as great as do litter mates adapted to a cool environment (65° F.), while mice in a control room at 70–75° F. fall midway between those in the hot and cold environment. This occurs when all other factors of life are held as constant as possible for all groups—same diet (Purina dog chow), similar lighting and ventilation, and the use of divided litters for the different groups to minimize the hereditary factor.

We have previously described the rooms and equipment used in this study[1] as well as the dominance exercised by ease of body heat loss over such basic physiologic functions as rate of growth and development, fertility and longevity. This dominance in man and animals seems to work through the internal combustion level allowed the individual. Energy for most physiologic functions can come only from this combustion, but body efficiency is not high, so that a large part of the combustion energy must be dissipated as waste heat. It is the ease or difficulty with which this waste heat can be dissipated that causes internal combustion rate to be dominated by external temperature levels. Men, as well as animals, show direct evidence of this dominance.[2]

Locke[3] has described a "fitness index" which he bases largely on the rate of oxygen consumption, resistance to infection being proportional to the rate of oxygen uptake. And in certain of man's infectious diseases, ability to survive seems definitely related to prevailing mean temperature level.[4] It therefore seemed important that a close analysis be made of all phases of this dependence on ease of body heat loss, the preliminary findings on resistance to infection being set forth in this brief note.

Using a 10-hour broth culture of hemolytic streptococcus kept at standardized virulence by the necessary mouse passages (so that 0.5 cc intraperitoneally kills healthy control mice within 16 hours), the estimates of M.L.D. given in Table 1 were obtained.

Although the M.L.D. was the same for control and cold-room animals, those from the control room died more quickly than did those from the cold. During the period of these tests, the control room temperature was about 70° F., only 5° above that of the cold room. Hot room mice succumbed with only one fourth the culture dosage needed to kill those of the other two groups.

When mice of all three groups were injected with the same amount of broth culture, 0.5 cc of a 1:20 dilution, then within 26 hours 100 per cent. of the hot room mice were dead, 60 per cent. of those from the control room, but only 30 per cent. of those from the cold. In another series injected with 0.5 cc of a 1:55 dilution of broth culture, 60 per cent. from the hot room were dead within 30 hours, but only 12 per cent. from the cold.

TABLE 1

| | Survival time in hours |
|---|---|
| Cold room mice (kept at 65° F) 0.5 cc of culture diluted 1–10 .................. | 12, 23, 23, 23, 30, 48, 48, 48 (2 did not die) |
| Control room mice (kept at 70° F) 0.5 cc of culture diluted 1–10 ............ | 7½, 11, 12, 12, 12, 23, 23, 23, 23, 23, 132 (1 did not die) |
| Hot room mice (kept at 90° F) 0.5 cc of culture diluted 1–40 .................. | 24,24, 30, 36, 50, 108 (1 did not die) |

There can be left little doubt, therefore, that difficulty in body heat loss and a lowered tissue combustion rate result in a sharply reduced ability to fight infectious invasion. This depressive effect on resistance to infection (also on growth, developmental rate and fertility) is evident within two weeks after the animals have been placed in the warm environment, and is almost complete by the end of three weeks.

The study is being broadened to include other pathogenic organisms and the appearance of various immune bodies in the blood. Undernutrition from dietary inadequacy, either qualitative or quantitative, has been known to make animals less resistant to infection.[5] It is likely that difficulty in body heat loss works in a similar fashion by making impossible the adequate utilization of even the most perfect diet when offered *ad lib.*

JOSEPH W. COLVIN
CLARENCE A. MILLS
LABORATORIES FOR EXPERIMENTAL MEDICINE,
UNIVERSITY OF CINCINNATI

[1] C. A. Mills and Cordelia Ogle, *Am. Jour. Physiol.*, 125: 36–40, 1939.
[2] C. A. Mills, *Am. Jour. Hygiene*, 29: 147–164, 1939.
[3] Arthur Locke, *Jour. Immunology*, 36: 365–380, 1939.
[4] C. A. Mills, "Medical Climatology," Chapter VII, Charles C Thomas, Springfield, Illinois, 1939.
[5] C. F. Church, *Am. Jour. Pub. Health*, 29: 215, 1939.

## THE MUSCLE HEMOGLOBIN OF SEALS AS AN OXYGEN STORE IN DIVING

IT is well known that the harbor seal, *Phoca vitulina*, can remain submerged for long periods without breathing. Dives of six minutes are common, while a maximum of 15 minutes has been recorded by Millais.[1] The seal's ability to hold its breath when submerged contrasts so strongly with the slight capabilities of terrestrial mammals that one is led to suspect an extra store of oxygen in the seal's case. The

[1] J. G. Millais, "The Mammals of Great Britain and Ireland," 3 vols. London, 1906.

extremely dark color of seal meat suggests that the oxygen store exists, at least in part, in the muscle hemoglobin.

The literature on muscle hemoglobin in aquatic mammals is both meager and contradictory. In a review paper on "Respiration in Diving Mammals" Irving[2] estimates the muscle hemoglobin of an aquatic mammal by analogy from Whipple's figures[3] for iron content of dog muscle, and shows that a 70 kg animal could absorb 335 cc of oxygen by this means. He concludes that such a store would, however, be only significant as a store for a fraction of a minute, whereas the endurance of divers requires provision for a number of minutes. But Theorell,[4] who observed that myoglobin occurs in concentrations of 5 to 10 per cent. in the juice pressed from seal meat, states that the necessary oxygen for prolonged diving comes with great likelihood in large part from the exceptionally great myoglobin content of the skeletal muscles, which are so strongly colored that they appear almost blue-black.

I have made some analyses to determine if muscle hemoglobin in the seal is present in concentrations high enough to serve as an oxygen store in diving. The work began with iron analyses of the tissues, as it was thought that the iron content would serve as a rough indication of the relative muscle hemoglobin concentrations. The method of iron determination followed that of Elvehjem and Hart.[5] All tissues analyzed were freed as far as possible from blood hemoglobin by washing in 0.9 per cent. NaCl solution. A single sample of seal meat gave an average of .229 mg Fe per gram of fresh tissue, compared with several analyses of beef muscle by the same method, giving an average of .048 mg Fe per gram of fresh tissue. This experiment indicated that a much larger amount of iron was present in the seal muscle.

In order to determine if the large excess of iron were really present as muscle hemoglobin, samples of tissue from a second seal were washed in 0.9 per cent. NaCl to remove blood hemoglobin, and the muscle hemoglobin was extracted by the dilute $NH_4$ method of Whipple.[6] The muscle hemoglobin in solution was converted to acid hematin and compared colorimetrically with a blood acid hematin standard. By this method a single sample of seal muscle yielded 7,715 mg of muscle hemoglobin per 100 grams of fresh tissue, compared with an average of 1,084 mg per 100 grams for several samples of beef muscle. In a 70 kg seal, if only 35 per cent. of the body weight represented muscle, there would be 1,890 grams of hemoglobin present, sufficient to combine with 2,530 cc of oxygen. As shown by Table 1, this might amount to 47 per cent. of the total oxygen stores of the animal.

TABLE 1

POSSIBLE OXYGEN STORES OF A 70-KG SEAL

| System | Oxygen stored |
|---|---|
| Lungs | 545 cc |
| Blood | 2,055 " |
| Fluids | 245 " |
| Muscle hemoglobin | 2,530 " |
| Total | 5,375 " |

SOURCES OF FIGURES IN TABLE 1

*Lungs:* Average lung capacity of two seals examined after death was 38.9 cc per kg. $38.9 \times 70 \times \frac{1}{5} = 545$.

*Blood:* Oxygen capacity of seal blood is 29.3 vol. per cent. (Irving, Solandt, Solandt and Fisher[7]). Blood represents 10 per cent. of the seal's body weight (Irving).[8] $70 \times 10 \times 29.3 = 2{,}051$.

*Fluids:* From Irving.[9]

*Muscle hemoglobin:* 7,715 mg Hb per 100 gm muscle. If 35 per cent. of the seal's weight is muscle, there are 24.5 kg of muscle. $24.5 \times 10 \times 7{,}715$ mg (7.715 grams) $= 1{,}890$ grams Hb. Muscle hemoglobin has the same combining power for oxygen as does blood Hb—1.34 cc per gram hemoglobin. $1{,}890 \times 1.34 = 2{,}532$ cc.

The resting metabolic requirement of a 70 kg seal would be 373 cc of oxygen per minute according to Irving, Solandt, Solandt and Fisher.[10] Assuming 100 per cent. utilization of all oxygen stores, it would be possible for the seal metabolizing oxygen at the basal rate to remain submerged for 14.4 minutes on a store of 5,375 cc of oxygen. This figure compares favorably with the common submersion time, when the animal is active, of about six minutes. But for active 15-minute submersions, such as recorded by Millais, there still seems to be no physiological explanation.

DOUGLAS ROBINSON

HARVARD UNIVERSITY

## THE ABSORPTION OF RADIO WAVES IN WATER

IN view of the recent submarine disasters, the question naturally arises as to the possibility of signaling from undersea craft by radio. Some years ago, Mr. Allen Bassett and the author carried out a series of tests in Lake Michigan which have a direct bearing on this problem. We chose for our task the determination of the law of absorption of radio waves in water.

A small transmitter with a loop aerial and an output of about one-tenth watt was set into operation, sealed into a water-tight box and lowered with a rope

2 L. Irving, *Physiol. Reviews*, 19: 112, 1939.

3 G. H. Whipple, *Am. Jour. Physiol.*, 76: 693, 1926.

4 A. T. H. Theorell, *Biochem. Zeitschr.*, 268: 81, 1934.

5 C. A. Elvehjem and E. B. Hart, *Jour. Biol. Chem.*, 67: 43, 1926.

6 G. H. Whipple, *Am. Jour. Physiol.*, 76: 693, 1926.

7 *Ibid.*, 6: 393, 1935*a*.

8 L. Irving, *Physiol. Reviews*, 19: 112, 1939.

9 L. Irving, *Physiol. Reviews*, 19: 112, 1939.

10 L. Irving, O. M. Solandt, D. Y. Solandt and K. C. Fisher, *Jour. Cell. and Comp. Physiol.*, 6: 393, 1935*a* and 7: 137, 1935*b*.

over the side of a boat to various depths. In the boat there was a loop aerial connected to a receiving set which was tuned to the transmitter and which operated a Wynn-Williams balanced vacuum tube voltmeter, rather than the usual loud speaker. The voltmeter gave a measure of the strength or intensity ($I$) of the radio wave. As the transmitter was lowered farther and farther into the water, thus increasing the thickness of the layer of water between the transmitter and receiver, the strength of the received signal decreased in the manner shown in Fig. 1. The different curves

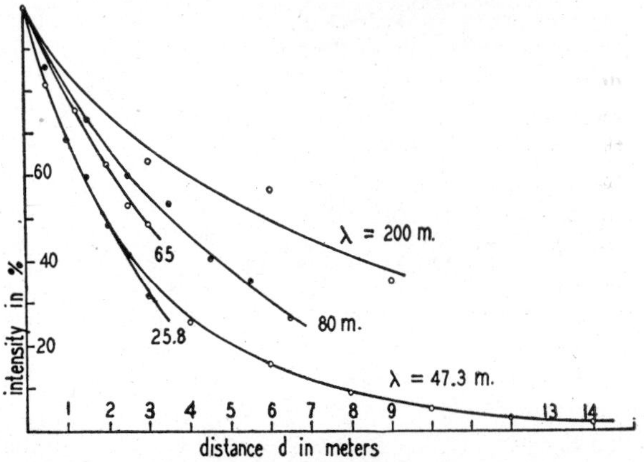


FIG. 1. The intensity $I$ of radio waves after passing through various thicknesses of fresh water. $\lambda$ = wave-length in meters.

refer to the indicated wave-lengths ($\lambda$) of the radio waves, as marked, and show that the shorter waves are more readily absorbed. Because of the rocking of the boat and the directional properties of the two loop aerials, the intensity of the received signal fluctuated considerably at any one separation of the transmitter and receiver. The intensity readings given in the figure are the maximum values at each point.

The form of the curves shown in Fig. 1 is typical of absorption processes in general and may be expressed by the well-known exponential law

$$I = I_0 e^{-ad}, \tag{1}$$

where $I$ is the intensity of the wave after penetrating $d$ centimeters of the absorbing material, $I_0$ is the original intensity at the transmitter, $e = 2.718$—, the base of the Naperian system of logarithms, and $\alpha$ is the so-called linear absorption coefficient. Large values of $\alpha$ indicate large absorption in unit thickness of the absorber and *vice versa*. If we take logarithms of both sides of equation 1 we have

$$\log_e I = \log_e I_0 - \alpha d, \tag{2}$$

or, changing to common logarithms,

$$\log_{10} I = \log_{10} I_0 + (-0.4343\alpha)d. \tag{3}$$

If, then, we plot log $I$ against $d$ we should get a straight line whose slope is negative and is numerically equal to $0.4343\ \alpha$. The straight lines in Fig. 2, obtained in

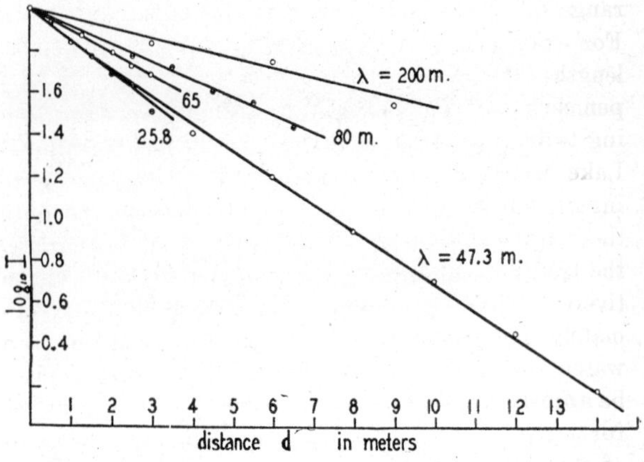


FIG. 2. Proof of the exponential absorption law and determination of the absorption coefficient $\alpha$.

this manner, prove that the radio waves are absorbed in the exponential manner of equation 1 in water. The values of $\alpha$ computed from the slopes of the straight lines are given in Table 1.

TABLE 1

| Wave-length in meters | Experimental $\alpha$ | Theoretical $\alpha$ |
|---|---|---|
| 200 | 0.00117 | 0.00126 |
| 80 | .00200 | .00198 |
| 65 | .00240 | .00220 |
| 47.3 | .00290 | .00260 |
| 25.8 | .00364 | .00350 |

By means of the electromagnetic theory it can be shown in a comparatively simple manner[1] that the absorption coefficient $\alpha$ is related to the permeability $\mu$ and conductivity $\sigma$ (e.m.u.) of the absorbing substance and to the frequency ($f$) of the radio wave in the following manner:

$$\alpha = 2\pi\sqrt{\mu\sigma f}. \tag{4}$$

The value of $\mu$ for water is unity. Our measured value of $\sigma$ for Lake Michigan water is $2.7 \times 10^{-14}$ e.m.u. Thus it is possible to calculate a value of $\alpha$ for each of the frequencies used in the experimental work. These theoretical values are given in the same table with those obtained from the slopes of the straight lines and show reasonably good agreement between theory and experiment. We are thus able to state with confidence that, over the range of wave-lengths tested (200 to 25.8 meters), the absorption per unit distance through fresh water increases as the square root of the conductivity

[1] A. Hund, "Phenomena in High Frequency Systems," p. 333. McGraw-Hill Book Company, 1936. G. P. Harnwell, "Principles of Electricity and Electromagnetism," p. 544. McGraw-Hill Book Company, 1938.

of the water and as the square root of the frequency of the radio wave.

We may now apply equation 1, with the known values of $\alpha$, to bring into evidence the shortness of the range of transmission of radio waves through water. For example, the intensities of radio waves of wavelengths 200, 80, 65 and 25 meters will be reduced to 10 per cent. of their value at the transmitter after passing through approximately 20, 11, 10 and 6 meters of Lake Michigan water, respectively. The corresponding distances for a reduction to one one-thousandth of the original intensity (irrespective of the strength of the transmitter) are 58, 35, 30 and 20 meters, respectively. Since the conductivity of sea water is approximately one thousand times as great as that of fresh water, the absorption coefficients of salt water will all be approximately thirty times larger and the distances, for a given ratio of intensities, will be only 3 per cent. of those in fresh water.

It may be concluded: (1) that radio waves can not be expected in appreciable intensity at any great distance from *deeply* submerged undersea craft unless the transmitter has considerable power; (2) that the longer wave-lengths will travel farther than the shorter ones, other conditions being the same; and (3) that greater distances will be reached in fresh than in salt water.

A test was also made in which the receiver was placed near the water, on the shore, while the transmitter was submerged a short distance under the water and moved parallel to the shore line, away from the receiver. Intensity readings were taken every 20 meters up to a distance of 140 meters when the transmitter was brought to the shore and then carried back on the land toward the receiver. Intensity readings were made on the return trip and gave practically the same shape intensity-distance curve as on the outward journey, lying slightly above the water values. Similar results were obtained with the receiver in one boat and the transmitter in or below a second boat. An intensity-depth curve for 47.3 meter waves, for $d$ from 0 to 2.6 meters, was made when the boats were 20 meters apart and yielded an absorption coefficient of 0.00260, in exact agreement (fortuitously) with the theoretical value.

The measurements in these latter tests were not made as carefully as those reported in the first part of this paper and, hence, can not be used with the same degree of conviction in drawing conclusions. We might assume, however, that the radio waves came to the surface within a comparatively short distance from the transmitter and, because of the comparatively high index of refraction of water (around 9, for these waves), were sharply refracted and traveled through the air to the receiver, rather than taking the shorter but much more absortive path directly through the water.

If these conclusions are valid, then it should be possible to signal to considerable distances from a submarine which is submerged only a *short* distance below the surface of the water.

The writer wishes to express his sincere thanks to Mr. M. Romberg for placing his power boat at our disposal and to the South Shore Power Boat Club for the use of its wharf and club house.

J. BARTON HOAG

RYERSON PHYSICAL LABORATORY,
UNIVERSITY OF CHICAGO

# SCIENTIFIC APPARATUS AND LABORATORY METHODS

## A SPECTROCOLORIMETER FOR COMPARING THE SPECTRA OF SOLUTIONS OF DIFFERENT DEPTH[1]

IN matching colors and absorption bands it is desirable to have a simultaneous reference. A hand spectroscope mounted immediately above the prisms of a standard colorimeter of the Duboscq type provides two spectra in immediate juxtaposition when the adjustable slit of the spectroscope is placed perpendicular to the line of division of the two fields of light. This allows the instrument to be used as a regular colorimeter with the added advantage that specimens having an interfering color, such as urine- or bile-stained blood, can be more accurately matched and a correction made for the increased absorption of light by these interfering colors. A quick and accurate method is provided

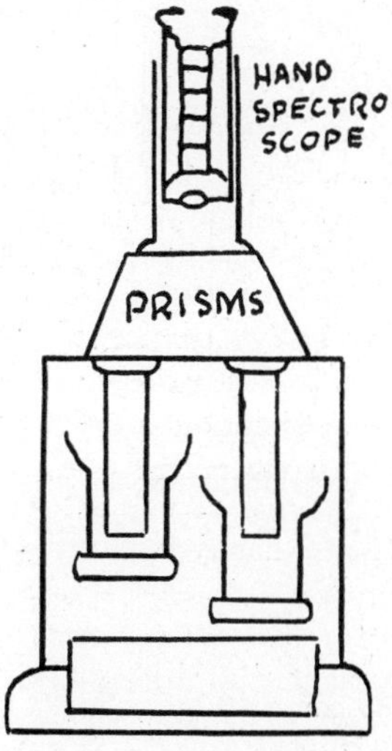


FIG. 1

[1] From the Littauer Pneumonia Research Fund, New York University College of Medicine, and the Medical Service, Harlem Hospital, Department of Hospitals, New York City, N. Y.

for identifying and determining the concentrations of substances having characteristic absorption bands, such as bilirubin, hematoporphyrin and methemoglobin.

ELY PERLMAN,
*Research Fellow, Pneumonia Service, Harlem Hospital*
NEW YORK UNIVERSITY COLLEGE
OF MEDICINE

## PERIODIC DISCHARGING OF LIQUIDS AND INTERMITTENT WASHING OF SOLIDS

A VERY efficient method of washing solids is an intermittent addition and draining of the solution. Also it is desirable in certain cases to add solution quickly for agitation but to drain slowly because of diffusion limitations from the surface or interior of the material being washed. Further, many substances such as shredded gels, being fragile, are partially lost in washing if agitation is done mechanically or by forcing gases through the bulk material.

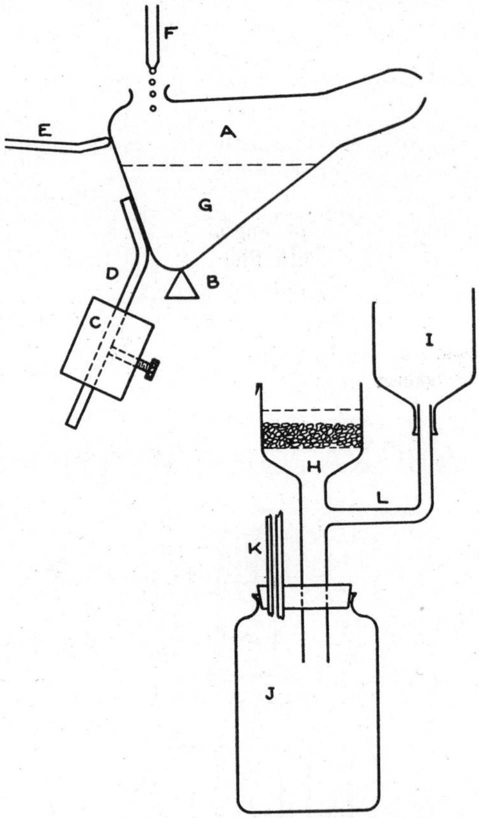


FIG. 1. Intermittent washing of solids.

We have devised a handy apparatus that can be set up in the laboratory. It is schematically shown in Fig. 1. A is merely an Erlenmeyer flask of appropriate dimensions with the mouth drawn down somewhat and a hole blown near the bottom. The flask rests on a fulcrum, B, and an adjustable weight, C, is attached to the flask by a rod D. B can include the holder for A, not shown in the diagram.

The sensitivity of the device depends on the unstable equilibrium, which in turn is influenced by the distance of the point of contact of the fulcrum from the center of gravity of the tilting flask containing liquid. With the appropriate dimensions the balance is maintained by moving C to the right position.

A stop bar, E, places the flask in the correct position for filling from a tube, F, and a slight adjustment of E also controls the amount of solution that will just dump. Obviously, the shape of the container is the cause of the mechanism shifting its center of gravity so that it functions on reaching a desired volume of wash solution. With a 500 cc flask the solution is delivered in 5 seconds.

The remainder of the figure is self-explanatory, H being a Buchner funnel and K a capillary that is adjustable. We have arranged that 500 cc drains in 3 minutes, while A fills in 5 minutes. The 111 mm inside diameter funnel will hold about 200 cc of material to be used. J is large enough to collect any sediment from the solid material so that K is not in danger of clogging.

The device is especially adaptable for washing such fragile material as shredded gelatin gels. The thinner the layer of material in the funnel the more uniform should be the washing. Funnels of larger diameter for the same weight of solid can be used for this purpose. No apparent difficulties are foreseen for making A any size desired.

C. L. GRAHAM
RAYMOND H. LAMBERT
RESEARCH LABORATORIES,
EASTMAN KODAK COMPANY

## BOOKS RECEIVED

*Bollettino di Pesca, di Piscicoltura e di Idrobiologia;* GUSTAVO BRUNELLI, Direttore. Anno XV, Fasc. 2, Marzo-Aprile 1939. Pp. 107–271. Illustrated. R. Laboratorio Centrale di Idrobiologia, Roma.

INGRAM, G. W. *Radio Interference Suppression.* Pp. viii + 154. 56 figures. The Electrical Review, London. 5/-.

National Geographic Society. *U. S. Navy Solar Expedition of 1937 to Canton Island.* Pp. 394. Illustrated. The Society, Washington.

OSEEN, C. W. *Johan Carl Wilcke, Experimental-Fysiker.* Pp. 397. Illustrated. Almquist and Wiksells, Upsala.

*Report of the First Scientific Expedition to Manchoukuo under the Leadership of Shigeyasu Tokunaga, June–October, 1933; Section V, Division I, Part I, Division II, Part IV.* Illustrated. Faculty of Science and Engineering, Waseda University, Tokyo.

SILVERMAN, ALEXANDER and ABRAHAM L. ROBINSON. *Selective Experiments in General Chemistry.* Pp. xi + 310. Illustrated. Van Nostrand.

VERZÁR, F. *Die Funktion der Nebennierenrinde.* Pp. 266. 16 figures. Benno Schwabe, Basel, Switzerland. Gebunden Fr. 25.

WINTERS, LAURENCE M. *Animal Breeding.* Third edition. Pp. viii + 316. 118 figures. Wiley. $3.50.

# SCIENCE

VOL. 90 — FRIDAY, SEPTEMBER 29, 1939 — No. 2335

*Non-aqueous Solutions:* PROFESSOR CHARLES A. KRAUS ... 281
*Obituary:*
*Frederick Parker Gay:* DR. CLAUS W. JUNGEBLUT. *William R. Perkins:* PROFESSOR GLENN W. HERRICK. *Recent Deaths* ... 290
*Scientific Events:*
*The Evacuation of the University of London; Chemical Imports of the United States; Biological Abstracts; The Scientific Programs of the Chicago Medical Society; The Relations of Science to Society* ... 292
*Scientific Notes and News* ... 294
*Discussion:*
*Important Paleolithic Find in Central Asia:* DR. ALEŠ HRDLIČKA. *A Second Household Palm:* DR. O. F. COOK. *Fresh-water Medusae Found in Kiating, Szechuen, China:* H. ZANYIN GAW and L. H. KUNG. *Anthelmintic Activity of Fresh Pineapple Juice:* JULIUS BERGER and CONRADO F. ASENJO ... 296
*Quotations:*
*The Voice of Science* ... 300
*Scientific Books:*
*Electromagnetics:* PROFESSOR H. BATEMAN. *The Philosophy of Physics:* PROFESSOR R. B. LINDSAY. *Meadow and Pasture Insects:* DR. E. P. FELT ... 300
*Societies and Meetings:*
*Fungi and Fungous Diseases:* DR. J. GARDNER HOPKINS and PROFESSOR J. S. KARLING ... 303
*Special Articles:*
*The Role of Microorganisms in the Conservation of the Soil:* DR. SELMAN A. WAKSMAN and JAMES P. MARTIN. *On the Molecular Weight of the Tobacco Mosaic Virus Protein:* PROFESSOR VERNON L. FRAMPTON. *Upward Transport of Minerals through the Phloem of Stems:* PROFESSOR FELIX G. GUSTAFSON ... 304
*Scientific Apparatus and Laboratory Methods:*
*An Aceto-carmine Method for Bird and Mammalian Chromosomes:* PROFESSOR T. S. PAINTER. *A Simple Rocking Device for Carrel Flasks:* DR. HERBERT SHAPIRO ... 307
*Science News* ... 8

SCIENCE: A Weekly Journal devoted to the Advancement of Science, edited by J. MCKEEN CATTELL and published every Friday by

THE SCIENCE PRESS
New York City: Grand Central Terminal
Lancaster, Pa. — Garrison, N. Y.

Annual Subscription, $6.00 — Single Copies, 15 Cts.

SCIENCE is the official organ of the American Association for the Advancement of Science. Information regarding membership in the Association may be secured from the office of the permanent secretary in the Smithsonian Institution Building, Washington, D. C.

# NON-AQUEOUS SOLUTIONS[1]

By Professor CHARLES A. KRAUS
BROWN UNIVERSITY

## I. INTRODUCTION

I HAD hoped to discuss the chemical, as well as the physical, properties of non-aqueous solutions, but upon further consideration, it became clear that any such discussion would necessarily consume far more time than I have available on this occasion. I shall, therefore, limit my discussion to the physical properties of non-aqueous solutions and, indeed, to the physical properties of solutions of electrolytes. I shall first consider the influence of the physical properties of the solvent medium upon the properties of the solutions and, thereafter, I shall discuss the influence of constitution of the electrolytes upon the properties of their solutions.

[1] Address of the president of the American Chemical Society, Boston, September 14, 1939.

## II. PHENOMENA DEPENDENT UPON SOLVENT PROPERTIES

*Solubility.* The solubility of ordinary, inorganic salts is chiefly determined by the chemical nature rather than by the physical properties of the solvent medium. The dielectric constant of the solvent is of secondary importance as a determining factor of the solubility in the case of ordinary, inorganic salts. Many inorganic salts, for example, are readily soluble in ethylamine, whose dielectric constant is 6.2, while there are few, if any, that are readily soluble in nitrobenzene, whose dielectric constant is 35.

The solubility of salts is of great importance in the study of solutions of electrolytes. In order to investigate the phenomena of electrolytic solutions broadly, it is necessary to dissolve a given electrolyte in a wide variety of solvents. This may be accomplished by using suitable substituted onium salts. By introducing long hydrocarbon chains into the positive ions of onium salts, it is possible to obtain electrolytes that are soluble in practically all liquids at ordinary temperatures, even in the saturated hydrocarbons.

*Influence of Dielectric Constant.* In order to get a picture of electrolytic solutions from a broad point of view, it is necessary to examine the properties of solutions of a typical strong electrolyte in a great variety of solvents. There are, perhaps, no experimental observations that serve this purpose more effectively than the conductance measurements of Dr. Fuoss with mixtures of dioxane and water. With these mixtures, it is possible to work with a solvent medium whose dielectric constant may be varied continuously between 78.6, that of water, and 2.2, that of dioxane. In Fig. 1 are plotted values of the logarithms of equivalent conductance, as ordinates, against the logarithms of concentration, as abscissas, for solutions of tetra*iso*amylammonium nitrate in dioxane-water mixtures. Logarithms are employed in order that all the data may be brought together in compact form; the equivalent conductance varies over a range of 1 to 1,000,000 and the concentration over a range of 1 to 100,000.

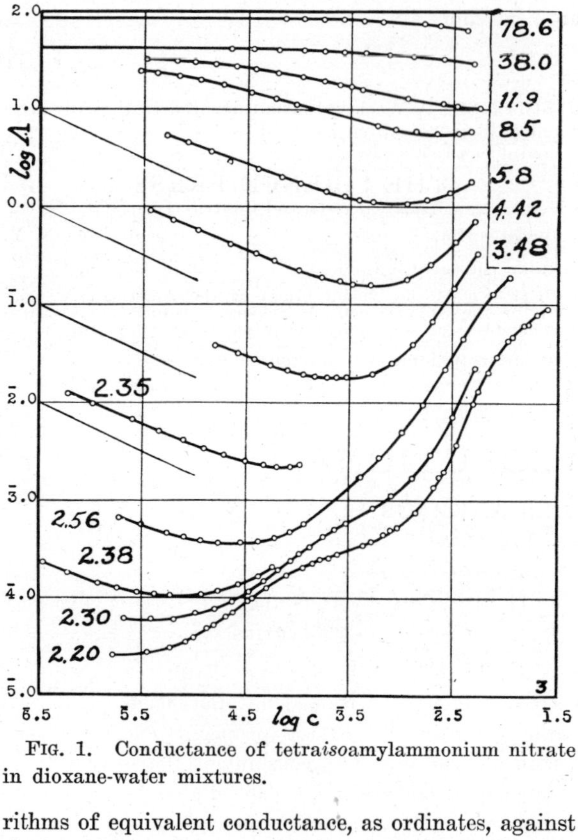


FIG. 1. Conductance of tetra*iso*amylammonium nitrate in dioxane-water mixtures.

I shall not attempt interpretation of the experimental results illustrated in the figure at this point, but the figure will serve to show the character of the phenomena with which we have to deal in solutions in non-aqueous solvents generally. Whether the two solvents be water and dioxane, or whether they be two other miscible solvents of widely differing dielectric constants, and whether the electrolyte be tetra*iso*amylammonium nitrate or some other salt, the general character of the conductance curves will closely parallel those of the figure just shown. We are clearly dealing with phenomena of perfectly general nature in which the dielectric constant of the solvent medium plays a predominant role.

*Solvents of High Dielectric Constant.* In solvents of high dielectric constant, such as water, typical strong electrolytes are completely dissociated into their ions and the properties of such solutions are accounted for in satisfactory manner by the ion atmosphere theory of Debye and Hückel and Onsager. According to this theory, there is a residual interaction between the ions, due to Coulomb forces, even though the solutions may be quite dilute. According to the theory, the equivalent conductance of an electrolyte should vary as a linear function of the square root of the ion concentration which, in the case of a completely dissociated electrolyte, is proportional to the total salt concentration. In Fig. 2 are plotted values

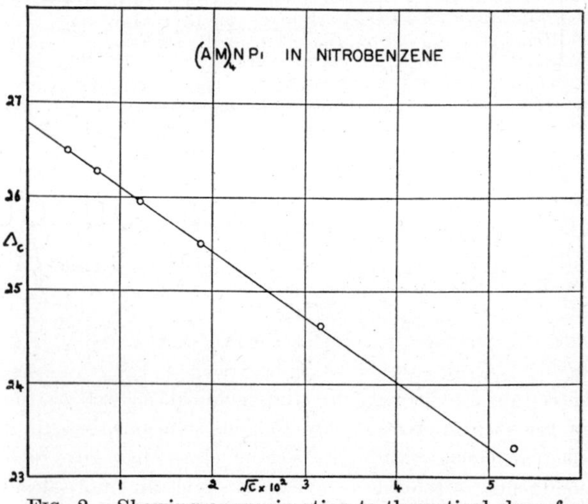


FIG. 2. Showing approximation to theoretical slope for tetra*iso*amylammonium picrate in nitrobenzene.

of the equivalent conductance for tetra-*n*-butylammonium picrate in nitrobenzene (D.C. = 35). As may be seen from the figure, the points at lower concentration approximate a straight line whose slope is predetermined by the physical constants of nitrobenzene. Obviously, in the case of this solvent, solutions of tetrabutylammonium picrate follow the same laws as do solutions of ordinary salts in water.

*Ion Association.* While the assumption of complete

dissociation of electrolytes in conjunction with the ion atmosphere theory of Debye and Hückel and Onsager gives an excellent account of the properties of electrolytic solutions at lower concentrations in solvents of high dielectric constant, it fails to account for the properties of electrolytic solutions in solvents of lower dielectric constant. This is well illustrated in Fig. 3,

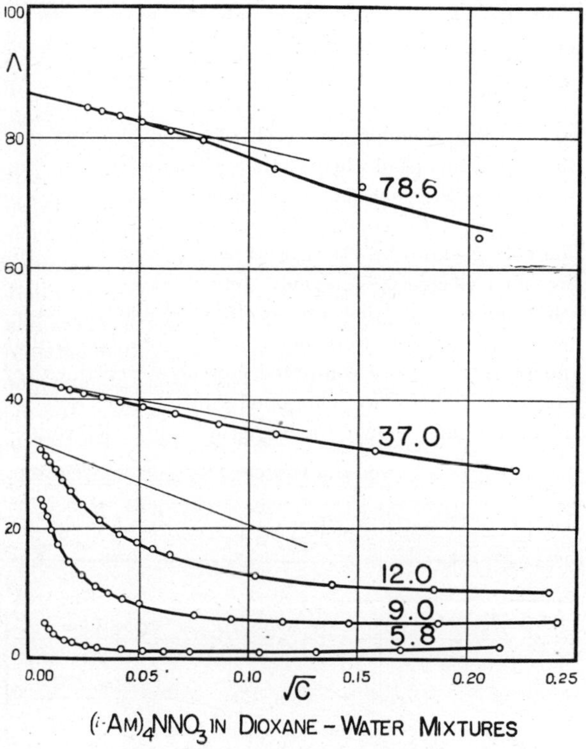


FIG. 3. Illustrating deviations from theoretical slope in solvents of lower dielectric constant.

where values of $\Lambda$ are plotted against values of the square root of total salt concentration for solutions of tetra*iso*amylammonium nitrate in dioxane-water mixtures whose dielectric constants range from 78.6 to 5.8. The values of the dielectric constant are shown on the figure. As may be seen from the figure, in the two uppermost curves for solvents having dielectric constants of 78.6 and 37.0, respectively, the conductance curves approach the theoretical slope tangentially in accord with the theory. For the solvent mixture having a dielectric constant of 17, the conductance curve fails to approach a limiting tangent. In solvents of still lower dielectric constant, the aberration from the simple ion-atmosphere theory is even more marked.

It is evident that in solvents of lower dielectric constant, a new phenomenon intervenes as a result of which the conductance diminishes much more rapidly with concentration than is called for by the ion atmosphere theory. What happens is that, in solvents of low dielectric constants, the energy of a pair of ions in contact becomes sufficiently great to render such a pair of ions measurably stable; in other words, complete dissociation of the electrolyte no longer occurs at measurable concentrations. It is, therefore, necessary to take into account an equilibrium between associated ions (ion pairs) and free ions in accordance with the equation:

$$M^+X^- \rightleftharpoons M^+ + X^-. \qquad (A)$$

This equilibrium is subject to the law of mass action, but, since the ions exist in the presence of other ions, their long-range interactions must be taken into account in accordance with the theory of Debye and Hückel and Onsager.

Assuming the associated ions, or ion pairs, to be normal in their thermodynamic behavior, while the free ions conform to the ion atmosphere theory, relations are readily obtained by means of which conductance data may be conveniently treated. In general, suitable functions are plotted such that if the assumed relations are correct, they lead to a linear plot. From the plots may be derived the value of the limiting conductance, $\Lambda_0$, and the dissociation constant, $K$, of the mass action equilibrium (A).

In Fig. 4 are shown such plots for solutions of

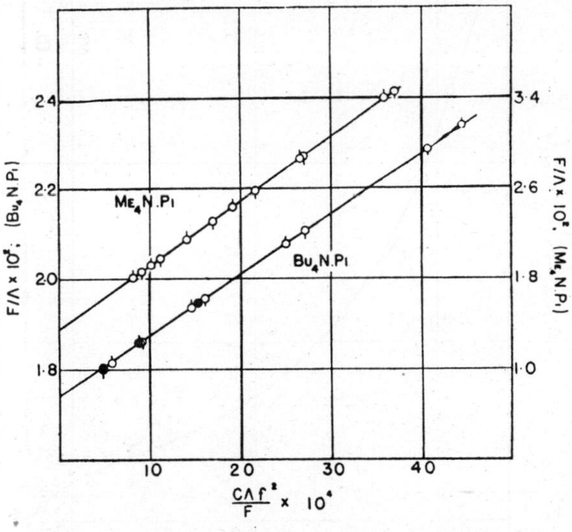


FIG. 4. Illustrating agreement of experimental and theoretical values for solutions in ethylene chloride.

tetramethyl- and tetra-*n*-butylammonium picrates in ethylene chloride (D.C. 10.3). As may be seen from the figure, the points, for both electrolytes, lie upon a straight line well within the limit of experimental error, which is less than 0.1 per cent. In the case of tetrabutylammonium picrate, concentrations have been carried as low as $1 \times 10^{-5}$ N.

*Bjerrum's Theory of Ion Association.* Some years ago, Bjerrum developed a theory of ion association.

Without going into details, it may be stated that he derived a relation connecting the association constant (reciprocal of dissociation constant) with the temperature, the dielectric constant of the medium and the sum of the ionic radii. The association constant stands in reciprocal relation to the product of these parameters, so that the dissociation constant is the greater, the larger the dielectric constant of the solution and the larger the radii of the ions. From the conductance data for solutions of tetra*iso*amylammonium nitrate in mixtures of dioxane and water, values of dissociation constants have been obtained by the method indicated above. Knowing the dissociation constants of the electrolyte for the different mixtures and the value of the dielectric constant for these mixtures, it becomes possible to make a test of Bjerrum's theory. While the ion diameters of the electrolytes of these solutions are not known, ion diameters may be assumed of such value as to pass the theoretical curve through one of the experimentally determined $K$-values. If the theory is correct, the curve should then pass through the remainder of the experimental $K$-values within the limit of experimental error. In Fig. 5 is shown a plot of

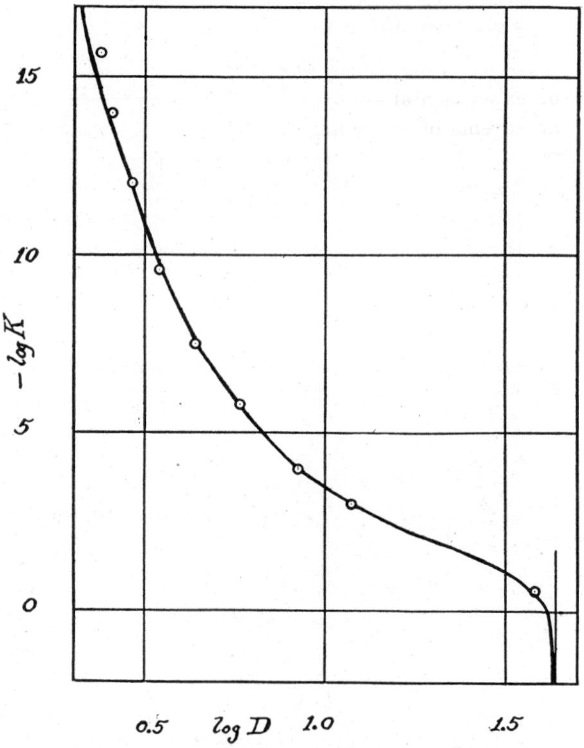


FIG. 5. Experimental and theoretical values of dissociation constants compared.

the negative logarithm of the dissociation constant (-log $K$) against the logarithm of the dielectric constant of the solvent medium (log $D$). The continuous curve is based on a value of 6.4 Å for the sum of the ionic radii. Inspection of the plot will show that the theoretical curve passes through all experimental values well within the limit of experimental error. The plot also shows that at a certain value of the dielectric constant, the curve turns sharply downward and crosses the axis of log $D$. For mixtures having dielectric constants in this region, the dissociation constant of the electrolyte is very large, which means that for these mixtures and other mixtures of higher dielectric constant, the electrolyte is completely dissociated into its ions.

*Mixtures of Electrolytes with a Common Ion.* If, in a solvent of lower dielectric constant, we have two salts with a common ion, each of which conforms to the requirements of theory, then it should be possible to compute the conductance of a mixture of these two electrolytes if the conductance curves of the pure compounds are known. In Fig. 4 were shown plots for two such electrolytes, namely, tetramethyl- and tetra-$n$-butylammonium picrates, in ethylene chloride. Values of $\Lambda_0$ and $K$ were determined from these plots and therefrom were computed conductance values for mixtures of these two components in the same solvent. In Fig. 6 are shown the experimentally determined

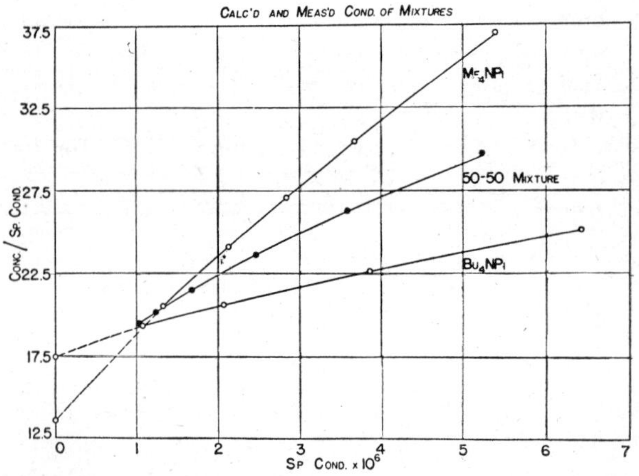


FIG. 6. Showing agreement of experimental and computed conductances for mixtures of electrolytes.

values (open circles) for the pure components. The continuous curves passing through these points are the theoretical curves. Between these curves is shown the computed curve for a 50-50 mixture of the two electrolytes; the experimental values are indicated by black circles. The experimental and computed values are in agreement within the error limit of 0.1 per cent.

*Triple Ion Equilibrium.* As shown in the first figure, for solutions of tetra*iso*amylammonium nitrate in mixtures of dioxane and water, all conductance curves in mixtures of lower dielectric constant exhibit a minimum. This phenomenon is a very general one and can only mean that in the region where the conductance increases with increasing concentration, the relative number of ions which carry the current is likewise increasing. This may be accounted for by assuming a further interaction due to Coulomb forces, namely, an interaction between the ion pairs and simple ions. The ion pairs are electrical dipoles and have a measurable electric moment. If, therefore, an ion comes into the neighborhood of an ion pair, a force acts between them which varies inversely as the cube of the distance. In solvents of lower dielectric constant, the energy due to this interaction becomes sufficiently great to render systems of this type stable. We thus have equilibria in accordance with the equations:

$$\begin{aligned} M^+X^- + M^+ &= M^+X^-M^+ \\ M^+X^- + X^- &= X^-M^+X^- \end{aligned} \qquad (B)$$

The complex ions, called triple ions, $M^+X^-M^+$ and $X^-M^+X^-$, carry, each, one unit of charge. As a result of the existence of these equilibria (B), the number of ions in solution at a given concentration will be greater than it would be if only the simple equilibrium (A) were involved. In solutions of a weakly dissociated electrolyte, the fraction of electrolyte present as triple ions increases with increasing concentration and a point is ultimately reached where the increase in the number of triple ions exceeds the decrease in the number of simple ions. It is evident, therefore, that, as a result of these equilibria, the conductance curve will exhibit a minimum.

In Fig. 7 are shown conductance curves for tetra-

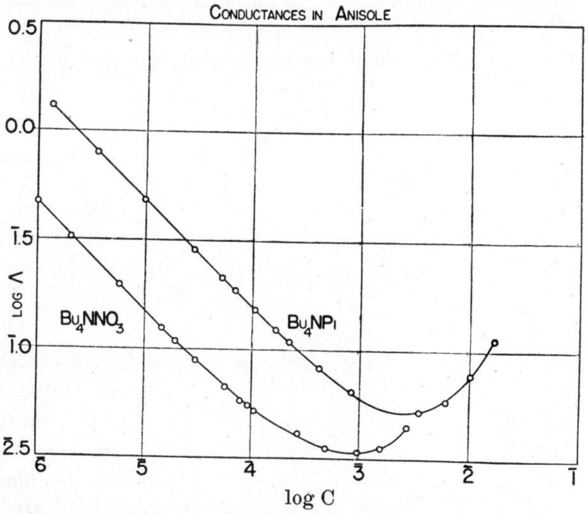


FIG. 7. Typical conductance curves in solvents of lower dielectric constant.

butylammonium thiocyanate and tetrabutylammonium nitrate in anisole (D.C. 4.29). The form of these curves is characteristic of solutions of binary electrolytes in solvents of lower dielectric constant. The slope of the curves at lower concentrations is characteristic of the equilibrium between simple ions and ion pairs for a weakly dissociated electrolyte.

Taking into account the equilibria (A) and (B), together with the ion atmosphere effect for the free ions, simple as well as triple, functions may be plotted, such that if the theory is applicable, the experimental points will lie upon a straight line. Such a plot is shown in Fig. 8 for solutions of tetrabutylammonium

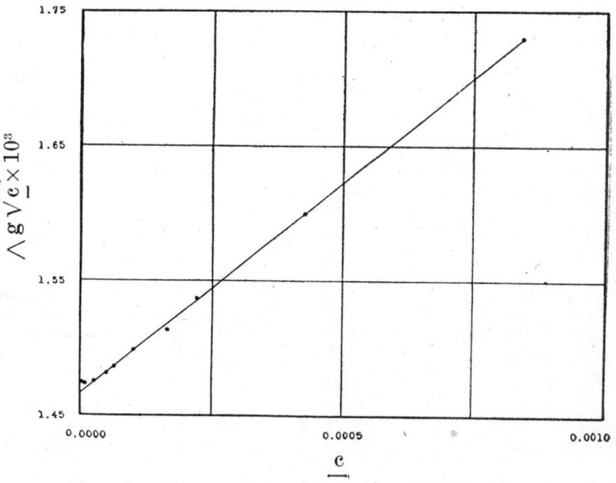


FIG. 8. Test of the Triple Ion Equilibrium.

picrate in anisole. As may be seen from the plot, the points approximate a straight line within the limits of experimental error. There seems little doubt that in solvents of lower dielectric constant, interaction between the ion pairs and free ions comes into play.

*Concentrated Solutions.* In solvents of very low dielectric constant, interactions of still higher type occur. This is illustrated, for example, by the complexity of the conductance curves at higher concentrations. Depending upon the nature of the electrolyte, the conductance curves may or may not exhibit several inflection points in the concentrated region. In Fig. 9 are shown plots of the logarithms of equiva-

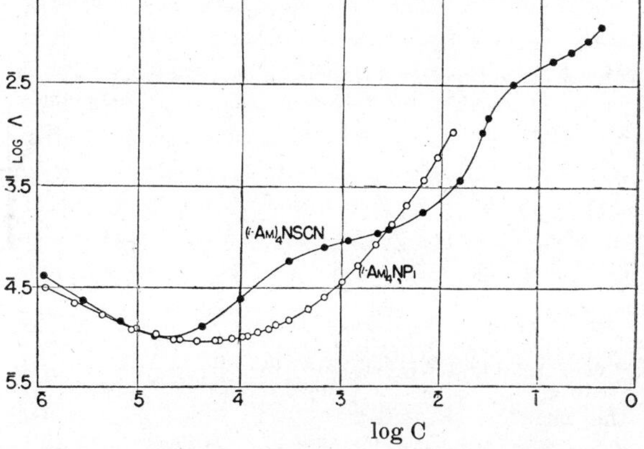


FIG. 9. Typical conductance curves in benzene.

lent conductance and of concentration for solutions of tetra*iso*amylammonium picrate and thiocyanate in benzene solution. As may be seen from the figure, the curve for the picrate is everywhere concave upward, while that for the thiocyanate exhibits several inflection points. The latter type of curve is the more common.

A study of the molecular weight of electrolytes in benzene solution gives further evidence indicating the complexity of the interactions in concentrated solutions of electrolytes in benzene. In Fig. 10 are shown

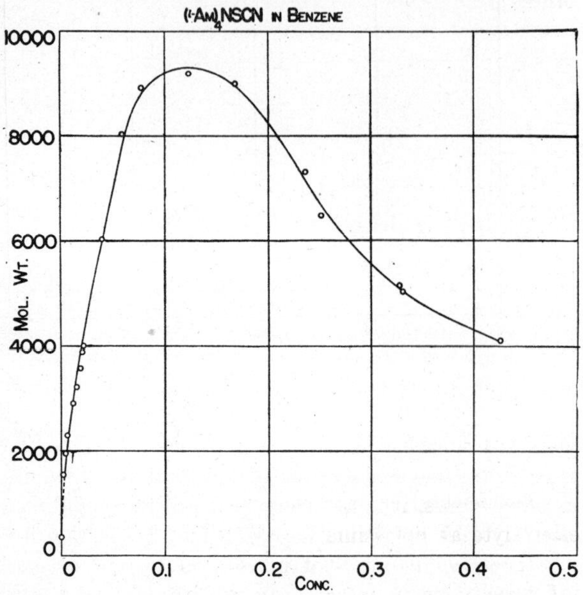


FIG. 10. Molecular weight of tetra*iso*amylammonium thiocyanate in benzene.

values of the apparent molecular weight as a function of concentration for solutions of tetra*iso*amylammonium thiocyanate in benzene. The formula weight of this electrolyte is 356.4; at approximately $1 \times 10^{-3}$ N, the molecular weight is 1,500, and thereafter it increases with increasing concentration until it reaches a maximum of 9,200 at a concentration of 0.12 N. Thereafter, the molecular weight diminishes with increasing concentration, reaching a value of 4,100 at a concentration of 0.425 N.

*Ion Dipoles.* From conductance measurements, there is obtained evidence of the existence of ions, but information relating to uncharged molecular species depends upon inference. If ions associate to form ion pairs, such ion pairs must have relatively high polar moments. If, therefore, an electrolyte is dissolved in a non-polar medium, the dielectric constant of the solution should be markedly greater than that of the pure solvent. Experiment has shown that this is actually the case. From dielectric constant measurements with solutions of electrolytes in benzene, molecular polarization values have been computed; these values are shown in Fig. 11. As may be seen, these polarization values are high, ranging all the way from

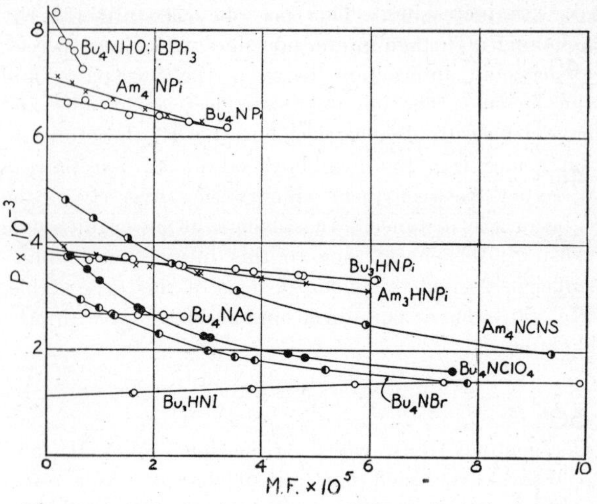


FIG. 11. Polarization curves of electrolytes in benzene solution.

1,500 to 8,000 cubic centimeters. The polar moments range from 8 to 20 Debye units. Ordinary, highly polar molecules, such as nitrobenzene, have molecular polarization values in the neighborhood of 500 cubic centimeters. The properties of dilute solutions of electrolytes in benzene, therefore, give direct evidence of the existence of ion pairs.

## III. INFLUENCE OF CONSTITUTIONAL FACTORS

*Size and Configuration.* Having discussed the behavior of solutions of electrolytes in various solvents without regard to the constitution of the ions themselves, we may now briefly consider the influence of such constitutional factors upon the properties of electrolytes. According to theory, an electrolyte should be the stronger in a given medium, the larger its ions. Since the conductance of an electrolyte is the lower, the larger its ions, we should expect that as the conductance of an electrolyte is lower, in a given medium, its dissociation constant will be greater.

TABLE I

ION CONDUCTANCES AND K-VALUES OF PICRATES IN ETHYLENE CHLORIDE

| Ion | $\Lambda_o^+$ | $K \times 10^4$ |
|---|---|---|
| $Me_4N^+$ | 42.6 | 0.326 |
| $Et_4N^+$ | 38.2 | 1.59 |
| n-$Pr_4N^+$ | 31.5 | 1.90 |
| n-$Bu_4N^+$ | 26.2 | 2.18 |
| n-$Am_4N^+$ | 23.3 | 2.38 |

In the second column of Table I are given conductance values of tetramethyl-, tetraethyl-, tetra-*n*-propyl-, tetra-*n*-butyl- and tetra-*n*-amylammonium ions, in ethylene chloride at 25°. In the third column are given values of the dissociation constant of picrates of the same ions.

In Fig. 12, these values of the ion conductances and

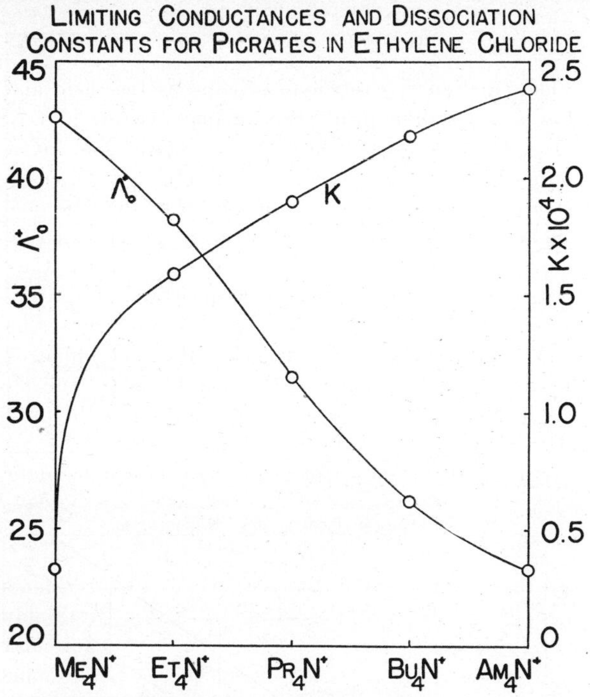


FIG. 12. Illustrating dependence of dissociation constant on ion size.

dissociation constants are shown graphically as functions of the number of carbon atoms in the substituent alkyl groups. It may be seen from the figure, as from the table, that as an ion is more complex and its conductance is lower, the dissociation constant of its salt is greater. The greatest increase of dissociation constant per carbon atom takes place between the tetramethyl- and the tetraethylammonium salts. This regularity, which has been found to hold in ethylene chloride solutions, likewise holds in all other solvents that have thus far been investigated.

If we consider a series of salts of various negative ions, we again find similar relationships, namely, that the larger the ion, the greater the dissociation of the electrolyte. In the case of unsymmetrical ions, that is, ions where the central negative charge is asymmetrically located with respect to the structure of the ion as a whole, we must take into account, not merely the size of the ion, but also its configuration. In Table II are given values of $\Lambda_0$ and $K$ for sodium salts of a number of negative ions in liquid ammonia at its boiling point.

TABLE II

CONSTANTS OF SODIUM SALTS IN LIQUID AMMONIA

| Salt | $\Lambda_0$ | $K \times 10^4$ |
|---|---|---|
| $NaOC_6H_5$ | 279.4 | 3.82 |
| $Na\beta\text{-}OC_{10}H_7$ | 268.1 | 6.50 |
| $Na\alpha\text{-}OC_{10}H_7$ | 265.3 | 8.08 |
| $NaSC_2H_5$ | 281.4 | 22.5 |
| $NaSC_6H_5$ | 275.1 | 36.0 |
| $NaSn(C_6H_5)_3$ | 220. | 150. |

It will be noted that sodium β-naphtholate is a markedly stronger electrolyte than sodium phenolate. The larger dissociation constant of the naphtholate is due to the greater size of the naphthyl group. With the phenolic oxygen atom in the α in place of the β position, the strength of the electrolyte is further increased by about 30 per cent. It is not alone the size of the group attached to the oxygen atom that must be considered but also the relation of the oxygen atom to other atoms in the ion.

It is interesting to compare the dissociation constant of sodium phenolate with that of sodium thiophenolate. In the case of the thiophenolate ion, the charge is localized on the sulfur atom, which is markedly larger than the oxygen atom. As a result, the dissociation constant of the thiophenolate is nearly ten times that of the phenolate. Even sodium ethylsulfide is a markedly stronger electrolyte than sodium phenolate. In this connection, it may be stated that the dissociation constant of potassium chloride is $8.73 \times 10^{-4}$. By localizing the charge of the negative ion on still larger atoms and by associating large groups with such atoms, it is possible to build up electrolytes that are even stronger than those already considered. Sodium triphenylstannide $NaSn(C_6H_5)_3$ has a dissociation constant of approximately $150 \times 10^{-4}$ in liquid ammonia; in other words, it is nearly twenty times as strong an electrolyte as potassium chloride.

*Choline Salts.* It is of interest to determine what influence elements other than carbon and hydrogen may have on the strength of electrolytes when introduced into the positive ion. For example, a hydroxyethyl group may be introduced into a quaternary ammonium ion in place of an ethyl group. The hydroxy group of a compound of this type may be replaced by halogens and other suitable groups and, in place of an ethyl group, methyl or other organic groups may be employed. In Table III are given values of the dissociation constant for a series of electrolytes of this type, dissolved in ethylene chloride.

TABLE III

CHOLINE SALTS IN ETHYLENE CHLORIDE AND NITROBENZENE

| Salt | $K \times 10^4$ | |
|---|---|---|
| | $C_2H_4Cl_2$ | $C_6H_5NO_2$ |
| $Et \cdot Me_3NPi$ | 0.460 | 575.0 |
| $HOC_2H_4 \cdot Me_3NPi$ | 0.0659 | 67.0 |
| $CH_3OCH_2 \cdot Me_3NPi$ | 0.254 | 262.0 |
| $BrC_2H_4 \cdot Me_3NPi$ | 0.132 | .... |
| $BrCH_2 \cdot Me_3NPi$ | 0.078 | .... |

It will be noted that hydroxyethyltrimethylammonium picrate (choline picrate) has a dissociation constant about one seventh that of ethyltrimethylammonium picrate. Throughout the series of salts appearing in the table, the dissociation constants are markedly lower than those of corresponding salts in which only hydrocarbon groups are present in the positive ions.

*Partially Substituted Ammonium Salts.* If, in place of the quaternary ammonium salts, partially substituted ammonium salts are employed in ethylene chloride or nitrobenzene, it is found that these substances uniformly behave as weak electrolytes. In general, their dissociation constants are approximately 1,000 times smaller than those of the corresponding completely substituted salts. In Table IV are given values of the limiting conductances and the dissociation constants of a series of butylammonium picrates dissolved in nitrobenzene at 25°.

TABLE IV

CONSTANTS OF PARTIALLY SUBSTITUTED AMMONIUM SALTS IN $C_6H_5NO_2$

| Salt | $\Lambda_0$ | $K \times 10^4$ |
|---|---|---|
| $NH_4Pi$ | 34.3 | 1.46 |
| $BuNH_3Pi$ | 32.79 | 1.50 |
| $Bu_2NH_2Pi$ | 30.36 | 1.51 |
| $Bu_3NHPi$ | 28.86 | 1.90 |
| $BuNH_3ClO_4$ | 37.75 | 25.2 |
| $Bu_3NHI$ | 33.48 | 0.943 |
| $C_5H_{10}NH_2Pi$ | 33.27 | 1.55 |

On examining the table, it will be noted that ammonium picrate and monobutyl- and dibutylammonium picrates have dissociation constants of approximately $1.5 \times 10^{-4}$; tributylammonium picrate has a slightly higher constant, $1.9 \times 10^{-4}$. Tetrabutylammonium picrate is a very strong electrolyte with a constant greater than $2000 \times 10^{-4}$. The strength of a partially substituted ammonium salt depends but little upon the nature of the positive ion. Thus, the constant for pyridonium picrate is $0.53 \times 10^{-4}$, that of piperidonium picrate is $1.55 \times 10^{-4}$ and that of ammonium picrate is $1.46 \times 10^{-4}$. The negative ion, however, has a marked influence on the dissociation constant. For butylammonium picrate, the constant is $1.50 \times 10^{-4}$, while for butylammonium perchlorate it is $25.2 \times 10^{-4}$.

The presence of hydrogen attached to nitrogen in the positive ion appears to introduce an energy term as a result of which the dissociation constant of the electrolyte is smaller than that of an electrolyte in which Coulomb forces alone are involved. Seemingly, there is an interaction between the proton attached to nitrogen and the negative ion. This view is supported by the fact that the partially substituted ammonium salts, including ammonium salts, are normally strong electrolytes in pyridine. Interaction between the proton and the negative ion is also indicated by the dependence of the dissociation constant upon the nature of the negative ion as exemplified by the picrate and the perchlorate in Table IV.

*Acid-Base Dissociation.* In the case of salts of weak bases, dissolved in non-basic solvents like nitrobenzene and ethylene chloride, an acid-base dissociation occurs. For example, in solutions of pyridonium picrate, we have to consider the two equilibria:

$$C_5H_5NH^+Pi^- \rightleftharpoons C_5H_5NH^+ + Pi^- \quad (C_1)$$

$$C_5H_5NH^+Pi^- \rightleftharpoons C_5H_5N + HPi \quad (C_2)$$

The fraction of electrolyte existing as free acid and base is in constant proportion to that existing as free ions. If the conductance data for solutions of pyridonium picrate are plotted in the usual way, the curve extrapolates to a value of $\Lambda_0$ much below the true one. The acid-base equilibrium may readily be repressed by adding an excess of either picric acid or pyridine. Carrying out a series of conductance measurements in the presence of an excess of acid or base, the true value of $\Lambda_0$ may be obtained. Knowing this, the value of the dissociation constant for the equilibria $C_1$ and $C_2$ may be obtained from the conductance data of the pure salt.

In Fig. 13 are shown plots of the conductance data

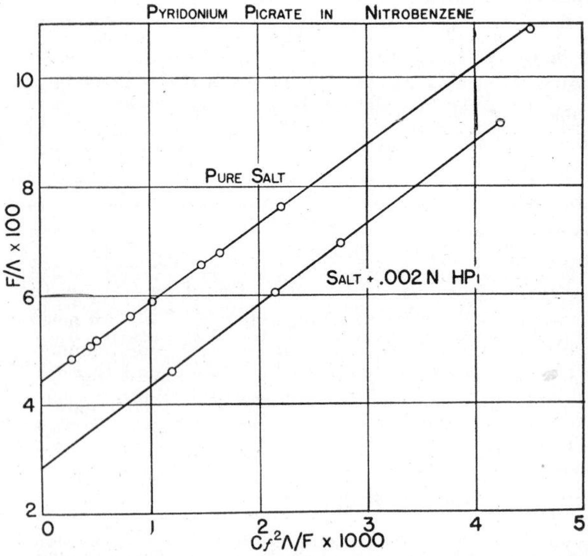


FIG. 13. Illustrating repression of ion-base dissociation in nitrobenzene.

for solutions of pyridonium picrate in pure nitrobenzene and in nitrobenzene containing 0.00203 N picric acid. The ordinates are proportional to $1/\Lambda$ and the intercepts on the axis of ordinates are the values of $1/\Lambda_0$. As may be seen from the figure, the value of $\Lambda_0$ obtained for pyridonium picrate in pure nitrobenzene (upper curve) is 22.52, while that in the presence of picric acid is 35.1. A series of measurements carried out with the addition of picric acid and of pyridine to solutions of pyridonium picrate yields 35.0 as the most probable value of $\Lambda_0$ and $0.551 \times 10^{-4}$ as the most probable value of the dissociation constant for the pure electrolyte. These yield a value of $1.74 \times 10^{-5}$ for the dissociation constant of the acid-base equilibrium $C_2$. In Table V are given values of $\Lambda_0$ and of the dissociation constant for pyridonium picrate in the presence of varying amounts of picric acid and of pyridine.

TABLE V

CONSTANTS OF PYRIDONIUM PICRATE IN THE PRESENCE OF VARYING AMOUNTS OF PICRIC ACID AND PYRIDINE

| Conc. HPi | $\Lambda_0$ | $K \times 10^4$ | Conc. Pyridine | $\Lambda_0$ | $K \times 10^4$ |
|---|---|---|---|---|---|
| 0.0 | 35.0 | 0.551 | 0.00095 | 34.76 | 0.580 |
| .00077 | 35.6 | .524 | .0101 | 34.19 | 0.876 |
| .00203 | 35.1 | .545 | .0272 | 34.00 | 1.34 |
| .00420 | 35.8 | .524 | .0528 | 33.80 | 2.21 |

The $\Lambda_0$ values obtained on addition of the acid are subject to experimental errors of the order of one-half unit, due, in part, to the conductance of picric acid itself. It is safe to conclude, however, that both $\Lambda_0$ and $K$ are independent of the amount of picric acid added in the concentration range of the table. In the presence of pyridine, the values of both $\Lambda_0$ and $K$ are functions of the concentration of excess pyridine. There is a rather marked decrease in the value of $\Lambda_0$ with increasing concentration of pyridine, which seems to be a real effect and is not due to change in the viscosity of the solutions. The dissociation constant, upon addition of pyridine, increases markedly. This constant is very nearly a linear function of concentration of pyridine and extrapolates to a value of $0.551 \times 10^{-4}$ for the dissociation constant of pyridonium picrate in pure nitrobenzene. This value of the constant harmonizes with the value of 35.0 for $\Lambda_0$.

*Proton Interaction.* The influence of bases upon the dissociation constant of electrolytes that have an active proton in the positive ion is quite a general phenomenon. In the case of the partially substituted ammonium salts, the investigation of the phenomenon is limited to a base identical with that of the salt. It is possible to investigate the phenomenon more advantageously, however, with salts of the quaternary type in which an OH group is attached to the nitrogen of the ammonium ion. In solvents such as ethylene chloride and nitrobenzene, these hydroxyammonium salts are even weaker electrolytes than are the partially substituted ammonium salts. In Table VI are given values of the dissociation constant of hydroxytrimethylammonium picrate in pure nitrobenzene and in nitrobenzene to which have been added varying amounts of different bases.

TABLE VI

INFLUENCE OF BASES ON THE CONSTANT OF HYDROXYTRIMETHYLAMMONIUM PICRATE IN NITROBENZENE

| Base | $K \times 10^4$ | Base ($C_5H_5N$) | $K \times 10^4$ |
|---|---|---|---|
| 0 | 0.169 | 0.00104 | 0.353 |
| $C_5H_{11}N$ 0.010 | 11.0 | .0101 | 1.19 |
| $(C_2H_5)_3N$ 0.038 | 10.0 | .037 | 3.33 |

As may be seen from the table, the salt has a dissociation constant of $0.169 \times 10^{-4}$. With addition of pyridine, the dissociation constant increases, reaching a value of $3.33 \times 10^{-4}$ for a pyridine concentration of 0.037 N. The stronger the base, the greater is the increase of the dissociation constant at a given concentration of base. Thus, in a 0.01 N solution of pyridine, the dissociation constant is $1.19 \times 10^{-4}$, while in a 0.01 N solution of piperidine, the dissociation constant is $11 \times 10^{-4}$. In other words, while a 0.01 N solution of pyridine increases the dissociation constant of the electrolyte approximately seven times, a 0.01 N solution of piperidine increases it nearly seventy times. Triethylamine is intermediate in its effect on the dissociation constant; at a concentration of 0.038 N, the constant is approximately three times that of a pyridine solution of the same concentration.

The influence of bases upon the dissociation constant of salts of the type here under discussion is largely, if not wholly, due to interaction of the base with the proton of the hydroxy group of the positive ion. When these electrolytes are dissolved in basic solvents they are normally strong electrolytes. For example, the dissociation constant of phenylhydroxydimethylammonium picrate in nitrobenzene (D.C. = 35) is $0.18 \times 10^{-4}$, while dissolved in pyridine (D.C. = 12.03), its dissociation constant is $12.5 \times 10^{-4}$.

## IV. CONCLUSION

The properties of solutions of typical strong electrolytes are little influenced by the chemical nature of the medium in which they are dissolved; they are chiefly, and very generally, determined by the dielectric constant of the solvent. In a solvent of high dielectric constant, electrolytes are completely dissociated into their ions. In solvents of somewhat lower dielectric constant, short-range ion interaction occurs and an equilibrium exists between simple ions and ion pairs; in solvents of still lower dielectric constant, ions and ion pairs associate to form triple ions. In solvents of very low dielectric constant, association becomes extremely complex at higher concentrations, leading to very complex relations between the concentration and the various physical properties of the solutions.

The association of ions to ion pairs depends, in the first place, upon the size of the ions. It also depends upon the geometrical structure of the ions and the distribution of charge among the various atoms of this structure.

Where interactions other than Coulombic occur between the ions or where special interactions occur between the ions and the solvent molecules, the properties of solutions depend upon the nature of the solvent medium. Certain acids, for example, are strong electrolytes in water but are very weak or non-electrolytes in nitrobenzene. In the case of nearly all the weak electrolytes, interactions other than Coulombic are present and the properties of their solutions are dependent upon the nature of the solvent medium as well as upon its dielectric constant.

# OBITUARY

## FREDERICK PARKER GAY

WHENEVER one of the really great men of science passes from our midst, not only are our hearts filled with sorrow for the loss of a dear and esteemed colleague, but our minds pause long enough to reflect upon a personality which has exercised such a tremendous influence on the time and sphere in which he lived and worked. These were the emotions and thoughts that came to the scientific world with the news of the death of Frederick Parker Gay on July 14, 1939.

Born in Boston, Mass., on July 22, 1874, he received a classical preparatory education at Boston Latin School and Harvard University. His career in research began early while he was still a medical student at the Johns Hopkins University. As assistant to Dr. Simon Flexner he traveled around the world with the Johns Hopkins Medical Commission, stopping in the Philippines to investigate cholera and dysentery. About thirty years later he was to return to the same Islands, this time in quest of leprosy, as a member of the Leonard Wood Memorial Commission.

By 1901, when Dr. Gay was graduated from medical school, the science of bacteriology was blossoming prodigiously and its spectacular achievements could not help but attract a man with Gay's intellectual curiosity and emotional drive. Because medical bacteriology began as a branch of morbid anatomy, the young bacteriologist naturally entrusted his early instruction to the pathologist. An award of the first fellowship by the new-born Rockefeller Institute opened a position as assistant demonstrator in pathology at the University of Pennsylvania from 1901–1903. For some years later Gay continued to call himself a pathologist; but as he advanced in age there developed in him a growing interest in the fundamental problems of microbiology which was to carry his activities far beyond the conventional lines of medical bacteriology. An inborn desire to elucidate principles rather than to record phenomena was probably the reason for his early association with the great theoretical genius of his time, Jules Bordet in Brussels. Here, during the years 1903 to 1906, his attention was fully absorbed by an investigation of the complexities of the alexin fixation reaction which was to initiate a long and fruitful series of contributions in the field of immunology. An important by-product of this period was his first book, a translation into English of the "Studies in Immunity" by Bordet and his collaborators, published in 1909. When he returned to this country, his scientific progress was one of uninterrupted activity and his career one of increasing momentum. During the years 1906 and 1907 he served as bacteriologist to the Danvers Insane Hospital in Massachusetts; between 1907 and 1909 he was assistant and later instructor in pathology at the Harvard Medical School. In 1910 he became professor of pathology at the University of California at Berkeley. Here he remained for thirteen years, except for a brief period of service as major in the Medical Corps of the U. S. Army during the World War. It was towards the end of his stay in California that he succeeded in developing bacteriology and immunology as independent sciences, separate from pathology, a division which led to his appointment, in 1921, as professor of bacteriology and director of the newly organized department. In 1923 he went to Columbia University as head of the department of bacteriology, a position which he occupied until his death.

His many contributions to bacteriology and immunology are known to all workers in the field and need no extensive review here. In roughly chronological order they included: studies of the serum reactions, particularly conglutination and alexin fixation (1905–10); anaphylaxis (1905–13); typhoid fever, both experimental studies of the carrier state in animals and immunization, vaccine therapy and skin tests in man (1913–18); pathogenesis and chemotherapy of hemolytic streptococcus infections (1919–39); tissue immunity, in particular the rôle of tissue macrophages (clasmatocytes) in enhancing local resistance and the relation of the reticulo-endothelial system to the formation of antibodies (1920–31); virus infections, especially the problem of the interrelationship of herpes and encephalitis (1929–39). He was also author of a number of papers on general topics in the realm of medical education and the historical development of bacteriology. Besides the translation of Bordet's "Studies in Immunity" he also wrote a monograph on "Typhoid Fever" (1918). In 1935 there appeared "Agents of Disease and Host Resistance," the most extensive American system of bacteriology, immunology and related aspects of the etiology of disease, which he planned and edited and of which he contributed the major part. His last book, "The Open Mind" (1937), was a monument to E. E. Southard, with whom he shared the bonds of a deep friendship as well as an intense interest in problems of psychiatry and sociology.

It may be taken for granted that a man who held such a key position in research and medical education should have shared generously in the honors and distinctions that science bestows on its outstanding exponents. Through his early affiliation with Bordet he belonged to the Société belge de Biologie. All prominent scientific societies in America counted him among their members, and often their president. From 1917 to 1918 he was a member of the Medical Section of the National Research Council, functioning first as its chairman and later as chairman of its Medical Fellowship Board. With the foundation of the American Commission for Relief in Belgium he was appointed exchange professor from Columbia University to Belgian Universities (1926–27); from 1932 to 1936 he served as chairman of the Advisory Committee on Research of the Leonard Wood Memorial. He was a Commander of the Order of the Crown of Belgium and received an honorary Sc.D. degree from George Washington University in 1932. At a meeting of the National Academy of Sciences in Washington, D. C., held in April, 1939, Dr. Gay was made a member of this society.

It would be difficult to say whether Gay's contributions to science, brilliant as they were, or the unforgettable part he played as an inspiring teacher and counselor were foremost in helping him to win the unique distinction that was his. A man of rare culture and outspoken personality, he would naturally imbue his lectures with an air of scholarly refinement that could not fail to make a deep impression on young medical students. But his presentation had also an unusual eloquence, an originality and facility of expression which made it an esthetic pleasure to listen to him. He was truly master of the printed and the spoken word. For there was in Gay's make-up a strong artistic impulse that often helped him to bridge the gap between intellectual skepticism and intuitive vision. This artistic talent, which found its natural outlet in literature and poetry, undoubtedly was a great creative force in Gay's productivity. At the peak of his life, it led him once to formally pose the question whether one good sonnet might, perhaps, not be worth more than a sheaf of scientific papers. A man with such gifts of mind and soul could not help but attract a wide circle of devoted friends and associates. This affectionate regard, which all who knew him intimately learned to share for Dr. Gay, was sometimes difficult to fathom for others whose contact with him was only brief. At first sight he often seemed cool and aloof, perhaps even introverted. His nature had in it a certain shyness, characteristic of all great men, which did not permit him the easy approach in establishing human relations. Coupled with this was an utter sincerity and fearless insistence on the rightness of certain principles—to which he sometimes referred as his New England conscience—which may occasionally have colored his decisions with an arbitrary note. Mistaken superficial impressions of this kind, however, can not do justice to the warm-hearted character that was capable of forging such strong bonds of affection with those who were close to him.

Had he lived but a little longer, there might have been a greater measure of outward perfection in his life even though his work was done, by his own decision. Earlier in the year he had made known to his associates his intention to retire from active service after a contemplated year's leave of absence. He had looked forward to a few quiet years at his beautiful country home, in pursuit of hobbies and in happy enjoyment of family life. Fate decided differently for him. He had not been seriously ill, except for recurring anginoid attacks during the last year or two. He passed away in his sleep, quietly, we hope painlessly. Death had gently shut the door upon a full life.

CLAUS W. JUNGEBLUT
COLLEGE OF PHYSICIANS AND SURGEONS,
COLUMBIA UNIVERSITY

## WILLIAM R. PERKINS

PROFESSOR W. R. PERKINS, vice-director, emeritus, of the Mississippi State Experiment Station, died on August 21 after forty-eight years of notable activity in agricultural work in three states, Mississippi, South Carolina and Louisiana. After graduation from the State College of Mississippi in 1891, he was employed as chemist in the Experiment Station until 1893, when he became agronomist in the Station and professor of agronomy in the college for the following seventeen years. In 1910 he was called to Clemson College, South Carolina, where he remained two years. For the next three years he determined to put in practice the facts which he had found in chemistry and in agronomy and to try out the theories which he had formulated during the years of his teaching and experimenting. Thus he returned to Mississippi where he demonstrated in the practical operation of a farm the soundness of his factual knowledge and of some of his theories. But the educational authorities would not let him follow his natural desires, and in 1915 he was called to the Louisiana State University as forage crop specialist for the extension department. Later, he became director of the extension department, a position which he filled with marked success until in 1928, when he came back to his native state as assistant director of the South Mississippi Experiment Station at Poplarville. In 1930 he was made director of the state system of branch experiment stations and, finally, vice-director of the State Experiment Station at the State College.

Professor Perkins retired from his administrative duties at the age of 70, but continued his activities until illness prevented further work. He was engaged in gathering data and compiling a history of the Experiment Station with which he became officially connected six years after its establishment in 1885.

Professor Perkins was of a modest and retiring disposition, but his knowledge of the different phases of practical agriculture was broad and profound. He was widely known in the southern states for his work as an agricultural chemist, agronomist and administrator in extension and experiment stations. He early recognized the economic futility of a one-crop system, cotton, and the distress to which it would finally lead southern agriculture. He saw the boundless possibilities in the growing of forage crops and the production of live stock under the most favorable climatic conditions in this country. In and out of season, he counseled conservation of the soil and diversification of agriculture.

He was much sought for his advice and counsel in all phases of agricultural work, for he was the kindliest of men, always ready to help to the full extent of his ability. He was a staunch and loyal friend to all who were earnestly striving to do their part in the world's work. The writer has known Mr. Perkins for more than forty years and during all that time we have known him to stand unflinchingly for the truth, even at times when it endangered his position to do so. If pressure to the contrary became too great he quietly stepped aside without recrimination, rather than to truckle to unwise dictators or to pernicious politics. Southern agriculture has lost a zealous advocate, an able administrator, a careful student and a just man.

GLENN W. HERRICK

## RECENT DEATHS

SIGMUND FREUD died in London on September 23. He was eighty-three years old.

CHARLES F. SHAW, professor of soil technology at the University of California, died suddenly on September 12 at the age of fifty-eight years.

THOMAS D. RICE, senior soil scientist of the Bureau of Chemistry and Soils of the U. S. Department of Agriculture, died on August 23 at the age of sixty-one years.

L. W. FORMAN, superintendent of experiments in soils and research assistant professor in the Agricultural Experiment Station of the Iowa State College, died on September 9 at the age of fifty-eight years.

ANDREW CLAUDE DE LA C. CROMMELIN, for thirty-six years a member of the staff of the Royal Observatory, Greenwich, known for his work on comets and minor planets, died on September 20 at the age of seventy-four years.

# SCIENTIFIC EVENTS

## THE EVACUATION OF THE UNIVERSITY OF LONDON

IN its issue for September 12, the London *Times* reports that next term students of the University of London will be scattered over various parts of the United Kingdom. Arrangements were almost complete for the evacuation of the whole of the university, and it was hoped to begin the new term early in October. Meanwhile the administrative offices will remain at the Royal Holloway College, Englefield Green.

An attempt has been made, wherever possible, to move the whole of each college to its new home, and other universities have cooperated with London in completing its arrangements.

University College is the only one which had been unable to find accommodations for all its students in one place. The men are going to the University of Wales, Aberystwyth; the women medical students to Sheffield, and other women students to Wales.

King's College, which has decided to discontinue its courses in Spanish, journalism, psychology and chemical engineering and its evening classes, is going to Bristol.

Other colleges are going to the following places:

King's College of Household and Social Science, Wales.
Queen Mary College, Cambridge.
Institute of Education, University College, Nottingham.
School of Oriental Studies, Cambridge.
Goldsmiths' College, Nottingham.
Westfield College for Women, Oxford.
College of Pharmaceutical Society, Wales.
Bedford College. Not yet decided.
Imperial College of Science and Technology, Edinburgh.
The Mining Department is moving to Camborne, Cornwall.

The medical schools are going to the following centers:

St. Bartholomew's Hospital and College, London, and the London School of Hygiene and Tropical Medicine to Cambridge.
Guy's and St. Thomas's to Oxford.
Middlesex to Bristol.
St. Mary's to Manchester.
London School of Medicine for Women to Aberdeen and St. Andrews.
King's College Medical School to Glasgow.

## CHEMICAL IMPORTS OF THE UNITED STATES

IN the United States, according to a report of the Chemical Division of the Department of Commerce, imports of chemicals and related products, including gums, resins, drying oils and drying seeds, increased steadily during the first half of the current year and recorded a gain of 18 per cent. over receipts of such products in the corresponding months of 1938.

Receipts for these materials reached a total value of $90,000,000 in the current year period, against $76,473,000 in the corresponding months of 1938, with fertilizer materials making up 24 per cent. of the total;

drying oils and drying oil seeds, 21 per cent.; medicinal materials and crude drugs, 10 per cent.; and gums, resins, balsams and waxes, 8 per cent.

Imports of fertilizer materials, not including tankage, showed little change in the first half of the current year, compared with the same period of 1938, remaining at about 800,000 tons valued at about $19,000,000, but imports of tankage increased sharply to 33,072 tons valued at $1,224,000 from 13,648 tons valued at $432,000 in the first half of last year.

Some changes occurred in the drying oil and drying oil seed group, due to disturbances in China, which reduced that country's exports of tung oil, but the aggregate for the whole classification advanced approximately 13 per cent., due to heavier imports of perilla and oiticica oils and flaxseed. In this group imports of tung oil decreased from 50,400,000 pounds in the first half of 1938 to 39,500,000 pounds in the current year period; but receipts of flaxseed increased from 7,383,000 to 10,763,000 bushels; perilla oil, from 15,571,000 to 23,000,000 pounds, and oiticica oil, from 1,360,000 to 9,019,000.

Among the medicinal and related product materials, receipts of cod-liver oil increased from 2,381,500 to 2,896,500 gallons; crude drugs, including cinchona bark, from $3,906,000 to $4,744,000 in value; and medicinal materials, including cinchona products, from $2,323,000 to $2,593,000, according to preliminary statistics.

Imports of coal-tar products increased sharply in the first half of the year to $10,742,000 in value from $7,330,600 in the same months of 1938, due to the heavy receipts of dyes, colors and stains from Germany.

Other items on the chemical and related product import list recording gains in the first half of the current year, compared with the 1938 period, included beeswax, receipts of which increased in value from $298,000 to $447,500; gums, resins and balsams, from $4,825,000 to $5,828,000; carnauba wax, from $2,494,000 to $2,844,000; vegetable wax, from $152,000 to $347,000; essential oils, from $2,285,000 to $2,755,500; vegetable dyeing and tanning materials, from $2,466,000 to $3,573,000; industrial chemicals, from $7,822,000 to $9,899,000; and soap and toiletry raw materials, from $1,132,800 to $1,310,000.

Other items recording decrease included glue stock, imports of which declined in value from $1,539,500 to $919,680; agar-agar, from $201,000 to $158,000; and industrial explosives, from $475,500 to $270,000.

## BIOLOGICAL ABSTRACTS

*Biological Abstracts* is undertaking a more complete abstracting and segregation of the current research literature in bioclimatology and biometeorology. The section Bioclimatology-Biometeorology will appear within the section Ecology, and will be under the editorship of Robert G. Stone, of the Blue Hill Observatory of Harvard University.

Attention is called to the increasing interest in climatic and meteorological factors in their relation to biology, medicine and agriculture. It is pointed out that ecologists have long appreciated the importance of temperature, humidity, radiation, barometric pressure, wind movement and meteorological factors generally as important factors in controlling the distribution and abundance of animals and plants, and that foresters, horticulturists and entomologists have likewise been concerned with the interrelationships of climatic and meteorological factors to the organisms with which they work. The developments of air conditioning and aviation have brought other research groups into the field, including individuals and groups the results of whose work frequently appears in periodicals not commonly consulted by biologists. The announcement reads:

> In all civilized nations diverse research groups have sprung into being which, though they often devote much attention to the same fundamental natural forces, still work in practical isolation from each other, with a different background of training and associations, belonging to different societies meeting at different times and places, publishing in different journals, reading different literature, investigating different types of things. These groups, however, are beginning to apply common ideas and common methods to the study of situations that are basically similar. For example, techniques and concepts derived from a study of the influence of weather factors on the spread of influenza or the common cold are likely to have a very high transfer value as applied to the study of the spread or survival of plant disease or economic insects. Conversely, it should be possible for research workers in the field of public health to make use of many findings of the entomologists, foresters, ecologists, plant pathologists and other biological groups.
>
> The abstracting journals of broad scope, like *Biological Abstracts,* are admirably suited to the sort of synthesis of fundamental knowledge that this situation demands. In inaugurating this service *Biological Abstracts* will be fulfilling one of the functions for which it was originally intended: that of providing an effective tool for research workers by coordinating the literature of border-line fields.

Under the sectional publication plan this material will be found, at present, not only in Section A, General Biology, but also under section B, Experimental Animal Biology; Section D, Plant Sciences, and Section E, Animal Sciences.

## THE SCIENTIFIC PROGRAMS OF THE CHICAGO MEDICAL SOCIETY

THE Chicago Medical Society is planning a series of all-day programs for the consideration of various diseases to be held on the third Wednesday of each month from October through April. In the morning and afternoon, there will be clinics, demonstrations, lectures and round table discussions on the general subject selected, certain aspects of which will be presented at the evening meeting. The day-time part of the program will be held in one or another of the teaching institutions of the city, but will be a program of the society presented in the institution, rather than a program of the institution presented to the members and guests of the society. The evening meetings will be held at 8:30 P.M. at the Chicago Woman's Club Theater on Eleventh Street near Michigan Boulevard. Detailed programs will be furnished each month.

The topics to be considered at these meetings are as follows:

October 18—Fractures at the Cook County Hospital; The Treatment of Skull Fracture, Harry E. Mock, Chicago.

November 15—Nutritional Deficiency Diseases at Thorne Hall on the Chicago Campus of Northwestern University; The Vitamin B Complex and Pellagra, Tom D. Spies, Cincinnati, Ohio.

December 20—Cardiovascular-Renal Diseases at One of the Institutions in the West Side Medical Center; Arteriosclerosis Obliterans: The Modern Conception of its Social Significance, Diagnosis and Treatment, Irving S. Wright, New York City.

January 17, 1940—Industrial Medicine and Traumatic Surgery at St. Luke's Hospital; The Evaluation of Disability Due to Cardiovascular Disease.

February 21—Topic and speaker to be selected.

March 20—Endocrinology at the University of Chicago Clinics; The Misuse of Biologicals in Medical Practice.

April 17—Obstetrics and Care of the New Born; Maternal and Infant Mortality in Chicago, 1935–39.

A luncheon for members and guests will be arranged at or near the institution in which the clinical program is to be presented, and a dinner will be held at the Chicago Woman's Club before the evening meetings.

## THE RELATIONS OF SCIENCE TO SOCIETY

THE American Association for the Advancement of Science has adopted two minutes on the relations of science and scientific men to the social order, which are here reproduced. The first was adopted at the Boston meeting in December, 1933, the second at the Indianapolis meeting in December, 1937.

The American Association for the Advancement of Science feels grave concern over persistent and threatening inroads upon intellectual freedom which have been made in recent times in many parts of the world.

Our existing liberties have been won through ages of struggle and at enormous cost. If these are lost or seriously impaired there can be no hope of continued progress in science, of justice in government, of international or domestic peace; or even of lasting material well-being.

We regard the suppression of independent thought and of its free expression as a major crime against civilization itself. Yet oppression of this sort has been inflicted upon investigators, scholars, teachers and professional men in many ways, whether by governmental action, administrative coercion or extra-legal violence. We feel it our duty to denounce all such actions as intolerable forms of tyranny. There can be no compromise on this issue, for even the commonwealth of learning can not endure "half slave and half free." By our life and training as scientists and by our heritage as Americans we must stand for freedom.

WHEREAS, Science and its applications are not only transforming the physical and mental environment of men, but are adding greatly to the complexities of their social, economic and political relations; and

WHEREAS, Science is wholly independent of national boundaries and races and creeds and can flourish permanently only where there is peace and intellectual freedom; now, therefore, be it

*Resolved*, By the Council on this thirtieth day of December, 1937, that the American Association for the Advancement of Science makes as one of its objectives an examination of the profound effects of science upon society; and that the Association extends to its protype, the British Association for the Advancement of Science, and to all other scientific organizations with similar aims throughout the world, an invitation to cooperate not only in advancing the interests of science but also in promoting peace among nations and intellectual freedom in order that science may continue to advance and to spread more abundantly its benefits to all mankind.

# SCIENTIFIC NOTES AND NEWS

A TESTIMONIAL dinner marking the completion of the first ten years of the administration of Dr. Alexander G. Ruthven as president of the University of Michigan will be given on October 27. Two thousand, six hundred alumni and others are expected to be present. Dr. Ruthven was from 1911 to 1929 professor of zoology at the university.

DR. LEE DE FOREST was honored at the New York World's Fair on September 22 at ceremonies marking Radio Pioneers Day. He addressed scientific men in Paris, via a short-wave broadcast from the French Pavilion. He was the guest of honor and made an address at a luncheon at the Ford exhibit.

THE *Journal* of the American Medical Association reports that the American Legion of South Carolina will confer its 1939 plaque for distinguished service to the state on Dr. Robert Wilson, dean and professor of medicine at the Medical College of the State of South Carolina, Charleston.

THE French Academy of Medicine has awarded the

Grand Prix Prince Albert I de Monaco to Dr. Jules Lefèvre, professor of general agriculture at the Institute of Agronomy, Paris, for his work on biology during the past fifty years.

OFFICERS of the National Association of Science Writers have been elected as follows: William Laurence, of *The New York Times, president;* Robert Potter, Science Service, *vice-president;* Jane Stafford, Science Service, *secretary;* Stephen J. McDonough, Associated Press, Washington, *treasurer.*

V. K. BROWN, director of recreation for the Chicago Park District, was elected president of the American Institute of Park Executives at the recent Philadelphia meeting. He succeeds Samuel N. Baxter, of Philadelphia.

S. F. MARKHAM was elected president of the Museums Association of Great Britain at the recent Cheltenham meeting; Lord Leverhulme and Sir Evan Charteris were elected vice-presidents. The annual meeting in 1940 will be held in Liverpool.

G. ARNOLD, of the National Museum of Southern Rhodesia, has been elected president of the African Museums Association. The meeting in 1940 will be held at Capetown.

AT the annual meeting of the American Neisserian Medical Society held in Milwaukee on June 22, it was voted that the name of Dr. P. S. Pelouze, of Philadelphia, be suggested to the Amory Fund Committee for consideration in connection with the 1940 award. Owing to a misunderstanding it was reported in SCIENCE that the award had been made to Dr. Pelouze.

DR. W. R. HORLACHER, head of the department of animal industry at the University of Arkansas, has become dean of the College of Agriculture and director of the station and of the extension service. H. E. Thompson, head of the Farm Security Administration in Arkansas, has been appointed assistant director of the extension service.

IN the department of zoology of the University of Illinois, Professor Victor E. Shelford has been appointed acting head of the department. New appointments include Assistant Professor C. Ladd Prosser, of Clark University, in charge of general physiology, and Dr. Hurst H. Shoemaker, instructor. The following promotions have been made: Frank B. Adamstone, to an associate professorship; B. Vincent Hall, to an assistant professorship, and Lester Ingle, to an associateship.

DR. WALTER H. BUCHER, professor of geology and chairman of the department of geology and geography at the University of Cincinnati, and Dr. Stephen P. Burke, consulting engineer at Washington, D. C., have been appointed visiting professors at Columbia University. Dr. Bucher will conduct courses in geology, and Dr. Burke will have charge of classes in chemical engineering.

DR. RALPH W. PHILLIPS, physiologist in the Division of Animal Genetics of the Bureau of Animal Industry at Beltsville, Md., has been appointed head of the department of animal husbandry at the Utah State Agricultural College. He will conduct research on the physiology of reproduction and nutrition of range live-stock animals. Dr. Phillips expects to take up the work on November 1.

AT the University of New Hampshire, C. Floyd Jackson, professor of zoology and entomology and dean of the College of Liberal Arts, has been appointed director of the newly established biological institute; Dr. A. F. Yeager, assistant professor of horticulture at the Michigan State College, has become head of the department of horticulture, and Dr. Daniel Clark Lewis, instructor of mathematics at Cornell University, has been appointed assistant professor of mathematics.

DR. THOMAS A. SHALLOW, of Philadelphia, has been elected to the Samuel D. Gross chair of surgery at Jefferson Medical College, Philadelphia. Dr. Shallow is neurological surgeon of the Philadelphia General Hospital and head of the surgical department of Jefferson Hospital. Dr. George P. Muller has been appointed Grace Revere Osler professor of surgery.

DR. ORREN W. HYMAN, dean of the College of Medicine, has been appointed dean of administration at the University of Tennessee. Dr. Conley H. Sanford, associate professor of medicine, has been made professor and head of the department of medicine to succeed Dr. James B. McElroy, who resigned recently because of ill health. Dr. Robert H. Miller, associate professor of anatomy, has been made assistant dean; Dr. Lathan A. Crandall, Jr., associate professor of physiology and pharmacology at Northwestern University, has been appointed head of the department of physiology, and Dr. Lucius C. Sanders, of Memphis, assistant professor of medicine.

THE reorganization of the School of Medicine of the Louisiana State University has resulted in the following appointments: *Dean,* Dr. Beryl Iles Burns; *Assistant to the Dean,* Dr. John Rudolph Schenken; other members of the executive committee are: Drs. Urban Maes, Edgar Hull, Richard Ashman and James T. Nix.

DR. ARTHUR KORN, formerly professor at the Technische Hochschule, Berlin, known for his work in phototelegraphy, has been appointed professor of electrical engineering at the Stevens Institute of Technology. Professor Korn's experiments are said to have led to the first transmission of a photograph on a telephone line and to the first wireless transmission of a photograph from Europe to America.

DR. HERBERT SHAPIRO, of Clark University, who was in 1937 Guggenheim Memorial Foundation fellow at the University of London, has been appointed instructor in physiology at Vassar College.

DR. J. M. WATKINS has been made assistant professor of agronomy and assistant research agronomist at the University of Delaware.

DR. JOSEPH CHANDLER MORRIS, of Princeton University, has been named visiting professor of physics at Newcomb College, Tulane University, for the present academic year. He will fill the temporary vacancy caused by the absence of Dr. Rose L. Mooney, who was recently appointed a Guggenheim fellow and who is now studying in Holland.

AN Associated Press dispatch dated September 22 reports that Dr. Ferdinand Augustus Silcox, chief of the U. S. Forest Service, had been offered by Secretary Harold L. Ickes the post of Under Secretary of the U. S. Department of the Interior, but that he had refused, writing, "that under the circumstances I should remain where I am." The report states that the long-standing Congressional controversy over the transfer of the Forest Service from the Department of Agriculture to the Department of the Interior influenced both the offer and the refusal.

DR. FOREST RAY MOULTON, permanent secretary of the American Association for the Advancement of Science, and Mrs. Moulton reached New York on September 18 on the American Republic liner *Brazil* after spending some weeks in South America.

DR. MELVILLE T. COOK, plant pathologist to the Agricultural Experiment Station of the University of Puerto Rico, has been granted leave of absence until June 30, 1940. He will spend the time in the United States.

DR. FRANK E. EGLER, assistant professor of botany at the New York State College of Forestry, Syracuse, has returned from Martinique, where he spent the summer in ecological investigations with the cooperation and support of the French colonial government. Problems with which he was directly concerned included the growing of mahogany, the restoration of the mangrove forests and the management of arid cattle ranges and watersheds.

APPLICATIONS must be on file with the United States Civil Service Commission at Washington, D. C., not later than October 10 for the positions of principal statistician, at a salary of $5,600 a year; senior statistician, $4,600; statistician, $3,800; associate statistician, $3,200, and assistant statistician, $2,600. Optional subjects for the examinations are: economics, mathematics, public health, sociology, social service, public administration, biological science and engineering and physical science. Further particulars can be obtained from the Civil Service Commission, Washington, D. C.

THE twenty-eighth meeting of the Italian Association for the Advancement of Science is scheduled to meet at Pisa from October 8 to 15.

ANNOUNCEMENT is made that the twenty-sixth French Congress of Hygiene will be held at the Institut Pasteur, Paris, from October 9 to 12. Dr. X. Leclainche is the general secretary of the congress.

THE eighth National Symposium for Organic Chemistry of the American Chemical Society will be held on December 28, 29 and 30 in the auditorium of St. Louis University. The speakers will include: Roger Adams, A. H. Blatt, F. F. Blicke, A. C. Cope, E. A. Doisy, Louis F. Fieser, Henry Gilman, Harold Hibbert, John R. Johnson, W. M. Lauer, Randolph T. Major, Rudolf Schoenheimer, Lee I. Smith and Wm. G. Young.

ACCORDING to the *Journal* of the American Medical Association, the School of Medical Sciences of Wake Forest College will be moved to Winston-Salem, N. C., and will become a four-year school. Funds adequate to develop the school to a capacity of two hundred students have been provided by the Bowman Gray Fund from the estate of the late Mr. Gray, of Winston-Salem.

# DISCUSSION

## IMPORTANT PALEOLITHIC FIND IN CENTRAL ASIA

A DISCOVERY of early human remains of outstanding importance has been made in the latter part of the previous summer (1938) by A. Okladnikov and his wife, young energetic Russian scientists, and may now be definitely reported. It is no less than a find of a Neanderthal child, with characteristic Mousterian implements and an old fauna, in a cave near Baisun, Uzbekistan, Central Asia.

The skeleton of the child lay in a regular burial, in a cave which, located in cliffs, had suffered no disturbance. The long and other bones were largely gone, but the skull and the lower jaw, while in pieces, were found capable of almost a perfect reconstruction, which was ably carried out, under Professor M. Plissetzky's direction, in the Anthropological Institute of the University of Moscow.

The writer was enabled to examine the remains, with the photographic and other records relating to the find, and to get additional information from the discoverers themselves. The skull, with its lower jaw and all the teeth, is the most complete and in general the best Neanderthal cranium yet recovered. It belongs to a normally developed child 8 to 9 years of age. The vault is as well developed as that in the La Quina and Gibraltar children, the supraorbital region, face, lower jaw and teeth denote all unequivocally a Neanderthal specimen. The implements found with the body are typically Mousterian; and the photographic record of the work shows a highly creditable procedure.

Thus, unexpectedly, Central Asia furnishes a first-rate piece of evidence of early man, which is bound to have a great bearing on the concepts of human prehistory in the Old World, and will necessitate a material revision of notions relating to the Neanderthal phase of human antiquity. The easternmost localities of Neanderthaloid remains hitherto known were Palestine, Crimea and the Caucasus—the Uzbekistan find extends the territory far beyond this, and halves the distance from the western Neanderthalers to Peking Man.

Before the writer's departure from Russia Dr. Okladnikov furnished him with the essential details of the find, the first notice of which he published, under the title "Nakhodka neandertalca v Uzbekistanie," in the *Viestnik Drievnei Historii,* 1939, No. 7, pp. 256–7. They are briefly as follows:

In 1938, I was charged by the Marr Institute for the History of Material Culture, and the Committee for Conservation and Study of Cultural Remains attached to the Council of the People's Commissaries of the Uzbek SSR, to search for remains of the Stone Age in the Bukhara District, Uzbekistan, and to check information received about finds of stone implements of the neolithic type in the Daria River Valley. The exploration showed that caves and rock-shelters containing remains of prehistoric man exist in the Valley, and systematic excavations were made in one of the newly found caves, the "Teshik-Tash."

This cave is situated in the upper part of the Shirabad-Daria Valley, near the village Machai, 18 km NW of the town of Baisun. The Turgan River cuts here through the Baisan Tau Mountains, which reach a height of about 8,000 to 9,000 feet above sea-level, and are a part of the Gissar Mountain Range.

The Baisun-Tau Mountains consist of Jurassic limestone. They present many canyons, caves and rock-shelters, with a well-developed Karst landscape.

The Teshik-Tash cave is situated on the NW-slope of the Baisun-Tau, in one of the left-bank canyons of the Turgan-Daria River and high above its level. Above it, the juniper growth runs out, leaving high mountain steppes and subalpine lawns. The cave is dry. Its dimensions are $20 \times 21$ metres, height at the entrance 7 metres. Excavations of its floor showed that it had been inhabited by man only in the paleolithic time. We uncovered five strata with remains of ancient culture, separated by sterile layers. The total depth of the cultural deposits approximated 1.5 metres.

There were many splintered bones in the deposits. They belonged to deer, leopards, wild horses, wild goats (*Capra siberica*), wild boars (*Sus scrofa*), marmots, creepers and birds. Many bones showed scratches and cuts, others had evidently served as anvils for making stone implements. The latter were made on the spot, and mostly of local siliceous limestone. The finest tools were made of jasper, but good materials were scarce, and the inhabitants used also quartzite and even rough quartz.

With the animal bones were found typical mousterian-like discoid nuclei, characteristic flakes, cutting implements and scrapers of mousterian form, small pointed implements chipped on one side, and chips. Most of these objects were related to fireplaces—patches of ashes and carbonaceous matter with underlayer of intensely burnt clay.

The ancient inhabitants of the cave dwelt under the massive roof, by their fires. They made there their implements. They got their living mainly by hunting wild goats. Goat bones prevail in the osteological materials from the cave. Whole horns of huge size, often in pairs and conserving their junction, were found almost in all the layers.

But the most interesting find was that of a human skeleton. This was found directly beneath the first (from above) layer containing cultural remains, being covered by it and embedded in the underlaying sterile stratum. The bones were in a fragmentary state, and many parts of the skeleton had disappeared. What remained were portions of some ribs and of a few limb bones, and finally a skull with the lower jaw. The human bones were surrounded by five pairs of goat horns, three of them united, placed approximately in a circle. Evidently this was a regular burial.

The skeleton belonged to a child. The study of the skull, perfectly restored by M. M. Gerasimov, and that of the other bones, by the anthropologists of the Moscow Anthropologic Institute, shows that they possess all the characteristic features of the Neanderthal man, and approach closely the European Neanderthal remains of similar youth.

The find in the Teshik-Tash cave establishes for the first time the existence of artifacts belonging to the Mousterian period, and the presence of remains of Neanderthal man, in Central Asia.

The exploration of the Uzbekistan caves was resumed by Okladnikov and his wife towards the end of July, this summer. Meanwhile upper paleolithic and extensive neolithic sites have been found by these same two explorers (and in part seen by the writer) along the Angara River up to 75 miles north of Irkutsk; while other paleolithic finds of different ages are being signalled by other Russian explorers in the Urals, in the Crimea and in other western parts of the country.

The USSR authorities deserve the thanks of science for furthering these researches more actively than is now possible or done in any other country.

ALEŠ HRDLIČKA
U. S. NATIONAL MUSEUM

## A SECOND HOUSEHOLD PALM, OMANTHE COSTARICANA

A NEAT little palm brought home in 1902 from mountain forests of eastern Guatemala was described in SCIENCE for August 6, 1937, as *Neanthe bella,* the first member of the palm order to prove well adapted for domestication as a house-plant, flowering and fruiting readily in living rooms, classrooms or laboratories, and opening this group to study as never before. The flowers of the two sexes are specialized and borne on separate plants, but simple methods of pollination have been devised, breeding-stocks are being established at several universities and experiment stations, and additional seeds or young plants are being supplied for educational, experimental or commercial propagation. Two detailed accounts have appeared, with photographs, "A Diminutive Palm from Mayaland," in *The National Horticultural Magazine* for January, 1938, and "Neanthe, a Palm for Genetic Study," in *The Journal of Heredity* for March, 1939.

Another attractive small palm obtained at San Jose, Costa Rica, in 1903, is related to Neanthe and tolerant of household conditions, but of cespitose habit, forming clumps like a bamboo. The creeping root-stocks may be divided, or cuttings may be rooted like "slips" of house-plants, a striking departure from Neanthe, which grows only from seeds. Other obvious differences are larger size and later fruiting, long-jointed trunks, closed leaf-sheaths, strongly veined pinnae and floral adaptations not previously reported. The principal diagnostic characters of the new genus Omanthe are the crassate style, accrescent perianth, excavate embryo, separate triangular male petals, sessile stamens, attenuate pistillode, plicate pinnae, evittate rachis and auriculate petiole-base.

The name Omanthe, meaning shoulder-flower, refers to the remarkably thickened upper part of the pistil, filling the female corolla and raising the stigma to the entrance of the flower, between the narrow recurved angles of the wide overlapping petals. The thickened shoulder may be described as a stylar cushion and compared with the large staminal cushion of Neanthe, the two structures doubtless serving similar functions in retaining moisture, but obviously not homologous. The staminal cushion of Omanthe is very small, the filaments obsolete and the anthers much exceeded by the tall conic-prismatic pistillode.

The type species is *Omanthe costaricana,* described by Oersted in 1858 as *Chamaedorea costaricana,* from the volcano Turrialba. The genus is represented in the U. S. National Herbarium from numerous localities in Costa Rica, including Guanacaste and Nicoya, also from Nicaragua and from the Chiriqui volcano in Panama. Outdoor plants at San Jose reach a height of 8 to 10 feet and form striking clusters of bright green foliage.

The leaf-sheaths are longer than in Neanthe, the petioles shorter and the leaf-blades larger; the pinnae, 17–20 on a side, more widely spaced, longer and more tapering, more curved and drooping and more prominently 5-veined, a single intermediate vein on each side stronger than the others, though weaker than the submarginal vein. The rachis and petiole uniform green underneath, lacking the pale stripe of many related palms. The mouth of the leaf-sheath has a triangular stipule-like tooth on each side, at the base of the petiole.

The inflorescences are developed below the leaves, the peduncle slender with 7 or 8 joints, the second extremely short, 5 or 6 joints with narrow scarious spathes; the axis emergent, relatively short; branches 20–35 in the male, 10–15 in the female, the male branches longer and the flowers closer together, though not crowded; base of branches often decurrent, the subtending bracts represented by broad short rims. Female calyx and corolla accrescent and persistent, yellow with brown margins. Staminodes minute, usually 3, opposite the petals, oblong or tapering, the apex thin and pale, truncate or retuse, doubtless a rudiment of the anther.

Fruits broadly oval, nearly round, turning black from green, only the point of attachment yellow like the branches; exocarp firmly fleshy, forming a rather tough rind coarsely wrinkled in drying, lined with a thin green pulp and a close network of fine mesocarp fibers. Seeds spherical, marked on each side by a widely arcuate groove, the embryo subbasal, the cavity protected by a specialized operculum minutely apiculate outside and an endosperm lining with a central prominence accommodated by a cavity in the base of the embryo. Seedling with first leaf simple, broadly v-shaped.

A single large inflorescence had somewhat larger fruits and more accrescent perianths, many of these with four calyx-lobes and only two petals, a notable example of metaphanic variation or replacement in a group generally adhering regularly to its basic number three. The petal that subtends the stigma often is smaller than the other two, and where only two petals are present the stigma usually is exposed, though not in all cases. On a greenhouse plant of Omanthe two forms of abortive fruits were developed from pollination with Neanthe and another related palm, as shown in the *Journal of Heredity.*

Only a few clusters of Omanthe, without flowers or seeds, were seen at San Jose in June, 1903, and only a female plant obtained, but now this palm has become a popular ornamental, variously used in open plantings, hedges, screens and arbors. "Pacaya" is the local name, though also applied to related kinds, more properly to those that have edible inflorescences. The present status of the palm in San Jose was observed by Mr. Loren G. Polhamus, of the U. S. Department of Agriculture, in December, 1938. Flowers of both sexes were collected, but no seeds were found, and even in March, 1939, when another visit to Costa Rica was made, only green fruits had developed. A rather definite seasonal habit is indicated, flowering in December and ripening its fruits in May, the fleshy pericarp doubtless attracting birds and the seeds scattered before the summer rains.

Through the kindness of Mr. W. E. Klippert, of the Goodyear Rubber Plantations Company, it was possible to arrange for ripe fruits to be sent, and a generous shipment reached Washington in May, 1939. The seeds were in excellent condition, were planted at once and germinated promptly. By the middle of July many seedlings had appeared, and a few had reached the stage of opening their first leaves. Thus adequate tests are in prospect at field stations and with private growers, to determine the value of the palm for household use with Neanthe and also for outdoor planting in Florida and California.

O. F. COOK

U. S. DEPARTMENT OF AGRICULTURE

## FRESH-WATER MEDUSAE FOUND IN KIATING, SZECHUEN, CHINA[1]

Two species of fresh-water medusae were found in a pond along Tatu River, Kiating, Szechuen, China, in association with tadpoles, green algae, diatoms, protozoa, rotifers, small Crustacea and other aquatic forms. The pond is about four hundred meters long, thirty meters wide and two meters deep, the bottom of which is covered by sand and gravel. The water is fairly clear, and at the time of the discovery of the medusae its temperature and hydrogen ion concentration were 12° C and 7.2, respectively.

One species, possibly a variety of *Craspedacusta sowerbii,* was found on January 14, 1939. A large number of them has been found since then, mostly on sunny days. The average diameter of the umbrella measures about 2.2 cm during expansion and 1.6 cm during contraction, although much smaller young and un-mature forms were observed. The manubrium is rather long; its ratio to the diameter of the umbrella is about 1:1.5. The height of the umbrella varies, of course, with the diameter as well as the activity of the animal, whether it is in expansion or in contraction. The number of tentacles is not constant, being variable from 259 to 272. They are of seven kinds in respect to their length, arranged radially around the margin of the umbrella with more or less regularity. Located at the base of the velum and inside of the small canals (which are in direct connection with the circumferential canal) are sense organs whose number varies from 129 to 146. The gonads as four greenish pocket-like outgrowths are situated at the junction of the gastrovascular cavity and the four radial canals.

The other species found in the same pond on February 12, 1939, is much smaller, whose average diameter is about 7. cm during expansion and .45 cm during contraction. The manubrium is relatively shorter. Its ratio to the diameter of the umbrella is about 1:2. The number of tentacles varies from 44 to 115, and they are of four kinds in respect to their length. Sense organs and gonads are located at the same positions as those of the preceding species, but the number of sense organs is less, only 29 to 71. So far, only four such specimens were found.

It might be interesting to note, in view of the observations made by Powers,[2] that the medusae we collected on January 14 have been living since in our unaerated aquarium, in which, however, the water is constantly changed, without showing any visible abnormality.

H. ZANYIN GAW

L. H. KUNG

NATIONAL WUHAN UNIVERSITY,
KIATING, SZECHUEN, CHINA

[1] The detailed description of the organisms will appear shortly in the Biological Science Series of the Science Reports of National Wuhan University.

[2] Edwin B. Powers, SCIENCE, 88: 498, November 25, 1938.

## ANTHELMINTIC ACTIVITY OF FRESH PINEAPPLE JUICE

THE use of latexes from Ficus species as anthelmintics has been known for a very long time. Robbins[1] and Walti[2] as well as others have shown that the enzyme ficin which they obtained from some of these latexes was the active agent responsible for the digestion of the parasites.

Since ficin, papain and bromelin belong to the class of so-called papain enzymes, it occurred to the authors that the bromelin of pineapple juice might exhibit anthelmintic activity similar to that of the ficin of the latexes. On looking over the scientific literature on pineapple juice no reference was found on the matter. However, it has been reported that the juice has been used in folk medicine as an anthelmintic.[3]

Living *Ascaris lumbricoides* and *Macracanthorynchus hirundinaceus,* obtained from hog's intestines, were incubated at a temperature of from 35° to 40° C. with pineapple juice freshly squeezed from a Cuban

[1] B. H. Robbins, *Jour. Biol. Chem.,* 87: 251, 1930.

[2] A. J. Walti, *Jour. Biol. Chem.,* 119, *Sci. Proc. Soc. Biochem.,* 31. Ci., 1937.

[3] K. M. Nadkarni, "The Indian Materia Medica," p. 62. Bombay, 1927.

pineapple. At the end of 24 hours both parasites were completely digested, while controls incubated in heat-inactivated pineapple juice and in saline solution were very lively and active.

The results obtained indicate that the juice possesses enzymatic activity similar in nature to that of some Ficus latexes, and therefore there is some scientific basis for its use as an anthelmintic.

The much wider availability and cheapness of fresh pineapple juice suggest it as a more practical source of non-toxic, ficin-like anthelmintic.

JULIUS BERGER
CONRADO F. ASENJO,
*Guggenheim Memorial Fellow, Latin-American Exchange*
UNIVERSITY OF WISCONSIN

# QUOTATIONS

## THE VOICE OF SCIENCE

ONCE more the burden of war is laid upon us. Once more, as in 1914, the cynical disregard of Germany for the rights of small nations has constrained the British people to take up arms in the cause of justice and fair dealing in international relations. The challenge of the German Reich has been accepted reluctantly, and with no illusions as to the nature of the glories of modern warfare, only after every effort to secure a peaceful but equitable settlement of the differences between Germany and Poland has failed. It has been accepted with full realization of the gravity of every implication of the decision. But in turning to war as the last resort, the British people has acted with a unanimity such as never before in its history, and with a grim determination that no effort shall be spared in the endeavor to ensure that the cause which it holds just shall prevail.

From 1914–18, the Allies opposed dynastic ambitions in the interests of the freedom of peoples. No longer were the people to be the pawns of the political intrigues of their rulers. The world, it was said, was to be made safe for democracy—words that now have a mocking ring. In 1939, the canker has sunk deeper. It is not merely political liberty that is at stake, though that too is jeopardized. It is the spirit of man.

In no previous war has science played so great a part as that which will be demanded of it in the struggle that is at hand. For a time, while the issue hangs in the balance, it is the duty of the man of science to lay aside his just misgivings whether the greatest force of the human intellect should thus be harnessed to the forces of destruction. For the moment, the interests of pure science as an intellectual pursuit and discipline must remain in abeyance. The energies, the abilities and the knowledge of each and every individual with scientific training must be directed without remission to the service of the Allied cause. Nevertheless, the end to be attained, and the end which science should hold ceaselessly before the eyes of the Allied peoples, is not destruction, but a constructive ideal—to ensure in the future such conditions as will make possible the advancement of all the peoples of the world without discrimination, according to the status and the traditions of each, in the light shed by reason and scientific knowledge. To keep alive the aims of science in furthering the pursuit of truth in the universe and the relation of that truth to the developments of man's nature, without regard to tribal and racial distinctions, should be, indeed, must be, the ultimate function of the scientific thinker, whatever may be his more immediate preoccupations.

As to the form in which that ideal will find embodiment, at the moment, in the turmoil of initial operations, it is too soon to attempt a forecast; but that it is no idealist's dream is certain. The failure of the League of Nations as a political organization has cast discredit in the popular mind on such forms of international cooperation. Possibly the League of Nations came before its time, and this has obscured in the popular verdict the enormous value of its scientific work in the study of social and economic problems, and the progress which has followed, where the practical application of the solutions suggested has not conflicted with the trends of nationalist development. To extend the fields in which such cooperation between peoples may be applied is the task of the future, when the time comes, as it surely will, for reconstruction.—*Nature*.

# SCIENTIFIC BOOKS

## ELECTROMAGNETICS

*Electromagnetics; a Discussion of Fundamentals.* By ALFRED O'RAHILLY. xii + 884 pp. Longmans Green and Co., 1938. 42/– net.

ANY one who has attempted to write a logical presentation of electromagnetics is quite aware of the difficulties and so should welcome this essay in constructive criticism published by the Cork University Press.

A good amplified presentation is given of the usual mathematical analysis and the existence of different views is shown by numerous quotations from the writings of prominent authors. In some cases the views of a writer are only partially expressed in the sentence quoted, and it is not clear what part the quotation is intended to play in the discussion. In some other cases the quotation serves as a definition; as, for instance, when a physical theory is defined, after Duhem, as a system of mathematical propositions deduced from a small number of principles whose object is to represent a group of experimental laws as simply, completely and exactly as possible. Such a definition makes constructive criticism a natural part of theoretical physics, for every presentation of a theory must be examined to ascertain how far the desired perfection has been obtained. Duhem's "sole test of a physical theory" is mentioned and reiterated in the following quotation from Dirac's "Principles of Quantum Mechanics," p. 7. "The only object of theoretical physics is to calculate results that can be compared with experiment; and it is quite unnecessary that any description of the whole course of the phenomena should be given." This statement, taken alone, seems too restrictive unless there is an intention to distinguish between theoretical physics and mathematical physics. The chief aim of the mathematician is to find out how to make calculations and to construct a language of symbols which will make it possible to think clearly about physical phenomena and to formulate the conventions under which the comparisons with experiments are to be made. The way to make calculations is often far from evident; it is important, moreover, to be able to choose an expeditious way and to be able to judge whether it is worth while to make the calculations. Mathematicians are glad to welcome any device or means of representation that may help them in their difficulties.

In an attempt to clarify the situation produced by the use of the word aether in at least three different senses the author recommends the use of the word schesis to denote the framework of reference used in the formulation of the electromagnetic equations. The absolute velocities occurring in these equations are then described as schesic velocities. With this proposition the reviewer is wholly in sympathy. The term absolute seems too drastic for the velocities in the scheme of representation that has been found most convenient. It should be emphasized also that relative velocity can only be defined when a scheme of representation has been chosen.

The reviewer would go further and recommend that the word aether should now be restricted to the sense in which it has become associated with the ideas of Heraclitus, who regarded everything as being in a state of flux and compared matter with a flame which burns or transforms the aether. As Heraclitus emphasizes the idea of force and the present author endeavors to found electromagnetics on the force formula between two moving electrons he may be regarded as a follower of Heraclitus who has an open mind with regard to the exact law of force, since he discusses the law of Ritz as well as that of Liénard and shows that Ritz's law accounts for some phenomena quite well.

Some writers may, of course, prefer to still associate the word aether with the "indeterminate" of Anaximander or the starry firmament. Thus Livens says in a portion of the passage quoted on page 630. "What happens in the space between (space is that something which can be occupied by matter) we do not and can not know."

The idea of space seems, however, to be inseparably connected with some scheme of representation. Any one familiar with the theory of geometrical transformations knows that two points which are contiguous in one representation may be separated in another. It is unlikely that there is an exact one to one correspondence between the descriptions of the universe obtained in different laboratories when, according to one description, there is an acceleration of one laboratory relative to the other. In actual life correspondences are seldom exact over a great range. The mathematical estimate of the closeness of fit of a correspondence may well play a part in an attempt to define pleasure and pain, good and evil.

The idea of empty space is just as difficult as that of an indeterminate aether. A distance between two points can only be measured by placing a yardstick or other measuring device in the "vacant region," in one sense, then, the interval has no existence until the yardstick is in place.

The fundamental electromagnetic equations do not require time to be associated permanently with each point of the framework arbitrarily chosen for a scheme of representing location. The equations merely state that when *a* time has been associated with each point according to some continuous law, then two flux relations hold. The equations do not even involve the velocity of light. This enters only when an attempt is made by the introduction of constitutive relations between the four electromagnetic vectors to account for observed physical phenomena.

A theoretical physicist is sometimes satisfied with a physical theory when calculated results agree with experiment. In some cases, however, the calculated results depend only on the characteristics of the partial differential equations used in the theory and may be the same in innumerable other theories in which the partial differential equations have the same characteristics. The mathematician can not then be satisfied by a simple agreement with experiment. He must scrutinize a theory carefully to ascertain what features of the theory are really confirmed by experiment.

The book under review contains discussions of many matters. Relativity and other recent theories are discussed. The ideas of Einstein and Maxwell are criticized. The author has little respect for authority, and this alone may entice readers to buy the book. The idea of localized energy is regarded as useless except in the case of radiation and the idea of stress in a medium is regarded as not helpful. The idea of contact action is just as difficult to comprehend as that of action at a distance.

H. Bateman

## THE PHILOSOPHY OF PHYSICS

*On Understanding Physics.* By W. H. Watson. Cambridge University Press, 1938.

This book is one more indication that interest in what has been variously termed the philosophy of physics or the logic of physics continues unabated. Sooner or later every physicist succumbs to the temptation to probe more deeply into the foundations of physical theories in the attempt to associate more meaning with what he is doing. The ultimate advantage of this procedure is not that it settles anything but that it does place certain problems in a clearer light. In some measure it also affords physicists an opportunity to clarify their philosophical tastes.

The author of the present volume believes that philosophy has great value in clarifying physical problems, but he also makes clear his opinion that the only kind of philosophy valuable for this purpose is that confined to the study of the logic of language. This sort of philosophizing has recently received much attention through the work of Wittgenstein and also the so-called Vienna circle of logical positivists. The author acknowledges his debt to Wittgenstein for the original stimulus to the present work. The first two chapters of the book are largely devoted to an expression and defense of the view-point that "the function of philosophy . . . is to clear up an understanding of the use of symbolism" and that psychology has little or nothing to do with the logic of physics.

The rest of the volume consists of four not completely integrated essays embodying the application of the author's ideas to various physical theories. There is indeed a common thread running throughout the discussion, namely, the emphasis that in its description of experience physics employs various methods of representation depending on the problem in hand. Unfortunately since the author does not make precisely clear what he means by a "method of representation," the reader will be forced to place his own interpretation on the treatment. The reviewer has the impression that *any* physical theory is an attempted representation of nature. On this view the author appears to be trying to say that whenever we have constructed a physical theory, in every application of the theory we must be careful to preserve consistency with the definitions and postulates of the theory and not try to mix in ideas from another and different theory. It is unlikely that physicists will disagree with this view.

In an interesting chapter on the "Nature of Mechanism" the author makes a few trenchant remarks about causality and points out that the wide-spread belief that quantum theory has abandoned causality is based on a misconception of the physicists' interpretation of this concept. It should perhaps be emphasized that to the author mechanism means simply the determinateness of physical theories, *i.e.,* the fact that theories make *precise predictions* from their postulates. It is not confined to mechanical or dynamical theories as commonly understood.

The last two chapters contain discussions of the concepts of substance and motion and certain aspects of the use of symbolism in mechanics and electricity. Most of the applications here are to classical physics.

The book as a whole is by no means easy reading. The reviewer feels that a closer integration of the various chapters would have enabled the reader better to grasp the gist of the author's admittedly carefully considered opinions and analysis of fundamental questions in the logic of physics.

R. B. Lindsay

Brown University

## MEADOW AND PASTURE INSECTS

*Meadow and Pasture Insects.* By Herbert Osborn. pp. i + viii, 1 + 288, 100 text illustrations. The Educators Press, Columbus, Ohio, 1939.

The meadow and pasture lands of the country are an important part of the agricultural area of the country. They comprised in the West in 1909 over 80 per cent. of the area and about 60 per cent. of the value of all crops in that part of the country.

This volume presents the first comprehensive account of the part insects play in reducing forage crops, especially grasses. There have been a number of excellent publications upon some of the more injurious species affecting these crops. It has remained for the author to bring together the results of his studies of grass-infesting species extending over a period of more than fifty years. He has been led to conclude that a reduction of nearly 50 per cent. in the forage after land has been in grass three or four years is largely due to insect levies. This is certainly of much practical importance to all owners of grazing land and all owners of live stock, particularly since the author discusses conditions which favor the multiplication of these pests and outlines practical methods for reducing losses of this character.

The ecologist will find much of interest in the volume in the extended discussion of the ecology of the meadow.

The author deals first with the physical factors of the meadow environment and secondly biological factors, the two producing a most important and far-reaching complex, admirably presented in diagrammatic form on page 41. It is necessary to give these factors careful study if practical methods for the reduction of injuries are to be worked out. The summary account of the animal groups of the meadow fauna is another interesting and practical phase.

The entomologist, aside from the general discussion of injuries, ecology and control, will find the accounts of different groups of insects occurring in meadows and pastures comprehensive and suggestive. This is particularly true of the Hemiptera-Homoptera, the group with which the author is most familiar. The book contains excellent illustrations and biographical data concerning numerous species, much of the information resulting from the author's investigations. This book is a handy source of information concerning these numerous important and largely unknown forms. The more technically minded will find here and there long lists of insects taken in various environments. There is also an extended bibliography and an excellent index which adds much to the value of the book.

The book is a valuable contribution to our knowledge of meadow and pasture insects. The author is to be congratulated upon the admirable and convincing presentation, while the publisher has done much to present this information in an attractive form.

E. P. FELT
BARTLETT TREE RESEARCH LABORATORIES,
STAMFORD, CONN.

# SOCIETIES AND MEETINGS

## FUNGI AND FUNGOUS DISEASES

FOR the first time at an International Congress for Microbiology a special section was organized to consider fungi and fungous diseases. Dr. R. A. Harper, emeritus professor of botany at Columbia University, and Dr. Fred D. Weidman, professor of dermatological research at the University of Pennsylvania, were copresidents of this section. Dr. B. O. Dodge, of the New York Botanical Garden, served as convener. Seventy-seven papers were presented. In spite of the fact that many foreign delegates were prevented from attending by the outbreak of the European war, twelve papers were read by foreign delegates representing Belgium, Brazil, Canada, Ceylon, England, Holland, Scotland, Sweden and Uruguay. The large number of papers submitted made it necessary to divide the section into two divisions, and eight sessions were held. Interest in the programs was evidenced by the large attendance at the meetings, and at one session on "Growth Substances" there was "standing room only."

As this was one of the first scientific meetings in which students of animal and veterinary medicine and students of plant pathology participated, a symposium was held on host parasite relationships for the purpose of comparing the processes of fungus infections of plants and animals. It was organized from the point of view of the animal kingdom by Dr. Fred Weidman, of Philadelphia, and the point of view of the plant kingdom by Dr. E. K. Stakman, of St. Paul. Papers were presented discussing: (1) Etiology of pathogenesis; (2) tissue reactions; (3) natural resistance, including immunity. It was apparent that further exchange of views of this sort would prove stimulating to workers in both fields.

On two mornings joint meetings were held with Section II (microbiological chemistry and physiology) on the subject of growth substances for microorganisms. These concerned mostly the effect of various elements in the nutrition of fungi and bacteria. Under the able direction of Dr. W. J. Robbins, of the New York Botanical Garden, speakers from the fields of chemistry, physiology, bacteriology and mycology were brought together for the discussion of the effects of these elements on the growth of organisms.

Under the direction of Dr. B. O. Dodge another program was devoted to sex, variation and genetics of the fungi, while Dr. M. Levine, Montefiore Hospital, New York City, sponsored a third session on the effects of microorganisms and chemical substances on atypical growth in plants. The latter papers concerned chiefly the production of plant tumors by bacteria or chemical agents. Another session was held jointly with Section I (Variation in Taxonomy) at which the classification and nomenclature of the Actinomycetes and yeast-like fungi were discussed in a number of papers. As a result of this discussion it was recommended that a committee be appointed to report at the next congress on the possibility of adopting some uniform nomenclature for the pathogenic fungi.

A number of papers were presented discussing various fungus diseases of man, including four papers on the ringworm infections and two on histoplasmosis. Dr. Carrion, of Puerto Rico, presented a study of the fungi of chromoblastomycosis, and Dr. W. A. E. Karunaratne reported a series of 104 cases of Rhinosporidiosis.

Dr. B. O. Dodge presented one of the main addresses of the general session of the congress on the subject of "Some Problems in the Genetics of the Fungi."

J. GARDNER HOPKINS
J. S. KARLING
*Secretaries*

# SPECIAL ARTICLES

## THE ROLE OF MICROORGANISMS IN THE CONSERVATION OF THE SOIL

CONSIDERABLE public attention has been focussed in recent years upon the problem of soil conservation, largely because of the effort made by the Federal Government to initiate large-scale investigations and to establish soil conservation agencies and special experiment stations in all parts of the country. Most of the investigations in this field have been largely based upon agronomic approaches and practical methods for preventing soil and water losses. Although some attention has been paid to the physical and chemical soil conditions, comparatively little consideration has been given to the possible role of the numerous soil-inhabiting microorganisms in the process of soil conservation. It is also generally recognized that soil organic matter, with which the soil organisms are intimately connected, plays an important part in conserving the soil; however, little is known as to whether this phenomenon is due to the organic matter as a whole or whether only a certain fraction of the organic matter is involved in the process.

A consideration of this important national problem, from a microbiological point of view, brings forth several phases which deserve careful investigation, namely: (1) the function of the cells of microorganisms, especially the mycelium of the fungi and actinomycetes, as soil-binding agents; (2) the production by microorganisms, notably by bacteria, of specific substances, such as slimy materials, which aid in binding the soil particles; (3) the specific stage of decomposition of organic matter added to the soil when it is most active in bringing about a binding or aggregation of the soil particles; (4) the formation, as a result of decomposition, of chemical complexes, comprising certain humus constituents, such as the so-called "humic acid" compounds, which exert a physical or perhaps even chemical effect upon the inorganic soil particles.

In a series of studies carried out at the New Jersey Agricultural Experiment Station, an attempt has been made to throw light upon some of these problems. These studies comprise both laboratory and field investigations.

Because the soil microorganisms differ in the type of growth and in the nature of the substances synthesized, it is logical to suppose that some organisms will affect the physical properties of the soil to a different degree or in a different manner from others. In order to ascertain the extent of soil binding and aggregation brought about by microorganisms, artificial soils were employed consisting of sterile sand-bentonite and sand-clay mixtures. Sucrose or cellulose were used as sources of energy, and nutrient salt solutions were added. The artificial soils were adjusted to optimum moisture and inoculated with pure cultures of fungi and bacteria or with a soil infusion. After various periods of incubation, the contents of the flasks were analyzed, using certain procedures designed to show relative differences in the binding effect upon the soil particles.

Certain typical results are presented in Table I.

TABLE I

BINDING EFFECT OF MICROORGANISMS UPON THE FINE PARTICLES IN SAND-BENTONITE MIXTURES[1]

| Energy source | Organism | Pipette method | | Slope method | |
|---|---|---|---|---|---|
| | | Unbound material in 50 gm | Bound | Unbound material in 50 gm | Bound |
| | | gm | per cent. | gm | per cent. |
| Sucrose | Control | 2.12 | 0 | 1.1 | 0 |
| " | *Rhizopus nigricans* | 2.07 | 3 | 0.7 | 36 |
| " | *Aspergillus niger* | 1.60 | 25 | 0.3 | 72 |
| " | *Azotobacter indicum* | 1.57 | 26 | 0.45 | 60 |
| " | *Bacterium fluorescens* | 1.90 | 10 | 0.7 | 36 |
| " | Soil infusion | 1.76 | 17 | 0.6 | 45 |
| Cellulose | Control | 1.86 | 0 | 0.8 | 0 |
| " | *Trichoderma köningi* | 1.54 | 18 | 0.6 | 26 |
| " | *Trichoderma + A. fumigatus* | 1.61 | 14 | 0.65 | 21 |
| " | *Trichoderma + Penicillium* | 1.48 | 21 | 0.6 | 26 |
| " | Soil infusion | 1.11 | 41 | 0.45 | 45 |

[1] Incubation period, 23 days for sucrose cultures and 55 days for cellulose cultures.

They show beyond a doubt that soil microorganisms exert an important binding effect upon the fine soil particles and that the degree of binding depends on the organisms involved. The contents of the flasks containing the fungi showed that the whole mass of artificial soil was held together by an extensive mycelial network. When the material was dried, it fell apart in a granular state. The contents of the flasks inoculated with *Azotobacter indicum* were held together by the slimy substances produced by the organism. Similar results were obtained by the use of sand-clay mixtures.

It is well established that when fresh or decomposed organic matter is added to the soil it brings about favorable changes in the physical properties of the soil, with a tendency to decrease soil erosion. The favorable effect is believed to be due primarily to a mechanical binding of the soil particles by the organic matter and to an increased aggregation of the soil brought about by physico-chemical interactions between the organic matter and the soil constituents. Increased moisture-absorbing and moisture-holding capacities might also be a factor. These changes increase percolation and infiltration, which in turn decrease run-off and erosion. If there were no microorganisms in the soil to decompose the organic matter the effect would be largely mechanical. However, when fresh organic matter is added to the soil countless organisms immediately begin to decompose it. Decomposition products and substances synthesized by the organisms interact with the fine soil particles, causing them to aggregate. The organisms themselves also tend to bind the soil particles.

Since plants and humus deposits differ in chemical composition, it is likely that organic matter from various sources will not affect the physical properties of the soil alike. In certain experiments designed to determine the effect of various typs of organic matter on the physical properties of the soil, related to soil erosion, a field soil was treated with alfalfa, straw, manure and peat material. At various intervals the total organic carbon, moisture-holding capacity, infiltration capacity and dispersion ratio were determined. The results showed that all four types of organic matter increased the infiltration capacity, with peat being most effective. Alfalfa, straw and manure brought about a rapid increase in the number of water-stable aggregates, as measured by the dispersion ratio, with alfalfa producing the greatest increase. Peat caused only a small increase in aggregation. After three months' decomposition, under favorable moisture and temperature conditions, the increase in aggregation had almost disappeared in the case of straw and peat; it was still apparent to some extent in the case of the manure and was quite marked in the alfalfa-treated soil.

In conclusion it may be stated that the role of microorganisms in soil conservation is highly important and is closely associated with the transformation of the organic matter added to the soil.

The detailed results of these experiments and the methods employed will be published in *Soil Science*.

SELMAN A. WAKSMAN
JAMES P. MARTIN
NEW JERSEY AGRICULTURAL EXPERIMENT STATION,
NEW BRUNSWICK

## ON THE MOLECULAR WEIGHT OF THE TOBACCO MOSAIC VIRUS PROTEIN

IN recognition of the unreliability of the value of 17 million for the molecular weight of the tobacco mosaic virus protein, as calculated from the sedimentation constant[1,2] of $170\text{–}200 \times 10^{-13}$, Stanley[3,4,5] and his co-workers have recently attempted a correction for the molecular weight by a combination of the data obtained by means of the standard Ostwald viscometer and the Kuhn, the Eisenschitz and the Perrin equations. The assumptions were that one could estimate the value for the relative dimensions of the elongated particles from viscosity data, and that these relative dimensions could be used in calculating the asymmetry constant to be used in conjunction with the data obtained from the ultracentrifuge. It has been protested[5] that the failure of the protein-water system to follow the Poiseuill's and Fick's law is not of sufficient importance to impair the usefulness of these methods in determining the asymmetry constant, and that all the data relative to the size and shape of the virus protein molecule are in good agreement.

An appreciation of the extent to which sols of the virus protein deviate from Fick's law may be obtained from Fig. 1. The data presented were obtained from a

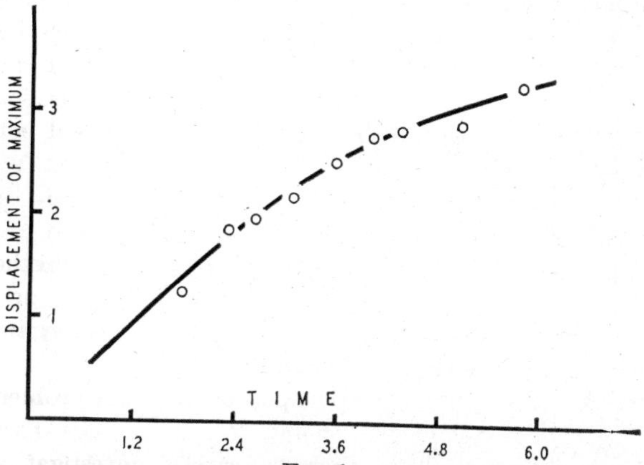


FIG. 1.

diffusion study, using the refractory method of Lamm,[6] of a sol containing .87 per cent. electrodialyzed protein dispersed in distilled water. As has been pointed out,[7,8] the curves obtained by plotting the displacement of the scale lines against the original line positions in the case of the virus protein are skewed, and the point of maximum displacement is shifted toward the solvent side. The rate of drift of the point of maximum displacement is shown in Fig. 1. The abscissa is in $10^5$ seconds; the ordinate is in millimeters. The ratio of the distance from the midpoint of the diffusion cell to the lens to the distance from the midpoint of the cell to the scale was .78. Substances that obey the normal laws of diffusion yield curves that are symmetrical with the maximum displacement at the original interface.

The normalized curves deviate markedly from the ideal. The maximum ordinates in normalized coordinates obtained after 1.78 and $5.85 \times 10^5$ seconds respectively were .62 and .74. The ordinate of the maximum for the ideal curve

$$y = \frac{1}{\sqrt{2\pi}} \quad e^{\frac{-x^2}{2}}$$

is .40. Following the "maximum height" method of

[1] Eriksson Quensel and T. Svedberg, *Jour. Am. Chem. Soc.*, 58: 1863, 1936.
[2] R. W. G. Wyckoff, S. Biscoe and W. M. Stanley, *Jour. Biol. Chem.*, 117: 57, 1937.
[3] M. A. Lauffer, SCIENCE, 87: 469, 1938.
[4] H. S. Loring, M. A. Lauffer and W. M. Stanley, *Nature*, 142: 841, 1938.
[5] M. A. Lauffer and W. M. Stanley, *Chem. Rev.*, 24: 303, 1939.

[6] O. Lamm, *Zeit. Physik. Chem.*, Abt. A 138: 313, 1928.
[7] V. L. Frampton and A. M. Saum, SCIENCE, 89: 84, 1939.
[8] H. Neurath and A. M. Saum, *Jour. Biol. Chem.*, 126: 435, 1938.

Lamm,[9] in calculating the diffusion constant, and neglecting the viscosity, values of 2.0 and $2.1 \times 10^{-8}$ were obtained from the initial and final photographs. It seems fair to state, however, that one is justified in calculating the molecular weight of the virus protein from these data, providing he can account for the peculiar diffusion behavior in a quantitative manner.

In Fig. 2, values for the ratio of the short to the

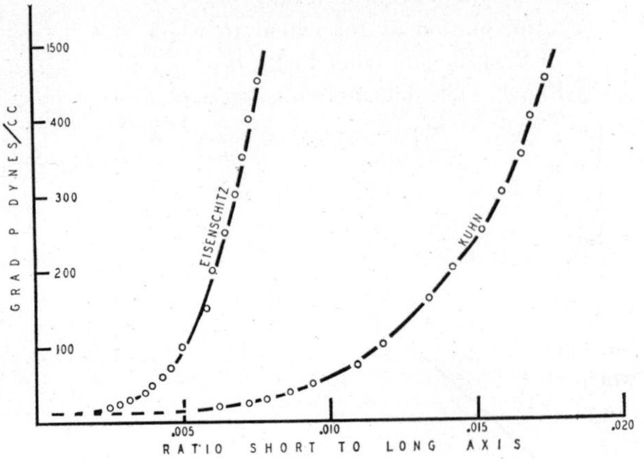


FIG. 2.

long axis of the virus protein at various shearing stresses, as calculated from Frampton's[10] data using the Kuhn and Eisenschitz equations, are plotted against the pressure gradient along the capillary of the capillary viscometer. These two equations may legitimately be used for solutions of elongated particles that obey Poiseuille's law in the case of a random orientation of the particles—ostensibly for a solution at rest. The extrapolated value of the short to long axis is zero; that is, the extrapolated value for the ratio of the long to the short axis for the quiescent fluid is infinite. In the Perrin equation

$$\frac{1}{R} = \frac{\left(\frac{a}{b}\right)^{2/3}}{\sqrt{1-\left(\frac{a}{b}\right)^2}} \log \frac{1+\sqrt{1-\left(\frac{a}{b}\right)^2}}{\frac{a}{b}},$$

where a/b is the ratio of the short to the long axis and R is the asymmetry constant, as a/b becomes smaller and smaller, the value of

$$\frac{\left(\frac{a}{b}\right)^{2/3}}{\sqrt{1-\left(\frac{a}{b}\right)^2}}$$

approaches zero more rapidly than

$$\log \frac{1+\sqrt{1-\left(\frac{a}{b}\right)^2}}{\frac{a}{b}}$$

approaches infinity. That is, in the limit, 1/R is zero, and R is infinite. Substituting the value of R in the well-known equation

$$R = \frac{M(1-\zeta v)}{6\pi\eta_0 NS_{20}\left(\frac{3Mv}{4\pi N}\right)^{1/3}}$$

where M is the molecular weight, we see that in the legitimate use of these methods the corrected value for the molecular weight of the virus protein, as determined by ultracentrifuge means, is infinite. From a similar consideration, the corrected value for the molecular weight as determined by means of diffusion is zero.

VERNON L. FRAMPTON

CORNELL UNIVERSITY

## UPWARD TRANSPORT OF MINERALS THROUGH THE PHLOEM OF STEMS

IN 1937 Gustafson and Darken[1,2] showed that radioactive phosphorus was conducted upward in the stem of a plan through the bark. In the second paper it was suggested that to get a quantitative comparison between the conduction in the xylem and the phloem the part of the plant above the cut of xylem or phloem should be ashed and the total activity determined. This has now been done with *Bryophyllum calycinum* and *Salix* sp.

The experiments were conducted as before, except that the activity was determined with a Geiger counter. Usually three plants as alike as it was possible to select were used in each experiment; one was used as control, the second had a section of the xylem removed and the third plant a girdle of bark removed. In some plants the xylem was separated from the bark for a distance of several centimeters, but a piece was not removed, only a cut was made at the lower end of the xylem-phloem separation. The lower end of this bare xylem was kept in a test-tube of water during the experiment to supply the top with an abundance of water, as it was found in some experiments, where a portion of xylem had been removed, that the leaves wilted soon after the experiment was set up.

At the end of the experiment the plants were cut off at the level where the girdle had been made and the two parts ashed separately. The lower part has been designated roots, even though several inches of the base of the stem was included. The ashing was done in a muffle furnace at 650° C.

The ash was dissolved in 10 to 20 ml of 10 per cent. HCl, depending upon the amount of ash. An aliquot (.2 to 1.0 ml, depending upon the activity of the phosphorus) was allowed to be absorbed by a piece of blot-

9 O. Lamb, *Zeit. Physik. Chem.*, Abt. 143: 177, 1929.

10 V. L. Frampton, *Jour. Biol. Chem.*, 129: 233, 1939.

1 F. G. Gustafson and Marjorie Darken, SCIENCE, 85: 482–493, 1937.

2 F. G. Gustafson and Marjorie Darken, *Amer. Jour. Bot.*, 24: 615–621, 1937.

ting paper somewhat smaller than the window over the target of the counter. This piece of blotting paper was then placed on the window over the target. The number of counts were noted for a certain length of time and the counts per minute calculated, and from this was subtracted the background count to give the number of counts due to the plant material. This count per minute was multiplied by the proper factor to obtain the count for all the ash, per minute. The total active phosphorus in the tops or roots was determined only in experiment 37, but as determined the activity in the different parts is strictly comparable and the figures in the table denote the number of counts that would have been observed per minute if all the ash of the particular part of the plant had been placed above the target of the counter.

Table 1 gives the number of beta particles originating in the irradiated phosphorus of the ash that would have hit the target of the Geiger counter per minute if all the ash had been placed above the target.

TABLE 1

| Plant and experiment number | Hours in solution | Control | | Conduction through xylem | | Conduction through phloem | |
|---|---|---|---|---|---|---|---|
| | | top | roots | top | roots | top | roots |
| Bryophyllum | | | | | | | |
| 16 .... | 41 | 310 | 1020 | 350 | 1030 | 15 (2) | 1100 |
| 20 .... | 48 | 360 | 1920 | 550 | 990 | 27 (1, 3) | 350 |
| 21 .... | 48 | 365 | 860 | 447 | 770 | 30 (1, 3) | 593 |
| 22 .... | 46 | 87 | 548 | 103 | 254 | 20 (1, 3) | 684 |
| 36 .... | 69 | 6100 | 6300 | 4200 | 4450 | 375 (3) | 5900 |
| 37 .... | 42 | 10200 | 10850 | 5880 | 6950 | 60 (1, 3) | 6950 |
| | | | | | | 820 (3) | 15400 |
| 48 .... | 47 | ..... | ..... | 1100 | 2460 | 500 (1) | 2040 |
| Willow | | | | | | | |
| 52 .... | 22 | 195 | 720 | 300 | 810 | 40 (2, 4) | 300 |
| | | | | | | 20 (1, 3) | 585 |
| 53 .... | 48 | 3060 | 765 | 135 | 345 | 45 (2) | 825 |
| | | | | | | 0 (1, 2) | 540 |
| 54 .... | 7 | 40 | 580 | 112 | 920 | 0 (2) | 720 |

*Note:* (1) Lower end of xylem in a tube of water; (2) leaves wilted badly long before the end of the experiment; (3) partly wilted at end of experiment; (4) plant was in solution only 5 hours.

Table 1 shows clearly that if the top was supplied with water through the cut end of the xylem rather than through the phloem, when the xylem was removed, there was much less phosphorus in the top than when all the water had to pass through the phloem and there was a transpiration stream connecting the top with the root.

The actual amount of active phosphorus in the tops of the plants in experiment 37 was 0.0024 g for the control, 0.0012 g for the plant carrying on conduction only through the xylem, 0.0002 g for the plant with phloem as the conduction element and only 0.000014 g when the conduction of the mineral took place through the phloem, but most of the water was supplied to the leaves through the cut end of the xylem.

From these experiments it would seem that not as much minerals are conducted through the phloem as Gustafson and Darken had supposed. Nevertheless, there is undoubtedly some upward conduction of minerals in the phloem under normal conditions.

FELIX G. GUSTAFSON

UNIVERSITY OF MICHIGAN

# SCIENTIFIC APPARATUS AND LABORATORY METHODS

## AN ACETO-CARMINE METHOD FOR BIRD AND MAMMALIAN CHROMOSOMES

EXCELLENT aceto-carmine preparations, either temporary or permanent, can be made of bird and mammalian chromosomes (and no doubt of other animals) by the simple procedure described below. The method is applicable to any tissue which can be readily subdivided by teasing with needles prior to fixation.

The tissue—usually young embryos, embryonic ovary or adult testis—is removed with the greatest possible speed and with the usual precautions to insure that the cells are living and normal, and quickly dissociated by teasing with needles for four or five seconds and then plunged in one of Carnoy's fixatives, where it can be further teased apart. Both the 3:1 and 6:3:1 solutions give excellent results with bird embryo somatic cells and ovaries, and with adult rat testes. (3 parts absolute alcohol and 1 part of glacial acetic acid, or 6 parts of absolute alcohol, 3 parts of chloroform and 1 part of glacial acetic acid.)

The tissue is fixed for 20 minutes to several hours and then placed directly into aceto-carmine, where it should stain for half an hour, more or less, depending on the tissue. *Small* bits of tissue are next removed with a pipette, along with aceto-carmine, and placed on a clean slide and covered with a coverglass. The preparation is now treated just as you would a salivary gland. The excess aceto-carmine is blotted off with filter paper and the soft tissue mashed out with considerable pressure from the finger tips. If necessary, complete spreading of the cells may be accomplished by rubbing a blunt needle over the coverglass. During this whole process the coverglass must not be allowed to slip about. For temporary mounts, the coverglass is sealed with vaseline or some other like agent and studied at once. For permanent slides the coverglass is left unsealed and the slide is placed at once into a jar saturated for alcohol vapor. (This is Bridges's alcohol-euparal method.) After standing in alcohol fumes for a few hours, the slides are placed in 95 per cent. alcohol, where they should remain for several hours or longer. If the coverglass doesn't loosen and come off it should be pried off with a spade-shaped needle in a Petri dish filled with 95 per cent. alcohol. When this is done part of the cells adhere to the slide, others to the coverglass and some are lost, especially when too much tissue was used in the first place. The slide is next removed from the Petri dish, the excess alcohol quickly drained or wiped off, and the adhering tissue is covered at once with a liberal amount of euparal or its equivalent. Next the excess alcohol is drained from the coverglass and the latter is placed back on the slide, face down and in its original position. Excess euparal is blotted off and after shifting the coverglass to as near its original position as possible, the preparation is ready for study.

The advantage of the method is its simplicity and speed and the excellent preservation and staining of the chromosomes. Meiotic chromosomes are especially well shown in the rat. The alcoholic-acetic fixation leaves the tissue so soft its cells can be separated by mashing after staining with aceto-carmine. The other preliminary fixatives tried so far (Flemming, Nawaschin, etc.) leave the tissues too hard or tough to be mashed out.

In studying any aceto-carmine preparation it is desirable to use green filters, Wratten filters Nos. 61 and 62 being especially recommended with artificial light. In a pinch, a piece of green eye-shade will do.

T. S. PAINTER

AUSTIN, TEXAS

## A SIMPLE ROCKING DEVICE FOR CARREL FLASKS[1]

IN experiments on the artificial parthenogenesis and development of rabbit eggs *in vitro,* we have usually placed the eggs in rabbit serum in a Carrel flask and left them stationary in an incubator at 37.5° C. When the eggs are removed from the Fallopian tubes within 15 hours after the final ovulating injection of pituitary has been given, each one is found covered by several layers of granulosa cells adhering closely to the protein layer immediately surrounding the egg, and the eggs as a whole are embedded in a much larger mass of loose material of similar nature. While standing in the incubator, these cells tend to fall away from the eggs, disintegrate and spread over the bottom of the flask. While this in itself may not be deleterious, it appears to be instrumental in causing the eggs as well to adhere to the glass substratum. To avoid this, we have found the shaker, of which a side elevation is sketched in the accompanying figure, to be of definite value. Not only does it in general prevent the sticking and disintegration of this material, referred to above, but it assists the adequate and uniform oxygenation of the culture, and helps prevent local accumulation of carbon dioxide. On the whole, the condition of the eggs is definitely an improvement over that when they are left stationary. It may be of use also in oxygenating tissue cultures with large quantities of fluid, which adhere firmly after an initial growth period.

[1] Aided by a grant from the Penrose Fund of the American Philosophical Society.

The construction is simple. On a baseboard (B), 42 × 20 cm a Telechron motor (T), giving four revolutions per minute, is mounted and attached by a 10 cm shaft (S) on the eccentric to the platform P, 8.5 × 25.5 cm, and 15 cm above the base. Seven Carrel flasks (C)

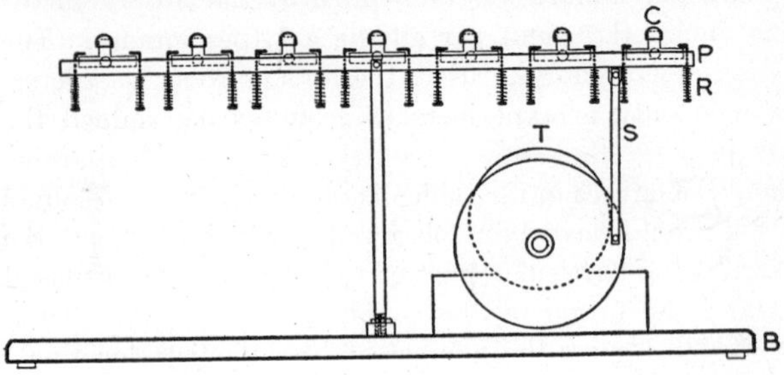


are shown held in place in depressions on the platform, by brass rods (R) bent at right angles, and fitted with springs under the platform. Each rod is covered with a short length of rubber tubing where it fits snugly against the top of the flask. The entire assemblage is kept inside the incubator during an experiment, which may last 24 to 30 hours. During this time it is regularly tilted back and forth about 30° from either side of the horizontal. The size of platform and number of flasks may of course be extended.

HERBERT SHAPIRO

CLARK UNIVERSITY

## BOOKS RECEIVED

ALBERT, A. ADRIAN. *Structure of Algebras; American Mathematical Society Colloquium Publications, Vol. XXIV.* Pp. xi + 210. The Society, New York.

AMBERSON, WILLIAM R. and DIETRICH C. SMITH. *Outline of Physiology.* Pp. vii + 412. 177 figures. Crofts. $4.00.

BEAUCHAMP, WILBUR L., JOHN C. MAYFIELD and JOE Y. WEST. *Science Problems for the Junior High School; Basic Studies in Science, Book 3.* Pp. x + 756. 610 figures. Scott, Foresman. $1.68.

CARROLL, FRANKLIN B. and others. *Interpreting Science; Book One, Understanding our Environment.* Pp. x + 438. Illustrated; *Book Two, Understanding our World.* Pp. xi + 554. Illustrated; *Book Three, Understanding the Universe.* Pp. xx + 712. 574 figures. Winston.

KURTZ, ALBERT K. and HAROLD A. EDGERTON. *Statistical Dictionary of Terms and Symbols.* Pp. xiii + 191. Wiley. $2.00.

MANGELSDORF, P. C. and R. G. REEVES. *The Origin of Indian Corn and Its Relatives; Texas Agricultural Experiment Station Bulletin No. 574, May, 1939.* Pp. 315. 95 figures. Agricultural and Mechanical College of Texas, College Station.

SMYTH, HENRY DE W. and CHARLES W. UFFORD. *Matter, Motion and Electricity; a Modern Approach to General Physics.* Pp. xiii + 648. 296 figures. McGraw-Hill. $3.75.

STEVENS, BERTHA, Editor. *Thoreau, Reporter of the Universe; a Selection of his Writings about Nature.* Pp. xiv + 229. Illustrated. John Day. $2.50.

THOMPSON, HOMER C. *Vegetable Crops.* Third edition. Pp. xi + 578. 68 figures. McGraw-Hill. $5.00.

# SCIENCE

VOL. 90 FRIDAY, OCTOBER 6, 1939 No. 2336



*Science and Social Pioneering:* DR. ISAIAH BOWMAN 309

*Obituary:*
*Arthur Edwin Kennelly:* PROFESSOR CHESTER L. DAWES 319

*Scientific Events:*
*Public Health in Germany in 1938; The Hall of Man at the World's Fair; Mead Johnson and Company "B-Complex" Award; Recent Appointments at Columbia University; Changes and New Appointments at Harvard University; Semi-centennial Celebration of the Founding of the Medical School of the University of Minnesota* 321

*Scientific Notes and News* 324

*Discussion:*
*Atmospheric Contamination:* PROFESSOR A. H. PFUND. *Oxidation-Reduction Potentials and the Mode of Action of Sulfanilamide:* DR. RICHARD O. ROBLIN, JR., and PAUL H. BELL. *Structure and Synthesis of a Plant Wound Hormone:* DR. JAMES ENGLISH, JR., DR. JAMES BONNER and A. J. HAAGEN-SMIT. *The Plasmodium of Hemitrichia vesparium (Batsch) Macbr:* LLOYD G. CARR. *Literature Service for Chemists:* DR. NEIL E. GORDON 326

*Scientific Books:*
*Recent Botanical Books:* DR. R. F. DAWSON, PROFESSOR G. W. KEITT, PROFESSOR C. L. WILSON. *Annual Review of Physiology:* DR. CARL J. WIGGERS 330

*Reports:*
*Scientists and the Press* 333

*Special Articles:*
*The Structure of the Red Oxidation Products of Tocopherols and Related Substances:* PROFESSOR LEE IRVIN SMITH, WILLA B. IRWIN and HERBERT E. UNGNADE. *Appearance of Fermentable Polysaccharide in the Blood and a Simple Method for Its Detection:* PROFESSOR THEODORE E. FRIEDEMANN and DR. WHEELAN D. SUTLIFF. *Listerella from a Premature Bovine Fetus:* DR. ROBERT GRAHAM, H. R. HESTER and NORMAN D. LEVINE. *Solute Transport in Plants:* DR. A. S. CRAFTS 334

*Science News* 10



SCIENCE: A Weekly Journal devoted to the Advancement of Science, edited by J. MCKEEN CATTELL and published every Friday by

THE SCIENCE PRESS

New York City: Grand Central Terminal

Lancaster, Pa. Garrison, N. Y.

Annual Subscription, $6.00 Single Copies, 15 Cts.

SCIENCE is the official organ of the American Association for the Advancement of Science. Information regarding membership in the Association may be secured from the office of the permanent secretary in the Smithsonian Institution Building, Washington, D. C.


# SCIENCE AND SOCIAL PIONEERING[1]


By Dr. ISAIAH BOWMAN

PRESIDENT OF THE JOHNS HOPKINS UNIVERSITY


THE classic tale has man witless until he receives the Promethean gift of fire. Light and fire are the age-old symbols of the mystery of the creative force in man or of what some would call the divine beginnings of man's discovery of a forward way. We talk less of mystery to-day for, if the source of the light of understanding is still unknown, man himself has successfully trimmed the wick. Reflected, dispersed and recombined from thousands of mental and spiritual facets, the light reveals ever-new possibilities of adventure, experiment and stimulating insight for the self-conscious creature, half angel, half brute, who talks endlessly about his elusive destiny. Whatever their own genius may be, all thoughtful persons borrow or reflect enlightening fact wherever they find it, and observe with alternating hope and anxiety the endless search by other men for that object of faith and labor called progress.

Reflecting in this fashion, it seemed to me presumptuous to express only my limited individual opinion in this opening address in an annual exchange between the British and the American Associations for the Advancement of Science. It seemed better to inquire of others what they would choose to say. Because scientists are apt to praise the children of their brains, the views of non-scientists were sought on the contribution of science to social welfare and to that uniquely human process of consciously planned advance across the threshold of experience which we may call social pioneering.

To that end I invited one hundred men who are not engaged in either physical or biological research or teaching to express their opinions. For special rea-

[1] The first British and American Association Lecture, Dundee meeting, 1939.

sons two exceptions were made. The opinions are almost wholly American; I have included those of but a few English and French friends. The list includes lawyers, teachers, artists, poets, government officials, historians, economists, preachers, industrialists, left-wing and right-wing publicists, military men, bankers and railway executives, as well as a member of the United States Supreme Court, a member of the President's Cabinet, public institutions of many kinds, men with power of command over others and men who exercise power only through ideas. With few exceptions they are men whose names are well known on both sides of the Atlantic.

Each person was asked to set down not his studied or rationalized opinion, but rather his quick and customary response to the idea that science has or has not added to man's cultural possibilities, given him a better way of thinking through his difficulties, raised his hopes for a more ethical civilization. Was his *habitual mode of thought* with respect to these propositions positive or negative?

To keep my promise to contributors the following twenty numbered statements, which combine the one hundred opinions, are given without references to sources. They are arranged in three groups—those which emphasize the gains (12), those which express qualified approval (5), and those which point to losses (3). No attempt has been made to give them consistency (compare, for example, items 10 and 5).

### Emphasizing the Gains

(1) Science is to-day the most excited front of human enterprise, and such excitement is a good in itself. The fact that tens of millions of people are interested in scientific discovery and theory is one of the hopeful things in this Pandora's box of a time. Conceivably these tens of millions are or might become interested in a wider view of human affairs.

(2) The light that science has thrown on religion has made the difference between fearing God and believing in God, for it brings God within the sphere of personal experience. It has done this mainly through the removal of the fear of the supernatural. It has not lessened the force of religion by weakening the force of orthodox religion. There is neither an Acheron nor a seat of torture of souls: the shades are peaceful abodes.

(3) Science has enabled us to understand many catastrophic forces though we control or combat, with limited success, but a few. Thereby it has reduced the areas and much of the strain of ignorance, superstition and myth. Forecast in several fields has entered so effectively into civilized man's thinking that it tends to stabilize both mind and act to a remarkable degree, giving a sense of permanence or at least assurance in the midst of obvious change. We no longer cower before "the forces of nature," at least intellectually.

(4) Science has encouraged specialization, and specialized knowledge is the mother of invention. Both have greatly complicated life by making us all increasingly interdependent. In the past half century a multitude of new occupations has grown up employing millions whose livelihood is dependent upon multiplied wants and the complexities of specialization and interchange that feed them. Science and invention, and commerce between the less civilized and the more civilized peoples, have encouraged a phenomenal increase in world population. "Back to the simple life" would mean starvation for many of these millions: it would also mean additional manual toil for almost all of us as well as diminished comfort and security. There can be no *Erewhon*.

(5) Science serves an expanding civilization, but we do not know anything at all about our ultimate fate: the future is beyond conjecture: "the end is forbidden." If science has introduced dangers it has also made a net addition to human welfare by greatly expanding man's identification and use of natural resources. Humboldt's dream of "enlarging the outlook of mankind" through geographical study has been realized: the diversities of the earth have enriched life immeasurably. Synthetic chemistry has supplied a host of new products and opened gateways to still wider conquests afield. Like animal and plant breeding, it has changed the human potentiality in, and therefore the significance of, large parts of the natural environment. It has not destroyed geographical diversity, but it has become a factor in the rearrangement and revaluation of diversified resources.

(6) Science insists that *facts* are indispensable in the ordering of social change or reform. Though we proceed by trial and error to a large extent, it is science, especially the analytical use of statistics in the social field, that ruthlessly exposes error and helps to restrict the areas of prejudice and uninformed preconception. Sentiment and emotion have their place in the evolution of society from lower to higher, but in themselves they are fallacious guides. Social programs are put forward as tentatives or hypotheses if the scientific method is followed. In earlier times one could give categorical answers to all questions of objective and meaning. Science has eliminated much of the categorical.

(7) The effect of the doctrine of evolution upon modern thought in many fields has come to be incalculably great. It has revealed a far more complex universe than had been conceived under the assumptions of fixed numbers and kinds of species that in turn accorded with the simplicities of the geometry and the idealized astronomy of the Greek climax. It destroyed in time the over-generalized doctrine of universals in

nature. It weakened the hold of metaphysics upon observational significances. It showed up the limitations of abstract logic in discovering or assimilating truth that is either essentially irrational or subject to change as new facts emerge and men are driven to make "a fresh examination of particulars," as Francis Bacon phrased it. It gave new meanings to both science and society by its revelation of a body of knowledge that drew its ordering from the historical record of the origins and evolutions of types correlated with the geological time-scale on the one hand and with experimental results on the other.

(8) Many of our social problems are ethical, and in this respect the common man is perhaps the equal of the intellectual in balance, temperament and insight, or even surpasses the insulated and stylized man who has the protective walls of an institution around him or the assurances of recognized social position or wealth. In these days of exaggeration, when mere political mechanisms tend to be worshipped as golden calves, the scientist at least knows that there is no collective salvation of souls and no final order. It is the business of science to discover truth, not salvation. In many instances salvation comes through the emotions and they are generally inaccessible to reason: it is also in large part an inner process, as Mazzini observed: "You will not have things better until you are better yourselves."

(9) Historically, the indebtedness of economic study to natural science is two-fold: replacement of the naïve premises of classical deduction by positive data and the use of such data in facilitating the much-neglected but indispensable step in economic deduction, namely, verification. The methods and objectives of political science have been re-examined under the inspiration of scientific influence. A healthy inconoclasm has ensued and the positive approach has become dominant. Historical writing has come to have greater accuracy and objectivity, less emotion, prejudice and prepossession, and more convincing conclusions, but might not these qualities have been gained without the example of science?

(10) Public health has been promoted by progress in biology and biochemistry and by public acceptance of or demand for appropriate administrative measures. Out of the disaster of the Asiatic cholera in the thirties of the last century arose the office of Registrar-General in England over which William Farr presided for a time. Concerning that event Dr. Parkes, an English hygienist, wrote: "It is impossible for any nation, or for any government, to remain indifferent when in figures which admit of no denial, the *national amount of health and happiness, or disease and suffering, is determined* (our italics). The establishment of the Registrar-General's office in 1838 and the commencement of the system of accurately recording births and deaths will hereafter be found to be, as far as the happiness of the people is concerned, one of the most important events of our time." During a discussion in Parliament in 1875 on the Public Health Act, described as the most complete code of sanitary law in existence, Disraeli said: "The public health is the foundation on which repose the happiness of the people and the power of a country. The care of the public health is the first duty of a statesman."

(11) The scientific attitude of mind is indispensable to further social progress, but scientists should be more modest in their claims. However closely one investigates and measures there is always a gap at the end to be jumped by the imagination. The gap can be narrowed considerably by careful thought, but after that one wants just knack or nose. Truth is deep down, said Democritus. In social applications of science one should be mindful of the precipitate of human experience which tradition represents as well as of the conflicting solutions and assumptions which we have inherited. Science itself does not supply adequate motivation for dedicated and unselfish living, living on a high level. If a scientist has these qualities it is because he is something more than just a scientist. Science has given a vast number of material satisfactions, but where has it left public thinking with respect to the heroic struggle without which a people has no fiber, no victory?

(12) Humanitarianism and democracy stand in the way of wider applications of science to social problems: they have permitted an enormous increase of population, with a rising proportion of biologically unfit and a rising standard of care for the unfit. Civilization may be too much for *Homo sapiens,* but at least we keep on trying, and science is one of the ways of trying. At times the growth of large corporations has also stood in the way of wholesome social change. In the absence of any clear philosophy of control by society they grow past the bounds of public knowledge. While they have had well-known beneficial effects they also permit a modern form of ruthless raiding. A democracy is required that not only gives economic and political opportunity but also treats men as ethical and spiritual beings.

### Qualified Approval

(13) Science, largely by its emphasis upon the freest and widest inquiry, has aided in the diffusion and acceptance of the principle of religious and racial toleration, but there is grave doubt of the strength and permanence of this gain.

(14) Lord Kelvin's remark that "you do not know much about a subject until you have tried to measure it" is clearly applicable only to that which can be measured. Science deals quantitatively with measurable material things and less with *quality* which sup-

plies the essence of culture. With its emphasis upon a mechanistic theory of inevitable law, science has acquired a prestige that can be a real danger. The crucial question is, what has science done to enable the individual to *see* the pattern of his ideal more clearly and to *fulfil* his new vision? Measurement and accuracy do not touch even the fringe of social questions. The totality of human affairs (ideas, beliefs, conduct, habits, institutions, etc.) can not be reduced to deterministic sequences. Knowledge of facts does not tell us what to do about them. *Social action is based upon assumptions, expressed or implied, respecting human values.* Science helps indispensably, however, in its zest for truth, for careful observation, for an even-tempered attitude.

(15) Science has shrunk the planet, close-knitted civilization, and practically revolutionized life. Once we thought it remarkable that *news* from all over the world got to us each morning; now the distant trouble itself is at our door. While our curiosity has been widened, will any one claim that our sense of responsibility has been enlarged? Are we usefully informed or only distracted? A high degree of accuracy has been attained by news services if methods and time limitations are taken into account, with the result that "public opinion" has gained a status not unlike that of a world conscience. The dictators always lay hands first upon radio, cable and newspaper. They wish the rest of the world to be unaware! Two chief difficulties delay the realization of a better international order: (1) the increasing dependence of individual welfare upon a limitlessly expanding number of other individuals unknown to him as persons; and (2) the creation of an unbelievably complex web of human ordering beyond our present means of guidance.

(16) Very few people know anything about or care about science in a fundamental sense. The better a product becomes and the more widely it is used the less public interest is shown in its origins and mechanism. It is the esthetic factor that now counts most in a motor-car: all cars run well. The public will continue to accept the findings of science but, if pushed too fast in the direction of new social schemes called "scientific," they will become frightened. Our time span for social change is now much shorter than formerly. In an earlier day more time was given to absorb change without conscious direction. Hair-trigger thinking is now fashionable in the social field, with action but an instant behind, and the revisionary habit of science applied to such thinking would have a desirable sobering effect. At present, applications are left to mediocre minds. Shamefully little progress is made towards the solution of basic social problems such as housing, access to medical care, stabilization of employment.

(17) Universal education offers the only hope of establishing in the minds of the people the minimum conclusions of science that bear on social welfare most directly, or appear to do so. These minimum conclusions can become the blueprint of social engineering only if they are kept within the range of mass thinking. That range, in turn, is limited because human desires are dynamic and simple, while human intellect is telic and complex. Desires propel, intellect can only feebly guide. "People" see the *things* of science and forget the *discipline*. Their minds are littered by ideological concepts and dogmas, incapable of verification, that stand in the way of acceptance of a scientific approach to social problems.

### LOSSES

(18) We live in "the dark hour of a gifted age." Science has made war more terrible; it has debased mankind by its growing disregard for helpless and innocent non-combatants; it has forced the whole of civilization to adopt the most horrible methods of destruction. Men have tried to agree not to use the worst instruments of warfare, as the Church once tried (1139) to anathematize the use of "the deadly and hateful art of crossbowmen and archers in wars against Christians and catholics"; but in the end each new frightfulness triumphed.

(19) It is a clever, cynical and hard-bitten world that science is making, one in which the idealistic and the spiritual are bound to have a diminishing place. Viewed against a background of classical education science has been a disadvantage to our society. If the most important questions of mankind are those concerning spiritual relations with one another and with God, then science is not to be taken seriously. Through dazzling discovery and successful practical application science gives a sense of power that is both demoralizing and dangerous. We are given an enormous driving force that does not permit us to be as bad or as foolish as we could be with impunity down to the middle of the eighteenth century. The impact of science on our morality, individual and national, is evil unless we rise successfully to the test of our character and moral traditions. Science has taught us analysis, but we have had as yet no large-scale and equally successful synthetic constructions that bear on human conduct. The mass mind seizes and acts upon perverted ideas of scientific generalization. Darwin's "survival of the fittest" encourages men to be brutal; Freud's "don't repress," to indulge their passions; Einstein's "relativity," to think that truth doesn't exist and doesn't matter.

(20) The fickle wishes and caprices of men, in economics and government particularly, have been given weight and apparent rationality by the adoption of unsuitable methods devised by technocrats accustomed to weighing material objects. To limit oneself to

"data" in social studies is to parody society. Human science must think of life as a whole. The riddle of life is not in objects or discoveries without, but in conscience and mind within. A man's "destiny" is what he can make out of his own character.

### "SCIENCE" IS NOT A UNIVERSAL

In weighing these responsive observations one does well to keep in mind that what we call "science" is largely though by no means wholly a conscious intensification of methods and results that had exceedingly remote origins. Science is a part of human life, not something separate and distinct. Farmers of all centuries, fishermen and especially sailing folk—all have developed science of a sort: empirical observation, limited analysis and generalization, confrontation of theory (idea) with fact, as well as revision or modification (with much myth and nonsense built in too). The methods were not labelled or systematized, cause and effect were often wrongly ascribed, but the result was progress by taking thought.

It does no good to vaunt science as if it were something that stood above the rest of knowledge—independent, self-sufficient, worshipful. As human experience, science is not a universal, a summation of knowledge applicable and useful to the whole of life; it is rather a thing of limited categories. Science gains nothing by the decline of humanism: it is itself a special form of humanism. One asks, what is its net worth in the sum of human interests? What does it add to education, to outlook, to citizenship? And especially what does it add to human possibilities, to spiritual incandescence?

No claim for science may be set up without pointing to the limitations of scientists as individuals in responding to prejudice, group opinion, and the like. To most scientists, science is only a specialized form of experience. When a scientific man turns to the social framework which contains his science, conditions it, encourages or discourages it, he is bound to take account of other elements of society than his own, other tastes, other judgments of value in life. Individual scientists are often affected by the source of their support. They will tend to approve the policies of the companies that supply them with a living. They will measure a social program by the yardstick of company prosperity. The company may be a profit-making concern or a university.

A scientific career, so-called, does not necessarily make its devotees broadminded, cautious of the word, modest in spirit. It takes more than science to widen a narrow man's sympathies! Science does not in itself "turn the common thoughts of life into gold." Few scientists have the power of persuasive exposition; many have "the gift of infrigidation." Scientists have no monopoly of the power to discard dogma, the courage and intelligence to win territory from superstition. Do they call attention to the merits of scientific method "to protect their banners and slogans" or to improve society?

### THE CONCEPT OF CHANGE

In so far as the methods of the physical and natural sciences teach patience, establish the value of both imagination and doubt, enhance analytical power, and provide training in observation, they are of value in any study—crime detection, historical inquiry or the rise of contemporary social movements. But these are not powers newly acquired by scholars in our scientific age. They have always marked all research and insight, in antiquity as in recent times. The poet shares them with the scientist. What biology and geology have done is far more distinctive and new in thought than these qualities denote. They have made the Greek "all flows" not only a matter of time, but also a matter of form and function—change as *the mode of the universe.* How and why things change is at the core of scientific inquiry, not alone how things are.

One of the greatest achievements of science is its emphasis upon free inquiry—the mind itself in command, driven by curiosity and the sense of intellectual adventure. The motive force in an earlier day was faith which removed "not mountains only but the whole material environment." Facts and events were removed from the realm of human action to that of divine grace. Theology and philosophy have since been modified, largely by the light of modern science. Evolution has required every intelligent religion to reshape its view of man. Recent pragmatic philosophy would have little substance if the evolutionary concept were subtracted. After 1860 historical writing clearly showed the effect of the evolutionary approach; and economic theory dealt increasingly with the problems of a dynamic society. The doctrine of evolution involved the minds of men in what can be conservatively described as an overwhelming revolution. In the eighty years since the "Origin of Species" was published no thinking man has escaped its influence.

The concept of evolution influenced some areas of thought long before the modern doctrine of biological evolution was formulated. It was a maxim of Roman law that the limit of the law is its greatest injustice. To codify the law and put it into "tables" represented progress; but it was greater progress to take it out of the tables again, so to speak. Precedents had been proven to be not enough; ethics and public utility were asked to determine forms, and ethics and public utility change with time and circumstance. The whole body of Roman law reflects an effort to apply reason and fairness to a changing society to be accommodated by an elastic set of rules in which the danger of definitions was pointed out. Principles were made to rest on experience; they were "rooted in a philosophic consideration of human life."

In the natural world no such progress was made in Roman times, and indeed we do not see how it was then possible. Lucretius showed what science (as he understood it) could do, but he was unable to make practical proposals for social applications. An understanding of nature would drive fear out of the world, said he, and a better knowledge of both nature and the gods would help bring peace and honor to men. Only as late as our time could the principle of evolution be so variously documented that the idea became accessible and interesting to all men, not the vision of a few. Each specialist came to see fruitful applications in his own field. Dynamic change displaced ideal pattern, fixity and immutability. Lawyer, economist, historian, geographer, priest, chemist and statesman could speak a common language of movement, of continuing adaptation, through nature and through interactive society.

### Diversities and Contradictions

Civilization may be usefully considered as an adventure in change. New forces are generated through the evolution of tools, the domestication and subsequent breeding for quality of animals and plants, through age-long folk experiment and through the occupation of new lands with their diversifying possibilities. Each people carries on the adventure in a different way because of its distinctive regional environment, its unique aptitudes and its variant objectives and philosophies.

The diversities of time, place and race may also raise barriers to understanding. Confluent in trade and travel we are nationally divergent and often discordant with respect to philosophies and ethics. Our rules are not the same, in Asia and America. Our languages are no more unlike than our systems of logic or our definitions. Our ethics and our judgments also change in time. It is sometimes said that ethics and manners are matters of geography. In this fluctuant world the geography changes rapidly also, because as man changes his techniques, his tastes and his systems, so also does he change the *significance* of much of his environment.

The main job of some schools of agriculture is to raise food-production per acre. This is condemned by those who say that we grow too much food already. It is praised by those who, as in over-populated Puerto Rico, are trying to get the value of food crops per acre raised to the level of the sugar crop, now 800 per cent. above food crops in value! The Netherlands East Indies tries to meet the reduced demand of world markets for her staple crops (rubber, sugar, coffee) by new crops—tung oil from plants imported from China, tanning material from an Acacia imported from South Africa, wood-pulp from imported pine trees. The ultimate values and distributions of men and resources are unknown to us: we suspect there are no ultimates. We keep learning in the hope of achieving net improvement for the time being. We have also learned that to learn is generally to change.

Most public discussion is babble about agriculture, industry, health, education, security, employment, taxes, war. The voter is asked to express opinions on a jumble of political and social programs by casting *one* ballot. One item in the bundle may be desirable, another highly undesirable. What effect will an act in one field have upon desired ends in another field? The whole must be dealt with, and the individual knows only a small part.

### Specialization Increases Satisfaction

Science and much dependent invention has added to our material equipment to so great a degree that it has given "standard of living" the magnitude of a major social force. The individual desires to possess maximum satisfaction, and nature is explored, invention hastened, productive techniques refined to that end. Public health is improved and education made general, in order that life may be more *satisfying.* Fabrics of high utility and pleasing color and design are now available at more generally attainable prices than formerly. The illustrative arts have opened new worlds of enjoyment to millions. Photography alone has vastly increased the satisfactions of mankind. The gains in food production are revolutionary. Quick-ripening wheat and rust-resistant wheat represent two epic breeding struggles with billions of dollars worth of human welfare at stake in the empire of the Canadian Northwest alone.

Let no one dismiss the gains of science lightly with the word "material," as if that didn't matter! We can not overlook the unrelenting fact that all but a few of the people in the world *must* think about food and clothing and power, muscular and otherwise, in order first of all to live. Only a protected life provides the time and strength for continuous thought about meanings, discovery, philosophy, esthetics. The genius alone may be an exception—the miller's son who became Rembrandt, the ploughman Burns.

The scientist no less than the humanist sees the smallness of the spiritual gains in deplorable contrast to the material benefits. What we are trying to do, said one who helped develop Crater Lake National Park, about the forested rim of a high circular bowl in which lies one of the loveliest of the blue waters of the world, is to offset speed. When it took a day to reach the place, people enjoyed it, after earning their enjoyment. Now they rush up to the top in an hour in swift motor-cars, dash to the rim, gasp, "My God, how blue it is!" and rush right down again!

### The Edge of the Possibilities

Science has become one of the greatest of the adventures of our time partly because it deals with the edge of the possibilities. Man was always working to push past limits, but much new knowledge, and vast organizations in our day have speeded up the process. Man has also discovered that he is changing his own possibilities as well as those of his world as he goes along. He is at the center of his own creative experiment. He has found that what science supplies is not at all an addition, positive and beneficial, until men have proved it so. The whole of that proof is in man himself and not in admiring regard for new facts and inventions. Things and forces, social and natural, good and bad, are added to himself, with the result that ever new possibilities are emerging.

Land pioneering to-day illustrates two such interacting forces—the edge of the possibilities (marginal land) and the desire for an acceptable standard of living. The limits of land cultivation are being traced farther and farther afield. But what is left of pioneer land in the twentieth century is marginal land whose conquest requires both knowledge and better material equipment. The pioneer, seeing himself as part of a wider community, asks for a share in the total benefits. If he is to be empire builder he wants his reward here and now. So, let government do it. Roads, schools, telegraph lines, favorable freight rates, market facilities, low taxes and security from undue risks to health on the frontier are demanded! The protection of children brings restrictions, limitations, conservatism. Things must get better in time or too many families will become habited to the backward look to optimal regions.

Science here serves as a supplement to marginal nature—what crops are adapted to uncertain rains, or late-spring and early-autumn frosts, long haulage and distant demand. If the frontier environment can not be supplemented, social deterioration will take place. It is not enough to push people out upon the land if the land is marginal, risky, remote. Civilization must accompany the settler. Finally, the intending settler must have the will to succeed and he must have the capacity to adapt his musculature to new physical tasks, his mind to the possibilities of new cultural (social) experiments on the frontier, his enterprise to the potentials of the land and the region. If spirit is wanting, if security and accustomed ways are indispensable, if adventure is dead within him, the frontier is no place for him, with or without science.

### New Frontiers in Old Communities

In the United States applied science has increased agricultural production per worker, through machinery and fertilizers chiefly, and speeded transport, with the result that agriculture has become dominantly commercial and competitive, with marked changes in crop production and type of farming in many regions. Civilization has become increasingly urban, with resulting weakening of both family ties and the neighborhood bond. Machinery has helped create more commerce, more striking and more numerous economic successes and a much higher standard of living for certain classes. Billboards on the highways tell youth that it is "entitled" to a good car, good clothes, a good time. Whether or not that entitlement was earned, what responsibilities go with it, what the advertised product will do to strengthen character or enfeeble it—these things are not put upon the billboards.

We have learned how to feed and breed animals to a high level of efficiency. We expect six thousand pounds of milk a year from a single cow to-day, whereas a hundred years ago two thousand pounds was the average. We know how to preserve food for long transportation. We successfully combat many plant enemies. We have done work upon the grasslands to preserve and improve them, upon soils to determine their rate of wastage and the extent of their need for conservation, upon fisheries as a food source for man. We have calculated the amount of ocean that will be required to sustain a man: a volume of sea water approximately equal to that of a football field covered five feet deep with water and requiring two and a half hours to filter out the zooplankton. If the result seems economically not feasible, science may yet find a way to strain sea water in the likeliest places and provide additional food. Here taste and preference may step in. Will a breakfast of copepods become popular even though we know that they are equal to the best meat in nutritive value?

The triumphs of a scientific age have coexisting population problems of a disturbing character. In the large cities of America there are now about 7 children to 10 adults. If our present reproduction rate remains stationary these 7 children would raise 5 children and the 5 in turn would raise about 3½. The middle class in the cities consistently diminishes its stock. By contrast, the farm population raises about 14 children to 10 adults; the 14 would have at the present reproduction rate about 20 children and the 20 about 28. In 1937 and 1938 the "farm-baby crop" increased, the total for 1938 being the largest since 1926. How long and with what stock will the farm help populate the city? Not enough children are being born to maintain the existing level of the population of the United States. Already the enrolment in the first grade of the public schools has fallen about 100,000 a year since 1930. In the six elementary grades it is declining about 200,000 a year.

It is not easy to point out offsetting conditions to

farm population decline. The electrification of farm operations, the development of credit unions and producers and consumers cooperatives may restore a sense of mastery to and lay a basis for cultural participation by those who are drawn into the struggle that tends to pull good stock to the cities, there to confuse and devitalize it culturally, morally, economically. Between 1790 and 1930 our rural population increased twenty times, while our city population increased three hundred times!

The play of the forces involved in these far-reaching movements and cultural changes, whether self-initiated and free or guided by government, denote a pioneer fringe of high interest in the social field. The situation needs vital leadership, courage and local pride as well as equipment and the experimental point of view. These are old-fashioned virtues and they imply the hard way. Can our entire population rise to such Spartan levels, to self-denying activity, to ideals of independence and strength that evoke dynamic enthusiasm?

### Individual and Group

It is a fallacy to suppose that *group energy* is the sum of the individual energies in the group. A man does not make war: a nation or a tribe makes war. A citizen with a gun and no license and a soldier with a gun have two quite different social prospects. A group approves group action which it may condemn in the individual. Our social ethics are not consistent with our personal standards. We are caught up by our generation in the world at large—its ideas, its wars, its conflicting loyalties.

Our culture has developed dysgenic rather than eugenic qualities. Success and its social rewards, implying unusual intellectual and other social capacities, have become linked with diminished fertility. The well-endowed are not reproducing on an adequate scale. This means a steady diminution in the supply of the inherited qualities that brought success. In so far as success is spurious or anti-social the loss of these inherited qualities need not be regretted. In so far as it represents socially valuable qualities it means continued erosion of human character and loss to the race and to civilization.

We are wanting in general acceptance of categories of socially useful qualities. "Eureka, I have found it" means nothing socially until all have found it. "The genius raids . . . the common people occupy and possess." Whatever we gather of scientific knowledge concerning society and how it might be improved is one thing; to persuade or to exercise control in order to bring about desired ends is quite another.

We say that youth should be taught to acquire power to adjust itself to associative living. To a large extent this means the acceptance of the standards of contemporary society, the routine encouragement in oneself of that which society encourages. To carry this out to the fullest extent might be to destroy individual gifts and powers. Social living is not all! Will society foster or permit the not-understood individual variations that include the genius?

The supposition that scientific discovery can be made to bear immediately upon social change, the scientist remaking society, seems faulty doctrine. "Society" is built upon beliefs, traditions, prejudices, suppositions and philosophies, as well as facts, institutions, inventions and materiel—all supported by power or force exercised through *time*. Every advance in applied science calls for a tighter and more inclusive social organization, and it is the state which inevitably controls that organization. In exercising its controls, the state (consisting of determined *groups of men* who hold power, no less than accepted but precarious forms of controls, institutions, and the like) may introduce only those discoveries that suit its book. The holders of power, to whom power is the first law, will scarcely legislate themselves out of office. Moscow, Berlin, London and Washington are alike in this respect.

What is unlike in these four countries is a far more profound thing—the relative degree of freedom for the individual in finding and proclaiming scientific discoveries and in *advocating* their social applications or acceptance. The fight for adoption or rejection of ideas is in the open social arena in democratic countries. If there are dangers we are free to denounce them: no philosophic theory of society stands in the way. By contrast, if it suits the dictator to rest his social argument upon the powerful effects of an improvised environment he rejects the findings of geneticist and eugenist and even a Vavilov loses his job. To be secure as a scientist in a totalitarian country one must first ask a political bureau what is sound.

Let no one suppose, however, that democracy ensures continued freedom. Only when democratic social control of economic life is fully extended shall one be able finally to test the hypothesis that freedom of learning can live in the house of democracy. If the gap between "knowledge" and folk thinking gets too wide we shall all have to turn to the forging of a common method of thought, with no small risk to be run that a sterile generalizer with power may impose a philosophy. This makes the conservation and freedom of the minority a vital need: how often has a single vigorous challenge saved a human situation!

### Planning Involves Risk

The tentative nature of social conclusions is often a deciding factor in the rejection of scientific findings. Rightness is not proved except through social experiment that is jeopardized by too short a period of trial, by misrepresentation and misunderstanding of effects, by the fact that the objects of experiment, men and women, care for different kinds of outcome and such caring may change the outcome. Speed in social reform itself creates a kind of road hazard because of unpredictable turns and their effects, unforeseen impacts and disturbances.

The long view and the short view are difficult to distinguish—a further complication. To preserve our civilization we strengthen our nation, pointing to the competitive situation in the world at large. Through national planning we seek to raise the level of health and strength, to solidify national interest. This will inevitably have the effect of intensifying international competition. Commerce is increasingly competitive and necessarily implies inequality of opportunity in specific lines. In a wide sense commerce is the mother of all wars.

In the international field the triumphs of increased home production, ersatz and autarchy, hailed one by one as proof of growing independence and enhanced welfare—all are advantages that are bought at the price of dislocations elsewhere. Many a national triumph implies a setback for some other nation.

## Identification of Causes Precedes Control

Social pioneering has to do with culture in the making, with environment that becomes understood by thinking about the conditions of trial and the effects of error. It deals with inevitably new social forms or old forms adapted to new situations, and becomes ever more complex and overpowering for the individual. Faced by an emergency we develop emergency measures only to find ourselves shackled indefinitely by the emergency forms which we set up, "thereby covering up the conditions that necessitate them."

The first duty of an intelligent society in the modern scientific period is to get at the causes of things. The increase in the general consciousness that wonders exist, that science can create marvels, and that science supplies valuable elements in social living is a gain of the first importance. It has taught whole peoples to look for causes or to expect that causes will be found. Man's greatest hope lies that way to-day. Once causes are located there is no guarantee that a situation produced by a given cause may come to human control. But there is at least *a chance!* Any gains made in this field have appealing potentialities: a basic discovery generally leads to a host of derivative discoveries.

The scientific method is needed nowhere so much as in the sorting of causes and the delimitation of the action of forces supposed to be at the root of our troubles. The United States Bureau of Investigation reminds the Boy Scouts that though they number 1,281,000 they are outnumbered four to one by the 4,750,000 murderers, thieves, burglars, embezzlers, arsonists, kidnappers, extortionists and other criminals. Equally the criminal hosts outnumber the college population of 1,200,000. The director of the bureau does not find the cause of this appalling condition in science: he points to the skulking despoilers and modern-day pirates, "the venal and corrupt politicians" who place personal profit above the rights of decent citizens. But what does he find in the decent citizens themselves? Apathy, lack of interest in honest law enforcement, laziness in the exercise of the power of the ballot. The underworld counts upon these qualities!

A recent advocate of "glandocracy" contends that a society is as good or as bad as its nervous system and its glands, which together make an integrating mechanism whose character profoundly conditions the individual and his attitude towards the society of which he is a part. Given a harmoniously integrated development and the instinctive reactions to good social conditions are more likely to be adaptive and harmonious. Too simplified and mechanical an explanation, one may say. But in any event science deepens the understanding of basic conditions, and searches endlessly for causes in the hope that once they are found a clue to control may follow.

## Breaking the Frame

In man's endless adventure in progress, are the objectives to be great works of art, literature and science, or the development of personal health, strength and hardihood joined to national conquest, thereby exalting the nation at the expense of the individual? Or is it sufficient to promote the glory of God by confession, by religious adoration?

Modern science is not without its infective transcendentalism. "Our destiny is in our hands . . . develop all [our] potential activities . . . reject all systems," says Carrel, who believes we can achieve almost illimitable social advance if we but give scope to feeling and genetic possibilities. He advocates resistance to "the tyranny of the quantitative." He would break the frame of the school, the factory and the office, and reject the very principle of technological civilization: mechanical inventions but hinder human development. This seems to overlook certain prime and as yet ineradicable troubles of mankind, such as divergent and conflicting aims, faults of organization, lack of wide social participation in the findings of science.

How resolve the conflicts between classes, reduce the arrogance of nationalism and diminish the chances of war? Which class is to benefit most from a given program, which nation? Are these questions any nearer settlement because of our present wealth of scientific knowledge? Would more scientific knowledge decide the correct and just apportionment of advantages and privileges and accessions to the forces that raise the standard of living? Without modern scientific knowledge would acceptable solutions be any nearer?

Justice to conflicting groups requires either agreement between them or a universal judge. Our sympathies are weak when we try to put ourselves in the places of men who are far away. We rationalize our own acts to make them good to us and those of the enemy to make them bad. When we fight for the good against the bad it is war nevertheless. Science should provide an even-tempered attitude, but it seems almost superhumanly difficult to cultivate it in society.

We believe in scientific progress, but we reject the findings of science if they disturb an existing going concern, a satisfied community, an assured communication method. We can see only a little way ahead. This produces caution in some. Others exclaim, "if there are remote consequences let our progeny struggle with them." To feed unemployed people we incur a debt. We assume that the fed are worth feeding, knowing that a good deal of unemployment is non-discriminatory. We say that a minimum degree of support is required for an unemployed person, but is not "minimum" determined by worth? If we needed more people would not "worth" rise? Will our children be willing to use the lesser wealth of their time to pay for the judgments of our time? Or do we act like the worker wasp that, when the food supply runs low, bites off the tail of the grub to feed to its head?

In the midst of our troubles, the endless search for simplicities goes on! The despairing layman's answer to the complexities of phenomenonology and doctrine is to set up or accept a new doctrine that is simple and clear and based on authority. There is a clamor for simplicity in economics, politics and education. One hundred books will educate you, and all educated men will then talk alike; a formula can surely be found to break down the barriers to unemployment; if all nations would embrace the principle of world cooperation we should have peace. Editorials, columnists' comment, articles, adjuration, philosophies, tend toward simplicities: ha! here at last is the prophet who has found a way!

There seems to be no straight path to a social goal; evolution seems chancey; progress is only a fitful byproduct, says the despairing observer. Our loyalties waver, our beliefs change, our confidence in accepted democratic methods is impaired as we observe the wide variation of intelligence, the difficult task of sustaining interest in community affairs, the low level of individual satisfaction, the little knowledge we have of our leaders, the prime difficulty of bringing democratic method down from a glowing historical abstraction to a concrete activity, the inevitable performance of many functions of government by individuals employing their own judgment, the large element of guesswork in all forms of experiment, including social pioneering, the difficulty in distinguishing between true and false results in short or long periods of time, the haphazardness, the waywardness, the *lack* in democratic judgments, perceptions and actions. To offset these tendencies we offer education, more science rather than less, and "a documented call for action" based upon agreement as to facts by social scientists. Little enough, one must admit.

### Analysis and Advance

Social forms can not keep pace with creative thought. A time lag is inevitable because we have found no way to teach and test ideas except through time-consuming and often inconclusive experience. No one subject of study is capable of solving the total array of problems of a people. Science is no more deficient in this respect than social studies themselves. Hear an economist: "Economics is not the science of welfare . . . it is concerned with the relationships of scarce means to given ends." Economists may formulate economic policies through the application of reason and systematic thought to a limited field of human relations; but economics can not provide a total social program, continues Mackintosh. Even the data and hypotheses of economics are limited to a particular age. The subject tends to become less general in its application, a doctrine rather than a science.

In the last quarter of the nineteenth century, modern economic analysis (Marshall, Jevons, Menger and Walras) found a tool of investigation whose focus is the principle of equilibrium and its use has been continuously extended "to attack equally problems of disequilibrium." When the economist is finished with his statistical analysis, he adds imagination, experience and reason to create and test his hypotheses. Are there institutions to carry out an indicated policy? Will the democratic group for which it is designed understand it, accept it and expand it to fit changing conditions? The ends that society has in view are constantly changing and only rarely are they precisely defined. The problems themselves are complex and so, too, are the methods by which they will be solved, whereas public attention is short-lived and public analytical power is extremely limited.

### Directives and Limits

From the evidence of paleontology chiefly it was discovered that life from the first had both plasticity and the potentiality of change. Whatever the underlying causes and mechanisms, increasing complexity of form and function has been life's mode. Both muscular and psychological complexity has given organisms increased power (efficiency) in the *use* of the physical environment. Will the process stop with defeat at the physical and psychological assembly known as man, or will the conscious human turn his unique power of understanding upon himself, both as an individual and as part of a social mechanism?

Faith and method joined to imagination and curiosity still lead us on. Science is the greatest inciter of hope that we know—rational hope that the triumphant methods that have given us deeper understanding and increased efficiency as biological and social mechanisms will one day give us a still deeper insight into who and what we are and what we may become when rational control is extended. As in art and religion so in science—new meanings evolve as the mind continues its unshackling process. The eternal is not brought down from aloft only: it is also sought out and raised up among men. Science is one way of acquiring a knowledge of meanings or of adapting or inventing meanings that give deep human satisfaction —for a time.

# OBITUARY

## ARTHUR EDWIN KENNELLY

With the death on June 18 of Dr. Arthur E. Kennelly, professor emeritus of electrical engineering at Harvard University and the Massachusetts Institute of Technology, electrical engineering lost one of the pioneers who began his professional work when the only practical application of electricity was its use in simple telegraph circuits, but who lived to see the art reach its present highly developed form. His unusual ability, his industry, his gifted personality and his many important contributions to the development of electrical engineering gave him international recognition as a scientist and a teacher. His career was contemporaneous with those other great contributors to electrical engineering such as Heaviside, Edison, Steinmetz, Elihu Thomson, Sprague, Houston, Brush, with all of whom he was more or less closely associated in his professional work.

Dr. Kennelly was born at Colaba, near Bombay, India, on December 17, 1861, his parents being David Joseph Kennelly and Katherine Heycock Kennelly. He was educated in private schools in Great Britain, France and Belgium, and especially at the University College School, London. He was definitely attracted to a telegraph engineering career by attending a public lecture in 1874 at Albert Hall, London, by Mr. Latimer Clark on "Submarine Telegraphy." In 1875, at the age of 14, he was appointed assistant secretary to the Society of Telegraph Engineers (later the I. E. E.), London. In 1876 he entered the submarine cable service of the Eastern Telegraph Company and for several years was engaged in the laying and repairing of submarine cables between England and India, rising to the position of senior electrical engineer in 1886. In 1887 he became associated with Thomas A. Edison in his electrical laboratory at Orange, N. J., remaining his principal electrical assistant until 1894. In 1893 he was made consulting electrician to the Edison General Electric Company and the General Electric Company of New York. From 1894 to 1901 he was a member of the firm of "Houston and Kennelly," consulting engineers. In 1902 he was engineer in charge of laying a submarine telegraph cable for the Mexican Government from Vera Cruz to Campeche. The same year he was appointed professor of electrical engineering at Harvard University, which position he held until 1930, when he retired as professor emeritus. He was also professor of communication engineering and director of electrical engineering research at the Massachusetts Institute of Technology from 1913 to 1923, becoming professor emeritus in 1930.

In 1903 he married Julia Grice, of Philadelphia, who died early in 1935. A son, Reginald Grice, a chemist, of Springfield, Massachusetts, survives.

During 1918 Dr. Kennelly was a civilian liaison officer for the Signal Corps for the U. S. Army in France. He was chosen as the first exchange professor in engineering and applied science at French universities from seven cooperating American universities. Also, he was the first Iwadare lecturer to Japanese universities (1931).

Dr. Kennelly has been honored by many professional and scientific societies and has been the recipient of several medals and similar honors. Space permits the mentioning of only a few.

He served two terms (1898 to 1900) as president of the American Institute of Electrical Engineers, in 1911 was president of the Illuminating Engineering Society, and in 1916 was president of the Institute of Radio Engineers. He held either active or honorary membership in the American Institute of Electrical Engineers, the British Institute of Electrical Engineers, Société Française des Electriciens, Royal Astronomical Society, American Association for the Advancement of Science, the German Elektrotechnische Verein, the National Academy of Science, the Japanese Institute of Electrical Engineers, the American Academy of Arts and Sciences, of which he was vice-president, and many others. In 1935 he was honorary president of Union Radio Scientifique Internationale and in 1938–1940 he was vice-president of the Edison Pioneers.

Among the several awards accorded him were the Edward Longstreth Medal and the Howard Potts Medal of the Franklin Institute, for electrical research; the medal from the Société Industrielle de l'Est; the

Cross of Chevalier de la Légion d'Honneur from the French Republic; the annual medal of the Institute of Radio Engineers; the Edison Medal of the American Institute of Electrical Engineers; the Mascart Triennial Medal of the Société Française des Electriciens. He was a member of Tau Beta Pi.

In 1895 he received the honorary degree of doctor of science from the University of Pittsburgh; in 1906 the honorary degree of master of arts from Harvard University, and in 1922 was made doctor of the Faculty of Science, University of Toulouse, France. In 1936 he received the honorary degree of doctor of engineering from the Technische Hochschule of Darmstadt, Germany, on the occasion of the centenary celebration of that Hochschule. In 1939 he was elected a member of the Royal Swedish Academy of Sciences.

One of his chief contributions to applied science is a paper on "Impedance" presented in 1893 before the American Institute of Electrical Engineers. This was the first publication of the extension of Ohm's law to the complex plane and is the basis of the application of complex quantities to alternating-current circuit analysis. Another of his outstanding contributions is the application of hyperbolic functions to the solution of electrical-engineering problems. In 1891 Heaviside had given in terms of hyperbolic functions the fundamental steady-state equations for potential and current along a line, but in alternating-current cases he showed only lengthy scalar methods for their solution. In 1894 Dr. Kennelly gave the first solution in terms of complex hyperbolic functions and at the same time introduced the polar notation for complex quantities, which has come into extensive use. He has since expanded the use of complex hyperbolic angles to alternating-current lines, such, for example, as expressing the equivalent $\Pi$ or T of a smooth line in terms of a complex angle $\theta$ and two other quantities. His publications, including tables of complex hyperbolic functions and charts, have long been in extensive use for the solution of line problems, by both students and practising engineers. Early in his career he developed an electrical method of localizing faults in submarine cables by varying the current strength, and he also originated the center of gravity method for loads on electric circuits. In illumination, he developed a diagram, known by his name, for determining the mean spherical candlepower of a lamp from its zonal distribution curve without the use of a planimeter.

In March, 1902, Dr. Kennelly advanced the theory that the conducting properties of the ionized rarefied upper atmosphere might reflect back electromagnetic waves, and later in the same year Heaviside also offered the same theory. This theory has been verified experimentally, and the reflecting upper atmosphere has become known as the Kennelly-Heaviside layer. In 1912, he worked out jointly with Dr. G. W. Pierce the motional impedance circle for a telephone receiver. This discovery is highly important, as it gives a method for evaluating the performance of a telephone receiver and the method is applicable to other vibrating apparatus having an electromechanical system.

Dr. Kennelly has published some twenty-eight books of which he is the sole author of ten. Among these are "Wireless Telegraphy and Telephony," "The Application of Hyperbolic Functions to Electrical Engineering Problems," "Chart Atlas of Complex Hyperbolic and Circular Functions," "Electrical Vibration Instruments," "Electric Lines and Nets." In addition he was the author of over three hundred and fifty technical publications.

Realizing the many advantages of the international metric system, as past president of the American Metric Society and after 1915 as officer of the Metric Association, he worked arduously to effect the adoption of the system in the United States; as a result it has already been adopted in many industries and laboratories, and has come to be used in athletic events.

He was always deeply interested in electrical units and standards. He was secretary of the Standards Committee of the American Institute of Electrical Engineers at its inception, and later became the chairman; likewise, at its inception in 1908, he was secretary of the U. S. National Committee of the International Electrotechnical Commission (I.E.C.), at one time was president and in 1938 was made honorary president. The I.E.C. always was one of his deepest interests and most continuous activities. In 1932 he was United States delegate and "chef de délégation" from the United States to the Paris Congress. On several occasions he was a delegate to international conferences on electrical units and standards and he assisted materially in the devising of the Meter-Kilogram-Second (MKS) system of electrical units which has recently been adopted internationally. At one time he was also chairman of the Sectional Committee of Definitions of the American Standards Association. For a number of years he was a member of the National Research Council, to whose work he made many valuable contributions.

He was deeply devoted to electrical engineering and its allied subjects and worked indefatigably for their advancement. To him this was not only a vocation, but in a large measure it was his recreation as well. His extensive contributions were made possible only by long hours of work and by planning and using his time with a high degree of efficiency.

The many who knew Dr. Kennelly were impressed by his versatility and resourcefulness and his breadth of interests. For example, in 1929 he presented a paper, "Meteorological Units Adopted by Various Countries." Also he has shown (1929) that an approximate law of fatigue underlies all the world's racing animals (and human beings) such that all the series of events plot as substantially parallel straight lines on logarithm paper. The writer has heard him give a lecture on Macaulay, the historian, that would do credit to an arts professor. He was also a natural linguist and could converse fluently in French, German and Italian.

He was an excellent teacher as well as investigator and scientist. He not only had a clear conception of the intricate relations that often exist in electrical circuits, but he was able to present them in direct and simplified form that is characteristic of the good teacher. He was held in the highest esteem by students and colleagues alike, and at all times was most congenial and courteous. The hospitality of Dr. and Mrs. Kennelly to students and the younger members of the instructing staff was long a tradition at Harvard.

Nothing was more delightful than an informal conversation with him, for he had a wealth of the most interesting experiences from which to draw, and the quiet humor that was always innate in him would inevitably come to the surface. He was a most interesting and resourceful speaker and his services as such were always in great demand, both in the United States and abroad.

When he retired as professor emeritus in 1930 his eyesight had begun to fail, and although operations served to prolong it, during the last year or two of his life he could barely distinguish even large objects. However, in spite of this and of rapidly failing health, he pluckily refused to give up the work to which his life had been devoted. Assisted by a chauffeur, he went regularly to his office each morning, and with the assistance of a secretary attended the considerable correspondence and other matters that came to him. Current technical literature, frequently in foreign languages, was read to him. At times a graduate student in electrical engineering assisted him in interpreting and making drawings, which he was unable to do himself because of his eyesight. It was under such difficulties that he wrote several recent papers dealing largely with electrical units and systems, particularly the MKS system. He continued thus to carry on until stricken down in his last illness. With the passing of Dr. Kennelly the world has lost a great scientist, teacher, scholar and gentleman.

Chester L. Dawes

# SCIENTIFIC EVENTS

## PUBLIC HEALTH IN GERMANY IN 1938

The Berlin correspondent of the *Journal* of the American Medical Association states that the report of the Public Health Service contains information regarding public welfare. Of those intending to marry, 47 per cent. made use of public consultations (36 per cent. in 1937). Of these, 38 per cent. received a marital loan, that is to say an addition to the expenses incidental to getting established. Maternity advice was sought by 6 per cent. of pregnant women. Infant welfare stations were available to the public in the ratio of one for seventy-seven infants born and were actually consulted on the average by sixty mothers per station. Consultation for pre-school children was offered in the proportion of 718 per hundred thousand inhabitants. More than 3,000,000 children of school age received attention, that is, about 4,545 per hundred thousand inhabitants. The schools of almost all districts, with few exceptions, were furnished dental supervision.

The care of tuberculous patients was extended during 1938. About 1,500,000 patients, against 1,250,000 in 1937, received attention. The number of roentgen treatments rose from about 1,250,000 to about 1,750,000. Hospitalization in public institutions increased from 45,000 to 49,000. Average x-ray examinations were 100 to thirteen patients. Somewhat greater facilities were provided for the treatment of venereal diseases, but the number of individual cases decreased (192,000 in 1938 against 200,000 in 1937). Consultation stations for cripples were increased and, on the average, 242 persons were advised per hundred thousand inhabitants. The increase in stations for alcoholic persons is more than counterbalanced by the decrease of the individual's consulting. However, other agencies not identical with these cooperated in the care for alcoholic patients, and their reports are not included in these figures. About 107,000 persons with psychic troubles were advised against 91,000 in 1937. The care for the infirm and aged is likewise organized according to regions. It is pointed out that these facts should not be regarded as completely evaluating the achievements of public health welfare in Germany, because there are other agencies besides the official health stations connected with public health bureaus.

## THE HALL OF MAN AT THE WORLD'S FAIR

The American Museum of Health, which has offices at 30 Rockefeller Plaza, New York City, and a series of exhibits at the World's Fair, will have, according to *Museum News,* the cooperation of Mayor La Guardia in the endeavor to acquire a permanent building for the museum at the close of the fair. At the dedication ceremonies of the museum on the Theme Plaza of the fair on June 17 the mayor announced that he had in mind to assign for this purpose the court house building now occupied by the Appellate

Division, at Madison Avenue and 25th Street. This plan would depend on the working out of a project to build a new court house.

The museum has created or acquired the exhibits in the Hall of Man in the Medicine and Public Health Building of the fair. It includes in its installation the Oberlaender Trust exhibits portraying all the functions of the human body associated with walking, breathing, digestion, the senses and reproduction, many of them visitor-participation exhibits. The seven sections of the hall deal with walking and working, blood and air, eating and drinking, the skin, the five senses, demography (study of statistics of births, marriages, deaths, etc.), and the retreat of death. A model of a man 20 feet tall with blood-red heart, the beat of which can be heard throughout the hall, dominates the entire scene. This hall is a gateway to the Hall of Medical Science, which has exhibits illustrating up-to-date information on diseases and their treatment, also on social hygiene, public health administration and allied subjects sponsored by public health and philanthropic organizations. *Museum News* reports that these exhibits have been among the most popular at the fair.

The Carnegie Corporation of New York, the Rockefeller Foundation and the Oberlaender Trust have contributed to the support of the museum.

## MEAD JOHNSON AND COMPANY "B-COMPLEX" AWARD

NOMINATIONS are solicited for the 1940 award of $1,000 established by Mead Johnson and Company to promote researches dealing with the "B-complex" vitamins. The recipient of this award will be chosen by a Committee of Judges of the American Institute of Nutrition, and the formal presentation will be made at the annual meeting of the institute at New Orleans on March 13, 1940.

The award will be given to the laboratory (nonclinical) or clinical research worker in the United States or Canada who, in the opinion of the judges, has published during the previous calendar year January 1 to December 31 the most meritorious scientific report dealing with the field of the "B-complex" vitamins. While the award will be given primarily for publication of specific papers, the judges are given considerable latitude in the exercise of their function. If in their judgment circumstances and justice so dictate, it may be recommended that the prize be divided between two or more parties. It may also be recommended that the award be made to a worker for valuable contributions over an extended period but not necessarily representative of a given year. Membership in the American Institute of Nutrition is not a requisite of eligibility for the award.

To be considered by the Committee of Judges, nominations for this award for work published in 1939 must be in the hands of the secretary by January 5, 1940. The nominations should be accompanied by such data relative to the nominee and his research as will facilitate the task of the Committee of Judges in its consideration of the nomination.

L. A. MAYNARD,
*Secretary of the American Institute of Nutrition*
CORNELL UNIVERSITY,
ITHACA, N. Y.

## RECENT APPOINTMENTS AT COLUMBIA UNIVERSITY

TWENTY appointments to professorships have been made by the trustees of Columbia University. The appointments of four visiting lecturers and the promotion of two faculty members are also announced. Three of the new faculty members are clinical professors, five are assistant clinical professors, two are associate professors, and eight are visiting professors. Appointments in science and medicine include:

Dr. Joseph E. Mayer, associate professor of chemistry at the Johns Hopkins University, associate professor of chemistry.

Dr. Stephen P. Burke, director of the Industrial Science Division of West Virginia University, visiting professor of chemical engineering.

Dr. Tracy J. Putnam, professor of neurology at the Harvard Medical School and neurologist-in-chief of the Boston City Hospital, professor of neurology and neurosurgery.

Dr. Vernon W. Lippard, director of the Commission for Study of Crippled Children of the City of New York, assistant dean of the College of Physicians and Surgeons.

*School of Medicine*

Dr. Gregory Shwartzman, bacteriologist to the Mount Sinai Hospital, New York City, clinical professor of bacteriology.

Dr. Max Pinner, chief, Division of Pulmonary Diseases, Montefiore Hospital, New York City, clinical professor of medicine.

Dr. Kaufman Schlivek, ophthalmic surgeon to the Mount Sinai Hospital, clinical professor of ophthalmology.

Dr. Paul F. A. Hoefer, assistant in neurology, Harvard Medical School, and junior visiting neurologist, Boston City Hospital, associate professor in neurology.

Dr. John L. Nickerson, professor of physics, Mt. Allison University, Sackville, N. B., Canada, assistant professor of physiology.

Dr. James W. White, director of the service of ophthalmology, New York Post-Graduate Hospital and Dispensary, promoted from associate clinical professor to professor of clinical ophthalmology and executive officer of the department of ophthalmology.

Dr. George Anopol, chief of clinic and attending orthopedic surgeon in the dispensary, New York Post-Graduate Hospital, promoted from associate clinical professor to clinical professor of orthopedic surgery.

Dr. Erik J. Kraus, formerly professor of pathology and director of the Institute, University of Prague, visiting professor of pathology.

*School of Tropical Medicine*

Dr. John Scott Andrews, assistant zoologist, U. S. Department of Agriculture, at the Puerto Rico Agricultural Experiment Station, assistant professor of parasitology.

Dr. Esteban G. Cabrera, director, San José Hospital, Santurce, Puerto Rico, and attending syphilologist of the University Hospital, associate professor of urology.

Dr. David B. Dill, professor of industrial physiology at Harvard University, visiting professor of physiology.

Dr. William B. Porter, chief of medical service, Hospital Division of the Medical College of Virginia, visiting professor of medicine.

Dr. William H. Taliaferro, dean of the division of the biological sciences in the University of Chicago, visiting professor of parasitology.

## CHANGES AND NEW APPOINTMENTS AT HARVARD UNIVERSITY

*The Harvard Alumni Bulletin* gives the following account of changes in the scientific departments of the university.

Dr. Richard de Mises, formerly professor of applied mechanics at the University of Berlin, has been appointed lecturer on applied mechanics and will give instruction in the new course on aeronautical engineering which the Graduate School offers this year. Professor William C. Graustein, of the department of mathematics, has been appointed assistant dean of the Faculty of Arts and Sciences.

The *Bulletin* points out that the European war will react on the academic program for the current year, and its full effects may not be known for some time. Dr. George D. Birkhoff, professor of mathematics and recently dean of the Faculty of Arts and Sciences, was appointed Harvard exchange professor to France, and Dr. Albert Pauphilet was appointed French exchange professor at Harvard University, but it is not certain that this exchange will take place. Holders of foreign fellowships and scholarships have been recalled or kept in this country, and foreign students who intended to go to Harvard University this year are not expected.

It is stated that at the time of going to press of the *Bulletin* there was doubt that Dr. Reginald P. Linstead, of the University of Sheffield, England, who late last year was appointed professor of chemistry, would be able to take up his work.

Visiting lecturers to the university from American institutions include Victor A. Conrad, of the Pennsylvania State College; Kurt Lewin, professor of child psychology at the State University of Iowa; Leslie Spier, associate professor of anthropology at Yale University; Hurd C. Willett, associate professor of meteorology at the Massachusetts Institute of Technology; and George de Santillana, of the New School for Social Research, New York City.

## THE SEMI-CENTENNIAL CELEBRATION OF THE FOUNDING OF THE MEDICAL SCHOOL OF THE UNIVERSITY OF MINNESOTA

THE fiftieth anniversary of the Medical School of the University of Minnesota will be celebrated on October 12, 13 and 14. Addresses and papers to be presented will be concerned with trends in medical progress, with particular reference to chemistry in medicine. According to the program those participating in the exercises will be:

*October 12*

*Morning Session, 9:00 o'clock.* "Progress in the Application of Physical Chemistry to Medicine." George E. Fahr, professor of medicine, University of Minnesota, *chairman.* Speakers: Herbert M. Freundlich, distinguished service professor of colloid chemistry, University of Minnesota; Maurice B. Visscher, professor of physiology, University of Minnesota; John P. Peters, professor of medicine, Yale University; Thomas Parran, Jr., Surgeon-General, U. S. Public Health Service.

*Round-table Discussion, 12:30 o'clock. Chairman,* Ancel Keys, professor of physiology; Hal Downey, professor of anatomy; Elexious T. Bell, professor of pathology; Gaylord W. Anderson, professor of preventive medicine and public health, all of the University of Minnesota.

*Afternoon Session, 2:30 o'clock.* "Some Recent Investigations in Metabolism." Clarence M. Jackson, professor of anatomy, University of Minnesota, *chairman.* Speakers: Lee I. Smith, professor of organic chemistry, and George O. Burr, professor of physiological chemistry, University of Minnesota; George H. Whipple, professor of pathology and dean of the School of Medicine and Dentistry, University of Rochester; Charles H. Best, professor of physiology, University of Toronto.

*Evening Session, 8:00 o'clock.* Medical Education. Harold S. Diehl, dean of the medical sciences, University of Minnesota, *chairman.* Speakers: The Honorable Harold E. Stassen, Governor of the State of Minnesota; Guy Stanton Ford, president, University of Minnesota; Anton J. Carlson, distinguished service professor of physiology, University of Chicago.

*October 13*

*Morning Session, 9:00 o'clock.* "Some Aspects of Immunity and Chemotherapy." Winford P. Larson, professor of bacteriology, University of Minnesota, *chairman.* Speakers: Robert G. Green, professor of bacteriology, University of Minnesota; Perrin H. Long, associate professor of medicine, the Johns Hopkins University; Henry F. Helmholz, professor of pediatrics, the Mayo Foundation, University of Minnesota.

*Round-table Discussions, 12:00 noon. Chairmen:* Arthur D. Hirschfelder, professor of pharmacology; Frank C. Mann, professor of experimental medicine (the Mayo Foundation); Owen H. Wangensteen, professor of surgery; J. Charnley McKinley, professor of nervous and mental diseases; A. T. Henrici, professor of bacteriology, all of the University of Minnesota. Leaders of the discussions will be Perrin H. Long, associate professor of medicine, the Johns Hopkins University; Walter B. Cannon, professor of physiology, Harvard University; Anton J. Carlson, distinguished service professor of physiology, University of Chicago; Detlev W. Bronk, professor and director, Institute of Neurology, University of Pennsylvania; Michael Heidelberger, professor of biochemistry, Columbia University.

*Afternoon Session, 2:00 o'clock.* "Some Approaches to the Nervous Control of the Organism." Andrew T. Rasmussen, professor of neuro-anatomy, University of Minnesota, *chairman.* Speakers: Irvine McQuarrie, professor of pediatrics, University of Minnesota; Herbert S. Gasser, director, Rockefeller Institute for Medical Research; Detlev W. Bronk, professor and director, Institute of Neurology, University of Pennsylvania; Walter B. Cannon, professor of physiology, Harvard University.

*Evening Session, 6:30 o'clock.* Harold S. Diehl, dean of the medical sciences, University of Minnesota, *chairman.* Speakers: Harold S. Diehl, dean of the medical sciences, University of Minnesota; Olaf J. Hagen, class of 1906, Moorhead, Minn.; Donald C. Balfour, director, the Mayo Foundation, University of Minnesota; Dr. George Earl, president of the Minnesota State Medical Association; Richard E. Scammon, distinguished service professor, University of Minnesota.

*October 14*

*Morning Session, 9:00 o'clock.* "Anniversary Clinics." William A. O'Brien, director, Postgraduate Medical Education, University of Minnesota, *chairman.* Speakers: Alfred W. Adson, professor of neurosurgery (the Mayo Foundation); Owen H. Wangensteen, professor of surgery; Arlie R. Barnes, professor of medicine (the Mayo Foundation); John L. McKelvey, professor of obstetrics and gynecology; Albert M. Snell, associate professor of medicine (the Mayo Foundation); Cecil J. Watson, associate professor of medicine, all of the University of Minnesota.

# SCIENTIFIC NOTES AND NEWS

DR. CHARLES F. SCOTT, professor emeritus of electrical engineering at Yale University, recently celebrated his seventy-fifth birthday. The celebration occurred at New Haven, Conn., under the sponsorship of the Connecticut section of the American Institute of Electrical Engineers. Dr. Scott graduated from the Ohio State University in 1885, and has recently completed a two-year term as president of the national alumni organization. He is the son of the late Dr. William Henry Scott, one-time president of both Ohio and Ohio State Universities.

DR. BRONISLAW MALINOWSKI, professor of anthropology in the University of London and chairman of the Board of Studies, has been appointed visiting professor of anthropology at Yale University for the current college year. Dr. Harold St. John, head of the department of botany at the University of Hawaii, is Bishop Museum visiting professor.

IN the Cornell University Medical College in New York City, Dr. William H. Chambers has been promoted to the rank of associate professor of physiology and Dr. Kendrick Hare to that of assistant professor of physiology. As has been announced in SCIENCE, Dr. Joseph C. Hinsey, who has served as professor of physiology and head of the department since 1936, will succeed the late Dr. Charles R. Stockard as professor of anatomy and head of that department. During the present academic year he will also serve as acting head of the department of physiology.

DR. ALBERT B. SABIN, formerly associate of the Rockefeller Institute for Medical Research, has taken up his new work as associate professor of pediatrics at the University of Cincinnati and as fellow of the Children's Hospital Research Foundation. He will continue his studies on viruses and the filtrable microorganisms of the pleuropneumonia group. One of Dr. Sabin's assistants will be Dr. Joel Warren, of the department of bacteriology of Columbia University, who will be a research associate in the Children's Hospital Research Foundation. Dr. Sabin will receive the Theobald Smith Award of the American Association for the Advancement of Science at its annual winter meeting.

DR. W. H. RIDDELL, associate professor of dairy husbandry and dairy products at Kansas State College, has become head of the department of dairy husbandry at the University of Arizona and at the Experiment Station.

FRANK COLLINS BAKER, since 1918 curator of the Natural History Museum of the University of Illinois, retired on September 1. He plans to devote his time to research. Dr. Leverett Allen Adams has been appointed his successor as curator of the museum and has been promoted to a professorship of zoology.

DR. CHARLES A. STONEBURG, formerly assistant in biochemistry and pharmacology in the Medical School of the University of Rochester, has been appointed instructor in pharmacology at the Medical College of the State of South Carolina to succeed Dr. S. Carl Werch, who has resigned.

DR. LEONARD WING has been appointed assistant professor of game management at the State College of Washington, Pullman. He will be in charge of the wildlife conservation work in the college. This work has been offered at the college since 1927 on a cultural basis. It has been expanded so that in recent years a full four-year professional curriculum in wildlife conservation has been given.

Dr. Konstantin V. Pestrecov, who for the past two years has been working in the nuclear research laboratory of Columbia University, has been appointed research associate to Dr. Peter V. Karpovich at Springfield College, Massachusetts.

Dr. Horace C. Bold is a visiting lecturer this year in the department of botany of Barnard College, Columbia University. He will carry on the work of Professor Tracy E. Hazen, who retired last summer after thirty-six years of teaching at the college.

Dr. Harry M. Hines, professor of physiology in the School of Medicine of the University of Iowa, is on leave during the academic year of 1939–40. He is spending the year in the Cornell University Medical College, New York City, where he has been appointed research associate in physiology for the year of 1939–40. Dr. Jane Snow likewise has an appointment as research associate in physiology. Dr. Hines and Dr. Snow are cooperating in investigations which are being made possible by the interest of Dr. John Staige Davis, Jr., of New York City.

The Rockefeller Foundation has made a grant of $5,000 in support of the work of Dr. Paul L. Kirk, associate professor of biochemistry in the University of California at Berkeley, for his work in microchemical analysis and its application to biological problems.

The Committee on Scientific Research of the American Medical Association has made a grant to Dr. Owen H. Wangensteen, professor and head of the department of surgery at the University of Minnesota Hospitals, for a study of the physiologic rationale of operations performed for the relief of duodenal and gastric ulcer.

Dr. Robert P. Fischelis, executive secretary and chief chemist of the Board of Pharmacy of the State of New Jersey, has been appointed a member of the New Jersey State Board of Health. The appointment comes at a time when a new State Food, Drug and Cosmetic Act, similar to the Federal Food, Drug and Cosmetic Act, goes into effect in New Jersey. Because of the more complete control over the manufacture and distribution of drugs, devices and cosmetics provided in the new state law, the legislature amended the State Health Act to add a pharmacist to the Board of Health, and Dr. Fischelis is the first pharmacist to hold this appointment, which is for a four-year term under the amended act.

Dr. Robert D. Coghill, assistant professor of chemistry at Yale University, has been appointed chief of the Fermentation Division of the Northern Regional Research Laboratory, Peoria, Ill. He will direct research involving the utilization of bacteria, yeasts and molds as agents for converting wheat, corn and agricultural waste products into chemicals such as alcohols, glycerol acetic and other acids, acetone and other products which may be of industrial or agricultural interest.

P. Burke Jacobs has been appointed senior chemical engineer in the Agricultural Motor Fuels Division of the Northern Regional Research Laboratory, Peoria, Ill. He will be responsible for that part of the work of the division dealing with the production of industrial alcohol from agricultural materials grown or produced in the United States.

*Museum News* states that Dr. Walter B. Jones, director of the Alabama Museum of Natural History, has been appointed director of the newly established State Department of Conservation, and W. G. Lunsford chief of the Division of State Parks, Monuments and Historical Sites.

Dr. Carl E. Guthe, lecturer in anthropology, chairman of the Division of Social Sciences and director of the University Museums at the University of Michigan, has been elected a member of the Board of Trustees of the Cranbrook Institute of Science, Bloomfield Hills, Mich.

Dr. Horace W. Stunkard, professor of biology at New York University, has returned after a year's leave of absence, most of which was spent in the Institut für Schiffs- und Tropenkrankheiten at Hamburg, with short visits to Italy, France and England. He returned to attend the third International Congress of Microbiology held in New York on September 2 to 9, one section of which, protozoology and parasitology, had been organized by him.

Dr. Claude E. ZoBell has returned to the Scripps Institution of Oceanography after spending a year in studying research methods in water biology, during which time he was research associate in limnology at the University of Wisconsin for two semesters and fellow at the Woods Hole Oceanographic Institution for two months.

Professor Enrico Fermi, of the department of physics of Columbia University, will address a meeting of the New York Branch of the American Chemical Society on October 6 on "Atomic Disintegrations Produced by Neutrons."

Dr. Harald U. Sverdrup, director of the Scripps Institution of Oceanography at La Jolla, will give on October 9 one of the annual series of faculty lectures of the University of California at Los Angeles. His subject will be "The Sea off the Coast of California and Its Influence on our Climate."

Dr. C. B. van Niel, professor of bacteriology at

Stanford University, spoke at the Iowa State College on September 28 on "Bacterial Photosynthesis."

The Hepsa Ely Silliman Lectures will be given at Yale University, beginning on December 4, by Dr. Richard Goldschmidt, professor of zoology at the University of California. The subject of the lectures will be "The Material Basis of Evolution." There will be eight lectures as follows: December 4, "The Neo-Darwinian Conception and its Taxonomic and Genetic Background"; December 5, "Microevolution within the Species"; December 7, "Are Subspecies Incipient Species?"; December 8, "The Species"; December 11, "Macroevolution by Large Steps"; and December 12, 14 and 15, "Evolution and the Potentialities of Development, I."

The Conference on Methods in Philosophy and the Sciences, in celebration of the eightieth birthday of Professor John Dewey, has arranged a symposium on his contributions to method in the philosophy of the arts and sciences, which will be followed by a discussion. This meeting will be held at the New School for Social Research, 66 West 12th Street, New York City, on October 22, at 1:30 P.M. The program is as follows: Professor Arthur E. Murphy, University of Illinois, "Dewey's Work in Philosophy and Logic"; Dr. Hu Shih, Chinese Ambassador to the United States, "Some Further Aspects of Dewey's Philosophy"; Dr. Albert Barnes, the Barnes Foundation, "Dewey's Esthetics," and Professor Walton Hamilton, Yale Law School, "Dewey and the Social Sciences."

The 1939 convention of the Association of Land-Grant Colleges and Universities will meet on November 15, 16 and 17 at the Willard Hotel, Washington, D. C.

The annual meeting of the Carolina Geological Society will be held at Spruce Pine, N. C., on October 21 and 22, under the presidency of Professor L. L. Smith, of the University of South Carolina. J. H. Watkins, the Citadel, Charleston, S. C., is vice-president, and Professor Willard Berry, of Duke University, is secretary-treasurer. The pegmatites and associate mineral deposits of that area will be visited under the direction of B. C. Burgess, of the Tennessee Mineral Products Corporation of Spruce Pine.

A symposium on Temperature, its Measurement and Control in Science and Industry will be held in New York City at the Pennsylvania Hotel, on November 2 to 4, by the American Institute of Physics, with the cooperation of the National Bureau of Standards, the National Research Council and officers and committees of many technical societies. The program is in charge of representative committees of authorities in various fields, who have arranged for a program of a hundred or more papers on scientific and technical subjects, which will be presented in concurrent sessions of selected groups. All those active in science or engineering are cordially invited to attend the sessions and to take part in the discussions of papers. A complete program containing full abstracts of the papers to be presented will be mailed in advance on request to the institute. It is suggested that those who expect to attend will inform the institute and make their hotel reservations early. There will be a registration fee of $1.00. The chairmen of the committees are Gustav Egloff, A. W. Ewell, C. O. Fairchild, J. D. Hardy, H. F. Mullikin, F. H. Norton, R. B. Sosman, C. B. Veal, H. T. Wensel and G. B. Wilkes. H. A. Barton, director of the institute, is chairman of the main committee.

According to the *British Medical Journal* delegates from all parts of Scotland are being invited to attend a conference, dealing with nutrition and education, which is to be held at the rooms of the British Medical Association in Edinburgh on Saturday, October 14, under the auspices of the Scottish Committee against Malnutrition. There will be an afternoon and evening session. Sir John Boyd Orr, director of the Rowett Research Institute, Aberdeen, will be one of the speakers. It is expected that about forty organizations will be represented at the conference. The afternoon session will be devoted to a discussion of "Existing Nutritional Conditions as Compared with Minimum Health Requirements." The evening session will deal with "Malnutrition as it Affects Education."

The Council of the American Chemical Society has announced that "Alpha Chi Sigma having presented to the society a definite pledge to sponsor the Award in Pure Chemistry in 1940, and having pledged $1,000 therefor with the expectation that they would shortly be able to assume the obligation for a period of three years, it was moved, seconded and carried that their offer be accepted with thanks and appreciation, and that the regulations heretofore used be continued with the additional proviso that there should be no restrictions as to the 'status of employment of the candidates under consideration.'"

# DISCUSSION

## ATMOSPHERIC CONTAMINATION

The purpose of this discussion is to present physical methods for evaluating the concentrations of certain gases and vapors when admixed with atmospheric air. These methods are limited to compounds such as $CO_2$, CO, $CH_4$, etc., which have characteristic absorption bands in the infrared. In view of the fact that some time must elapse before portable apparatus suitable for use in mines, tunnels, etc., shall have been developed, it seemed advisable to present a preliminary account of the work. Due acknowledgements will be made in a later, more detailed, publication.

The principles involved may, perhaps, be set forth more clearly by considering $CO_2$ as the contaminating gas. It is well known that $CO_2$ has narrow regions of strong absorption and emission near 2.7 and 4.4 $\mu$ in the infrared. According to the first procedure tried, radiations from a jet of hot $CO_2$ are passed through an absorbing chamber and are focused on a thermopile. Since the radiations from hot $CO_2$ are largely absorbed only by cold $CO_2$, it is evident that $CO_2$ in the absorbing chamber would reduce the intensity of the radiations falling on the thermopile—other gases and vapors in the chamber being ignored. The actual apparatus is sketched in Fig. 1, where J is a small

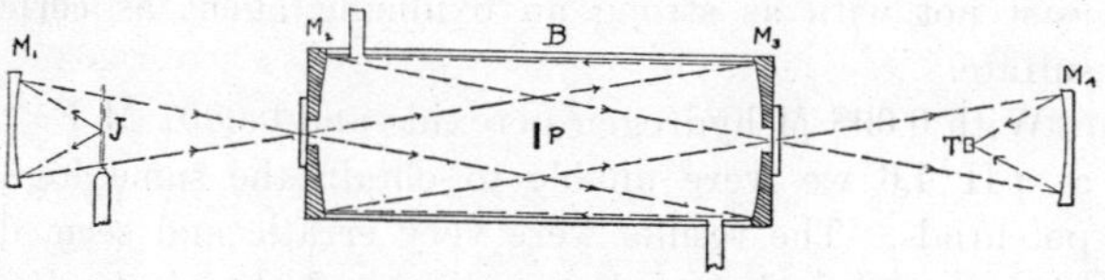


FIG. 1.

jet of hot $CO_2$ whose radiations, after leaving the concave mirror $M_1$, are focused on the absorbing chamber B. This consists of a brass tube (30 cm long and 6 cm in diameter) whose ends are closed by the concave mirrors $M_2$ and $M_3$—each supplied with a central hole 1 cm in diameter. As is evident, these mirrors make it possible to send the radiation through the tube three times. Direct transmission through the tube is prevented by the introduction of a small baffle at P. The system is made gas-tight by waxing windows of fluorite or rock-salt over the holes in the mirrors. The mirror $M_4$ focuses the emergent radiations on a thermopile T, which is connected to a sensitive galvanometer.

The results obtained are confined largely to $CO_2$. Using as source the radiations emitted by the hot $CO_2$ found in the non-luminous portion of a small gas-jet (burning in a water-cooled jacket) it was found that less than one part of $CO_2$ in a million of air could be detected. By employing a jet of hot $CO_2$ as the source, water-vapor in the absorbing chamber was completely ignored.

This procedure was soon found to suffer from a number of serious defects such as (1) lack of constancy of the source, (2) inability to heat all gases and vapors to a sufficiently high temperature without bringing about decomposition, (3) lack of exact agreement of the spectral regions of emission of the hot gas and of absorption of the cold gas.

Accordingly, a second procedure was evolved. Here, radiations from an incandescent nichrome spiral at J are passed through the absorbing chamber and are allowed to fall on a closed but (infrared) transparent receiver T filled with $CO_2$. As long as the absorbing chamber is free from $CO_2$, the gas in the receiver will be heated, due to the selective absorption of the radiations near 2.7 and 4.3 $\mu$. If, however, some $CO_2$ be admitted to the absorbing chamber, this gas will absorb, prematurely, some of the radiations which, previously, had heated the receiver. As a result, the temperature of the latter will drop. The first of these selective receivers consists of a brass capsule whose ends are closed with plates of rock-salt. After filling with $CO_2$ through a suitable side tube, this is connected to an improvised stethoscope. By mounting a phonic wheel at $M_2$ and raising the rate of interruption to about 200 per sec. a fairly loud sound is heard by applying the stethoscope to the ears. Evidently the $CO_2$ in the receiver is periodically heated by the direct absorption of radiant energy. Eventually this sound is to be amplified so that, upon replacing the loudspeaker by a portable galvanometer, sound-intensity may be translated into galvanometer deflections.

A second and more immediately useful receiver was constructed on the idea that if a polished thermopile were introduced into an infrared-transparent receiver filled with $CO_2$ and if the thermopile junctions were shielded from direct radiation, then the adjacent $CO_2$ would be heated by radiation and would, by diffusion, heat the junctions of the thermopile.

This receiver showed high sensitivity as well as selectivity. Having filled the receiver with $CO_2$, ordinary illuminating gas, free of $CO_2$, was allowed to fill the absorbing chamber to atmospheric pressure. In spite of the fact that illuminating gas contains methane and carbon monoxide, both to the extent of 20 per cent. or more, no measurable absorption could be detected. When, on the other hand, the receiver was filled with $CO_2$-free illuminating gas, the effect was enormous.

Obviously, the highest degree of selectivity is achieved by using as source a jet of hot gas or vapor x whose radiations fall on a selective receiver filled with x; the presence of x between source and receiver will be recognized decisively.

A. H. PFUND
JOHNS HOPKINS UNIVERSITY

## OXIDATION-REDUCTION POTENTIALS AND THE MODE OF ACTION OF SULFANILAMIDE

THE report by Shaffer[1] concerning a possible relationship between the potentials developed by certain

[1] SCIENCE, 89, 547–50, June 16, 1939, and Cold Spring Harbor Symposia on Quantitative Biology, 7, 1939, to be published.

oxidation products of sulfanilamide and its therapeutic activity contains much that is suggestive. Certainly it is reasonable to suppose that some oxidation of sulfanilamide occurs in the body. Furthermore, it is possible that the oxidation products account for the therapeutic effect. But that the high potentials reported by Shaffer are due to oxidation products of sulfanilamide and are responsible for the activity of the drug is open to question.

We believe that these apparently abnormally high potentials are attributable not to any oxidation products of sulfanilamide, but to the oxidizing agents used. For example, if to a dilute solution of sulfanilamide a dilute solution of ceric sulfate is added gradually as in a titration, some cerous sulfate will be formed almost immediately. As a result, a potential due to the cerous-ceric system will be established. Eventually all the ceric sulfate from any one addition will be reduced by the sulfanilamide. The reaction would be very slow in dilute solutions, however, and, if fresh additions of ceric sulfate were made before all the previous portion was reduced, a fairly steady potential would result. This should be particularly true if the rate of addition of ceric sulfate approximated its rate of reduction. Since the $E_0$ of the cerous-ceric system is $-1.46$ volts,[2] it would not be surprising to find high potentials. Most of the other effective oxidizing agents mentioned by Shaffer show potentials of the same order of magnitude.

The method used in our experiments was briefly as follows:

A standard Beckman Model G pH meter was used to record oxidation-reduction potentials. The cell was equipped with a saturated calomel half-cell, gold and platinum electrodes, a mechanical agitator, nitrogen inlet tube and 50 cc burette. Before, and at intervals during the course of the work, this set-up was checked with quinhydrone at various pH values. The results in all cases checked to within the limits of the instrument ($\pm 3$ millivolts).

A typical experiment involved the titration of 100 cc of 0.001 M sulfanilamide dissolved in 1.0 N sulfuric acid (pH 0.8) with 0.001 M ceric sulfate in 1.0 N sulfuric acid. By plotting observed potentials against cc of ceric sulfate added, curves were obtained which showed the same "plateau potentials" reported by Shaffer. If, however, the rate of addition of ceric sulfate was varied, differences in the "plateau potential" of as much as 70 millivolts were obtained. The same drift in potentials was also observed. This could be demonstrated more strikingly when 0.01 M ceric sulfate was employed. No "plateau potential" was obtained in this case, the potentials falling very rapidly to a limiting value.

It was possible to plot potentials against the time following the addition of a given amount of 0.01 M ceric sulfate. Smooth curves were obtained which appeared to be a direct indication of the rate of oxidation of sulfanilamide. With some refinements, it is possible that this method might be applied to a quantitative study of the rate of oxidation of aromatic amines. Preliminary studies on several compounds, including sulfapyridine, p,p′-diamino diphenyl sulfone and o- and m-amino benzene sulfonamide were made by means of this technique. This work was carried out with the idea that rate or ease of oxidation might be a factor in chemotherapeutic activity. However, no significant difference in the rate of oxidation of the above compounds could be demonstrated by this method, at least not with as strong an oxidizing agent as ceric sulfate.

With 0.008 M hydrogen peroxide and 0.0001 M $Fe^{++}$ at pH 4.6 we were unable to obtain the same high potentials. The results were very erratic and seemed to depend largely on the condition of the electrodes. Potassium permanganate gave much the same results as ceric sulfate except that no definite end-point could be established. For the results on potassium permanganate we are indebted to Dr. A. Moos, of the Lederle Laboratories, Inc., Pearl River, N. Y.

It might be argued that the rapid drop in potential when higher concentrations of ceric sulfate were employed was due to the rapid disappearance of the intermediate oxidation products of sulfanilamide responsible for the potentials. However, when a reverse titration was carried out, by adding 5- or 10-cc portions of 0.001 M sulfanilamide to 100 cc of 0.002 M ceric sulfate, the potentials at equilibrium were in good agreement with those calculated for a cerous-ceric system on the basis of four equivalents of ceric sulfate to one of sulfanilamide. The number of equivalents was determined by the normal titration method as described by Shaffer and was close to four.

Finally, we found that, on standing for 48 hours, a solution of 100 cc of 0.001 M sulfanilamide in 1.0 N sulfuric acid, to which was added 15 cc of 0.01 M ceric sulfate, developed a single electrode potential which was close to $-0.6$ volt. Since the gold and platinum electrodes checked as usual, we have assumed that this was a true equilibrium potential. The value obtained in this way was of the same order of magnitude as the potential reported by Conant and Lutz[3] for the system phenyl hydroxylamine-nitrosobenzene. We have determined this equilibrium potential for several therapeutically active and "inactive" compounds. Of the

[2] Kunz, *Jour. Am. Chem. Soc.*, 53: 101, 1931. The sign convention of Lewis and Randall, "Thermodynamics," McGraw-Hill Book Company, New York, N. Y., Chapter XXX, 1923, is used in this report.

[3] *Jour. Am. Chem. Soc.*, 43: 1059, 1923.

active substances, the potentials of sulfanilamide, sulfapyridine and p,p'-diamino diphenyl sulfone were measured. The potentials of these fell within a range of 20 millivolts. o- and m-amino benzenesulfonamide were the "inactive" compounds examined. These two substances gave potentials about 50 millivolts lower than the active compounds.

It must be emphasized that, until more is known about the blood levels obtained and the rate of absorption and excretion of "inactive" compounds, it is not possible to accept them as inactive in theoretical considerations. When an attempt is made to correlate activity, only compounds known to be present in the blood stream for intervals of time and in concentrations comparable with sulfanilamide or sulfapyridine, and under these conditions showing no therapeutic effect, should be considered as inactive. Strangely enough, for this type of work, some well-studied inactive compounds would be highly desirable. It seems possible that attempts of this sort to use some fundamental physical property as a stepping-stone in attacking the problem of correlating chemical structure with chemotherapeutic activity may lead to a more rational basis for the selection of new chemotherapeutic agents. Further work of this general nature will be reported later.

We conclude, on the basis of the following facts, that the "plateau potentials" of Shaffer are a function of the oxidized and reduced forms of the oxidizing agents employed, rather than of the oxidation products of sulfanilamide:

(1) In the presence of excess sulfanilamide the potentials fall rapidly as the oxidized form of the oxidizing agent is exhausted.

(2) Equilibrium potentials are established if partially oxidized solutions of sulfanilamide are allowed to stand for 48 hours.

(3) When an excess of ceric sulfate is present, the equilibrium potentials agree with those calculated for a cerous-ceric system.

(4) The "plateau potentials" can be varied within wide limits, depending on the rate of addition of the oxidizing agent.

RICHARD O. ROBLIN, JR.
PAUL H. BELL
AMERICAN CYANAMID COMPANY,
STAMFORD, CONN.

## STRUCTURE AND SYNTHESIS OF A PLANT WOUND HORMONE

IN an earlier publication the isolation of a crystalline substance possessing wound hormone activity has been described.[1] This substance, which was isolated from the water extract of green string-beans, possesses the property of eliciting renewed growth activity in the parenchymatous cells of the bean mesocarp, and its activity may hence be quantitatively determined by the bean test which has been described elsewhere.[2] Elementary analysis of the crystalline product, together with its molecular weight (by m.p. depression in camphor) leads to the formula $C_{12}H_{20}O_4$, and the equivalent weight by titration indicates a dibasic acid.[1] Upon catalytic hydrogenation a crystalline dibasic acid, $C_{12}H_{22}O_4$, identical with decane-1,10-dicarboxylic acid was obtained. After oxidative degradation of the natural wound hormone, sebacic acid was obtained in good yield. The substance must therefore be 1-decene-1,10-dicarboxylic acid:

$$HOOC \cdot CH{=}CH \cdot CH_2 \cdot CH_2 \cdot CH_2 \cdot CH_2 \cdot CH_2 \cdot CH_2 \cdot CH_2 \cdot CH_2 \cdot COOH.$$

This structure has been confirmed by synthesis of 1-decene-1,10-dicarboxylic acid. The resulting product was found to be identical with the natural product both in chemical properties and in physiological activity.

1-decene-1,10-dicarboxylic acid is capable of evoking intensive wound periderm formation in washed discs of potato tuber. It would seem probable therefore that the material with which Haberlandt[3] dealt in his early investigations of wound hormone activity in the potato was at least in part 1-decene-1,10-dicarboxylic acid. It would seem appropriate and convenient to refer to this substance as "traumatic acid"[4] (from Greek τραῦμα = wound). A detailed report of these investigations will appear elsewhere.

JAMES ENGLISH, JR.
JAMES BONNER
A. J. HAAGEN-SMIT
CALIFORNIA INSTITUTE OF TECHNOLOGY

[1] J. English, J. Bonner and A. J. Haagen-Smit, *Proc. Nat. Acad. Sci.*, 25: 323, 1939.

[2] J. Bonner and J. English, *Plant Physiol.*, 13: 331, 1938.

[3] G. Haberlandt, *Sitzungsb. d. Königl. Preus. Akad. d. Wiss.*, 16: 318, 1913.

[4] Report of work carried out with the aid of the Works Progress Administration, Official Project No. 665-07-3-83, Work Project Number 9809.

## THE PLASMODIUM OF HEMITRICHIA VESPARIUM (BATSCH) MACBR

SCLEROTIUM collected from a partially decayed log furnished the source of material used in studying certain cytoplasmic elements in the plasmodium of a Mycetozoan species that had been treated with mitochondrial methods of technique.

When exposed to a humid condition in a large dish, the revived sclerotium issued a bright yellow stream of plasmodium on the woody substratum that had been thoroughly moistened. At this stage of development it was impossible to make an accurate determination of the species involved. For over four months the plasmodium was active under the stimulus of food, moisture and slight light, but when exposed to a bright, artificial light for a continued period, immediate fruiting resulted. On examining the fruiting bodies, it was possible to classify the species as *Hemitrichia vesparium.*

A survey of the taxonomic history of *Hemitrichia vesparium* discloses that the color assigned to the plasmodium has been purple-red with no reference to the conspicuous yellow color observed in this study. It is of interest to record this color observation, since the recent monographs of Lister (1925) and Martin and Macbride (1934) assign a shade of red or purple to the plasmodium, evidently in accordance with the descriptions of the earlier workers. Whether the early descriptions of the form are inadequate as to the color status of the plasmodium or whether the plasmodium under certain physiological conditions assumes a purple-red, while under others a bright yellow color, are interesting questions. However, it appears from previous observations that plasmodia in relation to species are distinctly constant in color aspect.

LLOYD G. CARR
UNIVERSITY OF VIRGINIA

### LITERATURE SERVICE FOR CHEMISTS

BEGINNING on October 1 the Hooker Scientific Library, Fayette, Missouri, inaugurated a new literature service for chemists. Dr. Julian F. Smith is leaving the du Pont Company, where he has been doing chemical literature work, to become associate director of the "Friends of the Hooker Scientific Library," of which Dr. Neil E. Gordon is director.

Through Dr. Smith the library will offer translations and literature searches, backed by facilities for providing filmstat or photostat copies of any matter in the more than twenty thousand volumes comprising the collection. To his chemical education (B.S., Illinois 1916; M.S., California 1920; Ph.D., Chicago 1922) and his long experience in chemical literature work Dr. Smith adds linguistic skill acquired by years of practice in translating from German, French, Spanish, Italian, Portuguese, Dutch, Scandinavian, Polish and Russian.

The combination of a specialist in technical literature and one of the most comprehensive chemical libraries ever assembled is unique in chemical reference service. It offers an unprecedented opportunity to all chemists to have technical literature or patents clearly and accurately translated by a chemist, and to have the literature on any problem skilfully combed by an experienced searcher who is not hampered by language barriers.

The Hooker Scientific Library will render these services at cost (on a self-supporting but not a profit basis) to members of the "Friends of the Hooker Scientific Library." The minimum fee for an individual life membership is $10; for a permanent corporation or institutional membership, $100. All who are interested are invited to write to Dr. Neil E. Gordon, Central College, Fayette, Missouri.

NEIL E. GORDON
CENTRAL COLLEGE,
FAYETTE, MO.

## SCIENTIFIC BOOKS

### RECENT BOTANICAL BOOKS

*Protein Metabolism in the Plant.* By ALBERT C. CHIBNALL. xv + 306 pp. 21 figs. 9 plates. Yale University Press, New Haven. 1939. $4.00.

THE Silliman Memorial Lectures in Yale University for 1938 are here presented in an expanded form. It is fortunate that our knowledge of the physiological chemistry of the proteins in plants should be summarized for the benefit of plant physiologists and biochemists by one whose researches have led him far into the field. Drawing from his own extensive experience and from a wealth of historical and present-day literature, Professor Chibnall has succeeded in presenting a thought-provoking account of the problems and the progress of this field of plant science. The first three chapters are devoted almost entirely to a historical survey of many of the earlier contributions to the protein metabolism in seedlings from the point of view of their relationships to contemporary protein chemistry. Since they include commentaries upon the works of many of the original investigators of the natural amino acids, these chapters should be of additional interest to all present-day students of biochemistry. The classical studies of Pfeffer, Schulze and Prianischnikow receive special consideration and are interpreted in the light of more recent knowledge. One chapter discusses the formation of asparagine and glutamine in seedlings, with emphasis upon the origin of the ammonia and of the carbon precursors. Another deals with the mechanism of amino acid and protein synthesis in plants, and stresses the rôle of the α-keto acids. The preparation of proteins from leaf tissues and the application of the author's own methods to extensive studies of the composition and nutritive value of the proteins of forage plants are described at some length. Three chapters explore the protein metabolism of leaves and the rôle of proteins in the respiration of detached leaves. Evidence for the existence of a protein cycle in leaves is critically discussed, and the interrelationships between organic acids, carbohydrates and fats and proteins in leaf respiration are considered.

The contents of these three chapters are of particular importance in the sense that major developments in plant physiology seem to be here foreshadowed. The final chapter is concerned with the regulation of protein metabolism in leaves. The factors which determine when and to what extent proteins are synthesized and decomposed during the various stages of development of the plant are discussed in so far as present knowledge permits. Three appendices present valuable data on the hydrolysis and constituent analysis of leaf protein preparations.

The lectures represent the author's interpretations of a very large number of uncoordinated researches in an especially difficult field of investigation. Nevertheless, they present as a unit the most extensive and stimulating commentary yet available on the state of our knowledge of the metabolism of amino acids, amides and proteins in the green plant.

R. F. DAWSON
COLUMBIA UNIVERSITY

*Elements of Plant Pathology.* By IRVING E. MELHUS and GEORGE C. KENT. vii + 493 pp. 259 figs. The Macmillan Company, New York. 1939. $4.00.

THIS book is designed for an elementary course of one quarter or semester for students training for various aspects of agriculture. The authors have placed emphasis on phenomena of parasitism and principles of disease control and have condensed or omitted mycological and morphological considerations. Citations to literature are omitted, save for a list of books on or directly relating to plant pathology; and references to individual investigators are usually restricted to instances of classical contributions.

The first 113 pages deal with general aspects or principles, including chapters on plant pathology and human affairs, development of plant pathology, disease in plants, parasitism, the influence of environment on plant diseases and principles of control measures. The following 336 pages are devoted to specific parasitic diseases, grouped according to the systematic relations of the pathogens. Non-parasitic diseases are treated in 14 pages. A glossary of 7 pages follows.

The authors have made an excellent selection of material and presented it clearly and forcefully. The chapter on plant pathology and human affairs strikes at the outset a note of vitality that is maintained throughout the book. The reader with imagination is constantly reminded of the important contributions of plant pathology in the struggle of the race for an adequate physical basis to support its life and culture. The sharp restriction of the mycological, morphological and bibliographical treatment will be regarded by some as a disadvantage. Furthermore, the mode of treatment that the authors have chosen sometimes implies a finality that they would scarcely wish to maintain in a more advanced course. If these are disadvantages, they are largely imposed by the plan of treatment, which was thoughtfully developed by the authors in the light of their extensive teaching experience in both plant pathology and general botany.

The book is excellently printed and illustrated and will be welcomed as a valuable contribution to elementary teaching of plant pathology.

G. W. KEITT
UNIVERSITY OF WISCONSIN

*The World of Plant Life.* By CLARENCE J. HYLANDER. xxii + 722 pp. 249 figs. 195 plates. The Macmillan Company, New York. 1939. $7.50.

THE author has attempted a somewhat unusual work, a synoptical survey of the plant kingdom for popular consumption. The first 121 pages are devoted to an account of the groups usually included under the Thallophyta (here divided into 7 phyla), together with chapters on the Bryophytes and Pteridophytes. The bulk of the book consists of an enumeration of the larger families of flowering plants, arranged in an order which includes some rather puzzling departures from any current systems of classification. The plants dealt with include the more outstanding, curious, interesting and economically important forms, not only of the United States but of the world. Particular emphasis is laid upon food and ornamental plants, their origin and use. The magnitude of the work may be appreciated by the fact that the check list of species mentioned in the text includes nearly 2,000 scientific names. The numerous and on the whole excellent illustrations will aid materially in the recognition of many of these forms.

The author states that the book is planned primarily for the layman, and secondarily for college students who have had some introduction to the field of botany, for the semi-professionals such as gardeners and members of horticultural societies and for specialists in some small field of botany. Certain chapters should indeed appeal to the layman; among these is the introductory chapter, which deals with such topics as the nature of plants, a comparison of plants with animals, physiology, reproduction, classification, the significance of plant life to mankind, and the chapters on plant epiphytes, saprophytes and parasites, the orchids, the cacti, carnivorous plants and the beverage plants. While the book may appeal to one who has already had considerable experience and contact with plant life, and therefore constitutes a welcome addition to the shelves of plant-minded people, it is not, in the opinion of the reviewer, a book for the general reader. It is too bulky and too technical, and its encyclopedic account of the families of angiosperms belongs rather in a work of reference than in the type of book likely to be favored by one unacquainted with plant life.

Any attempt to popularize a subject is certain to bring forth criticisms of over-simplification from professional workers in the field. The book in general is not open to such criticisms, although it may be hoped that the term "breathing pores" as applied to stomates may eventually disappear even from popular literature. Here and there careless statements and minor errors occur, together with confusion and mislabeling in connection with the illustrations. Perhaps there are no more errors than might be expected in a volume of this size.

The author writes well, with many a happy turn of phrase, and demonstrates that he has mastered many of the aspects of presenting scientific subject-matter to the public, but his zeal and industry have caused him to fall short of his main purpose in this case.

C. L. WILSON

DARTMOUTH COLLEGE

## ANNUAL REVIEW OF PHYSIOLOGY

*Annual Review of Physiology.* JAMES MURRAY LUCK, Editor. VICTOR E. HALL, associate editor. American Physiological Society and Annual Reviews, Inc., Stanford University P. O., California, 1939. Pp. 705. $5.00.

THE first volume of Annual Review of Physiology—a sister publication to the well-established Annual Review of Biochemistry—comes as a welcome addition to the field of scientific publications. It is the only attempt to present in the English language a survey of contemporaneous work in physiological sciences, and the only publication in any language which accomplishes the task well, in concise and inexpensive form. This, of course, is largely due to the enthusiastic and conscientious efforts of the various contributors, each an authority in the field covered.

It is impossible to give a synopsis of a volume such as this, but mention of a few items selected at random may be allowed. Needham's review of Developmental Physiology calls attention to the importance of bringing embryology into the physiological field. The development of form depends on metabolic changes, and further understanding of embryological changes will be more and more determined by a better understanding of the energetics of cell growth and differentiation and of the chemical and physical excitants concerned. Burton's review of Temperature Regulation is characterized by explicit emphasis on the most significant lines of advance, *e.g.,* the evidence dealing with the more exact localization of the heat-regulating center in the hypothalamus and the highly discriminating power of peripheral temperature receptors. The extensive work of Winton, DuBois, Burton and their associates on ultimate factors concerned in heat loss, and their relation to clinical fevers, climatic adaptation, air conditioning, etc., are all reviewed. Murlin, in a section devoted to Energy Metabolism, gathers together in an authoritative way much new work relating to such old subjects as normal standards of basal metabolism, the importance of racial and hormonal factors, etc.

Bazett reviews the Peripheral Circulation, devoting considerable space to the subject of aortic elasticity. The control of the peripheral circulation by nervous and local metabolites has received renewed attention during the year that has passed, but one wishes it were possible to sift the material more critically. Some overlapping of subject-matter, with a subsequent chapter by Eyster on Heart occurs, a difficulty that will perhaps always exist in the artificial subdivision assigned to reviewers. Eyster's review includes new work on the course of impulses in the heart, electrocardiography, vectorcardiograms, etc. Limitation of space has prevented the expansion of subjects that the reviewer would have liked to see.

Gesell offers a charming review of Respiration, but is too inclined to fit all work into his own mold of thought. Bozler gives a good review of Muscle, and Ivy and Gray of the Digestive System. Newer work seems to relieve the gastric sphincter somewhat of its age-long function of guarding the pyloric gate, and nerves seem to have a subsidiary responsibility for secretion of bile. The reviewers properly stress the difficulty of drawing conclusions from experiments in which nerves are sectioned or stimulated, for, in control of secretion and motility, separate fibers rather than whole nerve trunks are undoubtedly activated. Mann and Bollman edit the complementary chapter which surveys the multifold functions of the liver. Hope is renewed that the moot problem of the fatty liver may soon be completely solved as a result of the application of experimental methods. It emphasizes the need of doing something more than looking at tissues through a brass tube with pieces of glass at its ends.

The contributions that have been made by means of action potentials in our understanding of the activity of nerve, spinal cord and brain are authentically analyzed by Bronk and Brink, Jr., Eccles and H. Davis, respectively. Hinsey reviews the work on the autonomic nervous system in his usual conservative manner, giving particular attention to the importance of the afferent pathways. The new work on posterior root afferents is included.

Homer Smith reviews the newest developments in renal secretion and calls attention to the possible intrarenal regulating mechanism for the control of blood flow, to the possibility of extraglomerular blood supply to the tubules, and to the action of the posterior pituitary and adrenal cortex on renal function.

Applied physiology is reviewed by Dill. This is restricted to such fields as muscular exercise, high temperature, low and high partial pressure of oxygen, etc. One wonders whether the term Applied Physiology should be allowed to be preempted for such a narrow field. The applications of physiology to medicine must not be forgotten and should form a topic for discussion in future reviews.

H. Evans gives his usual complete and lucid discussion of certain Endocrines—Gonads, Pituitary and Adrenals. In the great whirlpool of real and apparent contradictions, it is always refreshing to have Evans aid us in regaining another hold on the problems.

In conclusion, an ample index of authors and subjects covering 52 pages adds greatly to the value of the work as a reference medium. The sphere of usefulness of the Annual Review of Physiology should be large. A casual reading of any section—or of the whole volume for that matter—provides the reader with a good perspective of the trends that recent investigations are taking. The style is terse, crisp and pleasingly devoid of useless verbiage; but nevertheless reads like a connected narrative.

The reader who cares to delve deeper into particular problems is provided ample opportunity for doing so. The preface states that the aim is to furnish breadth rather than depth of information. But, correctly used, depth is there, too. Each section contains sufficient references to serve as leads for other work, past and present, so that the doubting reader need not necessarily accept the interpretations of contributors. However, the latter, on the whole, seems to be fair and impartial, but generally can not be regarded as overcritical. The question remains whether categorical statements of discoveries claimed or a little more separation of wheat from chaff is the more desirable form of review.

Carl J. Wiggers

Western Reserve University
Medical School

# REPORTS

## SCIENTISTS AND THE PRESS

A committee of the Boston and Cambridge branch of the Association of Scientific Workers, consisting of five scientists and three journalists, has examined in some detail problems of science news reporting. The following statement has been prepared in the hope of stimulating consideration of this matter, and eliciting comment and criticism.

Arrangements for reporting scientific work in the press are at present largely haphazard. The selection of science news is left almost wholly to journalists, who obtain it from a variety of sources, competent and otherwise. In these circumstances science reporting is inevitably scattered, superficial and centered about prominent personalities. Frequently it has been grossly inaccurate, or so poorly designed as to be almost certainly misleading.

Yet many scientists believe that wider and more dependable distribution of scientific information should benefit both science and the public. It should help to educate a large body of laymen in scientific objectives and accomplishments. It should mobilize aid for research, by interesting individuals and industrial organizations and by enlisting popular support for the governmental maintenance of science projects. Widespread and accurate news reports should help to counteract the flood of pseudo-scientific commercial propaganda in our newspapers; and equally the pronouncements of a few individuals who are popularly supposed, not always justly, to speak for science as a whole. Science is but one of many social activities, and particularly in a democracy the public should be kept well informed of its methods and purposes. Such knowledge constitutes a strong defense both of the public and of the future of free scientific activity.

Occasional scientists, however, feel that science should be withheld from newspapers, that they distort it in fact and spirit. In this light the recipients of newspaper publicity are sometimes regarded with suspicion and disapproval. Yet this position grows increasingly weaker. If only because the scientist can not control newspaper accounts of his work, which often appear without his knowledge or cooperation, the stigma sometimes associated with publicity is unreasonable and dangerous.

This is perhaps the crux of the matter. Scientists can neither suppress nor restrict science news. Usually they do not initiate it. Yet they are held responsible for it by the public and by many fellow scientists. A policy of passive resistance in the past has helped only to produce a chaotic press which seriously injures science and the individual worker.

A positive alternative is for scientists to recognize in the press a valuable agency for liaison with the public, and to attempt through active cooperation to improve its effectiveness. Such an approach admittedly offers difficulties. Important steps toward their solution already exist in Science News Service, the American Chemical Society News Service and similar institutions created by scientists; and the press has cooperated to a degree by employing specialists in science news, such as those who form the Association of Science Writers. But such agencies can use only what they are given. The general problems of initiation and critical supervision of science news can be solved by scientists alone.

As a first experimental approach to this situation we are testing the following plan at certain of the Harvard University science departments.

At our suggestion each of these departments has appointed an informal representative to deal with press problems. These men aid in preparing news reports from their departments and act as clearing agents for press inquiries. About once every month they meet with representatives of the University News Office and Science Service to discuss common problems and anticipated news situations.

The usual spot news report is handled as follows. The departmental representative discusses a potential science story with his directly interested colleagues. If the latter decide to issue a report, a trained journalist from the University News Office is introduced for an interview. He writes the story and returns it for correction and criticism.

The completed story is distributed by the University News Office to local papers, Science Service and the national press services.

In this way an accurate account written in newspaper style is made generally available. A complete record of the scientist's connection with it also exists within the university. Of course the story as finally issued may be changed by individual newspapers. We have urged that any serious inaccuracy or distortion of a science report be corrected in a letter to the responsible editor. Such letters are frequently published, and in any case tend to decrease the further garbling of science news.

However, in our short experience there has been little occasion for such action. The stories which we have sponsored, scientifically authoritative and written in newspaper fashion, have appeared with remarkably little distortion, usually almost verbatim. By issuing such reports more promptly and comprehensively than newsmen alone could possibly prepare them, scientists rather than reporters can select the news which issues from science departments.

It is hoped that these procedures may possess some general interest and validity. Communications may be addressed to the committee secretary, Mrs. B. J. Bok, care of Harvard College Observatory, Cambridge, Mass.

COMMITTEE ON PUBLIC RELATIONS OF SCIENCE, A.A.S.W., BOSTON AND CAMBRIDGE BRANCH

# SPECIAL ARTICLES

## THE STRUCTURE OF THE RED OXIDATION PRODUCTS OF TOCOPHEROLS AND RELATED SUBSTANCES[1]

WHEN tocopherols, 2,2,5,7,8-pentamethyl-6-hydroxy chroman (I) and similar substances are oxidized under suitable conditions, the products are yellow para quinones (II).[2] When, however, silver nitrate or nitric acid is used as the oxidizing agent and the action of the reagent is prolonged, brilliant red solutions are obtained[2a, 2b, 3] and Furter and Meyer[4] have developed a photometric method of analysis for tocopherols based upon the reaction with nitric acid.

We have obtained the same red crystalline compound, m.p., 109–110°, from the chroman I using either silver nitrate or nitric acid as the oxidizing agent. Photometric examination of solutions of this substance and of solutions obtained from I by the procedure of Furter and Meyer shows that this red substance is responsible for the color developed in the latter case.

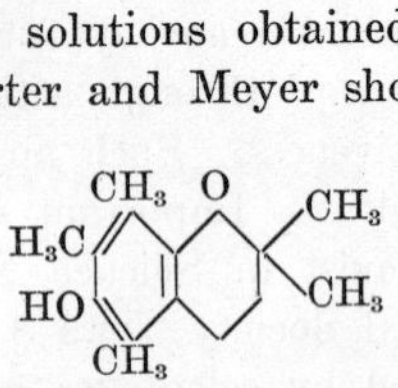

I

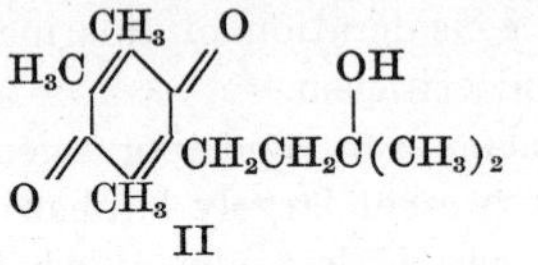

II

John and his associates[2a] established that the red compound $C_{13}H_{16}O_3$ from I differed in composition from the quinone II by one carbon and four hydrogen atoms; and Karrer and his associates[2b] showed that a similar difference in composition resulted when 2,5,7,8-tetramethyl-6-hydroxy chroman was converted into the analogous red compound $C_{12}H_{14}O_3$. Karrer also showed that the red compound was a quinone, and a tentative structure was proposed, which by analogy would become III when applied to the red

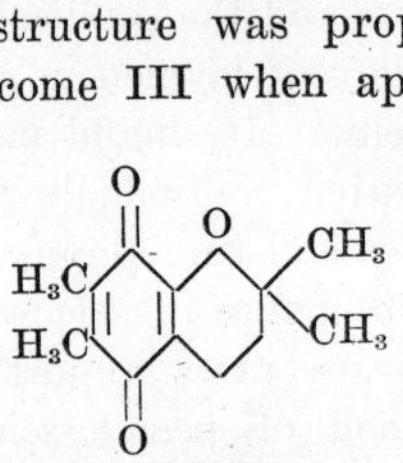

III

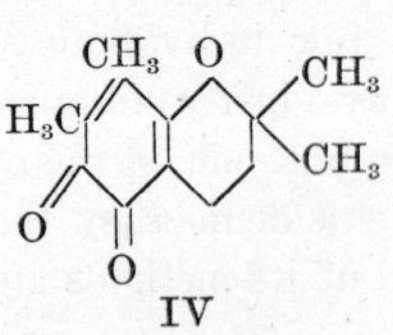

IV

[1] This communication is paper XVI in a series on "The Chemistry of Vitamin E." Paper XV, *Jour. Org. Chem.*, 4: in press, 1939.

[2] (*a*) John, Dietzel and Emte, *Zeitschr. physiol. Chem.*, 257: 173, 1939; (*b*) Karrer, Fritzsche and Escher, *Helv. Chim. Acta*, 22: 661, 1939.

[3] Evans, Emerson and Emerson, SCIENCE, 88: 38, 1938.

[4] *Helv. Chim. Acta*, 22: 240, 1939; see also ref. 2*b*.

compound from I. The red substance, however, is not a para quinone, but is an ortho quinone, and it has the structure IV. The substance forms a phenazine, m.p. 151–152° with o-phenylene diamine and this phenazine shows a strong greenish yellow fluorescence in ultra-violet light, a property shown by the phenazines of the lapachol group of compounds, similar in structure to IV.[5] That the methyl group in position 5 of I is the group lost in the conversion of I to IV was shown by the fact that the condensation products of o-xylo hydroquinone and isoprene (V, VI and VII), in which the group in position 5 is not methyl, all gave the same red compound IV, m.p. 109–110°, when subjected to the action of nitric acid or silver nitrate.

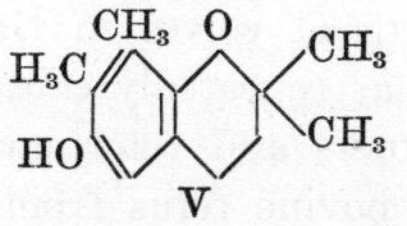

V

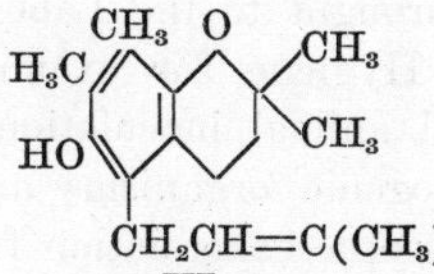

VI

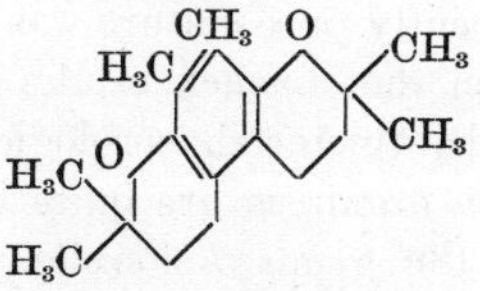

VII

A careful comparison of the absorption curves obtained from IV with absorption curves of known o-quinones also leads unmistakably to the conclusion that the red compounds can not be para quinones, but are ortho quinones.

The red o-quinone from α-tocopherol is an oil. Unfortunately, although it reacts with o-phenylene diamine, the phenazine is also an oil. However, solutions of this phenazine show the same strong greenish fluorescence as is shown by the phenazine of IV, and there can be little doubt but that the tocopherols are also converted into analogs of IV by nitric acid or silver nitrate.

The formation of red o-quinones is not confined to 6-hydroxy chromans, but occurs also with 5-hydroxy coumarans and other related substances. Catechol also produces a red color in the Furter and Meyer reaction, a fact which may be of importance in the examination of natural products by this method, since catechol derivatives are fairly common among natural products.

In these reactions, the mechanism is obscure, although it appears that an alcohol, preferably a primary or secondary alcohol, must be used as the solvent, and the results indicate that the alcohol is probably a reagent as well as a solvent.

Full experimental details of this work will be published elsewhere.

LEE IRVIN SMITH
WILLA B. IRWIN
HERBERT E. UNGNADE

SCHOOL OF CHEMISTRY,
UNIVERSITY OF MINNESOTA

[5] Hooker, *Jour. Chem. Soc.*, 63: 1376, 1893.

## APPEARANCE OF FERMENTABLE POLYSACCHARIDE IN THE BLOOD AND A SIMPLE METHOD FOR ITS DETECTION[1]

ALMOST 40 years ago Besançon and Griffon,[2] Huber,[3] Neufeld[4] and Wadsworth[5] noted that certain bacteria grow more abundantly in the sera obtained from pneumonia patients than in normal sera. When inoculated with pneumococci, a voluminous white precipitate is obtained, while normal sera develop only a slight cloudiness. E. C. Rosenow[6] and Longcope[7] showed that this is due not to bacteria and bacterial debris, as was previously supposed, but to the production of unusually large quantities of acid which precipitate the serum proteins. Longcope noted this phenomenon in sera from patients with pneumococcic and streptococcic infections, from cases of gonococcus endocarditis, acute articular rheumatism, chronic nephritis and uremia. He concluded that "there is . . . some substance which makes its appearance in the blood stream under certain conditions and from which the pneumococcus is capable of forming large quantities of acid." Until the present study was undertaken in 1934, no further work has appeared, and the literature contains scant reference to this very striking phenomenon.

The following simple procedure was adopted early in this work. One cc of the clear sterile serum is transferred to a small sterile test-tube. Serum from strongly hemolyzed blood should not be used. It is inoculated with one drop of an 18-hour culture of a *rapidly growing strain* of pneumococcus. It is then incubated at 37.5° C. The precipitation becomes apparent in about 12 hours; it reaches its maximum in about 36 hours. Normal sera become faintly cloudy. Sera from patients with abnormal states may become opalescent (+), almost opaque (++), opaque with small amount of precipitate (+++) or they may contain a voluminous precipitate (++++). In order to rule out

[1] This study was aided by grants from the Bartlett Memorial Fund and the Douglas Smith Foundation for Medical Research of the University of Chicago.

[2] F. Besançon and V. Griffon, *Ann. Inst. Pasteur*, 14: 449, 1900.

[3] F. O. Huber, *Centralbl. innere Med.*, 23: 417, 1902.

[4] F. Neufeld, *Zeit. Hyg. Infectionskrank.*, 40: 54, 1902.

[5] A. Wadsworth, *Jour. Med. Res.*, 10: 228, 1903.

[6] E. C. Rosenow, *Jour. Inf. Dis.*, 2: 280, 1904.

[7] W. T. Longcope, *Jour. Exp. Med.*, 7: 626, 1905.

any effect due to abnormal quantities of free sugar, it is advisable to determine the reducing sugar in the zinc hydroxide[8] filtrate prepared from 1 to 2 cc of serum. Results from sera which contain more than 125 mg of free sugar per 100 cc should be discarded.

The acids which are produced in normal sera can be accounted for entirely by the free sugar which is consumed. Growth of the organisms appears to stop when the sugar is used up; from 40 to 80 mg of lactic acid are produced. The average yield of lactic acid is 72 per cent.

Unlike normal sera, however, growth continues in positive (+++ or ++++) sera at an apparently undiminished rate after the free sugar is consumed, until a terminal acidity of about pH 5.5 is reached. *The quantity of lactic acid is always greater than can be obtained from the free sugar.* For example, a serum, which contained 104 mg of free sugar, yielded 233 mg of lactic acid. Approximately 75 mg of the acid were derived (by calculation) from the free sugar; 158 mg of lactic acid were therefore derived from some other source.

As has long been known, normal sera contain considerable quantities of protein-polysaccharides.[9–12] By using a standard technique[13] throughout (increase of reducing sugar after 6 hours of hydrolysis with acid), we have invariably obtained higher results in +++ and ++++ sera than in normal ones. None of the sera contain measurable quantities of glycogen. The polysaccharide content is not perceptibly decreased by the growth of the organisms in the normal serum, but large quantities may be rapidly removed in the serum in which precipitation is noted. The production of acids parallels the consumption of the hydrolyzable sugar. Our results therefore indicate that *the phenomenon is due to the presence of abnormal quantities of a polysaccharide which supports rapid growth and which is readily fermented by the pneumococcus.* It thus differs from the normally present polysaccharide, which is not apparently metabolized by the microorganism, since growth stops in normal sera when the free sugar is consumed.

Besides the conditions mentioned by Rosenow and by Longcope, the phenomenon can be noted in sera from many other diseases. We have most often observed it in acute bacterial infections which are associated with a sustained high temperature. Negative results were obtained from the majority of sera from chronic osteomyelitis. Of sera which were obtained from 9 patients with tuberculous infections, 5 were negative. The polysaccharide appears also in the serum in some conditions in which there is no direct evidence of an infection. It is present in the majority of sera in acute nephritis, in about one half of the sera from hypertension in pregnancy and in about one half of the sera taken during parturition in human subjects.

THEODORE E. FRIEDEMANN
WHEELAN D. SUTLIFF
DEPARTMENT OF MEDICINE,
UNIVERSITY OF CHICAGO

[8] M. Somogyi, *Jour. Biol. Chem.*, 86: 655, 1930.
[9] B. Glassmann, *Zeit. physiol. Chem.*, 158: 113, 1926.
[10] C. Rimington, *Biochem. Jour.*, 23: 430, 1929; *Nature*, 126: 882, 1930.
[11] H. Bierry, F. Rathery and Mlle. Levina, *Paris Medical*, 83: 137, 1932.
[12] L. F. Hewitt, *Biochem. Jour.*, 32: 1554, 1938.
[13] T. E. Friedemann, *Jour. Bact.*, 35: 527, 1938.

## LISTERELLA FROM A PREMATURE BOVINE FETUS

PREMATURE birth of calves in Bang's disease free herds in Illinois has repeatedly caused concern on the part of cattle owners and veterinarians. Recently a seven months-old bovine fetus from a Bang's disease free herd was brought to the Laboratory of Animal Pathology and Hygiene for examination. Cultural examination and animal inoculation proved negative to *Brucella,* pyogenic organisms and mycoses. The results of microscopic examination for *Tritrichomonas foetus* were negative. However, a gram positive organism in apparently pure culture was isolated on liver agar plates from the stomach of the fetus. The cultural, pathogenic, tinctorial, serologic and biochemic characters of the organism are quite indistinguishable from those of the genus *Listerella.* There was no definite history of encephalitis in the herd in which the fetus originated. Unfortunately, no study could be made of the aborting cow since she was sold for slaughter immediately after aborting.

The organism is a hemolytic gram-positive rod. It is slightly motile in semisolid agar stabs and in hanging drop preparations. Acid, but no gas is produced in dextrose, maltose, levulose, rhamnose, and salicin. Slight acid is produced in lactose and very slight acid in inosite after ten days, while sucrose is not fermented. A rabbit inoculated subcutaneously with the stomach contents of the calf fetus died ten days later, and the organism was recovered from its heart blood. A rabbit and two chickens were inoculated intravenously and a guinea pig was inoculated intraperitoneally with a saline suspension of the organism. The rabbit died two days later, and the organism was recovered from the heart blood and brain. The guinea pig died six days after inoculation, and the micro-organism was recovered from both heart blood and brain. It has been recognized that ocular instillation of Listerella cultures may cause a transitory conjunctivitis in different species of animals, and Julianelle and Pons[1] suggest that the production of conjunctivitis in rabbits

[1] L. A. Julianelle and C. A. Pons, *Proc. Soc. Exp. Biol. and Med.*, 40: 362, 1939.

is of value in the identification of *Listerella*. To determine if the organism under investigation could cause conjunctivitis a drop of a heavy suspension of the bacteria was placed in the eye of a rabbit and a guinea pig. Two days later a severe conjunctivitis appeared in both animals. While the pathogenesis of this organism is thus established, its abortifacient properties, if any, are not established.

The results of agglutination tests are of particular interest. Julianelle and Pons[2] found two serological types of *Listerella* among the strains they studied. Type I was composed of two rabbit and two human strains, while Type II comprised one strain each from cattle, sheep, goats, and man. The strain herein reported, when set up against antisera of these two types kindly furnished by Dr. Julianelle, was partially agglutinated by the ruminant type antiserum in a titer of 1–25, while with the rodent type antiserum it was completely agglutinated at a titer of 1–1600. Apparently the serological and host relations of *Listerella* strains are more complex than heretofore believed.

Jones and Little[3] first mentioned the relation of *Listerella* to bovine encephalitis. Olafson, according to Udall,[4] also recognized the spontaneous disease in cattle and sheep in New York State, while more than a year ago encephalitis and encephalomyelitis in both cattle and sheep associated with *Listerella* were recognized in Illinois.[5] More recently Biester and Schwarte[6] reported spontaneous bovine listerellosis in Iowa. During the past few months two unreported outbreaks in cattle and one unreported outbreak in sheep have come to our attention, but so far as we know the presence of *Listerella* has not been reported heretofore in the tissues of a prematurely born calf. However, Burn[7] reported Listerella infection in a day-old infant and a prematurely born child. His findings and our own observation suggest the desirability of further study to determine the significance of *Listerella* in the premature bovine fetus. The possible extended role of this pathogen heretofore regarded as an encephalitic and/or encephalomyelitic factor in cattle is further suggested by an apparent artificially induced abortion in a healthy pregnant heifer. This heifer originated in a small Bang's disease-free herd, and proved negative to the agglutination test for Bang's disease immediately preceding exposure to *Listerella*. Ten days following intravenous inoculation of the *Listerella* culture isolated from the bovine fetus described herein, abortion occurred. From the aborted fetus, *Listerella* was regained in pure and abundant culture from the brain stem, cerebrum, heart blood, thymus gland and bone marrow.

ROBERT GRAHAM
H. R. HESTER[8]
NORMAN D. LEVINE[8]
UNIVERSITY OF ILLINOIS

## SOLUTE TRANSPORT IN PLANTS

THE problem of water and solute movement in plants periodically appears for reconsideration. Though work of Strasburger, Dixon, Ursprung, Renner and others, resulting in the cohesion theory of water movement, and its corollary, the upward transport of mineral nutrients in the transpiration stream, satisfied many, Curtis contends that salts ascend the stem in the phloem, and Priestley, Peirce and others question the cohesion mechanism as explaining the rise of water.

Work by Maskell and Mason[1] and Clements and Engard[2] clearly indicated upward transport of salts in the xylem. Even more convincing are results by Stout and Hoagland[3] and Bennett and Snell[4] with radioactive elements showing that salts absorbed by the roots ascend unringed as well as ringed stems in the xylem.

Though described years ago, certain details of the cohesion mechanism continue to elude clear interpretation. Micro-dissection studies conducted in connection with the translocation of herbicides in plants have thrown light on a number of obscure points. When transpirational water loss exceeds absorption by the roots, the water balance soon becomes negative, and hydrostatic pressure in the xylem lowers until, crossing the zero point, a state of tension is developed in the conducting tracts. When in this state of tension, liquid, contrary to popular opinion, displays tensile strength as would a solid. And the degree of tension may reach many atmospheres and the state persist for long periods.

In the tensile condition xylem sap is virtually a superheated liquid in a metastable state, and the stability of the system depends upon the fact that there are no unwet surfaces upon which the vapor phase may become initiated. As Dixon, Askenasy and others have shown, this situation may be demonstrated in a strictly physical system and depends not upon the form

[2] L. A. Julianelle and C. A. Pons, *Proc. Soc. Exp. Biol. and Med.*, 40: 364, 1939.

[3] F. S. Jones and R. B. Little, *Arch. Path.*, 18: 580, 1934.

[4] D. H. Udall, "The Practice of Veterinary Medicine," p. 113, Ithaca, New York, 1936.

[5] Robert Graham, G. L. Dunlap and C. A. Brandly, SCIENCE, 88: 171, 1938.

[6] H. E. Biester and L. H. Schwarte, *Jour. Inf. Dis.*, 64: 135, 1939.

[7] C. G. Burn, *Am. Jour. Path.*, 12: 341, 1936.

[8] Assigned by the State Department of Agriculture to the Animal Pathology and Hygiene Laboratory to assist in diagnosis and research.

[1] E. J. Maskell and T. G. Mason, *Ann. Bot.*, 43: 205, 1929.

[2] H. F. Clements and C. J. Engard, *Plant Physiol.*, 13: 103, 1938.

[3] P. R. Stout and D. R. Hoagland, *Amer. Jour. Bot.*, 26: 320, 1939.

[4] J. P. Bennett and A. Snell, private communication.

or structure of plant cells but upon the properties of water.

In the dissection experiments made by the author, both intact and cut stems of plants growing in soil tubes were studied under the dissecting binocular. When a stem with tensile sap columns is cut, air immediately enters all the severed vessels, and the liquid columns recede from the cut end. However, if the deficit is not excessive, menisci in the smaller vessels soon reverse their movement, and these tubes are refilled. Meanwhile liquid in the large vessels continues to recede, supplying water for the refilling ones as well as that lost by transpiration. As expected from laws of capillarity, competition for water by various-sized tubes results in readjustment, the larger vessels losing and the smaller gaining. As the larger ones become depleted, successively smaller elements lose their contents until finally all conductors are sucked dry. During the various stages of readjustment, and particularly immediately following cutting, columns of sap, water vapor and air may be seen moving in opposite directions in the xylem—a fact that seems clear in terms of capillary action, yet one that has confused many students of translocation.

As might further be predicted, when tensile sap columns in intact xylem vessels are jarred or deformed by flattening the elements with a rounded instrument, they break and the vapor columns expand until they reach the limits of the elements in which they are formed, or until the pressure rises somewhat above the zero point. This proves the tensile state of the water columns, for the vapor phase would not continue to expand if the pressure was above that of saturated water vapor at the temperature of the experiment. As in the cut stem, if vapor is formed in several vessels and the stem is not further disturbed readjustment follows with the vapor columns in the smaller elements contracting and those in the larger continuing to expand. That the columns are water vapor and not air is proved by their rapid collapse under increased pressure. The forcing of air into solution by the surface forces of the bubble would require much more time, as is proved by similar tests with the Askenasy apparatus.

Though the above experiments provide satisfactory evidence of the existence and characteristics of tensile sap columns in plants, the old experiment on subaqueous transpiration performed by Dixon in 1897 has never been explained on a purely physical basis. As recently reported,[5] Smith, Dustman and Shull[6] failed to account for this phenomenon, for Dixon was able to obtain a rise of eosin after saturating his test shoots by immersion for twenty-four hours.

[5] H. H. Dixon, *Bot. School of Trinity Coll., Dublin, Notes*, 4: 319, 1938.

[6] F. Smith, R. B. Dustman and C. A. Shull, *Bot. Gaz.*, 91: 395, 1931.

The fact, recently confirmed by the writer, that subaqueous transpiration occurs only in the light suggested the following explanation: The pressure flow mechanism of solute transport in the phloem requires the osmotic absorption of water from the xylem in regions of active synthesis. Assimilates in solution move to regions of utilization where water is lost to the xylem or to expanding tissues.

Though a recirculation of water in the xylem will not explain the rise of eosin in subaqueous water movements, there are other places that the water might go. All growing cells of the cambium or expanding leaves of the shoot tips require water. Some liquid might also be lost to the intercellular spaces of leaves which often show a partial flooding. Uptake of water from the xylem would in all cases be a function of phloem activity rather than a secretory process of mesophyl cells as originally suggested by Dixon.

To substantiate these deductions, the writer has recently shown that when experiments on subaqueous water movement are set up using forked branches of *Syringa vulgaris,* ringing one of the branches will favor eosin movement up the unringed branch, especially if there is an appreciable portion of bare stem below the fork to provide an adequate differential of living tissue to consume the moving assimilates. These results indicate that the rise of sap in the non-living conduits of the xylem can be accounted for on purely physical grounds, and they explain the single exception made by Dixon to this assumption. On the other hand, they reemphasize the complexity of the over-all processes of translocation and point out the essential part played by living cells and tissues.

A. S. CRAFTS

UNIVERSITY OF CALIFORNIA, DAVIS

## BOOKS RECEIVED

ADRIANCE, GUY W. and FRED R. BRISON. *Propagation of Horticultural Plants.* Pp. ix + 314. 182 figures. McGraw-Hill. $3.00.

ENGELDER, CARL J. *Calculations of Quantitative Analysis.* Pp. viii + 174. Wiley. $2.00.

HALL, WILBUR, Editor. *Partner of Nature.* By LUTHER BURBANK. Pp. xi + 315. Illustrated. Appleton-Century. $3.00.

KAGAN, SOLOMON R. *Life and Letters of Fielding H. Garrison.* Pp. xvi + 287. Illustrated. Medico-Historical Press, Boston.

LEVY, HYMAN. *Modern Science; A Study of Physical Science in the World To-day.* Pp. x + 736. 160 figures. Knopf. $5.00.

METCALF, C. L. and W. P. FLINT. *Destructive and Useful Insects; Their Habits and Control.* Second edition. Pp. xvi + 981. 584 figures. McGraw-Hill. $7.50.

PELTIER, GEORGE L., CARL E. GEORGI and LAWRENCE F. LINDGREN. *Laboratory Manual for General Bacteriology.* Second edition. Pp. viii + 275. Illustrated. Wiley.

TUCKER, S. MARION. *Public Speaking for Technical Men.* Pp. xv + 397. McGraw-Hill. $3.00.

WHITMAN, W. G. *Household Physics.* Third edition. Pp. vii + 436. 412 figures. Wiley. $3.00.

# SCIENCE

VOL. 90 FRIDAY, OCTOBER 13, 1939 No. 2337

*Addresses at the Opening Assembly of the International Union of Geodesy and Geophysics:* DR. RICHARD M. FIELD, THE HONORABLE CORDELL HULL, PROFESSOR S. CHAPMAN, DR. CLOYD HECK MARVIN, DR. FRANK B. JEWETT and DR. D. LA COUR ... 339

*Obituary:*
*Warren Plimpton Lombard:* DR. ROBERT GESELL. *Recent Deaths* ... 345

*Scientific Events:*
*The Arnold Arboretum Expedition to Northwestern Canada; The Bishop Ornithological Collection; The Lalor Foundation Fellowship Awards; Symposium on Cryogenic Research of the American Chemical Society; Scientific Lectures of the College of Physicians of Philadelphia; Medical Education at the University of Chicago; Grants in Aid of Research of the American Association for the Advancement of Science* ... 347

*Scientific Notes and News* ... 350

*Discussion:*
*The Origin of the Human Races:* PROFESSOR A. B. DROOGLEEVER FORTUYN. *The Floating Population of the Air:* PROFESSOR T. D. A. COCKERELL. *A Request to Mathematical Geneticists:* DR. HARRISON R. HUNT. *The Range of Hearing of Canaries:* A. R. BRAND and DR. P. P. KELLOGG ... 352

*Scientific Books:*
*Plane Topology:* PROFESSOR R. L. WILDER. *The Physiology and Pharmacology of the Pituitary Body:* PROFESSOR PHILIP E. SMITH ... 354

*Special Articles:*
*The Sensitizing Properties of the Nucleic Acids and Their Derivatives:* DR. WALTER L. WICKENWERDER, DR. MARY V. BUELL and JOHN EAGER HOWARD. *A Possible Relation between Manganese, Sunlight and Winter Hatchability of Hen's Eggs:* J. B. CHRISTIANSEN, PROFESSOR J. G. HALPIN and PROFESSOR E. B. HART. *The Electrophoretic Analysis of Antipneumococcus Horse Sera:* DR. D. H. MOORE, DR. J. VAN DER SCHEER and DR. R. W. G. WYCKOFF. *The Physiological Changes Produced in Yeast by Ultra-violet Light and by Heat:* DR. THOMAS F. ANDERSON and PROFESSOR B. M. DUGGAR ... 356

*Science News* ... 6

SCIENCE: A Weekly Journal devoted to the Advancement of Science, edited by J. McKEEN CATTELL and published every Friday by

THE SCIENCE PRESS
New York City: Grand Central Terminal
Lancaster, Pa. Garrison, N. Y.

Annual Subscription, $6.00 Single Copies, 15 Cts.

SCIENCE is the official organ of the American Association for the Advancement of Science. Information regarding membership in the Association may be secured from the office of the permanent secretary in the Smithsonian Institution Building, Washington, D. C.

# ADDRESSES AT THE OPENING ASSEMBLY OF THE INTERNATIONAL UNION OF GEODESY AND GEOPHYSICS[1]

THE following addresses were delivered at the official opening of the Seventh Triennial Assembly of the International Union of Geodesy and Geophysics in the Departmental Auditorium, Washington, D. C., on Wednesday evening, September 6, at 8:30.

In opening the assembly, Dr. Richard M. Field, president of the American Geophysical Union, stated that: "Through the courtesy of the Government of the United States of America, the American Geophysical Union, with the cooperation of its parent body, the National Research Council, has both the privilege and the honor of acting as host to one of the most significant international organizations in the promotion of science among the nations of the earth—the International Union of Geodesy and Geophysics. In differentiating the work of this international body from that of national scientific societies, it is the peculiar province of this Union to devote itself to furthering the knowledge of the sciences of the earth in those particular fields where international cooperation is most necessary.

"The program of this seventh assembly now gathered in Washington includes those fundamental aspects of the sciences which deal with the problems of the earth's crust, its oceans and its atmosphere; problems that can not be solved without the cooperation of the many nations to whom are entrusted the various territories of our globe.

"We recognize that this assembly is called at a time of unusual stress, and the Executive Committee of this Union is therefore especially conscious of its

[1] September 6, 1939, Washington, D. C.

responsibilities since both our foreign colleagues and the Department of State have expressed the hope that we may continue our meetings essentially as scheduled in spite of disturbed conditions abroad. I am sure that I express the unanimous feelings of our American Geophysical Union, as an adhering unit of the International Union, when I state that the pursuit of science recognizes and includes those individuals of all races and nationalities whose devotion to extending the frontiers of knowledge make for international good-will and for the enlightenment of mankind.

"May I now introduce the Honorable Hugh R. Wilson, who will read an address of welcome by the Secretary of State, the Honorable Cordell Hull."

Mr. Hull's address was as follows: "I am pleased to have this opportunity to greet and welcome on behalf of the Government and people of the United States the distinguished delegates to the Seventh General Assembly of the International Union of Geodesy and Geophysics. It is regretted that recent events in Europe have prevented the attendance of many of your colleagues, and we all sincerely deplore the circumstances which have made their absence necessary. We deeply appreciate your selection of Washington as the seat of this important conference and we are honored by your presence. I offer to you our warmest hospitality.

"You have assembled not only as official representatives of your respective governments but also as the representatives of one of the most eminent of scientific bodies. The fruits of your tireless efforts are everywhere evident and universally enjoyed. All humanity benefits directly from your findings.

"The discussions at past general assemblies have contributed immeasurably to the store of knowledge of the earth's sciences. Delegates have brought to these international meetings important scientific facts growing out of their researches and experiences and in a spirit of true unselfishness have imparted this knowledge to their colleagues in all parts of the world. This free exchange of scientific information is a practical demonstration of the interdependence of science and a recognition of the benefits accruing to the entire world through the wide dissemination of significant professional truths.

"The work of a number of our governmental bureaus and private institutions is influenced directly by the discoveries and decisions made by members of your international organization. This Government constantly avails itself of the valuable publications of the International Union of Geodesy and Geophysics which could be duplicated by any one government or private organization only with great cost and difficulty. Your studies in the fields of geodesy, seismology, volcanology, meteorology, terrestrial magnetism and electricity, oceanography and hydrology are of daily interest and importance not only to our governmental agencies responsible for official activities in those spheres but also to innumerable private organizations and individuals whose economic existence is dependent upon your efforts. Millions of persons throughout the world owe in a large measure their comfort and livelihood to your notable contributions to the improvement of scientific aids to transportation by water, land and air, of building methods designed to minimize danger from earthquakes, of agricultural practices utilizing knowledge of surface and subterranean water supplies, of geophysical methods of prospecting and of the study of underground formations. It is the good fortune of the Government and people of the United States to have the opportunity of serving as hosts to those distinguished scientists who have labored diligently and unostentatiously in these fields so that the lot of their fellow men may be improved.

"This evening you meet as friends and colleagues to inaugurate the seventh in this series of scientific discussions. Through modern international cooperation science has progressed with strides which would have been impossible if restricted within national and economic borders. This cooperation is made possible through international gatherings such as we are opening this evening. Individually and collectively, your work is facilitated through the knowledge that your fellow scientists throughout the world are friends whose unselfish efforts are directed toward the creation and clarification of knowledge that can be utilized in every-day life to the advantage of all. The prevailing spirit in this assembly is one of friendliness, good-will and mutual understanding and respect. It is my fervent hope, which the people of this country share, that the day may soon come when the statesmen of the world will take a leaf from the book of the scientists and solve international political problems in the same dignified and friendly spirit."

Professor S. Chapman, chairman of the British National Committee, replied as follows: "As representing the nation which last received this Union, at its Edinburgh Assembly, I have been privileged by the American Organizing Committee and by the United States Government with the invitation to respond, in the name of the International Union of Geodesy and Geophysics, to the address of welcome, on behalf of the Government of the United States of America, with which we have been favored by the Honorable Secretary of State, Mr. Cordell Hull.

"During its twenty years of life now past, the Union has hitherto always met in one or other of the historic national capitals of Europe—in Rome, in Madrid, in Prague, in Stockholm, in Lisbon and in Edinburgh. At these assemblies an important share in the activities and the success of our meetings was taken by the large and influential American delegations which came to meet with us in Europe. On the occasion of this assembly the direction of travel has been to and not from these shores. Across the Atlantic and Pacific oceans we have come to meet together with a still greater number of our American colleagues in this no less historic capital of Washington.

"We are indeed glad to be present in this home of the greatest of all national societies for the study of geophysics, the American Geophysical Union—a society which has grown and flourished under the long-fostering care of its secretary, Dr. Fleming.

"The hospitable good-will shown by the United States Government toward our Union, in making the necessary provision for these arrangements, is further testified by the cordial address of welcome which we have to-night heard from Mr. Wilson on behalf of the Honorable Secretary of State. For this welcome I wish in the name of the Union to express our hearty thanks, and I would also affirm our confident hope that, despite the shadow of war which has fallen upon us while we have been gathering together here, this Washington meeting will prove to be one of the most harmonious and successful of our assemblies."

Dr. Cloyd Heck Marvin, president of George Washington University, then welcomed the International Union in the name of the local institutions as follows: "On behalf of the City of Washington, and on behalf of the George Washington University, I greet you. The Commissioners of the District of Columbia bid me transmit to you their personal welcome to the Nation's Capital. We of the University count it an honor and a privilege to have you assemble within our halls.

"Probably never before in its history has the Union met under conditions so difficult as those that confront it to-day—deprived of the collaboration of some of its member nations; its delegates harassed by thoughts of what is transpiring beyond the seas.

"Yet these very circumstances serve to emphasize the transcendent importance of what you are doing and what you represent. The Union has, indeed, become a symbol, standing for those enduring values, those fundamental phases of human activity that will continue even during the present crisis, and that will resume in full force when the stress of these days shall have passed. It is inspiring to know that those delegates who were called back to their countries have so earnestly desired and requested that the Assembly be not interrupted, and that you who remain—many of you in the face of deep personal anxieties—are going forward so splendidly.

"The earth sciences—there is something in the very phrase suggestive of eternal verity. If the disinterestedness, the selflessness, of the scientific discipline could be carried over into the management of human affairs, then might the peoples of the earth be enabled to live together in accord, directing their energies not toward destruction, but toward human betterment.

It is for this reason that at this hour we are peculiarly glad to have you in our midst, because for us you connote Science—Science that knows no national boundaries, no ideological frontiers, but that calls to all men of intelligence, everywhere."

Dr. Frank B. Jewett, president of the National Academy of Sciences, spoke as follows: "I feel it an honor to have been asked to participate in this official welcome to you who come as representatives of many countries of the world to form the Seventh General Assembly of the International Union of Geodesy and Geophysics. This is your first general meeting in the United States, and, speaking for American science, I trust that it will prove both pleasant and profitable. I know that we shall enjoy having you in our midst.

"It is a difficult thing to phrase a welcome to an international gathering at this time when the world of yesterday and to-day is being plunged headlong into the unknown world of to-morrow. All we can know is that the horror, devastation and destruction of a world war is beyond human imagining. How it will affect us individually or as nations no one can know—probably it is well that we can not.

"Nor can we sense in what way it will affect science—particularly fundamental science. We do know from the experience of twenty years ago that certain sectors of applied science were tremendously stimulated and that the drain of research men into some phase or other of the maelstrom retarded temporarily certain advances. Whether the retardation was not more than overcome during the 1920's and since none can say, however.

"Because of all that war on a world scale portends; because I am low in my mind at the thought that man after untold thousands of years has not yet evolved any better way of settling his mass difficulties than by mass murder; and because I do not even know how many of our foreign friends have been prevented from coming, my remarks are not at all those I had originally planned to give. If they seem quite inadequate I trust you will be charitable and remember that they are given against the background of an experience I dread having to face again.

"You are here as the guests of the American Geophysical Union acting with the cooperation of the National Research Council. It is therefore my pleasant duty to-day to represent what in reality is the parent of your host. As most of you doubtless know, the National Research Council, technically a committee of the National Academy of Sciences, is in reality a sort of business organization subsidiary to it. I need scarcely explain to you how such an arrangement is at times a very convenient one. For instance, it permits the parent to do certain things of which he imagines the child will remain ignorant; but actually, as in family life, the child is seldom so unobservant. It also permits the child to indulge in many liberties, ostensibly without the parent's being aware of what is going on. Let me assure you, however, that when the academy's offspring, the National Research Council, joined in inviting the Seventh General Assembly to convene in Washington, it was not one of those childish tricks of waywardness which the parent found it convenient to overlook. On the contrary, I am here to-day as president of the National Academy and I assure you that both the academy and American science as well feel honored by your visit.

"It seems inevitable and also fortunate that as the bounds of our knowledge expand, there should be increasing occasion for international cooperation in scientific endeavor. Just as mathematics and music are already international languages, the work of organizing to advance science is based upon a community of interest which can scarcely be expected to bear much relation to such accidentally conceived things as geographical boundaries. From the standpoint of science, lines of political separation can scarcely measure up in significance to the lines of demarcation which we arbitrarily and solely for the sake of convenience create when we speak, for instance, of physics, chemistry and biology as different departments of science. We know from the present-day activities which we label by such hyphenated terms as bio-chemistry and chemical-physics how fruitful the eradication of boundaries can be. Further, as one looks around at the present scene in world politics, he is tempted to venture a guess that if there were some way short of mass killing to eradicate the other kind of boundary we might all also stand to gain by the process.

"But history discloses many periods during which one or another department of science has lain fallow or quiescent. And perhaps the least that we can expect is that, from time to time, there will arise such sets of circumstances as to throw the international aspects of science into the background. In many respects we have been passing through such a period for the past half dozen years, and now that national issues have been joined in war, it will be accentuated. No one can say that it is an irretrievable loss however. After all, there is much sound philosophy in that line from Shakespeare which now amounts almost to a proverb, that by indirections we find directions out. I need not recall to your minds that science itself, although actuated only by the most enlightened of motives and guided solely by the most rigorous of logic, has on many occasions had to resort to indirections, finding the correct course finally by the method of trial and error.

"While your cooperative efforts and your sessions may be somewhat handicapped by the lack of political understanding which now manifests itself between nations, you are, relatively speaking, fortunate in another regard. So far as I can see, you are unembarrassed in your deliberations by the hoard of economic and sociological quandaries which at the moment beset the applied scientist either when he looks backward to contemplate his past achievements or forward in an attempt to plan the constructive contributions to the future.

"From the dawn of the human race man has existed in an environment which, if it changed at all, changed by only imperceptible amounts. But science has upset this provision of nature, and a creature which through the centuries was called upon to adapt itself only to slow changes finds itself in a veritable maelstrom. It helps not that the maelstrom is largely of his own making, no more than it helped Pandora to know that she herself had opened the troublesome box.

"As you have doubtless noticed, whenever applied scientists and engineers congregate these days, their discussions sooner or later veer over into the sociological and economic fields. I foresee no such anticlimax for your present deliberations. By refining the measurement of an arc of the earth's circumference or by adding another significant figure to the acceleration of gravity or another region of ionization to the upper atmosphere, your conscience need not—at least for the moment—trouble you with any thought that you are enspiriting that famous bugaboo known as technological unemployment. Your researches appear to be at least one stage removed from such sociological considerations. I therefore envy the air of detachment which, for the next few days at any rate, you are at liberty to indulge in.

"Whatever the future has in store for the world and its inhabitants, it is, I think, safe to say that every increment to our store of real knowledge is potentially an increment added to a better way of life. It may be a long way off, but the possibility of its attainment justifies our continuing the quest. The field you represent is one of the most important in the whole domain because it is concerned with the very foundation on which all else rests.

"On behalf therefore not only of the National Academy of Sciences and of the National Research Council but of American science in its entirety I wish you an outstandingly successful conference."

Dr. D. La Cour, of Denmark, then delivered his presidential address.

### Address of Dr. D. La Cour

In the name of the International Union of Geodesy and Geophysics I have the privilege to express the sincere thanks of the Union to the speakers who have so kindly welcomed the Union at this meeting. We are greatly honored by what you have said and enjoy the feeling of having your sympathy, and we are grateful for your contribution to the festival opening of our Assembly.

It proceeds from my heart when I express the very sincere thanks of the International Union of Geodesy and Geophysics to our hosts for the very great preparatory work they have undertaken in order to make us feel comfortable and to be among friends in this magnificent capital of the United States, but, particularly, we are grateful to the Local Organizing Committee for the great care taken on every point in order to further facilitate our work under your hospitable roofs.

Although this Congress is the seventh General Assembly of the Union, this meeting is the first to be held in the New World. Several of us have never been here before, although we have always been attracted to this country by its greatness and by admiration for what has been done here. Never could fate have guided the Union better than in leading us to meet just this time in the New World, where, thanks to your careful and thoughtful arrangements and with the help of so many distinguished American colleagues, the Union can carry through the great program for scientific work, drawn up by the Associations, in spite of the gales which sweep the world.

However, we all strongly feel that the American Organizing Committee merits more than words of thanks for what the committee has done in order to receive and help us. The most adequate expression of our gratitude would be not words but useful results from the discussions and the deliberations of the forthcoming days. It is our sincere hope that the results of this meeting may be so fertile for the growth of the sciences of geodesy and geophysics that this Washington Assembly will stand forever in the history of the International Union as a meeting of outstanding importance.

You will also allow me, in my capacity as president of the union, at this inauguration of the General Assembly, to thank all delegates and guests of the International Union present to-night, for having listened to the call and to welcome them to the meetings of the union and of the associations. Especially, I heartily welcome the great number of American colleagues who take part in our assembly at a very critical moment and fill out our ranks in such an excellent way. It is the hope of the International Union that our American colleagues who now for the first time attend a meeting of the union, will enjoy making our acquaintance as we enjoy their presence and are interested in their work and counsel.

I also wish on this occasion to send a friendly greeting to those of our colleagues who, on account of the unfortunate conditions in the world, are prevented from being present here. We know that wherever they are, at home or on their way back from here, every one of these distinguished men will look forward with longing to meet us again as we are longing for the moment when we can join them again and resume friendly and fruitful cooperation.

But there are some colleagues whom we shall never meet again. I beg you to rise from your seats, my dear colleagues, in commemoration of Professor Charles Lallemand who died 18 months ago after a long and active life. We shall always feel deep gratitude towards Lallemand, the founder of this union, for what he did when among us, and we heartily wish that the spirit and enthusiasm of this noble man of science may stand as guiding stars before the army of the union. Honneur soit à sa mémoire! Thank you.—

Many other colleagues have passed away since the last meeting of the union. The associations with which their work has been connected will individually recall their labors. On this occasion we remember with reverence all these who have passed away after lives devoted to the search for truth.

Since Benjamin Franklin undertook the truly dangerous, but permit me to say local experiment in Philadelphia, in order to try whether it was possible by means of a kite to fish the mysterious electric spark out of a thunder-cloud, and up to the present day when cosmic rays of still unknown origin are caught in strong American steel bombs, not only locally in America but also in other countries, the whole world knows that geophysical work made *in* America, or elsewhere *by* Americans, has been one long uninterrupted and always increasing activity of the greatest influence upon the development of both geophysics, pure physics and allied sciences, and for the opening of the fountains of the earth's riches.

The activities of the United States of America in geophysics have not been limited to investigations of electricity of the atmosphere; the exertion of energy has spread over all branches of geophysics and over geodesy, and the advancement of the whole of these sciences in other countries rests to a very large extent on discoveries and progress first made in the United States of America. Our host, the American Geophysical Union, is an ideal model of a body for coordination of researches. The American union is by far the greatest of the National Committees which have joined the International Union of Geodesy and Geophysics. The list circulated shows that the number of members of the American Union is no less than 1,095. Only a great country, the soul and power of which are based upon the pleasure of its inhabitants to unite their forces, can raise and maintain such an army of scientists and provide this army with instruments and other expedients necessary for working in the first line on all fronts. The regular reports of the American Union, recording the activities of Americans, are generally recognized as a most valuable source of information and stimulus to the whole world. In other countries we can admire your Union, but never reach you on this point. The International Union of Geodesy and Geophysics heartily congratulates the United States on having this army, as the Union congratulates itself upon its close collaboration with this efficient American organization. The collaboration, on an equal footing, of the American Union with National Committees even of small countries, is a remarkable evidence of real brotherhood between nations.

When I spoke to you about Franklin's historical experiment with his kite and about the strong American steel bombs for catching cosmic rays in various places on the earth, I referred to the expansion over the world of the spiritual forces of the United States. It is just as reasonable when foreign scientists meet in your country to remember also the great material support which over and over again has been given by America to assist science in other countries. This readiness of American institutions to further scientific activity wherever in the world science is germinating, has often meant a great stimulation to scientists, and many flowers grown abroad adorn the name of this nation, which has risen above the narrow walls of egoism in order to help other nations to attain prosperity and health through science. From my own field of work I can testify to the great encouragement it meant to numerous countries taking part in the undertaking known as the "International Polar Year" some years ago when institutions and men of science of the United States joined the work and took a leading part in it. Similar personal testimony as to precious help in other scientific fields of work generously extended to other countries by the United States, could be given by many other colleagues present here to-night and by a still greater number of those working in other branches of science.

Naturally, in declaring this seventh General Assembly of the International Union of Geodesy and Geophysics to be opened, I must refer to the actual unfortunate political situation.

Dark clouds have shadowed for a time the sunshine in which the union would like to work. During these very days of our meeting we have had sad evidence of the use of man's knowledge for the injury of human beings and the devastation of civilization. But it is a profound reason for great encouragement to know that truth, friendship and mutual understanding are germinating and growing within the walls of the union whether the sun shines or not. Truth, friendship and mutual understanding are all precious fruits of human virtue, and they are just the medicinal plants the world needs for its sickness that it may become the bright home for mankind, and for peace, we all would like to see. Scientific work is work done for the benefit of all peoples, and the union labors to increase that common fortune. At this very moment there are on each sides of the frontiers between fighting countries remarkable men, our colleagues, who are near friends, who continue to collaborate and who pay homage to the same truths. By proceeding along that path, common sense and brotherhood among the peoples must ultimately rule the world. During the coming days we shall remember with satisfaction that colleagues and friends, prevented from taking part in the assembly, will direct their eyes with sympathy towards our meeting and share our wishes for the success of the congress to the benefit of all.

No gloomy cloud is everlasting, and at this festival occasion it is well also to rejoice in the role the union has to play. I shall not go into details, for one thing because the work in the seven associations will be elucidated in presidential addresses during the coming days. Nor are details necessary to indicate the importance of international collaboration within geodesy and geophysics. The field of work of the union is not limited to the very thin shell round the globe where life is possible. The interests of the union stretch down through the deeps of the oceans, down to the sea-bed, and still further through fiery masses right to the center of the earth. Our interests also stretch upwards far beyond the blue of the sky, up into the crystal heavens where billions of ions are produced in bright sunshine and swarm by day as by night under the stars of heaven. Which empire on the earth rules these regions? Which empire rules the winds and the drifting clouds? Only organized international scientific collaboration can solve the problems of this marvelous globe.

The future of the union is bright because great results lie on our way. Modern science and technique have devised valuable instruments for our work, and their results are more wonderful than even authors of fairy-tales could have imagined. Not very many years ago, tedious and troublesome mountain ascents were necessary to gain but a slight knowledge of the temperature and humidity of the air at a few kilometers height. Nowadays it is possible with radiosondes to measure in less time than an hour those meteorological elements from the ground upwards to the air-streams flowing far above the highest mountains, and to get such measurements in the atmosphere made not only in places where mountains can be found and climbed but everywhere, also over the oceans; geodesists and seismologists can now get time-signals by wireless to a hundredth of a second wherever they are on the earth; high-going planes carry photogrammetrical instruments of high standard for quick and exact mapping of even the most inaccessible regions; naval submarines can do peaceful geophysical work under the waves of the seas and give information about the material below the oceans; seismologists have found improved instruments for exact records of the moments of the earth's crust and of the earthquakes, the sound-waves of which pass through the interior of the earth and reveal the inner structure and properties of the globe—somewhat as a doctor does when he examines the inner organs of a human body by means of his stethoscope. Instruments for counting in less than a second how many ions swarm in each cubic centimeter of the air several hundred kilometers above our heads, and methods of analyzing the properties of large and small ions or even of small subdivisions of these ultra-microscopic particles, have been made available; certainly the tools which geodesists and geophysicists have to work with nowadays are not only useful, they are simply wonderful.

And now, gentlemen, the union is going to take up its pleasant work. We shall enjoy and profit from the personal contact with each other, we shall unite our forces in the study of scientific problems pertaining to the welfare of the 2,000 millions people who now live on the earth and of the unknown millions who will follow us, we will in a time of trouble give an example of the great value of collaboration among men, we will contribute to the conquest for mankind of the bounties of this beautiful earth, handsomely decorated as it is with radiant crowns of polar lights, with deep blue oceans, and with snow-covered volcanoes raised on its surface as signs of the fervency of its interior and as memorials of the birth of our star.

Expressing once more our most hearty thanks to our hosts for their hospitality and for the excellent arrangements of this meeting, and conscious that the union is now, *as ever*, going to work for truth, friendship and mutual understanding, I have the honor to declare this congress, the Seventh General Assembly of the International Union of Geodesy and Geophysics, to be opened.

La Septième Assemblée Générale de l'Union Géodésique et Géophysique Internationale et ouverte!

# OBITUARY

## WARREN PLIMPTON LOMBARD

On July 13 America lost one of her early leaders in the field of physiology, for Warren Plimpton Lombard was among the small adventurous group who introduced experimental physiology to this continent. With that same death was lost a leader in humanity, for Dr. Lombard stood head and shoulders above his fellows in the better traits of man. He was truly a great gentleman.

A son of Israel and Mary Ann Plimpton Lombard, both descendants of early New England settlers, Dr. Lombard was born at West Newton, Mass., on May 29, 1855. It was here that he grew up and received his preparatory education in the Boston and West Newton public schools. This period of Lombard's life was a happy one, for his father had vowed that no son of his would experience the pangs of sorrow of his own childhood. This early training in happiness became a philosophy of Lombard's and guided him in his later life.

In 1878 he graduated from Harvard and continued there three years longer to receive his medical degree. Lombard realized how meager the facilities of this country were for physiological investigation and left for Europe to work in the laboratory of Ludwig. Three years later he returned to America to accept an assistantship in physiology in the College of Physicians and Surgeons in New York City. He left again for a short period of study abroad and then returned to become assistant professor of physiology at Clark University in 1889. In that same year Henry Sewall, who was then professor of physiology at Michigan, departed for the more friendly climate of Colorado. William Howell took Sewall's place. In 1892 when Howell accepted the professorship of physiology at the newly organized Johns Hopkins Medical School, Lombard was called to fill the chair of physiology at the University of Michigan. Here he remained in active charge for a period of 31 years, when he retired.

Dr. Lombard's appointment at Michigan was an important one, as may be gathered from his account of Henry Sewall and the department of physiology:

> When Sewall came to this university the whole method of teaching physiology changed. Not only did he know the subject as it is taught in the textbooks, but he was thoroughly acquainted with the most advanced methods of physiological investigation. . . . Nor did Sewall neglect the laboratory side of the subject. In the catalogue of 1884–1885 we read: "The equipment of the physiological laboratory contains most of the more essential instruments used in physiological demonstration and research." Then follows a list which is quite imposing, an equipment which was greater than that of any laboratory in the country, with the exception of the older laboratories of Harvard Medical School and the biological departments of Johns Hopkins. . . . This was the first laboratory course in physiology offered in any medical school in the country.

Under Lombard's directorship of the department

there were many changes, for physiology was prospering. With the growth of the Medical School at Michigan the physiology department was moved to larger quarters, which it shared with pharmacology. In this building Dr. Lombard's ingenuity stood him in good stead in developing an effective equipment for teaching and research. Lombard's main contributions were in the field of muscle and nerve physiology, reflexes, particularly the knee-jerk, the finer mechanics of muscles, tendons and joints in coordinated contractions, blood pressure, the pulse and the cardiac cycle and sensory endings. One of Lombard's first pieces of research appeared from Ludwig's laboratory in 1885. It dealt with the sequence and strength of contraction of the muscles of the lower extremity of the frog following on various forms of irritation applied to the skin. The simultaneous recording of contractions of as many as twenty muscles with the aid of a most ingenious mechanical system led to significant findings on the integration of spinal reflexes. Later studies of a purely mechanical nature complemented his earlier finding on nervous integration and revealed many unexpected uses of muscles, *e.g.*—"The fact that a two-joint muscle can make use of the tendon action of another two-joint muscle on the opposite side of the leg accounts for the paradox that a two-joint muscle, when in a position to have a stronger extensor than flexor leverage, may extend a joint of which it is a flexor." These studies were followed by the construction of models showing various complicated actions of two-joint muscles. Lombard was the first to construct a sensitive balance large enough to record the minute changes in weight accompanying each respiratory act in man, a method of investigation which has proven to be of value and of continuing promise. Another outstanding contribution was the visual inspection of the capillary circulation of man, a forerunner of innumerable important investigations in the field of circulation. The topographical localization of sensory endings in the skin with tattoo marks and plaster of paris impressions and their later identification at the original location is a striking example of the precision of his methods.

Historically Lombard's name will always be linked with American physiology. He not only brought the newer methods of investigation from abroad, but he was one of the charter members of the American Physiological Society. These incidents in his life were of unending satisfaction to him.

Dr. Lombard was married to Caroline Cook, of Staten Island, N. Y., on June 21, 1883. She died in 1923, the year that he retired. Her death was a great blow to him. He dropped physiology. He gave his valuable library to the Department of Physiology, set aside sufficient endowment to continue the subscriptions to the journals and turned his thoughts to art—drawing, water color and etching. Etching was his favorite, which he mastered with extraordinary ability. Those of the art colony at Monhegan, Maine, who saw his work each summer marvelled at his progressively increasing skill. Those who knew of his experimental ability understood. His work was shown in general exhibits and in one-man shows. In his later years art became his absorbing interest.

Friends who had the good fortune to know Dr. Lombard intimately will never forget his friendly and generous nature, which remained with him to his very last days. In "The Musings of an Old Man," written at the age of 84 and presented to a small scientific club at the University of Michigan, he makes the following statement:

> I have always been an optimist, and I can not claim to have ever been religious. I have thoroughly enjoyed life and feel that the finest one can do is to bring pleasures into the lives of others. In this I find a worthy reason for living, and shall be glad to live as long as I can enjoy life and help others to do so.

To those who admit the mechanistic forces of life and have faith in evolution, men like Warren Plimpton Lombard shine as rays of hope for the future happiness of mankind.

ROBERT GESELL

UNIVERSITY OF MICHIGAN

## RECENT DEATHS

DR. HARVEY CUSHING, Sterling professor of neurology at Yale University from 1933 until his retirement with the title emeritus in 1937, died on October 7 at the age of seventy years. Dr. Cushing was Moseley professor of surgery at Harvard University from 1912 to 1932, when he was made Moseley professor emeritus.

DR. CHARLES STAPLES MANGUM, successively professor of physiology and materia medica, pharmacology and anatomy and from 1933 to 1937 dean of the Medical School of the University of North Carolina, died on September 29. He was sixty-nine years old.

DR. OSCAR HENRY PLANT, professor of pharmacology and head of the department at the State University of Iowa, died on October 2 at the age of sixty-four years.

DR. E. VICTOR SMITH, professor of physiology at the University of Washington, died on September 28 at the age of seventy-two years.

PROFESSOR JOHN RAYMOND LAPHAM, dean of the department of engineering of George Washington University, died on October 3 at the age of fifty-three years.

F. L. MUSBACH, professor of soils in the University of Wisconsin, who had charge of soil investigations at the branch experiment stations, was killed in an automobile accident on September 14. He was sixty-three years old. Professor Musbach was a member of the American Association for the Advancement of Science and other scientific societies.

DR. CHARLES JASTROW MENDELSOHN, of the College of the City of New York, cryptographer, known for his work on the mathematics of code-word structure and the theory and structure of the cable codes, died on September 27 at the age of fifty-eight years.

# SCIENTIFIC EVENTS

## THE ARNOLD ARBORETUM EXPEDITION TO NORTHWESTERN CANADA

THE Arnold Arboretum expedition of 1939 to the Mackenzie basin of northwestern Canada returned to Boston on September 28. It left for the field on May 20, and arrived on June 9 at Fort Simpson on the Mackenzie River. On June 16 a chartered airplane was used for the journey to Brintnell Lake, approximately 200 miles west of Simpson. This lake lies at about 2,600 feet above sea-level and is surrounded by mountains ranging from 6,000 to 9,000 feet above the sea. Its position is in lat. 62° 5′ N., long. 127° 35′ W. The party remained there until August 20, when they returned to Simpson by plane. The boat journey southward was begun on September 8.

Approximately 1,000 field numbers of vascular plants, 620 of lichens and 60 of fungi, altogether about 15,000 herbarium specimens, were collected, mainly at Brintnell Lake and in the vicinity of Fort Simpson. The chief objectives of the trip were collections and notes on local vegetation in the Mackenzie Mountains of the South Nahanni River region, in which Brintnell Lake is situated. The lake is at the margin of the Snyder Range, a group of high mountains about the headwaters of the South Nahanni, and lies in one of the least known regions, biologically speaking, in boreal America. In fact, practically no botanical material from the whole Mackenzie Mountain system had been collected prior to this summer; and it was especially desirable in view of projected plans for a new floristic work on the northern parts of the continent.

The 1939 expedition was supported by the Arnold Arboretum and by liberal grants from the Milton Fund of Harvard University, the American Academy of Arts and Sciences and the National Academy of Science. The National Museum of Canada contributed substantially by the loan of field equipment. The party consisted of Dr. and Mrs. Hugh M. Raup, their two sons and James Soper, of Hamilton, Ontario.

HUGH M. RAUP

## THE BISHOP ORNITHOLOGICAL COLLECTION

THE Field Museum of Natural History, Chicago, has recently concluded arrangements to acquire the Bishop collection of more than 50,000 North American birds, one of the largest and most important private collections ever assembled and the last of its kind which had not passed to a public institution. The negotiations to obtain this collection were recently completed by Dr. Wilfred H. Osgood, chief curator of the department of zoology, on a visit to Dr. Louis B. Bishop at Pasadena, California. Dr. Osgood is an old friend of Dr. Bishop's, and in 1899 they conducted an expedition together to the Yukon and Alaska.

The Field Museum will obtain possession immediately of the major part of the collection, which is now housed at New Haven, Conn. The rest of it will remain in Los Angeles, where Dr. Bishop will continue work towards its improvement. It includes representatives of nearly all known forms of birds found in every section of North America north of Mexico, representing forty years of constant and intensive effort, both on the part of Dr. Bishop and of numerous professional ornithologists who have been associated with him at various times. According to Rudyerd Boulton, curator of birds at the museum, the specimens are distinctly superior to the average in quality of preparation. An important item is the inclusion of thirty type-specimens. Included also are specimens of various birds which are now extinct, such as the Carolina parokeet, the ivory-billed woodpecker, the Eskimo curlew and the passenger pigeon. Many others are of species which have become scarce and difficult to obtain.

Hitherto the principal efforts in ornithological research made by the museum have been devoted to the birds of Central and South America, Africa and other foreign localities. Although it has a collection in the North American field, this has been left largely to other institutions. The acquisition of the Bishop collection now gives to the museum one of the most comprehensive North American bird collections either in this country or abroad. It is estimated that it has cost its owner nearly $100,000, and it is doubtful if it could be reproduced at this time for double this amount.

## THE LALOR FOUNDATION FELLOWSHIP AWARDS

THE Lalor Foundation has announced its fourth series of fellowship awards, authorizing grants of $20,000 for the academic year 1940–41. The individual awards range between $1,800 and $2,500 or according to the special needs of the candidate.

Six fellowships of the 1939–40 series are being administered by the foundation, which was organized in 1935. The work of the holders of present fellowship awards is in the fields of physical chemistry, biochemistry and biophysics, and the institutions at which the researches are being conducted include the University of Oxford, Cornell University, Princeton University, the Johns Hopkins University, the Massachusetts Institute of Technology and the Johnson Institute of Biophysics of the University of Pennsylvania. The present war has caused almost complete abandonment of fundamental research in the belligerent countries, but the fellows who originally planned to work abroad have been able to make other plans for the coming year.

The awards in the 1940–41 series will be given for fundamental research work in any field of chemistry. Support for industrial research is not intended. The awards are open to both men and women and for work anywhere in the United States or abroad. Men and women in academic service who may be on leave of absence are among those eligible for appointment. Attainment of the degree of Ph.D. or training equivalent thereto is a requirement for candidacy. The final selections will be based on previous training, demonstrated competence and the promise of the candidates in their special fields of work.

It is pointed out in the official announcement that one of the important needs in science is to develop men who have a thorough background and training in fundamental chemical research and who have also adequate experience in the biological and medical sciences, qualifying them to attack with basic understanding research problems in the fields of biochemistry and chemotherapy. Accordingly, for a part of the Lalor awards, preference will be given to candidates directing their research toward applying the principles and discoveries of physical and organic chemistry to problems within these latter fields.

The qualifications of candidates will be passed upon by a selection committee consisting of Drs. C. A. Kraus, of Brown University; Arthur B. Lamb, of Harvard University; Roger Adams, of the University of Illinois; Hans T. Clarke, of Columbia University, and the secretary of the foundation.

Inquiries and requests for application forms for awards should be addressed to C. Lalor Burdick, Secretary, Lalor Foundation, Wilmington, Delaware. Applications should be in his hands by December 31, and appointments will be announced early in March, 1940.

## SYMPOSIUM ON CRYOGENIC RESEARCH OF THE AMERICAN CHEMICAL SOCIETY

ON September 11, the week of the Boston meeting of the American Chemical Society, the Division of Inorganic and Physical Chemistry sponsored a symposium on Cryogenic Research, held at the George Eastman Laboratories of the Massachusetts Institute of Technology. It was at the Rochester meeting two years ago that the first symposium held in the United States for the presentation of papers and discussion on low temperature methods and research took place. The recent meeting furnished convincing evidence of an astonishing increase in interest, equipment and volume of research over the two-year interval. Our scientific colleagues from the Cryogenic Laboratory of the University of Toronto, H. Grayson Smith and J. O. Wilhelm, contributed two papers, and the Mond Laboratory of Cambridge, England, was represented by Dr. D. Shoenberg, who contributed a paper on super-electrical conductivity. Papers were presented also by representatives of the cryogenic laboratories of the National Bureau of Standards (F. G. Brickwedde, R. B. Scott, H. J. Hoge), the University of California at Berkeley (W. F. Giauque and J. W. Stout), the Pennsylvania State College (J. G. Aston and G. H. Messerly), the Johns Hopkins University (W. T. Ziegler), the California Institute of Technology (Alexander Goetz and A. Dember), Columbia University (H. A. Boorse, V. W. Cohen, C. Williams, S. L. Quimby), Cornell University (J. G. Kirkwood) and the Massachusetts Institute of Technology (S. C. Collins, R. B. Jacobs, C. Starr, C. C. Stephenson, J. G. Hooley, J. A. Beattie, B. E. Blaisdell, J. Kaye, C. A. Johnson and H. T. Gerry).

The symposium was in part devoted to the consideration of techniques and methods adapted to improving the precision and scope of a wide range of types of measurements at the lowest temperatures. The bulk of the day, however, was occupied with reports on the peculiarities of the heat capacities and thermodynamic properties of a variety of substances, the velocity of sound in liquid helium, its viscosity and flow peculiarities, phase transitions of the second kind, electrical superconductivity as related to conductor size, x-ray reflection intensities, thermal and magnetic properties of the para-magnetic salt nickel sulphate heptahydrate, among other items.

Professor Alexander Goetz gave a survey drawing attention to the remarkable advantages for many purposes which the special properties of matter at very low temperatures possess. The low temperature preservation of cell life, for example, should be of immediate practical interest in preserving many kinds of cells—blood corpuscles of varied types, for instance.

The most serious present obstacle to the rapid development of a more detailed and profound knowledge of the properties of matter and associated phenomena lies in the expensive equipment and the danger attending the manipulation of hydrogen and gases generally under high pressure. In this connection the report by the Massachusetts Institute of Technology group (S. C. Collins and R. B. Jacobs) of progress in the attempt to develop inexpensive mechanical means for continuously maintaining sub-hydrogen temperatures was of general interest. If the difficulties of design and operation of a really low temperature engine (10° K level) can be solved, a substantial advance will have been made in promoting the conditions for larger scale and safer operations in a fascinating world of strange and as yet imperfectly understood phenomena.

The enthusiasm and greatly widened interest manifest throughout the course of the symposium warrant the belief that the United States in a very short time will be contributing cryogenic research results commensurate with the resources of the country.

F. G. KEYES

## SCIENTIFIC LECTURES OF THE COLLEGE OF PHYSICIANS OF PHILADELPHIA

THE first of the annual scientific lectures of the College of Physicians of Philadelphia was the Mary Scott Newbold lecture XLV, which was given on October 4 by Dr. Alfred Blalock, professor of surgery at Vanderbilt University. He spoke on "Shock."

The lectures for 1939 to 1940 are given at 8:30 P.M. on the first Wednesday of each month from October to May. The program follows:

November—James M. Anders Lecture XIV. Rolla E. Dyer, chief, Division of Infectious Diseases, U. S. Public Health Service. "Animal Diseases Transmissible to Man, with Special Reference to Typhus Fever, Spotted Fever, Undulant Fever and Tularemia."

December—Thomas Dent Mütter Lecture LII. Howard T. Karsner, professor of pathology, director of Institute of Pathology, Western Reserve University. "Certain Ovarian Tumors Associated with Sexual Endocrine Dysfunction."

January—James M. Anders Lecture XV. Charles Armstrong, senior surgeon, U. S. Public Health Service. "Recent Developments in Central Nervous System Virus Infections, with Special Reference to Lymphocytic Meningitis and Poliomyelitis."

February—Mary Scott Newbold Lecture XLVI. Tom D. Spies, associate professor of medicine, University of Cincinnati. "Clinical and Laboratory Studies on the Avitaminoses, with Special Reference to Nicotinic Acid, Thiamin and Riboflavin."

March—Mary Scott Newbold Lecture XLVII. Alvin F. Coburn, assistant professor of medicine, Columbia University. "Factors in the Initiation of Rheumatic Activity."

April—Balduin Lucké, professor of pathology, University of Pennsylvania. "Tumors in Cold-Blooded Animals; Their Significance in the Experimental Investigation of Cancer." Joseph McFarland, emeritus professor of pathology, University of Pennsylvania. "The Pathological Diagnosis of Cancer in Man."

May—Nathan Lewis Hatfield Lecture XXIII. Lecture and subject to be announced.

The following lectures for the general public are announced:

November 17, 1939—O. H. Perry Pepper, professor of medicine, University of Pennsylvania. "Medical Problems of Advancing Age."

January 19, 1940—J. Parsons Schaeffer, professor of anatomy and director of the Daniel Baugh Institute of Anatomy, Jefferson Medical College. "The Human Constitution and Some of Its Problems."

April 12—W. Edward Chamberlain, professor of radiology and roentgenology, Temple University. "The X-Ray as an Aid in Diagnosis."

## MEDICAL EDUCATION AT THE UNIVERSITY OF CHICAGO

DECISIONS affecting medical education on the west side of Chicago have been announced by President Robert M. Hutchins, of the University of Chicago, and John McKinlay, president of the Board of Managers of the Presbyterian Hospital. The university has decided to terminate undergraduate medical education at the Rush Medical College. The Board of Managers of the Presbyterian Hospital has voted that the hospital remain as at present on the west side of Chicago.

As a result of these decisions, the university will establish a program of graduate medical education at the Rush Medical College and committees will be appointed to formulate plans for a Graduate School, which it is hoped will be opened in the near future. It will emphasize research in medical science and provide training for graduates of medical schools in the various fields of specialization.

Undergraduate work will continue, however, at the Rush Medical College till July, 1942, to provide completion of training for the class entering next autumn. Undergraduate training also will continue at the south side medical school and after 1942 will be offered there exclusively.

The decision to establish the Rush Medical College as a center of graduate medical training terminates discussions as to its ultimate status which have been carried on intermittently since 1916. In that year the university approved plans for the south side school, which was opened in the autumn of 1927.

Rush Medical College, chartered in 1837 and in operation since 1842, was the pioneer medical school of the Middle West. It was merged with the university in 1924 after twenty-six years of affiliation.

## GRANTS IN AID OF RESEARCH OF THE AMERICAN ASSOCIATION FOR THE ADVANCEMENT OF SCIENCE

AT its annual meeting each year the council of the American Association votes a number of grants in aid of research. In order that applications for such grants may be examined and passed on by the committee on grants in time for the annual meeting, they must be filed in the office of the permanent secretary before November 1 on forms that will be supplied upon request. These forms contain full instructions respecting the information that must support the applications.

The funds from which the grants are made are derived from the income of endowments of the association by various gifts, from investments of reserve funds and from the income from the life membership fees of deceased life members. Although the income available for the support of research is as yet very limited, it fortunately has been increased in recent years by gifts from a friend of the association.

As a rule grants are not made to pay salaries of investigators or traveling expenses or for printing reports of the results of investigation. They are generally made for assistance in completing research projects that are well under way and for which valuable conclusions within limited periods may reasonably be expected. Often they complete the requirements for funds which have been partly met by the institutions with which the applicants are associated or from other sources.

F. R. MOULTON,
*Permanent Secretary*

# SCIENTIFIC NOTES AND NEWS

AT the meeting of the National Academy of Sciences to be held at Brown University, Providence, R. I., on October 23, 24 and 25, there will be three general addresses. At 4:30 on the afternoon of October 23, Dr. Frank B. Jewett, president of the academy, will give an address over the coast to coast network of the Columbia Broadcasting System on "How Science Could be Mobilized in the United States." In the evening, Dr. Harvey Fletcher, of the Bell Telephone Laboratories, will give a public lecture on "Auditory Patterns—a Demonstration Lecture." At the dinner on the evening of October 24, Dr. Albert D. Mead, of Brown University, will speak on "Episodes and Personalities in the Development of Biology at Brown."

THE eightieth birthday of John Dewey, which occurs on October 20, will be celebrated on October 20 and 21 by a conference at the Hotel Pennsylvania, New York City, under the auspices of the Progressive Education Association. There will be fourteen sessions, in which many leaders in philosophy and education will participate.

DR. GANO DUNN, president of the J. G. White Engineering Corporation and of Cooper Union, has been chosen as the 1939 recipient of the Hoover Medal, "awarded by engineers to a fellow engineer for distinguished public service." John V. W. Reynders, of New York, is chairman of a board of award representing the four national societies of civil, mining and metallurgical, mechanical and electrical engineers. "The medal signalizes great unselfish, non-technical service by engineers to their fellowmen." It will be formally presented to Dr. Dunn under the auspices of the American Institute of Electrical Engineers during the annual convention in New York City on January 22 to 26, 1940.

THE Roosevelt Memorial Association has awarded one of its Roosevelt Medals to Dr. George Washington Carver, of the Tuskegee Institute, distinguished for his work in agricultural chemistry.

DR. C. B. HUTCHISON, dean of the College of Agriculture of the University of California at Berkeley, has been awarded the degree of doctor of agriculture, *honoris causa,* by the University of Sofia, Bulgaria. The degree was awarded on the occasion of the fiftieth anniversary of the founding of the university. Dean Hutchison received the honor in recognition of the aid he gave to the university from 1924–27 while acting as a member of the European Mission of the International Education Board of the Rockefeller Foundation.

DR. PETER DEBYE, professor of physics at Berlin, has been elected honorary member of the Indian Academy of Sciences at Bangalore, of the Chemical Society of the Netherlands and of the Physical Society, London.

A DINNER was given on October 12 by colleagues and former students in honor of Dr. Evarts A. Graham, since 1919 professor of surgery at the School of Medicine of Washington University, St. Louis.

DR. WARREN H. MCBRYDE, of San Francisco, Calif., has been elected president of the American Society of Mechanical Engineers. He will take office at the sixtieth annual meeting to be held in Philadelphia from December 4 to 8. This is the first meeting to be held other than in New York City since the year 1890.

DR. HARDY A. KEMP, professor of bacteriology and preventive medicine at the College of Medicine of Baylor University, Dallas, Texas, has become dean of the College of Medicine at the University of Vermont. Dr. Kemp is also head of the reorganized department of bacteriology, hygiene and preventive medicine.

DR. ROBERT S. SHANKLAND has been appointed acting head of the department of physics at the Case School of Applied Science. He succeeds Dr. Dayton C. Miller, who retired in June, 1938.

DR. CARL WALDEMAR HAGQUIST, who served as acting professor of biology at the University of Richmond during the last session, has been appointed professor of biology at Albany College, Portland, Oregon.

Dr. Gerald F. Tape, graduate assistant in physics at the University of Michigan, has been appointed for the current year instructor in physics at Cornell University.

Dr. Alfred S. Lazarus, of the Hooper Foundation of the University of California and of the Connaught Laboratories of the University of Toronto, has been appointed instructor in the department of bacteriology and public health at the University of Colorado School of Medicine at Denver.

Dr. Clarence F. Hiskey has been appointed instructor in chemistry at the University of Tennessee. He will continue the research on rhenium in which he has been engaged at the University of Wisconsin.

Dr. Charles F. Rogers, assistant biochemist for the Minnesota Agricultural Experiment Station, has been appointed associate in biochemistry in the department of agronomy at the Ohio Agricultural Experiment Station at Wooster, to succeed Dr. Morris. He will continue in cooperation with plant physiologists on the biochemistry of corn.

Arthur Folger, since 1919 member of the Division of Animal Husbandry of the College of Agriculture at Davis of the University of California, has resigned to accept the post of regional director of the Farm Security Administration.

Dr. Alfred Fröhlich, formerly professor of pharmacology at the University of Vienna, has been appointed pharmacologist to the May Institute for Medical Research of the Jewish Hospital, Cincinnati, Ohio.

Gordon Gunter, of the department of zoology of the University of Texas, has been appointed marine biologist for the Coastal Division of the Texas Game, Fish and Oyster Commission.

Dr. J. H. Sandground, formerly assistant professor of helminthology in the department of tropical medicine at the Medical School and the School of Public Health of Harvard University, has joined the staff of the Lilly Research Laboratories at Indianapolis. He has recently returned from the Netherlands East Indies where, as a fellow of the John Simon Guggenheim Memorial Foundation, he spent a year working in the Pathologische Instituut of the Geneeskundige Hoogeschool at Batavia.

Dr. Arne Tiselius, professor of biochemistry at the Fysikalisk-Kemiska Institutionen, University of Uppsala, will deliver on October 19 the first Harvey Society Lecture of the current series at the New York Academy of Medicine. He will speak on "Electrophoretic Analysis and the Constitution of Native Fluids."

Dr. A. A. Bitancourt, sub-director of the Institute of Biology, São Paulo, Brazil, gave three lectures at the Iowa State College on October 2, 3 and 4. The titles of his lectures were: "The Influence on Agriculture of Destructive Insects and Plant Pathogens in Brazil," "The Coffee Borer and Its Control in the State of São Paulo" and "The Elsinoaceae as Plant Parasites in Brazil."

It is reported that Rear Admiral Richard E. Byrd will sail for the Antarctic about November 1 despite the withdrawal of one of his three vessels by the Government. The decision to keep the cutter *Northland* in home waters during the foreign crisis will necessitate a change in the plan of the expedition. The *Northland* was to have accompanied the *North Star* to New Zealand and then to Little America, while the old barkentine *Bear* put in at Valparaiso to pick up supplies. It will now be necessary for the *Bear* and the *North Star* to go to New Zealand and Antarctica first and then to return to Valparaiso to get the equipment and personnel waiting there.

It is announced in the *British Medical Journal* that owing to the war there will be no annual meeting of the British Medical Association in 1940. It was to have been held at Birmingham.

*Science Progress,* which is issued quarterly and which is now in its thirty-fourth volume, has suspended publication on account of war conditions.

It is reported that Germany is closing all but four of her universities; they are Berlin, Vienna, Munich and Jena.

Applications are being received for Benjamin Peirce instructorships in mathematics at Harvard University for the academic year 1940–41. Candidates should ordinarily have the doctorate or its equivalent. Applications should be sent to, and further information may be received from the chairman of the department of mathematics.

The City Service Commission of Milwaukee will hold an examination for the position of curator in "lower zoology" in the Milwaukee Public Museum to fill a vacancy caused by the retirement on pension of Thomas E. B. Pope. It will consist of a questionnaire in training and experience and in the submission of exhibits, particularly scientific publications. Candidates must have had at least one year of experience in a museum and at least three years of experience in either a museum, university, scientific bureau or other institution. The position is open to men only.

The second annual instrumentation contest with a first prize of $200 is announced by the Industrial Instrument Section of the Scientific Apparatus Makers of America. Twelve prizes in all, amounting to $500, will be awarded. The contest is open to any person not employed by an instrument manufacturer. Two themes are specified: instruments save money; instrumentation makes jobs. The contestant is to submit either an original report or an original essay in support of either theme. No manuscript should cover both themes. The contest will be judged by the following Jury of Award: M. F. Behar, editor, *Instruments;* C. S. Redding, president, Leeds and Northrup Company; H. B. Richmond, treasurer, General Radio Company; P. T. Sprague, president, The Hays Corporation, and chairman, Industrial Instrument Section S. A. M. A; L. G. Wilson, president, Precision Thermometer and Instrument Company; F. K. Taylor, vice-president, Taylor Instrument Company; Clemann Withers, treasurer, Sperry Gyroscope Company. The contest closes on November 15, 1939, and the judging will be held promptly. Copies of the rules of the contest and of the official entry forms can be obtained from the Scientific Apparatus Makers of America, 20 North Wacker Drive, R.3014, Chicago, Ill.

The twelfth annual Science and Engineering Fair of the American Institute of the City of New York will be held in 1940 from April 14 to 20, inclusive. Ten thousand students of science are members of the institute. All exhibits are the actual creations of the student participants, and cash prizes amounting to more than two thousand dollars will be awarded for the best displays. Working models, experiments, live animals and plants, technical and mechanical projects and miniatures are but few of the types of exhibits which have been designed and executed for this year's fair. It is the annual fair of New York County, a continuance of the annual industrial fairs of the institute which began in 1828.

The United States Sugar Corporation at Clewiston, Fla., has made a gift of $1,000 to establish the Napoleon B. Bernard Fellowship for research at the University of Florida. This marks the fourth gift by that organization to the university since 1937, the others being a similar $1,000 fellowship and two $2,000 scholarships. The new fellowship provides awards for "graduate study of the soil, climate and agriculture of the Everglades."

Dearborn Observatory of Northwestern University is being moved 600 feet south and east to clear the site for the erection of the new Technological Institute. Under the direction of Dr. Oliver J. Lee, chairman of the department, astronomers at the university have stored the telescope lenses in underground vaults, lashed the telescope to the walls and moved the most delicate instruments out of the building. The 125-ton brick pier on which the telescope rests will be moved with the building. Using 700 jacks, each of 25-ton capacity, the entire structure has been raised about three feet, placed on rollers, and is being taken away on tracks, using two teams of horses and a tractor. Test borings indicate tha the new site of the observatory is directly over an old creek bed, which will give the building a firm foundation on a dense clay substratum.

# DISCUSSION

## THE ORIGIN OF THE HUMAN RACES

Mankind may be divided into a number of races and, whereas various authors have different opinions about the question as to how many races there are, they are fairly unanimous in considering them to be the products of some natural force or forces. Presumably agencies similar to those responsible for the production of groups of nearly related species would be the cause of the human races.

It is a well-known fact that members of different races in all possible combinations may have fertile offspring. Therefore, there must be isolating factors which keep the races separated, as otherwise mankind would be a thorough mixture of a great many types, such as observed when studying a population, said to be of one race.

These isolating factors are thought to be natural, as opposed to human, in the same sense in which a house may be called a human and not a natural product, although in the last instance man, and all that which belongs to him, is part of nature. Here, in my opinion, a grave mistake is made. The human races are not maintained by an act of nature, but by human, that is, social, discrimination.

Proof for this lies in the nature of the qualities by which the races differ. They are all superficial and readily impress an untrained observer. The color of the skin, the shape of the eye or nose, the form of the hair which constitute the basis for the recognition of human races are visible to every one at the first glance and may therefore be subject to social selection. This causes their occurrence in large coherent sections of the human population.

The variations upon which the human races are based are by no means the only ones existing. Professor Komai has published a list of more than 80 inheritable variations common to the white race and the Japanese, although not occurring with the same frequency. Some of these, like color blindness, the presence of supernumerary fingers or toes and harelip are unobtrusive and free from social taboo. Others, like the blood groups, refer to inner organs or chemical substances and are invisible as such. None of them could serve as basis for the distinction of a human race. There are color-blind people among all races, but there is no race of color-blind men, because without a scientific investigation no one is able to select his mate in regard to this quality.

The human races, such as they are, would never have developed in nature in the absence of man's own social actions, the results of which are not restricted to the differentiation between the major races of mankind. Differences between tribes, some of them counting only a few hundred individuals, are due to the same cause.

The races of mankind are no less a product of man than the races of his dogs and horses. Here, too, a certain potential variability is a prerequisite for the creation of a number of races. In the case of the dog this must have been present in the wolf and the other wild species of carnivores which went into the crosses from which the various types of dogs were bred. This original variability is natural and not due to human action, but it need not show and may lie hidden in a comparatively uniform animal like the wolf.

The origin of this primary variability need not be discussed at present and is, as yet, uncertain. Only, it may be stated that the natural forces responsible for this variation have not necessarily long ago ceased to be active. There is reason to believe, for instance, that in man the character which is designated as blood group *A* has originated only a few thousand years ago.

Whatever the nature of this primary variability it does not lead to a distinction between races, if not accompanied by isolation of the various types in one way or another. Many recognize various environmental factors, as, for instance, the climate, as such isolating agencies. The various climates, it is said, would produce the human races. However, it is not clear why the climate would only affect the dispersal on earth of visible characters and not that of the more numerous characters which are more or less invisible.

Each of the human races, if inhabiting the earth alone, might spread over a somewhat different area, and factors like climate, or physical barriers obstructing migration, may have something to do with the segregation of mankind into groups with different types. But the social motives in regard to mate selection are much stronger than any motive to select a certain climate or other environmental condition. Generally speaking, members of the white race are willing to live all over the earth, but not to marry into other races.

If the idea discussed above is correct the problem of the human races is one to be more studied by sociologists than by biologists. It also gives hope that race differences will be viewed with less superstition and that race problems will be recognized as being more amenable to humane solutions than they appear to many at present.

A. B. DROOGLEEVER FORTUYN
PEIPING UNION MEDICAL COLLEGE

## THE FLOATING POPULATION OF THE AIR

IN my recent studies of the biota of the islands off the coast of Southern California I have found that the endemic insects appear to be mainly confined to certain groups, especially the more or less bulky Tenebrionid beetles, which can not fly. Excluding the species certainly or probably introduced by man, there is still a very large population of flying insects, as well as spiders, quite identical with species of the mainland. It might at first appear that these species were very constant in their characters, with little tendency to form distinct races or species when isolated. The true explanation, however, appears to be that they are constantly arriving through the air. The floating population of the air has not been sufficiently understood in the past, but the essential facts are admirably presented by Mr. P. A. Glick in his recently published work on "The Distribution of Insects, Spiders and Mites in the Air" (U. S. Department of Agriculture, Technical Bulletin 673, May, 1939). In this paper full details are given of the collections made by aeroplane in Louisiana and Durango, Mexico, the specimens secured having been carefully sorted and so far as possible identified. The work at Tallulah, Louisiana, involved 1,314 aeroplane flights, during which the insect traps were in operation for 1,007 hours. There were 44 flights in Durango, Mexico. In Louisiana, by day, 24,559 insects and arachnids were taken in 51,178 minutes. By night, 3,955 were taken in 6,790 minutes. Two hundred and twenty-five were taken in 2,455 minutes at altitudes over 5,000 feet; one spider at 15,000 feet. In Mexico, 1,294 specimens were taken in 2,120 minutes. There were numerous small wingless forms, carried upward by the air currents. All the various aspects of the work and its significance are most ably discussed by Mr. Glick, the bulletin extending to 150 pages. It is evident that the islands must be constantly receiving insects, spiders, and also spores and some seeds, through the air. Only a very small percentage of these can survive, but the constant supply enables the available environments to be populated, so that even recently introduced plants are often infested as they would be on the mainland. Thus at the Rancho Escondido, Sta. Catalina, I found the cocklebur, *Xanthium spinosum,* swarming with the trypetid fly which attacks it elsewhere. The introduced *Diaspis* scale of the prickly pear, at the same place, was infested by chalcidoid parasites. At the present time, the manner of arrival of the various species can only be guessed, but if the very numerous planes constantly flying about the islands could be utilized (with no inconvenience to the service or the pilots) for studies like those of Mr. Glick, we should soon have a mass of positive information. We may leave it to mathematicians to calculate, on the basis of the work done, the probable number of insects in the air, but the figure must be surprisingly large. There is also another aspect of the matter, which I have not seen referred to. The sea in the vicinity of the coasts (how far out, we do not know) must be constantly receiving a rain of small arthropods, which must represent a not inconsiderable food supply for the marine animals.

T. D. A. COCKERELL
BOULDER, COLORADO

## A REQUEST TO MATHEMATICAL GENETICISTS

THE lack of clarity in many papers dealing with theoretical genetics will probably retard to some extent the development of the science. Some of these are valuable contributions, but their merit is unnecessarily limited by the inadequate presentation of the mathematical materials. Much of the mathematics is simple algebra, but the lines of reasoning are frequently very hard to pursue, because many crucial equations are omitted. Sometimes lengthy and rather involved processes must be followed from one printed equation to the next, and there is not the slightest hint in the text as to what these processes are. Geniuses may have little difficulty with these papers, but such geneticists are scarce. Among the rank and file of animal and plant breeders one of the following courses is likely to be followed:

(1) The papers are ignored. Attempts to analyze a few of them bring the conviction that it is useless, and one can "get by" without them anyhow!

(2) The conclusions are accepted, but the reasons for them are not understood. It is obvious that such a state of mind is scientifically unsound.

(3) An enormous amount of time is expended in reading and analyzing the paper—very much more than would be required if a few crucial equations were added. A busy teacher is likely to give up through sheer need of sleep and revert to class (1) or (2)!

We teachers are training the geneticists of the future, and if we are not provided with reasonable opportunities for understanding the advances in mathematical genetics, such contributions may be too little known in the next generation. Genetics will not advance as it should. It is sometimes claimed that editors will not accept papers with too much mathematical material, for such printing is expensive. In reply, it may be said that there is little reason for publishing a paper if it is so brief that it can not be understood. Furthermore, mathematical clarity can usually be attained by adding such a small number of "clew" equations that the costs of printing would not be materially increased.

Biometricians should always remember that they are not writing for mathematicians, but for biologists who know the elements of mathematics, yet are not very familiar with many devices used in mathematical procedure. Please don't leave out so many equations!

HARRISON R. HUNT
MICHIGAN STATE COLLEGE

## THE RANGE OF HEARING OF CANARIES

TESTS[1] on starlings, English sparrows and domestic pigeons show that the range of hearing of these birds is considerably more restricted than human hearing. Their ranges cover about five octaves; normal human hearing is about ten octaves.

The method used in testing the canaries was the same as in the earlier experiments. The investigation of the hearing of five birds was conducted by means of conditioned reflexes to a range of sound which, during the conditioning of the experimental birds, had been followed by a mild electric shock from the feeding tray. The canaries' range was similar to that of the earlier birds experimented on but was even more restricted. Canary's range, 1,100–10,000 c.p.s., is only slightly over three octaves. Low and moderately high sounds are not heard. However, the bird undoubtedly hears all the sounds produced in its own song.

A. R. BRAND
P. P. KELLOGG
CORNELL UNIVERSITY

[1] A. R. Brand and P. P. Kellogg, 1939. *Wilson Bulletin*, 51: 38–41, 1939.

# SCIENTIFIC BOOKS

## PLANE TOPOLOGY

*Elements of the Topology of Plane Sets of Points.* By M. H. A. NEWMAN. Cambridge: At the University Press; New York: The Macmillan Company, 1939, viii + 221 pp., 93 figs. $3.50.

ACCORDING to the publisher's jacket, this book "has the double purpose of providing an introduction to the methods of Topology, and of making accessible to analysts the simple modern technique for proving the theorems on sets of points required in the theory of functions of a complex variable." It is divided into two parts. The first, occupying slightly less than half the volume, opens with some calculus of abstract sets, and investigates properties in metric spaces of closed and open sets, continuous mappings and connected sets.

The second part is devoted specifically to the subject-matter indicated by the title and utilizes the "combinatorial" approach through cells and complexes selected from "gratings" formed by lines in the plane or sphere of analytic geometry. The basic material is essentially an elaboration and adaptation to the plane of a celebrated paper of J. W. Alexander which appeared in the *Transactions* of the American Mathematical Society in 1922, but proceeds much further than such matters as the Jordan Curve Theorem. For example, many of the results of Schoenflies are derived, and a number of the properties of plane domains to be found in the work of American set-theorists are included. For the analyst, the author gives a proof of Cauchy's Theorem based on the topological methods introduced.

The book is modern, well illustrated, very readable and typographically appealing. Numerous exercises are provided. The final 22 pages of the volume contain supplementary bibliographical and mathematical notes and a good index. However, the bibliography seems weak; although in the case of some topics adequate references are given both to their origin and to their more extensive treatments in the literature, in other cases such references are entirely lacking. It is to be hoped that in a later edition this will be corrected in what seems otherwise a work well suited to fulfilling the purposes stated.

R. L. WILDER
UNIVERSITY OF MICHIGAN

*The Physiology and Pharmacology of the Pituitary Body.* By H. B. VAN DYKE. Volume II. University of Chicago Press. Pp. xiv + 402. 28 figures. $4.50.

THREE years have elapsed since the appearance of the first volume of this series. In the first volume the author reviewed and discussed the important work on the hypophysis from 1920 through part of 1935, although the background laid by earlier investigations was not ignored. In the new volume the literature for that part of 1935 not covered in the earlier volume and 1936, 1937 and a part of 1938 has been reviewed. All papers relating to the pituitary gland that appeared during this period are not included in the text or listed in the voluminous (80 pp.) bibliography, however. The author has selected, as in the first volume, what seemed to him to be the best and most informative of the publications. According to the author these constitute 78 per cent. of the articles considered. This is a severe but just indictment of recent endocrine literature. That even this percentage should be included is due to the fact that the reviews were limited to the anatomy, physiology and pharmacology of the pituitary body.

The text of this volume is only one hundred pages less than that of the first volume, although the period covered is but one fifth as long. An opportunity was thus afforded the author to be rather more critical in his comments than he was in the earlier work, and to add summaries at the end of each chapter.

The number of chapters has been cut from twelve to ten. This was accomplished by omitting the chapter on the effect of hypophysectomy and by devoting but one chapter, instead of two, to the physiology of the neural lobe. Otherwise, the chapter headings remain essentially unchanged. There are a generous number of illustrations, but none are used which appeared in volume I. They are well selected but, in contrast to the earlier book, are all copies from the literature. This has been an advisable change, in the opinion of the reviewer. A color plate is given to show the relationships of the cells of the pars glandularis. It might be questioned why a colored figure was necessary since the cell lineage given is identical with that described by Trautmann in 1912, whose description of cell relationships has been generally confirmed by cytologists.

The arrangement of the topics is logical and easily followed. Their range is broad, and includes, in addition to those which would obviously be discussed, topics such as the effect of the pituitary hormones and the chorionic gonadotropic hormones on neoplasms, the nervous control of the secretion of gonadotropic hormones, vitamins and minerals in relation to the gonadotropic hormones, to mention but a few. In the review of these subjects and in the chapter summaries an unprejudiced view-point is maintained and optimism in regard to the achievements of endocrinologists is notable by its absence. In regard to the number and action of the pituitary gonadotropic hormones, he holds that the only reasonable position to take is one of suspended judgment, unwelcome as this may be to many readers. He only provisionally and for convenience of discussion accepts a specific "growth-promoting" hormone. Yet he freely acknowledges that notable advances have been made in certain subjects, as for example in the studies on the physiology of the neural lobe.

An index sufficient to enable the reader to locate various subjects is appended. The full titles of the articles in the bibliography are given, which adds to the convenience and usefulness of the book. The opening sentence in the foreword, written by Professor A. J. Carlson, succinctly states what the author has accomplished: "Dr. van Dyke has again rendered a valuable service to biology and medicine in presenting in this second volume his critical digest of the experimental and clinical literature on the pituitary body that has appeared since 1935."

PHILIP E. SMITH
COLLEGE OF PHYSICIANS AND SURGEONS,
COLUMBIA UNIVERSITY

# SPECIAL ARTICLES

## THE SENSITIZING PROPERTIES OF THE NUCLEIC ACIDS AND THEIR DERIVATIVES

THE chemical relationships between the nucleic acids and their physiological degradation products have been intensively studied; the part that these compounds may play in immunological phenomena, however, has never been investigated. Preliminary studies indicate that they may bear a fundamental relationship to pollen sensitization. The authors have found that individuals who gave positive skin reactions, when injected intradermally with ragweed pollen extract, likewise gave positive reactions when similarly tested with dilute solutions of nucleic acids and many of their derivatives. These reactions, so far demonstrated in a series of fifty ragweed pollen-sensitive human beings, appears to parallel the sensitivity of these individuals to ragweed pollen, regardless of the occurrence of symptoms of hay-fever. Only an occasional reaction has been observed in a group of forty non-allergic control cases, most of whom were normal individuals but some of whom were patients suffering from a variety of unrelated diseases. Likewise, five cases who gave positive reactions to animal danders, dust and foods, but not to ragweed pollen extract, also failed to react to the nucleic acid group of compounds.

The skin reactions elicited by the nucleic acids and their derivatives were the typical, immediate, wheal-erythema type. Such reactions were obtained uniformly upon the intradermal injection of $8_{\gamma}$ (.008 mg) of either thymus or yeast nucleic acid (neutralized before injection). Three crystalline nucleotides prepared from yeast nucleic acid, namely, adenine, guanine and cytosine nucleotides, gave positive reactions in doses of $2_{\gamma}$ (.002 mg). Likewise, crystalline adenine nucleotides prepared from beef heart muscle, beef pancreas and tea leaves reacted in the same manner. The simple purine salts, adenine sulfate, guanine chloride, hypoxanthine nitrate, xanthine nitrate and sodium urate all gave positive reactions in doses of $1_{\gamma}$ (.001 mg), as did also the simple pyrimidine uracil. Allantoin, the chief end product of purine metabolism in most mammals except man, likewise gave positive reactions. The simple compound urea has also given typical reactions.

The compounds mentioned above, with the exception of urea, are all concerned in the metabolism of the nucleic acids and all contain a purine or pyrimidine ring structure. The alkaloid caffein (which contains the purine ring) and the amino acid d.l. histidine mono-hydrochloride (which contains the imidazole ring) gave consistent reactions, but the amino acid l. proline (which contains the pyrrolidine ring) reacted less frequently.

A skin-sensitizing antibody to yeast nucleic acid, muscle and yeast adenine nucleotides, caffein, allantoin, histidine and urea has been demonstrated so far in the serum of ten individuals reacting to these compounds.

Severe constitutional reactions were produced in two patients, when only 0.02 mg of two adenine nucleotides, prepared from yeast nucleic acid and from beef muscle, respectively, were used. For this reason only the small doses described above were employed in skin testing sensitive individuals.

WALTER L. WINKENWERDER
MARY V. BUELL
JOHN EAGER HOWARD
THE JOHNS HOPKINS UNIVERSITY

## A POSSIBLE RELATION BETWEEN MANGANESE, SUNLIGHT AND WINTER HATCHABILITY OF HEN'S EGGS

IT has been observed at this station (unpublished data) that slipped tendon occurs more frequently in the heavy breeds of chickens that are raised in batteries in contrast to those that are raised out-of-doors on wire screens. Since the discovery of the relation of manganese to slipped tendon, little attention has been given to the effect of sunlight on this condition. Evidence that the manganese requirements of laying hens may be increased in the absence of sunlight is indicated by hatchability records obtained during the past two years.

It was found that a mash consisting of 45 parts of yellow corn, 15 of wheat bran, 15 of middlings, 5 of alfalfa leaf meal, 1.5 of granite grits, 1.5 of limestone grits, 1 of cod liver oil and 16 parts of soy-bean oil meal was improved for egg hatchability by the addition of 85 parts per million of manganese. This ration contained adequate amounts of vitamin D; however, during the fall and winter months (September to April) the average per cent. of hatchability of the fertile eggs laid by the hens fed this ration without added manganese was 48.1. The corresponding groups which received added manganese produced eggs having an average hatchability of 62 per cent. When there was adequate sunlight during the late spring and early summer, there was little significant difference in the egg hatchability between these two groups. The increase in hatchability of the eggs from the group on the basal ration appears to be correlated with increased sunlight. Hatchability of these eggs increased to an average of 70 per cent. as compared to 75 per cent. hatchability of the eggs from the manganese-fed group. The effect of sunlight on the hatchability of the eggs from the basal group is shown very clearly in Fig. 1.

The bi-monthly hatchability of eggs laid by the first group (low manganese) was compared with the corresponding variations in temperature and hours of

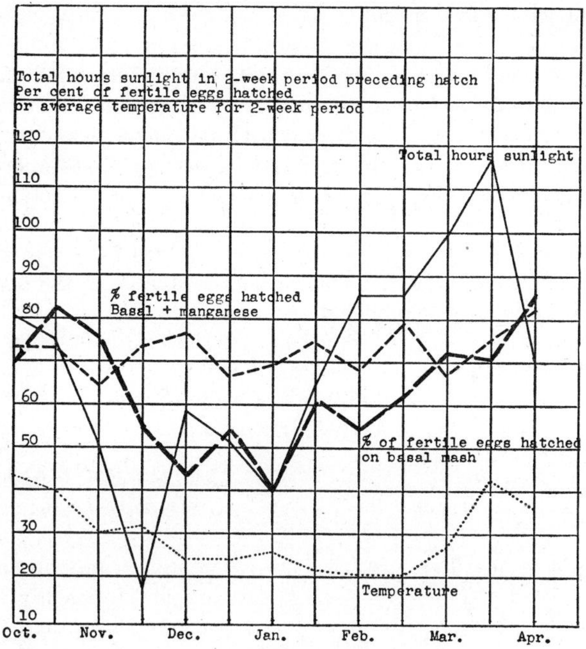


FIG. 1. The effect of manganese, sunlight, and temperature on hatchability of hen's eggs.

sunlight. The correlation was found between the total hours of sunlight during the 2-weeks period preceding the time the eggs were laid and the hatchability of the eggs. The period of diminishing per cent. of hatchability followed shortly after the period during which the total hours of sunlight diminished. Likewise the improvement in hatchability followed the increase in sunlight. There was no correlation between the fall or rise in the mean temperature and the per cent. of hatchability. Byerly, Titus, Ellis and Nestler[1] also have reported that hatchability of eggs from hens on a high soy-bean oil meal ration was markedly improved when the hens had direct access to sunlight. Since there was no fall in the hatchability of eggs from groups receiving added manganese, there must have been a borderline deficiency in the manganese content of the ration. During the spring, when there was adequate sunlight, this deficiency was eliminated, as was shown by the nearly equal hatchability of the two groups. That the vitamin D of cod liver oil was not a factor in the effect of sunlight has been shown by a number of experiments.

What explanation can be given for this apparent sparing action of sunlight on a hen's requirement for manganese can not be stated at present.

J. B. Christiansen
J. G. Halpin
E. B. Hart

University of Wisconsin

[1] T. C. Byerly, H. W. Titus, N. R. Ellis and R. B. Nestler, *Jour. Poultry Sci.*, 16: 323, 1937.

## THE ELECTROPHORETIC ANALYSIS OF ANTIPNEUMOCOCCUS HORSE SERA

Recent work has indicated that the antibody activity of antipneumococcus horse serum is associated with proteins which differ from the principal globulins of normal horse serum in both molecular weight[1] and electrical mobility.[2] These antibodies are heavier than the principal globulins and electrophoretic observations have indicated that they move with a velocity intermediate between those of the β and γ components of normal sera.[2]

We have made electrophoretic[3] measurements upon a number of antipneumococcus horse sera and of antibody concentrates from them. Our results differ from the foregoing in showing that the antibody activity in all our preparations has the same electrical mobility as the ordinary γ-globulin. This is illustrated in Fig. 1, which reproduces the Longsworth[4] mobility-concen-

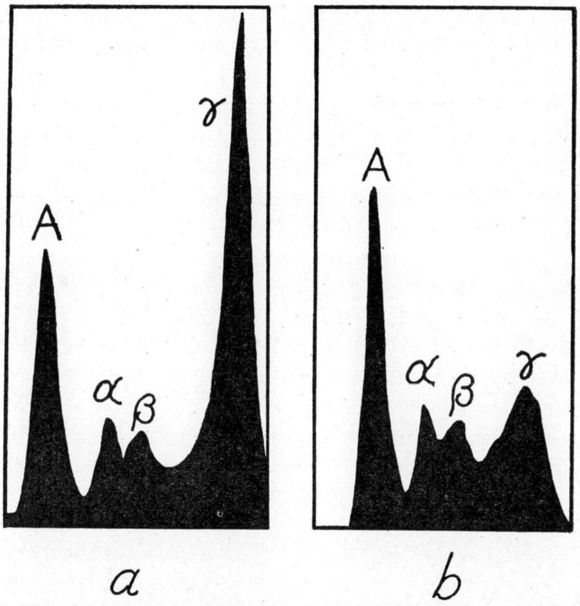


FIG. 1. Longsworth patterns of (a) unabsorbed and (b) absorbed antipneumococcus horse serum No. 6639. The albumin peak is designated by A, the globulin peaks by α, β, γ. The decrease in area of the γ-peak on absorption is evident.

tration patterns of an antipneumococcus horse serum before and after absorption of the serum with specific polysaccharides. This photograph was made with a bivalent Types I and II antiserum; similar results have been obtained with a bivalent serum against Types IV and VIII pneumococci. The measured mo-

[1] J. Biscoe, F. Hercik and R. W. G. Wyckoff, Science, 83: 602, 1936; M. Heidelberger and K. O. Pedersen, *Jour. Exp. Med.*, 65: 393, 1937.

[2] A. Tiselius and E. A. Kabat, Science, 87: 416, 1938; *Jour. Exp. Med.*, 69: 119, 1939.

[3] A. Tiselius, *Trans. Faraday Soc.*, 33: 524, 1937.

[4] L. G. Longsworth, *Jour. Am. Chem. Soc.*, 61: 529, 1939.

bilities of the various components in these sera are listed in Table 1; except for the absence in our photographs of the extra component with $-2.1 \times 10^{-5}$ cm$^2$ sec$^{-1}$ volts$^{-1}$ which had been identified as antibody, our measurements agree well with earlier ones.[2]

We have measured the areas under the globulin portion of the Longsworth photographs of sera before and after absorption with specific polysaccharides. This loss of area, limited to the $\gamma$-component, has paralleled the antibody content as determined by direct chemical[5] analysis (the last column of Table 1).

TABLE 1

| Serum | Type | Mobility | | | | | Decrease in globulin area on absorption | Antibody per cent. of total globulin |
|---|---|---|---|---|---|---|---|---|
| | | A | $\alpha$ | $\beta$ | Antibody | $\gamma$ | | |
| | | $-\mu \times 10^5$ cm$^2$ sec$^{-1}$ volt$^{-1}$ | | | | | % | % |
| 6639 | I and II | 5.3 | 4.0 | 3.0 | — | 1.0 | 37 | 32 |
| 8617 | IV and VIII | 5.1 | 3.7 | 3.0 | — | 0.8 | 32 | 33 |
| Tiselius and Kabat | ....... | 5.5 | 3.7 | 3.0 | 2.1 | 0.9 | | |

We are not yet able to explain in satisfactory fashion the differences between our results and those of Tiselius and Kabat. Both sets of experiments were made at the same pH (7.7) and with similar buffers (0.15M NaCl, 0.02M total phosphates). All our accurate electrophoretic measurements have been made on sera diluted 1:4, but a few photographs of undiluted sera and of sera diluted 1:2 have given the same results. Though there is as yet only fragmentary evidence[6] to support the hypothesis, it is possible that the antibodies in a horse become smaller under prolonged immunization. The sera available for the present experiments were all from horses which had been producing antibodies for many years, and their antibodies may be different from those in the sera examined by Tiselius and Kabat.

D. H. MOORE
J. VAN DER SCHEER
R. W. G. WYCKOFF

LEDERLE LABORATORIES, INC.,
PEARL RIVER, N. Y.

5 M. Heidelberger and F. E. Kendall, *Jour. Exp. Med.*, 61: 559, 1935.

6 See for instance, E. A. Kabat, *Jour. Exp. Med.*, 69: 103, 1939.

## THE PHYSIOLOGICAL CHANGES PRODUCED IN YEAST BY ULTRA-VIOLET LIGHT AND BY HEAT

As part of an extensive investigation in these laboratories[1] of the effects of salts and lethal agents on biological systems an occasion has recently been found to make a comparative study of the effects of ultraviolet light and of heat. A single cell isolation of a strain of *Saccharomyces cerevisiae* was used as the test organism. Of the physiological functions studied, the ability of the cells to divide, thus forming colonies on agar, was found to be the most sensitive to both agents. The aerobic respiration of the cells was quite sensitive to heat, but proved to be relatively unaffected by ultraviolet light, that is, λ2650. Likewise, the resistance to staining with methylene blue is decreased by heat, but within comparable time limits is relatively unaffected by λ2650.

One of the more striking observations is that irradiation with λ2650 followed by heat treatment is two to five times as lethal as the treatment of the organisms in the reverse order. This is manifest in both the ability of the cells to form colonies and the resistance of the cells to staining.[2] Both functions are thus sensitized to heat by this wave-length. On the other hand, the rate of respiration is not sensitized, but is reduced by the same amount whether radiation is followed by heat treatment or *vice versa*.

The details of these experiments and the significance of the results in a general understanding of the nature of the lethal action of heat and ultra-violet light will be published shortly. In addition, the results give certain indications as to the mechanisms of the physiological processes studied and establish that certain of them are relatively independent of each other, *e.g.*, the ability of the cells to form colonies and their rate of respiration.

THOMAS F. ANDERSON
B. M. DUGGAR

UNIVERSITY OF WISCONSIN

1 B. M. Duggar and A. Hollaender, *Jour. Bacteriol.*, 37: 219–239, 241–256, 1934; A. Hollaender and B. M. Duggar, *Proc. Nat. Acad. Sci.*, 22: 19–24, 1936; A. Hollaender and W. D. Claus, *Jour. Gen. Physiol.*, 19: 753–765, 1936; A. Hollaender and B. M. Duggar, *Jour. Bacteriol.*, 36: 17–37, 1938.

2 W. T. Bovie and G. A. Daland (*Amer. Jour. Physiol.*, 66: 55–66, 1923) have reported a similar sensitization of *Paramecium caudatum* to the lethal action of heat by irradiation with the short ultra-violet rays transmitted by fluorite (λ < 2000Å). The relation between our work and that of various investigators on the (small) temperature coefficient of the lethal action of ultra-violet light is probably rather remote.

## BOOKS RECEIVED

JELLINEK, KARL. *Kurzes Lehrbuch der Physikalischen Chemie.* Heft II. Pp. xii + 292. Illustrated. A. E. Kluwer, Deventer, Holland.

MANGHAM, SYDNEY. *Earth's Green Mantle; Plant Science for the General Reader.* Pp. 322. Macmillan. $3.50.

MULLER, H. J. *Bibliography on the Genetics of Drosophila.* Pp. 130. Oliver and Boyd, Edinburgh.

*Recent Marine Sediments.* A symposium. Pp. 736. Illustrated. American Petroleum Geologists, Tulsa, Oklahoma.

SHRADER, JAMES H. *Food Control; Its Public-Health Aspects.* Pp. ix + 513. Wiley. $4.00.

ZAHL, PAUL A. *To the Lost World.* Pp. x + 268. Illustrated. Knopf. $2.75.

# SCIENCE

Vol. 90 — Friday, October 20, 1939 — No. 2338

*The Broadening Horizons of Medicine:* Dr. Winfred Overholser ... 359

*Obituary:*
*Henry Chandler Cowles:* Dr. George D. Fuller. *Recent Deaths and Memorials* ... 363

*Scientific Events:*
*Bird Protection in the British Empire; The New Milford Laboratory of the Bureau of Fisheries; The Thomas R. Baker Museum of Rollins College; Mathematical Reviews; The United States Antarctic Expedition; Visiting Physicists at Cornell University; Award of the William H. Nichols Medal; Dr. Ames and the National Advisory Committee for Aeronautics* ... 364

*Scientific Notes and News* ... 368

*Discussion:*
*Vocal Mimicry of the Starling and the Mockingbird:* H. A. Allard. *Hibernation of Anopheline Eggs in the Tropics:* Dr. Wm. S. Stone and Lieutenant-Colonel François H. K. Reynolds. *Distribution of Artifacts Made From Chalcedony of Cerro Pedernal, New Mexico:* Dr. Louis L. Ray. *The Presence of Non-oxygen-combining (Inactive) Hemoglobin in the Blood of Normal Individuals:* Dr. Esther Ammundsen ... 370

*Scientific Books:*
*Matter and Light; Wavelength Tables:* Dr. W. F. G. Swann. *Magnetism; Radioactivity:* Dr. C. G. Montgomery ... 373

*Special Articles:*
*The Pathogenic Action of Phymatotrichum Omnivorum:* Dr. G. M. Watkins and Matilde Otero Watkins. *Urine Chloride Concentration in Patients with Cushing's Syndrome:* Dr. Abraham Cantarow. *Essentiality of Primary Amino Groups for Specific Activity of the Lactogenic Hormone:* Dr. H. M. Evans and Others. *Multiple Nature of the Rat "Filtrate Factor"—A Component of Vitamin $B_2$:* Dr. H. M. Evans and Others ... 374

*Scientific Apparatus and Laboratory Methods:*
*An Electric Sterilizer for the Culture Room:* Dr. Ernest E. Hubert. *The Influence of Centrifugation on the Agglutination of Pneumococci:* Dr. Paul F. de Gara ... 377

*Science News* ... 6

SCIENCE: A Weekly Journal devoted to the Advancement of Science, edited by J. McKeen Cattell and published every Friday by

THE SCIENCE PRESS
New York City: Grand Central Terminal
Lancaster, Pa. — Garrison, N. Y.

Annual Subscription, $6.00 — Single Copies, 15 Cts.

SCIENCE is the official organ of the American Association for the Advancement of Science. Information regarding membership in the Association may be secured from the office of the permanent secretary in the Smithsonian Institution Building, Washington, D. C.

# THE BROADENING HORIZONS OF MEDICINE[1]

By Dr. WINFRED OVERHOLSER

PROFESSOR OF PSYCHIATRY, GEORGE WASHINGTON UNIVERSITY SCHOOL OF MEDICINE; SUPERINTENDENT, SAINT ELIZABETHS HOSPITAL, WASHINGTON, D. C.

We meet this morning in the midst of a troubled world, a world troubled perhaps more than it has ever been in the history of mankind. For ten years this country, along with the rest of the world, has been going through the throes of an economic depression of greater intensity and greater duration than any previously recorded, a depression which has disorganized commerce among nations and which has affected profoundly the lives of almost every one. During this same period of time we have seen many of the fruits of man's struggle for liberty sacrificed in the rise of political authoritarianism. The freedom of speech, the freedom of thought, the freedom even of physical movement, have been completely abolished in several portions of the globe. Fortunately this tide of authoritarianism has not yet engulfed this country; although it behooves every one to be on the alert, we need not fear that the ideals for which so many of our forefathers struggled will be easily given up. And now added to the depression and the rise of authoritarianism, we have before us the spectacle of war, a war which threatens the very foundations of civilization, and which is unleashing truly awful forces of aggression and hatred throughout the world. The troubled state of mankind and the inexpressible folly of war have seldom been summed up more pungently than in the words of Professor Albert Einstein in a letter addressed to posterity which was deposited a year ago in the five thousand year capsule at the New York World's Fair. The letter reads:

[1] Address presented at the opening session of George Washington University School of Medicine, September 25, 1939.

Our time is rich in inventive minds, the inventions of which could facilitate our lives considerably. We are crossing the seas by power, and utilize power also in order to relieve humanity from all tiring muscular work. We have learned to fly and we are able to send messages and news without any difficulty over the entire world through electric waves. However, the production and distribution of commodities is entirely unorganized so that everybody must live in fear of being eliminated from the economic cycle, in this way suffering from the want of everything. Furthermore, people living in different countries kill each other at irregular time intervals so that also for this reason anyone who thinks about the future must live in fear and terror. This is due to the fact that the intelligence and character of the masses are incomparably lower than the intelligence and character of the few who produce something valuable for the community. I trust that posterity will read these statements with a feeling of proud and justified superiority.

I hope that I may be pardoned for starting these few remarks with what may appear to be a pessimistic note. I have, however, stated the facts and hope further to use them perhaps as a backdrop against which the prospects of medicine may stand out a little more clearly and brightly in relief. To a psychiatrist the present troubled state of the world emphasizes more than ever before the need of a balanced mind in an unbalanced world; the need for confidence, for the use of intelligence, for the restraint of emotion. The need for sanity and for its application to the affairs of life has never been greater.

Many of those present here to-day are taking their first step or steps along the road which leads to the practice of medicine. The road is a difficult one. Even those who are present here to-day for the first time have already spent two years or more in college studying pre-medical subjects. They must spend four years of study, and not particularly easy study either, in the medical school, after which there will come a period of interneship before actual practice is essayed. I am one of those bold enough to question the wisdom of some of the required pre-medical work. There is a tendency to-day, I believe, to require specialism altogether too early and to leave out of the equipment of the medical man what were known in the old days as the humanities. Although the field of medicine has developed almost unbelievably, there are still, however, other things in life which make life worth living and to which the medical man should not be inattentive. Let us hope that the day is not gone forever when the field of medicine can produce such litterateurs as Oliver Wendell Holmes, S. Weir Mitchell, Sir William Osler and Harvey Cushing. I recommend as a decided contribution to that balanced mind of which I have spoken earlier the development of hobbies, of other interests to which one can occasionally flee from the practice of medicine. This is not to say that medicine itself has not many facets and many satisfactions. If those of us here did not believe that, we should not be practicing or study medicine to-day.

In the midst of a cynical world it is well occasionally to reaffirm one's faith in the existence of such a thing as altruism, the desire to serve one's fellow men. I may perhaps be pardoned another quotation by referring to the tribute paid to the physician by that brave spirit, Robert Louis Stevenson. The physician, as a rule, he comments, stands above the common herd, shares as little as any in the defects of a period and most notably exhibits the virtues of the race; he then goes on to say:

> Generosity he has such as is possible to those who practice an art, never to those who drive a trade; discretion tested by a hundred secrets; tact tried in a thousand embarrassments; and what are more important, Heraclean cheerfulness and courage. So it is that he brings air and cheer into the sick-room, and often enough, though not as often as he wishes, brings healing.

Perhaps at this time when much is being said as to the nature of medical practice, it is well to give some heed to what we mean by a learned profession as distinguished from a trade or business. The professional man is, or should be, something of an idealist. He is guided by the ideals of his profession, rules of conduct which have been handed down and which for instance are embodied for the medical man in the Hippocratic oath. The professional man is primarily a learned man, a man who depends upon his knowledge as his stock in trade. He has specialized knowledge over and above that of the common man in relation to some particular topic, be that law, theology, accountancy, teaching or medicine. Perhaps the thing that distinguishes him more than anything else is the peculiarly personal relation to the client or patient which he enjoys, a confidential relationship, a situation in which he is adviser, guide and friend, a situation in which his interest does not cease when the particular transaction is concluded. It follows as a corollary that he is an individualist, one who functions far more efficiently without regimentation or coercion, but rather requires the opportunity to utilize freely his own initiative and judgment within the limits of his professional code of ethics.

He has, too, an interest in the results of this relationship in which he is called to advise, which is over and above the cash recompense which he receives; in fact, in the practice of medicine it is all too often the case that no monetary recompense is received at all, and more frequently the recompense is wholly inadequate to the value of the services rendered. The physician does not consider that he is receiving a *quid pro quo* when he is paid by his patient. It is not that he sells his opinion at so much a yard. He is entitled to a living, yes, but more than that he takes a satisfaction in seeing that the results of his advice have brought aid and comfort to the person who sought it.

Another feature is, or should be, the disregard of fixed hours, the readiness to be of service whenever called upon. It is a matter of regret to some of us in the medical profession to see certain other professional aides at times somewhat disinclined to regard this fundamental principle of the profession. The professional man is not a "clock-watcher." He does not count on regular hours. He realizes when he takes up the study of medicine that his sleep will often be interrupted, that his time will not really be his own, and he rejoices to feel that he may be called upon when others are in need regardless of his own comfort. One other point of distinction may be mentioned, and that is the principle as laid down in the Hippocratic oath that he will teach this art to others if they wish to learn it "without fee or stipulation." The physician, and indeed any professional man, should emulate the Clerk in the Canterbury Tales of whom Chaucer said: "And gladly would he learn and gladly teach."

Such are a few of the distinctions which set off the learned professions, and particularly the profession of medicine, from business. Our earliest prototype, the priest in primitive society, was the guide, counsel and friend, the original professional man. We belong to one of the oldest professions, and we may feel confident that when in years to come we prepare to retire from active practice we may still be looked upon as the members of a profession.

We have all been greatly pleased and deeply touched by the presentation this morning of the oil portrait of Dr. William Alanson White, the gift of the faculty to the school, and the few but eloquent words of Dr. Mallory which have accompanied this presentation. The faculty knew Dr. White well and some few of the student body probably came under his direct influence, though it is now two and a half years since he ceased to be among us. I like to look upon Dr. White as the ideal medical man. He embodied, certainly better and more fully than almost any one I have ever known, what we may look upon as the ideals of the physician. He was a student; he always wished to learn. He was a teacher, always happy in imparting his knowledge to others, a gift which he had in rare measure. He was deeply interested in the patient and desired first to understand the nature of the disorder. Whether or not he brought healing (and he often did bring about restoration to health), he always brought comfort. At the same time he remained a human being, a man in close touch with his fellow men, a man of wide and scholarly interests. To have known him is a benediction.

I shall speak later concerning Dr. White's influence on the development of psychiatry. For the present I should like to add a few words about the sphere of his personal influence and the devotion which he inspired in those who came into contact with him. It was a source of great personal satisfaction to Dr. White that the students of George Washington University School of Medicine, a school in which he had had a very close and vitalizing influence during his entire stay in Washington, a period of thirty-four years, showed not only a sufficient interest in psychiatry and its problems, but had sufficient personal respect and admiration for him to organize in this school the William Alanson White Society. This society was founded for the purpose partly of recognizing those students who had special interest and proficiency in psychiatry, and also for the consideration of what might be termed extra-curricular problems in psychiatry; that is, the broader applications of psychiatry to social problems. It is my earnest hope that this society will be long continued by the students as a tribute to the memory of this great man whom we are honoring to-day. Likewise, during Dr. White's life there was established in Washington the William Alanson White Psychiatric Foundation, which not only publishes a quarterly magazine entitled *Psychiatry,* but which is sponsoring this year for the first time a series of William Alanson White Memorial Lectures, to be given by an admirer of Dr. White and an outstanding psychiatrist, Dr. Harry Stack Sullivan, of New York. Such memorials to Dr. White are perhaps even more effective and closer to us than portraits such as this and such as the one which hangs at Saint Elizabeths Hospital. These portraits, however, are tangible reminders of the appreciation and affection which was felt for this fine physician, teacher and friend.

Certainly while we are paying tribute to the memory of Dr. White we should be remiss if we failed to remind ourselves likewise of another significant physician, a close personal friend and admirer of Dr. White who did much for this school. I refer, of course, to our late dean, Dr. Earl B. McKinley, an outstanding scientist, a man of high ideals, of great imagination and tremendous energy, who performed valuable services in developing this school to its present high plane of efficiency and reputation. His untimely death was a great loss to the cause of bacteriology, of medical education and this school. We all wish for our new dean, Dr. Bloedorn, the greatest of success in keeping George Washington University Medical School on the same high plane of standing. He may feel confident that the faculty shares his enthusiasm for the possibilities of the school and his desire to keep it a leader among the medical schools of North America.

If one were merely to enumerate the significant advances which have been made in medicine in the last century, he would have to be provided with a rather bulky book in which to record them. When we consider that less than one hundred years ago the benefits of anesthesia, the germ theory of disease and consequently the possibilities of preventing infection were not known, you can realize that some of the very elementary items of modern-day practice are relatively new.

Consider the advances of bacteriology; the significant work not only of Morton, Lister and Pasteur, but more recently of Banting and his epoch-making development of insulin; the work of Theobald Smith and McKinley in bacteriology; the work of Folin in chemistry and of Cannon in physiology; the development of the knowledge of the vitamins and of the endocrine glands, and of surgery in all its aspects—and we have achievements worthy of record indeed. Perhaps even more important is the aspect of preventive medicine for which Walter Reed did so much. To-day diphtheria, typhoid and many other diseases are virtually unknown. New horizons are being discovered daily in the field of allergy, and indeed there is much reason to think that the work of medicine is just beginning. The pessimist may say that much has been discovered, that there is nothing more to discover. Such an attitude, of course, is far from the fact. Each discovery lays the groundwork of a group of further discoveries. How could we have all the wonders of radio and television to-day had it not been for the painstaking work of Marconi years ago?

There is a story going the rounds that a long time ago a Commissioner of Patents of the United States advised closing the Patent Office because everything worth-while had already been discovered. Being curious as to the basis of this story I appealed to my friend, Mr. E. W. Chapin, librarian of the Patent Office, and am indebted to him for giving me the actual facts upon which the story is based. As is so often the case, there was a little fire, although a great deal of smoke, and this story illustrates very well how stories grow. The study of gossip and its development, indeed, would make an interesting topic of discussion for psychiatrists. It appears that in the year 1843 the Commissioner of Patents said in his report: "The advancement of the arts from year to year taxes our credulity and seems to presage the arrival of that period when human improvement must end."

Let us not be deceived into thinking that human improvement is nearly ended. Heaven knows that there is ample room for much improvement in many fields, including that of the conduct of individuals and of groups. Much more is to be learned concerning the possibilities in the field of heredity and constitution. Much remains to be learned in the field of bacteriology with particular reference to the virus diseases and the development of biological tests. The field of chemotherapy is only beginning. The almost miraculous effects of sulfanilamide and sulfapyridine in the treatment of certain infections lead one to the belief that perhaps we may be on the path toward that dream of the old physicians, the *therapia magna sterilisans*. Surgery is on the threshold of new developments, and the development of the newer anesthetics in the field of obstetrics has really revolutionized the practice of that specialty within the past few years. There is one field, however, on which medicine has hardly yet begun—medicine is just discovering man! So much in the past has been devoted to the parts of man, to his various organ systems and to his specific functions, that altogether too little has been thought about man himself, the social animal whose principal significance is his relations with other men. Dr. William A. White probably did more than any other medical man in this country to emphasize the importance of the individual, the "organism-as-a-whole," as he called it, a something which is greater and more important than the sum of all its parts, and indeed something different from the sum of its parts.

He emphasized the fact, now just beginning to be recognized in a general way, that the influences which impinge upon one from the outside, as well as the conflicts which arise from one's unconscious, have much to do with the physical functioning of the organism. To use Dr. White's own words, "The concept that considers the organism as a whole, and the necessary correlate thereto, that there is a psychological factor in every illness, bids fair to cause a revolution in medical thinking that will be of as great significance and as radical in its results as the revolution that has recently come about in the thinking of the physicists and the astronomers."

Although the physical manifestations of embarrassment such as blushing have long been recognized, the analogue of blushing which might be exhibited in palpitation or in spastic colitis as a result of emotional factors was overlooked. So much attention was focused upon the gastro-intestinal and circulatory tract that it was forgotten that they were parts of an individual who was perhaps expressing in this particular way and by these particular symptoms his emotional conflicts. The field of psycho-somatic medicine is in its infancy. It is encouraging to note recently in articles in the *Journal* of the American Medical Association moderately frequent references to the psychic factors in disease; during the coming year it is planned that considerable attention will be paid to these factors in the clinical instruction given in this school. Dr. White also emphasized what he called the language of the psychoses; namely, the fact that even the individual whose mental disorder is so marked as to require his commitment to a mental hospital is endeavoring in his way to meet a situation and is, perhaps in a highly symbolic manner, attempting by what we call his "jargon" to express what is going on in his mind;

after all, our language is but a symbol anyway, whether we be called psychotic or normal! Dr. White did much through his early espousal of the teachings of Freud to bring about an understanding of the unconscious mental mechanisms. The existence of these mechanisms is not denied to-day by many psychiatrists, and numerous happenings in everyday life emphasize the truth of the teachings of Freud. One of these truths, which may well be borne in mind in these parlous times of international name-calling, is that there is no such thing as pure reason, but that emotion colors every act and thought. A prominent English psychiatrist, Dr. Wilfred Trotter, has stated the case recently in a few telling words: "We can not separate off the reasoning process as such and set it to work in an emotional vacuum." He adds that if one says, "I am looking at it without prejudice," we may be sure that the statement is untrue—"We should do well on these occasions to inquire closely by what precise mechanism this supernatural purgation has been effected." A tremendous expansion in the psychiatric approach to medicine may confidently be looked for, and in this field we shall be constantly indebted to the contributions of Dr. White. Through his profound philosophical insight he adumbrated many things which have perhaps yet to be demonstrated, but as time goes on developments corroborate his keen intuition, aided by his scholarship and deep humanity.

We need have no fears that the development of medicine is at an end. Even though the world be troubled, we may confidently look for peace and satisfaction in the field of medicine, a field which is only at the beginning of possibilities of service and benefit to mankind. That medicine will continue as a profession in the hands of men possessed of individual initiative and of professional ideals, we likewise need have no doubt.

# OBITUARY

## HENRY CHANDLER COWLES

Henry Chandler Cowles was born at Kensington, Conn., on February 27, 1869. He died at his home in Chicago, Ill., on September 12, 1939, after a prolonged illness. He received his early education in the public schools and in the New Britain High School. He entered Oberlin College and was graduated with the degree of A.B. in 1893. He taught natural science at Gates College during 1894–95, and held a fellowship at the University of Chicago during 1895–96. His graduate studies were begun there in geology, but upon the appointment of the late John M. Coulter as professor of botany, he became a member of the first group in that science at the University of Chicago. While Cowles was a graduate student, the appearance of Warming's celebrated text-book of plant ecology inspired and guided him in becoming a pioneer leader in ecology in America. He received the degree of doctor of philosophy in 1898, presenting as his thesis his classical paper on the vegetation of the sand dunes of Lake Michigan. He then attempted to apply the principles of dynamic vegetation, so evident in sand dunes, to vegetation in general. The resulting "Physiographic Ecology of Chicago and Vicinity" formulated a philosophy of vegetation in which the central principle was that classification to be valid must be genetic and dynamic. In this monograph the concepts of succession and climax were for the first time adequately expressed. The principles thus enunciated were so vital and so fundamentally important that scores of graduate students were later guided in their researches by these two early publications.

In 1897 he became an assistant in the newly organized department of botany in the University of Chicago. From that time onward he was advanced repeatedly in rank until in 1911 he became professor, and in 1925 chairman of the department, a position he held until his retirement in 1934. In 1926 he became editor of the *Botanical Gazette,* a task in which he had assisted for many previous years and relinquished only at his retirement. His alma mater, Oberlin College, gave him the honorary degree of Sc.D. in 1923.

As a leader in plant science, particularly in dynamic plant ecology, he was enthusiastic but never dogmatic. He formulated no rigid system with complex classification and formidable new terminology, preferring to use non-technical language except when new ideas demanded new terms. From the beginning of his university work he was inspiring with facts, processes and principles, the basis of his stimulating teaching. He soon gathered about him a group of men and women who effectively spread the knowledge of dynamic ecology throughout the land. In 1914 the Ecological Society of America was organized, largely through the efforts of Cowles and his former students. One of these students, V. E. Shelford, now a leader in the field of animal ecology, became the first president of the new society. Cowles was its first secretary-treasurer, its president in 1917 and always a wise counselor regarding its welfare.

His world-wide leadership in the field of plant ecology was recognized in 1930, when at the International Congress, meeting at Cambridge, England, he was made president of the section of phytogeography and ecology.

In 1911 appeared the "Chicago Text Book of

Botany" in two volumes, afterwards expanded to three. Cowles contributed the volume dealing with ecology covering the branch of the subject known as autecology. In it, the theory of mechanical causation was stressed rather than teleology and adaptation which had previously been somewhat widely accepted.

No teacher brought his students more directly to nature than Cowles. Field trips, varying in length from one day to many weeks, inspired others to use the out-of-doors classroom. This led to his useful activities in all lines of conservation. No one was more influential than he in establishing the State Park system of Illinois and the Forest Preserves of Cook County, Ill. For many years he was president of the Chicago Academy of Sciences and a charter member and an active supporter of the Illinois State Academy of Science. He was also a patron and trustee of the Geographic Society of Chicago and president of the society for a term of years.

A member of many other scientific societies he served as president of the Association of American Geographers in 1910, as president of the Botanical Society of America in 1922 and vice-president of Section G of the American Association for the Advancement of Science in 1913.

In 1935 the July issue of *Ecology,* the official journal of the Ecological Society, was dedicated to Cowles by his students and friends. It was filled with articles from students and colleagues from America and from several European countries. From an appreciation of their friend and teacher, written for that issue of *Ecology* by W. S. Cooper, we quote the following paragraph:

"A man may be a great scientist and a great teacher and yet inspire in his colleagues and students little affection or none at all. With Cowles it was far otherwise. Something more than mere respect for high scientific attainment is necessary to account for the fact that, when the plan of this special number of *Ecology* was made public, more than three hundred persons responded. With almost every contribution came a letter expressing admiration for Cowles as a scientist, as a teacher, and above all, as a man. These facts speak for themselves; formal tribute is superfluous. And yet, merely because it is a joy to do so, we make mention of a few of his many lovable traits—his unfailing good humor, his far-famed ability in telling a story, his readiness to give ungrudgingly of time and effort in the service of students and friends, his eagerness to discover and commend whatever was meritorious in the work of a fellow scientist or admirable in the man himself.

"He relinquished his active labors secure in the consciousness of work well done, confident of achievement beyond the ordinary lot. He laid the foundation for a new and useful branch of science, he constructively influenced the thought of hundreds of investigators and teachers, and in his professional and personal contacts he made for himself a multitude of devoted friends."

George D. Fuller
The University of Chicago

### RECENT DEATHS AND MEMORIALS

John Allen Fulton, director of the Mackay School of Mines of the University of Nevada, who at one time was Republican nominee for Governor of Nevada, died on October 9 at the age of sixty-one years.

Dr. H. O. Knight, professor and head of the department of anatomy at the University of Texas, died on October 5 at the age of fifty-eight years.

Dr. Robert Alexander Craig, since 1904 professor of veterinary science at Purdue University, died as the result of a motorcycle accident on October 12. He was sixty-seven years old.

John Stuart Campbell, assistant professor of optics at the University of Rochester, died by suicide on September 26. He was thirty-five years old.

Frederic Theodore Bioletti, professor of viticulture at the University of California, died on September 12. A correspondent writes: "He was one of a group of young men who in the 1890s at Berkeley developed under the influence of Professor Edward L. Greene a permanent interest in botany. He made many critical plant collections which have been cited in Engler's 'Pflanzenreich' and other works. His vocation was viticulture. In this subject he was for nearly fifty years instructor and professor in the College of Agriculture of the University of California, save for an interruption of two years' teaching in South Africa. He published many papers in his field."

A picture of Dr. Warren P. Lombard, a member of the faculty of the Medical School of the University of Michigan from 1892 to 1923, was recently presented to the Medical School library in honor of his memory by a close friend, Colonel Ambrose Pack. Dr. Lombard was eighty-four years old at the time of his death last July. An obituary appreciation by Dr. Robert Gesell appears in the issue of Science for October 13.

## SCIENTIFIC EVENTS

### BIRD PROTECTION IN THE BRITISH EMPIRE

Reports on the present state of legislation for the protection of birds and its effectiveness in more than twenty different countries are printed in the fifth bulletin of the International Committee for Bird Preservation. The London *Times* gives an account of several relating to countries in the British Empire.

Writing of Australia, A. H. Chisholm expresses the opinion that lyre-birds, despite the fact that they lay only one egg in a season, are increasing throughout their range, which is from southern Victoria to southern Queensland. Certain other species, notably several beautiful parrots, have, however, decreased considerably, though, with the exception of the small varieties of emu, no Australian bird is known to have become extinct since the white occupation of the country. In Canada, according to Hoyes Lloyd, the insectivorous birds protected by the Migratory Birds Treaty with the United States are in no serious danger, and the attitude of children towards birds is, owing to better education, showing a great improvement. The shooting season for ducks and geese has since 1936 been limited to two months, and the shore-bird family is almost totally protected. The extension of bird sanctuaries has continued in Canada, but some of the prairie waterfowl sanctuaries are at present useless owing to drought.

E. V. Sanderson reports on the position in New Zealand, where the Forest and Bird Protection Society "is now a powerful and well-to-do organization." Unfortunately moose and other introduced mammals have done much damage by destroying natural vegetation in such reserves as the Fiordland National Park, which covers 2,600,000 acres. In New Zealand the upland game-birds have decreased greatly, leaving the grey duck to face most of the shooting, with the result that this bird is now becoming rapidly scarcer.

In an "informal report" on what is happening in South Africa, Dr. E. Leonard Gill says that wild birds seem to him to be better treated there than in most parts of the world, largely because in Africa sportsmen have shot big game and have not troubled much to shoot birds.

The bulletin also contains reports from Argentina, Mexico, Japan and many European countries, as well as the minutes of the meetings held at Rouen last year.

## THE NEW MILFORD LABORATORY OF THE BUREAU OF FISHERIES

CONSTRUCTION of a new laboratory for the Fisheries Service at Milford, Conn., according to the bulletin issued by the service, is now under construction as a Public Works Administration project. When completed, it will serve as a center for oyster-cultural research for the New England area and may be used also for investigations on other aspects of fishery problems.

The new laboratory will be housed in a two-story, fireproof building, 70 by 35 feet, constructed of brick and cinderblocks. The building is to rest on yellow-pine piling driven 35 to 40 feet into the ground. The first floor will contain the director's office and laboratory, one laboratory room 21 by 16 feet, two small rooms for investigators, a room for meetings, lectures and displays, 22.7 by 22 feet, rooms for the heating plant and mechanical equipment, lavatories and a carpenter shop.

Chemical, physiological and biological laboratories, each about 23 by 16 feet, will be placed on the second floor, together with the chemical stock room, balance room, photographic room and library. All the laboratories will be provided with standard equipment, *i.e.,* gas, electricity, cold and hot fresh water, sea water, compressed air and the necessary furniture. The chemical room is to be equipped with standard chemical tables and two large fume hoods with forced draft. The sea-water system consists of a non-corrosive pump of suitable capacity, a large steel rubber-lined tank in the attic and lead pipes delivering the sea water to drain tables placed in each of the laboratory rooms. With the exception of the director's office and display room, the floors are of concrete covered with rubber matting. The building will be steam-heated by means of an automatic oil burner.

There will be a series of large concrete outdoor tidal tanks, about eight feet deep, built along the water line. Each tank is individually filled with sea water through tidal gates and the depth of the water can be maintained at three different levels. Seven of these tanks have been erected and have proved useful for keeping animals for various experiments.

Before designing the laboratory and selecting its equipment, a careful study was made of existing biological stations, and efforts were made to introduce the necessary up-to-date equipment, yet at the same time to avoid expensive structural features. This work benefited from a detailed examination of plans and buildings of the Marine Biological Laboratory and the Oceanographic Institution at Woods Hole, Mass. Many of the architectural features proving useful in these institutions were incorporated in the plans. To conform with its surroundings, the Milford Laboratory is of simple design and colonial in style of architecture.

The Bureau of Fisheries has conducted oyster investigations in Long Island Sound from headquarters at Milford for nearly twenty years. The work to be conducted in the new laboratory will be devoted principally to the study of improved methods of oyster culture, and special attention will be given to the possibility of controlling the propagation of oysters and other commercial mollusks.

## THE THOMAS R. BAKER MUSEUM OF ROLLINS COLLEGE

LAST spring Rollins College received by deed from the City of Winter Park, Fla., a property known as the Aloma Golf Club to be developed by the college as an enlarged and more useful Natural Science Museum. The property consists of a large and attractive building and three acres of land about one and a half miles from the college campus. The Club House was built in 1926 at a cost of about $35,000. It consists of a large room suitable for exhibition cases, a library, a curator's office and laboratory, shop room, rooms for storage and preparation of specimens, laboratory space for visiting biologists and living quarters for caretakers. While the museum is a division of Rollins College, the trustees have appointed a large committee, consisting of officers and faculty of the college and other local residents interested in the development of the museum, to manage its affairs. The present plans include development along the following lines: Exhibition of and information concerning Florida fauna and flora; development of a library of general treatises on natural history and also special papers dealing with Florida plants and animals; educational work with students of all ages and finally laboratory facilities for visiting biologists. It will depend for its support on gifts of which several have already been made. It will strive to be of service to the thousands of residents of Central Florida and others. Further information can be obtained from Edward M. Davis, curator, Rollins College, Winter Park, Fla.

G. G. SCOTT

## MATHEMATICAL REVIEWS

A NEW international journal, to be known as *Mathematical Reviews,* will be edited at Brown University this year under the sponsorship of the American Mathematical Society, with the support of other learned and philanthropic organizations.

The Rockefeller Foundation has granted the university $49,500 for a micro-film laboratory to be set up in connection with the new journal and with the mathematics library of the university. Professor Otto E. Neugebauer, formerly editor of the *Zentralblatt für Mathematik,* and Professor J. D. Tamarkin, of the university, have been made editors; Dr. Will Feller will be assistant editor.

The journal is planned to "review all fields of pure mathematics," and will be published regularly in four languages—English, French, German and Italian. It is expected to be a clearing-house of information for teachers and research workers in all parts of the world.

The Carnegie Corporation has appropriated $60,000 for the journal, and the Rockefeller Foundation has pledged $12,000. The American Mathematical Society and the Mathematical Association of America have given $1,000 each. The micro-film laboratory will be used to copy rare mathematical material for Brown's mathematics library. Film copies of out-of-print journals and other publications will be available to mathematicians throughout the world. Films of any article reviewed in the journal will be sent to subscribers at cost.

## THE UNITED STATES ANTARCTIC EXPEDITION

THE National Bureau of Standards reports that the United States Antarctic Expedition, which is expected to leave early in November, has need for many special kinds of devices and scientific apparatus. The various governmental agencies have been requested to cooperate with the members of the expedition to insure the accomplishment of the objectives. Because of the unusual conditions under which the scientific work must be done, special apparatus had to be designed for much of this work.

The bureau is supplying the equipment and apparatus for determining the temperature and density of the snow and ice at various depths. It is planned to install thermometers in the snow at the surface and at various depths down to 160 feet to determine not only the temperature at the various depths but also how these temperatures are influenced by the air temperatures during the different seasons. In addition, measurements will be carried out at different stations to determine the influence of the local topography on the subsurface temperatures.

The bureau is supplying 42 electric resistance thermometers and 2 wheatstone bridges with accessories, such as switches, extra galvanometers, etc. The instruments will be graduated from $+10°$ to $-70°$ C. ($+50°$ to $-94°$ F.). The thermometers will be located in holes about 2 inches in diameter. Especially designed drills for making the holes are being constructed in the instruments shops. Electric heating devices are also being provided to melt holes into the snow or ice, in case it is not possible to drill the holes to the full depth with the limited manpower available.

Apparatus and materials for determining the density of snow and ice and for determining the amount of communicating air spaces consist of the following: Balances; sampling devices for obtaining representative samples of snow; triethylbenzene to be used for filling the communicating air spaces in the density samples; and a number of density standards for determining the density of the various liquids, such as triethylbenzene, kerosene, etc., which will be used in determining the density of the snow.

Because it is difficult to estimate the accuracy which will be obtained with the apparatus at the extreme temperatures at which it will be used, numerous standards, such as resistance coils, freezing-point samples, masses, etc., are being provided for the purpose of testing and calibrating the apparatus under the conditions encountered in the Antarctic.

## VISITING PHYSICISTS AT CORNELL UNIVERSITY

During the academic year 1938–39 and summer of 1939 reports by non-resident speakers were presented at meetings of the faculty and graduate students in physics at Cornell University as follows:

September 26—*Photo-conductivity and the Theory of the Latent Image,* Professor N. F. Mott, University of Bristol.

October 20—*The Philosophical Interpretations and Misinterpretations of the Quantum Theory,* Professor Philipp Frank, German University of Prague.

November 7—*Some Metallurgical Problems from a Physicist's Point of View,* Dr. S. Dushman, General Electric Research Laboratory.

December 1—*The Separation of Isotopes by Chemical Methods,* Professor H. C. Urey, Columbia University.

January 16—*Behavior of Matter under High Pressure,* Professor Edward Teller, George Washington University.

March 6—*Design and Construction of the Large Westinghouse Electrostatic Generator,* Dr. W. E. Shoupp, Westinghouse Laboratories.

March 20—*Cloud Chamber Studies of Cosmic Rays,* Professor J. C. Street, Harvard University.

March 27—*Proton Reactions,* Professor L. A. DuBridge, University of Rochester.

May 1—*High Pressure Research,* Professor P. W. Bridgman, Harvard University.

May 15—*The Self-energy of the Electron,* Dr. V. F. Weisskopf, University of Rochester.

July 31—*Problems of the Pick-up Tube in Television,* Dr. E. G. Ramberg, Research Division, Radio Corporation of America.

August 7—*Some Significant Developments in Nuclear Physics,* Professor S. W. Barnes, University of Rochester.

## AWARD OF THE WILLIAM H. NICHOLS MEDAL

The William H. Nichols Medal of the New York Section of the American Chemical Society has been awarded for 1940 to Dr. John M. Nelson, professor of organic chemistry at Columbia University, "for important contributions to the chemistry of life processes." The official statement of the jury of award reads:

Professor Nelson is an internationally recognized authority on the isolation and purification of naturally occurring enzymes and the quantitative study of their mode of action. He is the author of seventy-five papers in scientific journals, and has devoted the major portion of his research to determining the characteristics and activities of enzymes, substances which accelerate chemical transformations in nature—carbohydrates, the organic compounds manufactured by green plants, and valence, the quality which causes elements to react.

Professor Nelson is noted as an investigator of those complex chemical substances, the enzymes, by virtue of which life processes are carried on. They are the catalysts, the lubricants for the wheels of the vital mechanism. His work has been concerned with two of these enzymes: invertase, which is typical of those involved in the digestive processes of animals and in related processes in plant life; and tyrosinase, which is typical of those involved in the respiratory process. The latter process is a reaction related to combustion by which foodstuffs and air produce heat and mechanical energy.

Since Professor Nelson undertook his research work, chemists have shown that enzymes are proteins, either simple or complex. Consequently, much of the work that he has directed has been closely related to molecules of proteins, the fundamental building blocks in nature. Until 1934, his research was actively centered on invertase, the enzyme that occurs in the small intestine of mammals and in the tissues of certain animals and plants. His many publications on the activity of invertase and on methods for preparing highly active and purified preparations established him as one of the authorities on enzymes in this country.

In 1934 Professor Nelson became interested in problems concerning the utilization of molecular oxygen in plants and animals. The investigations of several groups of workers, largely European, have shown that the use of oxygen in many respiration processes occurs through a series of reactions in which two types of enzymes function—dehydrogenases and oxidases. The action of the former enzymes has been fairly well defined, but the functions of the latter are still the subjects for extensive researches.

During the past year Professor Nelson succeeded in obtaining a crystalline protein which has characteristics similar to tyrosinase, an oxidase. The importance of this development is apparent from the fact that although thousands of enzymes are known to exist, only about ten have been crystalized in a pure form.

Professor Nelson was born in West Point, Neb., on October 19, 1876. He was graduated from the University of Nebraska in 1901, and during the next two years he was employed as chemist for the Nebraska Food Commission. During 1903–04 he was instructor in chemistry at the Rose Polytechnic Institute, Terre Haute, Ind. He received the Ph.D. degree from Columbia in 1907. In 1907–08 he was instructor in the Rensselaer Polytechnic Institute.

He joined the Columbia faculty in 1908 as tutor, becoming assistant professor in 1915, associate professor in 1916 and full professor in 1922. He has had charge of the instruction of organic chemistry in Columbia College and has directed graduate research. The medal will be presented at a dinner of the New York Section on March 8, when Professor Nelson will speak on the various phases of the research in which he has been engaged.

The Nichols Medal was founded in 1902 by the late Dr. William H. Nichols, a charter member of the American Chemical Society and chairman of the board of the Allied Chemical and Dye Corporation, to "stimulate original research in chemistry."

## DR. AMES AND THE NATIONAL ADVISORY COMMITTEE FOR AERONAUTICS

PRESIDENT ROOSEVELT appointed George Jackson Mead, aeronautical consulting engineer, vice-president and director of the United Aircraft Corporation at West Hartford, Conn., to membership on the National Advisory Committee for Aeronautics to succeed Dr. Joseph S. Ames, who has been chairman of the committee or its executive body for twenty-four years and whose resignation because of ill health was accepted by Mr. Roosevelt "with sincere regret."

Mr. Mead was appointed for the unexpired term of five years from December 1, 1938, to which Dr. Ames was named last year. Dr. Ames advised the advisory committee in September that because of his physical condition he "could not in justice to the committee or to myself accept another term as chairman."

In his letter accepting the resignation of Dr. Ames, President Roosevelt said:

Our republic would not be worthy of the devoted service you have rendered for over twenty-four years without compensation if it could not on this occasion pause to pay tribute where it is so justly due.

When you were first appointed by President Wilson in 1915, very little was known about the science of aeronautics. To you and to your colleagues were entrusted by law the supervision and direction of the scientific study of the problems of flight. For the past twenty-four years you have served as chairman of the National Advisory Committee for Aeronautics, or chairman of its executive committee. The administration and the accomplishments of the committee under your leadership reflect your great scientific attainments, professional courage and executive ability.

That the people generally have not known of your brilliant and patriotic service is because it has been overshadowed by your passion for accomplishment without publicity. But the fact remains, and I am happy to give you credit for it, that the remarkable progress for many years in the improvement of the performance, efficiency and safety of American aircraft, both military and commercial, has been due largely to your own inspiring leadership in the development of new research facilities and in the orderly prosecution of comprehensive research programs.

# SCIENTIFIC NOTES AND NEWS

PROFESSOR GEORGE R. HARRISON, director of the Research Laboratory of Experimental and Applied Physics at the Massachusetts Institute of Technology, was presented on October 11 with the Rumford Medal of the American Academy of Arts and Sciences in recognition of "his notable work in spectrum photometry and spectrum analysis." Dr. Harlow Shapley, director of Harvard Observatory and president of the academy, presided; the presentation was made by Professor Norton A. Kent, of Boston University. Dr. Harrison made an address entitled "New Methods in Spectroscopy."

THE Frederic E. Ives Medal of the Optical Society of America was presented on October 14 at the Lake Placid meeting to Dr. August Herman Pfund, professor of physics at the Johns Hopkins University, in recognition of his work with infra-red rays. Dr. R. C. Gibbs, of Cornell University, president of the society, made the presentation.

THE seventieth birthday of Dr. R. S. Woodworth, professor of psychology at Columbia University, was celebrated on October 17. At an informal luncheon held at the Faculty Club his colleagues presented to him an anniversary volume, "Psychological Issues," containing a collection of twenty-five of his publications, a copy of his portrait and a complete bibliography. A reception was held at the Faculty Club in the afternoon from four to six where he was greeted by officers of the university, his colleagues and students in psychology.

AT a special ceremony in connection with alumni day, Colgate University on October 15 conferred the doctorate of science on William S. Murray, consulting and analytical chemist of Utica, N. Y., and a trustee of the university. President George Barton Cutten conferred the degree after Dean Carl A. Kallgren had read the citation. Mr. Murray is chairman of the New York Republican State Committee.

DR. FRANK AYDELOTTE, president of Swarthmore College, has been elected director of the Institute for Advanced Study at Princeton, New Jersey. He succeeds Dr. Abraham Flexner, who has been director of the institute since its establishment in 1930.

DR. FRANKLYN B. SNYDER, formerly vice-president and dean of the faculties, will be installed as the eleventh president of Northwestern University on November 15. He succeeds Dr. Walter Dill Scott, formerly professor of psychology, who resigned recently after serving as president since 1920.

AT the Armour Institute of Technology, Chicago, Linton E. Grinter, director of the civil engineering curriculum and dean of the Graduate Division, has been appointed vice-president of the institute. He will continue as dean of the Graduate Division.

DR. HERBERT C. SADLER, Alexander Ziwet professor of engineering at the University of Michigan, has retired because of ill health. Resolutions were adopted at a meeting of the Regents on October 7 expressing their appreciation of his services and conferring on him the titles dean emeritus of the College of Engineering and professor emeritus of naval architecture and marine engineering.

Dr. Royal N. Chapman, director of the Pineapple Producers Association of the Agricultural Experiment Station and dean of the Graduate School of Tropical Agriculture of the University of Hawaii, has returned to the University of Minnesota as dean of the Graduate School. He takes the place of Dr. Guy Stanton Ford, now president of the university. Dr. Chapman received the degree of bachelor of arts and master of arts from the university, and was from 1916 until he went to Hawaii in 1930 associated with it as instructor, assistant and associate professor and professor of animal biology and economic entomology.

Dr. Clarence E. Bennett has been appointed head of the department of physics of the University of Maine; Dr. J. Robert Smyth has been made head of the newly established department of poultry husbandry in the College of Agriculture.

Dr. David A. Boyd, Jr., instructor in psychiatry and assistant physician in the Neuropsychiatric Institute of the University of Michigan, has been appointed head of the department of mental and nervous diseases of the School of Medicine and Medical Center of Indiana University. Dr. Larue Carter has been named chairman of the division of neurology.

Dr. Fritz London, of the Institute Henri Poincaré, one of the divisions of the University of Paris, has been appointed professor of chemistry at Duke University.

Dr. Richard W. Linton, who was engaged in research on cholera in India from 1931 to 1938 under the auspices of the Indian Research Fund Association, has been appointed assistant professor of pathology at Cornell University Medical College, New York City. Dr. Linton is carrying on research on tuberculosis.

H. W. Straley, III, formerly of the University of North Carolina, has been appointed associate professor and executive officer of the department of geology of Baylor University at Waco, Texas.

Dr. Clinton V. MacCoy, assistant biologist in the New Hampshire Department of Fish and Game, has been appointed assistant professor of zoology at the Massachusetts State College. He succeeds Professor Herbert E. Warfel, who has joined the faculty of the University of New Hampshire.

Dr. Witold Hurewicz, of the University of Vienna, is this year assistant professor of mathematics at the University of North Carolina. Other appointments include: Dr. Jonathan Williams, of Northwestern University, assistant professor of chemistry, and Dr. Harry Davis Bruner, of the University of Louisville, assistant professor of physiology. As already announced, Dr. Robert E. Coker, head of the department of zoology, has been named a Kenan professor, succeeding the late Dr. H. V. Wilson. Dr. I. H. Manning, formerly dean of the Medical School, has been named Kenan professor emeritus of physiology.

Dr. Louis G. Kress, of Buffalo, has been appointed the first director of the newly established Division on Cancer Control of the New York State Health Department. He will open an office in Albany to direct the statistical, clinical and educational work. Dr. Kress was director of the old departmental division of cancer control. Dr. Morton L. Levin, of New York City, has been made assistant director.

Dr. Elliott C. Cutler, Moseley professor of surgery at the Harvard Medical School and surgeon-in-chief at the Peter Bent Brigham Hospital, Boston, has been elected president of the Harvard Alumni Association.

Dr. James H. Hibben, of the Geophysical Laboratory of the Carnegie Institution of Washington, has become chief of the Chemical Division of the U. S. Tariff Commission.

Dr. Robert T. Conner, instructor in chemistry at Columbia University, has become associated with the Biochemical Division of the General Foods Company at Hoboken, N. J.

Professor Hugh O'Neill, of the Catholic University of America, has returned to Washington after an expedition to Labrador, to the islands north of Canada and to Hudson's Bay. Geological specimens were collected, as well as 600 cross sections of wood showing growth rates; motion pictures were taken.

Dr. Wilfred H. Osgood, chief curator of zoology at Field Museum of Natural History, sailed from New York on October 6 for Peru, where he will assume leadership of the Magellanic expedition, sponsored by Stanley Field, president of the museum. The expedition, which includes in its personnel Colin C. Sanborn, curator of mammals, and Karl P. Schmidt, curator of amphibians and reptiles, will proceed from Peru via central Chile to the Straits of Magellan for collecting and research which will continue throughout the summer season of southern South America.

Dr. Thomas H. Johnson, assistant director of the Bartol Research Foundation of the Franklin Institute, lectured on October 18 at a stated meeting of the institute. His subject was "Cosmic Rays, What has been Learned About Them."

Dr. Werner E. Bachmann, associate professor of chemistry at the University of Michigan, is lecturing during October under the auspices of the American Chemical Society. He planned to speak in sixteen cities in Wisconsin, Minnesota, South Dakota, Montana, Washington, Oregon, California, Utah, Colorado, Nebraska and Iowa. The titles of his lectures are: "The Synthesis of Sex Hormones" and "Cancer-Producing Compounds."

DR. SOMA WEISS, Hersey professor of the theory and practice of physic at the Harvard Medical School, will give an address at a joint meeting of the Institute of Medicine of Chicago and the Chicago Society of Internal Medicine at the Palmer House on the evening of October 27. His subject will be "Syncope, Collapse and Shock-Mechanism and Treatment."

DR. DAVID SARNOFF, president of Radio Corporation of America and chairman of the board of the National Broadcasting Company, gave an address at Albany on October 13 entitled "Radio and Education" on the occasion of the seventy-fifth convocation of the University of the State of New York.

AN astronomical conference, on "The Internal Constitution of the Stars," sponsored by the New York Academy of Sciences, is being held on October 20 and 21 at the American Museum of Natural History, with Dr. Harlow Shapley, director of the Harvard Observatory, as chairman. At the morning session on October 20 there is a discussion of "The Distribution of Density in Eclipsing Binaries," at which the speakers announced are Professor Henry Norris Russell, Princeton University; Dr. Theodore E. Sterne, Harvard University, and Dr. Zdenek Kopal, Czecho-Slovakia. In the afternoon the subject is "Sources of Stellar Energy" and the speakers announced are: Dr. Hans A. Bethe, Cornell University; Dr. S. Chandrasekhar, University of Chicago, and Dr. G. Gamow, George Washington University. On Saturday, October 21, the subject announced is "Opacity Problems," and the speakers, Dr. Donald H. Menzel, Harvard University; Professor Philip Morse, Massachusetts Institute of Technology, and Dr. Jaakko Tuominen, Finland.

# DISCUSSION

## VOCAL MIMICRY OF THE STARLING AND THE MOCKINGBIRD

THE introduced starling and the mockingbird are unsurpassed as versatile vocal mimics among our American birds. While the mimicry of the starling is delivered in a more quiet and less spectacular manner than that of the mockingbird, it is in many respects a more skilled and persistent mimic, and its mimicry may even be more varied in its range and in its methods.

I have spent much time with starlings close at hand by means of observation boxes and nesting boxes placed near my bedroom window. The faithfulness with which the starling can imitate complex sounds is remarkable; in the proper mood its repertoire is almost inexhaustible.

There are many interesting characteristics which enter into its mimicry. First almost all sounds seem to have registered themselves in its brain at one time or another, as the fuss-and-ado made by a hen after laying an egg, the weird calls of the disturbed guinea hen, the calling of the quail, the song of the wood peewee, the mew of kittens, and many others.

Some of the more remarkable exhibitions have extended to very special notes such as the immature chirp of young robins, as well as the clearer less throaty notes of the adults. One of the most interesting renderings was the portion of a whistled song by some boy, the whistled notes being delivered with surprising clearness.

I have never yet heard the clear flute-like notes of the wood thrush attempted, although these birds are everywhere common singers in the immediate vicinity. However, this affords no criterion that some day they will not come from a starling's throat.

Every out-of-door nature student is probably familiar with the drumming notes of the woodpeckers, produced by rapid taps of the beak upon a dead limb. I was convinced that this was one note, so specialized and mechanical in its production, that the starlings would never attempt nor be able to reproduce it. I was wrong, but it took a long period of time to establish this, since for many years the birds had dwelt by my bedroom window and elsewhere in boxes in my trees, with no hint of such accomplishments. In the spring of 1938 a starling began delivering the long monotonal *clip-clip-clip* of the flicker, in its usual low voice, but perfect in its rendering, and from time to time it used its beak to drum out a low, but very clearly reproduced and accurate tattoo of this bird on the top of its box. This note was delivered from time to time for weeks, but only occasionally.

To my mind this is one of the most remarkable instances of mimicry, since it has demanded an entirely new method of mechanical sound production on the part of the bird. I am still convinced, however, that the starling, marvelous mimic that it has proven itself to be, will never reproduce the queer booming sounds of the nighthawk, which follows the termination of the high dive of this bird toward the earth with closed wings. This accomplishment should be beyond its scope and power, it would seem.

A second feature in the starling's mimicry is an out-of-season production of the notes of our summer birds. For instance, the distinctive notes of the wood peewee for weeks have been produced in the dead of winter, months after the birds have gone far southward. In some manner these notes gleaned in summertime have been retained by the nervous mechanism of the starlings, to come out aimlessly, spontaneously, yet faithful in their vocal copy, when the starlings were in a voluble mood.

There is a third phase in the starling's mimicry which deserves mention. I refer to the persistence of a given note which will have a "run," or become a popular "hit," so to speak, over a considerable period of time, and become an element in the repertoire of a number of birds for the same period. At one time it will be the call notes of the quail, at another that of the wood peewee, then these will be abandoned, not to be heard for weeks, months or years. In this fundamental behavior, starlings are like humans, and novelty seems to have its temporary interest, but the novelty by constant repetition wears off, it would seem, and a new outlet of expression is resorted to.

The mockingbird, it may be said, is also one of our great mimics, but he is more of an original artist than the starlings. He sings loudly, loves dramatic display, as witness the conscious display he makes of the white spots in his wings as he hops along a level privet hedge with uplifted and outstretched wings, or springs up from the roof gable or chimney top in his voluble exuberance with extended wings, or sings with wild revelry the night long on moonlight nights.

Vocal mimicry may not be a simple matter. The mimic appears to plagiarize blindly, indulging in a wild and lawless flow of borrowed notes, repeating them rapidly from 2 to as many as 20 or more times, not infrequently, as the mockingbird does. It would be remarkable, indeed, if a starling or mockingbird delivered the entire song of a wood thrush in the calm, deliberate, phrased manner of this classic singer. While the individual note, call or phrase of a song may be reproduced with great fidelity, the mimic does not go so far as to reproduce the method of the song, its time relations or its structures. I may refer to the song of the common phoebe (*Sayornis phoebe* Latham). This is a simple song characterized by two phrases usually delivered in alternation in the typical song. The only obvious difference in the two phrases appear to be a lowered inflection in the one and a raised inflection at the end of the other, *i.e.*, pee-wee ↘ . . . . pee-wee ↗ . . . . pee-wee ↘ . . . . pee-wee ↗, etc.

Now the mockingbird has very frequently indulged in the first phrase *pee-wee* of this series, repeating it hurriedly, with a very faithful rendering of its innovations, 10 times or more, but at no time has it ever adopted the simple song as a whole and reproduced it structurally as an alternation song which the peewee has learned to deliver. This degree of mimicry is a very different and more technical sort of attainment than the birds seem to be capable of, it would seem.

The mockingbird is very apt at times in its mimicry of the whippoorwill, but it apparently never introduces the low cluck at the end of the phrase whip-poor-will which the whippoorwill itself delivers.

While vocal mimicry has attained a high degree of development in a few of our birds, it would appear to be only a maudlin accomplishment, satisfying only to the whims and moods of the individuals of the species. In the process of accomplishment there must be some degree of attention and memory involved, even if only of a subconscious sort. Surely, also, there are profound differences in the capacities of the brain of different species to absorb the sounds which impinge upon the bird's attentions, since one species is an excellent mimic and another is not. So far as actual mimicry is concerned it is apparently an aimless and useless art, and of no survival value to the species. Nevertheless, one must admit that our great mimics among the birds are geniuses in their art.

H. A. ALLARD
U. S. DEPARTMENT OF AGRICULTURE

## HIBERNATION OF ANOPHELINE EGGS IN THE TROPICS

THE methods of survival of anophelines through the dry season in Panama have caused a great deal of speculation. It is a recognized fact that a small amount of anopheline breeding continues throughout the dry season and probably a few adults survive this period, but the sudden increase in anopheline larvae and adults occurring 7 to 10 days after the onset of the rainy season does not seem to be wholly accounted for as coming from these sources. The numbers of adults and larvae encountered at this time would make one think that some other method of survival is utilized by the anophelines to tide the majority of them over the unfavorable period of the dry season.

We felt that hibernating eggs might be one of the factors involved in the survival of these species. As far as we know, the survival of anopheline eggs by hibernation has not been demonstrated in the tropics.

As the dry season was well advanced when it was decided to test this possibility, we were unable to accurately measure and study anopheline eggs being oviposited at the beginning of the dry season and compare them with eggs oviposited during the summer and fall. It is our impression, however, from observation of *Anopheles albimanus* eggs, studied superficially during the latter part of December, 1938, that they were larger than those secured during the summer. Many of these apparently larger eggs, instead of hatching in 24 to 48 hours, required 7 to 14 days to hatch, and some failed to hatch within the 14-day observation period, although they did not appear to be unfertile.

In the Canal Zone there are many seepage areas that persist for about one month after the beginning of the dry season. These areas then dry up and no water is present in them until the rains begin in the latter part of April or the first week of May. The earth in these areas is dry and fissured, except when fallen leaves and grass cover the ground, in which case the soil is slightly moist but crumbly and will not pack when squeezed by hand.

On April 10, 1939, the superficial earth from a number of these seepage areas in the vicinity of Chiva Chiva, C. Z., was collected. It was estimated that the areas in which the collections were made had been dry for at least one month and no rains had been experienced in this area during that time. The slightly moist earth was collected, placed in sterile pans and then covered with tap water containing a small amount of hay infusion. The water and hay infusion were carefully handled and protected inside a screened building to preclude any mosquitoes gaining access to them. Two days after the addition of the water, a number of first instar Culex, Aedes, Psorophera and four anopheline larvae were present in the pans. The anopheline larvae developed out to be three *A. punctimacula* and one *A. albimanus*.

Additional samples of earth were collected in the Fort Clayton, C. Z., area on April 17 and 26, and on May 1 at Fort Davis, C. Z. The same precautions were exercised in the collection and handling of these specimens as reported for April 10. Three *A. albimanus,* one *A. tarsimaculatus* and five *A. punctimacula* larvae were recovered from these specimens.

Considering the method of collection and handling of this material, we feel that the larvae found had to come from eggs present in the moist earth collected from the dry seepage areas. These findings are insufficient to generally conclude that hibernating eggs are one of the ways that anophelines survive the dry season in the tropics, but the evidence seems to indicate it as a possibility. Careful observations and tests will be made prior to and during the 1940 dry season to determine the significance of the findings reported in this communication.

WM. S. STONE
FRANÇOIS H. K. REYNOLDS

ARMY MEDICAL RESEARCH BOARD,
ANCON, C. Z.

## DISTRIBUTION OF ARTIFACTS MADE FROM CHALCEDONY OF CERRO PEDERNAL, NEW MEXICO

RECENTLY Kirk Bryan[1] has called attention to the chalcedony or chert bed on Cerro Pedernal and San Pedro Mountain in north central New Mexico. This distinctive pearl-gray chalcedony is in part flecked by red and yellowish splotches. Occasional small holes are scattered at random throughout the material.

This chalcedony seems to have been quarried and manufactured over a period from the historic past to a time of considerable antiquity. Any material as distinctive and suitable for the making of artifacts should have been carried far and have been regionally dispersed by trade.

A point of this chalcedony some 4.6 inches long and 1.5 inches wide, of the type usually considered to be a knife, has been found recently in the Moreno Valley in the Sangre de Cristo Mountains, some seventy miles east and north of the known outcrops. Three other artifacts, a broken, but large oval blade, a tanged point and an "end and side" scraper, all of "Plains" type, have been found in a collection gathered locally near Mora, New Mexico, on the eastern slope of the Sangre de Cristo Mountains.

These four artifacts are without question made from the chalcedony of Cerro Pedernal, and further examination of collections may reveal an even wider distribution of this material, which appears to have been used by Indians of both Pueblo and Plains affinities, as well as by more ancient peoples.

LOUIS L. RAY

CAMBRIDGE, MASS.

[1] Kirk Bryan, SCIENCE, 87: 343–346, 1938.

## THE PRESENCE OF NON-OXYGEN-COMBINING (INACTIVE) HEMOGLOBIN IN THE BLOOD OF NORMAL INDIVIDUALS[1]

IT is generally assumed that all the hemoglobin circulating in the blood is capable of combining with oxygen and carbon monoxide, so that the capacity of the blood for oxygen absorption may be taken as a measure for the amount of hemoglobin.

It is found, however, that on employment of van Slyke and Hiller's method—after which the ability of a specimen of blood to combine with carbon monoxide (the active hemoglobin) is determined, whereafter reduction is performed with sodium hydrosulfite followed by a new determination of the carbon monoxide fixation power (the total hemoglobin)—several cases show a not inconsiderable amount of a kind of hemoglobin that is capable of binding carbon monoxide only after this reduction.

In 82 examinations carried out on healthy persons and patients who had not taken any methemoglobin-producing remedies there was found an average amount of the above-mentioned substance corresponding to a carbon monoxide fixation of 0.64 vol. per cent. = 3.5 per cent. hemoglobin (Haldane), varying from 0–2.64 vol. per cent. (0–14.5 per cent. Hb. (Haldane)). In about two thirds of the cases the amount

[1] From the Medical Department B of the Rigshospital, Copenhagen (Physician-in-chief, Professor E. Warburg, M.D.).

of this substance was less than 5 per cent. of the total amount of hemoglobin; only in a few cases (four altogether) did it exceed 10 per cent. of the total hemoglobin.

It was not practicable to identify this substance by ordinary spectroscopic examination; for the present its composition and the cause of its appearance will have to be looked upon as unknown.

According to these findings, however, the so-called active oxygen fixation power must be considered a very unreliable measure for the amount of hemoglobin. Indeed, in fourteen comparative colorimetric (Hellige's universal colorimeter) and gasometric blood examinations the colorimetric values were found to deviate considerably more from the active values than from the total.

Thus it can not be recommended to standardize colorimetric hemometers by means of the oxygen capacity.

Esther Ammundsen

# SCIENTIFIC BOOKS

## MATTER AND LIGHT

*Matter and Light.* By Louis de Broglie. Translated by W. H. Johnston, B.A. 300 pp. New York: W. W. Norton and Company, Inc. $3.50.

We have here a book written by an author outstanding in his field and noted for the clarity of his expression. In these matters the volume leaves nothing to be desired.

The book can hardly be regarded as one for the general reader. While at the outset matters of interest to the layman and comprehensible to him are presented, the author soon reaches a degree of sophistication in which the subjects treated would only have significance to a physicist and, indeed, to one who had thought fairly deeply along the lines of the modern quantum theory.

The nature of the various sections is such that there is a great deal of overlapping. We do not have here one book written in an ordered sequence, but rather a number of articles dealing with more or less the same subject in different words. This has some advantages and some disadvantages. Its advantages lie in the fact that the subject is one which is developed rapidly and presents to the minds of many a picture of artificiality and abstractness. For this reason, even a repetition of the ideas in different words is helpful in gaining more complete understanding of the matter. On the other hand, the type of treatment cited is not, perhaps, the best one for a reader whose purpose is to seek an ordered development of the subject.

In conclusion, it may be said that the book ranks as a very important contribution to the literature of the subject and will be enjoyed by a fairly large group of scholars who have the necessary background to understand it.

W. F. G. Swann

Bartol Research Foundation of
The Franklin Institute,
Swarthmore, Pa.

## WAVELENGTH TABLES

*Wavelength Tables.* Measured and compiled under the direction of George R. Harrison. xxviii + 429 pp. Boston: The Technology Press, Massachusetts Institute of Technology. New York: Wiley and Sons, Inc. London: Chapman and Hall, Ltd. 1939. $15.00.

The book comprises a systematic survey of spectrum lines giving intensities in arc, spark or discharge tube of more than 100,000 spectrum lines most strongly emitted between 10,000 and 2,000 A by the atomic elements under normal conditions of excitation. The measurements and compilation have been made under the direction of Professor George R. Harrison by staff members of the spectroscopy laboratory of the Massachusetts Institute of Technology, assisted by the Works Progress Administration.

There is a clearly written introduction summarizing the scheme of the book, and the notation, and dealing with several other matters such as the precision of the wavelengths, the nature of the apparatus used in the Massachusetts Institute of Technology observations, sources of error, etc.

There is a table stating the numbers of lines included for the various elements, a table giving the sensitive lines of the elements compiled from combinations of empirical and theoretical data selected from the literature, the lines being listed according to the elements. Then follows a table in which the aforesaid sensitive lines are arranged in order of wavelengths. Next comes a key to the symbols for authors and references, and finally what comprises practically the whole volume of the book, a table of the lines in order of wavelengths extending over the ranges already cited.

The material is set forth in a clear form, and the volume is of a size such as to provide for absence of crowding and for convenience of handling. The work will undoubtedly be found of great value to those working in both the pure and applied fields of spectroscopy.

W. F. G. Swann

Bartol Research Foundation of
The Franklin Institute,
Swarthmore, Pa.

## MAGNETISM

*Modern Magnetism.* By L. F. BATES. ix + 340 pp. Cambridge: at The University Press. New York: The Macmillan Company. 1939. $4.50.

IN many universities, the study of the magnetic properties of matter is not strongly emphasized, and the study of the experimental work in this field is almost totally neglected. This volume by Professor Bates, of the University College, Nottingham, is particularly welcome to both the student and the teacher for its presentation of much material which is unavailable except in the original publications. Although written primarily from the experimental point of view, the underlying theory is not neglected, and the work is by no means a mere compilation of observations. Proceeding from definitions of elementary quantities with no attempt to discuss the subtleties here involved, a rapid survey is made of atomic structure in terms of the vector model, and of the elementary theories of susceptibility. This is followed by descriptions of the methods of magnetic measurements and a review of the results of susceptibility measurements on isotropic and crystalline material. The measured susceptibilities are tabulated together with the electronic structures of the elements. It is unfortunate that references to the sources of the quoted values are not given. The chapters on atomic beams and nuclear spins and magnetic moments are interesting, particularly in view of the fundamental theoretical significance of the results. After a description of the several gyromagnetic effects, the volume closes with three chapters which summarize the experimental results involving the complicated phenomena of the behavior of the ferromagnetic domains, the energy changes and magnetostriction. In view of the enormous complexity and our lack of complete understanding of these phenomena, this portion of the volume is as well organized and digested as is possible without adding considerably to the length and detracting from the book's usefulness. The volume has both name and subject indices and a particularly complete table of contents, making it possible to locate any subject with ease.

C. G. MONTGOMERY
THE BARTOL RESEARCH FOUNDATION
OF THE FRANKLIN INSTITUTE

## RADIOACTIVITY

*A Manual of Radioactivity.* By GEORGE HEVESY and F. A. PANETH. Second edition, xvi + 306 pp., translated by Robert W. Lawson. Oxford University Press. 1938. $5.50.

ALTHOUGH this is designated as the second edition, it is in reality the fourth, since extensive revision was done each time the volume was translated into English. The merit of this excellent text-book has been much enhanced by the inclusion of the recent rapid advances in the field, and a revision of the older material in conformance with modern concepts. Chapters have been much enlarged or new chapters added which deal with positrons and neutrons, artificial radioactivity, the transmutation of the elements, the use of radioactive materials as indicators and so forth; and an appendix describing the cyclotron has been added. The volume suffers, as did indeed the former editions, from attempting to cover so large an amount of material in a relatively short space. But this ambitious program is precisely what renders the work most useful. Besides the physical aspects of radioactivity, its relations to the fields of chemistry, geology and even biology are outlined, and these relationships form a structure which it is possible to embellish with all the details and elaborations which the lecturer cares to add. Sufficient references to other works and to original papers are provided. The work of the translator has been well done. As a whole, the volume is a worthwhile addition to any library.

C. G. MONTGOMERY
THE BARTOL RESEARCH FOUNDATION OF
THE FRANKLIN INSTITUTE,
SWARTHMORE, PA.

# SPECIAL ARTICLES

## THE PATHOGENIC ACTION OF PHYMATOTRICHUM OMNIVORUM

CYTOLOGICAL studies[1] of cotton roots attacked by *Phymatotrichum omnivorum* (Shear) Duggar have presented indirect evidence of the importance of chemical action in the process of parasitism by this fungus. The data from cytological preparations were not accompanied, however, by experimental evidence of the type so well known for various fungi that cause rotting of plant tissues.[2] Henderson[3] has described toxic action on cotton seedlings by thermostable substances in filtrates from cultures of the fungus on liquid media. She found that the decreased pathogenicity resulting from continued culture on artificial media tends to be regained after growth upon a suitable living host. In the present work pure cultures of the fungus have been maintained in successive

[1] G. M. Watkins, *Amer. Jour. Bot.*, 25: 118–124, 1938; *Phytopath.*, 28: 195–202, 1938.

[2] Summary by W. Brown, *Bot. Rev.*, 2: 236–281, 1936.

[3] L. Henderson, *Amer. Jour. Bot.*, 24: 547–552, 1937.

transfers on roots of living cotton seedlings. When a fragment of infected root was placed against the root of a healthy seedling, it usually caused within a few hours a shrinking and discoloring of adjacent host tissues. This was followed by the formation of an encircling and penetrating hyphal weft, which produced within two or three weeks a thoroughly soft decay of the cortex along the entire root system. The immediately destructive action observed in such cases, occurring before penetration had been accomplished, suggested that a transfer of tissue-destroying substances from rotted to healthy roots had taken place, and led the writers to test the action of hyphal exudates apart from the fungus. It was found that small pieces of decayed roots, when squeezed with forceps, generally yield one or two drops of clear, amber-colored liquid. In one series of tests this fluid was applied directly, in the form of drops, to the surfaces of normal cotton seedling roots; in a parallel series healthy roots were treated with drops of liquid expressed from decayed roots which had been subjected to the temperature of boiling water for one hour. Similar tests were made for the action of liquid pressed from germinating sclerotia which had been formed on nutrient agar without access to host tissue. Special care was taken to avoid mechanical injury to the healthy roots and to maintain aseptic conditions throughout all experiments.

Liquid from unheated, decayed roots was usually absorbed into healthy roots in 4 or 5 hours, and frequently imparted a moist, water-soaked appearance to the tissue at the points of application. After 24 hours the tissue thus affected had begun to shrink and turn yellow or light-brown, forming sunken necrotic areas which resembled the lesions caused by the fungus on roots of young cotton seedlings. In most cases the shrinkage progressed around the root and extended somewhat longitudinally until the root appeared to be girdled or ringed almost to the central cylinder. After three or more days a number of small lateral roots began to break through the necrotic cortex, which suggests that the tissue destruction did not extend beyond the endodermis. Stained sections of roots fixed in different stages of cortical necrosis show a gradual disorganization of protoplasts, followed by swelling and distortion of cell walls from the epidermis inward. Finally the epidermis and cortex collapse into a deeply staining, disorganized mass, which shrinks toward the endodermis. Simultaneously, abundant cell division in the pericycle initiates the formation of lateral roots.

Cotton roots treated with liquid expressed from heated decayed roots reacted in a different manner; the liquid was not absorbed as readily, and usually only a slightly discolored spot resulted. No considerable shrinkage or disruption of tissue continuity was observed, although sections of the treated roots show that toxic effects had been exerted on protoplasts near the places of application. The experiments with unheated and heated liquid from germinating sclerotia gave results closely parallel to those described above.

Attempts to recover the fungus by placing on nutrient agar various samples of roots to which unheated fluid had been applied failed, and sections of such roots show no mycelium. Both of these circumstances tend to indicate that viable hyphae are rarely, if ever, transferred with the expressed drops of liquid, and that the induced lesions resulted from the activity of fungous secretions. The consideration that the lesions might have been brought about by possible toxic products of the chemical breakdown of host tissues is minimized by the fact that similar lesions resulted from the application of unheated liquid from germinating sclerotia. The demonstration of chemical action as an important factor in the pathogenic mechanism of *P. omnivorum* is of interest in connection with biochemical studies of the basis of resistance in certain plants to the root rot caused by this fungus.[4,5]

G. M. WATKINS
MATILDE OTERO WATKINS
U. S. DEPARTMENT OF AGRICULTURE

## URINE CHLORIDE CONCENTRATION IN PATIENTS WITH CUSHING'S SYNDROME

MCQUARRIE, JOHNSON and Ziegler[1] and Anderson, Haymaker and Joseph[2, 3] recently reported changes in the serum electrolyte pattern and urinary excretion of sodium and potassium in patients with Cushing's syndrome that were in most respects diametrically opposite to those in patients with Addison's disease. These findings, together with the observation[2] that extracts of the blood of such patients prolonged the lives of adrenalectomized rats, suggested that Cushing's syndrome may be dependent upon or associated with a state of hypercorticoadrenalism.[1, 2]

Cutler, Power and Wilder[4] have demonstrated that under standardized conditions of low sodium and chloride and high potassium intake the presence of supernormal concentrations of sodium or chloride in the urine is suggestive of a state of adrenal cortical insufficiency. Theoretically, the opposite condition should obtain in hypercorticoadrenal states under conditions of high sodium and chloride intake. The fol-

4 G. A. Greathouse, *Phytopath.*, 28: 592–593, 1938; *Amer. Jour. Bot.*, 25: 743–748, 1938.

5 The senior writer's share of this work was done during his tenure of a National Research Fellowship in Botany, 1938–39.

1 I. McQuarrie, R. M. Johnson and M. R. Ziegler, *Endocrinol.*, 21: 762, 1937.

2 E. Anderson, W. Haymaker and M. Joseph, *Endocrinol.*, 23: 398, 1938.

3 E. Anderson and W. Haymaker, *Proc. Soc. Exper. Biol. and Med.*, 38: 610, 1938.

lowing procedure was adopted: The basic diet was identical with that employed in the procedure outlined by Cutler *et al.*,[4] containing 0.949 gm Cl, 0.592 gm Na and 4.062 gm K daily. On the first day of the study period the fluid intake was fixed at 20 cc per kilogram of body weight, and 10 gm of NaCl (in capsules) was given with the morning and again with the evening meal. The same régime was followed on the second day. On the third day the bladder was emptied at 8 A.M. and urine was collected for the subsequent four-hour period. On this day 5 cc of fluid per kilogram was given before 11 A.M. Under these conditions, the intake of Na and Cl on each of the first two days was approximately 8.6 and 12.95 gm, respectively.

Of the several chemical studies performed during the test period, I wish to mention here only the chloride concentration in the four-hour urine specimen obtained on the morning of the third day. Sixteen subjects were studied. Three of these were patients presenting the characteristic clinical picture of Cushing's syndrome, with normal urinary findings and normal renal function (urea clearance); one was a patient with excessive hirsutism; the remainder were patients with miscellaneous diseases, including rheumatic fever, convalescent, afebrile (2 cases), mild essential hypertension with normal renal function (2 cases), hypertrophic arthritis (2 cases), bronchial asthma (2 cases), maxillary sinusitis (1 case) and inguinal hernia (2 cases).

In the three subjects with Cushing's syndrome the Cl concentrations were 0.193, 0.243 and 0.357 per cent., respectively, with urine volumes of 475, 450 and 500 cc. The corresponding values in the patient with excessive hirsutism were 0.179 per cent. and 535 cc. In the twelve subjects with miscellaneous disorders with no evidence of endocrine dysfunction the Cl concentration ranged from 0.462 to 1,265 per cent. (mean 0.642) and the urine volume from 680 to 1,120 cc. It appears, therefore, that under the conditions of the experiment the subjects with Cushing's syndrome and with hirsutism (suspected hyperadrenalism) were unable to eliminate chloride in the urine in as high concentration as subjects with various disorders not apparently associated with endocrine dysfunction. This test procedure may prove to be of value in detecting states of hypercorticoadrenalism. It must be kept in mind, however, as demonstrated by Thorn and Harrop,[5] that various sex hormones may exert an effect upon the urinary excretion of sodium, chloride and potassium similar to that exerted by the adrenal cortical hormone.

ABRAHAM CANTAROW
JEFFERSON MEDICAL COLLEGE, PHILADELPHIA

[4] H. H. Cutler, M. H. Power and R. M. Wilder, *J. A. M. A.*, 111: 117, 1938.

[5] G. W. Thorn and G. A. Harrop, SCIENCE, 86: 40, 1937.

## ESSENTIALITY OF PRIMARY AMINO GROUPS FOR SPECIFIC ACTIVITY OF THE LACTOGENIC HORMONE[1]

THE primary amino groups are essential for the action of the protein hormone of pituitary origin which stimulates the formation of the pigeon crop gland. We have recently demonstrated this by treating the lactogenic hormone with ketene.[2] Philpot and Small[3] have shown that nitrous acid resembles ketene in first attacking the primary amino groups in the protein molecule. They found that on the treatment of pepsin with nitrous acid, nitrogen liberation was complete within one half hour and that the secondary reaction—diazo compound formation—was scarcely started by this time.[4]

TABLE 1

EFFECT OF NITROUS ACID ON LACTOGENIC HORMONE*

| Conditions of treatment | Total dose/squab (intra-muscular) mg | Number of 30-day-old pigeons | Crop gland reaction |
|---|---|---|---|
| Untreated | 1.0 | 3 | Pronounced |
| 22–23° C, 30 minutes | 1.0 | 3 | Negative |
| | 2.0 | 3 | Negative |
| 0° C, 30 minutes | 1.0 | 3 | Negative |
| | 2.0 | 3 | Negative |
| | 1.0 | 3 | Negative |

* L 250: potency, 10 systemic units per mg.

It therefore seemed desirable to treat lactogenic hormone with nitrous acid in an effort to confirm the findings with ketene. A 1.5 per cent. solution of a highly purified lactogenic preparation was dissolved in 0.5 M acetate buffer (pH 4) and was treated for 30 minutes with an equal volume of 2 M $NaNO_2$ at 22° C. and 0° C. The mixture was then adjusted to about pH 5, was centrifuged, and the precipitate was redissolved and reprecipitated isoelectrically. As can be seen in the table, the crop stimulating activity of the preparation was completely destroyed by nitrous acid in this period. The results therefore confirm those obtained with ketene, indicating the essentiality of the

[1] Aided by grants from the Research Board of the University of California, from the Rockefeller Foundation of New York and from Parke, Davis Company of Detroit. Assistance was rendered by the Federal Works Progress Administration, Project OP 665-08-3-30, Unit A-5.

[2] C. H. Li, M. E. Simpson and H. M. Evans, SCIENCE, 90: 140, 1939.

[3] J. St.L. Philpot and P. A. Small, *Biochem. Jour.*, 32: 542, 1938.

[4] This specific action of nitrous acid has recently been confirmed by us in a study of the gonadotropic hormones. Pituitary follicle stimulating hormone, interstitial cell stimulating hormone and pregnant mare serum are inactivated quickly (one half hour) by nitrous acid, whereas human chorionic gonadotrophin is only inactivated *very slowly*. The same results were secured with ketene. (To be published).

primary amino groups in the physiological activity of lactogenic hormone.

Choh Hao Li
William R. Lyons
Miriam E. Simpson
Herbert M. Evans
Institute of Experimental Biology and Division of Anatomy,
University of California, Berkeley

## MULTIPLE NATURE OF THE RAT "FILTRATE FACTOR"—A COMPONENT OF VITAMIN $B_2$[1]

In our attempt to purify the "filtrate factor,"[2] a dietary component of vitamin $B_2$ essential for rat growth, we have obtained evidence that this factor must consist of at least two entities, one of which is extractable from acid solution by diethyl ether; the second factor remains in the residue.

The methyl alcohol soluble fraction from cane molasses was adsorbed on fuller's earth. The filtrate was acidified and extracted for 72 hours with ether in a continuous extractor (Preparation I). The residue was subjected to a second 72-hour extraction (Preparation II). These extracts, as well as the residue (Preparation III), were fed to female rats maintained on a vitamin B complex-deficient diet supplemented with thiamin, riboflavin and a source of $B_6$ in the form of a wheat germ eluate. Each preparation was fed for 56 days at the equivalent of 3 gm daily of the original molasses. The gain in weight (above that of the controls) was: Preparation I, 60 gm; Preparation II, no gain; Preparation III, 58 gm.

At this point it may be noted that black, gray and hooded rats receiving Preparation I exhibited no change in pelage coloring, while those receiving Preparation III showed a marked graying of black hair and a lightening of gray hair, although the nutritive state and growth were essentially the same in groups I and III. This experiment was repeated with new preparations and again the graying was observed in the rats receiving the residue and the coat was normal in those receiving the ether extractable fraction, although again growth was comparable in both groups. The graying of fur in "filtrate factor"-deficient rats was first noted by Morgan, Cook and Davison[3] and by Lunde and Kringstad.[4] The present work would seem to indicate that the "anti-graying" activity goes with the ether extractable component of the "filtrate factor."

The evidence for a relationship between the "chick anti-dermatitis factor" and the "rat filtrate factor" is conflicting. Woolley *et al.*[5,6] and Jukes[7,8] have demonstrated that pantothenic acid (Williams) is the "chick anti-dermatitis factor."

Hoffer and Reichstein[9] and Subbarow and Hitchings[10,11] have shown that the fraction extracted with ether is in all probability pantothenic acid and is a component of the rat "filtrate factor"; however, El Sadr and co-workers[12] found that β-alanine did not replace the liver or yeast "filtrate factor." Woolley *et al.*[5] have reported that the "chick anti-dermatitis factor" is readily destroyed by alkali. We have prepared an iso-amyl alcohol extract from a rice bran preparation. Its activity was not destroyed by heating in 1 N NaOH solution at 100° C. for 1 hour. It would, therefore, appear that the factor extractable with iso-amyl alcohol is not identical with the "chick anti-dermatitis factor."

Ali Mohammad
Oliver H. Emerson
Gladys A. Emerson
Herbert M. Evans
Institute of Experimental Biology,
University of California, Berkeley

# SCIENTIFIC APPARATUS AND LABORATORY METHODS

## AN ELECTRIC STERILIZER FOR THE CULTURE ROOM

To avoid the use of an open flame in culture room or transfer case a small electric sterilizer has been used for a number of years and found to be highly satisfactory. The constant heating of the culture space resulting from the use of a gas jet or an alcohol lamp; the resulting convection currents of air carrying con-

[1] Aided by grants from the Board of Research and the College of Agriculture, University of California, from the Rockefeller Foundation, New York, and from Merck and Company, Inc., Rahway, New Jersey. Assistance was rendered by the Federal Works Progress Administration, Project OP 665–08–3–30, Unit A-5. The following materials were generously contributed: Betabion (Thiamin) by Merck and Co., Riboflavin by Hoffmann-LaRoche, molasses by Waialua Agricultural Co., courtesy of Mr. John Midkiff, wheat germ by General Mills, Inc., and rice bran extract by the Galen Company.

[2] S. Lepkovsky, T. H. Jukes and M. E. Krause, *Jour. Biol. Chem.*, 115: 557, 1936.

[3] A. F. Morgan, B. B. Cook and H. G. Davison, *Jour. Nutr.*, 15: 27, 1938.

[4] G. Lunde and H. Kringstad, Avhandl. Norske Videnskaps. Akad. Oslo I, Mat. Naturv. Klasse 1, 1, 1938.

[5] D. W. Woolley, H. A. Waisman and C. A. Elvehjem, *Jour. Am. Chem. Soc.*, 61: 977, 1939.

[6] D. W. Woolley, H. A. Waisman and C. A. Elvehjem, *Jour. Biol. Chem.*, 129: 673, 1939.

[7] T. H. Jukes, *Jour. Am. Chem. Soc.*, 61: 975, 1939.

[8] T. H. Jukes, *Jour. Biol. Chem.*, 129: 225, 1939.

[9] M. Hoffer and T. Reichstein, *Nature*, 144: 72, 1939.

[10] Y. Subbarow and G. H. Hitchings, *Jour. Am. Chem. Soc.*, 61: 1615, 1939.

[11] G. H. Hitchings and Y. Subbarow, *Jour. Nutr.*, 18: 265, 1939.

[12] M. M. El Sadr, H. G. Hind, T. F. Macrae, C. E. Work, B. Lythgoe and A. R. Todd, *Nature*, 144: 73, 1939.

taminating spores; the production of harmful gases and the fire hazards are all eliminated by substituting a low rectangular frame of transite containing a number of turns of nicrome wire connected to the lighting circuit.

The details of the sterilizer are given in the accompanying sketch (Fig. 1). When using the sterilizer a pedal switch operates to turn the electric current on

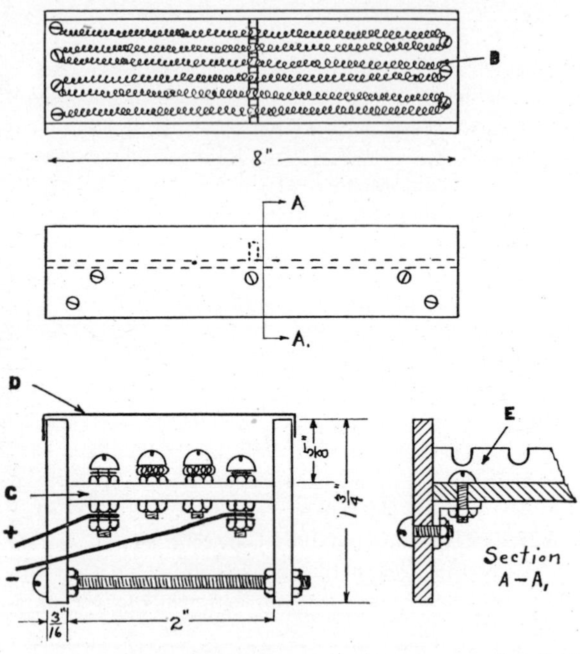


FIG. 1. Electric sterilizer, showing frame of 3/16″ transite which bears the coils of resistance wire B on a shelf C. The "12 to the inch" mesh galvanized wire screen D, covers the frame, prevents direct contact with the heating coil B and is used to hold various cultural instruments such as wire needles, special knives, scalpels, chisel forceps, long museum forceps and other instruments and materials during sterilization. In B the length of resistance wire from a cone-heating unit is looped around binding bolts at both ends and supported in the center by a slotted strip of transite E to prevent lateral contact between segments of the coil.

and off, keeping the heating coil hot only during the period when the culture instrument is being held over the mesh screen. The instrument is first dipped in alcohol and either held momentarily over the screen or laid upon it until the alcohol ignites and burns off. Glass rods used in special cultural technique for testing toxicity of preservatives in wood can be dipped in alcohol and a number of them placed over the screen for sterilization before placing them on the test fungus mat. The sterilizer is placed on a sheet of asbestos paper laid on the culture room table or the floor of the culture case in a position most handy for the worker.

The electric sterilizer is submitted for trial to those workers who desire, for one reason or another, to eliminate the open flame in the culture chamber.

ERNEST E. HUBERT

WESTERN PINE ASSOCIATION,
PORTLAND, OREGON

## THE INFLUENCE OF CENTRIFUGATION ON THE AGGLUTINATION OF PNEUMOCOCCI[1]

THE usual methods for detecting agglutinins (excepting the relatively crude slide agglutination), require 18–24 hours. Fleming,[2] stimulated by earlier observations of Gaehtgens[3] and of Gates,[4] employed centrifugation.

It was observed during observations on antigen-antibody balance in treated cases of pneumococcal pneumonias that centrifugation increases the rapidity and accuracy of agglutinin detection.

One half cc portions of the different antibody dilutions were mixed with 0.5 cc portions of bacterial suspensions. Readings were made after ½, 1 and 2 hours' incubation at the following temperatures: 4° C., 20° C., 37° C. and 55° C. and again after refrigeration at 4° C. overnight. The results obtained by this method were compared with those observed after immediate centrifugation of the antigen-antibody mixture for 5 minutes at 2,000 r.p.m. Immediate development of strongly positive reactions were observed in all tubes after centrifuging for 5 minutes. Reactions were always more definite than those obtained with water bath incubation for two hours and overnight refrigeration. The "inhibition-zone," observed after incubation in the water bath in tubes containing an excess of antibody, was eliminated.

PAUL F. DE GARA

[1] From the Medical Service of Harlem Hospital, Department of Hospitals, New York City, N. Y., and from the Littauer Pneumonia Research Fund, New York University College of Medicine. These studies received financial support from the Littauer Pneumonia Research Fund, of New York University College of Medicine, from the Metropolitan Life Insurance Company and from Mr. Bernard M. Baruch, Jr., Miss Belle N. Baruch and Mrs. H. Robert Samstag.

[2] A. Fleming, *British Jour. Exp. Path.*, 8: 231, 1928.

[3] W. Gaehtgens, *Munch. med. Woch.*, 53: 1351, 1906, and *Arch. Hyg.*, 56: 377, 1908.

[4] F. K. Gates, *Jour. Exp. Med.*, 35: 63, 1922.

## BOOKS RECEIVED

BALL, ALICE M. *Compounding in the English Language.* Pp. 226. Wilson.

*Science Reports of the Tôhoku Imperial University.* Fourth Series. (Biology.) Vol. XIV, Nos. 2 and 3. Pp. 121–326. Illustrated. Maruzen, Tokyo.

TAYLOR, JAMES H. Vector Analysis. Pp. ix + 180. Prentice-Hall. $2.85.

# SCIENCE

VOL. 90 FRIDAY, OCTOBER 27, 1939 No. 2339

*Some Problems in the Genetics of the Fungi:* DR. B. O. DODGE ... 379

*Chewing as a Technique of Relaxation:* PROFESSOR H. L. HOLLINGWORTH ... 385

*Scientific Events:*
*The British Association in War Time; The Australian National Research Council; Retirement Fund of the Field Museum of Natural History; A Biological Survey of the State of New Hampshire; Library for the History of Medicine at Yale University; The Research Council on Problems of Alcohol* ... 387

*Scientific Notes and News* ... 390

*Discussion:*
*Physiology of the Nervous System:* SIR HENRY DALE. *The Use of Prontosil as a Vital Dye for Insects and Plants:* DR. WALTER CARTER. *Formation of a Large Alcohol Bead:* DR. C. F. WINANS ... 393

*Scientific Books:*
*Recent Publications of the British Museum (Natural History):* PROFESSOR T. D. A. COCKERELL ... 395

*Special Articles:*
*Note on Water in Non-aqueous Solutions:* DR. W. J. V. OSTERHOUT and DR. J. W. MURRAY. *Cerebral Metabolism during Fever:* DR. HAROLD E. HIMWICH and OTHERS. *Crystalline Salmon Pepsin:* DR. EARL R. NORRIS and DANIEL W. ELAM ... 397

*Scientific Apparatus and Laboratory Methods:*
*Determination of the Velocity of Sound in a Gas; Application to Analysis of Mixtures of Helium, Oxygen and Nitrogen:* DR. WILLIAM B. DUBLIN, DR. WALTER M. BOOTHBY and DR. MARVIN M. D. WILLIAMS ... 399

*Science News* ... 8

SCIENCE: A Weekly Journal devoted to the Advancement of Science, edited by J. MCKEEN CATTELL and published every Friday by

THE SCIENCE PRESS
New York City: Grand Central Terminal
Lancaster, Pa. Garrison, N. Y.

Annual Subscription, $6.00 Single Copies, 15 Cts.

SCIENCE is the official organ of the American Association for the Advancement of Science. Information regarding membership in the Association may be secured from the office of the permanent secretary in the Smithsonian Institution Building, Washington, D. C.

## SOME PROBLEMS IN THE GENETICS OF THE FUNGI[1]

By Dr. B. O. DODGE

THE NEW YORK BOTANICAL GARDEN

### INTRODUCTION

NOT every one has had an opportunity, or the desire, to study the fungi critically. Most people, however, are more or less familiar with molds, mildews, mushrooms and yeasts. Those of you who were brought up in the country districts may remember how you enjoyed kicking over toadstools and puffing puffballs in each other's faces. The man who collects wild mushrooms in woodlands for food seldom thinks of them as plants. Botanists, on the theory that all living things must be either plants or animals, place the fungi in the plant kingdom. They say that if fungi ever had chlorophyll they have lost it through degeneration, and degenerates make little progress in evolution. It is a very common belief that the fungi are of little economic importance except as they cause decay and disease, and, since they show little evolution, their study would promise little as to throwing light on the great life processes. As a matter of fact, just to mention two examples, the fungi and bacteria are of incalculable value in building the soil and maintaining its fertility. Yeasts rival our boasted billion dollar corn crop, if we count the value of alcohol and other useful products of fermentation.

The old attitude is changing, as witness the interest in sex and genetics of fungi manifested during the past ten or fifteen years. This work will certainly be greatly facilitated in the next decade by the use of growth substances and sex hormones to bring into fertile cultures species of obligate parasites not now at all adapted for this type of genetic study. We may

[1] Presented at a general session of the Third International Congress for Microbiology, New York, September 6, 1939.

then hope to see a recognition of the fungi more in accord with their real importance in the great kingdoms of living things.

The farmer has known for sixty or seventy years that he should destroy the barberry because it is the alternate host of wheat rust. It is only very recently that a more important reason for destroying the barberry has been discovered, namely, it provides the opportunity, through mutation and hybridization, for the rust to develop new biologic races. Dr. M. B. Waite of the Department of Agriculture, who spent many years breeding pears for blight resistance, used to say that the real function of a plant pathologist was to turn plant breeder and develop new races of economic plants for disease resistance. It was suggested to him that while man was busy breeding up races of the host for resistance, mother nature was probably busy breeding up new races of the parasite for pathogenicity.[2] This brings us to the subject of this discussion—problems confronting those who are interested in resistance and immunity as well as those who would take up this rather new subject, mycogenetics.

### Genes in Diploid and Haploid Structures

In genetic studies of higher plants and animals the effects of factors of inheritance are usually manifest in connection with diploid structures, where each nucleus carries two sets of genes, one set contributed by each parent. The haploid mycelium of a fungus shows many variations as to color, types of growth and in the production of propagating bodies of all sorts. The foundation structures of the fruit bodies themselves are haploid. One is, therefore, enabled to observe in the fungi the effects of a single set of genes without the complications which are bound to arise when two different sets are present, as in diploids.

### Asexual and Sexual Stages of Fungi

At some time in the normal life cycle of a fungus there occur certain nuclear fusions. This phase is called the sexual stage, in contrast to the asexual stage which is a purely vegetative one where propagating bodies may or may not be developed. It was early found in all fungi where the story was complete, that the primordial reproductive structures both arose from a common stalk or branch of the mycelium. The classic text-book figures of *Aspergillus, Penicillium* and *Sporodinia* illustrate this type of development. This was accepted as proof that in the fungi each cell, or each nucleus, carried all of the inheritance of the species. Every individual was totipotent. Reproduction involving two different individuals was thought to be impossible. If a mycelium derived from a single spore did not produce zygospores, ascocarps or a mushroom, as the case might be, it was because the conditions were not suitable. This notion, held by our ultra-conservative leaders in botany, blocked mycological progress for years.

### Heterothallism and Homothallism

Blakeslee, in 1904, proved that in a number of species of the zygomycetes one can obtain zygospores only when two mycelia of opposite sex are mated. Gametangia are never produced on mycelia from single spores. Blakeslee suggested that such species be called *heterothallic*. Sexual reproduction requires mating what he called + and − races. Segregation of the sex factors is strictly bipolar and genetic. Species like *Sporodinia* are *homothallic,* because zygospores are produced on individual mycelia. Since that time heterothallism and homothallism have been found side by side in genera of all of the great groups of fungi, and this fact must be taken into account in all genetic studies involving the fungi, directly or indirectly.

### Mendelism in the Neurospora (Monilia) Bakery Molds

The salmon-pink bakery molds are of world-wide distribution, and are found especially in the tropics on burned-over sugarcane fields and on forest trees scorched by fires. The aerial branches bearing the monilioid conidia are also brightly colored. It was long thought that these molds had lost their power to reproduce sexually because they had evolved such an efficient method of propagating themselves asexually. The ascocarps, small pear-shaped fruit bodies about ½ mm in diameter, are obtained in culture only when two races of opposite sex are grown together. In three species the asci have eight spores each. These species are obligately heterothallic, so that four spores in an ascus are of one sex and four of the opposite sex, in their reaction. Three other species have 4-spored asci. They are not homothallic, although a single spore contains all of the essentials for reproduction. Each spore is originally provided with two nuclei of opposite sex.

### Mutations and Segregations

Medical mycologists in culturing skin disease fungi often find their old cultures "going pleomorphic" as they say. Sectors or spots of growth appear which are perhaps lighter in color, more fluffy and devoid of a certain kind of spores. This phenomenon probably does not differ from that to be observed in cultures of many other fungi. The question as to whether sectoring represents a true mutation or is a temporary phenotypic change due to cultural conditions is not

[2] We were just learning that we could cross races and species of the bakery molds just as easily as one could cross smooth and wrinkled peas, and with comparable results.

easily answered unless the sexual stage of a species is known. The application of growth substances and sex hormones here would be well worth trying out.

Mutations occur in these pink bakery molds as in other fungi and many different types of growth can be obtained in culture. We have one mutant albino non-conidial race which is stable. It may serve to demonstrate Mendelian segregation and how well these fungi are adapted for genetic study.

When we mate the albino race in culture with a normal salmon-pink race, hundreds of ascocarps mature within a few days. These are all exactly alike genetically, because every cell of a mycelium is potentially a gamete, and these must all be alike. The identical cross can be made over and over again through a term of years. We sometimes call these ascocarps developed from the mating, *hybrid* ascocarps, but it is only the individual young asci that are actually diploid and, therefore, hybrid, because their fusion nuclei do contain the inheritance contributed by both parents. Crushing out the ascus cluster from the fruit body, we find that the asci are all 8-spored and look alike. The ascus is a mother-cell in which the chromosomes undergo reduction, with segregations and new combinations of factors just as at maturation in animals and seed plants. When the eight spores are isolated one by one in order and are grown in tubes, we see a perfect demonstration of simple Mendelian segregation. Four races are albinos, the other four are orange-colored. By test it is proved that four races are of one sex and four of the other. We have now something new which has been obtained by hybridization, namely, a new albino race of the sex opposite to that of the one we started with. When there are four kinds of races it is possible to mate two albinos and find that all of their $f_1$ progeny are albinos, and so with the orange-colored races.

The mechanism by which the spores become so regularly distributed is very simple. The reduction division spindle and those of the second division are longitudinal, while those of the third division are transverse. When segregation for any pair of factors occurs in the second division the spores alternate two and two for these factors. If one pair of factors segregates in the first division and some other pair segregates in the second division, four kinds, and only four kinds, of spores can be found in one ascus. Lindegren was the first to suggest that second division segregation here is due to crossing-over. He has since proved, through the use of several linked genes, that second division segregation percentages are accurate measures of crossing-over percentages and he has constructed the first chromosome maps in the fungi on that basis. The eight spores from an ascus are comparable to the four eggs and four sperms in animals. Since, in *Neurospora,* gametes of both kinds are derived from a single mother cell the exact relationship of all eight is known. The closest possible inbreeding can be done without loss of three out of four gametes as is the case in animals and seed plants.

### MENDELISM IN YEAST FUNGI

Because of the great economic importance of breadmaking and the commercial value of alcoholic fermentation the yeasts have been the object of intensive research. Sexual reproduction with nuclear fusion at ascus formation has long been known for certain genera of yeasts. The common bakers' yeasts, wine yeasts and brewers' yeasts, however, were presumed to develop parthenogenetically, spores being formed without reduction of chromosome numbers. Hybridization of these most useful yeasts was deemed impossible on this account. Winge has shown how false this notion was, as he has made fourteen hybrids to date. He says that after spore germination a short period of budding occurs, then two of these small roundish buds fuse to form a larger ellipsoid cell which becomes diploid by nuclear fusion. This is a departure from what is known for other fungi where normally the vegetative phase is strictly haploid. Christiansen and Chilton have reported solo-pathogenic individual cases of corn smut where the mycelium is diploid, but at reduction normal haploid sporidia are formed, showing that this is merely a temporary aberration.

Winge and Laustsen have shown in a very simple way Mendelian segregation in the slime flux yeast *Saccharomycodes Ludwigii,* where the two spores at either end of the long ascus must be of opposite sex. Normally they germinate within the ascus and immediately fuse. Budding out of elongated diploid cells then occurs. By isolating the four spores from an ascus before they have germinated and fused in pairs, it is found that they will germinate in culture. One spore of each pair will give rise to a haploid yeast either with short buds or with long buds depending on its genotype. These haploid yeasts can be grown indefinitely in culture. The other two spores from the ascus, if they germinate, soon die.

It was assumed that two pairs of factors are operating to account for this behavior; $N/n$ control spore germination, and $L/l$ determine whether the growth shall be by long buds or short buds. Any spore containing the factor $n$ may germinate but it will always die. The authors are not clear as to the sex factors operating here. From their report one could assume that there is a very close linkage between the +/− sex factors, and the $L/l$, growth type factors. They later found that in one ascus, both spores of one pair germinated and produced haploid yeasts, one with short buds and the other with long buds. They allowed the other pair of spores to germinate in the ascus and they then proved by further analysis that the factor *n* had mutated to *N*. The diploid growth, when allowed to form new asci, showed that these asci were homozygous for the factor *N,* because all four of their spores germinated to produce haploid yeasts.

It looks as though *n* were a lethal factor that prevents germination and that it was originally itself a mutant which later *reverted* to the normal *N* or wild type. That is, in passing from *n* to *N* it represents a reversion to and not a mutation from the wild type.

Should we expect a wild yeast to be heterozygous for two such distinct specific types of growth? Mutations are apt to occur in fungi kept long in cultures. This point could be settled by analysis of other cultures of this species collected from the wild or from other sources. If, on the other hand, *S. Ludwigii* is heterozygous through previous hybridization, it could mean that fusions do occur between haploid cells outside of the ascus. Possibly the application of growth substances or sex hormones would bring on cell fusions and hybridization outside the ascus as in other yeasts where Winge has already obtained fourteen hybrids, as noted above.

As the result of a mutation or some other irregularity, a bisexual race of *Neurospora tetrasperma* appeared in culture in which the nuclei of one sex carried a lethal factor. This lethal operates to prevent an ascospore with a single nucleus from germinating to form a functional mycelium. If this lethal nucleus is carried in the same spore with a normal nucleus, that spore germinates normally to produce, under suitable cultural conditions, a functional mycelium which will mature ascocarps with asci. Then the situation is exactly comparable to that described by Winge.

### Sex-linked Characters

Haemophilia and color blindness are familiar examples of what are called sex-linked characters in humans, characters which are inherited by a man from his maternal grandmother. In genetic language this means that certain lethal factors are carried on the sex chromosome, *X*. In our heterothallic ascomycetes we have chromosomes which carry factors determining sex reactions. Any genes in these chromosomes would, in a sense, be sex-linked, although we do not have maleness and femaleness here as in animals.

*Saccharomycodes Ludwigii* is normally a diploid yeast, according to Winge, and always heterozygous for the sex factors which segregate at the formation of ascospores. If the growth-type factors, *L/l,* are so strongly linked with the sex factors that crossing-over is difficult or impossible, the yeast could very naturally exist in nature in a heterozygous condition for these factors and be a "balanced heterozygote." Here is a sex-linked differentiation which some will insist is a real sex difference. Of course, the larger and longer bud types are female, the smaller buds are male! That is, we have here male and female yeasts! Further work will no doubt disprove such a statement.

We have in *Neurospora tetrasperma* a similar example where certain factors are strongly linked with the sex factors. Races of one sex produce golden orange conidia; races of the other sex produce conidial masses more pinkish in color. We have never proved a cross-over. A culture of this species from Texas also showed a similar linkage. One can readily tell by their appearance which progeny races will mate and which will not. This situation is comparable to that found by Blakeslee and which led him to designate as "+," races that produced more sporangia than the others which he called "–." This is another good example of "sex-linkage" in fungi.

### "Hybrid" Mushrooms

The discovery of heterothallism and the secret of clamp formation in mushrooms by Bensaude and Kneip independently during the last World War, proved a great stimulus to genetic work in this type of fungi. Students have stated that they have obtained hybrids by uniting differently colored haploid races, say, pink and white of opposite sex, through anastomoses, to form a dicaryophytic growth of binucleate cells. Three questions arise here. (1) Are the cells of the dicaryophyte diploid? (2) Is the dicaryophyte heterozygous? (3) Is pink dominant over white? To all of these questions the answer is no. A diploid cell as defined by Strasburger is one in which its nucleus contains the double number of chromosomes. Such a diploid cell is to be clearly distinguished from a cell containing two haploid nuclei even though they are of opposite sex. Since only diploid nuclei can be heterozygous, pink could not be dominant over white. We can not think of a sperm as being heterozygous. The fertilized egg could be heterozygous. The basidia of the mushroom are diploid and normally they are the only cells in connection with which dominance could be expressed.

Dicaryophytes or mixochimeras are among the most interesting and important phenomena in the whole biology of the fungi. They occur in several groups of fungi. They are more interesting for what they *are* than for what they *are not*. If the two nuclei fused as they came into a cell to give us a true hybrid mycelium so that a true hybrid mushroom would result in the end, that would cease to be interesting because that is exactly what ought to happen, judging from the way embryos are developed in animals and seed plants. It is easy to understand what is meant by a diploid phase, but we have not yet opened our eyes to the beauty and significance of these dicaryophytic haploid partnerships. Dicaryophytes in general constitute one of the most important problems in the genetics of fungi.

It is difficult to see how one could obtain a true hybrid mycelium under normal conditions. The larger part of fruit bodies of mushrooms and ascomycetes are haploid; therefore we should not use the term hybrid to describe a mere intermingling of hyphae or nuclei of two different races to form the framework of such structures. If commercially valuable as mushrooms they could be propagated as spawn and given a trade name. They are a sort of chimera or graft hybrid, and any apparent dominance is a false one. After the fusion of two nuclei to form a hybrid basidium or an ascus, the spores that are produced after reduction may give rise to various sorts of mycelia because of new combinations of factors; but, as these new $f_1$ mycelia are haploid, they are not heterozygous and not hybrids.

### Dominance in Fungi

Real dominance in fungi is well demonstrated when one crosses an 8-spored species of *Neurospora* with a 4-spored species. All $F_1$ asci are 8-spored, although there is much spore abortion in these interspecific hybrid asci. Eight-sporedness is dominant over 4-sporedness. Real dominance is also shown when a race of smut with smooth spores is crossed with a race having rough spores and the $F_1$ spores are rough.

In *N. tetrasperma,* when both parents in a mating carry a certain recessive factor for ascus abortion, all of the $F_1$ asci from a mating, being homozygous, abort without spore formation. However, if one parent is normal and the other carries the lethal, all the $F_1$ asci are heterozygous and form spores normally. The wild type factor is dominant over the recessive lethal. In another race of this same species, asci that are heterozygous for a certain other lethal usually abort and become indurated. Here the lethal is dominant over the corresponding factor carried by the normal wild type race.

### Hybrid Vigor

Hugh Dixon, working with *Neurospora crassa,* has recently reported a race which he says shows hybrid vigor because the mycelium grows so much faster than does that of either parent. Since the mycelium must be haploid it could not show hybrid vigor. It is a new race which happens to have a different combination of factors that affect growth. These were contributed to it at the development of the spores in the $F_1$ ascus which was a real hybrid.

Winge and his associates have reported, as noted previously, that a number of our common yeasts of the industries are actually diploid. They point out, further, that some of their new races show a certain amount of hybrid vigor, or the effects of heterosis. This is clearly possible and no doubt true if their yeasts are actually diploid. This is the first time that an improvement of yeast strains has been undertaken by geneticists.

### Protoplasmic Streaming

Protoplasmic streaming in coenocytic fungi as well as in fungi with septate mycelia is often so vigorous in young growth as to carry vacuoles and other inclusions rapidly in the stream. The question arises: are the nuclei ever carried in the stream like other inclusions, or are the nuclear migrations in *Neurospora* and *Gelasinospora* due to sex attractions? Two races of opposite sex grown together in culture become heterocaryotic; but would intermingling of genetically different races of the same sex also give rise to a heterocaryotic mycelium because of nuclear migrations due to streaming?

### Phenotypic and Genotypic Sex Differences

No antheridia or archegonia are produced in one-spore cultures of *Ascobolus magnificus,* which is strictly heterothallic. When + and – races are grown opposite each other, antheridia and archegonia are produced in the zone where hyphae of both races intermingle. These organs always arise from different branches. Due to the maze of branching and anastomosing, it is impossible to trace their origin back very far one way or the other. This species ought to respond to the application of sex hormones to determine whether only antheridia are produced by one race and archegonia by the race of opposite sex reaction, proving that +/– relations are strongly linked with factors representing morphologically differentiated organs.

Blakeslee long ago made tests of +/– races of *Phycomyces* against hermaphroditic species of *Zygorhynchus* and *Absidia.* His results would indicate that mere size differentiations are not a reliable test for sexuality. If sex-linked genes are concerned, we must expect crossing-over, provided cell size factors and sex reaction factors are neither identical nor alleles.

Raper has added support for the theory that sex stuffs or sex hormones play an important part in sexual differentiations and sex reactions. This is not saying that I accept the statements by Moreau and his associates to the effect that a unisexual race of *Neurospora* derived from a single spore from an 8-spored ascus can be induced to mature ascocarps with asci and spores simply by the stimulus furnished by hormones produced by a mycelium of the opposite sex reaction. I have repeated their experiments many times without finding any evidence in support of their claims. I have faith, however, that growth substances and hormones will prove very useful in inducing a fungus race to develop to the full extent of its potentialities as represented by its factors of inheritance.

The theory of relative sexuality is being lifted above the realm of mysticism by Moewus and his associates and presented in a form that can be more generally accepted. They are studying the simple one-celled algae genetically. *Chlamydomonas Braunii* is a species having gametes of two different sizes, male and female, as they are called. It is strictly heterothallic genetically. Evidently the factors for heterothallism or +/− sex reaction characters, are very closely linked with the factors that determine cell size. *C. eugametos* occurs in several forms, one is isogametic and heterothallic. These sex factors segregate according to the Mendelian ration 50 : 50. By mating races of this species against ♀ and ♂ races of *C. Braunii,* Moewus proves that the "+" race of *C. eugametos* is female and the "−" race is male, and from this point on he discards the +/− symbols. This is interesting, coming from one of the foremost exponents of the theory of relative sexuality. He says in effect that two gametes morphologically exactly alike can be genotypically *male* and *female* because of the way they *function.* Other varieties of this species are hermaphroditic in the sense that sex differentiation is phenotypic so that each cell of the sporeling develops gametes, the progeny of which may fuse. Moewus explains this apparent anomaly by assuming that the realizators F and M are located on homologous chromosomes, but they are not alleles. Time does not permit further analysis of this work, but it should certainly prove illuminating and helpful to those who are working with similar problems in the fungi, such as species of *Glomerella* and other homothallic fungi.

Every mycelium of *Neurospora sitophila* develops: (1) incipient ascocarps with receptive organs; (2) small microconidia or spermatia and (3) large monilioid conidia. In earlier days I would have insisted that the receptive structures are female, the microconidia are male, and the monilioid conidia are asexual spores. To-day I am not so sure. If the spermatia are male because they can function in fertilization, then the monilioid conidia are super-males because they can do everything the spermatia can do and do it better. Suppose you take a little brush and wipe up some of the orange-colored powder from an infected loaf of bread, and then paint this on a culture of a mycelium of the opposite sex. Observe what follows after 24 hours and then sit down and write me definitions of sex, male and female, that will apply equally well to animals, higher plants and the fungi.

### Double Fertilization in Ascomycetes

The older mycologists assumed a nuclear fusion in the primordia of ascocarps to be the essential stimulus for further development. Such an assumption would seem logical if we again consider embryo and seed formation in animals and plants. The discovery, half a century ago, that two nuclei fuse at the origin of the ascus and the basidium, stimulated cytological research to find nuclear fusions in the ascocarp primordia. As a result of these studies double fertilization or two sets of nuclear fusions in the life cycle of a number of species of ascomycetes have been reported, the fusion in the primordia being the true fecundation, that in the ascus merely a compensating fusion. This has been supported by cytological evidence that a double reduction of the number of chromosomes occurs in the nuclear divisions in the ascus. Gwynne-Vaughan and her associates have reported double fertilization and double reduction in *Ascobolus magnificus* and *A. stercorarius.* From what we now know of the genetics of *Neurospora* and the phenomenon of crossing-over it would not be difficult to settle this old controversy once and for all by a genetic study of the two species of *Ascobolus* just mentioned. In crosses involving three pairs of genetic factors such as factors for sex, for spore color and for type of mycelial growth, we should find that the spores would alternate either *four* and *four* or *two* and *two* for any pair of factors, if there has been only one nuclear fusion. Regardless of how many pairs of factors should be represented in the mating no ascus should ever show over four kinds of spores.

Those who uphold the theory of a double fertilization and double reduction could prove their point absolutely by finding either that the eight spores alternate *one* and *one* for a certain pair of factors, or that sometimes eight genotypically different kinds of spores occur in an ascus. *Ascobolus carbonarius, A. geophilus* and *A. immersus* are also heterothallic. Analysis of spores from individual asci have been made by Betts for the first two species and by Rizet for the last one. They found no *"one and one"* alternation. Until this is done we must assume that in all ascomycetes, as in all other plants and animals, only one nuclear fusion occurs in a life cycle.

No genetic evidence has been obtained in *Neurospora* for such a double fertilization. All are agreed that no nuclear fusion occurs in *Neurospora* at the origin of the ascocarp.

### Conclusion

In closing I may point out that we should discuss topics arising in genetic studies of the fungi with the view to aid rather than to interfere with progress. Clearness of understanding of what one aims to accomplish in the end is certainly desirable and helpful.

Knowledge of the principles of inheritance in the fungi accumulated to date, should serve to warn those charged with breeding economic plants for resistance that they must first be informed regarding the stability or limits of variability of the parasites they seek to circumvent. We know now that new races of fungi are arising through natural hybridization. Hybrid structures have been obtained showing dominance and Mendelian segregations with crossing-over at reduction which is such an important feature in furthering evolution. We also find in the fungi: mutants, lethal factors, deficient chromosomes, sex-chromosomes, sex-linked characters and other genetic features. To repeat what I have said elsewhere: "The fungi in their reproduction and inheritance follow exactly the same laws that govern these activities in higher plants and animals."

I have tried to show that the fungi are not degenerate organisms which are on their way out in a scheme of evolution and so of little economic importance and scientific interest. The fungi, on the contrary, are progressive, ever changing and evolving rapidly in their own way, so that they are capable of becoming readily adapted to every condition of life. We may rest assured that as green plants and animals disappear one by one from the face of the globe, some of the fungi will always be present to dispose of the last remains.

# CHEWING AS A TECHNIQUE OF RELAXATION

By Professor H. L. HOLLINGWORTH

BARNARD COLLEGE, COLUMBIA UNIVERSITY

MOTOR automatisms in great variety have often been explained as "tension outlets." Tics and other accessory movements have been said to be the expression of "inner tensions" or perhaps to be the "symbolic release" of such tensions. Fidgeting, wriggling, pipe smoking, gum chewing, automobiling and various active sports have received a like extenuation. There has been, however, little precise definition of the character of these alleged "tensions," and experimental evidence of their relief by the collateral activities cited is not abundant. We present here a brief summary of a protracted series of experiments on this topic, conducted during the period of a year and involving the measurement of a considerable number of processes in 20 subjects during 20 experimental days.[1]

The experimental approach requires first of all specific measures of various forms of "tension," since this word has many meanings. It requires also a technique of producing collateral motor automatisms and maintaining them, under controlled conditions. Perhaps the most popular of the automatisms referred to is chewing. Our subjects have been studied under three conditions: (*a*) Normal—not chewing and having nothing in the mouth; (*b*) Chewing—the masticatory being ordinary confectioned chicle, sweetened and flavored; (*c*) Control—allowing a flavored candy wafer to melt in the mouth, as a control over such things as suggestion, sensory stimulation and like influences. The studies of the Carnegie Nutrition Laboratory have shown that the metabolism costs of chewing are the same, whether a gum or a rubber stopper be used.

The experimental schedules were so arranged as to equalize such factors as practise, fatigue and individual differences. In all cases a preliminary base was secured, and the experimental variations gave measures which could always be expressed in terms of the base for the particular working period. The subjects were throughout engaged in various types of standardized work, proficiency in which was always measured. Concurrently the various measures of tension were secured.

*Tension as Nervous Restlessness.* Without the knowledge of the subjects, special observers watched them throughout the working day and periodically rated each on a scale of motor restlessness. A restless movement was described as any motor activity irrelevant to the work being done at the moment. The units of comparison are steps on the rating scale, and since these may not be quantitatively equal the measures are relative only; but their direction is clear and consistent.

In one experiment (6 subjects, 6 full days of work and observation) a decrease of 9 per cent. in restless movement was found in the chewing periods. In another experiment (4 subjects, 4 days) a decrease of 10 per cent. was found. On the whole, therefore, there is a decrease of some 10 per cent. in restlessness while the masticatory is in use.

*Tension as Feeling of Strain.* After each round of work (about 45 minutes) the subjects rated on a linear rating scale their subjective feelings during the period. The linear scale was marked off into 20 equal steps, ranging from extreme strain at one end to extreme relaxation at the other. The rating was made by crossing this line with a pencil at some point between these two extremes. The units of comparison are again steps on the rating scale.

The workers unanimously report themselves as feeling more relaxed while chewing than during either of the other two conditions (normal and control). In

[1] The data are reported in full in the writer's recent monograph, "Psycho-Dynamics of Chewing," *Archives of Psychology*, No. 239, July, 1939, pp. 90.

one experiment (8 subjects, 6 days) subjectively felt relaxation increased 14 per cent. over control and 19 per cent. over normal, while chewing. In another experiment (4 subjects, 2 days) the decrease in felt strain amounted to 10 per cent.; in a third experiment (4 subjects, 4 days) the 10 per cent. strain reduction was again the average.

On the whole, then, tension in the sense of the subjective feeling of strain is reduced from 10 per cent. to 15 per cent., while the worker indulges in the collateral chewing movements.

*Tension as Fatigue.* If these two are not identical they are at least often closely related, the strain of fatigue being contrasted with the freshness of earlier hours of work. The problems involved in the measurement of fatigue are notorious. We have used an indicator which has been reported to have some general value—the rate of change of designs seen in equivocal perspective.

McDougall reports that fatigue decreases the rate of fluctuation of reversible figures (staircase, blocks, windmill) and that refreshing substances such as tea and coffee increase it. In one experiment (6 subjects, 6 days) we found no change in the rate of fluctuation (Scripture's blocks) when chewing or when using the control wafer. In a second experiment (4 subjects, 4 days, staircase figure) there was a definite increase of 11 per cent. in one-minute periods. In a third experiment (6 subjects, 6 days, staircase) the increase was over 7 per cent.; a fourth experiment with 2 observers also showed definite increase—the increased rate of fluctuation in all these cases being in the chewing periods.

The net evidence from these four experiments is that if there is any change in the rate of fluctuation of reversible figures while chewing it is by way of increase, this being the opposite of the effect said to be produced by fatigue. In so far then as fatigue means tension the indication is reduced tension when the masticatory is in use.

*Tension as Effort.* Tension as effort might be expected to show itself in the consumption of more energy and to be reflected in measures of metabolism and of pulse rate. We have carried through for one week metabolism measures on two workers, but the data are too complicated to summarize in this short review. They show, however, that such collateral activity as chewing may be carried with no actual cost to the organism, apparently because of the surplus due to reduced motor restlessness.

In the case of 4 subjects (2-day experiment) at sedentary work, pulse rate was found to increase 5 per cent. while chewing, this being only half that reported when a resting state is taken as the base. In another experiment (4 subjects, 4 days) when the main occupation was moderately active but far from strenuous, no change in pulse rate was found. It is clear that determination of energy costs of chewing, with a resting state as a base, can by no means be generalized to cover the situation when this motor automatism is added to a livelier initial activity level.

*Direct Muscular Tension.* Perhaps the best meaning of *tension* is the direct muscular strain existing in parts of the body not immediately occupied with the main occupation. Using a specially devised work chair we measured tension at the left elbow joint in the case of two subjects meanwhile occupied with the use of the right arm. Measures were taken 33 times during each hour of two working days, the subjects being occupied with such tasks as cancellation, addition and recording the changes in figures seen in equivocal perspective.

The apparatus releases, at the experimenter's wish, a weight which pulls against the unoccupied arm which lies on a hinged arm-rest. The rate at which the arm moves when the weight is thus applied is measured (in sixtieths of a second) by means of a kymograph and time line. The greater the tension existing in the arm at the moment, the slower is the movement produced in it by the fixed weight.

In this experiment conditions were varied each hour (chewing, not chewing, control wafer). Without exception, with both workers and during all three kinds of work, muscular tension is decreased during the chewing periods, the decrease amounting to an average of 5 per cent. in time units. While chewing, parts of the organism not occupied with the main task are appreciably relaxed. The relaxation thus found was greater in the case of the more "tense" of the two workers.

*Tension as Interference.* Any agent interfering with the proficient course of work might be said to result in strain or tension. In nine different varieties of work we have measured the output, for quantity and quality, during the three main experimental conditions. With the possible exception of work in which a wholly new performance is being learned chewing while working does not interfere with output. In some kinds of work, especially number checking and typing, the work is positively facilitated.

The suggested effect on new learning (not yet adequately demonstrated) is especially interesting. Some investigators have found that muscular contraction (tension) is an aid in learning tasks. But all our results show that sustained chewing results in a *lowering* of tension, however measured. We might therefore expect to find an indication of interference with new learning and such results would be an obverse confirmation of those showing more effective learning under conditions of greater tension.

*The Energy of Work.* In two ways we have measured the energy of the movements made in prescribed activities, while the workers were intent only on the accuracy and tempo of their work. In a variety of tasks the point pressure of writing was measured. In a specially devised set-up measure was secured of the energy of thrust in a "pin target" activity.

In all these cases more energy was put into the activities of the main occupation while chewing. The motor automatism not only reduces restlessness (nervousness), but some at least of the surplus energy thus resulting goes unwittingly into the main work. Whether or not this results in increased output obviously depends on the nature of the work.

*Conclusions.* All these results tell a consistent story. The collateral motor automatism involved in the sustained use of the conventional masticatory does result in a lowering of tension, and the tension thus reduced is muscular. In a sense this is only a confirmation of the testimony of the chronic pipe smoker, whistler, gum chewer and watch chain twiddler. His statement is likely to be that he does these things when he is "under strain" and that he gets from these collateral activities a "relief from tension." The results also give some support to the clinical inference that the motor automatism grows directly out of some tension, for which it serves as an outlet.

Perhaps these results also throw some light on the striking fact that during the past ten or more "tense" years the chicle processors have enjoyed their greatest prosperity. The results also suggest techniques which might be put to good use in "relaxation therapy."

These results can be fitted readily enough into almost any conception or explanatory scheme of neuro-muscular dynamics. Advocates of a "drainage" hypothesis could show how a collateral automatic activity such as chewing serves as an outlet for discharges that would otherwise take more devious, uncoordinated, and perhaps obstructive or interfering channels. At any rate it is apparent that such an activity may serve a neat regulative purpose and organize available energy more effectively. The subjectively felt gain in relaxation may be an introspective indicator of this organization. Effectual gains in some kinds of work output may be an objective sign of it as may also the increase in the energy of the working movements. Reduction of random restlessness may be the machinery through which it operates.

In the case of chewing particularly certain other considerations of a somewhat more subtle psychological type may be relevant. These are quite in line with certain systematic principles that have usefully guided our experimental program during the past dozen years. The primary function of chewing is of course the mastication of food. Eating is ordinarily a more or less "quiet" occupation. When we eat we sit; random restlessness is at a low point; we rest; we relax; and the general feeling tone is likely to be one of agreeableness and satisfaction.

An important item of the eating situation is chewing. It may well enough be that chewing, as a "conditioned stimulus," brings with it, whenever it is sustained, a posture of relaxation. Chewing, in other words, may serve as a reduced cue and some degree redintegrate the relaxation of meal-time.

# SCIENTIFIC EVENTS

## THE BRITISH ASSOCIATION IN WAR TIME[1]

SINCE the Dundee meeting of the British Association was brought to an untimely end, the office at Burlington House, London, has been reopened for the routine work which always follows upon the annual meeting, and a certain amount of official business is also being carried on at Down House, where the rooms normally open to the public are closed and dismantled, and Charles Darwin's former dining-room serves the valuable if regrettable purpose of an office-refuge. The first number of the new quarterly report, *The Advancement of Science,* will be produced, all being well, probably rather later than the announced date at the end of October, and in smaller bulk than was contemplated. As to its future, and, for that matter, the future of the association's work generally, obviously nothing definite can be stated. Preparations for the intended meeting next year in Newcastle-upon-Tyne have been suspended, by agreement with the authorities there. It is an unhappy coincidence that the last meeting in that city was the last to be held during the last war, in 1916. Conditions are so far different now that it is impossible to estimate whether any sort of meeting could or should be held next year, whether in Newcastle or anywhere else. Yet it is permissible to dream of the possibility of adapting the association's very flexible constitution to a meeting of four days or so, with science in war time as the leading theme, with sessions in three or four telescoped sections—physical, biological, anthropological and economic, for example—and of course the Division for the Social and Economic Relations of Science. No doubt before anything of this sort could be undertaken there would be need of careful and wide inquiry as to the amount of support which might be forthcoming for such an effort. But if this were favorable, such a meeting could be arranged at relatively short notice. "The minor humors of war" may be offered in advance as one subject on the anthropological side.

[1] From *Nature.*

## THE AUSTRALIAN NATIONAL RESEARCH COUNCIL

THE reorganization of the Australian National Research Council is announced in the *Australian Journal of Science.* The officers elected are: *Chairman,* Sir David Rivett; *Honorary Treasurer,* Professor O. U. Vonwiller; *Honorary Secretary,* Dr. A. B. Walkom.

The Executive Committee of the reorganized council consists of these three officers elected by the full council and two members from each state and from the Australian Capital Territory elected by the members of the council in that state or territory. The president, the honorary general treasurer and the honorary general secretary of the Australian and New Zealand Association for the Advancement of Science, if resident in Australia, are also *ex-officio* members of the executive committee. Any member of the executive committee not resident at the headquarters of the association has the right to appoint a proxy from among the members of the Australian National Research Council resident there.

The representatives of the Australian Capital Territory and of all states, with the exception of Tasmania, have now been elected, and the list is as follows, including proxies where such have been chosen:

*New South Wales:* Professor W. J. Dakin, Professor R. D. Watt.

*Victoria:* Professor E. W. Skeats (proxy, Mr. C. A. Sussmilch), Mr. W. E. Wainwright (proxy, Mr. A. J. Gibson).

*South Australia:* Sir William Mitchell (proxy, Professor J. P. Madsen), Sir Douglas Mawson (proxy, Dr. C. Anderson).

*Western Australia:* Professor E. de C. Clarke (proxy, Professor L. A. Cotton), Dr. G. L. Sutton (proxy, Dr. W. L. Waterhouse).

*Queensland:* Dr. D. A. Herbert (proxy, Mr. E. Cheel), Professor H. C. Richards (proxy, Mr. E. C. Andrews).

*Australian Capital Territory:* Dr. B. T. Dickson (proxy, not yet appointed), Dr. W. G. Woolnough (proxy not yet appointed).

Provision has also been made for the appointment of a deputy chairman when the chairman does not happen to reside in the state where the executive meets, and Professor R. D. Watt has been elected to that office.

The objects of the new Australian National Research Council are stated as follows:

1. In general to promote and assist the advancement of research in Australia, and in particular to obtain financial support for research work of a national character.

2. To act as a body which can advise the Commonwealth and State Governments as to the direction in which research is necessary and financial assistance advisable.

3. To advise the Commonwealth and State Governments as to suitable persons to undertake inquiry, investigation or research in certain national problems.

4. To act as the collective voice of scientific thought in Australia when it is considered necessary and advisable to bring under the notice of Governments, public bodies and organizations, matters in which scientific direction can affect the well-being and culture of the community.

5. To organize scientific bodies and workers into an effective unit for use in national emergencies.

6. To safeguard the interests and status of scientific workers throughout Australia.

## RETIREMENT FUND OF THE FIELD MUSEUM OF NATURAL HISTORY

DETAILS of a plan whereby retirement incomes will be provided for employees of Field Museum of Natural History have been made public. Because of the museum's status as an educational institution, its employees do not come under the provisions of social security legislation. The plan inaugurated independently by the museum management offers the employees benefits many times more generous than those provided under such laws.

Under the plan, which operates through a contract with the Metropolitan Life Insurance Company, and is now in effect, men employees will retire at age sixty-five years, and women employees at age sixty. All employees under those ages at the time the plan was instituted are eligible, and since the plan was announced a few weeks ago, and participation invited on a purely voluntary basis, it has been unanimously accepted by all those eligible.

The plan is outlined by Dr. Clifford C. Gregg, director of the museum, in the October issue of *Field Museum News,* as follows:

For many years it has been the desire of the management of Field Museum to establish a pension plan which might insure a regular retirement income for faithful employees after their period of active service had been completed. As early as 1916, Mr. Stanley Field, president of the museum, established a Museum Employees' Pension Fund, the proceeds of which gave to the employees the benefit of insurance protection for their dependents. While this benefit was greatly prized at the museum, it was still felt by those responsible for the operation of the institution that the employee himself was entitled to protection and leisure in his declining years, as well as some security for his dependents.

Recently Mr. Marshall Field, a trustee of the museum who always has been deeply interested in the welfare of the employees, provided the means by which such a pension plan might be established. Under the plan each employee pays approximately 4 per cent. of his salary to the pension fund. The museum contributes a much larger sum, and with the combined contributions purchases annuities amounting to 1½ per cent. of the employee's salary for each year of his membership in the plan. Annuities for past service, amounting to 1 per cent. of the current salary for each year of service prior to the beginning of the plan, will be purchased by the museum without employee contribution. Normal retirement ages have been set at 65 years for men and 60 years for women. Retirement will automatically occur at those ages unless the Board of Trustees requests that the employee continue longer in service, which invitation he may accept or decline.

It is impossible under any circumstances for an employee or his estate to receive from the plan less than he has put into it. Upon leaving the museum prior to retirement, the employee is entitled to the return of his money with interest compounded annually at the rate of $2\frac{1}{2}$ per cent. In the event of the death of an employee either prior to or subsequent to retirement, his estate is entitled to his entire contribution with interest compounded annually.

Another provision protecting the interest of the employee who leaves the institution after more than ten years of membership in the Pension Plan is the so-called ''vested interest'' provision. This provides that an employee after ten years of membership is entitled to receive at retirement age the full benefits of the pension thus far purchased for him by both his own and the museum's contributions.

The wide-spread approval of the employees is indicated by unanimous acceptance on the part of those eligible. Both the management and the employees rejoice in the assurance that a lifetime of faithful service at the museum may be followed by leisure and freedom from financial worries in the later years of life.

## A BIOLOGICAL SURVEY OF THE STATE OF NEW HAMPSHIRE

A BIOLOGICAL survey of the State of New Hampshire will be undertaken by the newly established Biological Institute of the University of New Hampshire, of which Dr. C. Floyd Jackson, professor of zoology and entomology and dean of the College of Liberal Arts, is director.

The survey, which is described by Professor Jackson as something which has long been needed, will be carried on by the staff members of the institute working in their respective fields. Mammals, birds, amphibians and reptiles, fish, insects, ornamental plants and shrubs, fungi and algae, trees and woods and rocks and minerals all will be included in the survey.

In connection with the work, a committee on taxonomy has been set up to assist teachers, nature study counselors and others interested in the biological sciences, in the identification of plant and animal specimens. Dr. Jackson states that the committee will receive any specimens sent in and will identify them. The plan works reciprocally, teachers and nature students will have identified for them plants and animals with which they are not familiar, and at the same time information will be obtained which can be used in the state survey.

A survey of the salt water regions of the state will be undertaken in the near future. Designed as a supplement to the water shed survey made some time ago by the state, the work will be conducted with the co-operation of the Fish and Game Commission. The Great Bay region and the coast from Portsmouth to Seabrook will be included in a compilation of biological specimens, their habits and their effects on the waters.

## LIBRARY FOR THE HISTORY OF MEDICINE AT YALE UNIVERSITY

THERE has been established in the Yale University School of Medicine a library devoted to the history of medicine. In making the announcement Dr. Charles Seymour, president of the university, said that it would constitute

a treasure house of the utmost importance to the medical profession and to scholars in the whole field of the history of science.

Well-known collections which will be brought together as the basis of this library are notably those formed by Dr. Harvey Cushing and Dr. John F. Fulton, of the Yale faculty. And word has been received from Dr. Arnold C. Klebs, of Les Terrasses, Nyon, Switzerland, that he is devising to Yale his magnificent library on the history of science and of medicine, including his unique apparatus for the study of early texts. The combined collections of these friends and collaborators happily supplement one another and by this assembly of materials a library of great strength has come into being.

These gifts to Yale are announced for the first time and there is promise that they will be joined by others when the library wing of the Medical School is extended to house them, for Dr. Cushing's decision to give his magnificent library to Yale has been the incentive for others to make similar gifts. Medicine may be regarded as the mother of the sciences and collections such as these will arouse the interest of the student in the scholarly aspects of his scientific profession, medical or otherwise.

To house the collections the library wing of the Sterling Hall of Medicine will be extended by funds set aside by the Yale Corporation from the estate of John W. Sterling. The extension, with room for 400,000 volumes, will take the form of a "Y" shaped building. In one prong of the "Y" will be the historical collections, in the other a working library for the school. Grosvenor Atterbury, of New York, is the architect; the Dwight Building Company of New Haven is the general contractor. Construction is expected to begin in the near future.

## THE RESEARCH COUNCIL ON PROBLEMS OF ALCOHOL

A PROGRAM for attacking the disease of alcoholism and the alcoholic psychoses based on research, approved by the newly elected executive committee of the Research Council on Problems of Alcohol, an associated society of the American Association for the Advancement of Science, has been announced by the chairman of the committee, Dr. Karl M. Bowman, director of psychiatry at Bellevue Hospital, New York City.

Three grants of financial aid to the council have been made. The Carnegie Corporation has appropriated $25,000 for a critical survey of all work done to date on the effects of alcohol upon the individual, a project sponsored by the Department of Psychiatry of the College of Medicine, New York University. It is under the supervision of Dr. Norman Jolliffee, associate professor of medicine, who recently directed a survey of alcoholic psychoses in Europe. The American Philosophical Society is financing a study of the toxic factors in alcoholism, conducted at the New York Psychiatric Institute under the direction of Dr. George A. Jervis, and the Dazian Foundation for Medical Research has granted funds for research on the role of alcohol in liver cirrhosis, a project being initiated by the College of Medicine at New York University. Some 200 patients with liver cirrhosis will be subjected to clinical, chemical and pathological study in an effort to reach a clearer understanding of the relation of alcohol to this disease.

The council proposes to concentrate upon alcoholism until the end of 1941. Three major measures will be employed: the evaluation and coordination of existing research; the development of a research program along lines inadequately investigated or not yet explored and the dissemination of the results of such research.

A statement issued by Dr. Bowman points out that the objective of the council is to discover the causes of alcoholism and better methods for its prevention and treatment. Prejudice, fear, secrecy and ignorance are among the obstacles to its control. The majority are disposed to think of alcoholism as a criminal or moral offense, instead of as a disease for which the patient is often not responsible. Alcoholism and the alcoholic psychoses constitute one of the great public health problems of modern times, perhaps the greatest not being systematically attacked. The council plans to deal with alcoholism in the same general fashion as other public health agencies combat tuberculosis, cancer, syphilis, heart disease and other major threats to human health.

The members of the executive committee are: Dr. Forest R. Moulton, permanent secretary of the American Association for the Advancement of Science; Dr. Winfred Overholser, superintendent of St. Elizabeths Hospital, Washington; Dr. Lawrence Kolb, chief of the Division of Mental Hygiene, U. S. Public Health Service; Dr. Hans T. Clarke, professor of biochemistry, Columbia University; Dr. Luther Gulick, director of the Institute of Public Administration; Leonard Harrison, director of the Committee on Youth and Justice; Dr. Nolan D. C. Lewis, professor of psychiatry, Columbia University; Austin H. MacCormick, commissioner of correction, New York City; Dr. A. T. Poffenberger, professor of psychology, Columbia University; Dr. Robert W. Searle, general secretary of the Greater New York Federation of Churches, and Albert W. Whitney, consulting director of the National Conservation Bureau. Dr. Bowman is chairman.

# SCIENTIFIC NOTES AND NEWS

DR. THEOPHILUS S. PAINTER, research professor of zoology at the University of Texas, has been appointed one of the four distinguished professors of the university. According to the official announcement, the title aims "to give nationally recognized professors an honor and an increase of $1,000 in yearly salary." Those in the sciences who hold the title are Dr. R. L. Moore, professor of mathematics, and Dr. J. T. Patterson, professor of zoology.

AT the Philadelphia meeting of the American College of Surgeons the Medical Records Prize was awarded to Dr. Don Wilbur McLean, of Detroit, Mich. Honorary fellowships were conferred on Dr. James Carre Magee, Surgeon-General of the United States Army; Dr. Ross T. McIntire, Surgeon-General of the United States Navy and physician to the White House; Dr. Thomas Parran, Jr., Surgeon-General of the U. S. Public Health Service, and Dr. Eugene P. Olya, of Budapest, Hungary.

ALEXANDER G. CHRISTIE, professor of mechanical engineering at the Johns Hopkins University and president of the American Society of Mechanical Engineers, and Henry Ford have been elected to honorary life membership in the British Institution of Mechanical Engineers. The certificates were to have been presented, together with the James Watt International Medal to Henry Ford, in New York on September 8, during the British American Engineering Congress, which was canceled a week before its opening because of the inability of the British engineers to come to the United States. The American Society of Mechanical Engineers expects to award the certificate and gold medal to Mr. Ford at its sixtieth annual meeting, to be held in Philadelphia from December 4 to 8.

THE presentation of the George Robert White Medal of Honor of the Massachusetts Horticultural Society has been made to Dr. George T. Moore, since 1912 director of the Missouri Botanical Garden, St. Louis, in recognition of "his work in developing the garden into one of the outstanding botanical centers in the world and for his success in the breeding of orchids."

THE Leslie Dana Medal for achievement in the prevention of blindness was presented on October 14 to Dr. Edward Coleman Ellett, of Memphis, Tenn., at a dinner given by the St. Louis Society for the Blind, in cooperation with the National Society for Prevention of Blindness. The presentation was made by Dr. Edward Jackson, of Denver, who in 1925 was the first recipient of the medal.

ON the occasion of the fiftieth anniversary of the founding of the University of Sofia, Bulgaria, Dr. Max Thorek, attending surgeon of Cook County Hospital and surgeon-in-chief of the American Hospital of Chicago, was made a commander of the Order of St. Alexander of Sofia for his contributions to surgical science. He had been decorated previously by the Italian and French Governments.

THE following officers were elected at the October meeting of the Indiana Chapter of the Society of Sigma Xi: *President,* R. J. Hartman, chemistry; *Vice-president,* R. E. Esarey, geology; *Secretary,* M. L. Lohman, botany; *Treasurer,* R. L. Kroc, zoology. The retiring president is Professor G. S. Snoddy, of the department of psychology.

DR. PERRY A. FOOTE, professor of pharmacy at the University of Florida, has been appointed acting director of the School of Pharmacy.

DR. CLAY B. FREUDENBERGER, professor of anatomy at the School of Medicine of the University of Utah, Salt Lake City, has been appointed acting dean during the absence, on account of illness, of Dr. Lyman L. Daines. Dr. Edward I. Hashimoto has been appointed to an assistant professorship of anatomy.

CHESTER RUSSELL, JR., professor of engineering at the University of New Mexico, has been appointed associate professor of electrical engineering at the University of Denver.

DR. LLOYD G. HUMPHREYS and Dr. Claude E. Buxton have been appointed to instructorships in psychology at Northwestern University. Dr. Humphreys was a national research fellow at Yale University last year, and Dr. Buxton was research associate at Swarthmore College.

DAVID J. MACK, of Purdue University, has been appointed assistant professor of chemical engineering at the University of Tennessee. He will be in charge of the metallurgical work of the department.

DR. ROBERT T. JACKSON, formerly assistant professor of paleontology at Harvard University, since 1928 curator of fossil echinoderms at the Museum of Comparative Zoology, has retired.

DR. WILLIAM COMBE WILSON has been appointed to the regius chair of surgery in the University of Aberdeen made vacant by the appointment of Professor James R. Learmonth to the chair of surgery in the University of Edinburgh.

DR. ROLAND K. MEYER, of the department of zoology at the University of Wisconsin, will conduct an investigation of the physiology of reproduction for which a grant has been made by the Lakeside Laboratories, Milwaukee. A similar grant from the same manufacturer has been made for an investigation of the physiology of sympathomimetic compounds to be carried out by Dr. Walter J. Meek, of the department of physiology. Dr. R. R. Greene, of Northwestern University, has received a grant for an investigation of the clinical use of estrogenic substances.

DR. PAUL W. WARD has been appointed associate secretary of the American Association of University Professors. He is on leave of absence as professor and chairman of the department of philosophy of Syracuse University, where he has taught since 1922. He is known to many members of the association as chairman of Committee T on the Place and Function of Faculties in College and University Government.

DR. MORRIS J. BLISH, head of the department of agricultural chemistry of the University of Nebraska and professor and chairman of the department of chemistry of the Nebraska Agricultural Experiment Station, has taken up his work as chief of the Protein Division of the Western Regional Research Laboratory of the Bureau of Agricultural Chemistry and Engineering at Albany, Calif. He will be engaged in the development of new industrial uses for the proteins of wheat, alfalfa, seeds and kernels.

DR. LUDWIG TELEKY, formerly of Düsseldorf, has been appointed technical adviser to the division of occupational hygiene of the Illinois State Department of Public Welfare, Chicago, where he will be associated with Dr. Milton H. Kronenberg, chief of the division.

PROFESSOR JOSHUA HAROLD BURN, professor of pharmacology at the University of Oxford, has been nominated to be for five years a member of the General Council of Medical Education and Registration in the United Kingdom in succession to Sir George Newman.

DR. WILLIAM BEEBE will spend the month of November on a lecture tour extending from Georgia and Texas to Idaho and Washington. His subject will be the life of the deep sea as studied by him on the Oceanographic Expeditions of the New York Zoological Society.

IN celebration of the hundredth anniversary of the founding of the American Statistical Association a special program is being arranged in connection with the annual meeting on the afternoon of December 29, and a joint dinner of the allied societies will be given in the evening. Dr. Raymond Pearl, professor of biology at the School of Hygiene and Public Health of the Johns Hopkins University, president of the association, will make the principal address.

DR. W. B. CANNON, professor of physiology in the Harvard Medical School and president of the American Association for the Advancement of Science, spoke at the University of North Dakota on October 11 under the auspices of the Society of the Sigma Xi, the Graduate Club, the Medical School and the District Medical Society. His subjects were the "Maintenance of Stable States in the Body," "Chemical Mediation of Nerve Impulses" and "Effects of Strong Emotions."

DR. JAMES B. CONANT, president of Harvard University, and Dr. Robert G. Sproul, president of the University of California, will be the principal speakers on November 1 at the academic centennial convocation of the University of Missouri.

DR. PERRIN H. LONG, associate professor of medicine at the Johns Hopkins University, gave a Mayo Foundation lecture at Rochester, Minn., on October 7. He spoke on "The Experimental and Clinical Use of Sulfapyridine and its Sodium Derivative in the Treatment of Pneumococcal Infections."

THE first Barnard Hospital Lecture on "Female Hormones and Genital Cancer" will be given by Dr. Edgar Allen, of the Yale University School of Medicine, in the auditorium of the St. Louis Medical Society on October 31.

IN an effort to interest the public in the problems faced by endowed colleges, the alumni of the Case School of Applied Science are sponsoring a nationwide radio-broadcast of a discussion of the endowed college of engineering. It will be heard over the coast-to-coast facilities of the Mutual Broadcasting Company on Saturday, October 28, from 1 to 1:30 P.M., Eastern Standard Time. The speakers will be Dr. Zay Jeffries, technical adviser to the General Electric Company; Randolph Eide, president of the Ohio Bell Telephone Company; Lee M. Clegg, executive vice-president of the Thompson Products Company; David Dietz, science editor of the Scripps-Howard Newspapers; Sam W. Emerson, president of the Sam W. Emerson Company, contractors, and George S. Case, chairman of the board of Lamson and Sessions Company, who will act as chairman for the discussion. Alumni of the college will hold luncheons simultaneously in about forty cities to listen to the discussion.

THE autumn general meeting of the American Philosophical Society, Philadelphia, will be held on November 17 and 18, in the hall of the society, Independence Square.

THE sixtieth annual meeting of the American Society of Mechanical Engineers will take place at the Bellevue-Stratford Hotel in Philadelphia, Pa., from December 4 to 8. Nevin E. Funk, vice-president of the Philadelphia Electric Company and chairman of the general committee, is making arrangements for the meeting. An attendance of more than 3,000 members is expected. Present plans call for 35 technical sessions at which 105 papers will be presented; a smoker and the introduction of the new officers of the society on the evening of December 5; the annual banquet and the conferring of medals and awards on December 6; college reunion luncheons and dinners on December 7.

SECTION I (Psychology) of the American Association for the Advancement of Science will meet in Columbus, Ohio, from Wednesday to Friday, December 27 to 29. Besides programs of special papers, there will be a symposium on Thursday morning on "The Internal Environment and Behavior" under the chairmanship of Dr. Ross A. McFarland, of Harvard University. There will also be a joint session with Section Q (Education) and a joint dinner with the same section, at which time Dr. J. F. Dashiell, of the University of North Carolina, will deliver one of the addresses. All members and fellows of the section are invited to send abstracts in duplicate (not more than 300 words in length) of papers which they wish to present. No paper presented can be allowed more than 15 minutes' time on the program. Abstracts should be sent to the Section Secretary, Dr. Leonard Carmichael, Tufts College, Medford, Massachusetts, not later than November 4.

A MEETING of the New York State Section of the American Physical Society was held at the Rensselaer Polytechnic Institute at Troy on October 21. The "Address of Welcome" was made by Dr. W. O. Hotchkiss, president of the institute. There were two sessions for the reading of technical papers and an exhibit of undergraduate projects in physics.

THE twenty-sixth annual meeting of the American Association of University Professors will be held in New Orleans on December 27 and 28. Headquarters for the meeting will be at the Jung Hotel. The program will consist of committee reports, addresses and symposia on subjects of professional concern to college and university teachers. Among these subjects are academic freedom and tenure, freedom of speech, policies and procedures of the association and place and function of faculties in college and university government. The meeting will be preceded and followed by sessions of the national council of the association.

# DISCUSSION

## PHYSIOLOGY OF THE NERVOUS SYSTEM

IN discussing some criticisms by Dr. Alexander Forbes of his book on the "Physiology of the Nervous System," Professor Fulton, in SCIENCE of August 4, 1939, makes the following statement with deliberate emphasis: "I know of no evidence fit for critical examination that would place the liberation of acetylcholine as a *primary* event essential for synaptic transmission, in any division of the nervous system, central or peripheral." In the case of the peripheral part of the system, with which the direct evidence yet available is almost entirely concerned, the statement seems to call for some comment.

The validity of the fundamental observation, that acetylcholine is released at ganglionic synapses by preganglionic impulses, was challenged by Lorente de Nó,[1] and Professor Fulton's book seemed to show that he had accepted its dismissal. I take the view that it has been effectively reinstated by MacIntosh,[2] whose evidence, as I think Professor Fulton would agree, must stand until it has been directly answered. If this fundamental observation is correct, it means that acetylcholine is released at the synapses by preganglionic impulses, in such concentration that it must directly excite the ganglion cells to the discharge of postganglionic impulses, or, to use Professor Fulton's phrase, its liberation must be a *primary* event essential for the synaptic transmission. It has rather hastily been assumed that, if acetylcholine were thus to act as transmitter, its disappearance during the refractory period, necessary to prevent repetitive discharge, could only be due to cholinesterase. Consequently, a whole literature has grown around observations on the ganglion with eserine, the largely negative character of which has, I think, been given undue importance by advocates of the electrical theory. The inadequacy of evidence for a particular mode of its disappearance does not, strictly, weaken that for the appearance of acetylcholine, in stimulating concentration, at the synaptic endings of preganglionic fibers. To dismiss such evidence, put forward by observers who are at least experienced and responsible, as not "fit for critical examination," might seem a little severe; but it will be noted that Professor Fulton's statement might mean, literally, not that he repudiates such evidence, but that he is not aware of its existence.

It may be admitted, further, that the possibility that the acetylcholine liberated at a synapse might act only as a sensitizer, necessary to render an electrical transmission effective, has been considered as an alternative, even in publications from my own laboratory. If I understand Professor Fulton, he might regard this idea as more worthy of consideration, since the function of acetylcholine in such a system, though essential, might be regarded as not *primary*—if, indeed, it would be proper to apply that term to one of several conditions essential to an effect. My chief concern, in any case, is with the evidence that the liberation and the activity of acetylcholine are in some way essential to transmission, at peripheral synapses and motor nerve endings. Even this, I think, would not be accepted by some of the distinguished contributors to the illuminating "Symposium on the Synapse,"[3] quoted by Professor Fulton in support of his own present belief. Through Professor Fulton's kindness I had an early opportunity of seeing this important document. Professor Erlanger and Dr. Lorente de Nó, in particular, there present a case for a purely electrical theory of synaptic transmission, which undoubtedly merits a critical examination. Dr. Bronk and Dr. Forbes make contributions to this in the same symposium, where they urge, from different points of view, the necessity of considering at least a chemical participation in, or a chemical aspect of, the synaptic phenomena. It is not likely, however, that either of them could have been fully acquainted with the number of facts now available, which suggest a singular significance in synaptic transmission for the release of acetylcholine, and for which a purely electrical theory appears to afford no explanation. Many of the observations in question are quite recent, and some, indeed, have not yet been published. Perhaps I may be allowed to offer a short list of some of them, as a footnote to the symposium and a modest contribution to the critical examination of the electrical theory.

(1) Nicotine (Feldberg and Vartiainen[4]) and Curarine (Brown and Feldberg[5]) annul the response of ganglion cells to preganglionic impulses and to acetylcholine, without affecting their response to K-ions in the case of Curarine, and without interfering with the release of acetylcholine by preganglionic impulses. These statements are equally applicable to the action of Curarine on voluntary muscle (Dale, Feldberg and Vogt[6]); Brown, Dale and Feldberg[7]; Brown[8]). Buchthal and Lindhard,[9] applying Curarine directly to the motor end plate of a lizard's muscle fiber, have found that it becomes insensitive simultaneously to motor nerve impulses and to application of acetylcholine, while K-ions similarly applied and direct electrical stimulation of the end plate are still normally effective in causing contractions of the fiber.

(2) After section of a preganglionic nerve, release of acetylcholine by preganglionic impulses and synaptic

[1] Lorente de Nó, *Am. Jour. Physiol.*, 121: 331, 1938.

[2] MacIntosh, *Jour. Physiol.*, 94: 155, 1938.

[3] "Symposium on the Synapse," *Jour. Neurophysiol.*, 2: 361–472, 1939.

[4] Feldberg and Vartiainen, *Jour. Physiol.*, 83: 103, 1934.

[5] Brown and Feldberg, *Jour. Physiol.*, 86: 10 P., 1936.

[6] Dale, Feldberg and Vogt, *Jour. Physiol.*, 86: 353, 1936.

[7] Brown, Dale and Feldberg, *Jour. Physiol.*, 87: 394, 1936.

[8] Brown, *Jour. Physiol.*, 91: 4 P., 1937.

[9] Buchthal and Lindhard, International Congress of Neurologists, Copenhagen, 187, 1939.

transmission disappear together (MacIntosh[10]), at a time when conduction in the preganglionic fibers is still unimpaired (Bacq and Coppée[11]).

(3) When Locke's solution containing no glucose is perfused through a ganglion, continued stimulation of the preganglionic nerve rather rapidly exhausts the mechanism of synaptic transmission, and the output of acetylcholine fails with it; both being promptly restored when glucose, lactate or pyruvate is added to the perfusion (Kahlson and MacIntosh[12]).

(4) Perfusion of a ganglion with Locke's solution lacking calcium, while it renders nerve fibers and ganglion cells abnormally excitable, in particular by K-ions, stops the release of acetylcholine by preganglionic impulses, and therewith synaptic transmission, both again being promptly and simultaneously restored by addition of calcium to the perfusion (Harvey and MacIntosh[13]).

Many observations by other workers could be cited, such as the important, though less direct, evidence of Cannon and Rosenblueth,[14] which Dr. Forbes mentioned. Even this limited selection, however, from those with which I have been directly in touch, seems to me to contain points worthy of critical examination by a supporter of a purely electrical theory, who, unless he can show that they are not valid as facts, should be prepared to explain how that theory accommodates them.

H. H. Dale
National Institute for Medical Research,
Hampstead, London, NW. 3
August 28, 1939

## THE USE OF PRONTOSIL AS A VITAL DYE FOR INSECTS AND PLANTS[1]

Recent studies by the writer on the effect of sulfanilamide compounds on a leafhopper vector of a virus disease have resulted in some incidental observations of some general interest.

One of these compounds, Neoprontosil,[2] has proved to be a useful vital stain for both plant and insect. Young corn seedlings, with or without the roots cut off, take up the dye with extreme rapidity, it being a matter of seconds for the leaves to be visibly streaked with red. After a few hours, the entire plant may show the red color diffused throughout or the lower leaves only may be entirely colored, with color on the upper leaves showing only as streaks in some of the fibrovascular bundles.

When nymphs and adults of *Peregrinus maidis* Ashm., the corn leafhopper, were caged on these dye-saturated leaves, the presence of the dye in the insect could be easily observed through the body wall, after feeding a day or two.

The experiment was tried of caging three or four of the insects in a cage which limited feeding of the group to a portion of the leaf tissue less than 1 sq. cm in area. Under these circumstances, great variation in the amount of dye visible in the individual insects could be observed, varying from no outward evidence at all to complete diffusion through the body of the insect. An insect showing no evidence of coloration from the outside may still have ingested the dye, as may be seen from colored defecations. This variation in amount of dye absorbed may be due either to variations in the amount of feeding by individual insects or to differences in the permeability of the intestinal tracts of individuals of the same species or to the specific plant tissues reached by individual insects. This last alternative is not confirmed by experiments wherein the insects were fed on solutions of the dye through membranes. Again, similar differences in amount of visible dye were to be found, insects caged on a single membrane showing all the degrees of color variation from none to a dense red diffused color.

Solutions up to 5 per cent. strength have been used, with one per cent. sucrose added for food, when the dye was administered through membranes.

Walter Carter
University of Hawaii

[10] MacIntosh, *Jour. Physiol.*, 92: 22 P., 1938.
[11] Bacq and Coppée, *Jour. Physiol.*, 92: 17 P., 1938.
[12] Kahlson and MacIntosh, *Jour. Physiol.*, 96: 277, 1939.
[13] Harvey and MacIntosh. In course of publication.
[14] Cannon and Rosenblueth. *Am. Jour. Physiol.*, 119: 221, 1937.
[1] Published with the approval of the director as Miscellaneous Paper No. 29 of the Pineapple Experiment Station, University of Hawaii.
[2] Winthrop Chemical Company, Inc., 170 Varick Street, New York, N. Y.

## FORMATION OF A LARGE ALCOHOL BEAD

A slight vacuum was applied to the residual lime mass in the preparation of absolute alcohol. The alcohol came over quite rapidly and formed a somewhat warm layer. As the rate of distillation became less, the drops of alcohol distillate were cooler and formed beads very readily on the surface of the liquid in the receiver. A short while later the surface of the alcohol had risen to touch the tip of the delivery tube, and a bead about 2.5 cm in diameter and hemispherical in shape was seen to be attached to the delivery tube. Distillation was proceeding at the rate of about 140 drops per minute, and the bead kept increasing in size, until at the end of 18 minutes it measured about 7.5 cm in diameter. The bead was in constant rhythmic pulsating motion, changing its shape from that of a wide shallow saucer-like object to that of a narrow deep bowl. It seemed to be much more highly refractive than the bulk of the alcohol distillate. Finally the bottle became so full of alcohol that distillation had to be stopped, and when the receiver was disconnected, the bead burst.

Thus, in the time during which the bead was observed, the volume increased from 4.1 $cm^3$ to 110.5 $cm^3$, and the total stable existence of this bead becomes about 19 minutes at a growth rate of 5.9 $cm^3$ per minute.

It would, doubtless, be quite interesting to develop a technique and grow a large bead to find just how large and how stable it could be. Several attempts to do this have failed, and the phenomenon must be viewed as a combination of happy probabilities.

C. F. Winans

The Goodyear Tire and Rubber Company
Akron, Ohio

# SCIENTIFIC BOOKS

## RECENT PUBLICATIONS OF THE BRITISH MUSEUM (NATURAL HISTORY)

The war of 1914–18 reduced the publication of zoological research to about half its normal amount, but in the last few years there has been a complete recovery, so far as the total output is concerned. Had it been possible to maintain peace and provide opportunities for scientific cooperation all over the world, it was to be expected that the biological sciences would continue to develop at a constantly accelerating rate, to a future which we can hardly imagine. Knowledge would not only increase rapidly, but would be so organized in catalogues, monographs and the like that in spite of its bulk and variety, it would be increasingly usable. Mankind would come to an understanding of living nature far beyond that which was possible even a few decades ago.

In this great work the British Museum (Natural History) has long been a leader. Its catalogues, at first designed to enumerate the specimens in the Museum, soon developed into monographs of the various groups of animals—the birds, reptiles, fishes of the world; or detailed and beautifully illustrated revisions of particular groups, such as Boulenger's four-volume work on the "Fresh Water Fishes of Africa." Few people have any idea of the magnitude and importance of the British Museum publications, because they are rarely seen assembled together, and no one has occasion to consult all the different works dealing with so many different topics. It must be said, however, that these revisions and monographs not only serve the needs of specialists, but also contain much of general interest for the biologist, if he has patience to dig it out. The present review deals with some of the most recent publications, quite inadequately, yet perhaps with sufficient detail to arouse interest.

(1) *The British Mosquitoes.* By J. F. Marshall. Pp. 341. 1938. The author of this work, finding mosquitoes exceedingly abundant about his home on Hayling Island, became interested in their study and organized a control scheme in 1921. This led to the establishment of the "now well-known British Mosquito Control Institute, which has been ever since a centre for both pure and applied research upon mosquitoes, and is in addition an admirable educational museum." The British mosquitoes had been so extensively and intensively studied that one might have supposed there was nothing more to be done, but Marshall's book, dealing with every phase of the subject and beautifully illustrated, is outstanding for its originality and marks a great advance in our knowledge, as may be seen by comparison with the "Handbook of British Mosquitoes" published by the British Museum in 1920. I can strongly recommend this new mosquito book for consultation in all entomological laboratories, especially as a model for those doing graduate work.

(2) *Mosquitoes of the Ethiopian Region.* Part 1: *Larval Bionomics of Mosquitoes and Taxonomy of Culicine Larvae.* By G. H. E. Hopkins, of the Department of Agriculture, Uganda. Part 2: *Anophelini, Adults and Early Stages.* By the late Dr. Alwen M. Evans, of the Liverpool School of Tropical Medicine. The first of these works (250 pp.) catalogues the species and records what is known of the larvae and their habits. The second book (404 pp.), by Miss Evans, has to do with the group which is concerned with the transmission of malaria and is therefore of prime importance in connection with public health. Miss Evans, long known as a keen student of mosquitoes, was fortunately able to visit Africa a few years ago, and after her return practically completed her monograph, and took it to the Museum. She was evidently ill at the time, and in August, 1937, she died, to the great regret of those who knew her or knew of her work. Dr. F. W. Edwards, of the Museum, saw the book through the press, adding some items to bring it quite up to date, and it was published in May, 1938.

(3) *Bombyliidae of Palestine.* By E. E. Austen. Pp. 188. 1937. Major Austen, who was keeper of the Department of Entomology in the Museum, took part in the Palestine campaigns of 1917–1918, and while engaged in military service was struck by the number and variety and also the beauty of the Bombyliidae or bee-flies of that country. He accordingly collected all he could and brought together those which had been collected by others, and when on his retirement he found sufficient leisure for the work prepared the detailed and beautifully illustrated volume published in 1937. The results were astonishing: out of 128 species or varieties, 46 proved to be new. These flies are of economic importance, being parasitic in the larval state on other insects, some of them on injurious locusts.

(4) *Monograph of the Genus Erebia.* By B. C. S. WARREN. Pp. 407 and 104 plates. 1936. This is a model treatment of an important genus of butterflies found in the Northern Hemisphere. The adult insects only are dealt with, as so little is known of the larvae, which are grass-feeders. The interest of the book for biologists in general centers in the detailed discussions of geographical distribution and the differentiation of species, subspecies and mutations. The author's views and results are provocative of lengthy discussion, which can not be attempted here.

(5) *A Monograph of the Pierine Genus Delias.* By G. TALBOT. In six parts, concluding part VI published in 1937, bringing the pages to 656 and the plates (several colored) to 71. These butterflies, abundant and varied in the Oriental Tropics, but absent from Africa, have been studied in great detail by the author who has examined the structural characters and so put the species on a firm foundation. Mr. Talbot was curator of the private museum of Mr. Joicey at Witley, Surrey. In 1932 Mr. Joicey died, and later his entire collection of Delias, numbering 6,800 specimens, was presented to the British Museum. The monograph is thus based on abundant material and constitutes a revision in the best sense of the word; a new vision would more literally describe it.

(6) *A Catalogue of the Ammonites of the Liassic Family Liparoceratidae.* By L. F. SPATH. Pp. 191 and 26 photographic plates. 1938. In Bristol, many years ago, when the fossil-collectors were seen going out with their hammers, it used to be a current joke to say: "Those are the Hittites, going after the Ammonites." The Ammonite fauna preserved in the rocks of Southern England is extraordinarily rich, and the said Hittites, over a period of many years, have accumulated very large collections, which show the evolution of types from one age to another. Dr. Spath's study of one group of these molluscs, published in the most sumptuous form, enables the reader to examine the evidence in detail and form his own opinions. After reading the work I felt that in some cases the interpretations given might be criticized, but could only admire the elegant presentation of the facts.

(7) *The British Rhaetic Flora.* By T. M. HARRIS. Pp. 84, 5 plates. 1938. A critical study of a small but important flora by the professor of botany in the University of Reading, who is especially known for his excellent work on fossil plants from Greenland. Botanists will be interested to find that one of the plants, an alga, is referred to the living species *Botryococcus braunii* Kützing. It has a variety of names based on fossil specimens, the oldest (from Esthonia) dating back to the Ordovician. Professor Harris declares that the abundant specimens agree perfectly with the living alga, but with no other organism, and he is not willing to treat them as distinct so long as he is unable to specify any distinguishing characters.

(8) *Fossil Orthoptera Ensifera.* By F. E. ZEUNER. Text pp. 321. Plates lxxx, in separate volumes. 1939. It has long been a reproach to European entomology that the various museums have contained great collections of fossil insects of prime importance for the understanding of the subject, yet almost wholly ignored by the taxonomists. It is difficult to understand why these precious and often beautiful specimens have not attracted many students, while even such papers as have been published have received scant attention. I recall my astonishment when, having found fossil tsetse flies in Colorado and placed a specimen in the Geological Department of the British Museum, I found that a leading authority on living tsetse flies, working in another department of the Museum, had not had the curiosity to look at it. Dr. Zeuner's fine work represents a breaking away from such apathy, and deals in a comprehensive manner with the grasshoppers, crickets and similar insects, having an extended ovipositor in the female. These insects are of great antiquity, and appear to have been the first musicians in the world. Some very striking types, after surviving through millions of years with comparatively little change have died out before the modern period. But the crickets, as we know them to-day, were singing in the forests and fields many millions of years ago, and have undergone no important change in the long interval.

In addition to such monographic or revisional works as are cited above, we have the reports of important expeditions, as follows:

(1) *Expedition to Patagonia and South Chile.* The flies (Diptera) were especially collected, very many new species being found. Part 7, fascicle 3, is before me, partly written by D. A. Hall, of the U. S. Department of Agriculture, and partly by John Smart, of the British Museum.

(2) *Ruwenzori Expedition of 1934–35.* This was a botanical-entomological expedition to the high mountains in the vicinity of the great African lakes, with F. W. Edwards and G. Taylor, of the Museum, as leaders. It was supported by grants from the Percy Sladen and Godman funds, the Uganda Government and Mme. de Horrack Fournier. Three volumes on the insects have been coming out in parts, each devoted to some special group. The first has to do especially with the blood-sucking flies; the second with other flies, and the third with various insects, including butterflies, caddis flies and fleas. The authors are mostly British, but one lives in Germany, another in Australia. The illustrations are numerous and excellent.

(3) *Great Barrier Reef (Australia) Expedition of 1928–29.* This has to do with marine life and the vari-

ous parts, though dealing with a remote region, are of great interest to American students. This will be understood from the citation of some of the titles, such as: Rock-destroying organisms in relation to Coral Reefs; The Zooplankton; Copepoda; Larvae of the Decapod Crustacea; Mollusca (a very large report, of which part 1 has appeared).

(4) *The John Murray Expedition of 1933–34.* Five volumes have been appearing in parts. The region surveyed was the Indian Ocean and the Gulf of Aden, full use being made of the echo-sounding machine, which made possible the detailed mapping of the ocean floor. In addition to the purely oceanographic work, very large collections of the marine animals were made, and I have before me detailed reports on such groups as the Cirripedia, pelagic Hemiptera, Pennatulacea, Amphipoda, Scyphomedusae, Polychaeta, Asteroidea, Phyllirhoidae, Pteropoda, Penacidae, Opisthobranchia, Astacura and Palinura, Pycnogonida and Corals.

The above account does scant justice to the activities of the British Museum, but the reader will get some idea of the volume of the work and the liberal policy with regard to publication. As I write, the news from Europe is extremely discouraging, and it is to be feared that the torch of science, if not extinguished, will be so dimmed as to shed little light or will blaze anew in creating means of destruction. Progress in human affairs, within the period of my recollection, has been so great and in most respects so admirable that it is hard to understand how any reasonable individual or group of individuals can fall under the influence of social pathology, nullifying the good that has been done, and might so easily continue in ever-increasing volume. The return to social health and sanity will no doubt eventually occur, but how soon and in what manner? In the meanwhile, scientific workers will carry on as circumstances may permit.

T. D. A. COCKERELL

UNIVERSITY OF COLORADO

# SPECIAL ARTICLES

## NOTE ON WATER IN NON-AQUEOUS SOLUTIONS

IN various models designed to imitate living cells the cell surface is represented by guaiacol, which acts very much like certain protoplasmic surfaces. In such models the behavior of water presents interesting features and it is desirable to ascertain to what extent they occur in the living cell.

The following example serves to illustrate the situation. To a two-phase guaiacol-water system at equilibrium at 25° C. we add increasing amounts of trichloroacetic acid and find that the concentration of water in the guaiacol phase steadily increases while its activity in this phase decreases.[1] When its concentration has increased 12 times its activity coefficient falls to less than 1/12 of its value before acid was added.[2,3] This indicates an attraction of the acid for the water.[4]

At the same time the activity coefficient of the guaiacol in the aqueous phase falls off nearly as much, indicating an attraction of the acid for the guaiacol.

Since the acid can attract both water and guaiacol it is able, when added in sufficient quantity, to make the two phases fuse into one.

A number of other systems follow this pattern, as is evident from the literature.[5] Substances which act like trichloroacetic acid (in other systems) are other organic acids, lower alcohols, acetone, phenols, aniline hydrochloride and pyridine.[5]

Trichloroacetic acid in diffusing through the guaiacol phase appears to carry water with it. Water moves from an aqueous solution where the concentration, mole fraction, vapor pressure and activiity of water are low to one where they are high. A variety of factors must be considered in this connection.[4]

One interesting feature is the following. Let us suppose that a diffusion cell is set up and that the diffusion reaches a steady state so that the concentration gradient of acid in the guaiacol phase may be represented by a fixed straight line, as in Fig. 1.

We may then represent the concentration gradient of water as in Fig. 1, since it is obvious in shaking experiments that for each concentration of acid there is a definite concentration of water.

The concentration gradient of acid is due to flux of acid, but that of water need not be due to flux of

1 This is shown by the fact that as the guaiacol phase takes up more water it comes into equilibrium with a series of aqueous solutions with decreasing vapor pressure of water.

2 The activity coefficient of water in the guaiacol phase before acid is added may be regarded as $f_w = a_w \div c_w$ where $a_w$ is the activity and the $c_w$ the concentration of water in the guaiacol phase. When acid is added the vapor pressure of the water in the guaiacol phase, $p_w$, falls to $p_w\ (x)$, where $x < 1$. When enough acid has been added to raise $c_w$ to 12 $c_w$ and to lower $a_w$ to $a_w\ (y)$, where $y < 1$, and $f_w$ to $f'_w$ we have $f'_w = a_w(y) \div (12c_w)$.

3 We have been unable to find similar calculations for other systems in our preliminary exploration of the literature, but data exist which might be employed for this purpose.

4 This will be discussed in a forthcoming article in the *Journal of General Physiology.*

5 *Cf.* "International Critical Tables," 3: 398 *ff.*, McGraw-Hill Book Co., Inc., New York, 1928, where various diagrams show that as the non-aqueous phase (which is not guaiacol) takes up more and more water it comes into equilibrium with aqueous phases containing less and less water just as in the guaiacol-water-trichloroacetic acid system.

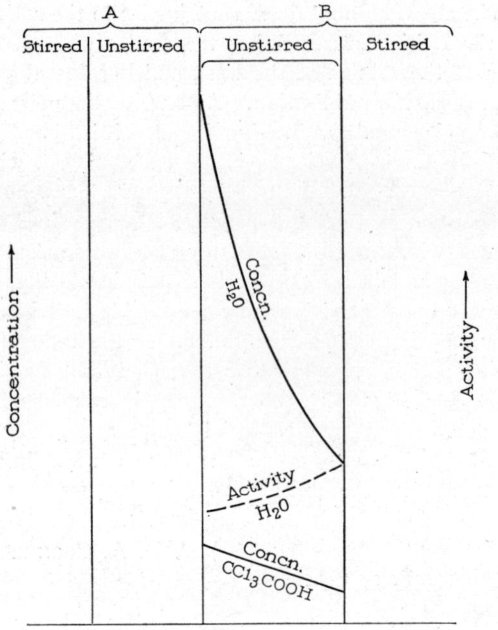


FIG. 1

water; there might conceivably be no flux of water or a flux in either direction.

Since the activity of water in the guaiacol phase falls off as its concentration increases it would seem that we may draw the activity gradient of water in the guaiacol phase as shown by the broken line in Fig. 1.

These considerations may help to explain some of the puzzling cases met with in the living organism.

W. J. V. OSTERHOUT
J. W. MURRAY
THE LABORATORIES OF THE ROCKEFELLER INSTITUTE FOR MEDICAL RESEARCH, NEW YORK

## CEREBRAL METABOLISM DURING FEVER[1]

THE treatment of general paresis with hyperthermia, initiated by Wagner-Jauregg in 1887, is now an accepted form of therapy. In some manner fever facilitates the action of specific treatment in the cerebral form of syphilis. In an attempt to elucidate this question, the brain metabolism of patients with general paresis was studied before and during fever produced by injections of typhoid vaccine and inductotherm therapy. Samples of arterial blood and of the return flow of the brain obtained from the internal jugular vein were analyzed for oxygen, carbon dioxide, glucose and lactic acid. The changes of cerebral blood flow were estimated from the variations of blood pressure and the velocity of the general circulation as determined by the objective cyanide method of Robb and Weiss.[2] The circulation rate through the brain is largely influenced by the changes of the general circulation.[3]

Complete studies were obtained on 7 patients after typhoid vaccine and 7 during fever therapy with inducto-therapy. Table I presents typical effects of

TABLE I

| Experiment | Temperature (°F.) | Oxygen A–V difference (Vol. %) | Velocity of blood (Sec.) | Mean blood pressure Mercury millimeter |
|---|---|---|---|---|
| 1. | 98.0 | 5.15 | 17.6 | 132 |
| | 100.4 | 6.55 | 11.0 | 126 |
| | 102.0 | 6.63 | 10.0 | 113 |
| | 104.4 | 7.61 | 13.0 | 101 |
| | 106.0 | 9.14 | 7.4 | 103 |
| 2. | 98.8 | 6.93 | 15 | 108 |
| | 105.4 | 7.88 | 11 | 79 |
| | 105.3 | 7.09 | 4 | 75 |
| 3. | 98.6 | 7.75 | 20 | 110 |
| | 105.0 | 15.82 | 17 | 112 |

fever on the oxygen A-V difference, velocity of the blood and mean blood pressure. In 11 of 15 observations the oxygen A-V difference rose from 2.0 volumes per cent. to 8.1 volumes per cent. In 12 of 15 experiments the blood velocity was also increased, as may be seen in a typical result (Experiment I). In 3 other results (one of which is presented in Experiment II), the oxygen A-V difference remained unchanged within the error of the method. Th velocity of the blood flow of the general circulation, however, was increased approximately 1½ and 3½ times. In these cases the more rapid blood flow was associated with the lower peripheral resistance, as indicated by a fall in blood pressure. One patient (Experiment III) reacted poorly and lapsed into a comatose condition. At this stage the oxygen A-V difference became huge, while the velocity of the blood revealed only a small acceleration. The small $O_2$ reserve in the venous blood indicated an insufficient $O_2$ supply to the brain. It is suggested that this relative anoxemia produced the coma.[4]

Thus in every instance an increase of cerebral metabolism during fever was indicated. This increase was evidence by a larger oxygen A-V difference, a faster blood flow, or both. The effect of the heightened metabolism of the brain on cerebral syphilis warrants further investigation.

HAROLD E. HIMWICH
KARL M. BOWMAN
W. GOLDFARB
JOSEPH F. FAZEKAS

[1] From the Department of Physiology and Pharmacology, Albany Medical College, Union University, and Bellevue Psychiatric Hospital, Department of Psychiatry, New York University Medical College. This work was aided by a grant from the Child Neurology Research (Friedsam Foundation).

[2] G. P. Robb and S. Weiss, *American Heart Journal,* 8: 1932–3, 650.

[3] H. S. Forbes and S. S. Cobb, *Brain,* 61: 221, 1938.

[4] Himwich, Bowman, Wortis and Fazekas, *Jour. Am. Med. Asn.,* 112: 1572, 1939.

## CRYSTALLINE SALMON PEPSIN*

A GLOBULIN type protein possessing high proteolytic activity has been isolated in crystalline form as colorless needles from the stomach mucosa of the Pacific Coast king salmon (*Oncorhynchus tschawytscha*). The specific proteolytic activity, as measured by the Hb method,[1] is comparable with that of crystalline mammalian pepsin. The activity decreases with lowering temperature, the decrease obeying the Arrhenius equation between 37° and 0° C., which more than covers the temperature range of the salmon's natural environment. The optimum pH for the digestion of Hb is near pH 2.2, which corresponds to that of Northrop's crystalline pepsin.[2] As determined by the minimum solubility of the amorphous form, the isoelectric point lies close to pH 1.9.

Identical potency and crystalline form are obtained either by direct acid extraction or by alkaline extraction of the zymogen and subsequent conversion to pepsin by acid. The latter method has been found to give a much greater yield and is now being used as follows: The ground mucosa is mixed with three times its weight of water and brought to a pH of 8.0–8.2 with $NaHCO_3$ for extraction. This mixture is strained through cloth and filtered; the extract is then acidified with 2N $H_2SO_4$ to a pH 1.8–1.9 and the solution filtered with the aid of Hyflow Super Cell to remove denatured proteins. Solid $(NH_4)_2SO_4$ is added to 0.6 saturation to precipitate the enzyme, which is filtered off. The precipitate is dissolved in M/10 acetate pH 4.2 and the solution clarified by filtration. Precipitation with $(NH_4)_2SO_4$ at pH 1.8–1.9 is repeated twice more. The final precipitate is dissolved in a minimum volume of M/10 acetate pH 5.0, centrifuged quickly, and allowed to stand at room temperature. Crystals begin to form in a few hours, the process being facilitated by seeding and stirring.

EARL R. NORRIS
DANIEL W. ELAM
OCEANOGRAPHIC LABORATORIES AND
DIVISION OF BIOCHEMISTRY,
UNIVERSITY OF WASHINGTON

* Contribution No. 89 from the Oceanographic Laboratories.

[1] M. L. Anson, *Jour. Gen. Physiol.*, 22: 79, 1938.

[2] R. M. Herriot and J. H. Northrop, *Jour. Gen. Physiol.*, 18: 35, 1934.

# SCIENTIFIC APPARATUS AND LABORATORY METHODS

## DETERMINATION OF THE VELOCITY OF SOUND IN A GAS; APPLICATION TO ANALYSIS OF MIXTURES OF HELIUM, OXYGEN AND NITROGEN

SINCE the weight of helium is approximately one seventh of that of nitrogen, variations in the volumetric percentages of these two gases in a mixture affect the density, hence are reflected in changes in the velocity of sound in the mixture. The amount of oxygen present in a mixture of gases can be determined by any standard method. Determination of the velocity of sound in a mixture of helium, oxygen and nitrogen, together with an analysis for oxygen, makes it possible to determine the volumetric percentages of all three gases in the mixture.

An apparatus for determining the velocity of sound in a gas has been constructed which is particularly suited for mixtures of helium, nitrogen and oxygen (Fig. 1). A glass tube 5 feet long, 1 inch in diameter, flared at the top to a diameter of 2 inches, is placed in the vertical position. The upper end is covered with tightly stretched rubber dam. Near the upper end are side tubes for inflow and outflow of gas. The lower end is sealed. Near the lower end is a side tube for inflow and outflow of water, to enable one to alter the length of the column of gas in the tube. A small jar for saturating the incoming gas with water vapor is placed in the side tube through which the gas enters. A rubber bag, provided with a rubber escape valve, is attached to the side tube for outflow of gas. Thorough flushing out of the apparatus is essential. If a sample

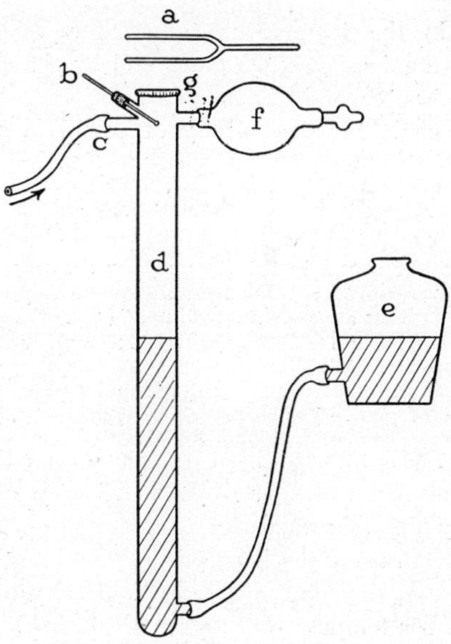


FIG. 1. Diagram of apparatus used in determining the velocity of sound in a gas. *a*. Tuning fork; *b*, thermometer, which can be placed either as indicated or adjacent to apparatus; *c*, side tube for inflow of gas which has been saturated with water vapor by passing it over water; *d*, glass tube. A slight increase in resonance is obtained if the upper end of this tube is flared to a diameter of approximately 2 inches; *e*, water reservoir, connected by rubber tubing to side tube at lower end of apparatus; *f*, rubber bag, provided with rubber escape valve; *g*, rubber diaphragm over upper end of glass tube.

of limited quantity is to be analyzed, the apparatus can be clamped shut at the proper moment. A tuning fork whose frequency of vibration per second is 512 is placed over the upper end of the tube. By striking the tuning fork and raising and lowering the column of water, points of resonance (accentuation of the hum of the tuning fork) are found. The distance between two adjacent points of resonance is half of one wave-length. This distance times two, multiplied by 512 (the frequency of vibration of the tuning fork) equals the velocity of sound per second. A small correction, which is rarely significant, is made in the velocity for variation in laboratory temperature (Table 1);

TABLE 1

CORRECTION OF VELOCITY OF SOUND FOR VARIATIONS OF TEMPERATURE FROM 24° C

| Velocity of sound, meters per second | to 650 | 750 | 850 | 900 and over |
|---|---|---|---|---|
| 1° C. equals (meters per second) | ± 0.5 | ±0.14 | ± 0.3 | special corrections (see below) |
| Add or subtract with rise in temperature | subtract | subtract | add | add |

*Special corrections for velocities of 900 meters per second and over:*

| 18° C. | 19 | 20 | 21 | 22 | 23 | 24 | 25 | 26 | 27 | 28 | 29 | 30 |
|---|---|---|---|---|---|---|---|---|---|---|---|---|
| −4.1 | −3.6 | −3.0 | −2.4 | −1.7 | −0.9 | 0.0 | +1.1 | +2.2 | +3.5 | +5.0 | +6.7 | +8.5 |

"−" indicates substraction for correction to 24° C.; "+" indicates addition.

changes in the temperature affect the velocity by changing the density of the gases and by changing the amount of water vapor in the mixture.

The formula for the velocity of sound in a gas is

$$V = \sqrt{\frac{\gamma P}{d}},$$

where

V = velocity of sound in centimeters per second;
$\gamma$ = Cp/Cv = ratio of specific heat at constant pressure to that at constant volume ($\gamma$ for oxygen is 1.401; for nitrogen it is 1.404; for helium it is 1.66);
P = pressure in dynes per square centimeter; and
d = weight of gas in grams per cubic centimeter.

A chart (Fig. 2) has been constructed on the basis of computation of the theoretical velocity of sound for many different mixtures of helium, oxygen and nitrogen. In using the chart one can read horizontally from the experimentally determined velocity of sound, corrected for temperature, to the determined percentage of oxygen, which may have to be interpolated, thence vertically to the percentages of helium and nitrogen in that portion of the gas remaining after deducting the oxygen. In practice, a large-sized replica of Fig. 2 on graph paper is used.

No attempt has been made to control all the sources of error, most of which are small and may offset one another. It is possible to determine the velocity of sound with our apparatus with an accuracy of ap-

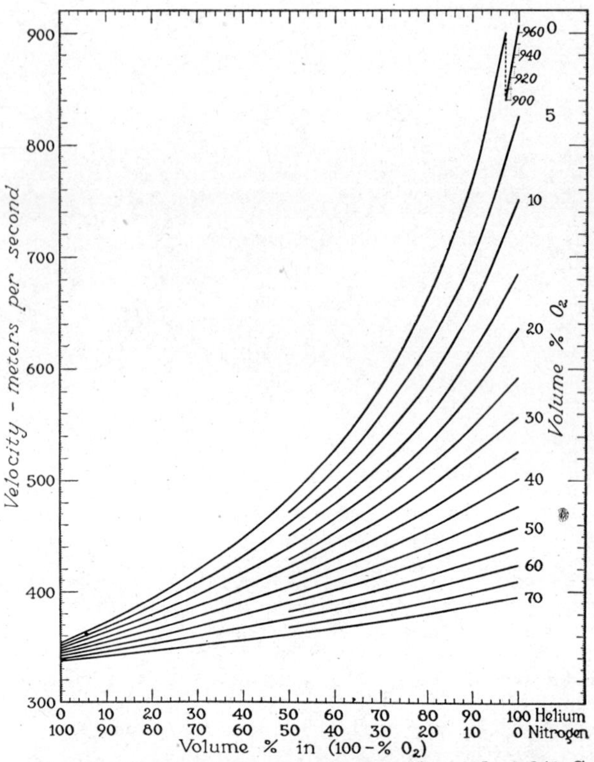


FIG. 2. Chart showing the velocity of sound at 24° C. in mixtures of helium, oxygen and nitrogen, saturated with water vapor.

proximately ± 0.5 per cent. (range of variability) and to determine the percentages of helium and nitrogen in the whole mixture with an accuracy of approximately ± 1.0 per cent. (range of variability). The apparatus and method are intended for practical use in medicine or industry where this degree of accuracy is satisfactory. The apparatus is inexpensive, mobile, simple and easy to use.

WILLIAM B. DUBLIN
WALTER M. BOOTHBY
MARVIN M. D. WILLIAMS

THE MAYO CLINIC

## BOOKS RECEIVED

ARNOW, L. EARLE. *An Introduction to Physiological and Pathological Chemistry.* Pp. 555. 143 figures. Mosby. $3.50.

CHARLES, BROTHER H. *Biology.* Pp. viii + 408. Illustrated. Bruce. $1.72.

EALES, N. B. *The Littoral Fauna of Great Britain; a Handbook for Collectors.* Pp. xvi + 301. 24 plates. Cambridge University Press, Macmillan. $3.50.

EDDY, SAMUEL, CLARENCE P. OLIVER and JOHN P. TURNER. *Guide to the Study of the Anatomy of the Shark, the Necturus and the Cat.* Pp. vii + 100. 15 figures. Wiley. $1.50.

PARKER, JOHN B. and JOHN J. CLARKE. *An Introduction to Animal Biology.* Pp. 503. 163 figures. Mosby. $3.75.

WHITEFORD, G. H. and R. G. COFFIN. *Essentials of College Chemistry.* Second edition. Pp. 534. Illustrated. Mosby.

# SCIENCE

VOL. 90 — FRIDAY, NOVEMBER 3, 1939 — No. 2340

*The National Academy of Sciences:*
*Remarks of the President at the Dinner:* DR. FRANK B. JEWETT ..... 401
*Abstracts of Papers* ..... 403

*Scientific Events:*
*The Exposition of Chemical Industries; The Tropical Flower Garden of the New York Botanical Garden; Reorganization of Laboratory Directors' Conference; In Honor of Dr. Evarts Ambrose Graham; Nominations for President-Elect of the American Chemical Society; Recent Deaths and Memorials* ..... 412

*Scientific Notes and News* ..... 415

*Discussion:*
*The War and Chronica Botanica:* PROFESSOR ROBERT F. GRIGGS. *Remarks on the Center of Population:* PROFESSOR RANDOLPH CHURCH, DR. C. B. READ. *The First Dating of Preserved Wood in New England:* PROFESSOR CHARLES J. LYON. *Notice of Possible Suspension of the Rules of Nomenclature in Certain Cases:* FRANCIS HEMMING ..... 418

*Scientific Books:*
*Quantum Mechanics:* PROFESSOR GEORGE H. SHORTLEY. *Uses of Chemicals:* PROFESSOR MARSTON TAYLOR BOGERT ..... 420

*Special Articles:*
*The Semiquinone Radicals of Methylene Blue and Related Dyestuffs:* S. GRANICK, DR. L. MICHAELIS and DR. M. P. SCHUBERT. *The Metabolism of Glutathione:* DR. H. WAELSCH and DR. D. RITTENBERG. *Synthetic Alpha-Tocopherol and Nutritional Muscular Dystrophy:* DR. STEWARD G. MORRIS ..... 422

*Scientific Apparatus and Laboratory Methods:*
*Student Apparatus for Analysis of Respiratory Gases:* J. MAX LITTLE and DR. HERBERT S. WELLS ..... 425

*Science News* ..... 10

SCIENCE: A Weekly Journal devoted to the Advancement of Science, edited by J. MCKEEN CATTELL and published every Friday by

THE SCIENCE PRESS

New York City: Grand Central Terminal

Lancaster, Pa. — Garrison, N. Y.

Annual Subscription, $6.00 — Single Copies, 15 Cts.

SCIENCE is the official organ of the American Association for the Advancement of Science. Information regarding membership in the Association may be secured from the office of the permanent secretary in the Smithsonian Institution Building, Washington, D. C.

# THE NATIONAL ACADEMY OF SCIENCES[1]

## REMARKS OF THE PRESIDENT AT THE DINNER

*Members of the Faculty of Brown University, Members of the National Academy of Sciences and Guests:*

THE National Academy of Sciences comes to Brown University with greetings to the scientific spirit that has always prevailed within its walls. The basis for this lies in the fact that since the inception of the Academy there has been a continuous liaison between Brown University and the Academy. One of your presidents, Alexis Caswell, was among the founders of the National Academy of Sciences, and members of your faculty have through the years of its existence been elected to membership in it.

In considering what it might be appropriate to say to you on this occasion, it seems to me that the custom established by my predecessors of saying first a word about the Academy, its origin and its functions is in order. This is an old story to members of the Academy and to those who have had close contact with its permanent committee, the National Research Council. To most people, however, it may not be clear as to just what the Academy is.

Although composed wholly of scientists, the Academy is *not* a scientific society in the ordinary professional sense as is the Physical Society, Chemical Society, etc. It is an organization of limited membership created by Congressional charter (the only one in the field of science) which has certain definite prerogatives and certain definite obligations to the state. These obligations in effect determine the qualifications of those elected to membership.

Principal among the obligations is the one which imposes on the Academy the necessity of giving to the government on request, and without remuneration, the best advice on scientific and engineering matters of major importance. It is this obligation which imposes the double requirement of a membership which covers

[1] Autumn meeting held at Brown University, Providence, R. I., October 23, 24 and 25.

broadly the entire field of fundamental and applied science and composed of men of established eminence in each field. It is an Academy in the true sense that every man or women elected to it has a record of proven creative accomplishment in his chosen field. It is consequently an organization of mature people.

The idea of an organization of some kind to give authoritative advice to the government in the field of science was not new at the time the Academy was chartered during the Civil War. It arose in colonial times because the question was continuously coming up with the settlers as to what could best be done with the abundance of natural resources at hand. Ways and means were considered and abandoned, only to be taken up again from time to time.

Benjamin Franklin thought the American Philosophical Society would be able to take care of investigations (that is, as to their value) and, if worth while, the members might be able to carry on the experimental work needed. Then the National Institute and later the American Association for the Advancement of Science were more or less thought of in their inception as advisory bodies to the National Government. None of them seemed to be just what was needed, however, and after considerable discussion between 1848 and 1862, the idea of founding a new body that would be recognized by Congress, to advise the Federal Government in scientific matters, to meet the needs of the time, began to crystallize. Combined with this and as a part of the broad consideration was the idea of honoring men of eminence by election to membership on the basis of their noteworthy contributions to knowledge in their fields of the natural sciences.

The Academy has had an eventful career over the seventy-six years of its existence, considering and reporting on many perplexing questions and problems which have confronted government, and the help given has fully justified the establishment of such a body.

This is neither the time nor the occasion on which to review the work accomplished in three quarters of a century of service as scientific adviser to the government. The problems have been as varied as the fundamental investigations required to adapt the magnetic compass to reliable use on ironclad vessels—a problem made patent at the time the *Monitor* and *Merrimac* battled; the geological investigations of the Panama Canal slides by a committee of the Academy on whose findings were based the methods of control adopted; the many problems of the World War days and in more recent and peaceful times the host of problems presented to the Science Advisory Board and the National Research Council.

The National Research Council, just mentioned, is a permanent operating agency of the Academy designed to broaden the base of its service to the nation. It originated in the vast complexities of major scientific problems of the war and post-war days. It was established by the Academy at the request of President Wilson and was made a permanent part of the Academy set-up in response to an executive order which he issued.

The Academy and Council together constitute an organization which is at all times and at short notice in position to bring to bear on any problems in the field of science the best talent that the nation has.

In addition to its advisory functions the Academy as a whole holds two meetings a year for the presentation of scientific papers and the conduct of its corporate affairs. The annual meeting at the Academy building in Washington each spring is also the time when new members are elected. The fall meeting is held at some scientific center, where brief summaries of the latest accomplishments in science are presented.

So much by way of explaining what the Academy is and how it came to be. Now a few words in a quite different vein but one which, it seems to me, is proper in a person of my antecedents.

In electing an applied scientist and engineer to its presidency, the Academy broke with the traditions of the past. Why, I do not know, unless it was because of a feeling that experience in the art of application might be helpful at this time in assisting the Academy to discharge its obligations as scientific adviser to the Government. Possibly my views on many matters concerned with science and its applications are not traditional ones, and in these concluding remarks I lay no claim to any considerable wisdom.

It is an old adage which counsels the shoemaker to stick to his last. In what I shall say to-night, I propose to take this maxim very much to heart. The American scene unfortunately suggests from time to time that this sage advice may have fallen into disrepute in certain quarters. If so, I suspect it is because of our own short-sightedness and not because of any obsoleteness in the adage. It is usually not a pleasant spectacle to behold a person who, having attained eminence in one field, casts a shadow across his own reputation by assuming to exhort his fellows in spheres of actions in which he has had no experience. It reminds me of a subtle combination of wit and wisdom which Sir Richard Gregory introduced me to while he was making his recent visit to this country. As I recall it, he said that a member of Parliament admonished the House one day that it was always a good plan to have an expert on *tap* but never on *top*.

Now, I am a specialist, an expert if you please—a fact for which I make no apology—and it is as such that I wish to stand before you to-day; *viz.*, one who is on *tap* but not on *top*.

As to my specialty, there is a great deal that could be said on such an occasion and at such a time as this. We live and, what is perhaps even more important, we *fight* in the midst of applied science, and with the tools and weapons which applied science has given us. This is certainly not the *fault* of science; neither does the responsibility for correcting the situation lie solely at the door of science. It is a problem as broad as society itself, and while the scientist very assuredly ought to have helpful suggestions which he can offer, he ought for his own sake to be cautious in delivering himself of panaceas. Perhaps our position is somewhat analogous to that of the chemist who synthesizes a new narcotic—he stands ready to advise regarding its making and its properties but leaves the matter of control in the hands of society through its appointed agents. To push the analogy farther than this would, I am afraid, be to risk the danger of overworking it. The narcotic problem is absurdly simple compared to that involved in the wise assimilation of science; more particularly the beneficent uses of the narcotic may be vanishingly small compared to its potentialities for harm, whereas we hope—perhaps we are incorrigible optimists in such hoping—that the contrary is true of science.

It is quite apparent that the administration of science has two very distinct aspects—one the national, the other the international—and that no competent agencies exist for dealing with either. This situation would on the whole appear to be a fortunate one. Certainly nothing could be more inimical with respect to future progress than an over-developed administrative agency which is insufficiently guided by wisdom, experience and accurate analysis of the problems to be met. Fortunately the affair is still largely fluid and such attempts at crystallization as have been made have as yet had little effect. But let us not drop into a state of indifference as a result of this. While we need scarcely fear that we are confronted at the moment with a condition of supersaturation or of supercooling, we must not forget that the National Academy bears a double responsibility. It is at the same time spokesman for the sciences collectively and the chief scientific adviser to the government. This, in itself, makes our position one calling for careful study. In the words of Pooh-Bah, the Lord High Everything Else, we may, as official representative of American science, declare in favor of untrammeled liberty for fundamental and applied research; or we may, as Lord High Councilor on Science to a Government which for a complex assembly of reasons and motives is drifting in the direction of socialization, make suggestions which might urge on the present drift.

Now, when I say that *we may* do these things, do not misunderstand me. I do not wish to imply that we ought to feel a special urge to do them now or even within perhaps the coming decade, nor do I mean to imply that we will so soon as this be asked for our advice upon this exceedingly complex matter. My thought is one solely of preparedness. There is abundant evidence that for a considerable period of time the tide has been drifting in the direction of increased intermeshing of social forces and increased centralization of control, and that the causes for the tide appear such as to suggest that as yet we have by no means reached the high-water mark. If this hypothesis is true—or, better, if it is not definitely known to be untrue—then I suggest that it is incumbent upon us, both because we are scientists and as such are eager to preserve the liberties of science, and because we are chief scientific adviser to the Federal Government and, therefore, in duty bound to give unprejudiced advice to this agency of the people as a whole, to give heed to the tide. In some way we must merge our collective talents so that to whatever extent is humanly possible, we will arrive at a long-range broad-visioned forecast of the sociological significance of our specialities when taken collectively and when integrated—as is steadily being done—into the fabric of our daily lives.

Let me caution again that I do not visualize this task as one which we can assume at a given moment and conclude at an equally definite but later moment. It is one with which, as I see it, we must be reconciled to living through the years to come. The objective of the present day will have been achieved if we accept the reality of the problem and regard it as one demanding conscious analysis and constructive thought to a degree greater than we as a body have accorded it in the past.

In conclusion, I return again to the adage of the shoemaker. We are all specialists and each must stick to his last. At the same time, as an Academy we are a single, although composite, expert, and as such we should be in possession of faculties at least as comprehensive as are anywhere else attainable. The future, even more than the present, promises to require cooperative effort—and in this problem, which we might denote as the socialization of science, we meet in transcendent form a challenge to our collective talents.

FRANK B. JEWETT

## ABSTRACTS OF PAPERS

*The sensory cortex of the chimpanzee's brain:* J. G. DUSSER DE BARENNE (introduced by W. R. Miles). Local strychninization, *i.e.*, strychninization of a few square millimeters, of the sensory cortex of an anesthetized animal results in typical changes of the electrical activity of this cortex, *i.e.*, the appearance of large and rapid voltage fluctuations, *strychnine-spikes*, in its electrocorticogram. These spikes not only appear in the electrogram taken at the site of strychninization but also in the electrograms from areas functionally related to the strychninized area. In this way it is possible to delimit the sensory cortex in the anesthetized animal. Thus, in collaboration with Dr. W. S. McCulloch, the location and extent of the chimpanzee's sensory cortex was determined. It proved to be a very large region, located both in front and behind the fissura centralis and subdivided in three major subdivisions: a face-, and arm- and a leg-area.

*Rhythmic electrical discharges from nerve cells in relation to their respiration:* HUDSON HOAGLAND (introduced by W. S. Hunter). Most nerve centers of both vertebrates and invertebrates show rhythmic voltage fluctuations at frequencies ranging roughly between one and thirty per second. The regular sinusoidal "alpha" brain waves (Berger rhythms) of about ten per second recorded from large areas of the human cerebral cortex furnish an outstanding example of the phenomena. It is probable, from what is known of other cells, that brain cells produce potential gradients as a by-product of their respiratory metabolism. These may be of the nature of diffusion potentials across the cell membranes which possess definite electrical impedance and which discharge when the potentials reach a critical value. In such a system the discharge frequency would depend on the speed with which the metabolic factor can load the capacities of the cell walls to their critical firing potentials. The absolute frequency would thus be determined by the rate of cellular respiration *and* by the electrical impedance of the cell walls. If this last be statistically constant for a particular group of cells under the conditions of the experiments the *frequency* should parallel and be a measure of changes in cortical respiration. To test this hypothesis of the mechanism of brain waves a number of studies have been carried out by the writer and his collaborators. Metabolic stimulants such as dinitrophenol and thyroxin increase the frequencies of alpha waves. Markedly lowering blood sugar, thus depriving the brain of its principal fuel, or markedly lowering the brain's oxygen consumption slows alpha frequencies. Studies of the effect of temperature on the frequencies of brain waves and, *in vitro,* temperature studies of the kinetics of simple enzyme systems known to be functional in brain respiration have furnished information as to how one or the other of the links in the chemical chain constituting cortical respiration may act as chemical pacemaker or master reaction. Under certain conditions, for example, we have been able to show that the dehydrogenation of succinate may be the pacemaker step; in other conditions it may be the cytochrome oxygen activating link. This work has been applied specifically to the analysis of chemical pacemaker changes in advancing brain syphilis (general paresis).

*The acquisition, extinction and spontaneous recovery of a conditioned operant response:* C. H. GRAHAM and R. M. GAGNÉ (introduced by W. S. Hunter). This study has been concerned with an analysis of the changes in strength of a conditioned operant response which occur as functions of reinforcement, non-reinforcement and spontaneous recovery. The apparatus consists of a simple runway, at one end of which is a starting-box and at the other end a food-box. The measure of response which we have used is termed the latent period. This is defined as the time taken by the animal to leave the starting-box before traversing the runway to food. The latent period for twenty-one male white rats was measured in fifteen reinforced trials, with a constant interval of 75 seconds between successive trials. A curve of acquisition is presented, revealing a response which begins with a log latent period value of 1.85 (corresponding to 71 seconds) and falls off with negative deceleration to reach a log value of 0.45 (2.8 seconds) at the fifteenth trial. The curve exhibits a nine-fold change in latent period from the second to the fifteenth trial. Changes in the latent period of response during extinction were recorded in forty-one rats, the trials being spaced at the same constant 75-second interval as in acquisition. The process of extinction is depicted in a curve showing the change in latent period of response during five unreinforced trials. This curve begins at a log latent period value of about 0.40 (2.6 seconds) and rises with negative acceleration to a log value of 1.33 (21 seconds). Thus during extinction the magnitude of the latent period increases in the ratio of nine to one. Spontaneous recovery of the response was measured after extinction had proceeded to a criterion of a 3-minute latent period. Recovery was tested in twenty rats, five at each of four recovery intervals of no stimulation. The intervals used were 1 minute, 3 minutes, 6 minutes and 10 minutes. The progress of spontaneous recovery in these intervals is shown in the form of a graph. Recovery is rapid during the first three minutes, but after 6 minutes the rate decreases rapidly. The recovery after 10 minutes is not complete, as indicated by the fact that latent period is still of the order of 35 seconds. A theoretical discussion of the results is presented. This considers changes in an internal condition of excitation which may account for a number of the processes involved in conditioning.

*Experimental modification of the polarity potential of the human eye:* WALTER R. MILES. The steady potential existing between the anterior and posterior poles of the eyeball has been measured by means of electrodes applied to the skin on either side of the eye. When the eye is turned the cornea is brought nearer to one electrode, which then becomes positive, while the other is negative. The potential registered under standardized objective conditions shows a rather steady value for a given individual but is influenced somewhat by the subjective factors of apprehension and relaxation. The present report considers the possibility of temporarily modifying the steady potential of the eye. For this purpose small amounts of sodium chloride solution were instilled into the conjunctival sac. Shortly after this application of hypertonic solution to the anterior portion of the eye a marked increase in the eye potential was found present and persisted for several minutes. The change, studied on 18 young women, showed an average increase which amounted to two times the standard deviation of the pre-salt mean value and is thus a highly reliable indication of an induced modification of the polarity potential. In some instances the hypertonic salt solution gave rise to a second phenomenon which may be interpreted as a "diffusion potential." This occurred when the eye was turned 30° laterally from the primary line of regard, and a part of the salt-soaked sclera thus came into contact with tissue of lower salt content. Diffusion potentials of this character were also found in rare cases (out of a population of 200 examinations) occurring spontaneously without the experimenter having instilled hypertonic solutions.

*The theory of the visual threshold.* W. J. CROZIER (introduced by W. S. Hunter). The physical interpretation of data of sensory excitability necessarily implies a theory of the nature of the effects responsible for threshold discrimination. The common assumption, sometimes only implicit, has been to the effect that in visual performance, for example, threshold effects are equal or equivalent. That they are really equivalent in any meaningful sense has never been demonstrated. A detailed examination of human visual thresholds ("absolute" and relative) shows that the interrelationships among the effects due to such variables as area, exposure time, intensity and wavelength, at a number of retinal locations, are such as to demonstrate that in homogeneous data the form of the quantitative dependence of the threshold intensity upon any one of the other variables depends upon the magnitudes of the rest. Before it can be attempted to provide a coherent account of the nature of the neural disturbance at the discriminatory threshold, means must be found for analytically separating the specifically statistical properties of the relevant elements of neural action from those which may reveal the physico-chemical character of the excitatory and discriminative processes. Indications can be given as to the directions which such analysis may take. The interrelations of time and intensity provide one illustration of the role of purely statistical considerations. It does not seem profitable to regard the data of intensity discrimination under fixed conditions as in general resulting from a physically fixed quantity of sensory disturbance.

*Localization of response in the cochlea as determined by electrical recording:* E. H. KEMP and PARKER JOHNSON (introduced by W. S. Hunter). Electrical responses from the cochlea of the guinea pig were studied by means of an amplifier, a cathode-ray oscillograph and a wave-analyzer. The guinea pig was anesthetized with dial and urethane, put under artificial respiration and placed in a "soundproof" room. A beat-frequency oscillator, attenuator and speaker provided tones which were delivered to the ear of the guinea pig through a rubber tube and a speculum which had been sewed into the external meatus. The cochlear response to frequencies of 100, 200, 400, 600, 1,000, 2,000, 4,000 and 6,000 cycles per second was recorded from selected positions on each turn of the cochlea. For each frequency a series of intensities was used and a log response—log relative sound intensity curve obtained. From these curves the relative intensity of sound of each frequency necessary to elicit a response of three microvolts was determined for each recording position. The data obtained make it possible to construct a map of the cochlea which meets the requirements of the place theory of audition, and which confirms a map of the cochlea previously constructed by Culler from data obtained by a somewhat different method.

*The effect of direct current stimulation on the contractions and the electrical behavior of the oyster heart:* IVON R. TAYLOR and EDWARD M. WALZL (introduced by C. A. Kraus). The makes and breaks of a direct current (4–13½ volts), applied to the ventricle of the excised, perfused oyster heart, were timed to occur at certain phases of the cardiac cycle as the mechanigrams and electrograms were recorded simultaneously. An action potential, due to a propagated wave, was produced when the break of the current occurred at full systole or later in the cardiac cycle, but no such effect was produced, in any phase of the cycle, due to the make. A slow electrical wave, probably due to local polarization of the tissues, was sometimes observed on the make. During contraction of the ventricle, a make caused a decrease in the amplitude and duration of systole, and a break produced the reverse effects. During relaxation, a make favored relaxation, but a break caused a contraction with amplitude and duration greater than normal. The above and additional results lend support to a previous report by Walzl to the effect that the make and the passage of a direct current cause inhibition but the break, excitation of the oyster ventricle. During the constant passage of the direct current, the spontaneous action potentials were markedly increased in amplitude, usually, although the ventricle was in a partly inhibited state. This effect is probably due to an increased polarization of the surface of the tissue. The amplitude of the spontaneous action potential appeared to vary parallel with the initial length of the ventricular tissue.

*The effects of biologically conditioned medium on the growth rate and population yield of certain ciliated protozoa:* GEORGE W. KIDDER (introduced by W. S. Hunter). Three species of holotrichous ciliates were used in this study, *Colpidium campylum*, *C. striatum* and *Glaucoma pyriformis*. They were grown in bacteria-free, particulate-free culture and tested as to growth rate and population yield in fresh broth (proteose-peptone), broth from which a previous population had been removed by centrifugation and broth from which a previous population had been removed by filtration. No significant difference was observed between the growth phases of the three species, but large and significant differences occurred between the different types of media. In fresh broth (control) growth proceeds logarithmicly for about 36 hours (initial inoculum of 100 to 150 cells) then levels sharply and continues in the stationary phase for weeks. When the same number of cells are inoculated into conditioned broth (from which a previous population has been removed by centrifugation) there is a significant acceleration of growth during the early periods with a gradual slowing of the growth rate. The maximum population yield is always lower than the control. When the same number of cells are inoculated into filtered conditioned broth (the previous population having been removed by a Seitz filter) there occurs a significant lag period with a final population yield similar to that of the conditioned broth. Both the accelerative and the depressive effects are destroyed by heat and the accelerative effect is decreased in direct proportion to the length of time the conditioning is carried out. We may postulate the elaboration of two substances within the culture medium as a result of the population growth, one an accelerator to growth which appears to be adsorbed on a negative filter and the other a depressor which, when allowed to act independently of the accelerator, produces a pronounced lag in the growth rate of a second population of ciliates. These two substances are thought of as being produced simultaneously but at different rates during any population growth.

*Analysis of variance applied to human genetics:* C. B. DAVENPORT. The analysis of variance as developed by "Student" and R. A. Fisher has been used hitherto to differentiate races of animals and plants but apparently not to compare intrafamilial with interfamilial difference to get a measure of the importance of heredity in human family traits. In 7 families containing 5 to 3 Nordic boys each, at age of 16 years at time of observation, the variation between families and within families of 14 dimensions was computed. The results are as follows: In all 14 cases, with degrees of freedom of 6 for the greater mean square and 17 for the less the F value ranges from 2.40 to 2.65 (2 cases), through 2.96 and 3.86 (2 cases) to over 4.10 (10 cases). The ratio that may be exceeded by chance 5 times in 100 trials is 2.70; by chance once in 100 trials is 4.10. Accordingly, the adjusted ratio of intrafamilial to interfamilial variation may be given, by chance, slightly more than 5 times in 100 trials in 2 cases; between 5 times and 1 time in 100 trials in 2 cases; and less than 1 time in 100 trials in 10 cases. Thus, in all families variation within families is significantly less than between families. The difference is much more significant (perhaps because the genetical factors are stronger) in the various head widths than in the elements of facial height.

*Bodily constitution and longevity:* RAYMOND PEARL and W. EDWIN MOFFETT. There were observed and measured 2,332 adult white males falling in six series on the basis of the eventual causes of their deaths. All were in a state of sound health when observed. In each cause-of-death series there were two groups of individuals separated upon the basis of duration of life. The Longevity (+) group in each series contained every individual in our total material for that series, without other selection, whose survival after observation was *greater* than the expectation of life for his age when observed as given by the Dublin and Lotka 1929–31 life table. The *average* ages at death of the Longevity (+) groups ranged from 75.0 years in the cancer series to 77.2 years in the nephritis series. The Longevity (−) group in each series contained the shortest-lived individuals to be found in that series who were, individual for individual, of the same age in years at observation and measurement as the individuals in the Longevity (+) series with whom they were paired. Their average ages at death ranged from 40.2 years in the accident series to 54.7 years in the diabetes series. The Longevity (+) group outlived the Longevity (−) by average amounts varying from about 21 years in the diabetes series to about 36 years in the accident series. The Longevity (+) group was not significantly differentiated from the Longevity (−) group in any series in respect of mean *stature* or in mean *chest expansion* at the time of disease-free observation. The same was true of mean *body weight* in the pneumonia series and in the accident series. But in the heart disease, and the nephritis series, the mean *body weight* and mean *chest girths* were significantly greater in the Longevity (−) group than in the Longevity (+) group. Mean *pulse rate* was higher in the short-lived (−) groups in all cause-of-death series, but not significantly so in the accident or pneumonia series. Further details regarding other constitutional differentiations between the long-lived and short-lived groups are given in the complete paper.

*Inheritance of internal morphological characters:* PAUL B. SAWIN (introduced by W. S. Hunter). Irregularities in the number of pairs of ribs and of presacral vertebrae and of other internal morphological structures are anomalous variations described in numerous species and in all classes of tetrapods. Evidence of inheritance has been presented by several investigators as the result of study of corresponding variations in the domestic fowl, the rabbit, mouse and man, but in none is a simple mendelian interpretation adequate to explain all the facts. In the rabbit our extensive breeding within three closely bred families shows that by selection in two of them (IIc and III) the proportion of 13-ribbed progeny has been increased from 86.6 per cent. and 76.3 per cent. to 94.7 per cent. and 97.7 per cent., respectively, whereas random mating within a third family (V) has induced but minor change over seven generations. Crosses of the two 13-ribbed families with the same 12-ribbed family reveal tendencies for the 12-ribbed type to dominate in the first generation and to segregate in subsequent backcross generations in expected mendelian manner but with aberrant proportions of 12- and 13-ribbed progeny roughly corresponding to the respective disproportion existing in the parental families. This is indicative of minor genetic differences between these two 13-ribbed families, although crosses between the two have produced only 13-ribbed young. A cross between one of the 13-ribbed families (III) and the 12-ribbed individuals of the unselected family V has produced 40 young, 66 per cent. of which are 13-ribbed, and which continue to breed as 13-ribbed. This could be explained on the basis of parental unifactorial hybridity of the family V parents. This interpretation is erroneous, however, since analysis of 134 matings within this family shows that segregation is neither unifactorial nor fortuitous. Similar studies of anomalies of the sternum and of the vascular branches arising from the aortic arch, dorsal aorta and inferior vena cava within the same families show patterns of incidence of anomalies typical for each family, but for which at present likewise no simple mendelian explanation is completely adequate. The author is inclined at present to consider a multifactorial explanation parallel to that suggested by several investigators for adult body size as the more likely, although body size itself is not directly correlated at least with the skeletal variations. The high familial incidence of these anomalies, which are associated with regions (branchial and urogenital) subject to great evolutionary vicissitudes, coupled with the regularity of their transmission in crosses, offers a new approach to problems in vertebrate evolution through the combined application of the principles of comparative anatomy and genetics.

*A study relating to cytoplasmic effects of uniparental inheritance in Daphnia:* A. M. BANTA and THELMA R.

WOOD (introduced by C. A. Kraus). In biparental inheritance reciprocal crosses between stocks of *Daphnia longispina* possessing either of the mutant characters studied, excavated head or sex intergradedness, it was found that when the eggs came from the mutant-bearing stock and the sperm from the normal (non-mutant-bearing) stock the sexually produced offspring, about 50 per cent. of which carried the character, produced a higher average manifestation of the character involved than when the cross was made in the reverse direction. The differences in reciprocal crosses appeared conclusive. Such a result may find explanation in that the factors for the mutant characters affect the cytoplasm of the egg previous to fertilization. Inasmuch as parthenogenesis in Daphnia is diploid, there theoretically being no opportunity for genic segregation during the one non-reductional maturation division of the eggs, all the parthenogenetic descendants of an individual should be genetically identical, except as a mutation occurs. However, with the two mutant characters studied, both of which are highly variable in their manifestation, there was strong presumptive evidence that even among parthenogenetically produced clutch mates, a mother phenotypically low for the character produced uniparental, diploid offspring with a slightly lower average manifestation of the character than did her clutch mates which themselves were phenotypically higher for the character involved. Only cytoplasmic influences would seem to account for such a result. In an attempt to get critical evidence concerning such cytoplasmic effects experiments were set up as follows: Clutch sisters having different grades of manifestation of the mutant character were reared in individual bottles of the same culture medium under as nearly identical conditions as could be provided. As many parthenogenetic young as possible were obtained from each mother. The offspring from each mother were graded with reference to the manifestation of the character. An average grade for all the offspring from each mother, in many cases 150 to more than 300 per mother, was thus obtained. The general average grade of offspring from mothers which were phenotypically of one grade of expression of the character was then compared with averages for offspring from mothers having other grades of expression of the character studied. The data thus obtained for the excavated head character reveal no evidence for a cytoplasmic effect in the inheritance of this character in parthenogenesis. On the other hand, extensive data (which will be presented) for the sex intergrade character appear to confirm the earlier evidence which suggested cytoplasmic effects in inheritance in parthenogenesis.

*The effect of calcium on potassium retention in skeletal muscle:* P. H. MITCHELL and L. SARIN (introduced by C. A. Kraus). Pairs of frog sartorius muscles were used as control and experimental material. They were immersed in Ringer solution or in Ringer modified as to its calcium concentration. The control was kept at rest; the experimental muscle was directly excited electrically to give tetanus contractions of one third second duration at intervals of 20 seconds. Confirmatory of previous work at this laboratory and elsewhere, potassium losses were noted from stimulated muscles only. If stimulation was continued during two hours, large potassium losses, amounting to about 30 per cent. of the total muscle potassium, were observed when the muscles were in Ringer solutions containing 12 to 24 milligrams per cent. of calcium chloride. With 36 milligrams per cent., the potassium losses fell to about 15 per cent. of the total muscle potassium. If stimulation was continued during only one hour the potassium losses became smaller as the calcium chloride concentration was increased. In the presence of 36 milligrams per cent. of calcium chloride, the losses were too small to be detected by the method of chemical analysis employed. It is suggested that increase in calcium concentrations may so affect the muscle cell surfaces as to alter the normal permeability relations and check or even prevent loss of potassium during excitation and contraction.

*The isolation, constitution and synthesis of Vitamin $K_1$:* E. A. DOISY, D. W. MACCORQUODALE, S. A. THAYER, S. B. BINKLEY and R. W. MCKEE. Evidence of the existence of an anti-hemorrhagic factor was first obtained by Dam in 1929; in 1935, he suggested the term Vitamin K for this factor. The difficult and laborious tasks of developing satisfactory bioassay procedures and of devising methods for purification of the vitamin were undertaken mainly by Dam and his collaborators in Europe and by Almquist and his co-workers at the University of California and by our group at the St. Louis University School of Medicine. Dried alfalfa leaf meal and putrefied sardine meal were found to be satisfactory sources of the vitamin. We have isolated an anti-hemorrhagic compound in a pure state from each source. Chemical reactions and ultra-violet absorption curves have indicated clearly that both of these compounds are derivatives of 1,4-naphthoquinone. By oxidation experiments it has been shown that Vitamin $K_1$ (alfalfa) is 2-methyl-3-phytyl-1,4-naphthoquinone. This structure has been confirmed by synthesis, and degradation experiments on the synthetic compound have given the same products that were obtained by oxidation of the natural compound. As soon as the quinonoid structure of Vitamin K was recognized various simple quinones were tested for Vitamin K activity. Only 1,4-naphthoquinones and compounds which upon oxidation in the organism might yield 1,4-naphthoquinones showed activity. 2-methyl-1,4-naphthoquinone is at least as active as Vitamin $K_1$. 1,4-dihydroxy-2-methylnaphthalene and 4-amino-2-methyl-1-naphthol possess approximately the same potency as Vitamin $K_1$. These two compounds are of great importance from a therapeutic standpoint, since they are soluble in aqueous media and therefore can be used for parenteral therapy. This is important because of the difficulty in securing absorption of the enterally administered natural vitamin, which because of its oily character can not be used intravenously.

*The medical cyclotron of the William H. Crocker Radiation Laboratory:* ERNEST O. LAWRENCE. The new 60-inch cyclotron of the William H. Crocker Radiation Laboratory, weighing over 220 tons, is the largest one yet built and has many important new features of design. The improvements have greatly increased the efficiency of the apparatus over smaller models, as evidenced by the fact that 100 microamperes of 16 million volt deuterons and 1 microampere of 32 million volt helium ions are obtained with only 50 kilowatts input to the radiofrequency oscillator. The first experiments with these atomic projectiles of considerably greater energies than heretofore available have given extraordinarily interesting results. It has been observed, for example, that the neutron yield per microampere of deuterons is 5 times greater at 16 million volts than at 8 million volts, while the yield of radioactive iodine is 20 times greater at the higher voltage. Moreover, bombarding bismuth and lead with 32 million volt helium ions gives rise to large yields of new alpha particle emitting radioactive substances. The gratifying initial performance of the new cyclotron, which indeed has surpassed expectations, makes it certain now that it is entirely feasible to build a 120-inch (2,000 tons) cyclotron capable of producing atomic projectiles of energies above 100 million volts. The rapid and successful construction of the 60-inch cyclotron, which is of great importance for medicine as well as for the physical sciences, was made possible through the joint efforts of all the members of the Radiation Laboratory and through the active interest and generous support of the Chemical Foundation, the Rockefeller Foundation and the National Advisory Cancer Council.

*Auditory patterns, a demonstration lecture:* HARVEY FLETCHER. For many years physicists have been devising methods and apparatus for accurately measuring hearing, and it is now possible to describe the ear in physical terms much as other machines are described. In more recent years, auditory research has been directed more toward obtaining the relation between such a physical description and the character of the sensation evoked by a sound. Sound waves entering the inner ear set into vibration a relatively long flexible membrane, which has distributed along its length the endings of the auditory nerve fibers. These endings are sensitive to the vibrations, and initiate a series of nerve impulses or tiny electrical currents, which travel along the nerve fibers to the brain. Such nerve messages contain the information that is used in forming the sensation of sound. By utilizing the discovery that human nerve fibers behave like busy telephone wires, relations have been obtained between the physical characteristics of a sound and the pattern of the nerve messages which it produces. When a nerve fiber is busy carrying messages for one sound it is unable to carry messages for a second sound. In order to be heard, the intensity of the second sound must be increased until nonbusy fibers can be found. From such busy tests, the fibers at different positions on the membrane that are excited by a given sound can be charted. Such a chart is called an auditory pattern, and portrays to the eye the information that the brain must utilize in order to form sensation. By choosing a sound which renders the fibers at different positions on the membrane uniformly busy, relations have been obtained between the pitch of a sound and the position of the excited fibers, the intensity of a sound and the rate at which messages are evoked and the changes in position and rate which accompany just noticeable changes in pitch and intensity, respectively. In the demonstration lecture, this complicated process is vividly depicted by creating sounds and portraying the corresponding auditory patterns by means of animated charts. Deafness is artificially created and the audience sees and hears sound in the roles of both the normal hearing and the deafened.

*A Raoult law study of chlorbenzene-symtetrachlorethane mixtures:* JOHN R. LACHER (introduced by C. A. Kraus). An equilibrium still is described which permits a fairly rapid determination of vapor-liquid equilibrium. The apparatus is flexible and enables one to determine whether or not the steady state set up is independent of the factors required to bring it about. Pressure composition isotherms of chlorbenzene-symtetrachlorethane mixtures were determined at 75° and 100° C. The deviations from the ideal solution law are small and negative. The measurements satisfy the Gibbs-Duhem-Margules' equation within experimental error. That the solutions should be nearly ideal is indicated by the fact that the molar volumes of the two pure liquids differ by only 4 per cent. at 30° C. Density measurements of the liquid mixtures show that there is a small decrease in volume on mixing. This shows that the attractive forces between the unlike molecules should produce small negative deviations from the ideal solution law, as were observed.

*Mixed copper-chromium oxide hydrogenation catalysts:* V. N. IPATIEFF, B. B. CORSON and J. D. KURBATOV. Pure copper does not hydrogenate benzene at ordinary pressure and 225°, but the presence of chromium oxide enables it to do so. As chromium oxide is added to copper, the hydrogenating activity rises abruptly to a maximum at 5 per cent. of oxide, and then falls with continued addition. The same is true for the hydrogenation of isopentene at ordinary pressure and of benzene at superatmospheric pressure. We have called this mixture of maximum activity the "eucoactic mixture." The presence of 0.1 per cent. of chromium oxide lowers the temperature requirement for the hydrogenation of isopentene from 225° to 75°. Copper is very susceptible to activation by traces of nickel, and the 95 per cent. copper-5 per cent. chromium oxide catalyst is even more susceptible. For instance, copper containing not more than 0.001 per cent. of nickel does not hydrogenate benzene at ordinary pressure and 225° in 90 seconds, whereas the presence of 0.005 per cent. of nickel raises the hydrogenation to 4 per cent. On the other hand, the hydrogenating activity of the 95 per cent. copper-5 per cent. chromium oxide catalyst is raised from 4 per cent. to 16 per cent. by the addition of 0.005 per cent. of nickel. Also, copper containing 0.2 per cent. of nickel hydrogenates benzene 19 per cent. in 12 seconds' contact time, whereas the 95 per cent. copper-5 per cent. chromium oxide catalyst, to which 0.2 per cent. of nickel has been added, hydrogenates benzene 62 per cent. In the absence of nickel, the copper-chromium oxide catalyst hydrogenates benzene only 2 per cent. in 12 seconds.

*Line absorption spectra of solid compounds:* JOHN P. HOWE and W. S. HERBERT (introduced by C. A. Kraus). Neodymium acetylacetonate has been chosen as a compound, the study of whose absorption spectra should give data bearing on the subject of energy levels in solids. It has been shown by various workers that the color of rare earth compounds is due to transitions between levels of $(4f)^n$ electronic configurations of the triply ionized rare earth ion. These levels being highly degenerate are split in the electric fields due to the charged groups surrounding the ion in a solid. The splitting pattern depends on the electronic level involved and the symmetry of the electrical field. The absorption spectrum of neodymium acetylacetonate has been photographed with the compound at 78°, 120°, 193° and 298° Kelvin. From the results, an energy level diagram has been constructed which is consistent with the assumption of a field of nearly octahedral symmetry about the rare earth ion. A small axial field is indicated. In addition, it was necessary to assume that a molecular vibration frequency couples with the electronic transitions. The splitting pattern of the ground state is similar to that observed in other neodymium salts. All the observed lines are accounted for except one group which appears to rise from transitions to two electronic states lying close enough together to mix up.

*Work functions of different faces of silver single crystals:* H. E. FARNSWORTH and RALPH P. WINCH (introduced by C. A. Kraus). The work required to transport an electron through the (100) and (111) faces of silver single crystals has been determined by a photoelectric method after extended outgassing of the crystals. The equilibrium value of this work function for the (100) face is 4.81 ± .01 electron volts. This value was obtained after 2,283 hours of heating at temperatures up to about 700° C; 356 hours of additional heating did not change this value. After the crystal had subsequently remained at room temperature for 2,130 hours, at a pressure of 1 to $3 \times 10^{-8}$ mm Hg, the work function decreased to 4.65 e.v. After 100 hours of additional heating of the crystal the work function increased to 4.79 e.v., and after an additional 118 hours of heating it returned to the equilibrium value of 4.81 e.v. The equilibrium value of 4.75 + .01 e.v. for the (111) face was obtained after 1,227 hours of heating at temperatures similar to those above. This crystal had been outgassed in two previous experiments so that a much shorter time was required to reach the equilibrium value of the work function than for the (100) face. The above equilibrium value was not changed by 407 hours of additional heating. At this time the crystal became slightly contaminated while heating a tantalum plate near it. The effect of the contamination was to cause a failure of the experimental results to fit the Fowler theoretical curve. Measurements on the contact potential difference between the two crystal faces by the Kelvin null method agreed with the difference of the photoelectric work functions to within + .01 volt until the results for the (111) face failed to fit the Fowler theoretical curve. We believe that these values are the best that can be obtained by heating, since silver crystals etch rapidly, thus exposing other faces, when heated at temperatures where appreciable evaporation occurs. The above values may be compared with 4.74 e.v., previously obtained by Winch (*Physical Review,* 37: 1269, 1931; 38: 45, 1931), for polycrystalline silver after heating for 1,200 hours with short intervals at temperatures as high as 850° C. where evaporation is rapid.

*The filtration of sound in non-homogeneous media:* R. B. LINDSAY (introduced by C. A. Kraus). Previous work (*e.g.,* Lindsay, Lewis and Albright, *Jour. Acoustical Soc. Amer.,* 5: 202, 1934) has indicated that when periodic compressional elastic waves pass through a stratified medium consisting of a series of alternating layers of two different substances, which may be either fluid or solid, not all frequencies are transmitted. In other words, the medium acts as an acoustic filter with alternate transmission and attenuation frequency bands. This analysis of the transmission characteristics of the medium was based on the assumption that the transition in acoustical properties (*i.e.,* density and sound velocity) from each layer to the next is *abrupt* and effectively discontinuous. The purpose of the present investigation is to examine the consequences of assuming that the transition in question is a *gradual* one. The interesting theoretical result is that for a gradual transition in which there are no discontinuous changes in either the acoustical properties or their gradients the stratified medium no longer acts as a filter but passes all frequencies equally well. In order to assure filtration for a gradual transition one must assume at least discontinuity in the gradients of the acoustical parameters. Certain special cases and their consequences are investigated.

*Excitation of fractional multiplets by electron capture:* GEORGE H. SHORTLEY and DONALD H. MENZEL (introduced by Harlow Shapley). Observations show that certain permitted multiplets of O III and N III are not completely represented in the spectra of gaseous nebulae. Some mechanism apparently acts to give selective excitation of some levels of a term without exciting the other levels. Bowen attributes the phenomenon to resonance absorption, principally of the ultimate line of He II, which happens to coincide with an ultimate line of O III. Certain questions and consequences of Bowen's mechanism are discussed. Another method of excitation of fractional multiplets, by direct electron capture by an ion in the ground level of a term (e.g., $^2P_{\frac{1}{2}}$ of O IV), is examined. The components predicted by quantum mechanics do not, however, agree with those observed in the nebulae. The conclusion is reached that Bowen is probably right, although a few discrepancies still remain unexplained. His method apparently requires inelastic electron impacts to be sufficiently frequent to maintain approximately a thermodynamic-equilibrium population of atoms in the levels of the ground term.

*The coronaviser, an instrument for observing the solar corona in full sunlight:* A. M. SKELLETT (introduced by F. B. Jewett). Special television apparatus has been developed to scan the region of the sky around the sun, to separate the component of the photoelectric current arising from the glare (mainly a d–c. component) from that arising from the scanning of the coronal features (mainly an a–c. component), and to amplify the latter component and to reproduce therefrom an image of the corona. The scanning follows a spiral path. The input scanner is mechanical and works on the image at the focus of the 15-inch horizontal refractor of the Cook Observatory at Wynnewood, Pa. The reproduction is effected entirely by electrical means and appears on the screen of a cathode ray tube. Numerous images of prominences have been obtained, and a number of the images showed features that apparently were of coronal origin. On one particularly clear day a bright jet or flare in the corona was photographed a number of times over a period of several hours. This feature turned about the optic axis of the telescope with time at the correct rate for a coronal feature.

*Southern clusters and galaxies:* HARLOW SHAPLEY and JOHN S. PARASKEVOPOULOS. In reporting on the work of the galactic bureau at the Harvard Observatory the following specific projects and objects in the Southern Hemisphere will be discussed: (1) A photometric survey of two new groups of galaxies, each involving many hundreds of individual systems. Distances and dimensions of these supersystems will be estimated, and the luminosity law (distribution of brightness) will be evaluated. (2) Two spirals without nuclei, both large and one possibly within the local supergalaxy. (3) A new "Magellanic Cloud" in Cetus, possibly a member of the local group of galaxies also. (4) The distribution of the periods of classical Cepheid variables in the Magellanic Clouds. The peculiar concentration of the longer periods to regions of higher frequency of stars suggests that we may have in this newly found phenomenon an indicator of the distribution of potential throughout a galaxy.

*The Egyptian picture of the sky:* O. NEUGEBAUER (introduced by C. A. Kraus). Egyptian and Babylonian astronomy are usually quoted as equivalent foundations for Greek, and therefore medieval and modern, astronomy. But in spite of this fact only very little was known about Egyptian astronomy. Since Brugsch published in 1883 his fundamental collection of different inscriptions of an astronomical character, detailed studies on the history of astronomical concepts in Egypt have been made in only two fields, namely Borchardt's investigations on Egyptian sundials and waterclocks and Pogo's studies on the so-called Decan-starlists on coffin lids belonging to the period *ca.* 2000 B.C. This situation is the more remarkable because in the meantime the impressive structure of the Babylonian theoretical astronomy has become more and more unveiled, showing clearly that Greek astronomy was based on Babylonian knowledge, leaving practically no space for an Egyptian influence. This situation has now, in the meantime, become understandable by the investigation of different Demotic astronomical texts, showing that the Egyptian methods of treating the moon-phenomena and the movement of the planets were only very approximate and without any consideration of details. This picture of Egyptian astronomy is now completed by a Demotic text recently purchased by the Egyptological Institute in Copenhagen, which shows us how the aspect of the sky, the setting and rising of the stars, was connected with religious myths. This text explains the famous picture of the star-goddess Nut, who is represented as bending over the earth, touching with her feet and hands respectively the eastern and western borders of the earth. We learn from this text how the Egyptians interpreted mythologically the invisibility of shifting groups of stars, and how the discovery that this invisibility of stars is merely due to the vicinity of the sun deeply influenced these religious concepts. On the other hand, the close connection of religion, especially as far as the underworld is concerned, with the changing aspect of the sky during the year explains that the main interest of Egyptian astronomy was not a mathematically detailed description of very complex effects, but merely a rough scheme, just good enough to reflect the main traces of the observed facts.

*On the decomposition of transitive permutation groups generated by the symmetric group:* J. S. FRAME (introduced by C. A. Kraus). Every subgroup $H$ of the symmetric group $G$ of degree $n$ generates a transitive permutation group $G_H$ on the cosets $HS_i$ of $G$ with respect to $H$, which orders to an element $R$ of $G$ the permutation $HS_i \rightarrow HS_iR = HS_j$. If we restrict $R$ to the elements of $H$, the cosets which are then permuted among themselves will form aggregates $HS_iH$ called double cosets. Now if $G_H$ is written as a group of permutation matrices and completely reduced, the sum of the squares of the multiplicities of the irreducible components is equal to the number of double cosets $HS_iH$. We show in this paper that the number of self-inverse double cosets, with respect to a subgroup $H$ of $G$ which is the direct product of symmetric groups, is equal to the sum of the multiplicities of the irreducible components of $G_H$. In the proof the double cosets are displayed in a series of squares each having a side equal to the multiplicity of an irreducible component of $G_H$ and having inverse double cosets symmetrically placed with respect to the diagonal. This generalizes a diagram of G. deB. Robinson in a recent paper "On the Representations of the Symmetric Group," in which the elements themselves (double cosets with respect to the identity subgroup) are similarly displayed. Use is made of the theory of lattice permutations introduced by P. A. MacMahon and developed by D. E. Littlewood, A. R. Richardson and G. deB. Robinson.

*On drawings composed of uniform straight lines:* G. D. BIRKHOFF. The question considered is a curious one, dealing with the kinds of drawings in the plane which can be made by a pen or pencil which makes many uniform rectilinear strokes of very narrow width. For instance, the depth of blackness may vary inversely as the distance from a fixed point, tending from black through diminishing grayness towards whiteness at remote points. The mathematics involved leads to a generalization of an integral equation, due to Abel.

*A new method in statistical mechanics:* NORBERT WIENER and BROCKWAY MCMILLAN. The authors integrate the differential equations of motion of a system of similar particles acted on by central forces in such a way as to give symmetric functions of these particles in terms of the time and of symmetric functions of the initial positions and velocities of the system. They then introduce a process of averaging with respect to the initial parameters which gives the averages of the symmetric functions in terms of the time alone. Finally they let the time become infinite and obtain asymptotic values of these averages. In this way they arrive at the equation of state of a gas. Similar methods can be used for liquids.

*Respiratory metabolism of mammalian eggs and embryos:* EDGAR J. BOELL and JOHN S. NICHOLAS (introduced by L. L. Woodruff). The respiratory metabolism of rat eggs and embryos during the earliest stages of development has been measured by means of a micromanometer based on the principle of the Cartesian diver in an attempt to discover possible relationships between morphological development and physiological activity. The delicacy of the method can be appreciated by the fact that the oxygen consumption of as few as six to ten eggs, corresponding to a dry weight of approximately 0.0002 milligram, can be measured with a fair degree of accuracy. The eggs were obtained by excising the oviducts of fertilized females at definite intervals after copulation. The oviducts, when cut into small pieces, extrude the ova by peristaltic activity. The embryos were obtained, by surgically freeing them from associated maternal and extraembryonic structures within the uterus. The preparation of eggs and embryos for respiratory studies was performed under approximately sterile conditions, and, as a rule, approximately one hour elapsed between the administration of anesthetic and the beginning of readings on respiration. The oxygen consumption averages 0.00073 cu mm per egg per hour. No significant differences have so far appeared in the respiration of one-cell and eight-cell eggs, for development at this time involves merely the division of the egg into a number of smaller units with no perceptible increase in the actual mass of respiring material. When embryonic growth occurs, the oxygen consumed accurately reflects the increase in embryonic mass. On the eighth day of development the oxygen used per embryo amounts to approximately 0.01 cu mm per hour, and during the next two days, during which embryonic organization occurs, this figure is increased twenty times. The influence of various metabolites on the maintenance of embryonic respiration *in vitro* suggests that carbohydrate is easily utilized as a primary energy source during early mammalian development.

*The eye in relation to chromatophoral color changes in animals:* G. H. PARKER. As a rule fishes with only one eye respond by color changes to differences in their environment as successfully as do those with two eyes. In this respect the trout has long been known to be peculiar, for on the loss of one eye it darkens contralaterally. The common catfish, *Ameiurus nebulosus,* when deprived of one eye conforms neither to the general rule for fishes nor to the special one for the trout. A one-eyed catfish is at first very dark, after which it may change slowly in tint according to its environment, though without ever becoming fully pale. Such fishes may finally assume in the same environment somewhat different tints and retain these with considerable individual persistence. This diversity appears not to be due to variations in the irritability of the orbital wound which might influence to various degrees the stumps of the optic nerve. The cause of these more or less characteristic color differences is unknown. In these respects one-eyed catfishes are unlike any other fish thus far described. The fact that intermedin, the secretion from the pituitary gland, plays a very important part in the color changes in catfishes and that in this fish chromatophoral nerves, both dispersing and concentrating, are less significant than the pituitary gland, may be the occasion of the difference between Ameiurus and most other teleosts whose chromatophores are often under almost exclusively nervous control.

*The effect of dissolved substances on regeneration in Planaria maculata:* J. WALTER WILSON (introduced by W. S. Hunter). Flatworms with heads removed by a transverse cut and placed in four fifths Ringer's fluid, fail to close the wound but regenerate a head by producing two lateral half heads, which are later united by a bridge of tissue which grows forward ventral to the wound. The result is a head, at first notched at the tip, but later normal in shape, with an open wound just behind the eyes. This is of interest because of its bearing on three problems: (1) wound closure; (2) source of the cells of the blastema; (3) origin of organization in the blastema. The following experiments were performed in an attempt to discover how the four fifths Ringer's fluid acts: Worms were cut transversely and permitted to regenerate. (1) In six tenths-, seven tenths-, and eight tenths-Ringer's fluid. The wound closed in some worms in seven tenths and most of them in six tenths. Previous experiments had shown that closure occurs in all lower concentrations. (2) In similar solutions after three days in the same concentrations. This exposure previous to the cut did not change the result. (3) In separate solutions containing the individual salts of Ringer's fluid in concentrations that they occur in the four fifths. (4) In four fifths Ringer with KCl, $CaCl_2$ or both left out, and also with KCl, $CaCl_2$ or both doubled. (5) In glucose solution isosmotic with four fifths Ringer's fluid. In all solutions approximately isosmotic with four fifths Ringer's fluid, the wounds failed to close and, if the worms lived, regeneration like that in the four fifths Ringer's fluid occurred. In all more dilute solutions the wounds closed and regeneration occurred as in water unless the solution proved toxic. It is concluded that the effect is due to the osmotic pressure of the solution and not to its chemical nature. It is suggested that it is produced because the isotonic solutions have a weaker stimulating effect on the exposed tissues than the more dilute solutions and water.

*Effect of induced polyploidy on doubleness and flecking in flowers of Portulaca grandiflora:* A. F. BLAKESLEE and H. E. WARMKE. In *Portulaca* the gene for double flowers (D) is dominant to the gene for singles (d). Full doubles ($D_2$) do not set seed; semi-doubles (Dd), however, are fully fertile. In diploids there are two types of doubles ($D_2$ and Dd); in tetraploids there may be four. The two new double types are $D_3d$ and $Dd_3$. The homozygous tetraploid ($D_4$) corresponds to the homozygous diploid ($D_2$) and does not set seed. The tetraploid $D_3d$ type is fertile. The tetraploid $D_2d_2$ corresponds in doubleness to the diploid Dd. The tetraploid $Dd_3$ has flowers with at most only a few extra petals. If segregation is in accord with random assortment of 4 chromosomes the plant-breeder could guarantee that all the seeds from selfing a $D_3d$ parent would be high-grade doubles. If segregation followed random assortment of 8 chromatids, there should be not over 0.13 per cent. singles. In certain races, red flecks occur on white flowers, due to dominant somatic mutations. In diploids the number of flecks per petal is from 2 to 6 times as frequent as in what appears to be comparable tetraploid material. Since there are twice as many chromosomes per cell in tetraploids one would expect twice as many mutations leading to an increased number of flecks per flower. This appears not to be the case, even if account is taken of the fact that there are slightly fewer cells per tetraploid flower. Our present interpretation is that tetraploidy in some way reduces the mutation rate in individual chromosomes.

*The genera of the Boletaceae:* WALTER H. SNELL (introduced by Charles Thom). The classification of the Boletaceae most widely accepted in Europe and America has contained four genera: *Strobilomyces, Boletinus, Boletus* and *Gyrodon,* with *Boletus* containing all but 14 of the species arranged in 13 subgroups. The genera and the subgroups of *Boletus* are separated on the basis of gross morphological features of the carpophore. Some of the subgroups of *Boletus* as now constituted differ more from one another than *Boletus* does from the other genera, especially *Boletinus.* In the belief that spore characters are more fundamental as a basis for classification and that the use of them will provide a more natural and usable arrangement of the species in this family, it is proposed to adopt the scheme of Gilbert with certain modifications and made up as follows: subfamily Boleteae, with smooth spores containing the following genera—*Phylloporus, Boletinellus* (a segregate from *Boletinus*), *Boletinus, Ixocomus* (the present Viscipelles), *Pulveroboletus* (the Pulverulenti), *Xerocomus* (the present Subpruinosi and Subtomentosi), *Boletus* (including the Calopodes, Edules and Luridi), *Tylopilus* (the Hyporhodii), *Trachypus* (the Versipelles), *Porphyrellus* (containing two pilose, reddish-spored species), *Gyroporus* (the Cariosi), *Gyrodon,* and a new genus for three species with very small spores; subfamily Strobilomyceteae, with ornamented spores, containing the genera *Strobilomyces* (with globose, reticulate spores), *Boletellus* (with large, elliptical spores longitudinally striated or verrucose spores), and *Polyporoletus* (with spherical, warted spores).

*Cytogenetic strains in certain species of grasses:* GEORGE L. CHURCH (introduced by Charles Thom). In studies correlating polyploidy with species differentiation and geographic distribution in three genera of grasses, some cases of cytological differences are found within the limits of the species. Most of the forms of *Spartina patens* (Ait.) Muhl. are hexaploids, as well as two allied varieties that are usually recognized as distinct species; *i.e., Spartina caespitosa* A. A. Eaton and *Spartina bakeri* Merr. However, a tetraploid form is occasionally found in Massachusetts and a tall, robust, octoploid type is reported from Florida. Coastal specimens of *Spartina pectinata* Link. are hexaploid, but a Nebraska strain is dodecaploid. It is thought that in New England the hexaploid *S. caespitosa* could arise as a cross between *S. pectinata* and *S. patens.* The early-flowering, strand forms of *Spartina alterniflora* Lois. are octoploid, while the taller, robust, late-flowering forms of tidal lagoons are decaploid. The widely distributed *Panicum virgatum* L. is tetraploid, but a smaller strain with pilose leaves from Oklahoma is octoploid. The latter occurred in a planting of a large tetraploid strain. In the genus *Andropogon,* western strains of *A. haillii* Hack. and *A. provincialis* Lam. are hexaploid, but specimens with an extra monoploid complement are found. The lack of polyploidy in the southern strains of *A. virginicus* L. thus far studied is attributed to the fact that the probable parents, typical *A. virginicus* L. and *A. glomeratus* (Walt.) B.S.P. are both diploids.

*Biographical memoir of Julius Stieglitz:* W. A. NOYES.

*Biographical memoir of Graham Lusk:* E. F. DUBOIS.

*Biographical memoir of Elihu Thomson:* K. T. COMPTON.

*Biographical memoir of Ernest William Brown:* FRANK SCHLESINGER and DIRK BROUWER.

*Biographical memoir of George Ellery Hale:* WALTER S. ADAMS.

# SCIENTIFIC EVENTS

## THE EXPOSITION OF CHEMICAL INDUSTRIES

THE seventeenth Exposition of Chemical Industries will be held at Grand Central Palace, New York, from December 4 to 9. Three floors have been reserved for the exhibit, and nearly 300 exhibitors, representing over forty industries, have engaged space.

Chemicals, chemical raw materials and fabricated materials will be shown in terms of their manufacture and use. One exhibit will be devoted to carbon monoxide and its use as a reagent in educational, industrial and commercial laboratories. In the field of drying agents a soluble anhydride, the result of research on the fundamental nature and behavior of hydrates of calcium sulfate, will be demonstrated. Applications range from refrigeration to the drying of cable splices in the telephone and telegraph industries, also a new large-scale process for the dehydration of serums from the frozen state.

Materials of construction will include acid and corrosion proof linings for tanks, towers, process equipment, also for electrolytic refining tanks and for acid water and oil-proof linings which will be demonstrated in their uses for pickling tanks and acid disposal equipment, also for electrolytic refining tanks, and for acid sludge in petroleum refineries.

The field of precision instruments will include the latest types of temperature and pressure measuring devices. There will be a vibration proof potentiometer controller, a recorder controller pyrometer for throttling fuel heat and a new line of rectangular-case indicating recorders and controllers with nine-, ten- and twelve-inch charts for temperature and pressure. Other instruments of precision will include a machine to determine plasticity. Measurement by this instrument is said to provide an accurate index to changes in the material caused by different temperatures, addition of ingredients or fillers, breakdown action of catalysts, etc. A new recording viscosimeter offers a spiral drive thermometer, the first of its kind to be manufactured, which governs a constant speed temperature increase of the suspension to be measured.

One exhibit will display meters for measuring and integrating accurately the quantity of liquids passed through closed pipes—to permit knowledge of the cost of liquids metered, to facilitate control of the use of liquids and to assure accurate manufacture of products containing a liquid.

There will be a complete range of process equipment, including steam jacketed kettles and tanks, made from stainless steel, monel metal and pure nickel. Glass-lined steel equipment will be demonstrated, and especially acid-resistant units will be offered for high-pressure work.

## THE TROPICAL FLOWER GARDEN OF THE NEW YORK BOTANICAL GARDEN

A NEW tropical flower garden in the main conservatories at the New York Botanical Garden will be opened to the public on the week-end of November 4. Members of the garden will attend a formal opening in a brief ceremony the preceding afternoon; on Saturday morning the public will have its first view of the completed garden, which, with the rest of the greenhouse, will be open daily without charge from 10 to 4.

Taking part in the ceremony will be Dr. William J. Robbins, director; Allyn R. Jennings, general superintendent of parks; Colonel Robert H. Montgomery, representing the board of managers of the garden, and Mrs. Elon Huntington Hooker, president of the advisory council.

The occasion will also mark the opening of the indoor floral displays for the 1939–40 season. These displays, in which from two to five thousand pots of flowering and foliage plants are used at a time, have brought nearly half a million people to the garden since the newly rebuilt conservatory range was opened less than a year ago.

The new tropical flower garden, which is one of fifteen units in the conservatory range, contains many plants with which travelers in the tropics are familiar, and also decorative plants which are rarely seen either in southern regions where they would grow outdoors or in northern conservatories. A few are cultivated only at the New York Botanical Garden.

The tropical flower garden is the tenth specially planted house to be opened since the large greenhouse was rebuilt by the city during 1937 and 1938. First to be seen in their new quarters were the cacti and other succulent plants which are natives of the great deserts of the world. The Botanical Garden has more than 2,000 different kinds, the true cacti in one house, the other New World succulents (which are plants with fleshy leaves or stems) in another, and the succulents of the Old World in a third.

Last year at Christmas time a tropical rain forest house was opened, and adjoining it a tropical fern house, both naturalistically planted. A special house, which was opened in the spring, contains plants of the Aroid family, including the spectacular genus Amorphophallus, one of whose members bears the flower known as the largest in the world. Adjoining it is the aquatic house, where a specimen of the royal waterlily, *Victoria regia,* now is in bloom. Other houses, containing palms, economic plants, begonias and other subjects, are open to the public, although the planting arrangement in them is not yet complete.

## REORGANIZATION OF LABORATORY DIRECTORS' CONFERENCE

A REORGANIZATION of the Conference of State Laboratory Directors was effected at its nineteenth annual meeting in Pittsburgh on October 16, when a constitution and by-laws were adopted changing the name and expanding the organization into a Conference of State and Provincial Public Health Laboratory Directors with full membership privileges limited to directors of official state and provincial public health laboratories. The committee on reorganization which proposed the constitutional changes was composed of the following members representing laboratories widely scattered geographically throughout the United States and Canada: E. M. Bramhall, Utah; L. F. Ey, Ohio; M. H. McCrady, Quebec; Dr. C. A. Perry, Maryland; Dr. E. S. Robinson, Massachusetts; Dr. T. F. Sellers, Georgia; Dr. H. J. Shaughnessy, Illinois; Dr. A. B. Wadsworth, New York, and Dr. Friend Lee Mickle, Connecticut, *chairman.*

Associate membership was made available to the responsible assistants of directors of state and provincial laboratories and to the directors and responsible assistants in municipal and other official public health laboratories in the two countries.

In the newly adopted constitution it is stated that the purposes and objects of the conference shall be to promote the development, improvement and effectiveness of public health laboratory service; to coordinate public health laboratory activities; to stimulate the interchange of experience among directors of official public health laboratories; to develop and maintain adequate standards for the professional training of public health laboratory personnel; to encourage constant effort toward the improvement and standardization of technical methods; to collect and make accessible to all persons in official administrative positions in public health laboratories such information and data as might be of assistance to them in the proper fulfilment of their duties.

It is proposed in the by-laws that the conference continue to meet annually at the place of the annual meeting of the American Public Health Association on the day preceding the opening date. Scientific and business meetings open to the entire membership have been provided for, as well as executive sessions limited to full members for action on matters of policy affecting state or provincial public health laboratories. The conference will continue issuing annually a mimeographed volume of proceedings which will be furnished to members and sold to others as in the past.

The officers and councilors elected for 1939–40, all directors of state laboratories, are: *Chairman,* Dr. Friend Lee Mickle, Connecticut; *Vice-chairman,* L. F. Ey, Ohio; *Secretary-Treasurer,* Miss K. E. Cox, West Virginia; *Councilors,* Dr. T. F. Sellers, Georgia, and Dr. E. S. Robinson, Massachusetts.

## IN HONOR OF DR. EVARTS AMBROSE GRAHAM

THE former and present pupils and associates of Dr. Evarts Ambrose Graham, Bixby professor of surgery at Washington University, Saint Louis, celebrated recently the twentieth anniversary of his professorship. Scientific sessions were held on October 11 and 12, and a dinner in his honor was given on the night of the twelfth.

At this dinner public tributes were given by Dr. Philip A. Shaffer, dean of the department of medicine at Washington University; Dr. Allen O. Whipple, professor of surgery, Columbia University, and president of the American Surgical Association; Dr. J. A. Hayden, of Melbourne, Australia, and by Dr. Malvern B. Clopton, clinical professor of surgery of Washington University and president of the corporation of this institution.

In addition to the presentation of a scrapbook and silver, there was announced the establishment of the Graham Lectureship to be given annually in Saint Louis. Dr. Graham received tributes by letter and telegram from all over the world. There were present about forty-five of his former pupils from scattered points. Several guests expected from abroad were prevented from attending by the war. An abstract of the proceedings is to be published in *Surgery.*

## NOMINATIONS FOR PRESIDENT-ELECT OF THE AMERICAN CHEMICAL SOCIETY

LOCAL sections of the American Chemical Society have proposed for nomination for president-elect the following members:

H. S. Booth, professor of chemistry, Western Reserve University.

Sidney M. Caldwell, director of Development Division, Tire Department, U. S. Rubber Company.

William Mansfield Clark, professor of physiological chemistry, the Johns Hopkins University.

M. L. Crossley, director of research, the Calco Chemical Company, Bound Brook, N. J.

Gustavus J. Esselen, president and treasurer, Gustavus J. Esselen, Inc.

William Lloyd Evans, professor of chemistry and chairman, the Ohio State University.

Francis C. Frary, director of research, Aluminum Company of America.

Per K. Frolich, director of the Chemical Laboratories, The Standard Oil Development Company.

Harry N. Holmes, professor of chemistry and head of the department at Oberlin College.

Henry G. Knight, since 1927 chief of the Bureau of Agricultural Chemistry and Engineering, U. S. Department of Agriculture.

Townes R. Leigh, acting vice-president of the College of Arts and Sciences, University of Florida.

R. E. Swain, head of the department of chemistry, Stanford University.

Floyd E. Bartell, professor of chemistry, the University of Michigan.

## RECENT DEATHS AND MEMORIALS

DR. MARGARET FLOY WASHBURN, professor emeritus of psychology at Vassar College, died on October 29 at the age of sixty-eight years.

HENRY CLAY ANDERSON, dean of the College of Engineering of the University of Michigan, died on October 14 at the age of sixty-six years.

PROFESSOR WILLIAM JORDAN SWEETSER, since 1915 head of the department of mechanical engineering at the University of Maine, died on October 15. He was sixty-five years old.

DR. RODOLPHO VON IHERING died in São Paulo, Brazil, on September 15, at the age of 56 years. At the time of his death he was chief of the Serviço Federal de Piscicultura, Rio de Janeiro.

R. S. TROUP, professor of forestry in the University of Oxford and fellow of St. Johns College, from 1924 to 1935 director of the Imperial Forestry Institute, died on October 1, aged sixty-four years.

DR. G. M. MURRAY, emeritus professor of medicine in the Victoria University of Manchester, known for his work on diseases of the thyroid gland, died on September 21.

DR. EDOUARD BUGNION, professor emeritus of the Medical Faculty and the University Faculty of Lausanne, died on July 4 in his ninety-fourth year. He was known for his work on the anatomy and histology of invertebrates.

PROFESSOR GIULIO SIROVICH, professor of chemistry in the University of Rome and director of the National Institute of Metallurgical Chemistry, was killed in an automobile accident on October 4.

A MEMORIAL meeting in honor of the late Dean Herman Schneider, of the University of Cincinnati, founder of the plan of cooperative technical education, will be held at the University of Cincinnati on November 5. President Raymond Walters will preside, and addresses will be made by Dr. Charles F. Kettering, vice-president of the General Motors Corporation; Dr. Parke R. Kolbe, president of the Drexel Institute of Technology, Philadelphia, Pa., and Dr. Frank W. Chandler, professor of English and comparative literature in the College of Liberal Arts.

# SCIENTIFIC NOTES AND NEWS

THE Nobel Prize for physiology and medicine for 1939 has been awarded to Dr. Gerhard Domagk, of the German I. G. Farbenindustrie, in recognition of his work with protonsil, forerunner of sulfanilamide and similar chemical compounds for the treatment of streptococcus infections. The prize for 1938, which was held over from 1938, has been awarded to Dr. Corneille Heymans, professor of pharmaco-dynamics at the University of Ghent, Belgium, in recognition of his work on the sinus aorta mechanism in breathing. Dr. Domagk is reported to be awaiting the approval of the German Government before accepting the prize.

DR. EDWARD A. DOISY, professor of biological chemistry and director of the department of the School of Medicine of the St. Louis University, received the seventh annual St. Louis Award, at a public ceremony held in the mayor's office on October 26. The award, $1,000 and a certificate, is the gift of an anonymous donor. The certificate states that Dr. Doisy was chosen: "For his brilliant investigations and research which resulted in the discovery, isolation and synthesis of the vitamin that checks hemorrhage."

THE Perkin Medal, given annually by the Society of Chemical Industry for "valuable work in applied chemistry," has been awarded to Dr. Charles M. A. Stine, vice-president in charge of research of E. I. du Pont de Nemours and Company. The Chemical Industry Medal has been awarded to Dr. Robert E. Wilson, president of the Pan American Petroleum and Transport Company.

THE annual Progress Medal of the Society of Motion Picture Engineers was presented on October 18 at the semi-annual dinner to Dr. Loyd A. Jones, since 1916 chief physicist of the laboratories of the Eastman Kodak Company, in recognition of his contributions to motion picture technology.

THE Franklin Institute of the State of Pennsylvania has made its first award of the Vermilye Medal "in recognition of outstanding contribution in the field of industrial management" to Lewis H. Brown, president of the Johns-Manville Corporation, New York. Presentation of the medal will be made in Philadelphia on November 14. It is named after its donor, William M. Vermilye, vice-president of the National City Bank of New York.

AT the graduation ceremony of the University of St. Andrews on October 6 the honorary degree of doctor of laws was conferred on Dr. Alexander Mackenzie, from 1914 until his retirement with the title emeritus in 1938 professor of chemistry in University College, Dundee.

THE Chicago Branch of the American Association of Scientific Workers at its October meeting elected the following officers and members of the executive committee: Professor Arthur H. Compton, *chairman;* Dr. Zelma Baker, *secretary-treasurer;* Professor Anton J. Carlson, Dr. Ralph W. Gerard, Dr. Victor E. Johnson and Dr. Benjamin F. Miller, *members.*

DR. LOUIS M. MASSEY, professor of plant pathology at Cornell University, was elected president of the American Rose Society at the recent Brooklyn meeting.

DR. P. S. BURGESS has returned as dean of the College of Agriculture of the University of Arizona and director of the Experiment Station, after spending a year in a similar capacity at the Rhode Island College. Dr. R. S. Hawkins, who has served as acting dean and acting director, has been appointed vice-dean and vice-director in addition to reassuming his position as head of the department of agronomy.

DR. WILLARD M. ALLEN, associate professor of obstetrics and gynecology at the Medical School of the University of Rochester, New York, has been appointed professor of obstetrics and gynecology in the Medical School of Washington University, St. Louis. Dr. Otto H. Schwarz, who for eleven years has been head of the department, has expressed his desire to be relieved of the administrative responsibilities of the conduct of the department in order that he may have time to engage in consulting practice.

*Nature* states that W. C. Wilson, director of the unit for clinical research in surgery at Edinburgh Royal Infirmary, has been appointed regius professor of surgery in the University of Edinburgh.

Dr. M. J. Murray, head of the department of chemistry, and Dr. Forrest F. Cleveland, head of the departments of physics and mathematics of Lynchburg College, have been appointed to assistant professorships of chemistry and physics, respectively, at the Armour Institute of Technology, Chicago. They will continue their joint research on the Raman effect and molecular structure.

Dr. Alfred Blalock, professor of surgery, Vanderbilt University School of Medicine, and Dr. Homer W. Smith, professor of physiology in the New York University College of Medicine, have been appointed members of the Medical Fellowship Board of the National Research Council for the period ending June 30, 1941.

Professor George Erle Beggs, of Princeton University, has been elected chairman of the Engineering Foundation. Dr. O. E. Buckley, executive vice-president of the Bell Telephone Laboratories, New York, has been elected vice-president; Otis E. Hovey has been reelected director, and John H. R. Arms has been reelected secretary.

Dr. Esmond R. Long, director of the Phipps Institute, Philadelphia, has been elected a member of the Medical Research Committee and of the Committee on Standards of Undergraduate Education of the National Tuberculosis Association.

Richard W. Jackson, associate professor of biochemistry at the Cornell University Medical College, has been appointed chief of the Protein Division of the Eastern Regional Research Laboratory at Wyndmoor, Pa., of the U. S. Department of Agriculture, where he will be in charge of research on the isolation and properties of proteins available from agricultural products.

Parke, Davis and Company have renewed their fellowships on Cascara and Vitamin C in the department of chemistry of the University of Pittsburgh. Robert W. Liddell, of the University of Pittsburgh, has been reappointed fellow, and Kenneth A. Kuiken has been appointed Vitamin C fellow. The Abbott Laboratories, Incorporated, also have provided a Vitamin C fellowship, to which Howard H. Fricke, of Washington State College, has been appointed. Dr. C. G. King, professor of biochemistry, is directing the researches.

Dr. George L. McNew, fellow at the Rockefeller Institute for Medical Research, Princeton, N. J., has been appointed chief of research in plant pathology at the New York State Agricultural Experiment Station.

Leonard J. Goss, pathologist for the department of animal pathology of the Kentucky Agricultural Experiment Station, has been appointed veterinarian at the New York Zoological Park.

According to *Nature* Professor Kanichi Terazawa, dean of the faculty of science of Tokyo Imperial University, has succeeded Professor Mishio Ishimoto as director of the Earthquake Research Institute. Professor Ishimoto will continue his work as a member of the institute.

Dr. Mortier F. Barrus, professor of plant pathology at Cornell University, sailed on September 29 for Venezuela to organize extension workers there and to help to overcome plant disease problems. Dr. Carlos S. Chardon, formerly president of the University of Puerto Rico, is one of his co-workers.

The Medical Aid Committee for Spanish Refugees announces that under its auspices Dr. Emilio Mira, professor of psychiatry in the faculty of medicine of the University of Barcelona, will spend two weeks in the United States prior to taking up his work as director of mental hygiene for the Cuban Government.

Dr. C. A. Elvehjem, professor of biochemistry at the College of Agriculture of the University of Wisconsin, will deliver the second Harvey Society lecture of the current series at the New York Academy of Medicine on November 16. He will speak on "The Biological Significance of Nicotinic Acid."

Dr. Edward R. Weidlein, director of the Mellon Institute of Industrial Research, gave the principal address at the dedication of the Paul Mellon Science Hall of the Choate School at Wallingford, Conn. The building is the gift of Paul Mellon, son of the late Andrew W. Mellon.

Dr. George B. Cressey, of Syracuse University, gave on October 25 an illustrated lecture on "China, Its Natural Resources and Their Significance" before the Smith College Chapter of Sigma Xi. During the afternoon he spoke to the members of the Department of Geology on "Pioneering in Siberia."

Dr. Ernest W. Goodpasture, professor of pathology at the Vanderbilt University School of Medicine, Nashville, gave a series of lectures before the Portland Academy of Medicine from October 23 to 25. His subjects were "Investigations of Virus Infections and Immunity by Means of Chick Embryo Technic"; "Experimental Bacterial Infections of the Chick Embryo" and "A Consideration of Pathogenesis of Virus and Bacterial Infection, with a Review of Some Virus Diseases."

Speakers at the ninth annual Forum on Current Problems of *The New York Herald Tribune* included Dr. James Bryant Conant, president of Harvard University; Dr. Arthur H. Compton, professor of physics at the University of Chicago; George Washington Carver, professor of chemistry at Tuskegee Institute; Dr. Perrin H. Long, associate professor of medicine at the Johns Hopkins University; Dr. Foster Kennedy, professor of neurology at Cornell University Medical College, and Dr. Francis Carter Wood, director of the Crocker Institute for Cancer Research, Columbia University.

DR. HARLOW SHAPLEY, Dr. Otto Glasser and Dr. Paul B. Sears are among the speakers announced by Cooper Union, New York City, in a series of lectures entitled "Adventures in Ideas" extending from October to April. They speak in the Sunday evening series, which will be held each week, with the exception of December 24 and 31, at 8:00 P.M., and which will be broadcast over station WQXR.

FELLOWSHIPS in the medical sciences, administered by the Medical Fellowship Board of the National Research Council, of which Dr. Francis G. Blake, of Yale University, is chairman, will be available for the year beginning July 1. These fellowships are open to citizens of the United States or Canada who possess an M.D. or a Ph.D. degree. They are intended for recent graduates and not for those already professionally established. Fellows will be appointed at a meeting of the board about March 1. Applications to receive consideration must be filed on or before January 1, 1940. Appointments may begin on any date determined by the board. For further particulars concerning these fellowships, address the Secretary of the Medical Fellowship Board, National Research Council, 2101 Constitution Avenue, Washington, D. C.

THE National Association of Manufacturers is planning to extend specific recognition to science, in the form of awards to "outstanding contemporary scientists who will be selected as modern pioneers." The first occasion on which these awards will be bestowed is at the celebration of the one hundred and fiftieth anniversary of the American Patent System on February 27. Dr. Karl T. Compton, president of Massachusetts Institute of Technology, has been elected chairman of a committee of six scientific men who will make the selection. The other members are Dr. Forest R. Moulton, permanent secretary of the American Association for the Advancement of Science; Dr. George B. Pegram, dean of the Graduate School, Columbia University; Professor John T. Tate, professor of physics and dean of the College of Science, Literature and Art and director of University College of the University of Minnesota; Dr. Edward R. Weidlein, director of the Mellon Institute for Industrial Research, Pittsburgh, and Professor Frank C. Whitmore, research professor of organic chemistry and dean of the School of Chemistry and Physics at the Pennsylvania State College. The association has asked its members and trade groups and scientific societies to send nominations to its offices at 14 West Forty-ninth Street before December 1. A special committee of eighty industrialists has been appointed to promote the search for "modern pioneers." The chairman is Robert L. Lund, executive vice-president of the Lambert Pharmacal Company.

THE twelfth annual Graduate Fortnight of the New York Academy of Medicine was opened on October 23 with an address of welcome by Dr. Malcolm Goodridge, president of the academy. This year the subject discussed is "The Endocrine Glands and Their Disorders." Seven hundred visiting physicians, in addition to the 2,300 fellows of the academy, registered. Twenty-two clinical conferences and demonstrations were arranged to be held in seventeen of the hospitals of New York City, and eight round table conferences have been organized. Ten evening meetings, during which addresses were delivered by twenty-three speakers drawn from the leading universities and research institutions of the United States and Canada, were held, at which the speakers included: Dr. H. M. Evans, director of the Institute of Experimental Biology of the University of California; Dr. J. B. Collip, professor of biochemistry, McGill University; Dr. Elmer L. Sevringhaus, professor of medicine, the University of Wisconsin; Dr. Walter B. Cannon, professor of physiology, Harvard University; Dr. Robert F. Loeb, professor of medicine, Columbia University; Dr. C. N. H. Long, Sterling professor of physiological chemistry, Yale University; Dr. R. T. Woodyatt, clinical professor of medicine, Rush Medical College; Dr. John F. Fulton, Sterling professor of physiology, Yale University; Dr. William G. MacCallum, professor of pathology, the Johns Hopkins University, and Dr. Philip E. Smith, professor of anatomy, Columbia University. The scientific exhibit, which covers many aspects of endocrinology, is in the building of the New York Academy of Medicine.

THE winter meeting of the Industrial Research Institute will be held in Chicago on Friday and Saturday, December 8 and 9. The institute, an affiliate of the National Research Council, has a membership made up of executives who manage scientific research for large and small industries in the United States. Members of the institute will be the guests of Swift and Company at its laboratories on Friday morning and afternoon. The Friday evening and Saturday sessions will be held at the Hotel Stevens.

THE policy to be followed by the Royal Institution during the war has been under consideration by the managers, who have decided to maintain its activities so far as possible. The libraries and reading rooms will be kept open as usual. Although the present lighting restrictions prohibit the holding of the Friday evening meetings, a series of afternoon lectures is being arranged.

THE Royal Society, London, will function normally

during the war; the administrative office has been moved to Trinity College, Cambridge, and it is probable that the meetings of the society will be held in that town.

THE celebration of the centenary of the Royal Microscopical Society in October has been postponed. It may be found necessary for the time being to curtail the number of ordinary meetings normally held in London during the session. Arrangements are being made to continue publication of the society's journal as usual.

THE new mechanical parts plant of the Spencer Lens Company was opened formally on October 26. The operations of each department were demonstrated, and there was an exhibit of scientific optical instruments.

# DISCUSSION

## THE WAR AND CHRONICA BOTANICA

THE impact of the European war on science has already been felt in the United States through the cancellation of foreign subscriptions to American scientific journals and to services like *Biological Abstracts*. The same is true in other neutral nations as well as among the belligerents, no doubt. An obligation rests upon every scientific society and association in this country to consider the effects of the war situation and to join forces in preserving, as far as may be possible, essential scientific publishing and abstracting services until normal conditions return.

A colleague permits the writer to quote from a letter from the editor of *Chronica Botanica,* the international plant science news-magazine. The letter is signed by Dr. Frans Verdoorn, who writes in September from Leiden, Holland (Postoffice Box 8) as follows:

> The present war which is expected to be a lengthy one makes it impossible for me to continue *Chronica Botanica.* About a fortnight ago my morning mail dropped from about 60 pieces to 12 and hardly any information or money is being received. I can still finish this year's *Chronica* and am doing so, but that will be all. This country of course is neutral and there is a fair chance that it will remain so, but that does not help me much as I am wholly dependent on information and subscriptions from countries now in war, from which I do not hear anything.
>
> My wife and I gave 5 years to building up the *Chronica* and we are in great distress that we should have to stop it. And I will have to do so as the post which I will have to accept under the circumstances in the very near future, is in Java, . . . but one can not do any international work there. It is out of question to continue the *Chronica* there.
>
> I feel, however, that it would be possible to continue the *Chronica* in some form in the States. Even if the States would be involved in a war, I could continue it there with the aid of North and South American editors, and it would still remain self-supporting. But I would need some kind of post for my own living, as—at least during the war—there will be hardly any profits on the *Chronica.* . . .
>
> Even if I had a minor post to start with, I would be able to continue my *Chronica* in the States during the war, and that is the only thing that matters at present.
>
> I am asking this not on behalf of myself, as there are for me personally suitable posts, but on behalf of the *Chronica* which during the past year has become a symbol to its 2,000 readers, a symbol of good will and cooperation, which I am most anxious to continue.

Any suggestions which may disclose possibilities for the continuance of *Chronica Botanica* should be sent immediately to Dr. Frans Verdoorn, Editor, *Chronica Botanica,* P. O. Box 8, Leiden, Holland. Dr. Verdoorn's ability as a plant scientist is widely recognized and the unique editorial services he has rendered to his professional colleagues all over the world through the medium of *Chronica Botanica* are deeply appreciated. It would be a permanent international scientific loss if *Chronica Botanica* should be forced to suspend on account of the war. Is there not a way out?

ROBERT F. GRIGGS

## REMARKS ON THE CENTER OF POPULATION

THIS note is written to draw attention to an erroneous statement made at the end of the paper on "Centers of Population of Learned Groups," by C. B. Read.[1]

In the paper referred to the center of a population the $n$ members of which have rectangular coordinates $(x_i, y_i)$, $i=1, 2, \ldots, n$, is defined as the point with coordinates

$$x=\frac{\Sigma x_i}{n} \qquad y=\frac{\Sigma y_i}{n}$$

that is, the point $(x, y)$ is the center of gravity of the distribution. A statement is made implying that the sum of the distances of the members from this point is minimum. This is not true in general; $(x, y)$ is the point for which the sum of the *squares* of the distances is minimum.

The distinction is clear in the special case of a population distributed on a straight line. The mean point is the center of population as here defined, while the median, a point such that the same number of members lie on each side of it, has the property that the sum of the distances from it is minimum. These points do not in general coincide; for many distributions the median is between the mean and a point of greatest population density, the mode. As a definite example consider the seven points having coordinates 0, 1, 2, 3,

[1] SCIENCE, 90: 61–63, July 21, 1939.

4, 10, 15. The median is at 3, with the sum of distances 26, while the mean is at 5 with the sum of distances 30.

If a point may be discussed when no direct means for obtaining it are given (at present), a point in the plane of a distribution such that the sum of the distances from it to the members is minimum may be called a median. An example of a triangle consisting of two nearby points and a third point remote from them shows that the median and the center of population do not in general coincide, and the difference can by no means be neglected. The special distribution on a straight line and simple examples of plane distributions make it seem reasonable to believe in the absence of more complete information that the median is frequently closer to the center of greatest population concentration than the center of population is.

RANDOLPH CHURCH
U. S. NAVAL ACADEMY,
ANNAPOLIS, MD.

THE criticism offered by Dr. Church is certainly justified, since the center of population as determined by the method described or by that of the Bureau of the Census does not give the point the sum of whose distances from the stated address of members of the group is a minimum. Without question it should have been clearly pointed out that the points determined are centroids and only roughly satisfy the minimum distance criterion. The actual determination of such points did not seem to be a feasible problem; the centers of population as determined do allow direct comparison with various positions of the center of population of the United States as determined by each federal census, the primary purpose of the study.

A method by which one might attempt to approximate the location of the point Dr. Church calls a median would be to locate what the Census Bureau designates as a "median point," that is, the point of intersection of a north and south line which divides the population into two equal parts, with an east and west line which likewise divides it into two equal parts. For the groups mentioned the median line running east and west is usually from ten to fifty minutes of latitude north of the center of population. The line running north and south may be through the center of population as with the American Speech Correction Society; about a degree and twenty minutes (roughly sixty or seventy miles) east as in the Mathematical Association of America; perhaps three degrees east in the American Association for the Advancement of Science; other groups range from no change to about two and a half degrees east. For exact determination of a mathematical point, these are large variations, but for locating a convention city various factors make the difference relatively unimportant.

Even if one knew the location of the ideal point with sums of straight-line distances of members from this point a minimum, if the problem of a proper place for a convention of the group is involved, air-line distances should be corrected to distances by a regularly traveled route (and, shall this be by rail, bus, plane, private car or steamer?). If this can be determined, there arises the need for some reasonably large city in the vicinity. The relatively small variation of median lines from centers of population make it seem probable that the centers of population determined give a sufficiently accurate general location from the point of view of minimum travel requirements. Such cities as Cincinnati, Columbus and Dayton seem well located; for most groups Chicago is to the northwest and Pittsburgh slightly to the northeast.

C. B. READ
UNIVERSITY OF WICHITA

## THE FIRST DATING OF PRESERVED WOOD IN NEW ENGLAND

THE principle of cross-dating wood of unknown age by comparing the sequence of its ring widths with that of an acceptable record of dated rings has not been hitherto applied in the New England area. An opportunity to test the method came in 1938, when the September hurricane felled some virgin white pine not far from Wolfeboro, N. H., where buried logs of the same species were uncovered in an excavation at the site of an ancient bridge abutment. The skeleton plot method of Douglass has given the date of 1806 for the last ring formed in the trees used to build the bridge. This solution is very reasonable in the light of Wolfeboro history.

Sections of three trees were removed from a level several feet below the water line at the bridge. The wood and bark had been very well preserved in the saturated soil. The rings of each tree were measured by methods previously described.[1] The mean ring width was calculated for each of the 153 years represented by at least two trees, while the third tree had 189 rings. The growth was semi-complacent but small minima and maxima in the composite graph, found also in two or more of the individual graphs, were located on the skeleton plot[2] for comparison with the sequence of dated rings.

A record of white pine ring widths for a 260-year period was obtained from three trees at North Sutton, N. H., 39 miles southwest of the bridge at an elevation slightly higher. A cross-identification was established between this record and that of the buried pine when the outer 128 rings of the latter overlapped the inner rings of the Sutton trees. Although not sufficient in

[1] C. J. Lyon, *Ecology*, 17: 457–478, 1936; *Tree-ring Bull.*, 5: 27–30, 1939.

[2] W. S. Glock, "Principles and Methods of Tree-ring Analysis," Part I., Carnegie Institution Pub. 486, 1937.

number to give a standard scale of white pine growth in the area, these Sutton pines gave a record that cross-identified well but not perfectly with nearby white pine records of the period 1867–1934.[3] The presence of 260 rings was notable for white pine and important for the problem because of the wide overlap made possible even with trees buried more than a century.

The accuracy of the cross-identification is shown by the following facts. Of the six wide rings in the buried wood, five checked perfectly with the Sutton pines, while each record for the 128 years showed one maximum not represented in the others. In the same way and for the same 128 years, of the 16 narrow rings in the buried trees, eight checked with lows in the Sutton trees, four checked with years marked by lows in the hemlock record of the Wolfeboro district and by drouths recorded in a diary, two missed agreement with the Sutton record by one year, while only two stand alone.

This relatively unimportant problem demonstrates the possibilities of the method for the area and the extent to which significant narrow and wide rings appear in sensitive trees of the New England area. The cross-identification is apparently less perfect here than in the Southwest, but valid solutions of archeological problems seem possible, particularly when the material includes a long series of rings from a native "softwood" tree.

CHARLES J. LYON
DARTMOUTH COLLEGE

[3] L. Goldthwait and C. J. Lyon, *Ecology*, 18: 406–415, 1937.

## NOTICE OF POSSIBLE SUSPENSION OF THE RULES OF NOMENCLATURE IN CERTAIN CASES (A.(n.s.) 1)

IN accordance with a resolution adopted by the International Zoological Congress at their ninth meeting held at Monaco in 1913, prescribing that not less than one year's notice is to be given by the International Commission on Zoological Nomenclature of all applications received for the "Suspension of the Rules," the attention of the zoological profession is hereby invited to the fact that requests for the "Suspension of the Rules" have been received by the commission in the undermentioned cases:

(a) ECHINODERMATA.—*Diadema* Humphreys, 1797 (type *Echinometra setosa* Leske, 1778) to be added to the Official List of Generic Names (see Mortensen, 1937, *Ann. Mag. nat. Hist.* (10) 19: 463–469) (reference Z. N. (S.) 52).

(b) INSECTA, Neuroptera.—To be added to the Official List of Generic Names with types as shown in brackets:—*Hemerobius* Linnaeus, 1758 (*Hemerobius humulinus* Linnaeus, 1758); *Chrysopa* Leach, 1815 (*Hemerobius perla* Linnaeus, 1758) (see Cowley and others, 1937, Generic Names of British Insects, Pt. 4) (reference Z. N. (S.) 42).

(c) INSECTA, Lepidoptera.—To be added to the Official List of Generic Names with the type as shown in brackets:—*Actinote* Hübner, [1819] (*Papilio thalia* Linnaeus, 1758) (see Hemming, 1936, *Proc. R. ent. Soc. Lond.* (B) 5: 56–57) (reference Z. N. (S.) 63).

(d) REPTILIA.—*Bitts* Gray, 1942 (type *Vipera* (*Echidna*) *arietans* B. Merrem, 1820), to be added to the Official List of Generic Names, and *Cobra* Laurent, 1768, to be suppressed (Stejneger, 1936, *Copeia*, 3: 140) (reference Z. N. (S.) 121).

In adopting the resolution referred to above, the International Zoological Congress expressly stated that their object was thereby to render it possible for zoologists, particularly specialists in the group in question, to present to the commission arguments for or against the suspension of the rules proposed. Any such representations should be furnished to the Secretariat to the Commission (British Museum (Natural History), Cromwell Road, London, S.W. 7) as soon as possible and in any case within one year of this day's date. Every such communication should be clearly marked with the commission's reference number as given above.

BY ORDER OF THE COMMISSION,
(Signed) FRANCIS HEMMING,
*Secretary to the Commission*
SECRETARIAT OF THE COMMISSION,
BRITISH MUSEUM (NATURAL HISTORY),
CROMWELL ROAD, LONDON, S.W. 7.
27TH JUNE, 1939

# SCIENTIFIC BOOKS

## QUANTUM MECHANICS

*Introductory Quantum Mechanics.* By VLADIMIR ROJANSKY. Prentice-Hall, Inc., New York, 1938. $5.50.

THE current literature of modern physics is of such a character that one can not in general appreciate the arguments without an understanding of the physical ideas, and in many cases the mathematical methods, peculiar to quantum mechanics. Hence it is necessary that a graduate student of pure physics acquire this knowledge early in his career. While the new physical notions can and should be presented in advanced undergraduate courses on the phenomena of modern physics, the mathematical treatment must perhaps in general wait for the fuller experience of graduate study, but should certainly be begun in the first graduate year if the doctorate is to truly represent a maturity of knowledge and ability. But at this stage the study and teaching of a subject as fundamental as quantum mechanics is greatly facilitated by the use of a textbook. This volume by Rojansky represents in the reviewer's opinion, the first suitable book of this sort. The few volumes designed for use as introductory text-books which have appeared in the past have been concerned almost exclusively with Schrödinger's differential equation. But very many, perhaps even a majority, of the applications employ matrices and operational methods. There are subjects such as theoretical spectroscopy in which the solution of Schrödinger's equation by the ordinary methods of the calculus of differential equations occupies only a small fraction of the papers and treatises. Hence it is undesirable to spend almost the whole of an introductory course on a detailed discussion of Schrödinger's equation, as such. This is especially true, since it seems to have the result that most students never grasp the general ideas of the quantum-mechanical method but cling to Schrödinger's differential equation as to a lone friend in a strange land. They try to write and employ horrible-looking differential equations where a few operational ideas would save many complicated pages. While this sort of thing has ample precedent in important early work of competent physicists, particularly in papers on spectroscopy, it should have been ended by the brilliant expositions of Dirac. But now for the first time do we have an introductory text-book which follows in Dirac's footsteps.

In examining this book one is appalled at the bulk, when presented in a truly introductory fashion, of the material which the student has to learn, has to have at his fingertips, before he is prepared to follow easily the literature employing quantum mechanics. The mathematical methods employed will seem to the student strange, but not more difficult than the courses in pure mathematics he is prepared to study. This is especially true since in an introduction to quantum mechanics, just as in an introduction to classical theoretical physics, neither too rigorous a mathematical treatment nor too logical a development of the physical postulates is necessary. In this connection Rojansky's book "makes little pretense to rigor and often aims to make plausible rather than to prove."

But in spite of the fact that the book succeeds in presenting very well and in a fashion as elementary as possible the tremendous machinery necessary to the understanding of the applications of quantum mechanics, it is not quite the ideal elementary text-book which one would advise a beginner to study by himself without benefit of lectures. For one is shocked at the idea of studying through the whole book and finding as little concrete physics as is there contained. As the book stands now it is a course in which one is taught to make many different mathematical manipulations on commands couched in physical terms, but has little idea as to why he is learning to make them. This is partly unavoidable, but can often be remedied by informal classroom discussion concerning the fields in which the various ideas are of particular use. Since this text makes no claim to logic or rigor, more of this informal discussion might well have been introduced to keep alive the student's interest. To give a few examples: the application to the nuclear vibration of molecules of the energy levels and transition probabilities found for a harmonic oscillator might have been discussed; the importance of the potential well for the study of metals and of gases might have been explained; cold emission could have been used as a second example (in addition to radioactivity) of the tunnel effect; and the diffraction of an electron beam passing through an idealized metal surface would have furnished an excellent application of de Broglie waves.

As we have noted, the book has practically nothing in the way of applications of the theory. It does get to the point of treating the hydrogen atom, including spin-orbit interaction and nuclear motion. But in general, as is proper, its function is to carry the student exactly to the point where specialized treatments of the applications of quantum mechanics are likely to begin. It discusses one-particle problems only, has no mention of the exclusion principle and practically nothing on radiation theory.

The commendable introductory chapter on classical mechanics is designed not so much for review as to introduce terms and notions fundamental in quantum mechanics but not usually employed in elementary classical mechanics. Thus the student, while still in familiar surroundings, encounters potential wells, distribution functions, expectation or average values, the uncertainty of the result of a measurement, the state of a system, probability packets.

This chapter is followed by an excellent formulation and discussion of the fundamental assumptions of quantum mechanics directly from an operational point of view; then a detailed treatment of the Schrödinger method in one dimension. One might refer to the particularly clear treatment of composite states, the brief but convincing exposition of the Heisenberg uncertainty principle, and the first treatment in an elementary book of the one-dimensional potential lattice.

Then follows an excellent treatment of operational and matrix methods. The student is gently introduced to the two sorts of matrices of particular interest—those representing Hermitian operators and unitary transformations—by a geometrical discussion of "mappings" and "frame changes."

At the end are chapters which treat the elements of motion in three dimensions, Pauli's theory of spin and Dirac's theory of the electron.

The book contains literally hundreds of carefully chosen problems which should be of great value in familiarizing the student with the employment of the quantum-mechanical methods.

The presentation of the subject is in general extremely clear and gives the impression of having been very carefully prepared. In this regard, the reviewer would have only one suggestion—that greater use might be made of graphical illustrations of the type so convincingly employed in Gurney's book. For example, for the case of hydrogen, a plot of $-1/r+l.(l+1)/2r^2$ for various values of $l$, with the radial eigenfunctions superposed on the respective energy levels, renders very plausible the coincidences of these levels in this case and the lack of coincidences if the central field departs in the least from the Coulomb value.

Finally one might remark that the typography of the book is very pleasing and should serve as a model for other American texts. It approaches the English and German books for beauty of format, avoiding the ugly fat radicals, the huge thick integral signs and the black summation signs which so clutter up the pages of most American physics books; and goes far toward making the cuts and equations fit into and become an attractive part of the page instead of standing out like trees in the middle of South Dakota. One even finds (p. 515) an equation pleasantly protruding into the margins, a thing unheard of in American typography. One still finds, however, too much blank space around short equations (*e.g.*, p. 355).

GEORGE H. SHORTLEY
THE OHIO STATE UNIVERSITY

## USES OF CHEMICALS

*Uses and Applications of Chemicals and Related Materials.* By THOMAS C. GREGORY. vi + 665 pp. New York: Reinhold Publishing Corporation, 1939. $10.00.

TWENTY-FIVE years ago, when we entered the World War, it became necessary for the Secretary of War to commandeer all supplies of various essential chemicals and allocate them according to our war needs. This allocation was made with the assistance and upon the advice of the Chemicals and Raw Materials Division of the War Industries Board. Even in a group of experts of this kind, it was not always possible to find men who were familiar with all the varied uses of a well-known chemical or the proportionate amounts required by various industries. For example, those not specialists had no idea of the quantity of arsenious acid required by the glass manufacturers or of saccharin by the tobacco industry.

Such a book as the one under review would have been very helpful, and it seems to the writer, therefore, that its appearance is opportune, now that we may be facing problems similar to those of 1917–18.

The volume describes, in alphabetical order, the current industrial uses, potential applications and sales possibilities of 5,167 chemicals and related products. It is based upon surveys made over a period of 15 years and published in the *Oil, Paint and Drug Reporter,* under the titles *"Where You Can Sell"* (up to and including the issue of September 9, 1935) and "Industrial Uses of Chemicals and Related Materials" (from the issue of September 16, 1935, onwards). The uses are classified under appropriate sub-headings, synonyms and foreign names are given, and patent references are frequent. At the close of the volume is an extensive "Synonyms and Cross References" index. The book is an encyclopedia of useful information.

MARSTON TAYLOR BOGERT
COLUMBIA UNIVERSITY

# SPECIAL ARTICLES

## THE SEMIQUINONE RADICALS OF METHYLENE BLUE AND RELATED DYESTUFFS

THE occurrence of free radicals, designated as semiquinones, as intermediate reduction products of reversibly reducible dyestuffs, was considered as an exceptional case when it was first discovered for pyocyanine and some related phenazin derivatives. Meanwhile, these radicals have been shown to exist for all the more familiar classes of reversible dyestuffs, except for the thiazines and oxazines. Since methylene blue, a thiazine, is the most frequently used dyestuff in biochemical research, the failure of any report about the existence of its semiquinone was somewhat puzzling. This problem is especially important with regard to the hypothesis of compulsory univalent reduction[1] which claims that no oxidation or reduction can proceed with any appreciable speed otherwise than in univalent steps. The faculty of acting as a catalyst for oxidation, especially respiration, should accordingly also be correlated with the faculty of the catalyst to be either a univalent oxidation-reduction system, such as the iron porphyrin compounds; or if it be a bivalent system, to be reducible in two successive, although more or less overlapping steps.

This note is to give a preliminary report on the discovery of the hitherto unknown semiquinones of these dyestuffs.

According to the theory on stability of free radicals, based on the theory of reasonance, the authors came to the conclusion that the radicals of thiazines should be most stable in a very strongly acid solution. This expectation has been verified by experiment. It is easiest to demonstrate the radical of thionin (Lauth's

[1] L. Michaelis and C. V. Smythe, *Ann. Review Biochemistry,* 1938.

violet). When a solution of the dye in 20 $NH_2SO_4$ is reduced, say by $TiCl_3$, the free radical appears as intermediate step of reduction. It is yellow and exhibits a series of distinct absorption bands in the blue part of the spectrum, recalling the bands of the triphenylmethyl radical. Analyses of the potentiometric titration curves, obtained by especially adapting the technique to the unusually high acidity of the solutions, showed that this yellow compound is a free radical, not a polymerized compound. The separation of the two steps rapidly diminishes with decreasing acidity but never vanishes entirely. Even in neutral solution an analysis of the potentiometric titration curves reveals that the dye solution in its half-reduced state contains the semiquinone to an extent that may be estimated as between 5 per cent. and 10 per cent. of the total dye. In such solutions the radical can no longer be detected, optically, for two reasons. Firstly, a few per cent. of a light yellow compound escapes optical detection when mixed with the large excess of the deeply colored blue dyestuff itself; secondly, it can be assumed from theoretical arguments that the radical is in a different state of ionization in extremely acid, than in less acid or neutral solution, and that the form existing in neutral solution should exhibit an extremely slight absorption, if any at all, in the visible range of wave-lengths.

The only difference between thionin and methylene blue is that the latter requires still a somewhat higher acidity than thionin in order to obtain the same degree of separation of the two steps of oxidation. The absorption spectrum of the methylene blue radical is quite similar to that of thionin.

Then, these dyestuffs, after all, fit very well into the theory of compulsory univalent oxidation. Any bivalent oxidation reduction system must be capable of forming a semiquinone radical to a measurable extent in order to behave as a reversible system; and any organic dyestuff can act as a catalyst for sluggish oxidations only by intermediation of the radical.

Another experiment should be mentioned with regard to the assertion that the catalytic action of a dye depends on its faculty to form a semiquinone radical. It has been shown recently,[2] that the first oxidation product of diamino durene (I) is a free radical, analogous to those designated as Wurster's dyes. It has been shown furthermore that any methylation at the

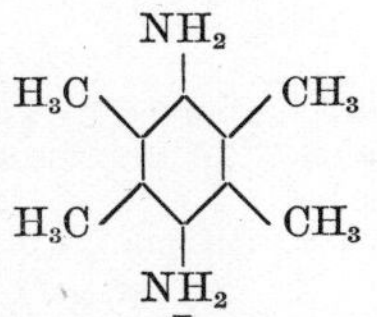


I

2 L. Michaelis, M. P. Schubert and S. Granick, *Jour. Am. Chem. Soc.*, 61: 1981, 1939.

amino groups destroys the faculty of forming this radical. In the latter case, the benzene ring, the two N atoms and all the atoms attached to the two N atoms are prevented from lying in one plane due to steric hindrance of the voluminous side chains. The steric possibility of such a coplanar arrangement is requisite for establishment of resonance. For this reason the methylated compounds can not form a radical. Now, the unmethylated compound increases respiration of erythrocytes to approximately the same extent as does methylene blue, but the methylated compound has no catalytic effect at all.

S. GRANICK
L. MICHAELIS
M. P. SCHUBERT
THE ROCKEFELLER INSTITUTE FOR
MEDICAL RESEARCH, NEW YORK

## THE METABOLISM OF GLUTATHIONE[1]

INVESTIGATIONS concerned with the fate of glutathione in the living organism have dealt almost exclusively with the behavior of the tripeptide as an SH-carrier. The methods used have been based on determination of the SH-group.

Little attention has been paid to the possibility that the combination of the three amino acids, glycine, cystine and glutamic acid in this peptide, GSH, has some special significance aside from its function as an SH-carrier. It is striking that these three amino acids are the ones which are found combined with compounds other than amino acids in the mammalian body, *e.g.*, bile acids and the products of detoxication. One of us has previously suggested that GSH may act as an amino acid donor in the formation of those compounds.[2] In support of this conception a decrease in the substances titratable with iodine in human blood was found after intake of phenyl acetic acid which is excreted as phenyl acetyl glutamine.[3]

It is now possible by the use of the isotope technique to follow directly the fate of the amino acids of GSH and to estimate its rate of turnover. Glycine containing 1.18 atom per cent. $N^{15}$ excess was administered to rats. After two hours the concentration of $N^{15}$ in the GSH of the liver and intestine, together with the $N^{15}$ content of the protein glycine and NPN of these organs, was determined. The GSH was isolated as follows: The frozen and ground livers were extracted with metaphosphoric acid. The GSH was precipitated as the cuprous compound and purified by reprecipitation. The method of isolation yields about 16 mg of copper glutathione per rat liver, correspond-

1 This work was made possible through a grant from the Friedsam Fund donated to the Division of Child Neurology, Neurological Institute, New York, N. Y.

2 H. Waelsch, *Arch. exper. Path. u. Pharm.*, 156: 356, 1930.

3 H. Waelsch and E. Weinberger, *ibid.*, 156: 370, 1930.

ing to 30 to 40 per cent. of the values given by titration procedures.

The results (Table I) show that within 2 hours an appreciable part (7.6 per cent.) of the nitrogen of the liver GSH was derived from the administered glycine. By contrast the nitrogen of the protein glycine and of the NPN of the liver represented only 1.6 and 3.4 per cent. respectively. A similar relationship was found in the intestine. In view of the short period of the experiment and of the finding by Braunstein and Kritzmann,[4] Bach[5] and others that the speed of deamination of glycine is slow it is probable that all the labeled N is in the glycine portion of the GSH. If this assumption is correct the concentration of $N^{15}$ in the glycine of the liver GSH would be $3 \times 0.09$ atom per cent. and the minimum rate of turnover of GSH would be 22.3 per cent. (intestine 9.6 per cent.) in two hours (Table I, column 4). By contrast in the same period only 1.6 per cent. (intestine 1.5 per cent.) of the protein-glycine of the liver was exchanged. This experiment establishes the fact that GSH is a very unstable and reactive compound in the living organism.

TABLE I

RATS GIVEN 75 MG. GLYCINE (1.18 ATOM PER CENT. $N^{15}$ EXCESS)

| Liver | $N^{15}$ excess atom per cent. | Dilution factor of labeled N | Dilution factor of labeled glycine |
|---|---|---|---|
| Cu glutathione | 0.09 | 1 : 13 | 1 : 4.3 |
| NPN | 0.04 | 1 : 29 | |
| Glycine (protein) | 0.019 | 1 : 62 | 1 : 62 |
| Intestine: | | | |
| Cu glutathione | 0.038 | 1 : 31 | 1 : 10.3 |
| NPN | 0.014 | 1 : 84 | |
| Glycine (protein) | 0.017 | 1 : 70 | 1 : 70 |

Rittenberg and Schoenheimer[6] administered benzoic acid and glycine labeled with $N^{15}$ to rats. One third of the glycine excreted as hippuric acid during the following 24 hours came from the glycine administered. To obtain further information concerning the synthesis of hippuric acid in relation to the turnover of GSH, benzoic acid and glycine containing 1.98 per cent. of $N^{15}$ excess were injected subcutaneously into rats. After five hours GSH was isolated from the liver. The GSH contained 0.151 atom per cent. $N^{15}$ excess. Assuming again that it represents an uptake of labeled glycine by the GSH the minimum rate of turnover of the GSH from the liver would be 23 per cent.

Hippuric acid isolated from the urine collected during the five-hour period contained 1.08 per cent. $N^{15}$ excess, indicating that 55 per cent. of the glycine of the hippuric acid was derived from administered glycine. Since the liver GSH glycine contained less $N^{15}$ (0.453 atom per cent. excess) at the time it was measured than did the excreted hippuric acid (1.08 atom per cent. excess) the experiment offers no support for the hypothesis that GSH furnishes glycine for hippuric acid formation.

Further work is in progress to determine whether the rapid turnover of GSH is indicative of its role as an intermediary in the metabolism of proteins.

H. WAELSCH

DEPARTMENT OF BIOCHEMISTRY,
NEW YORK STATE PSYCHIATRIC INSTITUTE
AND HOSPITAL, NEW YORK, AND
DEPARTMENT OF NEUROLOGY,
COLUMBIA UNIVERSITY

D. RITTENBERG

DEPARTMENT OF BIOCHEMISTRY,
COLUMBIA UNIVERSITY

[4] D. F. Braunstein and M. G. Kritzmann, *Biokhimiya*, 3: 590, 1938, C.A. 33, 2916, 1939.

[5] S. J. Bach, *Biochem. Jour.*, 33: 90, 1939.

[6] D. Rittenberg and R. Schoenheimer, *Jour. Biol. Chem.*, 127: 329, 1939.

## SYNTHETIC ALPHA-TOCOPHEROL AND NUTRITIONAL MUSCULAR DYSTROPHY[1]

RECENTLY Goettsch and Ritzman[2] found that alpha-tocopherol prevented the development of muscular dystrophy in young rats when alpha-tocopherol was fed from the tenth to the twenty-fifth day after birth. Control rats under similar conditions but without the supplement of alpha-tocopherol showed symptoms of muscular dystrophy at the end of the above test period. Their own criticism of the results was that it was conceivable that the alpha-tocopherol employed might have contained impurities that were active in preventing the muscular disease. The alpha-tocopherol was a natural product isolated according to the method of Evans, Emerson and Emerson.[3]

Mackenzie and McCollum[4] later showed that the natural alpha-tocopherol was effective in curing muscular dystrophy of rabbits on the Goettsch and Pappenheimer diet no. 13 plus 10 per cent. of ether extracted wheat germ.

In the present work with muscular dystrophy of rabbits, the writer has used a diet consisting of ground U. S. No. 3 grade alfalfa hay ad libitum, and 20 grams of a grain mixture daily per rabbit. The grain mixture is made up of 40 parts of whole yellow corn meal, 30 parts of wheat bran, 20 parts of soybean meal and 10 parts of linseed meal. One part of sodium chloride is added to the mixture. Each animal received daily 1 cc of a good grade cod liver oil, either placed upon

[1] This research was supported by an appropriation from Bankhead-Jones funds (the Bankhead-Jones Act of June 29, 1935).

[2] M. Goettsch and J. Ritzman, *Jour. of Nutrition*, 17: 371, 1939.

[3] H. M. Evans, O. H. Emerson and G. A. Emerson, *Jour. of Biol. Chem.*, 113: 319, 1936.

[4] C. G. Mackenzie and E. V. McCollum, SCIENCE, 2312, 370, 1939.

the grain or by mouth. Muscular dystrophy can be produced equally well when petroleum ether extracted No. 1 alfalfa hay replaces the No. 3 alfalfa hay.

The muscular dystrophy producing property of this diet is dependent upon the cod liver oil. This is in agreement with the report of Madsen, McCay and Maynard[5] that cod liver oil added to a synthetic diet increased the rate of development and early severity of the muscular dystrophy. The water-soluble factor associated with nutritional muscular dystrophy as indicated by Morgulis, Wilder and Eppstein[6] is not lacking in this diet.

In this laboratory feeding of alpha-tocopherol,[3] prepared from wheat germ oil[7] has cured muscular dystrophy of rabbits, confirming the findings of Mackenzie and McCollum. Recently 300 milligrams of synthetic alpha-tocopherol[8] were obtained. Six rabbits suffering from muscular dystrophy but still able to walk with difficulty were given doses of this synthetic material. Experience would indicate that each of these rabbits, if left untreated, would within 24 hours have been unable to stand or consume food.

The individual doses of the synthetic alpha-tocopherol in milligrams were as follows: 17, 18, 20, 26, 51 and 65. All animals were cured except the one receiving the 17 milligram dose. A seventh animal which received 30 milligrams also died, but it was in a much more advanced stage of collapse at the time of treatment.

It is apparent that 20 milligrams is near the lower limit as a single curative dose. An animal is considered as cured when it loses its stiffness and begins to gain in weight within 48 hours and continues to gain for 10 days or more. Although no attempt is made to establish the minimum curative dose with such limited amounts of material, it is definitely shown that synthetic alpha-tocopherol will cure muscular dystrophy in rabbits as produced experimentally under the conditions stated. The 5 cures become more significant when one considers that from several hundred dystrophic animals we have never observed spontaneous cure of an untreated animal.

STEWARD G. MORRIS
U. S. DEPARTMENT OF AGRICULTURE

# SCIENTIFIC APPARATUS AND LABORATORY METHODS

## STUDENT APPARATUS FOR ANALYSIS OF RESPIRATORY GASES

THE gas burette to be described was devised especially for medical students for whose instruction analyses of expired air are required of just sufficient accuracy to illustrate the general principles of respiratory exchange and metabolism. The usual complicated apparatus (*e.g.*, the Haldane-Henderson) is, we believe, poorly adapted to this type of instruction, for several reasons: (1) too much time is required to acquire proficiency with the method; (2) due to the excessive cost per unit insufficient apparatus is available; (3) the size of the equipment makes storage a problem; and (4) the difficulty of cleaning the apparatus when it becomes fouled, as so frequently happens, imposes a severe strain on the time and patience of the instructor.

By the simple method, here reported, an inexperienced operator may determine the $CO_2$ and $O_2$ of expired air with an error not often exceeding 0.1 volume per cent., corresponding to an error of about 5 per cent. in the calculated value of the metabolic rate. The time required for an analysis (30 to 60 minutes) may seem excessive, but students can actually make more determinations, during the limited period available for the work in respiration, than they can with the ordinary methods. It is suggested, in view of the low cost of the equipment, that each unit consist of two burettes, mounted together for simultaneous determinations. In this way the average time of an analysis will compare favorably with that required by the Haldane-Henderson method.

### APPARATUS

The burette[1] is of Pyrex glass, with replaceable stopcock of the type which requires little or no lubricant. The graduations, which extend from the cock to 10 cc by 0.05 cc intervals, should be calibrated to within 0.005 cc for total and partial volumes. The burette should be carefully cleaned to allow complete drainage of the reagents. The leveling bulb should contain approximately 35 cc, and it may be conveniently suspended by a cord wrapped once over a horizontal rod, and a large rubber stopper may be used as counterweight. A thermometer reading to 0.2° C. should be available to each group of students.

### REAGENTS

(1) Solution of NaCl (U.S.P.) 23.5 per cent. by weight, having a specific gravity of 1.18, to which is

[5] L. L. Madsen, C. M. McCay and L. A. Maynard, *Proc. Soc. Exp. Biol. and Med.*, 30: 1434, 1933.

[6] S. Morgulis, V. M. Wilder and S. H. Eppstein, *Jour. of Nutrition*, 16: 219, 1938.

[7] The wheat germ oil from which the tocopherol was prepared was kindly supplied by the Archer-Daniel-Midland Company, Minneapolis, Minn.

[8] The synthetic alpha-tocopherol was furnished by Merck and Company through the courtesy of Dr. J. M. Carlisle.

[1] A suitable burette may be obtained from the Scientific Apparatus Company, Bloomfield, N. J., or from the Fisher Scientific Company, Pittsburgh, Pa.

added 5 cc of 85 per cent. lactic acid per 1,000 grams of salt solution. Phenol red or other indicator may be added if desired. Approximately 150 cc of the acid-saline is required for each analysis. The solution may be dispensed from stock in 500 cc cylinders, for convenient filling of the apparatus.

(2) Solution of NaOH, 16.0 per cent. by weight, having a specific gravity and vapor pressure approximately the same as the salt solution, for absorption

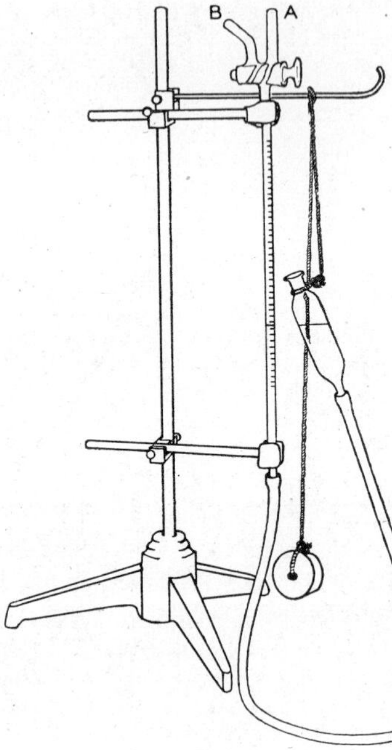


FIG. 1

of $CO_2$ and rinsing down of oxygen absorber. A single separatory funnel, with pipette-like tip, will allow the reagent to be conveniently accessible to the operators of 3 or 4 sets of apparatus.

(3) Oxygen absorber, consisting of 10 grams sodium hydrosulfite (Baker) and 1 gram sodium anthraquinone β sulfonate (Eastman) dissolved rapidly in 50 cc of 3N KOH, filtered through cotton and stored in a separatory funnel under paraffin oil. A single container should supply 6 to 10 students.

### PROCEDURES

Levelling bulb, tubing and burette are filled with salt solution and about 1 cc is run into the reagent cup "A," a gas sample is then introduced through the tube "B" to approximately the 10 cc mark. Most of the saline is run in from the cup, the cock is closed, and the burette tapped to dislodge traces of solution from the upper end. Levels are adjusted and readings recorded at intervals until drainage is complete, which may require 5 to 15 minutes. The room temperature should be noted to the nearest 0.2° C. in vicinity of the burette. It is essential that the gas sample should be protected from sunlight or other causes of sudden variation of temperature. To this end the operator should remain at least 3 feet distant from the burette except during necessary manipulations, for heat radiated by the body may elevate the temperature of the gas without affecting the thermometer. A water jacket will not assist in maintaining constancy of temperature, for the heat of neutralization and of dilution which is liberated during the analysis must be completely dissipated, a process which occurs most quickly by air conduction.

$CO_2$ is now absorbed by running in 2 cc of the alkali, during about a minute. Time for complete drainage of the alkali rarely exceeds 8 minutes. Levels should be adjusted for the new reading and the temperature should be recorded. The volume of the gas should be corrected in each instance for temperature changes greater than 0.5° C.

$O_2$ is absorbed by running in 3 to 4 cc of the hydrosulfite reagent during approximately 2 minutes. To facilitate complete drainage and to avoid errors due to vapor pressure differences, the hydrosulfite should be washed down with 4 to 5 cc of the NaOH solution. Complete drainage may require from 10 to 15 minutes. The temperature, corresponding to the final volume, should be recorded.

After each analysis the fluid is run out by lowering the leveling bulb to a container placed on the floor. The burette is then washed through the reagent cup with 5 to 10 cc of NaOH, followed by water, followed by saline. The leveling bulb is then raised and refilled with saline. If sulfur scum appears in the burette it may be necessary to discard the first filling.

Since incomplete drainage is the chief source of error of the method, scrupulous attention should be paid to this factor.

During changeable weather it is advisable to record the barometric pressure and to make appropriate corrections of the gas volume.

J. MAX LITTLE
HERBERT S. WELLS
PHYSIOLOGY DEPARTMENT,
VANDERBILT UNIVERSITY SCHOOL
OF MEDICINE

## BOOKS RECEIVED

ANDERSON, J. RINGLAND. *Hydrophthalmia of Congenital Glaucoma; Its Causes, Treatment and Cure.* Pp. xv + 377. Cambridge University Press, Macmillan. $7.00.

DICKSON, LEONARD E. *Modern Elementary Theory of Numbers.* Pp. vii + 309. University of Chicago Press. $3.00.

MORGAN, ALFRED P. *The Pageant of Electricity.* Pp. xxvi + 363. Illustrated. Appleton-Century. $3.50.

National Resources Committee. *The Structure of the American Economy; Part I, Basic Characteristics.* Pp. vii + 396. Illustrated. Superintendent of Documents, Washington, D. C. $1.00.

# SCIENCE

VOL. 90 — FRIDAY, NOVEMBER 10, 1939 — No. 2341

*Cancer and the Public Health:* SURGEON GENERAL THOMAS PARRAN, JR. ... 427

*A New Reaction in Organic Chemistry:* DR. GEORGE CALINGAERT ... 430

*Obituary:*
*Witmer Stone. Recent Deaths and Memorials* ... 434

*Scientific Events:*
*The Galton Laboratory; The Privately Endowed College of Engineering; The American Academy of Ophthalmology and Otolaryngology; Scientific Expeditions; Field Work of the U. S. Geological Survey* ... 436

*Scientific Notes and News* ... 438

*Discussion:*
*Vitalizing Historical Geology through Field Trips:* PROFESSOR ROBERT H. MITCHELL. *Endogone as Animal Food:* DR. WILLIAM W. DIEHL. *Muscle and Blood Hemoglobin in the Dolphin:* DR. LILLIAN EICHELBERGER and OTHERS. *Biography of Dr. Harvey Cushing:* DR. JOHN F. FULTON ... 441

*Special Articles:*
*The Action of Certain Hormones as Dietary Constituents:* DR. CASIMIR FUNK and IAN CASIMIR FUNK. *The Excretion of Cortin after Surgical Operation:* PAUL WEIL and DR. J. S. L. BROWNE. *Periodic Mitotic Activity in the Epidermis of the Albino Rat:* PROFESSOR C. M. BLUMENFELD ... 443

*Scientific Apparatus and Laboratory Methods:*
*A Device for Rapid Rinsing of Absorption Towers Used in Gas Analysis Studies:* N. F. CHILDERS, D. C. KIPLINGER and H. W. BRODY. *A New Culture Medium for Paramecia:* DR. BERTIL GOTTFRID ANDERSON ... 447

*Science News* ... 8

SCIENCE: A Weekly Journal devoted to the Advancement of Science, edited by J. MCKEEN CATTELL and published every Friday by

THE SCIENCE PRESS

New York City: Grand Central Terminal

Lancaster, Pa. — Garrison, N. Y.

Annual Subscription, $6.00 — Single Copies, 15 Cts.

SCIENCE is the official organ of the American Association for the Advancement of Science. Information regarding membership in the Association may be secured from the office of the permanent secretary in the Smithsonian Institution Building, Washington, D. C.

# CANCER AND THE PUBLIC HEALTH[1]

By Dr. THOMAS PARRAN, Jr.

SURGEON GENERAL, UNITED STATES PUBLIC HEALTH SERVICE

WITH parts or all of every continent at war, it is difficult even for neutrals to retain that dispassionate concentration upon *science* which is necessary for a fruitful discussion of the problems confronting this Third International Cancer Congress.

Devoting our lives, as we are, to the saving, the conservation of human life, it is inescapable that our first reaction to mass killing is one of frustration, of futility. How puny are our efforts to save compared with the effect of war. Four years of the World War nullified, wiped out, the results of probably forty years of medical progress. The lifetime of a hundred laboratories, a thousand scientists, tens, yes, hundreds of thousands of doctors and nurses gone for naught.

All of you, I am sure, share with me the fervent hope that we and our children will be spared the material, the physical, the mental, and above all the spiritual losses which follow a major conflict at arms.

Whether you thank or blame *science,* in these days no nation ever wins a war or profits by it—whether as a combatant or a neutral. Whatever its duration or costs, however, there is some consolation in the fact that every war is followed by peace.

Instead of becoming amateur strategists—as we are tempted to do—each of us must look forward even now to that peace, and consider in the meantime what we individually, in our chosen sector, can do to neutralize, to make up the losses which war entails.

Not counting other losses, if the material costs of the World War and the armament costs since then could have been spent to satisfy the basic needs of the people for peaceful living, the world to-day would be experiencing a standard of living beyond anything ever dreamed of. To attain a higher standard of national

[1] Address before the Third International Cancer Congress, Atlantic City, N. J., September 13, 1939.

health is an urgent need in this country—whether the future brings us continued peace or war.

In either event the nation can not afford the continued luxury of unnecessary disease, disablement and death. The public in this country is beginning to demand that its doctors and health organizations join hands to put their knowledge to work effectively—to prevent sickness, to improve health, to promote physical fitness, and to restore the sick to health.

The people have accepted the idea that a disease which takes a sweeping toll of lives each year from the productive ages of our population; a disease which knows no state or county boundaries; a disease which is so costly in its diagnosis and treatment that but few of its victims can pay the costs unaided—is a public health problem. Cancer is such a disease.

Each year more than 140,000 deaths from cancer occur in the United States—more than twice as many as live in Atlantic City. Irrefutable evidence indicates that skilled medical care is available only to a small proportion of the half million or more cancer sufferers in the United States to-day. Cancer death rates are highest among industrial workers and among the underprivileged economic groups.

There was a time when public health activities were limited to the control of epidemic diseases and basic measures to improve the sanitation of the environment. Health activities of to-day, however, are concerned with the prevention, alleviation, and cure of all of the major causes of disablement and death. Prompt restoration of the patient to health is equally important with the prevention of disease.

It is the realization among medical men of the *possibility* of *cure* for the cancer sufferer that motivates our modern cancer control activities. Some twenty-five years ago, professional groups and interested citizens joined to launch in the United States a movement which had as its objective the educating of physicians and the public to an effective understanding of the primary importance of early diagnosis and prompt expert treatment of cancer. This required a change in the traditional thinking of doctors. As has so frequently been the case in the advancement of health in this country, the private voluntary agency led the way to national action against cancer. The movement, initiated by the American Society for the Control of Cancer, has succeeded beyond expectations. Its future exceeds any of our present concepts.

Experience during the past twenty-five years, however, has clearly indicated that education alone is not enough to stem the mortality from cancer. We must know better how to prevent and cure it. Also, the advance of scientific knowledge and the improvement of technical skills and tools have placed cancer in the category of high-cost diseases. Organized services, special equipment and physicians highly trained in tumor pathology, radiology and surgery are the *sine qua non* of modern cancer therapy. For these reasons and because so many of the patients are unable to meet the costs of diagnosis and treatment, cancer has become one of our major health problems. Cancer deaths are increasing, and because of the aging of the population will continue to cause an increasing number of deaths if the present age-specific rates persist. Prior to 1937 only five states in the United States had recognized the importance of cancer as a public health problem, and had taken steps for the more wide-spread application of scientific knowledge of cancer. These states were: Massachusetts, New York, Connecticut, New Hampshire and Georgia.

An event possibly of great future significance in the growing anti-cancer movement in the United States was the passage by the Seventy-fifth Congress of the National Cancer Institute Act in August, 1937. Senator Homer T. Bone, who introduced the bill in the Senate, said at the laying of the cornerstone of the institute on June 24 of this year (1939): "Ninety-six members of the United States Senate attached their names to the bill creating this great institution. Never in the history of this Republic had the entire membership of either body of Congress sponsored a piece of legislation. Such an action reflected a great outpouring of sentiment and evidenced a grim determination to stamp out a disease that was threatening every home in America."

Two basic concepts underlie the Act: Research to develop more effective methods for the prevention and cure of cancer; and the better application of existing knowledge for the benefit of present cancer patients.

Experiments and investigations relating to the cause, diagnosis, and treatment of cancer are being conducted extensively. It is the function of the institute also to assist and foster approved research activities by other institutions, both public and private, by the distribution of funds and through cooperation.

Under the provisions of the National Cancer Institute Act, a National Advisory Cancer Council is created consisting of six members, selected from the ranks of leading medical or scientific authorities, who are outstanding in the study, diagnosis, or treatment of cancer in the United States.

This is a new venture in government policy. Never before has Congress authorized the distribution of tax funds to private institutions and individuals for medical research. We have been fortunate in the caliber of the members who thus far have served us on this council. Since so many scientific disciplines are important in the whole field of cancer research and treatment, it has not been possible to have representation of all of these disciplines on the council at any one time. We hope to seek advice and guidance broadly, however, from the various specialties concerned with any aspect of this problem through the appointment of special committees of the council.

The council is in effect a policy-making body. Specifically it is authorized: (a) to review research projects or programs submitted to or initiated by it; (b) to collect, coordinate, and then disseminate the information with regard to cancer which is available or which will come to light as research and investigation progress; (c) to review applications from any university, hospital laboratory or other institution, whether public or private, or from individuals for grants-in-aid for research projects relating to cancer and certify its approval of grants-in-aid in such projects as show promise, and (d) to recommend the acceptance of conditional gifts to the National Cancer Institute.

To date, upon the certification of the council, grants-in-aid in excess of $180,000 for research projects have been made to various institutions throughout the country. Thus, in augmenting research and supporting worthwhile and promising cancer studies already being carried on by other agencies, the National Cancer Institute has taken its place in the world-wide attack on the cancer problem.

Two other important functions of the National Cancer Institute are provided in the Act, both of which have a direct relationship with the application of existing knowledge of cancer in the saving of lives: namely, the loan of radium and the training of professional personnel.

Under the provisions of the National Cancer Act, the Public Health Service is authorized to purchase radium and to make it available on loan to institutions, including hospitals, for cancer research or for the actual treatment of cancer. In 1938 nine and one-half grams of radium, costing $200,000, were purchased by the National Cancer Institute. The entire amount has already been allocated to various hospitals and cancer clinics. As funds become available, more radium will be purchased. It should be understood, however, that radium is *not* loaned *unless* an institution can meet certain requirements as to qualifications of the personnel, equipment and organization. The importance of this function of the institute can readily be appreciated when we consider the statements of experts when the Act was passed, that the United States possessed only about 50 per cent. of the radium needed for research and treatment of cancer.

Availability of competent personnel is also of great significance in the fight against cancer. Under the National Cancer Act, young physicians who are interested in cancer as a specialty and who have had previous training may apply to the National Cancer Institute for financial assistance in obtaining special training offered by designated training centers in tumor pathology, radiology and surgery.

Physicians eligible for training must be graduated from an approved medical school, must have completed at least one year of internship in an approved hospital, and must be less than 40 years of age. These fellowship appointments are made for one year, and are subject to renewal if the trainee's work is satisfactory. During the past year and a half, 36 physicians have received appointments.

Twenty-three institutions in the United States have been designated as centers where training and instruction may be given under a National Cancer Institute "traineeship," in all technical matters relating to the diagnosis and treatment of cancer. These institutions include nineteen leading schools of medicine and four outstanding hospitals devoted exclusively to tumor and cancer patients.

In compliance with another provision of the Act, the institute has endeavored through cooperative activities, to stimulate the interest of state health agencies in the promotion of cancer prevention and control. At the present time nine states—New Hampshire, Massachusetts, New York, Connecticut, Georgia, Missouri, Vermont, Pennsylvania and South Carolina—have cancer control laws. The cancer programs in Massachusetts, New York, New Hampshire, and Connecticut have been in operation for a number of years; those in Georgia, Missouri, Vermont, Pennsylvania and South Carolina are of more recent establishment, having been initiated during the past three years.

As a basis for cooperative services to other states, the National Cancer Institute has made an analysis of the effective cancer legislation in these nine states. The institute is now able to advise, upon request, as to the principles which should be considered in framing cancer legislation. In fact, upon the recommendation of the State and Territorial Health Officers at their annual conference with the Public Health Service, April, 1938, the National Cancer Institute has prepared a model bill for the guidance of the states. Upon request from state medical societies and state boards of health, the institute is prepared to give technical advice in regard to cancer control legislation. Among other urgent needs for future advances in cancer research is an improvement in diagnosis and therapy, and a clarification of the present state of confusion surrounding cancer nomenclature and classification. The same unsatisfactory condition exists in regard to cancer record forms. To meet the need for uniformity of nomenclature and cancer case records, the National Advisory Cancer Council recommended the creation of a special committee to study these problems and to develop uniform nomenclature and uniform case records, including records of therapy and follow-up. Subcommittees have been formed. Organizations which are participating in the detailed study of these problems include: American College of Surgeons, American Board of Surgery, American Board of Radiology, American Society for the Control of Cancer, Memorial Hospital in New York City and the Massachusetts Health Department.

It is probable that many months will have to be devoted to the solution of the problem engaging the interest of these experts. That the most advanced thought and the ablest advice will be brought to bear upon the questions under study goes without saying. Regardless of the time spent, we may confidently expect a satisfactory clarification of the perplexities connected with terminology and clinical records in the cancer field.

That the health of the people is a responsibility of government is no longer a question. Educators, statesmen and business men realize *now* that our greatest national assets are the human resources of the nation. Again and again, health departments, insurance companies and private agencies have demonstrated that no investment yields surer returns than expenditures for the prevention of disease and the care of the sick. For example, the Metropolitan Life Insurance Company has spent over a period of 30 years, 120 million dollars in health education, in nursing the sick and in the general prevention of disease. "We who are used to actuarial methods," says Dr. Louis I. Dublin, vice-president of the company, "are entirely satisfied with our investment. Year in and year out we have increased our investments in the preservation of health because we felt that these investments paid."

What the National Cancer Institute will eventually mean to the nation in the saving of lives may only be conjectured at this time. This will depend upon the extent to which it merits the confidence and cooperation of the scientific institutions, the medical profession and the people themselves. It is hoped that the benefits to the people, however, will be both direct and indirect; not limited to the present, but promising much for the future. The provision of a more adequate supply of radium for the treatment of present and future sufferers from cancer; the training of personnel for the correct diagnosis and appropriate treatment of the disease in its early stages are the more tangible and immediate benefits.

We have not the slightest doubt that some day, maybe soon, the cancer problem will be solved. There is no reason to be pessimistic about cancer research. It is not likely that any individual worker will single-handedly conquer cancer. Scientific knowledge has increased and become so complex, that only through close coordination of research in the biological sciences with other disciplines can future advances in our knowledge of cancer be made. The National Cancer Institute of the Public Health Service hopes to demonstrate by the soundness of its policies, the extent of its cooperation and help, that it can attain an important place in this concerted warfare against the disease.

What we are discussing is no academic problem; cancer represents one important sector of a people's fight for life. You are engaged in a long-time struggle against one of mankind's oldest and most resourceful enemies; malignant growth of cells. If from this congress with its clashes of intellect and ideas, there should be generated the spark of understanding as to a means of ridding the world of the cancer menace, your contribution to humanity—to its happiness and future prosperity—might equal or even exceed the human losses of another world war.

On behalf of our government, therefore, I welcome your presence here. I wish you success in your deliberations. The one in ten of us in this country who, under the present rates, is doomed to die of cancer, pray that at least a beginning may be made toward unravelling the tangled skein, toward eradicating the menace of cancer.

# A NEW REACTION IN ORGANIC CHEMISTRY: THE REDISTRIBUTION REACTION

By Dr. GEORGE CALINGAERT

DIRECTOR OF CHEMICAL RESEARCH, ETHYL GASOLINE CORPORATION, DETROIT, MICHIGAN

THE chief difference between typical organic and inorganic compounds is the complete sharing of pairs of electrons in the bonds of the former, in contrast to the presence of electrostatic bonds in the latter. This results in profound differences in the behavior of these compounds. Electrostatic or ionic bonds are readily loosened in a suitable dielectric medium, such as water, for instance, and solutions result in which the two ions of opposite signs are in mass equilibrium with one another but where any one ion does not remain paired with one individual ion of the opposite sign. As a result, when two or more kinds of positive ions are introduced in a solution with two or more negative ions, separation of the salts from the solution will not necessarily yield back the particular salts which were originally introduced: the pairing of anions with cations will be governed primarily by solubility relationships, and appropriate manipulations of the conditions, primarily concentrations and temperatures, will effect predictable changes in the composition of these precipitated salts. Accordingly, we should not think of a solution as containing, say, sodium ions in equilibrium with chlorine and bromide ions:

$$NaCl + KBr \rightleftarrows Na^+ + K^+ + Cl^- + Br^- \rightleftarrows NaBr + KCl.$$

The covalent bond, as the sharing of a pair of electrons is called, is not readily dissociated either by solution in a dielectric solvent or by heat or other means. Thus, a solution of ethyl acetate and methyl butyrate still contains these two compounds in the proportions in which they were introduced, and they can be readily recovered unchanged by any appropriate method such as fractional distillation. In order to separate the two groups forming such a molecule, namely, the acid group and the alcohol group, it is necessary to resort to chemical means whereby one of these groups is replaced by one of similar chemical nature but of greater reactivity; for instance, treatment of an ester with sulfuric acid will liberate the organic acid, while the more reactive sulfuric acid then becomes combined with the alcohol. If it is preferred to liberate the alcohol, a base such as sodium hydroxide may be used, in which case it is the organic acid which is obtained in combined form:

$$EtOAc + H_2SO_4 = EtOSO_3H + HOAc$$
$$EtOAc + HaOH = EtOH + NaOAc.$$

A new reaction has now been found whereby the alcohol and acid groups present in such a mixture of esters can be caused to exchange freely between the two or more groups of the opposite type which are present in the solution. Thus, the above mixture will yield two new compounds, namely, methyl acetate and ethyl butyrate.

$$EtOAc + MeOBt \rightleftarrows MeOAc + EtOBt$$ [1]

This reaction takes place by the simple use of a catalyst without the observable expenditure or production of energy, and practically without side reaction of any kind. The result, therefore, bears a striking similarity to the distribution of ions in an aqueous solution.

The reaction is not limited to esters, and similar observations have been made in the case of alkyl halides such as ethyl chloride and ethylene dibromide, and even more strikingly in the case of organo-metallic compounds. The latter case is all the more remarkable because these compounds, in general, behave very much like hydrocarbons, and their organic radicals can hardly be called functional groups, like the acid and alkyl groups in esters, or the halogens in alkyl halides, which are all susceptible of being removed or reintroduced at will by the use of appropriate strong chemical reagents. Typical examples of this reaction are illustrated in Figs. 1, 2 and 3, which show the distillation curve of mixtures containing originally two compounds, and after reaction all the possible combinations of the two kinds of radicals or atoms present.

[1] Ac = acetyl: $CH_3 \cdot CO-$; Bt = butyryl: $CH_3 \cdot CH_2 \cdot CH_2 \cdot CO-$.

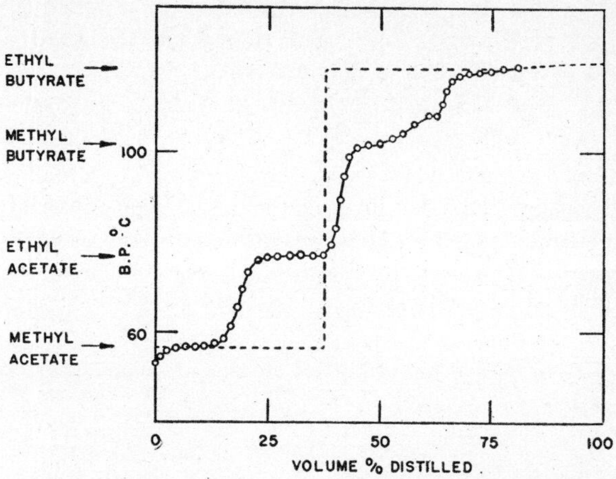


FIG. 1. Distillation of the reaction product of methyl acetate + ethyl butyrate. Dotted line represents distillation of same mixture before reaction.

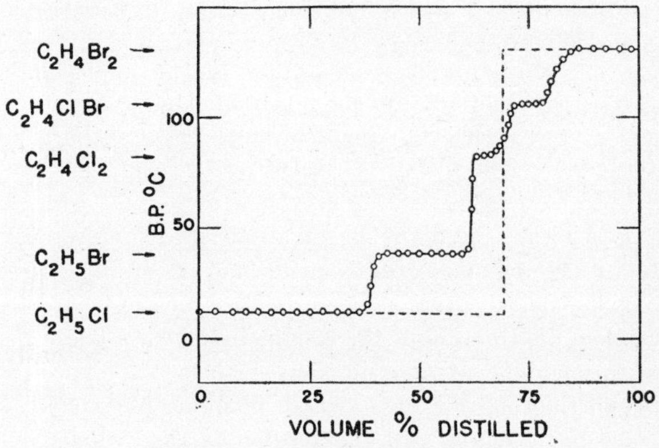


FIG. 2. Distillation of the reaction product of ethyl chloride + ethylene dibromide. Dotted line represents distillation of same mixture before reaction.

The organic chemist is apparently so steeped in the tradition that no reaction can take place between

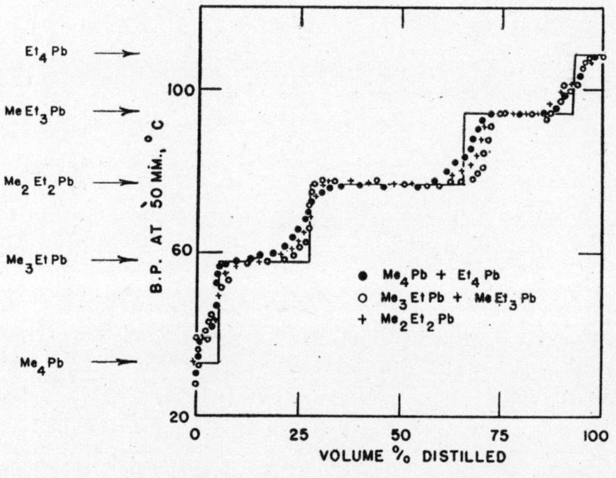


FIG. 3. Distillation of the reaction product of methyl and ethyl lead compounds. Solid line calculated for random equilibrium mixture having $r = 0.5$.

molecular groupings of the same type that no statement to that effect is found in the text-books; the notion becomes so obvious on the basis of our general chemical knowledge that it is subconsciously accepted. The present discovery seemed to strike so deeply at the foundation of our conception of organic chemistry that the investigation was soon directed toward an attempt to discern order in this seeming chaos. Systematic investigations have established the following characteristics of this unusual reaction:

(1) As far as has been ascertained, the reaction appears to be general within the classes of compounds investigated.

(2) The reaction is quantitative, and in some cases the most elaborate and precise methods of detecting by-products failed to find any.

(3) Little or no energy change is involved.

(4) The reaction is reversible, that is, the same final composition is obtained from any one or more starting materials as long as the bulk composition of the system is unchanged.

(5) The equilibrium composition is not appreciably affected by dilution with inert solvents, by temperature or any other commonly recognized independent variable in a chemical equilibrium, but is a function only of the gross composition of the system.

In view of the above observations, the simplest assumption was made regarding the nature of this equilibrium, namely, that it corresponded to the complete random distribution of the groups involved. The laws of probability express in simple form the expected proportions of all the possible combinations in systems of this kind. In the particular case which has been used most extensively for quantitative investigation in this field, namely, the case of tetraalkyllead compounds containing only methyl and ethyl groups, if we call $r$ the mole fraction of methyl groups in the mixtures of methyl and ethyl groups, *i.e.*, Me/(Me + Et), the concentration of the five possible compounds will be expressed by:

| | |
|---|---|
| $Me_4Pb$ | $r^4$ |
| $Me_3EtPb$ | $4r^3(1-r)$ |
| $Me_2Et_2Pb$ | $6r^2(1-r)^2$ |
| $MeEt_3Pb$ | $4r(1-r)^3$ |
| $Et_4Pb$ | $(1-r)^4$ |

Fig. 3 shows, as a solid line, the calculated distillation curve for such a system containing equal proportions of methyl and ethyl groups, *i.e.*, $r = 0.5$, and the three series of experimental distillation curves superimposed correspond to three systems for which $r = 0.5$ or nearly so, but in which the starting materials in each case were quite different, namely: $Me_4Pb + Et_4Pb$, $Me_3EtPb + MeEt_3Pb$ and $Me_2Et_2Pb$. Fig. 4 likewise gives corresponding calculated and observed distillation curves for two systems with high and low values of $r$, namely, $r = 0.345$ and $r = 0.776$. In each case, the agreement is remarkably good, showing that the distribution truly takes place completely at random.

These novel characteristics for a chemical reaction suggest the advisability of coining some new chemical terms and, accordingly, the reaction has been named "The Redistribution Reaction" and its final product a "Random Equilibrium Mixture."

The further investigation of the reaction was carried on principally in the field of organic metallic compounds, because these compounds react readily and with little or no side reaction and because the identity and exact concentration of the constituents of such systems are easily established.

Extended investigation of the reaction has shown it to take place in the case of alkyl or aryl groups, as well as with other metals than lead, such as tin, silicon and mercury, and complete random interchange of the radicals has been found to take place.

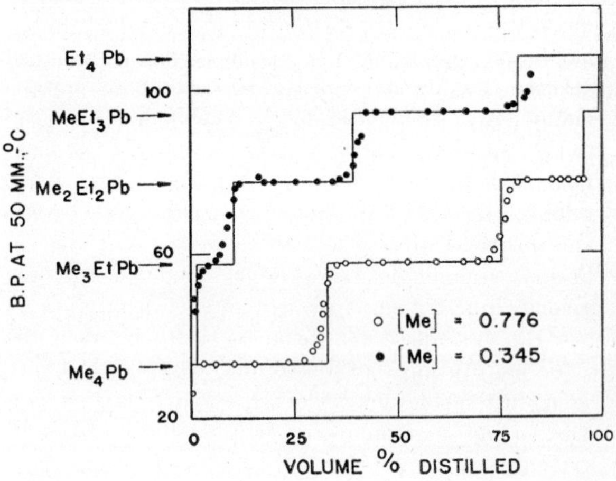


FIG. 4. Distillation of the reaction product of tetramethyllead + tetraethyllead. Solid lines calculated for ○ $r = 0.776$; ● $r = 0.345$.

Considering what we know of the instability of free radicals and their tendency to react with molecules or to rearrange yielding saturated and unsaturated hydrocarbons, it is remarkable to observe here a complete random mobility, without any loss of these groups through side reactions. This observed random distribution signifies that the bond strengths of the linkages involved are independent of the nature of the other linkages in the same molecule, that is, that the strength of a Me-Pb bond, for instance, is the same whether the other three linkages of the Pb are to methyl or to ethyl. This unexpected conclusion is likely to attract the attention of the chemists who spend considerable effort in attempting to determine bond strengths in atomic linkages. The systematic use of the redistribution reaction will be of considerable help in solving this key problem of molecular chemistry.

Another interesting application is in the study of relative affinities. When a system is investigated in which two or more groups of one kind, say alkyl radicals in organo-metallic compounds, are redistributed between two or more different "acceptors," as we shall call them, such as lead and mercury, a new factor enters into play. In this case, methyl and ethyl radicals wander not only from one lead atom to another, but also from a lead atom to a mercury atom. Although, as it has just been stated, when only one metal is involved, the methyl bonds are not affected by the presence of ethyl bonds and conversely, there seems to be no reason to assume that the same will hold when two metals are present. In this case, a methyl radical attached to a lead atom may interchange with an ethyl radical attached to a mercury atom, and the two metals need not necessarily have the same relative affinity for the two alkyl radicals involved. This can be tested experimentally: If a random equilibrium mixture is made, for instance, containing equivalent quantities of methyl and ethyl radicals, on the one hand, and mercury and lead atoms on the other, in the absence of different affinity relationships, the observed methyl-ethyl distribution on each metal will be equal to the over-all distribution, namely, $r = 0.5$. A greater relative affinity of one metal for one radical will be reflected by a shift of the value of $r$ up for one metal and correspondingly down for the other. The equilibrium so obtained will obey the mass action law and give an equilibrium which is expressed by:

$$K = \frac{[Me-Pb]\ [Et-Hg]}{[Me-Hg]\ [Et-Pb]},$$

where the brackets denote the concentration of the corresponding bonds in the total product. The result of such an investigation on the Me-Et-Pb-Hg system is illustrated in Fig. 5, where the same final equilibrium

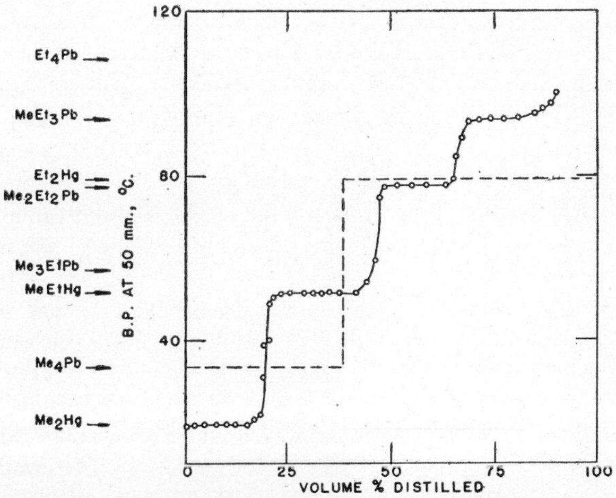


FIG. 5. Distillation of the reaction product from $Me_4Pb + 2\ Et_2Hg$, or $2\ Me_2Hg + Et_4Pb$. Dotted line represents distillation of the same mixture before reaction.

was reached from either end, that is, starting with $Me_4Pb + 2\ Et_2Hg$ as well as with $Et_4Pb + 2\ Me_2Hg$. By careful fractional distillation supplemented by analysis of each distillation cut for Pb and Hg, it was possible to tabulate the exact amount of each of the five lead and three mercury compounds formed. This corresponded in each case to a value of $r_{Pb} = 0.32$ and $r_{Hg} = 0.68$, giving a value of $K = 4.5$, showing that lead has a greater affinity for ethyl radicals, as compared to methyl, than has mercury.

Thus it is now possible by using the redistribution reaction to effect a direct measurement of the relative strengths of two kinds of bonds by actual observation under conditions of rigid equilibrium between the bonds involved, rather than by inference from the comparison of separate measurements, such as rates of reaction or the displacement of one radical by another.

The above quantitative observations clearly show the nature of the equilibrium. They throw, however, no light on the reasons for its existence or the mechanism involved. Reasoning by similarity with inorganic compounds, one might expect the mechanism to be through the formation of ions, while, on the other hand, the known existence of free radicals suggests the possibility of their playing a role in the redistribution reaction. Too much, however, is known about ions and free radicals as well as about the electronic nature of the covalent bond to make such explanations tenable. The organic compounds involved here are definitely not ionizable under the conditions used, and free radicals, if formed at all, would be bound to react with one another as well as with undissociated molecules, leading to the formation of large amounts of secondary products which are remarkably absent here.

The catalysts used in each case, although they may vary appreciably in chemical formulae, seem to have two characteristics in common, namely, (*a*) they contain one or more of the groups or atoms the redistribution of which they are capable of effecting, and (*b*) they are known or expected, on account of their electronic structure, to be capable of readily forming addition compounds with complete molecules of some kinds. This suggests that the mechanism of the redistribution reaction may be the reversible formation of a loose complex between a molecule of the catalyst and one or more molecules of the compounds to be redistributed. In this complex, the atoms or radicals to be redistributed are no longer identified with the particular molecule which has supplied them to the complex, but are shared in common by the residual parts of the catalyst as well as of the other molecule. When the complex breaks up, which probably occurs very frequently, each molecule, that is, the catalyst and the other compound, is reformed with its proper complement of groups, but these groups are taken at random from the common supply, and the final result of the repetition of this process is then the mathematical equilibrium corresponding to complete random redistribution. This is represented schematically by the equation:

$$R_2R'_2M + R'C \rightleftharpoons [R_2R'_3]\,[MC] \rightleftharpoons R_3R'M + RC$$

in which R and R′ are the groups to be redistributed, M is the carrier, such as Pb in the case of alkyllead compounds, and R′C or RC is the catalyst.

The information obtained so far on the redistribution reaction is in accord with such a mechanism, but does not yet include data which confirm its correctness. Kinetic studies of the reaction and investigation of the physical and chemical characteristics of the catalyst are, however, expected to throw light on this point. It seems fair to expect that a closer scrutiny of the mechanism of the reaction will lead to a better understanding of the exact nature of the covalent bond and particularly of the exact mechanism whereby it is loosened and reformed in ordinary chemical reactions.

Beyond these positive studies one may well speculate whether this heretofore unsuspected reaction does not often take place spontaneously in natural systems containing several kinds of similar compounds. It may well be that the aging of alcoholic beverages is due at least in part to the redistribution of the esters to which they owe their flavor, while some of the little understood changes which take place in the living cell may correspond to the random interchange of the amino acid groups between the molecules of protein.

Practical applications should also not be overlooked. Two groups already suggest themselves at first sight. One is the preparation of mixed compounds such as mixed esters of polybasic acids, for instance: instead of preparing these by successive esterification, they can now be prepared directly by redistribution between the two corresponding symmetrical esters. A second and perhaps less obvious line would be the opening of new fields of use for materials heretofore considered too inert to be of practical value in chemical syntheses. For instance, organic bromides are not usually thought of as brominating agents because the bromine can not be removed by ordinary methods. As shown in Fig. 2, appropriate double decomposition between ethylene dibromide and an organic chloride will yield the corresponding bromide. Bearing in mind the availability and ease of handling ethylene dibromide, it seems probable that its use will prove advantageous in the preparation of some organic bromides, especially where the corresponding chloride is readily available.

The scientific reader who is not directly concerned with organic chemistry will be interested to note that this discovery carries a lesson which reaches well beyond the confines of its field. The concept of the absence of reaction between similar organic compounds has been accepted without challenge because of its usefulness in introducing order in our chemical knowledge. The experimental evidence reported above proves once more that we should ever bear in mind that the validity of any concept depends on how strictly we have been able to subject it to experimental verification and not on how long we have had it or how easily it fits our mental processes.[1]

[1] A complete technical report on the subject will appear in the *Journal* of the American Chemical Society beginning in October, 1939.

# OBITUARY

## WITMER STONE[1]
### (1866–1939)

WITMER STONE was born a naturalist, nurtured a naturalist, and a naturalist he lived to the end of his days. Most of the many activities that filled his busy life flowed from his profound interest in nature. An instinctive collector, he loved to gather about him the objects that excited his admiration and curiosity. In naming and classifying his specimens he became a systematist and a scientist. Inevitably as he made and mastered collections his keen perceptions discovered new kinds of animals and plants and new facts relating to kinds previously known. He wrote of his discoveries so wisely and so well that he became editor of the foremost ornithological journal of America. As a master editor and through his technical papers he became known throughout the world and added to his fame and that of the institution which was his scientific home.

Stone's association with the Academy of Natural Sciences of Philadelphia was practically life-long. It began in a boyish fascination following a visit to the museum when he was eight or nine years old and became closer year by year until 1888, when he assumed charge of the bird collections for the Ornithological Section. From this nominal official connection he succeeded step by step through curatorial positions from conservator to director of the museum. His life became so merged with that of the academy that for many years it was difficult to think of them apart. During the half-century of his official connection the collections of the academy grew greatly. The number of birds alone increased from 26,000 in 1888 to 143,000 in 1939.

Apart from his curatorial duties but more or less closely linked with them Witmer Stone's activities may be placed under four heads: namely, (1) scientific research, (2) nomenclatural, (3) editorial and histori-

[1] Based on a Minute of Appreciation presented to the council of the Academy of Natural Sciences of Philadelphia, October 3, 1939.

cal and (4) educational. To a remarkable degree he possessed the diverse attributes that made him successful in each. That these successes were somewhat notable is perhaps best indicated by the opinions of competent contemporaries, who so often designated the field of their own specialty as that in which Stone had excelled. There is a wide-spread agreement among ornithologists concerning the importance of his contributions under 2 and 3. His book reviews in the *Auk,* of which he wrote about 1,500, are famous and widely read. Except for his "Bird Studies at Old Cape May," his papers on moult, plumages and migration and his "Plants of Southern New Jersey," his research publication seems to be less read, but its good quality is unquestioned. Concerning the value of his informal but effective educational influence, there is almost universal agreement. It was effected chiefly through direct personal contact. One prominent ornithologist writes, "I have never heard him open his mouth, either in private conversation or public speech without saying something significant and worthy of attention."

In each of his several activities Dr. Stone became by sheer ability and industry a recognized leader. He was a founder or a constructive member of several important biological societies. He became president or vice-president or both of the American Ornithologists' Union, the Delaware Valley Ornithological Club, the American Society of Mammalogists, the Philadelphia Botanical Club and the Pennsylvania Audubon Society. He was a vice-president of the Academy of Natural Sciences of Philadelphia and could have become president, following the death of Dr. Samuel G. Dixon, had he not declined. He was secretary of the Ludwick Institute since 1920 and a manager of the Philadelphia Zoological Society. Of the famous University of Pennsylvania Class of '87 he was secretary from undergraduate days to the time of his death. Many other unsought honors came to him. The University of Pennsylvania conferred upon him the Sc.D. and the Alumni Award of Merit. The National Committee of Audubon Societies established the Witmer Stone Wild Life Sanctuary at Cape May. The Hungarian Ornithological Society awarded him its Otto Hermann Medal and the American Ornithologists' Union its Brewster Medal posthumously. No other person received so many honors from the latter society as did he. Dr. Stone was elected to honorary or equivalent membership in many important foreign ornithological societies. After twenty years as editor of the *Auk* some 130 fellows and members of the American Ornithologists' Union presented him with a volume of testimonial letters, and on his seventieth birthday he was presented with a similar tribute from friends. The letters express the esteem in which he is widely held. When our front-rank ornithologists apply to him such terms as "dean of American ornithologists," "master workman in ornithology" and the like, it means that we have lived in the presence of a man of exceptional merit.

It may be permissible to venture a description of the historical niche in American ornithology which Witmer Stone occupies. Briefly, North American ornithology may be divided roughly into four periods. First was the pioneer period when the birds of the eastern United States were discovered and described. Second was the period of exploration and government surveys of the West, extending our knowledge of birds to the Pacific. Third was a period of consolidation and systematization, of organized effort, largely through the American Ornithologists' Union, to eliminate confusion by the adoption of exact concepts of species and subspecies and the attainment of a stable nomenclature. Dr. Stone was a dominant figure during much of this period, and its close may be placed in 1931 with the publication of the fourth edition of the A. O. U. Check List. One ornithologist has designated it as the "Stone Age" of American ornithology. Due to the arduous labors of Stone and his contemporaries it forms a solid foundation for the precise studies of the fourth or present period.

Of Dr. Stone it may be said that the seed within him on fertile soil grew into a sturdy tree of many branches, bearing fragrant flowers and nourishing fruit. Naturalist, scientist, faithful custodian of collections, biographer and historian of scientists and their science, interpreter of the rules of zoological nomenclature, protector of birds, writer of exceptional beauty and vigor, sometimes poetical, lecturer and teacher, helpful adviser, delightful companion and valued friend, Witmer Stone gave the best of his life and labor to this historic academy and of the riches of his personality to colleagues and associates.

His works and our memories are a fitting memorial, and may his spirit long abide in the lives of those on whom he spent it.

## RECENT DEATHS

DR. FLOYD KARKER RICHTMYER, professor of physics and dean of the graduate school of Cornell University, died on November 7 at the age of fifty-eight years.

DR. WALDEMAR LINDGREN, from 1912 until his retirement with the title emeritus in 1933 Rogers professor of economic geology at the Massachusetts Institute of Technology, died on November 4 at the age of seventy-nine years.

DR. FRANK ANGELL, emeritus professor of psychology at Stanford University, died on November 2 at the age of eighty-two years.

DR. ROBERT MACDOUGALL, emeritus professor of analytical psychology at New York University, died on October 31 at the age of seventy-three years.

DR. JOSEPH B. LINDSEY, from 1911 to 1927 head of the department of chemistry at the Massachusetts State College and from 1911 to 1932 Goessmann professor of agricultural chemistry, died on October 27 at the age of seventy-seven years.

DR. WILLARD BURR SOPER, associate professor of medicine at Yale University and medical director of the William Wirt Winchester Hospital, the tuberculosis unit of the New Haven Hospital, died on October 30 at the age of fifty-six years.

COLONEL GUSTAV J. FIEBEGER, Corps of Engineers, who for twenty-six years was head of the department of civil and military engineering of the United States Military Academy at West Point, died on October 18 at the age of eighty-one years.

# SCIENTIFIC EVENTS

## THE GALTON LABORATORY

DR. R. A. FISHER, Galton professor of eugenics at University College, London, writes under date of September 29 the following letter to the editor of the London *Times:*

The evacuation of London University has been represented as carefully planned and smoothly carried out in accordance with prior arrangements, and I am sure that the central officials of this loose federation have done what they can in difficult circumstances. The position in which the Galton Laboratory finds itself may be typical of other research departments in the university, or it may be, as I hope, exceptional, but it is scarcely what could have been intended by the careful planners.

The laboratory was founded on a generous bequest of the benefactor whose name it bears, and has, I presume, an unquestioned right to the provision of facilities for the prosecution of its researches. Nevertheless it has been ordered to evacuate the accommodation it now occupies at University College without alternative accommodation being provided. Worse than this, when in my difficulty I approached my former chief, Sir John Russell, Director of the Rothamsted Experimental Station, and he had helpfully and generously offered to provide alternative accommodation for my department and equipment rent free, I was informed that my assistants, while still in receipt of their salaries, are forbidden to continue their duties.

As the head of this department, therefore, the only determined policy which I can recognize on the part of the College Committee is that of suppressing research work and dispersing the research units such as that which it has been my work and, as I understood it, my duty to build up.

During the last war our administrators learned, though perhaps with some reluctance, that men trained in research were essential for the success of the national effort. The remaining nucleus of my department, if I may speak in its praise, constitutes a unit for heavy mathematical computations as efficient, both in machines and men, as the country can command. Obviously no work of first-class national importance can be found for such a unit at a few days' notice. I submit that it is almost equally obvious that in certain contingencies its continued existence might be of the greatest value, so long as the machines and the expert knowledge had been kept together. Can not a little patience be exercised before completing its demolition?

## THE PRIVATELY ENDOWED COLLEGE OF ENGINEERING

A BROADCAST sponsored by the alumni of the Case School of Applied Science was made on October 28 for consideration of the question, "What's Ahead for the Privately Endowed College of Engineering?" The program, which was given at a luncheon of the alumni in Cleveland, was carried nationally over the Mutual Broadcasting Company's system.

The consensus of opinion of the six participants in the radio discussion was that engineering colleges which depend on endowment and gifts need additional funds to overcome the decline in earnings from investments and to provide for new educational services. These funds should be sought from those benefited, directly or indirectly, from the work of the colleges, These comprise the alumni, industry, which depends on these colleges for their trained personnel, and society, which profits from the earnings of industry. The reasons why so few large gifts have been made to colleges of technology is due, the conferees believed, because of the inactivity of these institutions in placing their needs before persons of wealth.

Participants in the radio discussion were leaders in industry and scientific men, all residents of Cleveland. The speakers were: George S. Case, chairman of the board, Lamson and Sessions Company; Lee M. Clegg, executive vice-president, Thompson Products Company; David Dietz, science editor, Scripps-Howard Newspapers; Randolph Eide, president of the Ohio Bell Telephone Company; Sam W. Emerson, president of the S. W. Emerson Company, contractors, and Dr. Zay Jeffries, technical director, Lamp Department, General Electric Company.

In summing up the problem of getting funds for technological education, Dr. William E. Wickenden, president of the Case School of Applied Science, said:

Traditional motive makes it much easier to get money for religion, for hospitals, for medical research and for the fine arts, than for science and engineering. Our graduates are giving splendidly, out of loyalty, but I wonder if our big job is not to implant new motives in the minds of wealthy men.

One such motive is this: No man, no company, no industry can do business to-day without the aid of the priceless heritage of science and skill which has come down to it all the way from Tubal Cain to Arthur Compton without a cent of direct cost. Take away Faraday's work and where would the electrical industry be? There's a moral debt to be paid, and the best way to pay it is through the schools of applied science. Then, too, much of to-day's wealth is coming from natural resources we can never replace. Every pound of coal or iron, every gallon of oil, every foot of natural gas we consume makes it just that much harder for our children and their children to make a good life. This is going to hit Cleveland, which owes so much of its wealth and greatness to these resources, unless it builds up resources in science and skill to take their place. That is the way to make good to the future for what we are using up to-day, to build up science and skill.

An institute of applied science, such as Case, really asks nothing for itself. Every cent goes back to the community and the nation with its value multiplied, to make to-day's living better and to-morrow's future more secure.

## THE AMERICAN ACADEMY OF OPHTHALMOLOGY AND OTOLARYNGOLOGY

Dr. Frank R. Spencer, of Boulder, Colo., was chosen president-elect of the American Academy of Ophthalmology and Otolaryngology at the annual session held in Chicago on October 11. He will succeed Dr. Frank E. Brawley, of Chicago, when the latter becomes president of the academy on January 1. Dr. Spencer is a graduate of the University of Michigan Medical School and has been a member of the faculty of the University of Colorado School of Medicine since 1905.

The academy decided to act as sponsor for a proposed Pan American congress of ophthalmology and otolaryngology. South American physicians attending the meeting in Chicago will arrange for the attendance of delegates from their respective countries to such a congress to be held in connection with the next meeting of the academy. It is understood that invitations to each of the countries concerned will have the sanction of the Department of State and will be forwarded through diplomatic channels.

Other officers elected were Drs. Arthur W. Proetz, St. Louis, *first vice-president;* Joseph F. Duane, Peoria, Ill., *second vice-president,* and Charles T. Porter, Boston, *third vice-president;* Secord H. Large, Cleveland, *comptroller,* and William P. Wherry, Omaha, Nebr., *executive secretary,* reelected. Dr. Erling W. Hansen, Minneapolis, was elected secretary for public relations, succeeding Dr. Ralph A. Fenton, Portland, Ore., who resigned. The following secretaries were reelected: Drs. William L. Benedict, Rochester, Minn., for ophthalmology; John L. Myers, Kansas City, Mo., for otolaryngology; Dean M. Lierle, Iowa City, for instruction in otolaryngology, and Albert D. Ruedemann, for instruction in ophthalmology. Dr. Albert C. Snell, Rochester, N. Y., was elected a member of the academy's governing council, and Dr. Frederick C. Cordes, San Francisco, to represent the academy on the American Board of Ophthalmology.

The academy continued the following appropriations for research: Dr. Olof Larsell, University of Oregon Medical School, Portland, $400 for research on development of the internal ear; Dr. M. H. Lurie, Harvard Medical School, Boston, $400 for research on the balancing apparatus of the ear, and for the Army Medical Museum at Washington, D. C., $1,500 for maintaining collections of pathological specimens in diseases of the eye, ear, nose and throat. An appropriation of $1,500 was also made for the establishment under the supervision of the academy of reading courses for young physicians serving as residents in hospitals who are preparing for specialization in diseases of the eye, ear, nose and throat. A grant of $400 was made to Dr. Spencer for research on the action of drugs on tubercle bacilli in the nose and throat. The committee on physiological optics received $50 and the committee on orthoptics $200.

## SCIENTIFIC EXPEDITIONS

The expedition sponsored by the National Geographic Society and the University of Virginia with the U. S. Coast Guard cooperating, which was to have sailed from San Francisco on September 19 on the Coast Guard cutter *Hamilton* has been postponed. The *Hamilton* has been ordered to Atlantic waters as part of the coast patrol. In preparation for the expedition tons of scientific equipment had been shipped to the Pacific Coast to be loaded on the *Hamilton,* and members of the expedition had spent months of intensive work in preparing apparatus for studying geology, magnetism of the earth, variations in gravity, earthquakes, marine biology, weather, ocean currents, and for collecting samples of the ocean bottom from great depths. The expedition was planned to conduct the most extensive program of scientific work so far attempted in the region of the Pacific Islands. Professor Wilbur A. Nelson, leader of the expedition, is returning to his work as professor of geology at the University of Virginia, to await conditions better suited to scientific research on the high seas.

The second Fahnestock expedition to the South Seas of the American Museum of Natural History, organized by Bruce and Sheridan Fahnestock, will leave New York in the near future in the three-masted auxiliary schooner *Director II.* In addition to collecting material for six habitat studies for the new Whitney Memorial Bird Hall and specimens of fish, insects and minerals, islands out of position on existing charts will be remapped. It is expected that the expedition will take from eighteen months to two years. Later an entomologist, a geologist and a recording technician will be appointed from the American Museum staff and from Columbia University.

A SIX months' expedition to make a comprehensive collection of the plants of Guatemala for the herbarium of the Field Museum of Natural History left Chicago on September 27 under the direction of Dr. Julian A. Steyermark, assistant curator of the herbarium, who sailed on the steamship *Ulm* from New Orleans. The expedition is sponsored by Stanley Field, president of the museum. It is planned to explore the little known Oriente area in the departments of Chiquimula, Jutiapa and Jalapa. Work in the desert area around Zacapa will be carried out during the rainy season, and Dr. Steyermark expects to find a number of unusual species of plants. The expedition then plans to move into the Sierra Madre region of western Guatemala, in the provinces of San Marcos and Huehuetenango. Particular attention will be devoted to the flora of the Tajumulco volcano, and collecting is contemplated in the district around Mazatenango.

### FIELD WORK OF THE U. S. GEOLOGICAL SURVEY

AMONG the members of the Geological Branch who have recently returned to Washington, D. C., after completing their season's field work on the projects indicated, are the following:

S. R. Capps, who studied the structural history of west-central Idaho in its relation to the gold placer deposits.

H. G. Ferguson, who continued studies of structural and stratigraphic problems in Nevada and completed preliminary mapping of the western and central parts of the Sonoma Range quadrangle.

T. A. Hendricks and Paul Averitt, who investigated the geology and oil possibilities in the western part of the Ouachita Mountains, Okla.

A. A. Baker, who studied the phosphate and coal resources and oil and gas possibilities in the southern Wasatch Mountains, Utah.

W. P. Woodring, who examined the geology and oil resources in the Santa Maria district, Calif.

W. C. Warren, who, with the aid of aerial photographs, mapped about 1,150 square miles of coal lands in southeastern Montana.

D. A. Andrews, who completed his fourth season of study of the stratigraphy, structure, economic geology and geomorphology along the northeast flank of the Bighorn Basin, Wyoming and Montana.

C. B. Hunt, who completed his fifth and final season of investigating the geology of the Henry Mountains, Utah, and examined gold placer gravel deposits and unusual erosion features in the canyon of the Colorado River between Hite and Lee's Ferry.

Members of the Alaskan Branch have completed the season's field work in Alaska and have returned to Washington for the office and laboratory studies required to put their resulting maps and notes into shape for publication. F. H. Moffit examined the east-central part of the Alaska Range, embracing principally the country between Delta and Johnson Rivers. J. C. Reed carried on geological surveys in the northwestern part of Chichagof Island, southeastern Alaska. J. B. Mertie, Jr., investigated the potential tin fields of western Seward Peninsula. Gerald Fitzgerald made extensive topographic surveys in the vicinity of Porcupine River from Fort Yukon to the Canadian Boundary. T. V. Ranta revised much of the early exploratory mapping of the country between Nabesna and Chisana Rivers, near the head of Tanana River. Philip S. Smith inspected a number of the more accessible mining districts in central Alaska, and collected information as to new mining developments in progress.

## SCIENTIFIC NOTES AND NEWS

THE Royal Society, London, according to a wireless report in *The New York Times,* awarded on November 2 the Copley Medal to Professor Thomas H. Morgan, director of the William G. Kerckhoff Laboratories of the California Institute of Technology, for his work in genetics, and the Davy Medal to Dr. James W. McBain, professor of chemistry at Stanford University, for his work in colloid chemistry.

THE Sedgwick Memorial Medal, awarded for distinguished service in public health, was presented to Dr. Thomas Parran, Jr., Surgeon General of the United States Public Health Service, on October 17 at the sixty-eighth annual meeting of the American Public Health Association in Pittsburgh. Dr. Milton J. Rosenau, director of the Division of Public Health of the School of Medicine of the University of North Carolina, made the presentation.

DR. FRANCIS CARTER WOOD, director of the Institute of Cancer Research of Columbia University, was presented with the Clement Cleveland Medal for 1939 at the annual dinner of the New York City Cancer Committee.

A CITATION for distinguished service to agriculture was presented to Dean Emeritus F. B. Mumford, of the Missouri College of Agriculture, at the annual banquet on November 2 of the Association of Alumni and Former Students. The banquet was held on the last evening and formed part of the centennial celebration of the university.

THE Charles Frederick Chandler Medal of Columbia University will be presented to Thomas Hamilton Chilton, director of the Technical Division of the Department of Engineering in the E. I. du Pont de Nemours and Company, on the evening of November 16, when Mr. Chilton will deliver the annual Chandler Lecture. His subject will be "Engineering in the Service of Chemistry."

ACCORDING to press reports the Nobel Prize for physiology and medicine "has been regretfully declined" by Professor Gerhard Domagk, director of the research institute of the I. G. Farbenindustrie Laboratory at Elberfeld. It is said that he has written to the Stockholm committee, thanking them for the honor conferred on him, but pointing out that under the present law no German is allowed to accept a Nobel Prize.

SIR CHARLES SHERRINGTON, Waynflete professor of physiology at the University of Oxford, has been elected to an honorary fellowship in Magdalen College.

ARTHUR NUTT, vice-president for engineering of the Wright Aeronautical Corporation, has been nominated for the presidency of the Society of Automotive Engineers.

DEAN OLIN J. FERGUSON, of the College of Engineering of the University of Nebraska, has been elected president of the Society for the Promotion of Engineering Education for the year 1930–40. He succeeds Dr. Karl T. Compton, president of the Massachusetts Institute of Technology. The secretary is Dr. F. L. Bishop, of the University of Pittsburgh. The annual meeting will be held at the University of California from June 25 to 28, when it is expected that a thousand delegates will be in attendance.

PROFESSOR FRANK CYRIL JAMES, director of the School of Commerce of McGill University, will succeed Dr. Lewis W. Douglas as principal and vice-chancellor of the university. Mr. James, a native of London, is thirty-six years old and is a British subject. In 1924 he was appointed instructor of finance in the Wharton School of Finance and Commerce of the University of Pennsylvania, becoming full professor in 1935.

DR. GEORGE W. CORNER, since its establishment in 1924 professor of anatomy and chairman of the department in the School of Medicine and Dentistry of the University of Rochester, has been appointed director of the department of embryology at the Carnegie Institution of Washington. He succeeds on May 1, 1940, Dr. George L. Streeter, who since 1917 has been director of the department.

KENNETH H. CONDIT will succeed Professor Arthur Maurice Greene, Jr., as dean of the School of Engineering of Princeton University, Professor Greene, since 1922 dean of the school, having presented his resignation. Mr. Condit is at present assistant to the president of the National Industrial Conference Board. He was elected at the recent annual meeting vice-president of the American Society of Mechanical Engineers.

DEAN WILLIAM H. HALL has been made head of the new college of engineering at Duke University.

DR. WILBER E. POST, for the past twenty years clinical professor of medicine at the Rush Graduate School of Medicine of the University of Chicago, has been appointed dean.

DR. HOWARD Y. MCCLUSKY, of the University of Michigan, has been promoted to a professorship of educational psychology, mental measurements and statistics. He has also been made assistant to the vice-president in charge of university relations in the field of adult education.

DR. LEROY A. SCHALL, who has been instructor in laryngology at the Harvard Medical School since 1926, has been appointed Walter Augustus Lecompte professor of otology and professor of laryngology. He succeeds Dr. Harris P. Mosher, who has taught at the Medical School for more than thirty years and now becomes professor emeritus.

DR. S. ULAM has been appointed lecturer in mathematics at Harvard University for the academic year 1939–40.

DR. PETTUS HOLMES SENN, of the department of agronomy of the University of Florida, has been promoted to a professorship of agronomy and to the head of the department in the teaching division of the College of Agriculture.

DEPARTMENT chairmen at Queens College, New York City, who are elected by the faculty, have been chosen in the science departments as follows: Professor Donald E. Kirkpatrick, physics; Professor Anne Anastasi, psychology; Dr. John Dambach, health and recreation; Professor T. Freeman Cope, mathematics; Professor Roland Whittaker, chemistry; Dr. Hortense Powdermaker, anthropology and sociology, and Professor Donald E. Lancefield, biology. The appointments will be presented to the Board of Higher Education for formal approval.

DR. ELIOT G. MEARS, professor of geography and international trade at Stanford University, will be the general chairman of the seventeenth annual Institute of World Affairs, to be held under the auspices of the University of Southern California at the Mission Inn, Riverside, Calif., from December 10 to 15.

DR. DETLEV W. BRONK, director of the Eldridge R. Johnson Foundation for Medical Physics and of the Institute of Neurology of the University of Pennsylvania, has been appointed managing editor of *The*

*Journal of Cellular and Comparative Physiology* of the Wistar Institute of Anatomy and Biology, Philadelphia. He succeeds Professor E. Newton Harvey, of Princeton University.

SIR JOSEPH BARCROFT, from 1926 until his retirement in 1937 professor of physiology at the University of Cambridge; Sir Harold B. Hartley, chairman of the Fuel Research Board of the Department for Scientific and Industrial Research, and Sir Frank E. Smith, secretary of the department and a secretary of the Royal Society, have been appointed members of the Advisory Council to the Committee of the Privy Council for Scientific and Industrial Research. Lord Cadman and Sir James Jeans have retired from the council on completion of their terms of office.

DR. FOREST RAY MOULTON, permanent secretary of the American Association for the Advancement of Science, addressed members of the Academy of Medicine of Washington, D. C., on the evening of October 27. The title of his address was "A Jaundiced Look at the Human Machine."

DR. C. STUART GAGER, director of the Brooklyn Botanic Garden, gave an address at the three hundredth meeting of the Botanical Society of Washington, D. C., on November 7. His subject was "How Botany Advances." The address was preceded by "illustrated reminiscences," with portraits of former botanists of Washington.

DR. ELLIOTT C. CUTLER, Moseley professor of surgery at the Harvard Medical School, spoke before the Omaha Mid-west Clinical Society in Omaha on October 26 on "Incomplete Intestinal Obstruction" and on "Acute Appendicitis." On October 30 he spoke on the "Surgical Treatment of Gallstones" at the Inter-state Post-graduate Medical Assembly of North America in Chicago.

THE first of the 1939–40 series of Foster Lectures at the University of Buffalo was given on October 26 by Dr. Vincent du Vigneaud, professor of biochemistry at the Cornell University Medical College, New York City. His subjects were "The Metabolic Relationship of Choline and Methionine" and "Tracing Chemical Reactions in the Body by Means of Isotopes." During the week of November 13, Professor Kasimir Fajans, of the University of Michigan, will be in residence. He will give six lectures on the chemical aspects of crystal structure, adsorption indicators, types of chemical linkages, and refractometric investigations. The Foster lectures are provided by the proceeds of a fund given the university by the late Mrs. O. E. Foster in memory of her husband.

THE program for the New England Conference of the American Association of Museums at the Springfield Museum of Fine Arts has been arranged in outline, according to *Museum News,* as follows: Friday, November 24, registration, address of welcome and a business meeting; a special performance in the planetarium for delegates, followed by tea and a subscription dinner, with an address by Andrey Avinoff, director of the Carnegie Museum, Pittsburgh, on "The Relationship of Science and Esthetics in the Museum." Saturday, November 25, morning sessions by art and science groups meeting separately; a special program for the art group in connection with an exhibition of paintings and drawings by David and Ingres; luncheon at the museum; a joint session, at which questions raised by Mr. Avinoff's address will be discussed, and a tea and a gallery talk by Katherine Dreier in connection with the first showing of the collection of the Société Anonyme.

THE recently formed Sigma Xi Club of Hawaii held its first annual meeting in the new Union Building of the University of Hawaii on October 20. The election of thirteen new members raised the membership total to sixty-five. Officers elected for the ensuing year were: *President,* Dr. C. J. Hamre, associate professor of zoology in the University of Hawaii; *Vice-president,* Dr. Martha Potgieter, associate nutritionist in the Hawaii Agricultural Experiment Station; *Secretary-Treasurer,* Dr. S. S. Ballard, assistant professor of physics in the University of Hawaii; *Councilors,* Dr. H. E. Gregory, retired director of the Bernice P. Bishop Museum, and C. E. Pemberton, executive entomologist of the Experiment Station of the Hawaiian Sugar Planters' Association. The address of the evening was delivered by Dr. Hamre, who spoke on "Some Aspects of the Physiology of the Bone Marrow."

IN a statement made by Chancellor O. C. Carmichael, of Vanderbilt University, it is announced that more than $1,500,000 of a bequest from the estate of Frederick W. Vanderbilt has been received by the university.

BY the will of the late Henry W. Putnam, a New York manufacturer, who left an estate valued at over $21,000,000, Harvard, Yale and Princeton Universities will share the sum of $9,858,332 upon the death of four of his cousins. The sum of $3,000,000 is bequeathed to the Henry W. Putnam Memorial Hospital at Bennington, Vt.

ACCORDING to a press dispatch from Pasadena, Dr. John Martin Vincent, emeritus professor of European history in the Johns Hopkins University, who died in September at the age of eighty-one years, left his estate, said to be of the value of $1,500,000, to the department of history.

THE will of the late Richard Halliburton, the explorer, leaves an estate, believed to be worth about

$100,000, largely in trust to his parents with the provision that, following their death, it be turned over to Princeton University to establish a Richard Halliburton Geological Library.

The five million kronen collected on the occasion of the thirtieth year of the reign of King Gustaf of Sweden will be devoted to the establishment of a foundation for the study of paralytic diseases, especially poliomyelitis, and to the campaign against tuberculosis.

Formal exercises dedicating the Medical Building at the University of North Carolina will be held on December 4. The morning will be devoted to addresses by prominent physicians and experts in public health. The afternoon will be given over to inspection of the new building, and a banquet in the evening will conclude the program.

An Associated Press dispatch states that further Nobel Prize awards will be withheld this year, due to the European war. The literary, physics and chemistry prizes for 1939 may be awarded next year, but the 1938 chemistry prize, postponed last year, will be permanently omitted and the prize money, about $38,769, returned to the main fund.

The Statistical Laboratory of the Iowa State College, of which Professor G. W. Snedecor is director, has recently made an agreement with the Bureau of Agricultural Economics of the U. S. Department of Agriculture to provide for joint research in the statistics of agriculture and associated statistical theory.

# DISCUSSION

## VITALIZING HISTORICAL GEOLOGY THROUGH FIELD TRIPS

Field trips, if they are to constitute a part of a course in general geology, should make a vital contribution to the course. It frequently happens that this contribution can be made more easily when the work deals with physical geology than when it deals with historical geology. Since one or more of the geologic agents are continually at work in any given region it is not difficult to plan a field trip on which the student can observe some of the physical processes which they study in class. In some regions it is a little more difficult to plan a field trip that will make a vital contribution to the study of historical geology. In some localities only a limited geologic column is accessible to the students without the expenditure of an unreasonable amount of time and money. In such cases the field trip may resolve itself into a fossil-collecting expedition or a superficial study of the rocks of the region with little or no connection with the work of the classroom.

For several years the author has been attempting to remedy this weakness and to make the field work of his students contribute more than that to their work in general geology. An article recently published by Gwynne[1] describing his efforts to make the field trip a real teaching device, suggested to our mind that the plan we had tried this year might be interesting and helpful to other geology teachers.

It so happens that the rocks in the region around New Concord are in the Conemaugh series of the Pennsylvanian system. Most of the ridges of the region are high enough to include the lower part of the Monongahela series. Since this is the case it seemed desirable to make an effort to correlate the field trips with our class discussion of the Pennsylvanian system.

As early in the spring as weather conditions would permit field work the students were given a mimeographed schedule of observations and records that were to be made on field trips. Small groups of students were then taken into the field and together with the instructor observed and recorded a typical exposure of a succession of rocks of Pennsylvanian age found in a road cut near New Concord, Ohio. Each student contributed his observations, and the members of the group recorded the observations in their note-books. The instructor directed the activities and attention when necessary, making sure that all important points were observed.

After the group instruction in the field each student chose from a list of places previously selected by the instructor a road cut, ravine or roadside ditch near New Concord in which to observe and study a consecutive succession of rock exposures. The student was instructed to observe and describe the successive exposures and their contacts as carefully as possible and to collect whatever fossils they could find. The fossils which they collected were identified in the laboratory. Thus the field trip contributed to the work in the laboratory. When a student's observation was complete the record was presented to the instructor, who checked it for completeness and accuracy. In most cases it was necessary to send the student back over the area to make a more careful and detailed observation. All observations were to be completed and the records checked and accepted before the day on which the class discussion of the Mississippian period was finished.

On the day scheduled for the beginning of the class

[1] C. S. Gwynne, Science, November 11, 1938.

study of the Pennsylvanian period the selected sections described by the students were assembled and copied on the blackboard, and in so far as possible these sections were correlated. From these correlated sections, covering an area of about three square miles, a generalized cross section of the rocks of the New Concord region was made. This work was done largely by the students; the instructor, acting as a secretary, did the actual writing on the board.

From the information thus collected the class then reconstructed the geologic history of the region immediately surrounding New Concord. This offered an opportunity for the students to apply the scientific method in their study of the region. With the history of our own area in mind we then turned to the textbook for a more complete picture of the Pennsylvanian as a whole, keeping in mind the idea of tying up the region we had actually studied with the Pennsylvanian system as it is found in North America and tying the geologic history of the New Concord region as we had reconstructed it from our field study of the region with the history of the Pennsylvanian of North America.

This plan of procedure is not without its weaknesses, most serious of which is the fact that before the student starts out on his own to observe the rocks and record his observations he needs more field experience than we have given him. We plan to overcome this difficulty by beginning to observe and describe the rocks during the first semester in addition to the observation of the physical phenomena which heretofore has constituted most of our field work during the first semester. It is quite possible, too, that we will be able to find time for more than one conducted field trip early in the second semester field season before sending the student into the field on his own.

On the other hand, this procedure has several desirable features. The student develops a realistic idea of the Pennsylvanian and, indeed, the whole of the geologic column and of geologic history by actually studying, recording and interpreting his observations of a part of the rocks of the Pennsylvanian system. He arrives at a better appreciation of the work of the geologist through his own experience in working as the geologist works. His interest in geology is increased through active participation. He has had the experience of observing and recording evidence and in drawing inferences from the evidence. Thus he has actually had a concrete experience with the scientific method.

Robert H. Mitchell

Muskingum College

## ENDOGONE AS ANIMAL FOOD

Although the genus Endogone has received comprehensive taxonomic treatment little is recorded of the rôle which species of these hypogeous fungi may play in the economy of nature. It is to be expected that the small, truffle-like fructifications of *Endogone* might be eaten by some animals, but accounts of their use as food seem strangely lacking. It seems in order, therefore, to place on record certain instances where such materials have been found in stomach contents of shrews and mice.

Dr. W. J. Hamilton in August, 1938, sent to the U. S. Biological Survey specimens from Ithaca, N. Y., with the observation that "the small black objects . . . were often, but not invariably associated with earthworms in stomach contents" of *Blorina brevicauda*. The "small black objects" referred to the writer for identification proved to be zygospores with the abundant hyphal network characteristic of *E. macrospora* Tul. It was suggested that the black zygospores which often measured ¼ mm (250 μ) in diameter might have been ingested first by the earthworms and secondarily by the shrew. On consultation with Mr. H. C. Gauss, of Washington, who has had a vast experience in cultivating earthworms, the information was elicited that earthworms would have difficulty in swallowing refractory objects of that diameter and that he doubted the ability of any North American earthworms to ingest such material. It is, of course, likely that the shrew had developed a taste for this fungus as a condiment with the pièce de résistance.

Dr. Hamilton in correspondence, furthermore, reported the finding of these black bodies in stomach contents of two other shrews (*Sorex fumeus* and *S. cinereus*) as well as of three woodland mice (*Peromyscus leucopus novoboracensis, Clethrionomys gaperi* and *Synaptomys cooperi*) and pointed out that these findings in the small rodents which very seldom feed on earthworms supported the assumption that the shrews and mice may well have eaten the *Endogone* directly.

In this connection it is pertinent to note an older record of such fungi in stomach contents of a mouse (*Synaptomys cooperi gossi*) as attested by preserved microscopic preparations on file in the Mycological Collections of the Bureau of Plant Industry. These slides show zygospores of a distinctly different species of *Endogone* as yet undetermined specifically. The specimens studied and recognized as *Endogone* in 1926 by Miss V. K. Charles was collected by T. E. White in Douglas County, Kansas, in October, 1925, and examined first by C. C. Sperry, of the Biological Survey, who found the total stomach contents to be *Endogone* 5 per cent. and finely chewed vegetation, probably grass, 95 per cent. This latter information has been most kindly furnished by Dr. Clarence Cottam, of the Survey. In this case it is also notable that there is no reference to any accompanying earthworms.

William W. Diehl

Bureau of Plant Industry,
U. S. Department of Agriculture

## MUSCLE AND BLOOD HEMOGLOBIN IN THE DOLPHIN

Robinson[1] has recently reported the muscle hemoglobin of harbor seals (*Phoca vitulina*) as being 7.715 gm per 100 gm of fresh tissue. We are reporting our results for skeletal muscle and blood from dolphins (*Turciops truncatus*) studied during the past summer through the courtesy of the Marine Studios of St. Augustine, Florida.

Muscle and blood samples were obtained simultaneously from a living female dolphin which weighed 149 kg. Muscle hemoglobin was determined by the method of Whipple[2] and compared colorimetrically with the blood hemoglobin.

The oxygen capacity of the blood was 19.1 volumes per cent., or 14.25 gm hemoglobin per 100 cc. The hemoglobin content of the sacro-spinalis muscle was 3.534 gm per 100 gm tissue. The muscle hemoglobin concentration in the dolphin is thus less than that found in the seal by Robinson, but greater than that in the dog (0.85 to 1.00 gm per 100 gm rectus abdominis muscle).

It should be noted that the common submersion time of the dolphin is rarely over a few minutes; therefore the oxygen storage of the dolphin need not be as great as that of the seal. It will also be necessary to determine the amount of myoglobin in dolphin skeletal muscle in order to determine the oxygen storage more exactly; work on this problem is now in progress.

Lillian Eichelberger
Edwin S. Fetcher
E. M. K. Geiling
Bert J. Vos[3]

University of Chicago

## BIOGRAPHY OF DR. HARVEY CUSHING

Mrs. Cushing has requested me to prepare a biography of her husband, and I should be most grateful to any one who wishes to make letters, anecdotes or other memorabilia available.

Copies of all letters, no matter how brief, are desired, and if dates are omitted it is hoped that, when possible, these may be supplied (*e.g.,* from the postmark). If original letters or other documents are submitted, they will be copied and returned promptly.

A new Medical Library building is being erected at the Yale University School of Medicine to receive Dr. Cushing's library and collections, including his letters, diaries and manuscripts. Any of his friends who wish, now or later, to present correspondence, photographs or other memorabilia for permanent preservation among the Cushing papers will receive the appreciative thanks of the university.

John F. Fulton, M.D.

Yale University School of Medicine

# SPECIAL ARTICLES

## THE ACTION OF CERTAIN HORMONES AS DIETARY CONSTITUENTS

The present study was prompted by the following theoretical consideration.[1] We know that normal food contains small quantities of hormonic substances, which may exert certain activity and may perhaps be utilized by the organism as precursors of other hormones. On the other hand, a deficient diet may lack certain building stones from which the animal organism synthesizes its own hormones.

Judging from our present knowledge, the various hormones belong mainly to three chemical classes, *viz.,* simple nitrogenous substances, derived mostly from the amino acids of the diet, hormones belonging to the steroid group and finally hormones of protein nature. As far as the first two groups are concerned, it is obvious that the organism prepares these substances from material present in the food. More complicated is the origin of activity of the protein hormones. These substances when hydrolyzed do not seem to differ in structure and composition from the usual proteins; yet no known protein exhibits any definite hormonal activity. Whether the hormonal action is associated with a definite constituent or whether this activity depends on certain spatial configuration of the amino acids, must remain unanswered for the present.

Further, it seems possible that on deficient diets, the synthetic capacity of the organism may become impaired, even though the actual precursors are present. It is hoped that further work will give an answer to the problems outlined.

The present study deals with the action of estrin, testosterone propionate and gonadotropic hormone (of pregnant mare serum)[2] when added to the diet. The problem was approached in this way: a diet was chosen which causes a definite retrogression of the organs to be studied; then a regeneration was sought by inclusion in the diet of the corresponding hormone. It was soon found out, however, that most of the problems raised require special dietary studies: for instance, a diet which is responsible for marked retrogression of the female sex apparatus exerts no influence on the corresponding organs of the male.

In order not to complicate our task, we have used

1 D. Robinson, Science, 90: 276, 1939.

2 G. H. Whipple, *Am. Jour. Physiol.,* 76: 693, 1926.

3 These names are listed alphabetically because the work was carried out by the authors as a group. No indication of seniority is implied.

1 The present work was outlined by the senior author in an address given on November 10, 1938, at the Hotel Pierre, New York City.

2 We are indebted for the hormones to Roussel Laboratory, Paris, and Dr. André Girard.

TABLE I

EXPERIMENTS WITH ESTRIN*

| Diet | Nature of experiment | Number of animals | Duration days | Dose mg | Weight | Loss or gain per cent. | Food | Ovar. mg | Uteri mg |
|---|---|---|---|---|---|---|---|---|---|
| I | Controls | 8 | 26 | | 920 | 0 | 1,595 | 541 | 897 |
| I | Estrin | 8 | 26 | 17.6 | 928 | − 10.7 | 1,467 | 476 | *1,797* |
| I | Controls | 8 | 34 | | 1,151 | + 2.5 | 2,307 | 458 | 971 |
| I | Estrin | 8 | 34 | 10.27 | 1,126 | − 1.5 | 2,055 | 535 | *2,047* |
| I | Estrin plus Gonadotr. H. | 8 | 30 | 10.27 E<br>5.2 G. H. | 1,097 | + 0.4 | 2,021 | 555 | *1,674* |
| II | C. | 8 | 33 | | 1,069 | + 11.8 | 2,221 | 765 | 1,907 |
| II | Estrin | 8 | 33 | 6.3 | 1,049 | + 11.9 | 2,115 | 682 | 1,864 |

* The doses of hormones and other data are calculated for 8 rats for the whole period throughout all the tables.

largely a purified diet, to which only those vitamins were added which were available in a pure form. This procedure presented the disadvantage that the diet was incomplete and that the experiments had often to be interrupted before a complete exhaustion of the dietary reserves could be expected. This study was carried out on some 240 piebald rats and the composition of the diets used was as follows:

| | *Diet I* | *Diet II* | *Diet III* |
|---|---|---|---|
| Casein | Non-pur. 200 | Non-pur. 180 | Same as Diet I, but casein and starch washed with dil. HCl and extracted with alcohol. |
| Starch | " 500 | " 470 | |
| Lard | " 250 | " 250 | |
| Salts | 40 | 40 | |
| Cod liver oil | 20 | 15 | |
| Yeast | — | 60 | |
| Whole wheat | — | 200 | |
| Daily additions: | | | |
| $B_1$ | 5 $\gamma$ | | |
| Lactoflavin | 10 " | | |
| Adenosine | 50 " | | |
| Nicotinic ac. amide | 100 " | | |

From the above results we may conclude that a deficient diet, as used above, produces a marked retrogression of female sex organs; and that this is definitely influenced by an oral administration of estrin. On less deficient diet (Diet II), retrogression does not take place, and estrin *per os* has no effect. Estrin in female rats depresses the food intake and causes loss in weight. Simultaneous administration of estrin and gonadotropic hormone slightly inhibits the estrin action on the uterus. The activity of estrin incorporated into a deficient diet, and its inactivity on a more complete diet supports our view of the possible importance of this substance as a food constituent (as outlined in the introduction).

TABLE II

EXPERIMENTS WITH TESTOSTERONE PROPIONATE

| Diet | Nature of experiment | Number of animals | Duration days | Dose mg | Weight | Loss or gain per cent. | Food | Test. g | S.V. g |
|---|---|---|---|---|---|---|---|---|---|
| I | C. | 3 × 8 = 24 | 39 | | 1,001 | + 3.9 | 2,308 | 24.8 | 2.08 |
| I | Testost. | 3 × 8 = 24 | 39 | 17.5 | 1,002 | + 0.6 | 2,500 | 24.0 | 2.2 |
| II | C. | 8 | 40 | | 1,199 | + 43.4 | 3,593 | 23.9 | 7.9 |
| II | Testost. | 8 | 40 | 15.45 | 1,212 | + 52.7 | 3,716 | 24.4 | 8.5 |
| III | C. | 8 | 28 | | 1,146 | − 24.1 | 1,719 | 22.4 | 1.0 |
| III | Testost. | 8 | 28 | 16.75 | 1,147 | − 14.8 | 1,820 | *26.4* | *1.8* |

In discussing the Tables II and III we may conclude that a diet which produces sex organ degeneration in females, leaves the male practically untouched. No changes take place unless the animals lose considerable weight. The action of male and gonadotropic hormones seems to be fairly definite. In contrast to the estrin action in females, the male and gonadotropic hormones exert a rather beneficial action on the food intake and weight, which is perhaps another evidence of their value as food constituents.

Having established that the degeneration of the male sex organs takes place on purified casein and starch,

TABLE III

EXPERIMENTS WITH GONADOTROPIC HORMONE

| Diet | Nature of experiment | Number of animals | Duration days | Dose mg | Weight | Loss or gain per cent. | Food | Test. g | S.V. g |
|---|---|---|---|---|---|---|---|---|---|
| I | C. | 3 × 8 = 24 | 39 | | 1,001 | + 3.9 | 2,308 | 24.8 | 2.08 |
| I | G. H. | 3 × 8 = 24 | 39 | 22.3 | 1,008 | + 1.2 | 2,486 | 23.2 | 2.34 |
| III | C. | 8 | 28 | | 1,146 | − 24.1 | 1,719 | 22.4 | 1.0 |
| III | G. H. | 8 | 28 | 16.75 | 1,147 | − 21.5 | 1,676 | *26.2* | *1.4* |

we have initiated dietary studies in this direction, keeping in mind, however, that the above effect might be due to loss in weight, rather than to dietary deficiencies.

TABLE IV

INFLUENCE OF DIET ON SEX ORGANS OF THE MALE

| Diet | Nature of experiment | Number of animals | Duration days | Weight | Loss or gain in per cent. | Food | Test. g | S.V. g |
|---|---|---|---|---|---|---|---|---|
| I | C. ......... | 8 | 39 | 1,314 | +11 | 2,449 | 23.7 | 5.75 |
| I | 60 g. yeast per kg food .... | 8 | 39 | 1,241 | +46 | 3.359 | 22.8 | 8.33 |
| I | 200 g. whole wheat added to kg food.. | 8 | 39 | 1,327 | +27 | 3,246 | 22.6 | 7.31 |
| I | C. ......... | 8 | 32 | 1,070 | − 6.3 | 1.977 | 26.9 | 1.5 |
| I | Casein extr.* | 8 | 32 | 1,069 | − 5.2 | 2,297 | 28.7 | 1.8 |
| I | C. ......... | 8 | 35 | 841 | + 9.5 | 1,844 | 26.2 | 1.24 |
| I | Casein extr.† | 8 | 35 | 834 | + 1.6 | 1,710 | 22.6 | 0.85 |

* Acetone, acid alcohol and aqueous HCl extract added to imperfectly purified casein.

† Acetone and alcohol extract added to imperfectly purified casein.

From the above table we gather that the nature of dietary additions plays an important role in maintaining the normal aspect of the sex apparatus of the male rat. Additions and extracts containing undefined substances of yeast, whole wheat and aqueous casein extracts exert a favorable action on the food intake and weight, as well as on the picture of the seminal vesicles. Contrary to this, the only experiment with fatty extract of casein was unfavorable in these respects.

Finally, experiments were performed for the purpose of ascertaining the action of synthetic estrogens (dihydro-stilbestrol) which have nothing in common in chemical structure to natural estrogens. Further, we investigated whether testosterone can replace estrin as a hormonic dietary precursor.

Both groups of rats receiving dihydro-stilbestrol in their food showed continuous estrus. The action was practically the same on an incomplete and on a more complete diet. This is in marked contrast to the estrin action, which is only evident on an incomplete diet. As compared with the controls, testosterone initiated in several instances the beginning of an estrus, but it could not be substituted as a dietary estrin precursor. Stilbestrol on a more incomplete diet was somewhat toxic, but less so on a more complete dietary. Testosterone acted adversely in female rats regarding the food intake and therefore weight.

On a deficient diet female sex organs undergo a marked retrogression with cessation of estrus. Inclusion of estrin in such cases shows evidence of definite activity. On the other hand, a more complete diet causes no retrogression and estrin activity is not noticeable. Dihydro-stilbestrol, on the contrary, exerted the same activity on both types of food. Testo-

TABLE V

ACTION OF DIHYDRO-STILBESTROL AND TESTOSTERONE PROPIONATE ON FEMALE RATS

| Diet | Nature of experiment | Number of animals | Duration days | Dose mg | Weight | Loss or gain per cent. | Food | Ovar. mg | Uteri mg |
|---|---|---|---|---|---|---|---|---|---|
| I | C. ....... | 8 | 34 | | 779 | − 8.9 | 1,183 | 294 | 542 |
| I | Stilbestrol. | 8 | 34 | 4.7 | 774 | −27.9 | 906 | 273 | 1,779 |
| I | Testost. .. | 8 | 34 | 9.1 | 777 | −12.1 | 1,143 | 315 | 541 |
| I | Stilbcstrol. | 8 | 34 | 5.3 | 754 | − 5.8 | 1,319 | 369 | 1,716 |

SUMMARY

sterone can not replace estrin as a dietary hormonal precursor.

The sex organs of the male are more resistant to dietary deficiencies, the animals showing only retrogression along with a significant loss in weight. Testosterone and gonadotropic hormone (of pregnant mare serum) produce a small but definite restorative effect.

Oral administration of estrin to females depresses the food intake, while testosterone, and less so the gonadotropic hormone in males produces the opposite effect. This effect can be regarded as evidence of the dietary significance of these two hormones.

The expenses of the present investigation were defrayed by the U. S. Vitamin Corporation, of New York City.

CASIMIR FUNK
IAN CASIMIR FUNK

CASA BIOCHEMICA,
RUEIL-MALMAISON, FRANCE

## THE EXCRETION OF CORTIN AFTER SURGICAL OPERATION

A METHOD for the extraction and determination of cortin in human urine has been described.[1] The determination is based on a biological assay for cortin described by Selye and Schenker.[2] Using the method in a study of a group of cases, including one appendectomy, one dilatation and curettage, two gastric resections and one colostomy (none of whom developed post-operative shock), it was found that after operation there is an increased amount of cortin in the urine. Two cases are illustrated in the accompanying table. The excretion of cortin increases to a maximum between the third and fifth post-operative day and then gradually declines to pre-operative levels.

It had previously been shown[1] that cortin appeared in the urine during convalescence from influenza in persons who normally excrete none and that in the presence of chronic suppurative infection cortin is

[1] P. Weil and J. S. L. Browne, Proc. Am. Physiol. Soc., Toronto, 1939, Vol. 121, p. 652.

[2] Hans Selye and V. Schenker, *Proc. Soc. Exp. Biol. and Med.*, 39: 518, 1938.

TABLE I

| Date | | Units |
|---|---|---|
| June 9 | | 0 |
| 10 | | 0 |
| 11 | | 0 |
| 13 | Operation-Colostomy | |
| 14 | | 25 |
| 15 | | 25 |
| 16 | | 50 |
| 19 | | 75 |
| July 2 | | 50 |
| 4 | | 25 |
| 6 | Operation-Gastrectomy | |
| 7 | | 75 |
| 9 | | 125 |
| 10 | | 125 |
| 11 | | 100 |
| 12 | | 50 |

excreted. We believe that the increased excretion of cortin is a manifestation of the response of the organism to a damaging stimulus by an increased secretory activity of the adrenal cortex. It has been shown that the adrenal cortex of the laboratory animal hypertrophies after damage.[3] These experiments and the present investigation suggest that an increased secretion of the adrenal cortical hormone forms part of the protective mechanism against damage.

Paul Weil[4]
J. S. L. Browne

University Clinic,
Royal Victoria Hospital,
Montreal, Canada

## PERIODIC MITOTIC ACTIVITY IN THE EPIDERMIS OF THE ALBINO RAT

The knowledge that mitotic activity was periodic in some plants led Fortuyn-van Leyden to investigate this phenomenon first in various tissues of young kittens,[1] later, in young mice.[2] She found periods of maximum and minimum activity. Since then Ortiz Picón,[3] working with the epidermis of young mice, and Carleton,[4] studying the epidermis and hair follicles of young mice, have corroborated her findings as to periodicity, but have not agreed as to the time of maximum and minimum activity. More recently Cooper and Schiff[5] have demonstrated periods of greater and lesser mitotic activity in the epidermis of the prepuce of human male infants. The author[6] has reported a study of mitotic activity in the renal cortex of male albino rats. The curve plotted from the findings exhibited both periodic and rhythmic features (Fig. 1, broken line). Elliott,[7] as part of a study on the growth mechanisms of articular cartilage, obtained specimens during the day and night, but found no difference in rate of cell division.

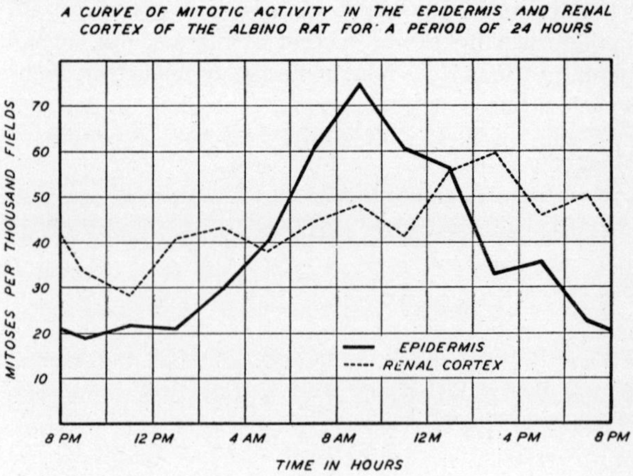


Fig. 1

The importance of such studies in the problem of normal and abnormal growth is obvious. The differences in results of various investigators may be due to the ages and orders of mammals employed, organ or region studied, inherited qualities or individual variation, character of environment or the small size of some of the samples. An addition to available data is here presented, a study of mitotic activity in the epidermis of the albino rat.

Materials and methods were as follows: from each of 96 male albino rats, 28 days old, killed in groups of 8 at intervals of 2 hours during a period of 24 hours, a square of skin was cut from the central ventral portion of the abdominal wall. The specimens were fixed in Bouin's, cross-sectioned at 8 microns, mounted serially and stained with hematoxylin and eosin Y. Every fourth section was studied to avoid counting the same mitosis twice. The number of mitoses observed in 1,000 consecutive fields was taken as an index of mitotic activity in a specimen. From the data obtained a curve was constructed and biometric studies made. To conserve space individual values are not presented.

The curve (Fig. 1, solid line) is composed of mean values for each 2-hour interval, placed at the mid-point of the interval. Each mean value is the average of 8 individual values. It will be seen that mitotic activity was greatest during the interval 8 a.m. to 10 a.m. (75 mitoses per 1,000 fields) and least during the interval 8 p.m. to 10 p.m. (19 mitoses per 1,000 fields); or, in other words, mitoses were almost 4 times as numerous in the morning interval as in the evening period. With few exceptions the skin was obtained from the same rats as were the kidneys previously studied. A

[3] Hans Selye, *Endocrinology*, 21: 169, 1937.

[4] Aided by a grant from the Banting Research Foundation.

[1] C. E. D. Fortuyn-van Leyden, *Proc. Akad. wet. Amsterdam*, 19: 38, 1917.

[2] C. E. D. Fortuyn-van Leyden, *Proc. Akad. wet. Amsterdam*, 29: 979, 1926.

[3] J. M. Ortiz Picón, *Zeitschr. f. Zellforsch. u. mikr. Anat.*, 23: 779, 1933.

[4] A. Carleton, *Jour. Anat.*, 68: 251, 1934.

[5] Z. K. Cooper and A. Schiff, *Proc. Soc. Exp. Biol. and Med.*, 39: 323, 1938.

[6] C. M. Blumenfeld, *Anat. Rec.*, 72: 435, 1938.

[7] H. C. Elliott, *Am. Jour. Anat.*, 58: 127, 1936.

comparison of the curve of mitotic activity in the epidermis with that of the renal cortex shows coincidence of the periods of minimum activity but an interval of 6 hours between periods of maximum activity. Nor does the curve for the epidermis have the rhythmic character of that for the renal cortex.

For biometric studies the 24-hour period was subdivided thus: first half of day, 8 A.M. to 2 P.M.; second half of day, 2 P.M. to 8 P.M.; first half of night, 8 P.M. to 2 A.M.; and second half of night, 2 A.M. to 8 A.M. Mitotic activity was found to be significantly greater during the first half of the day and significantly lower during the first half of the night than during the rest of the 24-hour period.

No explanation of these findings can be given as yet. If factors external to the cells have a part in determining periods of maximum and minimum mitotic activity they did not, in these animals, exert their influence in all parts of the body at the same time. A most valuable lead is furnished by the work of Huggins and Noonan[8] on the relation of temperature to red bone marrow activity and of Fay and Henny[9] and Smith and Fay[10] on the relation of temperature differences to normal and abnormal growth. This is one direction in which the present work is being continued.

C. M. BLUMENFELD

UNIVERSITY OF UTAH

# SCIENTIFIC APPARATUS AND LABORATORY METHODS

## A DEVICE FOR RAPID RINSING OF ABSORPTION TOWERS USED IN GAS ANALYSIS STUDIES[1]

WHERE an assembly of several glass absorption towers are employed for carbon dioxide or other gas determinations as, for example, in case of the Heinicke and Hoffman[2] photosynthesis apparatus, there is a special need for rapid and efficient rinsing of the towers after each determination. The simple device described below has these two advantages.[3] The whole system can be made from standard glassware in about a half day. The time necessary for each rinsing of the towers is reduced by more than one-half.

Details of this device, which has been used successfully for several months, are clearly shown in Fig. 1. The rinse water can be made to flow under pressure by connecting a blower pump or air-pressure line at A and applying pressure in the 10-gallon carboy, B, until the mercury in the manometer, C, indicates a level differential of about 12 inches. The pinch clamp, F, is a safety clamp employed between rinsings. It aids also in directing distilled water to the stationary stock water bottle, D, from the portable bottle, N. The same source of air pressure used at A can be attached at M, to force the water from bottle, N, to bottle D.

To rinse the towers after a determination, clamp F is released first (clamp G is open only during the filling of bottle D),[4] then clamp H is released with the left hand and clamp I (to another pair of towers) is released with the right hand. This allows the distilled water under pressure to squirt through the syringe-like bulbs at K and L as well as through the bulbs in another set of towers which is connected to the system at I. Thus, a set of four towers can be washed at one time. The water will flow evenly down the sides of the towers, provided they have been thoroughly cleaned in the beginning with a strong cleaning solu-

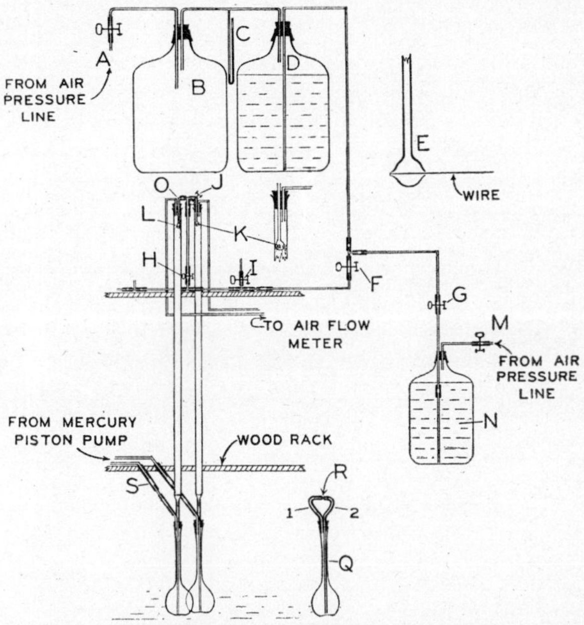


FIG. 1. Diagram showing system employed for rapid rinsing of gas-absorption towers.

[1] The authors are indebted to the Sherwin-Williams Paint Company, under whose fellowship part of this information has developed, and to F. W. Southwick, graduate assistant in horticulture, for helpful suggestions.

[2] A. J. Heinicke and M. B. Hoffman, SCIENCE, 77: 55–58, 1933.

[3] The removal and replacement of stoppers at the top of towers before and after rinsing is not necessary. They may be securely set and sealed about the edges with a mixture of grafting and sealing wax to obviate possible leakage of air at this point.

[8] C. Huggins and W. J. Noonan, *Jour. Exp. Med.*, 64: 275, 1936.

[9] T. Fay and G. C. Henny, *Surg., Gynec. and Obstet.*, 66: 512 (no. 2A), 1938.

[10] L. W. Smith and T. Fay, *Jour. Am. Med. Asn.*, 113: 653, 1939.

[4] Clamp J should be closed when air-flow records are taken. This prevents back-pressure from one tower to another of a pair.

tion to remove waxy and oily films, and provided the four or five perforations in each bulb are approximately the same size. The glass tubing used for the main water lines should be about 9 mm outside diameter, while leads to the individual towers may be smaller in diameter or about 7 mm outside diameter.

The bulbs, one of which is described at K, can be made easily without special technique in glass blowing. The following procedure is suggested: Heat the end of a five-inch glass tube which is approximately 7 mm in diameter until it has sealed; remove from the flame and blow immediately a bulb on the end, which is about one half inch in diameter. Allow to cool; heat again one side of the bulb and blow a pimple. Heat another side at a right angle to the first; blow another pimple and with a file gently file two holes at these points. The last two or three holes can be made quickly by inserting a rigid wire through the first holes and pushing out pimples on individually heated sides of the bulb, as shown at E. These pimples are filed off and the holes fire-polished.

Sometimes difficulty is encountered with loss of solution by bubbling over the tops of the towers, especially when about two drops of n-butyl alcohol[5] have been added to every 100 cc of alkali solution to increase the number of bubbles and decrease their individual size. When the solution in a tower threatens to overflow at the beginning of a run, this may be checked by removing the rubber tubing at 0 and with a medicine dropper allowing about two drops of capryl alcohol to settle to the base of the bulb. Capryl alcohol has the reverse effect of butyl alcohol on surface tension. When a mass of bubbles strikes the bulb, the foam immediately falls back.

The diagram at Q demonstrates how the rubber tubing on the two arms of a flask may be sealed from outside air before and after it is attached to the apparatus. This eliminates the expense and awkwardness of pinch-clamps. The three-inch glass tube, R, should be inserted further in the rubber tubing of arm 1 than arm 2. It thus will consistently, pull out of arm 2 more easily than arm 1, and will be ready for the rubber connection, S.

N. F. CHILDERS
D. C. KIPLINGER
H. W. BRODY
OHIO AGRICULTURAL EXPERIMENT STATION,
OHIO STATE UNIVERSITY

## A NEW CULTURE MEDIUM FOR PARAMECIA

VARIOUS devices have been suggested for slowing down and entangling Paramecia for microscopic study. The most satisfactory appears to be the addition of a small amount of fine cultural debris to the drop of medium on the slide. Cultures made up of hay infusions contain relatively little fine material. In order to increase the amount of fine debris we use the following method of raising Paramecia. 0.2 gram "Pablum" (an infant food manufactured by Mead Johnson and Company) is added to 400 cc of tap water in a wide mouth pint jar. This is covered by an inverted glass coaster and autoclaved at 15–20 pounds steam pressure for 30 minutes. After the mixture has cooled it is inoculated with Paramecia and allowed to stand at room temperature. In a week's time a dense culture of Paramecia is obtained. The "Pablum" concentration given above seems to be optimum.

To dispense the Paramecia to students we usually stir up the contents of a culture jar for a uniform distribution of Paramecia and fine cultural debris. On microscopic examination we find that most of the Paramecia are feeding and therefore easier to study. When greater concentrations of Paramecia are desired on a slide an unagitated drop of medium from the surface where the Paramecia aggregate, together with a small amount of debris from the bottom, may be used. Ordinarily one such culture as described above suffices for a hundred or more students.

BERTIL GOTTFRID ANDERSON
BIOLOGICAL LABORATORY,
WESTERN RESERVE UNIVERSITY

5 M. D. Thomas, *Ind. Eng. Chem., Anal. Ed.*, 5: 193–8, 1933.

## BOOKS RECEIVED

BOARDMAN, EDWARD T. *Field Guide to Lower Aquarium Animals.* Pp. 186. 51 figures. Cranbrook Institute of Science, Bloomfield Hills, Michigan.

CALEY, EARLE R. *The Composition of Ancient Greek Bronze Coins.* Vol. XI, 1939 of the *Memoirs* of the American Philosophical Society. Pp. viii + 203. Illustrated. The Society, Philadelphia.

*Collected Letters of Antoni van Leeuwenhoek, Part I.* Edited by a committee of Dutch scientists. Pp. 454. 39 plates. Swets and Zeitlinger, Amsterdam.

EGE, VILH. *A Revision of the Genus Anguilla Shaw.* Pp. 256. 53 figures. 6 plates. Carlsberg Foundation and Oxford University Press, London.

MACK, JULIAN E. and MILES J. MARTIN. *The Photographic Process.* Pp. xvii + 586. Illustrated. McGraw-Hill. $5.00.

STENGER, ERICH. *The History of Photography; Its Relation to Civilization and Practice.* Translation from the German by EDWARD EPSTEAN. Pp. xiv + 204. Mack Printing Co., Easton, Pa.

TANSLEY, A. G. *The British Islands and their Vegetation.* Pp. xxxviii + 930. 416 photographs, 179 figures. Cambridge University Press, Macmillan. $16.00.

THURSTON, ROBERT H. *A History of the Growth of the Steam-Engine.* Pp. xii + 555. 182 figures. Cornell University Press, Ithaca, New York. $3.00.

TURNBULL, HERBERT W., Editor. *James Gregory; Tercentenary Memorial Volume.* P. xi + 524. Illustrated. G. Bell and Sons, London. 25s.

WHYTE, R. O. *Research on Grassland, Forage Crops and the Conservation of Vegetation in the United States.* Herbage Publication Series, Bulletin 26. Pp. 113. Imperial Bureau of Pastures and Forage Crops, Aberystwyth, Great Britain. 5s.

WINKLER, JOHN K. and WALTER BROMBERG. *Mind Explorers; the Story of Mental Healing.* Pp. 378. Reynal and Hitchcock. $3.00.

# SCIENCE

VOL. 90 FRIDAY, NOVEMBER 17, 1939 No. 2342

*The Sixth Pacific Science Congress:* PROFESSOR ROY ELWOOD CLAUSEN ... 449

*The Structure of the Pacific Basin as Indicated by Earthquakes:* PROFESSOR B. GUTENBERG ... 456

*Scientific Events:*
*The City and Rural Health Conservation Contest; The Expedition to Hudson Bay of the University of Minnesota; The Importation of Foreign Books and Periodicals; Lectures in the Department of Physics at the University of Wisconsin; Award of the John Fritz Gold Medal; Recent Deaths and Memorials* ... 458

*Scientific Notes and News* ... 461

*Discussion:*
*The Allowed Directions of Cosmic Rays as an Existence Problem of Mathematical Analysis:* DR. I. OPATOWSKI. *Revision of Dental Symbols:* DR. BRUNO OETTEKING. *Possible Implications of Reptilian Thermal Tolerance:* DR. RAYMOND B. COWLES 463

*Scientific Books:*
*The Carnegie Institution of Washington and Dr. Merriam:* PROFESSOR WILLIAM K. GREGORY ... 466

*Reports:*
*Work of the Canadian National Research Council* 468

*Special Articles:*
*Effect of Ultra-short Radio Waves on Plant Growth:* DR. J. VAN OVERBEEK, DR. L. REED BRANTLEY and PROFESSOR G. W. POTAPENKO. *Bio-electric Potentials of the Hen's Egg:* PROFESSOR ALEXIS L. ROMANOFF and DR. CASPER L. COTTRELL. *Implants of Embryonic Tissue Inhibit Parturition in the Rat:* DR. ALFRED TAYLOR ... 470

*Scientific Apparatus and Laboratory Methods:*
*Apparatus for the Isolation of Monochromatic Light of High Intensity:* DR. LAWRENCE J. HEIDT 473

*Science News* ... 8

SCIENCE: A Weekly Journal devoted to the Advancement of Science, edited by J. MCKEEN CATTELL and published every Friday by

THE SCIENCE PRESS

New York City: Grand Central Terminal

Lancaster, Pa. Garrison, N. Y.

Annual Subscription, $6.00 Single Copies, 15 Cts.

SCIENCE is the official organ of the American Association for the Advancement of Science. Information regarding membership in the Association may be secured from the office of the permanent secretary in the Smithsonian Institution Building, Washington, D. C.

# THE SIXTH PACIFIC SCIENCE CONGRESS

By Professor ROY ELWOOD CLAUSEN

UNIVERSITY OF CALIFORNIA; SECRETARY-GENERAL OF THE SIXTH PACIFIC SCIENCE CONGRESS

THE sessions of the sixth Pacific Science Congress were held in the San Francisco Bay region from July 24 to August 12, 1939. The University of California, Stanford University and the Golden Gate International Exposition acted jointly as hosts to the congress. Most of the technical sessions were held either at the University of California or at Stanford University, but many of the social functions and public lectures were held at the Golden Gate International Exposition on Treasure Island.

The sixth Pacific Science Congress was organized under the auspices of the National Research Council, specifically under the general supervision of its Committee on Pacific Investigations, of which Dr. Herbert E. Gregory is chairman. The details of organization of the congress, however, were delegated to a local committee, the Committee on the Sixth Pacific Science Congress, with Dr. C. B. Lipman, of the University of California, as chairman; Dr. Roy E. Clausen, of the same institution, as secretary, and with representatives of Stanford University, the University of California and the Golden Gate International Exposition as members. Dr. Ross G. Harrison, chairman of the National Research Council, was president of the congress, and Dr. Roy E. Clausen, secretary-general. Dr. Frank R. Lillie, retiring president of the National Academy of Sciences, was honorary chairman; Dr. Robert Gordon Sproul, president of the University of California; Dr. Ray Lyman Wilbur, president of Stanford University, and the presidents of previous congresses were honorary vice-chairmen.

The sixth Pacific Science Congress was the first meeting of the Pacific Science Association to be held on the mainland of the United States of America.

The fifth congress was held at Victoria and Vancouver in 1933, and in the normal course of events, the sixth congress would have been held at some far eastern center; in fact, provisional arrangements had been made to hold it in French Indo-China, but unfavorable circumstances prevented the fulfilment of these plans. In this predicament, it seemed desirable to take advantage of the Golden Gate International Exposition, with its emphasis on Pacific relations and cultures, to continue the series. Accordingly, arrangements were made rather hurriedly to convene the sixth congress in the San Francisco Bay region during the time of the exposition.

Despite the short time available for preparation and the unsettled conditions, the sixth congress drew a small but representative attendance from countries of the Pacific region. The registered attendance at the congress was 492, about the same as that of the fifth congress, and twenty-eight countries were represented. Attendance at the congress was particularly satisfactory in view of the almost continuous procession of meetings in the San Francisco Bay region during the past summer. In a number of instances, when other meetings occurred concurrently, arrangements were made for joint sessions or for informal coöperation, without the requirement of registration for the congress, which no doubt contributed materially to the gratifying attendance at the technical sessions. Thus the tenth annual meeting of the Western Branch of the American Public Health Association was held in Oakland from July 23 to 28, 1939. Sessions of the section on public health and nutrition were arranged so as to permit participation by their membership, and abstracts of the papers to be presented in this section were made available to them. Similarly, the summer meetings of the Geological Society of America, the Paleontological Society, the Seismological Society of America and the Society of Economic Geologists were held in Berkeley from August 8 to 10, 1939. The sessions of the section for geophysics and geology of the congress were held in the previous week, in order to permit members of the congress to join in their activities. By special arrangement, members of the congress were also permitted to participate in a number of excursions organized for members of these societies. The Oceanographical Society of the Pacific suspended its usual summer meeting in order to cooperate fully with the section on oceanography, fisheries and marine biology.

### PUBLICATIONS

Before the congress opened, a number of announcements containing various kinds of information about the congress were circulated to a mailing list made up of institutions and organizations having some interest in the Pacific area and of individuals from lists obtained from section chairmen and other sources. The first of these, a preliminary announcement, setting forth the general purposes of the congress and outlining its organization, was issued in January, 1939. A second, supplementary announcement, containing chiefly a tentative outline of the program and the names and addresses of section chairmen, was issued in March. Finally, an advance announcement, containing information about accommodations, a detailed outline of the program, etc., was issued in June.

On registration, members received a copy of the General Program, a booklet of 160 pages, containing general information about the congress and full details of the technical sessions, including names of authors and titles of papers to be presented. They also received, on request, mimeographed sets of abstracts of the sections in which they were interested, as well as other miscellaneous material designed to acquaint them with some of the features of the San Francisco Bay Region and with activities and events in progress during the meeting. Ten sets of abstracts were issued; *viz.*, Geophysics, Pre-Tertiary Geology, Tertiary Stratigraphy, General Geology, Oceanography, Fisheries and Marine Biology, Pacific Climates Past and Present, Anthropology, Epidemiology, Industrial Hygiene and Nutrition.

As with previous congresses, the general records of the congress and the papers presented in its sessions will be published in a set of volumes under the title, "Proceedings of the Sixth Pacific Science Congress," which will be distributed by sale and subscription only. Copies of the General Program may be obtained, as long as they are available, on request to the Secretary-General, 205 Hilgard Hall, University of California, Berkeley, California.

### THE INAUGURAL SESSION

The formal opening of the congress was held on July 24, at the University of California. At the inaugural session, Dr. Herbert E. Gregory, president of the first congress and chairman of the Committee on Pacific Investigations of the National Research Council, introduced the president of the congress, Dr. Ross G. Harrison, chairman of the National Research Council. Messages of welcome were extended in behalf of the host institutions by Dr. Ray Lyman Wilbur for Stanford University and the Golden Gate International Exposition, and by Dr. Monroe E. Deutsch for the University of California. A message to the congress from Dr. Frank R. Lillie, retiring president of the National Academy of Sciences, was read, and the president of the congress delivered an address of welcome to the visiting delegates. Responses to the address of welcome were made by representatives of fourteen countries.

### BUSINESS SESSIONS

The congress held two plenary sessions for a consideration of business matters, the first dealing with organization of the congress and the second with matters referred to it by the Pacific Science Council, the executive committee of the Pacific Science Association. The council consists of one representative each from fourteen countries included in the Pacific region or having dependencies therein. For the present congress its membership consisted of Ross G. Harrison (United States of America), *chairman;* E. C. Andrews (Australia); R. C. Wallace (Canada); Y. R. Chao (China); Jules Rouch (France and French Indo-China); V. H. Blackman (Great Britain); C. Montague Cooke (Hawaii); Shinkishi Hatai (Japan); H. A. Brouwer (Netherlands); H. J. Lam (Netherlands Indies); Patrick Marshall (New Zealand); Walfrido de Leon (Philippine Commonwealth); and H. E. Gregory (United States of America). R. L. Pendleton (Thailand) was present by invitation, and only the Union of Socialist Soviet Republics was not represented.

### THE SEVENTH CONGRESS

The congress accepted an invitation extended by the Commonwealth of the Philippines to hold the seventh congress in Manila in 1943. In the absence of any permanent secretarial staff for the Pacific Science Association, informal arrangements were made to have Dr. Patrocinio Valenzuela, secretary of the National Research Council of the Philippines, act as interim secretary of the association for the period between the sixth and seventh congresses.

### STANDING COMMITTEES OF THE PACIFIC SCIENCE ASSOCIATION

The council gave special attention to the reorganization of its standing committees, looking towards more effective activity in the intervals between congresses. The list of committees and their chairmen, as approved by the congress, follows:

*Oceanography:* Dr. Thomas G. Thompson, University of Washington, Seattle, Washington.

*Protection of Nature:* Dr. Carl Skottsberg, Botanic Gardens, Gothenburg, Sweden.

*Volcanology:* Dr. Patrick Marshall, Public Works Department, Wellington, New Zealand.

*Soil Survey and Classification:* Dr. R. L. Pendleton, Bureau of Agriculture and Fisheries, Bangkok, Thailand.

*Classification and Utilization of Land:* Dr. J. W. Coulter, University of Hawaii, Honolulu, Hawaii.

*Mountain Structure:* Dr. H. A. Brouwer, University of Amsterdam, Amsterdam, The Netherlands.

*Forestry:* Dr. Arthur F. Fischer, Bureau of Forestry, Manila, Philippine Islands.

*Economic Entomology:* Dr. C. E. Pemberton, Hawaiian Sugar Planters' Association, Honolulu, Hawaii.

*Blood Groups:* Dr. Tanemoto Furuhata, Tokyo Imperial University, Tokyo, Japan.

*Distribution of Terrestrial Faunas in the Inner Pacific:* Dr. C. Montague Cooke, Bishop Museum, Honolulu, Hawaii.

*Pacific Plant Areas:* Dr. H. J. Lam, University of Leiden, Leiden, The Netherlands.

### RECOMMENDATIONS OF THE CONGRESS

The council also gave extended attention to the need for coordination of efforts in successive congresses and drew up a number of recommendations, which were adopted by the congress, on ways and means of promoting scientific research in the Pacific region. These proposals, as outlined herewith, are to be brought to the attention of the proper authorities by the interim secretary, Dr. Patrocinio Valenzuela: (1) advocating the establishment of additional seismological stations in the Pacific area; (2) advocating extension of observations of gravity values within the Pacific; (3) advocating the construction and operation of non-magnetic vessels for a more complete magnetic survey of the Pacific region; (4) advocating the extension of coastal surveys to inadequately charted coasts of the Americas and of the Pacific Islands; (5) recommending continued study of the configuration of the floor of the Pacific Ocean by sonic sounding; (6) recommending continuation and extension of the oceanographic program of the International Fisheries Commission; (7) recommending further studies of the nature and origin of coralline deposits; (8) recommending that island stations and ships in the Pacific be required to provide full synoptic weather reports four times daily; (9) recommending preparation of large-scale exhibits of geological columns of each country of the Pacific; (10) advocating preservation of a number of unique natural areas within the Pacific region; (11) recommending appointment of a Standing Committee on Plant Areas; (12) recommending prosecution of an extensive project of soil classification and survey to be coordinated with the activities of the Fifth Commission of the International Society of Soil Science; and (13) recommending inclusion of discussions on public health and nutrition in the seventh Pacific Science Congress.

### PUBLIC LECTURES

While the main emphasis of the congress was placed upon the technical sessions, arrangements were made for a number of illustrated lectures which were open to the public. Two of these lectures were given at the University of California in connection with the program on public health and nutrition, a series of seven was given at the Conference Room of the Pacific House on Treasure Island, and three were given at Stanford University. The names of speakers and the titles of their addresses follow:

At the University of California:

"The Present Status of Health Conditions in Canada." Dr. C. P. Brown, Canadian Department of Pensions and Public Health.

"The Progress of Health Work and Social Services in the British Colonies." Sir William McLean, representative of the British Colonies at the New York World's Fair.

At Treasure Island:

"Ocean Currents of the Pacific and Their Bearing on the Climates of the Coasts." Dr. H. U. Sverdrup, Scripps Institution of Oceanography.

"Public Health Conditions in China." Dr. A. Stampar, professor of public health, Zagreb.

"The Origins of Cultivated Plants in Relation to the Origins of Civilizations." Dr. Elmer Drew Merrill, Harvard University.

"Explorations in the Lesser Sunda Islands." Dr. H. A. Brouwer, University of Amsterdam.

"The Structure of the Pacific Ocean as Indicated by Earthquakes." Dr. Beno Gutenberg, California Institute of Technology.

"On Mimicry in its Relation to Other Forms of Protective Coloration." Dr. G. D. Hale Carpenter, Oxford University.

"The Government Botanic Gardens at Buitenzorg and the Mountain Garden at Tjibodas, Java." Dr. H. J. Lam, University of Leiden.

At Stanford University:

"Pithecanthropus and Sinanthropus and Their Relationship to Later Stages of Human Evolution." Dr. Franz Weidenreich, Peiping Union Medical College.

"The Biology of the Great Barrier Reef." Dr. C. M. Yonge, University of Bristol.

"The Flora of the Hawaiian Islands and the History of the Pacific Basin." Dr. Carl Skottsberg, Gothenburg Botanical Gardens.

### Radio Broadcasts

A number of radio broadcasts were arranged through the courtesy of Dr. Milton Silverman, director of the Hall of Science at the Exposition. A series of three round-table broadcasts under the general title, "Meet the Scientists," was given on Monday evenings, over W6XBE (now KGEI), the General Electric short-wave station and over the Blue Network of the National Broadcasting Company, through KGO. In this series, on July 24, Dr. Karl F. Meyer, of the Hooper Foundation, and Sir William McLean, representative of the British Colonies at the New York World's Fair, discussed with Dr. Silverman international aspects of the public health problems of the Pacific area; on July 31, Dr. E. D. Merrill, of Harvard University, and Dr. Carl Skottsberg, of Gothenburg, discussed botanical problems of the Pacific, and on August 7, Mr. E. C. Andrews and Dr. H. C. Richards of Australia participated in a discussion of geological problems of the region.

Besides these programs, which were released over a national hook-up, fifteen-minute broadcasts were arranged over W6XBE after each of the seven public addresses at Treasure Island. At these broadcasts Dr. Silverman interviewed the speaker of the evening in the general field of his subject.

### Social Events

The social program of the congress included a variety of events, some arranged by the congress through the services of Dr. Chauncey D. Leake and some by the officers of the Golden Gate International Exposition, particularly through the courtesy of the Women's Board of the Exposition and also through the active interest of Mr. and Mrs. Philip N. Youtz of the Pacific House. The congress is deeply grateful to the many persons who assisted in the preparation of these events, for they were all enjoyable, well-attended affairs which provided an unusual opportunity for members of the congress to meet and become acquainted with one another.

At Berkeley, the officers of the congress tendered a reception to members of the congress on Monday afternoon, July 24, at the university in the Women's Club Rooms of Stephens Union. On Wednesday afternoon, July 26, a short sight-seeing trip through the Berkeley Hills was followed by a reception and tea at the Women's Faculty Club of the university. On Saturday, July 29, an international tea and program was given at the Berkeley Women's City Club. On Wednesday afternoon, August 2, a sight-seeing trip through Marin County, including visits to the Muir Woods redwood grove and Mount Tamalpais, was followed by a reception and tea at the Pacific House on Treasure Island.

The formal banquet of the congress, in honor of visiting foreign delegates, was held at the Claremont Hotel on Friday evening, August 4. Dr. C. B. Lipman was toastmaster, and the speakers were Dr. Ross G. Harrison, president of the congress; Dr. Patrick Marshall (New Zealand), Dr. Y. R. Chao (China), Dr. Walfrido de Leon (Philippine Islands), Dr. Luis Patiño-Camargo (Colombia), and Dr. Carl Skottsberg (Sweden).

At Treasure Island, an elaborate special program of hospitality arranged by exposition officers began on Thursday afternoon, July 27, with a reception in the lounge of the San Francisco Building. Mayor Angelo J. Rossi and other officers of the city government extended greetings to members of the congress. On Friday afternoon, July 28, Mr. Koiti Tenniti, the Japanese Commissioner to the Exposition, tendered a reception to members of the congress at the beautiful Japanese Pavilion. A musical program was given and *tenpura* refreshments were served in the Japanese style. On Monday afternoon, July 31, Mr. George

Creel, United States Commissioner to the Exposition, tendered a reception to officers and delegates of the congress at the Federal Building, and on Tuesday afternoon, August 1, coffee was served to members of the congress at a number of pavilions in the Latin American Court, particularly in those of Brazil, Colombia, El Salvador and Guatemala. The Committee of the Pacific Area tendered a reception to members of the congress on Wednesday afternoon, August 2, at the Balcony of the Pacific House, following the sight-seeing trip to Marin County. Finally, on Thursday afternoon, August 3, the Women's Board of the Exposition received members of the congress at the Yerba Buena Club. Besides these events, arrangements were made by members of the Women's Board for individual entertainment of the speakers, together with invited guests, at Treasure Island at dinner preceding their evening addresses, and many smaller parties were entertained at week-end affairs. After each evening address, Mr. and Mrs. Youtz served refreshments in the Balcony at the Pacific House.

At Stanford University, a tour for ladies was given on Monday afternoon, August 7. Mrs. Herbert Hoover received the ladies at her home on the campus, and at the conclusion of the tour, tea was served at the home of Professor and Mrs. F. M. MacFarland. On Tuesday, August 8, many of the members of the congress participated in the excursion to Pacific Grove, which included a visit to the Hopkins Marine Station, a trip over the famed Seventeen-mile Drive on the Monterey Peninsula and a luncheon at the Peninsula Country Club arranged through the courtesy of Dr. W. K. Fisher, director of the Hopkins Marine Station. On Wednesday afternoon, August 9, a sight-seeing tour through the Peninsula District was followed by a reception and tea in the Patio of the Women's Gymnasium. On Thursday afternoon, August 10, Professor and Mrs. Bailey Willis entertained the members of the congress at their home on the campus.

### THE TECHNICAL SESSIONS

Only the briefest attention can be given to the technical sessions, which constituted the most important feature of the congress. About 125 sessions were held, and over 700 papers were listed for presentation. In some instances excursions, motion picture films, laboratory demonstrations and luncheons and dinners were scheduled as part of these programs.

The program was organized into eight sections with eighteen major subdivisions. In general a committee appointed by the National Research Council on nomination of the Committee on the Congress was placed in charge of each major subdivision, and to it was delegated the details of organization of the program and the duty of extending invitations to participate in it. In view of the short time available for this purpose, invitations to participate were extended not only to the national organizations of the countries of the Pacific but also directly to individual scientists in these countries who were known to have made significant contributions in the fields under discussion.

The program committees were allowed a considerable degree of freedom in conducting their activities. Usually, however, a program outline was set up, enumerating general topics for consideration, and then invitations to participate were extended to individuals who had made notable contributions to the subjects in question.

*Geophysics:* Beno Gutenberg, Perry Byerly, A. L. Day and N. H. Heck, in charge. On July 27, the subsection was invited to participate in a program on earthquake resistant design, arranged by the Structural Division of the American Society of Civil Engineers and held at the St. Francis Hotel in San Francisco. Sessions were held on magnetic data and the structure of the Pacific area; on shallow earthquakes in the Pacific area and structure; on deep focus earthquakes in the Pacific area; on gravity, tilt and displacement in the Pacific area; and on hypotheses on the development of the Pacific basin. One session was devoted to a general conference on geophysical problems concerning the Pacific area, and the subsection participated in sessions dealing with Pacific climates, as based on the fossil record, and with causes of climatic change. The standing committee on seismology also held a meeting under the *pro tempore* chairmanship of James B. Macelwane, of St. Louis University.

*Geology:* Eliot Blackwelder, Herbert E. Gregory and W. C. Mendenhall, in charge. The committee in charge of the subsection on geology outlined a number of topics and delegated the preparation of programs for these subjects to specialists in the fields. A program of six sessions on the Pacific basin and lands in pre-Tertiary times was arranged by C. E. Weaver, of the University of Washington. H. G. Schenck, of Stanford University, arranged a program of four sessions on Tertiary stratigraphy, paleontology and history of the islands in and the continents bordering on the Pacific Ocean. A fifth session was devoted to a round-table conference on procedure in stratigraphy; and two field trips were conducted; one to the south side of Mount Diablo, under the leadership of B. L. Clark, of the University of California, and another to inspect the southwest flank of the Pacheco syncline near Martinez, under the leadership of the chairman.

A one-session program on Antarctic Pacific, continental and marine problems was arranged by L. M. Gould, Carleton College; and a two-session program on the bottom deposits of the Pacific Ocean and processes of marine sedimentation by Parker D. Trask, of the U. S. Geological Survey. One-session programs were devoted to Pleistocene and Recent changes around the Pacific border, under the leadership of Eliot Blackwelder, of Stanford University, to changes of ocean level in the Pacific basin under J. E. Hoffmeister, of the University of Rochester, and to volcanoes of the Pacific region under the direction of Howel Williams, of the University of California.

*Oceanography and Marine Biology:* The section was organized under the general supervision of a committee consisting of Thomas G. Thompson, Martin W. Johnson, H. A. Marmer, Robert C. Miller, H. U. Sverdrup and W. F. Thompson. It was divided into three subsections—oceanography, fisheries and marine biology—for development of the program. General activities of the section included consideration of an extensive report drawn up by the Standing Committee on Oceanography of the Pacific, of which Thomas G. Thompson was chairman. The Oceanographical Society of the Pacific held its annual luncheon and business meeting in connection with these sessions on July 27, at the Berkeley Women's City Club.

*Oceanography:* H. U. Sverdrup, in charge. The first session was devoted to oceanographic reports from various portions of the Pacific region. It was followed by two sessions devoted to currents of the Pacific Ocean, their physical and chemical characteristics, and concluded with a session devoted to contributed papers.

*Fisheries:* W. F. Thompson, Harry A. Dunlop, Roger W. Harrison, George S. Myers, Paul R. Needham and W. L. Scofield, in charge. Seven sessions were held. The first dealt with the distribution and relationship of marine species, stressing those features which make them of international importance. The second was devoted to the life history of important species of fishes and the factors in their exploitation and conservation which make them of international importance. The third session dealt with the evolution of methods of exploitation and utilization, the scientific and practical principles involved and their relation to conservation or the national economy of the countries of the Pacific area. The fourth session considered management methods for inland waters, and the fifth discussed fisheries research programs. Two following sessions contained miscellaneous contributions on fisheries biology and technology.

*Marine Biology:* Robert C. Miller, Martin W. Johnson, Frederick H. Davidson, C. McLean Frazer, Trevor Kincaid, S. F. Light and Irene A. McCulloch, in charge. Two sessions were devoted to the distribution of plant and animal life in the Pacific and one each to the productivity of the sea, the microbiology of the sea, the tropical Pacific and the physiology of marine organisms. Round-table discussions in connection with the sessions were scheduled to deal with the present status of distributional studies in the north Pacific area, the utilization of "indicator" organisms in marine biological investigations, the objectives of future biological investigations in the tropical Pacific and the present status of investigations of the morphology and physiology of Pacific invertebrates.

*Past Climates of the Pacific:* Ralph W. Chaney, in charge. Two sessions were devoted to a consideration of Pacific climates as based on the fossil record in which evidence from the response of modern organisms to climate as well as evidence from the fossil record were considered. A third session was devoted to a discussion of causes of climatic change.

*Present Climates of the Pacific:* Charles F. Brooks, E. H. Bowie and J. B. Leighly, in charge. Two subsections, one dealing with meteorology and the other with climatology, were organized.

*Meteorology:* E. H. Bowie, N. E. Bradbury and E. C. Haynes, in charge. Five sessions were scheduled for a consideration of the synoptic meteorology of the Pacific. During these sessions a movie film on the artificial production of snow crystals, prepared by Professor Ukitiro Nakaya, of the Hokkaido Imperial University, and brought to the congress by Dr. K. Hidaka, was shown. Another feature of the program was a daily air-mass-frontal analysis of the weather chart of the north Pacific Ocean, presented by Messrs. H. B. Byers, R. C. Counts, Jr., and E. M. Vernon, of the U. S. Weather Bureau.

*Climatology:* John B. Leighly, in charge. Three one-session programs were arranged dealing with the maritime climatology of the Pacific, climatic fluctuations in California and climatic features of the western United States.

*Anthropology:* A. L. Kroeber and T. D. McCown, in charge. The program was divided into six sessions with the following topics of discussion: culture history; acculturation; regional contributions; ethnobotany; earliest man, his remains, his tools and the times in which he lived; and racial migrations in the Pacific region.

*Zoology:* F. M. MacFarland, H. Burrington Baker, Ernst Mayr and Karl P. Schmidt, in charge. Two sessions of the subsection, dealing with the general subject of faunistic studies of the Pacific area, were organized.

*Entomology:* E. O. Essig, C. P. Clausen, W. B. Herms, D. B. Mackie and E. C. Van Dyke, in charge. The several portions of the program were organized by different members of the committee. A two-session program on the faunal relations of the insects of the Pacific area was arranged by E. C. Van Dyke. A session dealing with economic problems was held under the leadership of D. B. Mackie. Four sessions under the leadership of C. P. Clausen were devoted to the general problem of biological control of insect pests; and one session on the terrestrial arachnids of the Pacific area which may affect the health and well-being of man and animals was organized by W. B. Herms.

*Botany:* E. B. Copeland, in charge. The general topic of discussion was the terrestrial floras of the Pacific area, to which three sessions were devoted. A fourth session was devoted to contributed papers on economic applications dealing particularly with plant breeding and forestry. The subsection also participated in a discussion of reports of the Standing Committee on Forestry, presented by F. W. Foxworthy and of the Standing Committee on the Protection of Nature, prepared by Carl Skottsberg.

*Plant Pathology:* E. C. Stakman, in charge. The program consisted of four sessions; one devoted to virus diseases of plants with a round-table discussion of virus problems led by Eubanks Carsner; a second dealt with variation in plant pathogens, with a round-table discussion on variation in pathogens and its importance, led by M. W. Gardner; a third considered the problem of dissemination and distribution of plant pathogens including physiologic races, led by J. H. Craigie; and the fourth, devoted to plant diseases caused by nutrient deficiencies, included a round-table discussion on diseases caused by nutrient deficiencies and mutual relationships between organisms in relation to pathogenicity.

*Public Health and Nutrition:* K. F. Meyer, L. S. McClung, F. A. Carmelia, L. R. Chandler, W. M. Dickie, C. E. Dolman, J. C. Geiger, Ira V. Hiscock, C. H. Kellaway, J. F. Kessel, C. D. Leake, G. W. McCoy, Agnes F. Morgan, R. R. Parker, Langley Porter, A. C. Reed, R. R. Sayers, W. P. Shepard and R. P. Strong, in charge. The inclusion of the section on public health and nutrition represented, in a sense, an innovation in the program of Pacific Science congresses, since the fifth congress, after considering the matter, abandoned plans to organize such a section, and previous congresses had laid little emphasis on the field. However, through the active services of Dr. K. F. Meyer and Dr. L. S. McClung, chairman and secretary, respectively, of the organizing committee, together with the associated efforts of a large group interested in the subject, an extensive program was prepared and presented. The section was so successful in its efforts that the congress endorsed its request for continuation of the section in subsequent congresses.

General activities of the group included arrangements for the three public lectures previously listed, given by Dr. C. P. Brown, Sir William McLean and Dr. A. Stampar. A dinner in honor of officers of the section and visiting participants was given at the Faculty Club of the University of California on Thursday evening, July 27. Moving picture films in color were shown on Tuesday evening, July 25, "A Trip to Panama; Possibilities for Nutrition Research in the Tropics," by Dr. George R. Cowgill, of Yale University, and on Saturday afternoon, July 29, films were exhibited by Dr. R. R. Parker on the "Life History of the Rocky Mountain Spotted Fever Tick, and Methods of Preparation of Rocky Mountain Fever Vaccine."

The technical sessions were organized under four subsections; epidemiology, industrial hygiene, nutrition and health education. As previously mentioned, the program was so arranged as to permit attendance of members of the Western Branch of the American Public Health Association, which met in Oakland from July 23 to 28. Members of the congress were also invited to attend the annual banquet of the association, which was held on Wednesday evening, July 26, at the Hotel Oakland.

*Epidemiology:* K. F. Meyer, in charge. The program consisted of sixteen sessions organized around specific topics, with 172 papers listed for presentation. An attempt was made to secure reports on these topics from as wide a territory as possible. One session dealt with the enteric infections; dysenteries, cholera and typhoid fever. It was followed by two sessions on insect-borne diseases; one covering tularemia and relapsing fever; the other, yellow fever and plague. Two sessions dealt with neurotropic virus infections; one with poliomyelitis, equine encephalomyelitis, St. Louis encephalitis and rabies; the second with undulant fever and leptospirosis. Two sessions on animal-borne diseases covered undulant fever, leptospirosis and psittacosis. One session was devoted to food poisonings and one to the history and influence of geographic and climatic factors on disease. Three further sessions on insect-borne diseases dealt with rickettsia and bartonella infections. A session was given over to fungus infections, another to newer knowledge on trachoma and two to leprosy.

*Industrial Hygiene:* Dr. R. R. Sayers, in charge. The program consisted of four sessions, with 34 papers listed for presentation. One session was devoted to a consideration of the present status of industrial hygiene; a second to public health problems relating to transportation and changes in barometric pressure; and two to organic solvents, insecticides, pest control agents and spray residues in relation to public health.

*Nutrition:* Agnes F. Morgan, C. L. Alsberg, L. S. McClung and K. F. Meyer, in charge. Eight sessions were held at which 64 papers were listed for presentation. The group also gave a luncheon at the Women's Faculty Club, University of California, on Tuesday, July 25. Two sessions dealt with the probable nutritional inadequacies of diets in common use by Pacific populations; the first with the white bread, sugar and meat diet of the Occident, and the second with the polished rice and fish diet of the Orient. These were followed by a session on vitamin requirements and vitamin content of foods of the Pacific area. One session was given over to the value of the soybean in supplementing deficient diets; one to the avitaminoses and alcoholism and metabolism; and one to fortification of foods with vitamins and hypervitaminoses. A further session dealt with nutrition as a factor in the geographical distribution of dental caries and paradentosis; and a final session was given over to a discussion of defective nutrition and public health.

*Health Education:* Dr. Ira V. Hiscock and Dr. W. P. Shepard, in charge. The sessions on health education were all joint sessions arranged by the Western Branch of the American Public Health Association. The sessions were opened by a symposium on health education at which addresses and reports upon various aspects of health education were presented. Following this session the program was divided into five sessions meeting simultaneously; three dealing with school health education (health instruction in the classroom, health service in schools and physical education and recreation), and two with health education of the public. The sessions continued with a résumé of the discussions on school health education and with further sessions on health education of the public. The sessions concluded with a general symposium on health education at which Dr. Walter H. Brown summarized the discussion on school health education, Dr. W. Ford Higby that on health education of the public, and Dr. Ira V. Hiscock discussed health education in the U. S. A.

*Soil Resources:* C. F. Shaw, S. W. Cosby, M. H. Lapham, R. E. Storie and W. W. Weir, in charge. This section, under the leadership of the late C. F. Shaw, was somewhat differently organized from the other sections. The main emphasis was laid on informal discussion of topics rather than upon formal presentation of papers. Included in the program were two two-day field trips; one to Placerville and way stations and one to Watsonville and Santa Cruz and way stations to inspect projects dealing with land use and methods of conservation and to serve as a basis for discussions at following sessions. Sessions were devoted to natural factors determining land use; soil, climate, water supply and topography, and to methods of study and mapping of the natural factors determining land use. A series of sessions were devoted to soil conditions and land use in various localities; in the foothills and interior valleys of California, in Oregon, in Washington, in the western Canadian provinces, in Central America, in Mexico, in China, in the tropical Pacific, in Australia and New Zealand, and in the Pacific coastal regions. The sessions closed with a general discussion of soil problems of Pacific lands.

# THE STRUCTURE OF THE PACIFIC BASIN AS INDICATED BY EARTHQUAKES[1]

By Professor B. GUTENBERG

CALIFORNIA INSTITUTE OF TECHNOLOGY, PASADENA

OUR earth originated about 2,000 million years ago. Great changes must have occurred in its early history, but even yet both gradual and sudden changes show us that it has not gained complete equilibrium. The sudden movements, which we call earthquakes, give us important information about the constitution of the earth.

The main features of earthquakes are fractures and displacements which occur usually at some depth, the focus of the earthquake, but which occasionally may extend to the surface and be visible there in the form of cracks, displaced roads or fences, etc. Such displacements frequently recur for long intervals in time and space in the same direction. A well-known example is the fault system in California, especially the San Andreas fault. The movements there occur in such a way that the eastern (continental) side moves southeastward relative to the western (Pacific) side. The same fact is proved by geologic measurements in Japan.[2] As mentioned already, movements occur gradually as well as during earthquakes. If in a certain region a block along one side of the fault moves gradually in one direction relative to the block on the other side, strains will be set up along the fault which finally lead to an earthquake at the time when the strain exceeds the breaking strength of the material and a break occurs. At this moment the material on one side of the fault "snaps" towards the unstrained position in one direction, that on the other side of the fault in the opposite direction. On both sides there is a compression in the direction in which the "snapping"

[1] Abstract of a public address at the Sixth Pacific Congress, Berkeley, Calif., August 1, 1939.

[2] During the meeting of the Pacific Science Congress Professor Ch. Tsuboi stated that in Japan, along all faults without exception, the continental (western) side is moving southward relative to the Pacific side; and, according to a statement by Dr. Bailey Willis, movements along the major fault in the Philippines occur in the same way, the continental side moves southward relative to the Pacific side. These results suggest the possibility of a general movement of Eastern Asia and Western North America to the south relative to the Pacific Basin. However, many more observations are needed before this can be considered a fact.

occurs and a dilatation in the opposite direction so that in such a simple case we should expect two quadrants about the source in which compressional waves are observed and two with dilatational waves. It is of interest that such patterns of compressions and dilatations are actually observed in earthquakes. More complicated patterns occur when the shock occurs at some depth and along a fault plane which is not vertical. The fact that thus far definite patterns have been observed in all earthquakes (no data exist for those produced by volcanic eruptions) regardless of their focal depth indicates that in all shocks the processes producing the waves are of the same type of "faulting" (shearing) and can not be due to a pure explosion or collapse in the interior of the earth.

The "shallow" earthquakes (less than 30 miles deep) show one belt of high activity around the Pacific Ocean, and another through southern Asia and the Mediterranean. The "great" earthquakes are more common around the Pacific. A still larger percentage of the "intermediate" shocks (depth 30 to 200 miles) and all very deep shocks which have been found thus far (maximum depth about 450 miles) originate in the circum-Pacific area. The boundary of the true Pacific Basin is outlined by the earthquake epicenters. On the west side it follows the "Andesite line," which separates regions of different petrologic and chemical composition, and runs east of Japan, the Marianne Islands, the Palau Islands, thence north of New Guinea and the New Hebrides towards the islands of Samoa which are on the Pacific side, and then turns southward, leaving the Kermadec Islands and New Zealand on the "continental" side. On the American side, the boundary is close to the coast. The fact that the foci of all earthquakes originating deeper than 200 miles have been found close to and on the continental side of this boundary indicates that the Pacific Basin has a unique structure.

The waves produced by an earthquake spread in all directions. There are different types, which are characterized by different modes of vibrations and different speeds. The fastest waves are of the "push-pull" (longitudinal) type and travel through the interior of the earth. They are followed by vibrations in which the particles vibrate sidewise back and forth. The last group are various types of surface waves, traveling exclusively along the surface of the earth. The speed of the first waves has been determined in various regions. The results indicate that certain granitic and basaltic layers exist in the continental regions down to a discontinuity at depths between 20 and 35 miles, depending on the locality. The data for the Pacific Basin are scant and agree with the assumption that the continental surface layers are missing there. On the other hand, in Japan and New Zealand, which we have considered already as belonging to the "continental" area, these continental surface layers clearly exist, though their thickness is relatively small; this is true also for the California coastal region.

The waves traveling along the surface lead to similar conclusions. They show, in addition, that the surface structures of the Atlantic and Indian Oceans are similar to those under the continents, but much thinner. Surface waves crossing the boundaries of the Pacific Basin lose a noticeable fraction of their energy, which indicates this boundary is a marked discontinuity between different structures. The fact that very long waves are not appreciably affected leads to the conclusion that the difference between these structures ends at a depth of noticeably less than 100 miles.

Finally, waves which are reflected at the surface of the earth can be used to deduce conclusions as to the conditions at the point of reflection. If the distance between the source of the shock and the recording stations exceeds a few thousand kilometers, the energy of the "echo" is stronger if the reflection has taken place within the continental surface layer than if this was absent at the point of reflection. Discussion of these observations has confirmed results from other sources and added some details as to the exact location of the boundary of the "Pacific Basin." It has added evidence in favor of a limited area with continental structure in the southeastern part of the Pacific and of Pacific type of structure in a part of the Arctic basin.

All evidence available agrees with the conclusion that the layers which form the uppermost crust in the continents are lacking in the Pacific Basin as defined above. The belt surrounding the Pacific Basin is characterized by faults in great number. Earthquakes originating at depths from close to the surface down to several hundred miles and the existence of relatively large gravity anomalies in many of the areas involved leave no doubt that this belt is the most active region of the world and that changes are going on in it extending from the surface to a depth of a few hundred miles at least. These processes, on which local changes are superimposed, seem to persist in their directional characteristics over long-time intervals and over large distances, at least notable fractions of the Pacific boundary. The source of the energy which produces these movements and the mechanism involved are not known exactly. It seems very likely that subcrustal currents, perhaps due to thermal processes, and the difference in structure between the Pacific basin and the surrounding regions play an important role.

However, another conclusion is unavoidable: There is no reason why the earthquakes around the Pacific belt should cease. While we can not predict the exact time or location of coming shocks, there is no doubt that there will be great earthquakes somewhere around the Pacific Basin during each coming year. As a matter of fact there is no day without small shocks in this narrow belt. However, there need not be any excessive damage connected with these shocks, even the greatest, as the science of engineering has made such progress during recent years that earthquake resistant structures can be built at a cost not exceeding much the cost of ordinary buildings. Just as large parts of California have been made "drought-proof," so that even in the driest years no lack of water is to be feared, all works of construction in the circum-Pacific belt should be made "earthquake proof," thus providing another triumph of science.

# SCIENTIFIC EVENTS

## THE CITY AND RURAL HEALTH CONSERVATION CONTEST

THE Chamber of Commerce of the United States in cooperation with the American Public Health Association has announced awards for the 1938 City Health Conservation Contest and the 1938 Rural Health Conservation Contest. These contests are said to be the most effective means of stimulating adequate health protection and health promotion services yet devised in this country.

Awards are made not necessarily to the healthiest communities, but rather on the effectiveness with which a community is meeting its health problems. Each city or county is appraised by a grading committee consisting of a group of carefully selected health experts from all parts of the country. Each community is appraised on what measures it takes: (1) to provide and safeguard its water supply; (2) to furnish adequate and safe sewerage disposal; (3) to reduce infant and maternal deaths; (4) to combat tuberculosis and syphilis; (5) to protect its citizens against other communicable diseases; (6) to insure healthy children; (7) to protect and safeguard its milk and other foods; (8) to promote effective cooperation with its physicians and dentists in furnishing necessary services to all those who need them; and (9) to enlarge and improve its lay-understanding of ways and means of preventing sickness and death and of maintaining good health.

The City Health Contest is financed by a group of life insurance companies. The Rural Health Contest is financed by the W. K. Kellogg Foundation of Battle Creek, Michigan. The contest in Canada is sponsored jointly by the Canadian Public Health Association and the American Public Health Association.

Two special contests, one on tuberculosis and one on syphilis, are carried on in conjunction with the City Health Contest. Awards are made to those competing cities which appear to have the most comprehensive and effective programs for combatting tuberculosis and syphilis as follows:

In Group I (cities over 500,000 population) Cleveland, Ohio, wins the first award. Awards of merit in this population group go to Buffalo, N. Y., and Pittsburgh, Pa.

In Group II (cities of 250,000 to 500,000 population) Providence, R. I., is the winner. Awards of merit in this group go to Memphis, Tenn.; Louisville, Ky.; Dallas, Texas, and Cincinnati, Ohio.

In Group III (cities of 100,000 to 250,000 population) the winner is Grand Rapids, Mich. Awards of merit go to Reading, Pa.; Yonkers, N. Y., and Erie, Pa.

In Group IV (cities of 50,000 to 100,000 population) the winner is Newton, Mass. Awards of merit go to Madison, Wis., Greensboro, N. C., and Evansville, Ill., tied.

In Group V (cities of from 20,000 to 50,000 population) the winner is Plainfield, N. J. Awards of merit go to Winona, Minn.; Orange, N. J., and Stamford, Conn.

In Group VI (cities of less than 20,000 population) the winner is Englewood, N. J. Awards of merit go to Hibbing, Minn., and Virginia, Minn.

In the 1938 Special Contest for Tuberculosis Control Hartford, Conn., and Newton, Mass., tied for first place. In addition a certificate of merit was awarded to New Haven, Conn. In the 1938 Special Contest for Syphilis Control the winner was Louisville, Ky.

## THE EXPEDITION TO HUDSON BAY OF THE UNIVERSITY OF MINNESOTA

THE University of Minnesota Expedition to Hudson Bay returned to Minneapolis on September 18. It left Senneterre, P. Q., by plane on June 25, arriving at its objective, Richmond Gulf, on June 26.

Richmond Gulf is a large, triangular body of salt water in Lat. 56° 15′ N. and Long. 76° 30′ W. It is surrounded by hills rising 800 to 1,500 feet above sea level, making this region relatively rugged for the east coast of Hudson Bay. The thoroughly glaciated hills are composed of sedimentaries of various kinds overlaid or penetrated by diabase trap, and also are composed in some cases of Archaean granites.

Botanically, the area is significant not only because it has needed thorough botanical exploration, but also because it has a great diversity of habitats and lies at the transition from coniferous forest to the barren grounds.

The members of the expedition collected flowering plants, ferns and some mosses, lichens and hepatics in the Richmond Gulf area until August 13. At this time the party left by canoe for Great Whale River. Collections were made in the vicinity of Great Whale River and along Manitounuck Sound until the arrival of the Hudson's Bay Company's vessel on August 22. The opportunity was taken to accompany the vessel on its annual visit to the Belcher Islands, where further collections were made. The return trip on the vessel was completed on September 11 upon arrival at the end of the railroad at Moosonee (Moose Factory), Ontario.

During the summer there were collected 1,336 numbers of flowering plants and about 400 numbers of lower plants, the number of herbarium specimens being about 8,000. In addition, about 250 tree borings and wood specimens from 80 trees were collected by John Marr for a study of tree growth climatic correlations.

The party was composed of Dr. Ernst C. Abbe, Mrs. Lucy B. Abbe and Mr. John Marr, a graduate student at the University of Minnesota.

The expedition was supported by funds from the Graduate School of the University of Minnesota, supplemented with liberal grants from the National Academy of Sciences (Bache Fund), the American Academy of Arts and Sciences, the Penrose Fund of the American Philosophical Society, the Smithsonian Institution, the Arnold Arboretum of Harvard University and the Minnesota Academy of Sciences.

ERNST C. ABBE

## THE IMPORTATION OF FOREIGN BOOKS AND PERIODICALS

THE Executive Board of the American Library Association on October 3 arranged for the appointment of a Joint Committee on Foreign Importations to act on behalf of the association and also of the Medical Library Association, the Special Libraries Association, the Association of Research Libraries and the Association of College and Reference Libraries. One or two other organizations may join in the project later. The following, of whom the first four form the executive committee, have accepted appointment to membership in the committee:

Harry Miller Lydenberg, New York Public Library, *chairman.*

Robert Lingel, New York Public Library, *vice-chairman.*

Keyes D. Metcalf, Harvard University Library.

Thomas Paul Fleming, Medical Library, Columbia University.

Dr. William Warner Bishop, General Library, University of Michigan.

Lawrence Heyl, Princeton University Library.

Bernhard Knollenberg, Yale University Library.

Harold L. Leupp, University of California Library.

Dr. Phineas Lawrence Windsor, University of Illinois Library.

Messrs. Lydenberg and Lingel conferred in Washington on November 4 with Dr. Archibald MacLeish, librarian of Congress, and B. L. Hunt, assistant legal adviser of the Department of State. Dr. MacLeish assured them of the willingness of the Library of Congress to aid American Libraries if it became necessary to lay their case before diplomatic authorities. Mr. Hunt is acquainted with the library situation. He agreed to consider on behalf of the Department of State any statements forwarded by the Library of Congress and to see that action was taken through appropriate channels as the circumstances might warrant.

Present conditions facing American libraries may be summarized as follows: publications of all kinds will be irregular because of war conditions; shipments are subject not only to wind and weather but to transportation irregularities both on sea and land. So far as the committee can learn, however, no embargo on shipments of books and periodicals has been laid. Restrictions on exports of books from Italy were limited to a short period after the war began. On September 28, the Department of State cabled to the American Embassy in London, with a view to making some general arrangement for the transmission of general publications from Germany. As soon as a reply has been received by the Department of State, the committee will be advised. There seems, however, at the present time, to be no difficulty in exporting books and periodicals from Germany in neutral vessels. The report states that agents seem so far to have been able to make their shipments with no more delays or difficulties than one must expect under such circumstances. Further announcements will be made by the committee which has its headquarters at 476 Fifth Avenue, New York City.

The American Documentation Institute of the library of the U. S. Department of Agriculture, Washington, requests that failure by a subscriber to receive European scientific journals be reported promptly. The cultural relations committee of the institute hopes to be able to surmount such war obstacles as interrupted transportation, embargoes and censorship, which seriously affected the progress of research during the last war. It is hoped that the principle will be established that materials of research having no relation to war shall continue to pass freely, regardless of the countries of origin or destination. Reports with full details of where subscription was placed and name and address of subscriber, volume, date and number of the last issue received should be addressed to the American Documentation Institute, Bibliofilm Service, U. S. Department of Agriculture Library, Washington, D. C.

## LECTURES IN THE DEPARTMENT OF PHYSICS AT THE UNIVERSITY OF WISCONSIN

DURING the academic year 1938–39 and the summer of 1939 the following speakers from out of town gave talks before faculty members and graduate students of the department of physics at the University of Wisconsin:

November 23, Dr. L. N. Ridenour, University of Pennsylvania, Artificial Radioactivities.

J. Schwinger, Columbia University, The $[\sigma_1\sigma_2 - 3(\sigma_1 r)(\sigma_2 r)r^{-2}]J(r)$ terms and the quadrupole moment of $H^2$.

December 2, Professor Otto Struve, Yerkes Observatory, Interstellar Absorption and Emission.

December 14, Professor S. Chandrasekhar, Yerkes Observatory, Stellar Structure and Stellar Energy.

December 16, Dr. K. K. Darrow, Bell Telephone Laboratories, History of the Mesotron.

January 6, Dr. D. P. Johnson, U. S. Bureau of Standards, Mercurial Thermometers.

April 4, Professor I. I. Rabi, Columbia University, Experiments with Molecular Beams on Nuclear Magnetic Moments.

Dr. M. Goldhaber, University of Illinois, Slow Neutron Boron Reaction.

April 14, Professor L. Brillouin, Collège de France, Spins and Statistics of Elementary Particles.

May 12, Professor R. S. Mulliken, University of Chicago, Intensities of Electronic Transitions and the Color of Organic Compounds.

May 19, Professor A. Ellett, State University of Iowa, The $D + D \rightarrow H_1 + H_3$ Reactions. Dependence of Angular Distribution and Cross Section upon Energy.

May 25, Professor A. H. Compton, University of Chicago, The Production and Disintegration of Mesotrons.

June 7, Dr. E. Feenberg, New York University, Canonical Transformations for Field Theories.

July 3, Dr. S. A. Korff, Bartol Foundation, Neutrons in Cosmic Radiation.

July 12, Professor Otto Struve and Dr. L. G. Henyey, Yerkes Observatory, Spectroscopic Evidence Regarding Interstellar Matter.

July 19, Professor T. W. Bonner, Rice Institute, Recent Work in Nuclear Physics at the Cavendish Laboratory.

## AWARD OF THE JOHN FRITZ GOLD MEDAL

THE posthumous award of the 1940 John Fritz Gold Medal to Dr. Clarence Floyd Hirshfeld, who until his death on April 19 of this year was chief of research of the Detroit Edison Company, has been announced.

The medal, given annually for notable scientific or industrial achievement by a board composed of sixteen representatives of the four national societies of civil, mining and metallurgical, mechanical and electrical engineers, was given to Dr. Hirshfeld "for notable leadership through research and development in power generation and electric traction, and for being a great teacher and friend of men both young and old."

Modernization of the electric street-car completely from trolley wire to track is among the many advances in engineering credited to Dr. Hirshfeld. His career extended over thirty-six years and included teaching, writing and direction of research work. He was born in San Francisco on January 30, 1881. From 1903 to 1914 he taught at Sibley College of Cornell University, becoming professor of mechanical engineering. In 1913 he organized for the Detroit Edison Company what is thought to be the first research department established and maintained by an electrical city supply company, where he became chief of research.

Dr. Hirshfeld was chief engineer of the Electric Railway Presidents' Conference Committee. He was the author of many books and articles on technical subjects, dealing principally with thermodynamics, steam power and problems of the transit industry. He was a member of the American Committee of the World Power Conference and of the U. S. National Committee of the International Electrotechnical Commission. He also served on the board of national councilors of the Purdue Research Foundation and on the advisory council of Yenching University. He was the first chairman of the Engineers' Council for Professional Development, and belonged to many scientific societies.

Dr. Hirshfeld was being considered as a candidate for the Fritz Medal at the time of his death. The award was, therefore, made posthumously.

## RECENT DEATHS AND MEMORIALS

DR. LIVINGSTON FARRAND, president emeritus of Cornell University, who was from 1903 to 1914 professor of anthropology at Columbia University, died on November 8 at the age of seventy-two years.

DR. WILLIAM H. BROWN, lecturer in botany at the Johns Hopkins University, previously from 1924 to 1933 director of the Bureau of Science at Manila, P. I., in charge of scientific investigations for the Philippines, died on November 9. He was fifty-five years old.

DR. FREDERICK ADAMS WOODS, formerly lecturer in biology at the Massachusetts Institute of Technology, who since 1927 has lived in Rome, died on November 5 at the age of sixty-six years.

DR. ALFRED ALEXANDER DIXON, professor of physics at the North Carolina State College of Agriculture and Engineering, died on October 15 at the age of fifty-three years.

WILLIAM ARTHUR COWAN, who served for forty years as chemist of the National Lead Company, died on October 27 at the age of sixty-five years.

DR. L. O. ELLISOR, assistant entomologist at the Louisiana Agricultural Experiment Station, died on October 21 at the age of twenty-nine years. Bullion A. Osterberger, also assistant entomologist at the station, died on May 20.

DR. RALPH ALLEN SAMPSON, Astronomer-Royal for Scotland from 1910 to 1937, professor of astronomy at the University of Edinburgh, died on November 10 at the age of seventy-three years.

TRIBUTE to the late Dr. W. E. Britton, Connecticut state entomologist from 1901 until the time of his death last February, was part of the program of the sixteenth annual conference of Connecticut entomologists that met on October 27 at the University of Connecticut at Storrs. The principal address was given by Dr. E. Porter Felt, formerly state entomologist of New York and now director of research at the Bartlett Tree Laboratories at Stamford.

THE *Journal* of the American Medical Association states that, in response to the request of many members, the council of the Minnesota State Medical Association sponsored a memorial pilgrimage to Rochester on October 27 to pay tribute to Drs. William J. and Charles H. Mayo. Every member of the association was invited to participate in the ceremonies at Plummer Hall in the Mayo Clinic and at Oakwood Cemetery. With Dr. George A. Earl, St. Paul, president of the state medical association, presiding, Dr. Edward L. Tuohy, Duluth, gave the address entitled, "An Expression from the Medical Profession of Minnesota." There followed a procession to the cemetery.

# SCIENTIFIC NOTES AND NEWS

THE Nobel Prize in physics for 1939 has been awarded by the Swedish Academy of Science to Dr. Ernest O. Lawrence, professor of physics and director of the radiation laboratory of the University of California, in recognition of his research into the structure of atoms and the use of radiation in problems affecting biology and medicine.

THE Nobel Prize in chemistry for 1939 has been divided between Professor Adolf Butenandt, director of the Kaiser Wilhelm Institute for Biochemistry at Berlin-Dahlem, and Professor Leopold Ružička, of the Technische Hochschule, Zurich, in recognition of their work on hormones. The prize in chemistry, which was withheld last year, has been awarded to Professor Richard Kuhn, of the Kaiser Wilhelm Institute of Berlin, for his work on carotinoids and vitamins. It is expected that if Professor Butenandt and Professor Kuhn are unable to accept the prizes the money will be returned to the Nobel Foundation.

THE University of Paris on November 9 conferred honorary degrees on Dr. Robert Andrews Millikan, chairman of the executive committee of the California Institute of Technology; on Sir Humphry Rolleston, who was from 1925 to 1932 regius professor of physic at the University of Cambridge, and on Dr. Philippe Roy, Montreal physician, since 1928 Minister to France from Canada. President Lebrun and the Minister of Education, M. Yvon Delbos, attended the ceremony.

THE Gordon Wilson Medal of the American Clinical and Climatological Association was presented at the meeting on October 10 at Saranac Lake, N. Y., to Dr. George R. Minot, professor of medicine at the Harvard Medical School. On that occasion he gave the Gordon Wilson Lecture before the association.

DR. LOUIS DAVIDSON RICKETTS, of Arizona, consulting engineer, has been chosen the James Douglas gold medalist for 1940 by the American Institute of Mining and Metallurgical Engineers, in recognition of his "inspirational leadership and distinguished achievements in the metallurgy of copper." Dr. Ricketts, who is now eighty years old, was at one time state geologist of Wyoming and was later associated with Phelps, Dodge and Company.

AT the meeting of the American Public Health Association in Pittsburgh, on October 18, the 1939 awards of the Pennsylvania Public Health Association were presented to Professor C. G. King, of the department of chemistry, University of Pittsburgh, in recognition of his research work in biochemistry and nutrition, and to Professor H. T. Price, of the School of Medicine, for his clinical and educational work in the field of pediatrics.

THE Royal Australian Ornithologists Union has elected Dr. Robert Cushman Murphy, of the American Museum of Natural History, a corresponding member in recognition of his active interest in the conservation of wild life.

DR. PERCY BARTLETT, for thirty-five years a member of the faculty of the Medical School of Dartmouth College, has retired with the title of professor emeritus of surgery.

DR. CARLO J. TRIPOLI has been appointed professor of medicine in charge of the department of medicine of the Graduate School of Louisiana State University.

DR. RAYMOND L. GREGORY, professor of medicine at Howard University College of Medicine, Washington, has been appointed professor and head of the department of medicine at the University of Arkansas School of Medicine.

DR. ROBERT M. DICKEY, since 1936 head of the department of geology and mineralogy of the Michigan College of Mining and Technology, has resigned to become an engineer with the Bucyrus-Erie Company. His headquarters are in Chicago. Dr. Thomas M. Broderick will serve as acting head of the department until a permanent successor can be named, probably about January 1. Dr. Broderick is chief geologist of the Calumet and Hecla Consolidated Copper Company, and has been also for some years a special lecturer at the college.

DR. JOHN G. B. CASTOR, assistant in plant physiology at Harvard University, has become a member of the Division of Viticulture at Davis of the University of California. He will work on the microbiology of wine.

DR. WILLIAM G. GORDON, for the past four years instructor in biochemistry at Stanford University, has been appointed Smith, Kline and French Laboratories research fellow in the department of agricultural biochemistry at the Pennsylvania State College. He will work in the field of milk protein.

DR. WALTER M. SCOTT, for the last nine years consulting chemist for G. J. Esselen, Boston, has been appointed chief of the Cotton Chemical Finishing Division of the Southern Regional Research Laboratory at New Orleans of the U. S. Department of Agriculture. He will be responsible for the scientific and administrative work of the division, which will involve research and development work to improve or modify by chemical treatment cotton fiber, cotton yarns, cotton textiles and cotton fabrics. Dr. Evald L. Skau, International Cancer Research Foundation fellow at Yale University, has been appointed senior chemist in the Oil, Fat and Protein Division of the laboratory. Dr. Skau's investigations will involve a study of various physical and chemical methods of separation of the fatty acids and glycerides, of cottonseed and peanut oils.

DR. ARLIE V. BOCK, Henry K. Oliver professor of hygiene at Harvard University, has been elected a member of the board of overseers of the Browne and Nichols School, Cambridge.

E. O. ESSIG, professor of entomology and entomologist of the Agricultural Experiment Station of the University of California, has been appointed advisory representative to the National Research Council from the Entomological Society of America. He also has become a director of the American Iris Society.

THE Committee on Scientific Research of the American Medical Association has made the following grants: To Dr. Wallace D. Armstrong, assistant professor of physiological chemistry at the University of Minnesota, to aid him in his work on the mechanism of the calcification process; to Dr. H. D. West, professor of biochemistry at Meharry Medical College, Nashville, Tenn., a renewal of the grant made last year for the continuance of his work on the synthesis of dl-threonine, and to Dr. H. P. Lankelma and Dr. B. S. Kline, of Western Reserve University, in aid of their work on the isolation of a substance in tissue extracts for use as antigen in tests for syphilis.

THE John and Mary R. Markle Foundation has appropriated a sum of $2,900 for an investigation of the viscosity of the blood to be carried out at Lafayette College under the direction of Professor Eugene C. Bingham. He continues the work begun a hundred years ago when Poiseuille made the first experiments leading to our knowledge of viscosity as a part of a study of the circulation of the blood.

THE Tuberculosis Institute of Chicago and Cook County, through the Theodore B. Sachs Memorial Fund, will support at the University of Illinois College of Medicine a study on bronchiectasis and pulmonary abscesses. This study, for which $1,000 is available, is being conducted by Dr. Felix Basch, of the department of pediatrics, and Dr. Paul H. Holinger, of the department of otolaryngology.

THE Elizabeth McCormick Child Research Grant of $1,000 for 1939–40 of the Institute of Medicine of Chicago will be used for the encouragement of research. Awards have been made to Dr. Mila I. Pierce for a program of research on leukemia; to Dr. Heyworth N. Sanford for a study of the role of the qualitative platelet factors in the coagulation of the blood, and to Dr. Clayton J. Lundy for a study of heart murmurs in children with rheumatic heart disease.

DR. A. A. BITANCOURT, sub-director of the Institute of Biology, São Paulo, Brazil, has completed a three-months official visit to the United States. He came as a delegate from the Brazilian Government to attend the third International Microbiological Congress held in New York from September 2 to 9. During his stay in the United States he visited various state agricultural experiment stations and colleges in Florida, New York, Wisconsin, Iowa, California and elsewhere, at some of which he made addresses on agriculture and plant pathology as related to Brazil. He also spent a month in Washington, conferring with members of the Department of Agriculture, and was for nearly two weeks at the Citrus Experiment Station, Riverside, Calif. On his way back to Brazil he planned to stop at Panama and several South American countries to make a study of citrus diseases.

DR. DENIS L. FOX, assistant professor of marine biochemistry at the Scripps Institution of Oceanography at La Jolla of the University of California, who has had a year's leave of absence as Rockefeller research fellow, has returned to the United States. He has been making a study at the University of Cambridge of pigments in lower plants and animals.

A DISCUSSION on "Science and the Press" will be held under the auspices of the New York chapter of the American Association of Scientific Workers in the Engineering Societies Building, New York City, on November 17 at 8:15 P.M. The speakers announced are: Dr. Waldemar Kaempffert, science editor, *The New York Times,* and Dr. Leslie C. Dunn, professor of zoology at Columbia University.

DR. VICTOR G. HEISER, consultant for the Committee on Healthful Working Conditions of the National Association of Manufacturers, formerly director for the East of the International Health Board of the Rockefeller Foundation, spoke on November 2 before the Lancaster Branch of the American Association for the Advancement of Science. His subject was "Adventures in International Health."

DR. ELLICE MCDONALD, director of the Biochemical Research Foundation of the Franklin Institute, made a report on the work of the foundation at a stated meeting of the institute on the evening of November 15.

DR. JOHN T. AUTEN, silviculturist at the Central States Forest Experiment Station, spoke at the Iowa State College on October 24, at a meeting of Sigma Xi on "Forests and Soils" and on October 26, under the auspices of the Research Council, on "The Significance of the Physical Properties of Forest Soils."

DEAN B. E. LISCHER, of the School of Dentistry of Washington University (St. Louis), gave a course of lectures on the "Diagnosis of Dento-facial Anomalies" to graduate students of the School of Dental and Oral Surgery of Columbia University, during the week of November 6 to 11.

THE forty-first annual meeting of the American Physical Society will be held in Columbus, Ohio, on Thursday, Friday and Saturday, December 28, 29 and 30, in affiliation with the section of physics of the American Association for the Advancement of Science.

THE fourth annual meeting of the Carolina Geological Society was held at Spruce Pine, N. C., on October 21 and 22. B. C. Burgess, of Tennessee Mineral Products, Incorporated, was chairman of the local committee, which arranged visits to mines and plants in the region. About twenty-five members and forty-five guests were present. The pegmatites with their associated minerals and the kaolins were studied and discussed in the field. The following were elected officers for the coming year: *President,* Major J. H. Watkins, Charleston, S. C.; *Vice-President,* W. J. Alexander, Bryson City and Spruce Pine, N. C.; *Secretary-Treasurer,* Professor Edward Willard Berry, Duke University; *Chairman Membership Committee,* Professor J. J. Petty, University of South Carolina.

THE American Association for the Advancement of Science is desirous of obtaining for its annual exhibition, which this year will be held at Columbus, Ohio, exhibits of recent advances in the various fields of pure and applied science. Space will be provided for exhibits of special interest to members of the association attending the meeting. Applications should be made to the Director of Exhibits, 3941 Grand Central Terminal, New York, N. Y.

ANNOUNCEMENT has been made by the Finney-Howell Research Foundation, Inc., that all applications for fellowships for next year must be filed in the office of the foundation, 1211 Cathedral Street, Baltimore, by January 1. This foundation was provided for in the will of the late Dr. George Walker, of Baltimore, for the support of "research work into the cause or causes and the treatment of cancer." The will directed that the surplus income from the assets of the foundation together with the principal sum should be expended within a period of ten years to support a number of fellowships in cancer research, each with an annual stipend of two thousand dollars, "in such universities, laboratories and other institutions wherever situated, as may be approved by the Board of Directors." Fellowships carrying an annual stipend of $2,000 are awarded for the period of one year, with the possibility of renewal up to three years; when deemed wise by the Board of Directors, special grants of limited sums may be made to support the work carried on under a fellowship.

THE 1939 award for achievement in chemical engineering of the American Institute of Chemistry has been given to the Standard Oil Development Company "for its work in developing processes for the large-scale production of new aviation fuels and other synthetic chemical products from petroleum." The award was established in 1933 by *Chemical and Metallurgical Engineering.* It will be presented by the publishers to a representative of the company on December 4 at the opening of the national exposition of the chemical industries in the Grand Central Palace.

# DISCUSSION

## THE ALLOWED DIRECTIONS OF COSMIC RAYS AS AN EXISTENCE PROBLEM OF MATHEMATICAL ANALYSIS

IT is a wide-spread opinion and a matter of fact that the physicist may be interested only in an actual solution of a mathematical problem, whereas the question of the *existence* of a solution is without interest to him, for the existence of a solution may be always easily inferred from the physical meaning of the mathematical formulation of the problem.

In spite of this well-known fact, the theory of cosmic rays, as developed by Professor M. S. Vallarta,[1] provides a very clear example (and probably a first one) in which the question of the existence of a solution is the only one of interest. The knowledge of the conditions under which the solutions exist is here the only one way available for an experimental verification of the theory, whereas the solution itself—represented by the trajectory of an electrical particle coming from far cosmic regions—is beyond experimental means.

Let this statement be explained in more detail. The theory of cosmic rays, considered as a motion of charged primary particles, is ruled by a system of three ordinary differential equations of second order in three unknown functions (the coordinates of the particle) and one independent variable, the time $t$. The solutions of this system are trajectories of the particle, so that the problem appears to be a boundary problem, the boundary conditions being expressed by the values of three coordinates of the point $P$ on the earth's surface, through which the trajectory passes, and by the infinite length of the radius vector for $t=\infty$. A fifth condition is given by the value of the energy of the particle, which is equivalent to the value of the velocity for instance at $P$. As a sixth condition, such a relation between the angles which the velocity vector in $P$ forms with two fixed axes is required that a solution exists. This condition geometrically interpreted leads to the allowed cone[2] of Vallarta.

By means of the Lagrange's function the problem can be reduced to an extremum problem of the calculus of variations.[3]

The method with which Professor Vallarta solved the problem is an inductive one, based on an actual evaluation of the solutions. A direct method for the determination of the existence conditions is unknown, and perhaps there is no one example in the Mathematical Analysis, in which the existence and non-existence conditions for a boundary problem are as completely known as is required by the theory of cosmic rays.

I. OPATOWSKI

THE UNIVERSITY OF MINNESOTA

1 See, for instance, the recent papers of M. S. Vallarta, "An Outline of the Theory of the Allowed Cone of Cosmic Radiation," The University of Toronto Press (1938) and "Present Status of the Effect of the Earth's Magnetic Field on Cosmic Rays," *Jour. of the Franklin Institute*, 227: 1, 1939.

2 Actually there is another supplementary condition due to the fact that the earth acts as an impenetrable body. However, the first step in the solution of the problem is that related to the pure boundary conditions.

3 T. Levi-Civita, *Archiv f. Mathem. og Naturvid.*, 31: 1911; and I. Opatowski, *Comptes Rendus*, 208: 638–640, 1939.

## REVISION OF DENTAL SYMBOLS

UNDER this heading there appeared in the issue of SCIENCE for April 7 an article by E. S. Riggs. No doubt, Mr. Riggs's suggestions aid in simplifying the typographical complexity of dental formulae used in various stages of paleontological and anthropological representations. It seems to the present writer that Mr. Riggs's proposition is not exhaustive enough to meet all the exigencies of the situation.

In his inventories and literary work, the present writer has availed himself of a system of listing dentures and individual teeth which he gradually developed in long years of practice and study and which has proven satisfactory in anthropological use and, in its fundamentals, should be adaptable without difficulty to any branch of the reptilian or mammalian sciences.

In his system, then, teeth are recorded with regard to their denomination and state of preservation as well as to their presence or absence in the dentures of the upper and lower jaws. The method employed by the writer of accounting for the teeth in cataloguing or describing a special skull or series of skulls is by numbers, which holds for both the adult or permanent and the infantile or deciduous generation of teeth, when for the former he uses the Arabic, for the latter, the Roman characters. The two schemes following here represent the conditions mentioned:

Adult (permanent) dentition:

| | | | | | | | | | | | | | | | | |
|---|---|---|---|---|---|---|---|---|---|---|---|---|---|---|---|---|
| 8 | 7 | 6 | 5 | 4 | 3 | 2 | 1 | \| | 1 | 2 | 3 | 4 | 5 | 6 | 7 | 8 |
| 8 | 7 | 6 | 5 | 4 | 3 | 2 | 1 | \| | 1 | 2 | 3 | 4 | 5 | 6 | 7 | 8 |

Infantile (deciduous) dentition:

| | | | | | | | | | | |
|---|---|---|---|---|---|---|---|---|---|---|
| V | IV | III | II | I | \| | I | II | III | IV | V |
| V | IV | III | II | I | \| | I | II | III | IV | V |

The figures in these schemes account for the number and denomination of teeth in each jaw-half, namely, eight (8) in the adult and five (V) in the infantile. In cases of gradual replacement of the deciduous by the permanent teeth or by the addition of the gradually erupting molars, the infantile scheme is to be varied by the substitution or addition of Arabic numbers according to the individual status of the developing dentures.

Counting from the cranial, *i.e.*, dental midline to either side of the orientation conforms to general topographic concepts, the left sides of the schemes representing the right dental halves, and *vice versa*. Incisor teeth, then, in these schemes are enumerated as 1 and 2 (I and II); canines as 3 (III); premolars, corresponding to infantile molars, as 4 and 5 (IV and V), and the permanent molars as 6, 7 and 8.

Customarily the individual teeth of the dental generations and in each jaw-half are symbolized by initial letters, capitalized for the adult or permanent teeth and indicated by small letters for the infantile or deciduous teeth, and in addition to their serial numbers either above or below the line indicative of their positions in the upper and lower jaws. Thus, $I^1$ signifies an upper permanent first incisor tooth; $Pm_2$ a lower permanent second premolar; $m^2$ an upper second infantile molar (to be replaced by $Pm^2$ of the permanent generation), and so forth. Right and left furthermore may be signified either by an additional *r* or *l*, so that $M_{1r}$ stands for a lower right first molar, $i^{2l}$ for a deciduous upper left second incisor. The canine as of single occurrence in the jaw-half requires no enumerative marks, so that $C^r$ stands for a permanent upper right, $c_l$ for a deciduous lower left canine. Symbols like these are preferably used in the description of individual teeth, deciduous or permanent, fossil or recent.

As regards their state of preservation, individual teeth may either be non-erupted, lost, pathological or in process of eruption. The following list in a summarized form accounts for these features, as also for those described above:

1 – 8, indicating the permanent teeth of an adult jaw-half in mesiodistal orientation;
I – V, indicating the deciduous teeth of an infantile jaw-half in mesiodistal orientation;

*I* = incisor, *C* = canine, *Pm* = premolar, *M* = molar — Symbols (capitalized initials) of permanent teeth

*i* = incisor, *c* = canine, *m* = molar — Symbols (small initials) of deciduous teeth

State of preservation of teeth in the dental schemes:

–, indicating non-eruption;
x, indicating post-mortem loss of tooth as shown by an empty alveolus, or a possible intra-vitam loss with a more or less obliterated alveolus or a more or less distinct gap remaining;
( ), indicating a pathological tooth, *e.g.*, (3);
○, a tooth in eruption, *e.g.*, (8).

Tentatively applying the last four symbols to the adult dental formula, the latter may individually occur as follows:

x x x x 4 3 (2) 1 | 1 2 3 (4) x 6 x 8
○7 6 x 4 3 2 1 | 1 – 3 4 5 6 7○

According to this formula and also using some of the other symbols, the state of dental preservation accounts in the right half of the upper jaw for a pathological $I^{2r}$ and a missing $Pm^{2r}$ and missing $M^{1-3r}$, in the left for a pathological $Pm^{1l}$ and a missing $Pm^{2l}$ and $M^{2l}$, while in the right half of the lower jaw $Pm_{2r}$ is missing and $M_{3r}$ in eruption, the left half accounting for a non-erupted $I_{2l}$ and $M_{3l}$ in eruption.

BRUNO OETTEKING
MUSEUM OF THE AMERICAN INDIAN,
NEW YORK

## POSSIBLE IMPLICATIONS OF REPTILIAN THERMAL TOLERANCE

INVESTIGATIONS into the thermal responses of the reptiles of southern California deserts have established a few facts that appear to be of particular interest since they suggest an alternative explanation for the sudden disappearance of their large Mesozoic predecessors.

The inhabitants of this extremely hot area show only moderate physiological adaptation to the maximum environmental temperatures to which they are subjected, achieving their survival largely through behavior in response to excessive insolation and heat.

The most heat-tolerant forms include the following diurnal lizards: *Sauromalus obesus, Dipsosaurus d. dorsalis, Uma notata, Phrynosoma platyrhinos* and *Phrynosoma m'callii.* These appear to be conspicuously thermophilous forms and yet, with ground-surface black-bulb thermometer readings as high as 87° C. common occurrences in their environment, they are characterized by optimum temperatures ranging between 37° C. and 38° C. The coastal lizards from appreciably cooler areas, *Phrynosoma b. blainvilii* and *Phrynosoma b. frontale,* as well as species from the higher or cooler desert areas, such as *Crotaphytus collaris baileyi, Crotaphytus wislizenii* and *Crotaphytus silus,* approach or equal these temperatures.

The most surprising fact relative to high temperatures is the characteristic reptilian inability to endure body heat much above the optimum, an increase of only 2° C. causing marked discomfort which seldom if ever will be tolerated voluntarily. Short exposures to higher temperatures cause death in from 60 seconds to an hour, the time element depending on ground heat, intensity of radiation, capacity for color change and volume of the lizard. Toward low temperatures these animals exhibit a far greater latitude, although 28° C. appears to be the lowest voluntarily tolerated temperature. These and other factors concerning the thermal relationships of desert lizards clearly suggest the possibility that high temperatures and increased insolation, rather than cold, may have been the chief element in bringing about the disappearance of the Mesozoic reptilian fauna, and it can be stated that if these forms were as notably susceptible to the lethal effects of high temperatures as our most heat-loving desert species of to-day, they could scarcely survive exposure to the direct sunlight of a hot summer day. Certainly it is notable that their successors were mainly homoiotherms or aquatic vertebrates, the terrestrial poikilothermous reptiles having disappeared with puzzling universality, especially from the viewpoint of encroaching low temperatures as the lethal agent.

In spite of our limited knowledge as to the actual density of vegetation during these important times it appears probable that exposure to direct sunlight was becoming increasingly unavoidable. The vegetational changes provide evidence of increasing aridity and suggest increasingly wide spacing of the trees and the development of savanna types of country, presumably resulting in serious exposures of the larger reptiles at least, to almost direct untempered insolation.

Although no information is available it is probable that in common with the terrestrial poikilothermous vertebrates of to-day, the early Mesozoic reptiles may have relied upon a suffusion of melanin or other comparable heat-absorbing pigment for temperature regulation, a characteristic which appears to be of vital importance in the survival of desert lizards in order to achieve and control the body temperatures requisite for the normal functioning of physiological activities. The necessity for pigmentation by heat-absorbing substances would seem to have been particularly necessary if the commonly accepted concept of dense vegetation, heavy blanketing clouds and abundant water vapor existed on and above the earth's surface during Triassic, Jurassic and early Cretaceous times. With such pigmentation and lacking the capacity for color change, progressive reduction in the amount of water vapor or clouds would be accompanied by a disastrous rise in the body temperature of exposed reptiles. It is notable that desert snakes with no known capacity for color change are almost altogether either crepuscular, nocturnal or subterranean in habitat. The diurnal racers appear to survive excessive heat through their capacity for swift retreat to shade and in hot weather the trend is toward a crepuscular existence.

Additional evidence for progressively higher temperatures appears to be provided through the thermal evolutionary sequence as seen in the changes exhibited from the fishes to mammals and birds in which there is a distinct tendency toward the adoption of progressively higher body temperatures with an increasingly unfavorable susceptibility to cooling. This trend toward the optimum temperatures of complete homoiothermism and its perfection in the birds may reflect a gradual development in the environment of conditions feasible for the initial steps toward thermal control without excessive expenditures of energy due to internal-external temperature discrepancies, that is, in a gradual increase in available heat.

A much confused but apparently similar thermal-evolution relationship among plants is highly suggestive.

RAYMOND B. COWLES

UNIVERSITY OF CALIFORNIA
AT LOS ANGELES

# SCIENTIFIC BOOKS

## THE CARNEGIE INSTITUTION OF WASHINGTON AND DR. MERRIAM

*Published Papers and Addresses of John Campbell Merriam.* Publication No. 500, The Carnegie Institution of Washington.

*Cooperation in Research.* Publication No. 501, The Carnegie Institution of Washington.

MANY readers of SCIENCE doubtless noted with interest that Dr. John Campbell Merriam, president of the Carnegie Institution of Washington since 1921, had retired on December 31, 1938, in order that he might be free to devote his time to research and writing, and that the board of trustees of that institution, in appreciation of his far-sighted leadership, had appointed him president emeritus, with provision for the support of his studies.

Soon afterward the trustees also made arrangements for the publication of a testimonial volume to Dr. Merriam (Publication No. 501). Previously to this, the trustees had authorized the republication of the "Published Papers and Addresses of John Campbell Merriam"; this publication (No. 500) fills four large volumes, comprising 2,672 pages, an index, a bibliography and many illustrations. Both publications are of exceptional importance not only because they contain a great mass of valuable scientific and educational records and results, but also because they afford abundant evidence, direct and indirect, of the development of the Carnegie Institution itself under the influence of Dr. Merriam's far-reaching and constructive methods and philosophy.

Neither Dr. Merriam nor the Carnegie Institution could ever be fairly classed with those who learn "more and more about less and less"; they stand indeed at the opposite pole from that famous senior wrangler who gloried in the practical uselessness of his subject. Professor Chester Stock's appreciative article at the close of Publication No. 501 makes it clear that Dr. Merriam, a student all his life, has never ceased to extend and develop his first-hand knowledge of many sciences: botany, paleobotany, invertebrate paleontology, geology, vertebrate paleontology, archeology, anthropology and related fields; also that as an administrator he has gained such an insight into the methods and objectives of the physical sciences, history and philosophy that he has achieved far-reaching success in organizing and integrating the activities of many otherwise disconnected agencies in these diverse fields.

With this clue in hand we may thread our way with rising enthusiasm through the far-flung labyrinth of his scientific papers and addresses. However, the future historian who desires to study the earliest published writings of Dr. Merriam will be disappointed when he turns to the bibliography and reads the statement: "Not listed are several short articles between 1889 and 1891," which articles one would naturally search for possible early indications of the trends which characterize Dr. Merriam's maturity. The first paper of Volume I is Dr. Merriam's doctorate thesis in the University of Munich: *"Ueber die Pythonomorphen der Kansas-Kreide."* This work by a young man of twenty-four is a finished piece of analysis, ending in an illuminating table of the contrasts of the three leading genera of American Cretaceous mosasaurs. It would do credit to a paleontologist of many more years of experience. At Munich he evidently found in his famous master, Professor Karl A. von Zittel, the clarity and precision in analysis and the insight that results in synthesis, which have always been the rocks upon which he has built. (We trust, by the way, that Dr. Merriam will not resent our analyzing him as he has analyzed his mosasaurs, ichthyosaurs and Tertiary mammals!)

The necessary limitations of space prohibit more than a mention of Dr. Merriam's papers (1895–1908) on the Triassic Ichthyosaurs of California and Nevada, culminating in his great monograph of 1908. This may safely be characterized as one of the major documents of vertebrate evolution and should be on the list of seminar discussions for all graduate students in that field. Regretfully we must pass over Dr. Merriam's intensive and extensive explorations and studies of the geology and paleontology of the John Day Basin of Oregon (Oligocene), of the late Tertiary and Pleistocene faunas of California, Nevada and Idaho (Vol. I and Vol. II in part) and his numerous papers on the Pleistocene mammalian fauna of the famous "tarpits" at Rancho La Brea, which the visitor to Los Angeles may now view both at Hancock Park and the Los Angeles Museum (Vol. II in part). Nor may we do more than refer to the "Tertiary Mammalian Faunas of the Mohave Desert," containing, with other papers in Volumes II and III, most important documents of mammalian evolution during the late Tertiary.

With his vast experience in the history of vertebrate and invertebrate life it was almost inevitable that Dr. Merriam should also take a special interest in the paleontological evidence bearing on the origin and emergence of man, especially in Western North America. All that may be said here is that he has succeeded, largely by direction of researches supported by the Carnegie Institution, in bringing to light much new evidence of the association of human artifacts of relatively advanced cultural stage with a mammalian fauna which has the aspect of late Pleistocene or early Recent provenience; the age of which in a recent memoir by Edgar B. Howard is tentatively estimated as of about 10,000 years. Thus Dr. Merriam's work tends strongly to confirm the relatively late arrival of man in America as compared with his history in Europe and Asia.

The fourth volume is devoted chiefly to Dr. Merriam's numerous addresses and papers relating to history, biography, problems relating to nature, research and publication, research and government, Carnegie Institution addresses and extracts from presidential Annual Reports.

When in 1936 Dr. Merriam was awarded the gold medal of the American Institute, the present writer referred to him as "both author and interpreter of an epic poem of unsurpassed grandeur. This poem is not written in verse but in the sober language of science. It is the epic of the history of vertebrate life on the Pacific coast, and the story is told in a long series of publications, chiefly in the bulletins of the Department of Geology in the University of California, but of late years also in the paleontological memoirs and papers of the Carnegie Institution of Washington. More than sixty localities scattered over California and the adjoining states have yielded the historical documents, in the shape of fossilized animal and plant remains, upon which this great epic has been built up."[1] With the fuller documents contained in Volumes I–IV of Publication 500 before us, the foregoing citation is seen to be even an understatement.

The volume "Cooperation in Research" (Publication 501), by staff members and research associates of the Carnegie Institution, comprises fourteen papers on the physical sciences, thirteen on the biological sciences, seven on history (mostly American archeology), five on paleontology and geology, three on philosophy and interpretation. In the first paper, entitled "An Adventure in Scientific Collaboration," Dr. Arthur L. Day, chairman of the Advisory Committee in Seismology, describes the large-scale cooperation between the Carnegie Institution as a whole and numerous other research foundations, the end being the development of the science of seismology from an "uninspiring status" to its present prominence and importance. During the course of this work the U. S. Coast and Geodetic Survey, the U. S. Geological Survey, the Navy Department and other government agencies collaborated with various universities, observatories and geological societies of California, and their work was supported and endorsed by still another group of organizations. The results have contributed greatly to the knowledge, not only of earthquakes and their causes, but also of the physical properties of the successive zones of the interior of the earth, of the conditions under which the oceans and the continents are held in equilibrium, as well as those under which severe disturbances of the rock strata take place.

For cooperation on a smaller scale among the members of a special group, one may turn to the paper by

[1] *The Scientific Monthly,* 42: 4, 377–380, April, 1936.

the editor of the publications of the institution, Dr. Frank F. Bunker, on "Cooperative Research, Its Conduct and Interpretation." As an example of the fruitful results that may be obtained by the functional integration of a closely cooperating group, the editor selects the story of the activities of the Division of Plant Biology, under direction of Dr. H. A. Spoehr, in research on photosynthesis from the year 1911 through twenty-eight years.

Dr. Bunker explains the success of scientific research in our times as due to the same principle of cooperation. He writes:

> Again, as never before, there is team work among investigators who recognize neither national nor group boundaries. Neither are there ''trade secrets'' in scientific research. Progress reports are continually being interchanged among the workers throughout the world and thus each shares what he has learned with all the others; so, also, each borrows from others and builds upon what he borrows.
>
> An army of investigators, then, trained for the tasks, relieved of economic worry, supplied with every facility required, and working in tacit cooperation, accounts for the epoch-creating achievements now being made in the various fields of scientific research.

In the Year Book of the Carnegie Institution for 1934 Dr. Merriam wrote:

> As yet comparatively little attention has been given to the idea that science may have made its most noteworthy contribution through influences which aid in determining attitudes of mind and objectives. In other words, we have been concerned more largely with discussion of the extent to which science affects our environmental conditions than with the possibility that it helps to give us new points of view and a bettered attitude toward life. The great significance of this difference becomes apparent when we consider that influences determining point of view and attitude furnish major sources of human initiative, and are among the most important guiding elements in life.

These sentences take on new and startling aspects when we consider to what extent diverse points of view and attitude have determined conflicting human initiative within the past few months.

Thousands of people have doubtless gained a wider perspective and "a bettered attitude toward life" both from Dr. Merriam's own writings and from the numerous scientific and educational activities that have been sponsored by the Carnegie Institution under his guidance. Meanwhile "Cooperation in Research" affords a small-scale model of a cooperating society of diverse groups working in harmony, toward which a war-torn Europe may yet turn.

WILLIAM K. GREGORY

# REPORTS

## WORK OF THE CANADIAN NATIONAL RESEARCH COUNCIL

THE twenty-first annual report of the National Research Council has been issued. The work of the council falls naturally into two main divisions: the research investigations carried out in the laboratories at Ottawa, and the activities of the numerous committees that have been organized by the council to investigate specific problems and sometimes to plan and direct research which may be carried on in the universities or other institutions having special facilities for studies in certain subjects.

Special mention is made in the current report of the formation of the Associate Committee on Medical Research under the chairmanship of Sir Frederick Banting, co-discoverer of insulin. The method of forming this committee may be considered as typical. Preliminary discussions by representatives of the Canadian Medical Association, Royal College of Physicians and Surgeons, the Department of Pensions and National Health and the National Research Council resulted in the calling of a conference for the consideration of all matters relating to medical research in Canada. At this conference a composite picture of medical research was presented when each institution represented at the meeting reported on the scope of the researches on which it was engaged. On the recommendation of the conference the Associate Committee on Medical Research was formed.

Since then the correlation of medical research in Canada has been fostered through interchange of visits by research workers and group-planning of investigations in many fields. A distinct contribution to the furtherance of organized research in the medical field has thus been made.

Similar committees function under the council in many fields: aeronautics, asbestos, coal classification and analysis, field crop diseases, fire hazard testing, forestry, gas research, laundry research, leather, magnesian products, market poultry, metallic magnesium, parasitology, plant hormones, potato research, radio, radiology, survey research, weeds and wool.

In the laboratories there are four main divisions: biology and agriculture; chemistry; mechanical engineering, including aeronautics and hydraulics; and physics and electrical engineering. Supplementing these are a section on codes and specifications and the research plans and publications section. In addition there are the general administrative services necessary to such an organization.

Direction of the National Research Laboratories is vested in the president and all matters of policy are decided upon by the National Research Council, a body of 15 men appointed on the recommendation of the Committee of the Privy Council for Scientific and Industrial Research, which in turn consists of seven members of the Dominion Cabinet, presided over by the Honorable W. D. Euler, Minister of Trade and Commerce.

In the Division of Biology and Agriculture, the development of equipment for malting tests and for cold storage purposes has occupied an important place. Development of special equipment has enabled the laboratories to provide improved service to breeders of malting barleys. Efforts are being made to combine high yield and disease resistance with the superior malting quality needed for enlarging the potential domestic and foreign market for Canadian barley.

The development of equipment to provide temperatures as low as $-40°$ F. in addition to ordinary storage equipment has simplified the study of cold storage of perishables. It is now possible to deal with produce by the quick-freezing method, instead of allowing it gradually to reach the temperature of storage. In cooperation with the industry a comprehensive study of the whole system of curing and pickling bacon is under way, with the object of improving the quality and uniformity of the Canadian output.

Plants elaborate certain substances which, in very minute amounts, have profound effects on plant growth. These have been referred to as "plant hormones." Efforts have been made to utilize these substances as aids to plant growth by treating seeds with them. A method has been developed in the laboratories in which the substance in very small amounts is applied as a dust. By this means root development of cuttings has been stimulated. Types of cuttings that foresters have found very difficult to root have responded well to this kind of treatment. Experiments also indicate that improved germination, root development and growth of leafy parts may be attained when the seed or small growing plants are treated with dust. The substance is cheap, very minute quantities are needed, and since farmers already use dust treatment for the control of fungi, the use of the hormone will involve little extra expenditure of money or labor.

The Division of Chemistry has organized relations for research with the laundry and dry cleaning industry, the asbestos industry, the leather industry and, to a less extent, with the wool manufacturing and sugar industries. Much other work has basic industrial importance, *e.g.*, work on paints, rubber and textiles.

One of the most striking pieces of work of the last few years relates to the utilization of waste natural gas. It has been found that by heat treatment in a furnace of a special but nevertheless simple design, the fraction of waste gas known as stabilizer gas can be made to yield three to four gallons of liquid motor fuel of the benzol type per 1,000 cubic feet of gas. The striking result has now been secured that the residual gas from such heat treatment will yield six to seven pounds of carbon black. This combination process seems to have attractive commercial possibilities.

A distillation column has been developed that is of great interest to the oil-refining, synthetic chemical and coal-tar industries, as well as to other industries using distillation as a process. Noteworthy results have been obtained in researches on starch. In the corrosion laboratory problems ranging from the corrosion of laundry hot water pipes to that of hydro-electric power dam gates are being investigated.

The work on magnesian products in the laboratories has been very profitable to Canada. The magnesian products laboratory has not only made available to the Canadian metal industry better refractories, and a greater range of them, but it has shown that these can be produced from Canadian materials. An investigation of various domestic barks as sources of tannin for the leather industry has been carried on in the leather laboratory. In the rubber laboratory much has been done on the bonding of rubber to metal, including particularly the application to the manufacture of automobile engine mountings of a bonding material previously developed in the laboratories.

In the Division of Mechanical Engineering there are available a wind tunnel for the testing of aeroplane models, streamlined locomotives and any other equipment in which air resistance is important, and a model-testing basin in which somewhat similar problems in regard to water may be investigated.

Five ship models have been tested during the year in the towing basin in connection with the design of private and government vessels. In two instances it was found possible to make major improvements in the propulsive characteristics. A one-hundredth scale model of a stop-log emergency dam was tested to ascertain the forces likely to be met in the operation of similar full-scale structures. Engines, aircraft instruments, gasoline and lubricating oils have been tested for various branches of the government service. Instruction is also given to members of the staff of the Royal Canadian Air Force in the testing, care and maintenance of the instruments used in their work.

In the division of Physics and Electrical Engineering, the normal fundamental phases of work on sound, light and heat, and the studies on electrical engineering are carried on concurrently with a steadily increasing amount of testing, examination and standardization of instruments. Advice has been given to a number of government departments in connection with such varied matters as the acoustical treatment of rooms and buildings, apparatus for depth-sounding purposes, forest fire hazards, collection of insects and methods of plotting results of aerial surveys. In the metrology laboratory, apparatus for the precise calibration of standard gauges for industry has been designed and built. A satisfactory heater for use in refrigerator cars in winter to prevent freezing has been developed and is being taken up commercially. New apparatus has been installed in the electrical engineering laboratory to provide high-voltage current, and progress has been made in the precise regulation of voltage. Thousands of aircraft castings are being examined by x-ray methods and a 600,000-volt apparatus has been constructed to permit expansion of this work and for standardization of equipment for hospital use. Type approval of meters is being continued. The cathode-ray compass and direction finder, detection of fires through haze, estimation of forest fire hazard, vibration in aircraft, ultrasonic generators for depth sounding, problems in camera design for air photography and spectroscopic analyses are some of the other matters under study.

Recent additions to equipment include an electric surge generator capable of developing a million volts for use in the testing of transmission line and other insulating material.

Radium preparations in large numbers are measured and certified in the radium laboratory. Recently a device for rapid testing of radium tubes for leakage was constructed and a method for measuring the radium content of barium-radium bromide preparations was developed.

# SPECIAL ARTICLES

## EFFECT OF ULTRA-SHORT RADIO WAVES ON PLANT GROWTH

A NUMBER of papers were published during the last few years on the effect of radio waves on plant growth. The results obtained were not quite clear, but in a few cases a definite stimulation of plant growth was observed after seeds or plants were radiated with ultra-short radio waves.[1]

The present article summarizes some of the results of our investigation of the effect of radiation of young corn seedlings with radio waves 2.5 m long.

The waves used were generated by a magnetron oscillator of about 25 watts of power, with a GE type FH 11 split anode magnetron in a conventional circuit.[2] The tube was operated with a DC plate voltage of 1,500 volts in an air solenoid with a magnetic field strength of about 750 gauss. The heating of the filament was such that the plate current was equal to 50 mA. The tank circuit consisted of a single loop of two parallel thin-walled copper tubings 3 mm in diameter and 32 cm long. These tubings were placed vertically 3.5 cm apart. Their lower ends were connected to the plate terminals of the magnetron, and their upper ends were short-circuited. At a distance of 3 cm above the plate terminals a condenser was connected to the tubings. It was made of two 1/16 inch copper strips 3 by 5.5 cm bent to form a split cylindrical condenser about 3.5 cm in diameter. The wave-length was determined with a Lecher system loosely coupled with the oscillator.

The following experimental procedure was followed. Corn seeds were germinated in moist sand in a physiological darkroom at 25° C and 90 per cent. humidity. After 2½ to 3 days the seedlings were dug out for treatment in a room illuminated with white light of moderate intensity. Radiation of the seedlings was accomplished by placing the shoot (excluding the seed and roots) between the plates of the condenser on a strip (7 mm wide and 2 mm thick) of "Victron," a material which shows a very slight absorption of the waves used. The controls were treated exactly like the experimental plants, with the exception of the exposure to the short waves. After radiation the seedlings were planted in moist sand and put back in the darkroom, where they were kept for the duration of the experiment.

Various exposures were tried. Those of 60 seconds and longer usually destroyed the upper part of the mesocotyl, which became limp immediately after treatment and the seedlings died. Exposures of about 10 seconds turned out to be too short to produce any appreciable effect. Therefore the exposures of between 20 and 30 seconds were used in the experiments.

The results of these experiments did not demonstrate any stimulation of growth. To the contrary we found that the waves used produced, at least as far as corn seedlings were concerned, a markedly reduced growth of the first internode,[3] whereas the growth of the coleoptile was far less affected.

It was discovered a few years ago by one of us[4] that

[1] G. Murray McKinley, "Biological Effects of Radiation," pp. 541–558. McGraw-Hill, 1936; K. v. Oettingen, *Strahlentherapie*, 41: 251–285, 1931; S. Sasada, *Nippon Elect. Comm. Engin.*, 7: 295–297, 1937; A. Denier, *Proc. Intern. Congress for Short Waves*, Vienna, 1937: 320–322.

[2] Complete description in General Electric pamphlet GEJ–239A; see also E. D. McArthur and E. E. Spitzer, *Proc.* IRE.,19: 1971–1982, 1931.

[3] The shoot of the seedlings of grasses consists of the first internode or mesocotyl and above it the coleoptile which envelops the primary leaf.

[4] J. van Overbeek, *Rec. trav. bot. neerl.*, 33: 333–340, 1936.

the growth of the first internode of young seedlings of maize can be considerably reduced if they were kept in an electric oven at 48° C for 30 minutes. It was shown at that time that this effect of reduction of growth depends upon the decrease in auxin (growth hormone) production due to heat treatment. The auxin is produced in the coleoptile tip and controls the growth of the first internode. Thus a decrease in auxin production could account for the decreased growth of the internode. This conclusion was proven experimentally when it was shown that the application of synthetic auxin (indoleacetic acid) immediately after the heat treatment made the internode grow normally again.

The present investigation similarly disclosed that plants having a reduced growth of the first internode, due to ultra-short wave radiation, had a reduced auxin production (See Table 1). The auxin production was determined by means of the diffusion method.[5]

TABLE 1

AMOUNT OF AUXIN, IN DEGREES OF CURVATIVE IN THE AVENA TEST, GIVEN OFF DURING HOURLY PERIODS BY 10 COLEOPTILE TIPS. THE TEST WAS MADE 20 HOURS AFTER THE SEEDLINGS HAD BEEN EXPOSED FOR 20 SECONDS (80929).

| | Radiated | Controls |
|---|---|---|
| First Hour | 6.3 | 11.5 |
| Second Hour | 3.5 | 6.9 |
| Third Hour | 1.9 | 6.5 |
| Length of mesocotyl (mm) | 34.6 | 44.8 |

In a number of cases additional auxin was applied to radiated plants. This was done with a paste of indoleacetic acid in lanolin applied to the tip of the seedlings immediately after the radiation. As experiments showed (see Table 2) such application of additional auxin restored the first internode to normal.[7]

TABLE 2

LENGTH (IN MM) OF THE COLEOPTILE (C) AND THE MESOCOTYL (M) OF CORN SEEDLINGS AFTER RADIATION WITH AND WITHOUT AUXIN TREATMENT. AVERAGES OF ABOUT 40 PLANTS (81007), (80924).

| | Time of exposure (sec) | Auxin concentration per cent. | Time after radiation (hours) 24 | | 48 | | 72 | |
|---|---|---|---|---|---|---|---|---|
| | | | C | M | C | M | C | M |
| Radiated, no auxin applied | 20 | .. | 11.2 | 13.0 | 20.3 | 30.8 | ... | ... |
| | 30 | .. | ... | ... | ... | ... | 40.7 | 35.6 |
| Not radiated, no auxin applied | .. | .. | 13.3 | 17.2 | 26.2 | 39.8 | 45.9 | 53.0 |
| Radiated, auxin applied | 20 | .02 | 12.8 | 25.0 | 20.0 | 50.3 | ... | ... |
| | 30 | 1.0[6] | ... | ... | ... | ... | 53.3 | 45.6 |

[5] J. van Overbeek, *Plant Physiol.*, 13: 587–598, 1938.

[6] An indoleacetic acid concentration of 1 per cent. turned out to be too high, causing the internodes to swell rather than to elongate.

[7] Both control plants and experimental plants were exposed to light when brought in the radiation room. The reduction in growth caused by exposure to light is also offset by auxin application.

From these results it follows that, at least under the condition of our experiments, the effect of ultra-short radio waves on young corn seedlings can be accounted for as a heat effect.

J. VAN OVERBEEK

WILLIAM G. KERCKHOFF LABORATORIES
OF THE BIOLOGICAL SCIENCES

L. REED BRANTLEY
G. W. POTAPENKO

LABORATORY OF PHYSICS
CALIFORNIA INSTITUTE OF TECHNOLOGY

## BIO-ELECTRIC POTENTIALS OF THE HEN'S EGG

THE possibility of detection of vital activity of the blastoderm of fertile eggs by physical means was suggested by Waller.[1] Also it was tried by Vorontzov and Serguijevski[2] to measure the electrical potential through the shell, between the top and the bottom of the egg on the equatorial plane. They observed that 3 to 4 hours incubated eggs gave an electro-potential difference of about 0.5 millivolt and 20 hours' incubation about 1.0 millivolt. But fresh eggs were almost isopotential, or electro-potentials were very small. Owing to that fact it is still a question whether there is a difference in electrical potentials in fresh fertile and infertile eggs. In an attempt to answer that question the present study of bio-electric potentials of the opened hens' eggs was undertaken.

The procedure followed was to apply a pair of physiological saline solution capillary electrodes to the opened egg. One electrode was touching the albumen several millimeters beyond the yolk, while the other electrode successively was placed on the top of the yolk in contact with points at various distances from the center of the blastoderm. To insure more intimate contact on the exposed surface of the yolk, the albuminous sac of the thick middle layer was ruptured and moved aside.

Potential differences existing between the electrodes were measured by a vacuum tube microvoltmeter similar to one described by Burr, Lane and Nims.[3] However, the circuit used by us was somewhat modified from that of Burr *et al.* A duotriode 6C8G tube was used with a pair of parallel filament resistances forming the grid biases close to floating grid potentials to partially offset A battery fluctuations. The input grid was brought accurately to floating grid potential by an additional C battery potentiometer control and the input was then applied across 10 megohms between the grid and ground.

[1] A. Waller, ''Signs of Life.'' London, 1903.

[2] B. S. Vorontsov and M. V. Serguijevski, ''L'electrophysiologie de l'oeuf de poule.'' Probleme der Tierzsucht No. 6, Moscow, 1933 (in Russian).

[3] H. C. Burr, C. T. Lane and L. F. Nims, *Yale Jour. Biol. and Med.*, 9: 65–76, 1936.

The electrodes proper were of Ag-AgCl prepared as described by Brown[4] and were constant to several microvolts during a run. The capillary electrodes were so arranged that fresh saline solution formed the contact for each measurement. Checks of the inherent electrode potential differences were made before and after each reading.

The sensitivity of the voltmeter and electrodes was slightly above 100,000 mm/volt with a wall galvanometer. Measurements were made inside a wire screen cage to reduce pick-up disturbances. Room temperature varied less than 2° F. from day to day. Fresh eggs having been collected from the nests in the morning were brought into the room and allowed to come to room temperature for at least four hours before being measured. Several groups of measurements were delayed until the following day and were found somewhat higher than those made on the day the eggs were collected.

The incubated eggs were measured immediately after having been removed from the incubator and opened. While being measured the eggs were close to the incubating temperature, which was maintained by a thermostatically controlled enclosure.

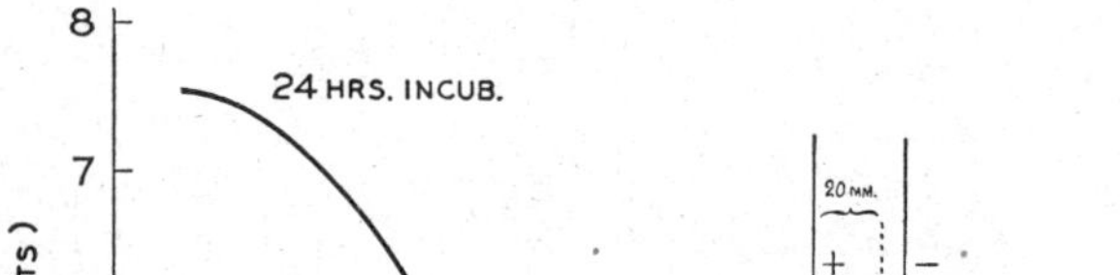


FIG. 1. The general trend of electrical potential differences of fresh and incubated eggs. One electrode was touching the albumen, while the other electrode was in contact with yolk at various distances from the center of the blastoderm.

[4] A. S. Brown, *Jour. Am. Chem. Soc.*, 56: 646–647, 1934.

The results of these observations are graphically shown in Fig. 1. There was evident an increase in potential differences with incubation, which was several times greater than through the shell.[2] On the same egg the differences decreased as the contact was moved away from the blastoderm, though some differences were still indicated at the margin of the yolk.

Most significantly in these measurements differences in electrical potential were found between fertile and infertile fresh eggs. Fertile eggs showed on an average of about 0.8 millivolt difference in potential, while with infertile eggs the difference averaged less than 0.2 millivolt.

ALEXIS L. ROMANOFF
CASPER L. COTTRELL

CORNELL UNIVERSITY

## IMPLANTS OF EMBRYONIC TISSUE INHIBIT PARTURITION IN THE RAT

MASAO[1] described a tumor-like teratoma which he produced in mice by the inoculation of embryonic tissue. Histologically these tumors appeared to be identical with naturally occurring teratomata. The writer has subjected numerous albino rats to this procedure in the last two years. The production of these artificial teratomata is very simple. Rat fetuses about 18 days old were crushed fine enough so that the tissues could be passed through a gauge 18 hypodermic needle. A little mammalian ringer solution was added, and about 2 cubic centimeters of this material was injected into the visceral cavity. Care was taken to complete the operation as rapidly as possible. So far the embryonic tissue implanted in this manner has continued to grow in every instance. The rate of growth is rather slow. A weight of 3 to 12 grams has been attained at the end of one year.

Recently seven females 11 months of age which had carried these teratomata for six months were bred to a normal male. Their response was normal in every way except that parturition was inhibited. The fetuses developed normally, attaining the maximum size which the placentae allow and then died unless removed by hysterotomy. This experiment has been repeated on a group of ten females, and the same results were obtained.

It has been noted, however, that the implant of embryonic tissue must have had time to develop to a certain degree before parturition is completely inhibited. One rat with this implant present was able with difficulty to achieve the birth of her young. The same animal six weeks later was unable to evacuate the uterus. At the latter period the implant of embryonic tissue weighed 1.1 grams.

[1] *Jap. Jour. Cancer Res.*, 22: 28, 1928.

In his review of the factors concerned with the duration of pregnancy Snyder[2] has pointed out that parturition is under endocrine control. King[3] and others have shown that an extract of pregnancy urine will prolong the gestation period in the rat. It has been known for some time that urine from women afflicted with certain tumors such as hydatidiform mole and chorionepithelioma reacts positively in pregnancy tests. Also urine from men suffering from teratoma of the skin of the testes gives positive results in this test. It would seem, then, that these embryonic implants also secrete a chemical substance which is similar to the prolan contained in pregnancy urine, and as a result the presence of this tissue in the body affects the gestation period in the same manner as the injection of pregnancy prolan.

ALFRED TAYLOR

OREGON STATE COLLEGE

[2] *Physiol. Rev.*, 18: 578, 1938.

[3] *Am. Jour. Physiol.*, 122: 455, 1938.

# SCIENTIFIC APPARATUS AND LABORATORY METHODS

## AN ARRANGEMENT OF APPARATUS FOR THE ISOLATION OF MONOCHROMATIC LIGHT OF HIGH INTENSITY AT λ, 254 mμ[1]

WHEN monochromatic light is isolated by a monochromator, focal isolation or an optical train using filters, the light available for photochemical work represents only a small fraction of the total light produced by the source at that wavelength. This has been overcome sometimes by placing the actinic system, to be studied, in a vessel which surrounded both the light source and a suitable filter. Such an ensemble, however, requires that the volume of the actinic system be large unless the absorbing layer is made unduly thin. Sometimes the filter has been dispensed with and the actinic system allowed to contact the light source; but then, temperature control has been troublesome. The arrangement of apparatus given in Fig. 1 overcomes some of these difficulties by working in from the light source—in this case, a mercury "resonance" lamp. Any other source, however, may be used if it operates in a similar environment.

The lamp was constructed of quartz tubing coiled cylindrically like one previously used at M. I. T. to produce Raman spectra.[2] It differed from that lamp by having the axis of the coil parallel to the electrodes rather than perpendicular to them. This modification permitted the lamp to operate in a conducting liquid, such as water, with the axis of the coil vertical and the electrodes dry. Stray light from the tubing extending beyond the coil was eliminated by wrapping these parts in aluminum foil. The coil consisted of four complete turns of 1 cm tubing, which formed a cylinder 7 cm i.d. and 8 cm high. The electrodes were iron cylinders coated with a mixture of the carbonates of Ba, Ca and Sr. These carbonates were subsequently decomposed by being heated in a vacuum with an induction furnace, followed by flushing the red-hot electrodes and quartz tubing with a discharge through hydrogen. The cold lamp was then filled with argon at a pressure of 1 cm of mercury, and after introducing about half a gram of mercury the lamp was sealed while a discharge was passed through. It was lighted by a transformer rated to deliver 120 milliamperes at 5,000 volts when connected to a 110-volt A. C. line. The leads from the secondary were made as short as possible and were well insulated.

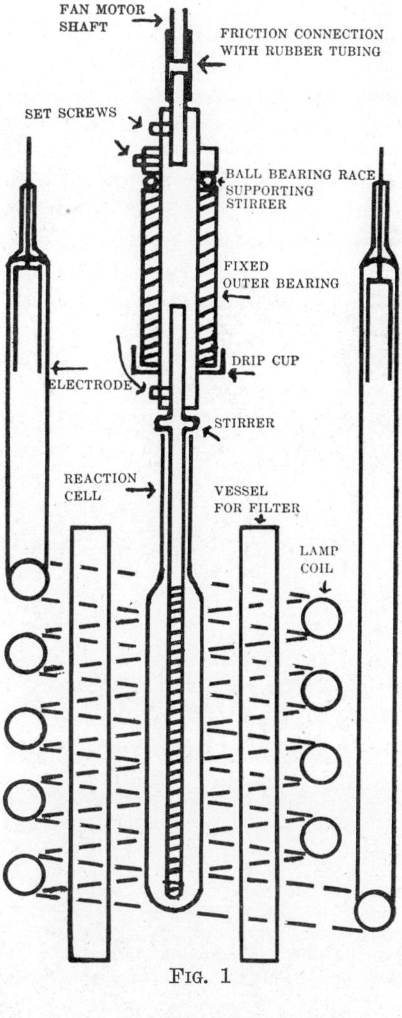


FIG. 1

[1] Contribution from the Research Laboratory of Physical Chemistry, Massachusetts Institute of Technology, No. 430.

[2] Harris, Ashdown and Armstrong, *Jour. Am. Chem. Soc.*, 58: 852, 1936.

Within the lamp coil was centered a cylindrical quartz vessel (3.5 cm i.d. and 10 cm high), which contained between its walls a 1 cm layer of dry chlorine at 1 atmosphere. This layer of chlorine absorbed 94 per cent. of 297 and 366 mμ and even more of the light between these wave-lengths.[3] Glacial acetic acid (reagent quality) was discolored when it was used as a filter for several days and then absorbed strongly λ, 254 mμ. It was not improved when refluxed over chromic anhydride (reagent quality) and then distilled in vacuum.

The system to be illuminated was placed in a quartz reaction cell centered on the axis of the light filter, so that the lamp light could reach the cell only by passing through the filter.

The lamp reached equilibrium with its surroundings after it had been lighted half an hour. When it was stopped momentarily to introduce a new cell, equilibrium was reestablished by relighting the lamp ten minutes before illuminating the photo-sensitive system. Subsequent fluctuations in the light intensity then remained within less than 5 per cent. over at least twenty hours.

Ultra-violet light reaching the reaction cell was over 95 per cent. of λ, 254 mμ, as observed from spectrograms of the light before and after it traversed the layers of chlorine and water. Other observations[4] have shown that a mercury resonance lamp emits light which is over 82 per cent. of λ, 254 mμ. When the lamp was operated in air, an odor of ozone was produced by light at λ, 185 mμ and shorter wave-lengths;[5] but the 2 cm layer of water, between the lamp and reaction cell, absorbed this light as well as most of the infrared.[6] Visible light reaching the reaction cell usually can be ignored by properly adjusting the concentrations of the light-absorbing species when their extinction coefficients are greater at λ, 254 mμ than in the visible.

The light flux was measured with the dilute solutions of uranyl oxalate recommended for use as actinometers.[7] These solutions were stirred with a thin ribbon of transparent quartz in the form of a screw turning at more than 500 r.p.m. Care was taken not to let a large fraction of the actinic light reach the stirrer in order to avoid the difficulties of evaluating corrections for scattered light, particularly when the reaction under investigation depended upon the light intensity. To realize this the stirrer was kept half a centimeter from the part of the cell wall holding the solution. Here, the cell was 1.3 cm i.d. and 8 cm long; one end was fuzed shut and the other end was fuzed to 6 cm of .7 cm quartz tubing to minimize evaporation of the actinic solution. The volume of the solution, in this case, happened to be 11 cc, but smaller or larger volumes also would have intercepted the light fluxes given below, merely by changing the diameter of the cell and, if necessary, that of the stirrer. A light-proof aluminum tube that slipped over the cell acted as a shutter. The temperature was controlled by regulating the temperature and rate of flow of the air or water surrounding the lamp, filter and the reaction cell.

When the ensemble was used in air, $5 \times 10^{19}$ photons of λ, 254 mμ were incident per minute on the actinometer; in distilled water there were $4 \times 10^{19}$ photons; and in running Cambridge tap water $10^{19}$. These values of the light flux in air and distilled water are over two hundred times greater than the light flux that has been obtained at λ, 254 mμ from a monochromator.[8] The light intensity was diminished further, when desired, by surrounding the filter with a wire gauze of the proper mesh, and could be increased by winding the lamp coils closer together and surrounding them with polished aluminum or some other suitable mirror.

LAWRENCE J. HEIDT

CAMBRIDGE, MASS.

[3] Gibson and Baylies, *Phys. Rev.*, 44: 188, 1933.

[4] Avery and Forbes, *Jour. Am. Chem. Soc.*, 60: 1006, 1938; and Cline and Forbes, *ibid.*, 61: 716, 1939.

[5] Flory, *Jour. Chem. Phys.*, 4: 23, 1936.

[6] I. C. T., 5: 271.

[7] Forbes and Heidt, *Jour. Am. Chem. Soc.*, 56: 2363, 1934. A more sensitive actinometer that can be used advantageously for very low light intensities has been studied carefully by Harris and Kaminsky, *ibid.*, 57: 1154, 1935.

[8] Forbes and Brackett, *Jour. Am. Chem. Soc.*, 53: 3973, 1931.

---

*Errata:* In the article by Dr. H. Waelsch and Dr. D. Rittenberg entitled "The Metabolism of Glutathione," printed in the issue of SCIENCE for November 3, the last line on the second column on p. 423 should read "6 mg" of copper glutathione instead of "16 mg."

In the article by Drs. Casimir Funk and Ian Casimir Funk printed in the issue of SCIENCE for November 10, on p. 445, the last line of Table V, "I" Stilbestrol should read "II" Stilbestrol.

---

## BOOKS RECEIVED

EVE, A. S. *Rutherford.* Pp. xvi + 451. Illustrated. Macmillan. $5.00.

LOWENBERG, MIRIAM E. *Your Child's Food.* Pp. ix + 299. Illustrated. Whittlesey House, McGraw-Hill. $2.50.

MCMINN, HOWARD E. *An Illustrated Manual of California Shrubs.* Pp. ix + 689. 775 figures. J. W. Stacey, Inc., San Francisco. $5.00.

Storrs Agricultural Experiment Station. *Studies of Suburbanization in Connecticut; 3, Wilton; a Rural Town Near Metropolitan New York,* by NATHAN L. WHETTEN. Pp. 132. 19 figures. Connecticut State College.

TWENHOFEL, W. H. *Principles of Sedimentation.* Pp. v + 610. 44 figures. McGraw-Hill. $6.00.

WHITTLESEY, DERWENT. *The Earth and the State; a Study of Political Geography.* Pp. iii + 618. 85 figures. Holt. $3.75.

# SCIENCE

VOL. 90 | FRIDAY, NOVEMBER 24, 1939 | No. 2343

*Harvey (Williams) Cushing:* DR. ELLIOTT C. CUTLER 475

*The Present State of Solar Activity and Associated Phenomena:* DR. HARLAN T. STETSON 482

*Scientific Events:*
*A Discussion of Franklin and His Times; The Eighth American Scientific Congress; Awards of the American Society of Mechanical Engineers; Award of the Willard Gibbs Medal. Recent Deaths* 484

*Scientific Notes and News* 487

*Discussion:*
*The Founding of a Department of Fishes in the Museo Poey of the University of Havana:* CORRESPONDENT. *A Noteworthy Aurora:* DR. S. STILLMAN BERRY. *Ozone in the '38 Hurricane:* PROFESSOR CHARLES A. PETERS. *The International Union of Chemistry:* PROFESSOR MARSTON TAYLOR BOGERT 490

*Scientific Books:*
*Recent Books in Geology:* PROFESSOR KIRTLEY F. MATHER 492

*Societies and Meetings:*
*The Semi-centennial Celebration of the Medical School of the University of Minnesota:* DR. M. B. VISSCHER 494

*Special Articles:*
*Toxic Effects of Desoxycorticosterone Esters in Dogs:* DR. ROBERT F. LOEB and OTHERS. *The Encephalitogenic Property of Herpes virus:* KATHERINE ANDERSON. *The Chemical Composition of Suckleyana:* DR. C. G. BARR, DR. H. W. REUSZER and DR. FRANK THORP, JR. *Experimental Chronic Cadmium Poisoning:* DR. ROBERT H. WILSON and DR. FLOYD DEEDS 496

*Science News* 10

SCIENCE: A Weekly Journal devoted to the Advancement of Science, edited by J. MCKEEN CATTELL and published every Friday by

THE SCIENCE PRESS
New York City: Grand Central Terminal
Lancaster, Pa. Garrison, N. Y.

Annual Subscription, $6.00 Single Copies, 15 Cts.

SCIENCE is the official organ of the American Association for the Advancement of Science. Information regarding membership in the Association may be secured from the office of the permanent secretary in the Smithsonian Institution Building, Washington, D. C.

# HARVEY (WILLIAMS[1]) CUSHING

## April 8, 1869–October 7, 1939

By Dr. ELLIOTT C. CUTLER

HARVARD MEDICAL SCHOOL AND PETER BENT-BRIGHAM HOSPITAL

Honour a physician with the honour due unto him for the uses which ye may have of him: for the Lord hath created him. For of the most High cometh healing, and he shall receive honour of the king. The skill of the physician shall lift up his head: and in the sight of great men he shall be in admiration.—*Book of Ecclesiasticus, Chapter 38, Verses 1–3. Being the First Lesson for St. Luke's Day.*

No other individual in modern medicine has revealed such a variety of accomplishments as Harvey Cushing: master-surgeon, neurologist, physician, critical investigator, medical bibliophile, inspiring teacher, litterateur, artist! His craftsmanship and technical performance in surgery were superb; his precise exploration of the nervous system made him an eminent neurologist; his care of and interest in his patients were an example for the most devoted family physician and brought to him the faith and love of patients above what is accorded most physicians; his curiosity led him to an interest in original sources and a love of books which resulted in his amassing a great medical library and becoming one of the leading medical historians of his day; his scientific medical contributions form an important background in neurophysiology and endo-

[1] The Williams, his maternal ancestor's name, was finally dropped after his settling in Boston in 1912, where his mail often became confused with that of a surgical colleague, Dr. Hayward Warren Cushing. But an even earlier episode had warned him of this difficulty, for in 1895 when he had taken the examination for house-pupil at the Massachusetts General Hospital, he failed to hear the result for a long time after the other candidates had been notified. Investigation revealed that his notice of successful application, which seemed all-important to him at that time, had been forwarded to the same Dr. Hayward Warren Cushing, one of the most promising younger surgeons of Boston. This first incident was probably a major influence in his dropping the use of his middle name in his publications as early as 1900.

crinology; his product in inspired and devoted pupils is exceptional; and his abilities as a writer both medical and otherwise are attested to by his being awarded the Pulitzer Prize in Letters for 1926.

Harvey Cushing was born in Cleveland, Ohio, on April 8, 1869, and died of coronary occlusion in New Haven, Connecticut, on October 7, 1939. He had long been a sufferer from peripheral vascular disease of the lower extremities and from gastric ulcer, disorders which he bore with a superb stoicism and courage. He is survived by his widow (Katherine Stone Crowell) and four children, Mary, Betsy, Henry and Barbara. William, another son, was killed in an accident while a student at Yale University in 1926. His first American ancestor, Mathew, landed at Hingham, Massachusetts, in 1638, and his ancestry contained a long line of doctor people whose roots were in New England. His great-grandfather, David (1768–1814), practiced medicine in Cheshire, Massachusetts; his grandfather, Erastus (1802–1893), was a teacher in the now defunct Berkshire Medical College; and his father, Henry K. Cushing (1827–1910), was the leading practitioner of his time in Cleveland, Ohio. During my years of residence in Cleveland (1924–1932) I often heard stories of both the ability and austerity of the father. His older brother, Edward, educated at Yale College, Harvard Medical School and the Massachusetts General Hospital, became in turn the leader of medicine in the Cleveland of his day. This brother was somewhat different from his forebears, more friendly and gregarious, loved by children, full of fun and, if the stories are correctly told, much like William Osler. And this brother was Harvey Cushing's direct stimulus and mentor. He took his brother Harvey on trips, talked to him about medicine, and filled him with aspirations and ideals. An early death robbed medicine of the full development of this older brother and Harvey Cushing of further influence from this source. This influence is attested to by the great admiration of the younger for the older brother, an admiration which endured throughout his life. Harvey Cushing liked to dwell on his brother's accomplishments and frequently spoke of his brother Ned's influence, when a house pupil at the Massachusetts General Hospital, in liberating the up-to-then starvation diet of the typhoid patient. It was apparent that the younger brother admired greatly the open and friendly nature of the elder brother and sought to emulate his characteristics. This emulation is seen again in his admiraton for Osler and others whose ease of personal contacts was of the same order. It is indeed a remarkable tribute to the breadth of Harvey Cushing's accomplishments and character that though similar traits were not his by nature, he actually did find time in his busy life for pleasantries and friendly contacts. These characteristics greatly endeared him to his young assistants and to his patients, and when in the later years the pressure of active clinical work had lessened, they became more prominent and brought him hosts of youthful student friends.

From school in Cleveland he went to Yale College (A.B., 1891), and then to the Harvard Medical School (A.M. and M.D. *cum laude,* 1895). A study of Cushing's grades as found on his record in the dean's office at the Harvard Medical School is of some interest. The eleven A's and three B's are in sharp contrast to three C's, especially when we find the latter in therapeutics, clinical obstetrics and clinical surgery (C minus). However, one should know that at that time the curriculum provided only a minimum of clinical work and often the better men deserted class exercises and by their own initiative obtained experience at hospitals. We can easily imagine Harvey Cushing rebelling in the course in therapeutics at the very idea of committing to memory the doses and action of drugs which he foresaw he would never use. Indeed this record itself expresses his early intellectual independence. While still a senior at the Harvard Medical School, his brother Ned took him to Baltimore to visit the Johns Hopkins Hospital and Medical School, though it is dubious whether he met at that time either Halsted or Osler.

Following graduation from the Medical School, he was house officer on the South Surgical Service at the Massachusetts General Hospital. There his unusual abilities were in evidence and his hospital records represent the diligence, care, precision and artistic accomplishments which were soon to flourish and bear fruit. From Boston he went to the Johns Hopkins Hospital (1896–1900) to work under the beneficent influence of William S. Halsted. The shift from the Boston surgery of that day, where speed of operating was still considered advisable and even used as a gauge of ability, to the painstaking, slow and gentle methods of Halsted was an everlasting inspiration to the pupil Cushing. He often told the story himself that, coming from Boston where a complete breast procedure was accomplished in twenty-eight minutes, he saw with misgivings a four-and-one-half-hour operation for the same undertaking. How amazed he was that stimulants were unnecessary and how horrified he was when told not to dress the wound for ten days! Recalling the wounds he had previously studied, he remarked to himself: "I may not see the wound, but I will smell it!" When in ten days the wound was dressed and found perfectly healed, his skepticism disappeared. Moreover, here he was first introduced to the experimental method, was taught the value of careful and detailed records whether in the laboratory or on the ward. From Halsted he learned that precise and thorough concentration on a small problem might yield more than great labors in routine work. Here, too, he learned the value of a meticulous and gentle technique that sought to spare each cell from being damaged, a technique which was to permit him later to create the surgery of the central nervous system. It is doubtful if Halsted had any other pupil who learned so rapidly and thoroughly the art of surgery as he, Halsted, conceived it.

Finally, his training as a general surgeon completed, Dr. Cushing went abroad (1900–1901), and in Berne through Kocher and Hugo Kronecker accomplished his first work in experimental neurology ("Physiologische und anatomische Beobachtungen über einige hiermit verwandte Erscheinungen." *Mitt. Grenzgeb. Med. Chir.,* 9: 773–808, 1902). This neurological field was to become his life work, and it is of interest to examine the stimulus which brought him to it. My notes made after conversations with Dr. Cushing led me to feel that Dr. Halsted suggested to him the field of neurological surgery, but recently Dr. Roy McClure, who worked with Dr. Cushing during the first year that the Hunterian Laboratory was open and who later became Halsted's resident surgeon, and others have made it certain that Harvey Cushing himself proposed the field to Dr. Halsted. Dr. Halsted's first reply was, "Why, Dr. Cushing, we had only two cases of brain tumor last year!" When Dr. Cushing persisted, Dr. Halsted remarked, "All right, the field is yours." And perhaps there were indications of this leaning even earlier, for the title of Dr. Cushing's second paper was "Haematomyelia from Gunshot Wounds of the Spine. A Report of Two Cases, with Recovery Following Symptoms of Hemilesion of the Cord" (*Amer. Jour. Med. Sci.,* 115: 654–683, June, 1898). This article was spoken of by Dr. Thomas, then professor of neurology at the Johns Hopkins Medical School, as the best investigation of superficial sensory supply carried out up to that time. In addition Osler may have influenced him in this selection. Speculation is incited when we know that Dr. Cushing, while a surgical interne at the Massachusetts General Hospital, had written to Dr. W. S. Thayer to ask if there might be an opening for him on Dr. Osler's staff. This letter to Thayer was never answered, and one can only imagine the consequences had this application received an affirmative answer!

During this early trip to Europe, Dr. Cushing also met Sherrington in Liverpool and in Pavia, Italy, picked up a clinical model of Riva-Rocci's blood pressure apparatus with inflatable armlet which he adapted for use in all his subsequent surgical procedures. The charts on which such records were kept represent the first anesthesia charts, though it should be known that Amory Codman and Harvey Cushing had a wager when house pupils at the Massachusetts General Hospital (1895) as to who could anesthetize without subsequent vomiting and kept records for this purpose. Their pioneer efforts to chart a patient's condition properly throughout a surgical procedure are now bound together in the Record Room of the Massachusetts General Hospital as evidence of a beneficent change in which the youngest members of a hospital staff played a rôle. This effort did not originate with these young men, but represented a desire of their visiting surgeon, Dr. Harrington, and was actually in use before Harvey Cushing went on service.

On his return from Europe, Cushing became the neurosurgeon of the Johns Hopkins Hospital group. It was a difficult and discouraging beginning. The mortality was terrific, though better than that obtained by other surgeons. Always there was extreme diligence and thoroughness. Autopsies were secured whenever possible. The reasons for catastrophes were thus explained and technical perfection thus secured. The happier field of the surgical treatment of trifacial neuralgia was reopened, studied and made safe. Laboratory efforts previously in the field of general surgery continued in this newer field, and soon he began to investigate the pituitary body. Tumors of it were studied; investigation of its functions grew apace; and by the time of his removal to Boston, his first book appeared, "The Pituitary Body and Its Disorders. Clinical States Produced by Disorders of the Hypophysis Cerebri. An amplification of the Harvey Lecture for December, 1910" (J. B. Lippincott Company, Philadelphia and London, 1912).

These formative years in Baltimore, when his work hardened entirely along neurophysiological lines, were the years when he discovered in William Osler a chief stimulus and mentor. They were next-door neighbors, and his footsteps were often turned to Osler's home, where he found the encouragement, guidance and leaven which only such a brilliant character could give. Here he began to acquire his love of books and his amazing information in the background of medical history. Here he gathered in acquaintances from many corners of the world to emerge a real cosmopolitan. Osler's departure to Oxford in 1905 seemed a great loss to Harvey Cushing, but by this time he was well started in his bibliophilic adventures and perhaps was really benefited by the independence of thought and action which this separation enforced. Anyway, the trail between these two was now well established and their correspondence formed a major tie of interest for each until Osler died.

In 1910 he was simultaneously appointed professor of surgery at the Harvard Medical School and surgeon-in-chief to the Peter Bent Brigham Hospital. It is clear that the trustees under the will of Peter Bent Brigham, who had died in 1877, had at last decided that the time was ripe to construct the hospital, which the donor had specified was to care for "sick persons in indigent circumstances residing in the County of

Suffolk." The new Harvard Medical School had been opened in 1906, and one can visualize the wise heads that brought together the Harvard authorities and the Brigham Hospital trustees. But it was not until August, 1911, that ground was actually broken, on a cow-pasture adjacent to the new Medical School, and the construction of the hospital was only partly finished when Dr. Cushing with his family moved to Boston in the summer of 1912. At this time his Medical School title was changed to that of Moseley Professor of Surgery, the position in surgery previously filled by Maurice Richardson. Now he began to organize his work in the Harvard Medical School laboratory and in the partly constructed hospital, which was to open its doors in January, 1913. The appointments of David Cheever and John Homans to the senior staff gave to the new hospital the most promising of the junior surgeons of Boston of that time, and his house staff, largely composed of Johns Hopkins men, contained a few Harvard graduates of the class of 1913.

Soon the work was in full swing, and the details of his accomplishments at the Brigham Hospital are readily accessible in the Annual Reports of the hospital. It is appropriate to point out here that Harvey Cushing and his colleague Henry Christian, put great emphasis on the value of professional hospital reports. Here they reviewed and prophesied the changing character of both medical education and medical practice and thus elevated hospital reports to a useful professional level. At first he kept his interest in the general surgical clinic, but his prominence in neurosurgery was so outstanding that gradually this field occupied all his energy and time. That his primary interest lay in neurophysiology and neurosurgery is perhaps better reflected in the laboratory efforts of his full-time assistants, which began with the work of Lewis Weed, his first Arthur Tracy Cabot fellow,[2] whose important contributions to the cerebrospinal fluid circulation appeared in 1914. Yet, in spite of these responsibilities, there was at first time for tennis and frequent discussions with the devoted members of his house staff. Indeed it was these informal meetings plus his weekly rounds on patients with other than neurological disorders and the influence of his great example in the care of his own neurological patients which permitted him to be the major influence for many years to come on many pupils whose interest lay in the field of general surgery. And from time to time he did take on the performance of some unusual task in the field of general surgery, and such procedures will long be remembered by the internes of the first few years of the Brigham Hospital as among their greatest moments of inspiration. Before the Great War was upon us, he had become one of the leading surgeons of our day, a matter attested to by the invitation to give the oration in surgery at the International Congress of Medicine in London in 1913, "Realignments in Greater Medicine; Their Effect upon Surgery and the Influence of Surgery upon Them." (*Brit. Med. Jour.* 2: 290–297, August 9, 1913. Also: *Lancet,* 2: 369–375, August 9, 1913.)

Then came war, and for Dr. Cushing two experiences, one with the French Army at the American Ambulance Hospital in Paris, April, 1915,[3] and later, after the United States had entered the war, with Base Hospital No. 5 in France, May 1917–May, 1919. His great abilities soon led to his removal from this Base Hospital group, of which he was the organizer and peace-time director, to become the senior consultant in neurosurgery of the American Expeditionary Force. During these experiences his tremendous labors under the severe physical strain of forward conditions brought comfort and life to many an injured soldier, but his unsparing devotion to the task eventually undermined his health and left him a sufferer from arterial disease for the remainder of his life. All through this period of immense physical strain, his publications continued. His contributions to the care of intracranial war-wounds set the proper methods in this field. Great as was his devotion to professional work, he found time to keep up his daily "Journal," a habit begun in youth and continued throughout his life whenever he traveled away from home. In 1936, excerpts from his daily "War Journal" appeared in book form, "From a Surgeon's Journal" (Boston: Little, Brown and Company, 1936). For his great works in France he was honored by his own country by the award of a "Distinguished Service Medal," by Great Britain by the Order of the "Companion of the Bath" and by France with the position "Officer of the Legion of Honor."

During this war experience there were several trips to England and each time the long-desired visits with Osler. On one of these occasions the writer was present and recalls as brightly as if it were but yesterday the witty and brilliant chaffing which flowed forth at

[2] This fellowship was endowed through the generosity of Dr. and Mrs. F. C. Shattuck in honor of Mrs. Shattuck's brother, who had been a leading surgeon in Boston and a visiting surgeon at the Massachusetts General Hospital when Harvey Cushing was a house-pupil.

[3] At the outbreak of the European War Americans in Paris organized the American Ambulance Hospital under the auspices of the American Hospital, a small incorporated hospital largely used by the American colony there. The French Government placed the new Lycée Pasteur in Neuilly at the disposal of this new Ambulance Hospital. One of the three services was organized to be staffed by groups which rotated every three months from American Medical School Hospitals. A unit under Dr. George Crile from the Lakeside Hospital, Cleveland, Ohio, began this service on January 1, 1915; the Harvard Medical School unit followed, April–June, 1915, and was in turn followed by a unit from the University of Pennsylvania Medical School. Dr. Cushing remained with his unit only for the month of April, 1915, returning via England, where he visited Sir William Osler.

the time. It was shortly before Revere Osler's death, and though the imminence of disaster seemed in the very air, the comfort and happiness of the guests was overwhelming. Conversation this time drifted from the first written medical document, a piece of stone covered with unknown writing, to how difficult it was for the British to learn the value of corn as food for man, having for centuries thought it fit only for pigs and chickens! All the time Harvey Cushing sat wrapped in devoted and appreciative silence.

After the war he became reestablished in Boston, and his labors in neurosurgery took on their final form. His interest in general surgery lagged, for there was no time for it. Assistants flocked to his side to work in neurology and neurosurgery, and the output of their work and influence is world-wide. In the midst of all this William Osler died, and at the request of Lady Osler he took up the writing of a biography. It was a labor of love, but it was accomplished with the same tools and vigor that surrounded all Harvey Cushing's works. First every possible source of information was gathered in and digested, the smallest references in daily newspapers were consulted and from this background the great two-volume biography appeared. Small wonder to those who knew of the sincere efforts that the product would be so universally acclaimed.

On the occasion of his sixtieth birthday, 1929, his pupils dedicated to him a collection of their writings. This "Festschrift" special number in honor of Harvey Cushing's 60th birthday; (*Arch. Surg.,* 18: 935–2045, 1929) emphasized his qualities as a teacher. The eighty-two papers were contributed by men then holding some of the most important medical and surgical positions not only in the United States of America but in Europe. And the contributions not only were in the field of neurology and neurological surgery but ranged over the entire field of medicine and included historical essays as well as experimental and clinical observations. The impact of Cushing's character and abilities is nowhere better pictured than in this affectionate tribute.

His effect upon the Harvard Medical School Faculty was considerable, even though he and the dean of the school during this period did not always agree in matters of policy and action. Cushing was greatly interested in the establishment of a common library, in the modification of the curriculum with its resultant reduction in didactic hours and was a leader in opposing the adoption of the "full time clinical teaching" in the strict Rockefellerian sense and in opposing a plan that the Medical School edit a text-book which purposed to infiltrate all departments of the school with preventive medicine.

The hospital regulation set by himself and Henry Christian automatically retires the professional members of the Brigham Hospital staff at 63, and this by custom is accompanied by resignation from the Medical School appointment. And so in 1932 arrived the date of retirement set by himself. It came at a time when Dr. Cushing was working as never before, though bothered with peripheral vascular disease and the signs and symptoms of gastric ulcer. The transition from his tremendously active life was great, but he made it abruptly, and surgery was given up. He refused the repeated requests of the Brigham Hospital trustees to remain in service as surgeon-in-chief, and attempts were soon made to entice him to many places, though it was hoped he would stay in Boston and work on his collection of brain tumors. He remained at the hospital for another year, however, and worked in uncomfortable quarters, for he insisted that his successor occupy immediately the quarters set aside for the surgeon-in-chief. The following year he went to Yale as the Sterling Professor of Neurology (1933–1937). Here he was offered an active post, not simply an honorary sinecure, and to a man in the full vigor of his years this opportunity and his natural devotion to his alma mater, which had the vision to utilize his great abilities, turned his footsteps away from Boston and Harvard. With him went his collection of brain tumor specimens and photostatic copies of the patients' records. At Yale he continued a thorough study of this great mass of material, the assembling of which represented such unusual physical efforts. Major fragments of this material had appeared either in book form, as the monograph on the acoustic neurinomas (1917) and the classification of the gliomata with P. Bailey (1926) or in separate smaller publications, notable among these being his final contribution in the field of pituitary disorders, "basophilism," a clinical syndrome which now bears his name. At Yale, the work continued in spite of frequent physical discomforts. Clinical, experimental and historical papers continued. But chiefly there was the continued study of his own experiences in the field of brain tumors, and always there went on the end-result letters and follow-up examinations.[4] Though the Yale professorship terminated in 1937, the work continued unabated, and he was as active from 1937 up to the time he died as at any time in the last five years. The great volume on the meningiomas did not appear until 1938.

On the occasion of his seventieth birthday, his publications were listed in book form ("A Bibliography of the Writings of Harvey Cushing, prepared on the occasion of his seventieth birthday, April 8, 1939, by

[4] As late as July, 1939, a chromophobe pituitary adenoma patient seen first by Dr. Cushing in February, 1926, turned up at he Brigham Hospital to show the writer a letter from Dr. Cushing inquiring about his condition with the request that the writer examine him and send the information to Dr. Cushing. This done, there was the immediate grateful reply, so characteristic of his correspondence with a pupil.

the Harvey Cushing Society." 1939. Charles C Thomas.)

The major books are:

"The Pituitary Body and its Disorders. Clinical States Produced by Disorders of the Hypophysis Cerebri." An amplification of the Harvey Lecture for December, 1910. Philadelphia and London: J. B. Lippincott Company, 1912.

"Tumors of the Nervus Acusticus and the Syndrome of the Cerebellopontile Angle." Philadelphia and London: W. B. Saunders Company, 1917.

"The Story of U. S. Army Base Hospital No. 5. By a Member of the Unit." Cambridge, Mass.: University Press, 1919.

"The Life of Sir William Osler." Oxford: At the Clarendon Press, 1925.

"A Classification of the Tumors of the Glioma Group on a Histogenetic Basis with a Correlated Study of Prognosis." (With P. Bailey.) Philadelphia, London and Montreal: J. B. Lippincott Company, 1926.

"Studies in Intracranial Physiology and Surgery. The Third Circulation. The Hypophysis. The Gliomas." London: Humphrey Milford, Oxford Press, 1926.

"The Pathological Findings in Four Autopsied Cases of Acromegaly with a Discussion of their Significance." (With L. M. Davidoff.) New York: Rockefeller Institute for Medical Research (Monograph No. 22), 1927.

"Tumors Arising from the Blood-Vessels of the Brain. Angiomatous Malformations and Hemangioblastomas." (With P. Bailey.) Springfield, Ill.: Charles C Thomas, 1928.

"Consecratio Medici and Other Papers." Boston: Little, Brown and Company, 1928.

"Intracranial Tumours. Notes Upon a Series of Two Thousand Verified Cases with Surgical-Mortality Percentages Pertaining Thereto." Springfield, Ill.: Charles C Thomas, 1932.

"Papers Relating to the Pituitary Body, Hypothalamus and Parasympathetic Nervous System." Springfield, Ill.: Charles C Thomas, 1932.

"From a Surgeon's Journal 1915–1918." Boston: Little, Brown and Company, 1936.

"Meningiomas. Their Classification, Regional Behaviour, Life History, and Surgical End Results." (With L. Eisenhardt.) Springfield, Ill.: Charles C Thomas, 1938.

The addresses, papers in journals and reports number three hundred and five and, though largely in the field of neurosurgery, neurophysiology and endocrinology, include a large leaven of historical items of great importance.

Honors came to him in profusion. He held twenty-three honorary degrees, and honorary fellowships, membership or corresponding membership in most of the medical societies of the world. He was a past president of the American College of Surgeons, 1922, the American Neurological Association, 1923, and the American Surgical Association, 1927. These honors seemed to please Harvey Cushing, and particularly one of the last he was to receive. He crossed the Atlantic as late as 1938 to receive the degree, doctor of science, "honoris causa," from Oxford.

Death came through coronary disease; first a severe attack that necessitated hospital care and three days later final rest. It came after seventy years of fruitful, vigorous labors for the good of others. The end was perhaps foretold in his long-standing suffering with peripheral vascular disease, which for twenty years gave him great discomfort, though this was known only to his intimates.

It is difficult to analyze and estimate Dr. Cushing's accomplishments, for he reminds us of the great characters of the Renaissance, such as Leonardo da Vinci, who achieved success in many fields. However, Dr. Cushing's accomplishments seem to flow from a single characteristic. This was his *extraordinary capacity for sustained work*. By nature he was essentially *a perfectionist* and *an aristocrat*. Everything was good or bad; there was scant room for mediocrity or in-betweens. His naturally artistic temperament made his technical surgery a work of art, and his abiding desire for accuracy and perfection brooked no compacts with mediocrity. Behind this craving for accomplishing everything that came to hand in a complete and artistic fashion, lay his enormous energy. It was as if he he had a dynamo within him which was unaffected by use. This is visualized better in his unseen activities, the writing of his journal each night, the hours spent in reading pupils' manuscripts, the immense breadth of his bibliophilic forays, only meagerly reported, rather than in his physical labor at the operating table or the publications for which he is so widely known.

A further natural characteristic was his *insatiable curiosity*. He was not content to see something; he must know all about it. This was revealed as well with books as with patients. Thus when he acquired a new book, he was not content just to read the book and show it to others; he had to know all about the man who wrote it, all about the previous owner, about the press it came from and the other works of the printer. Thus an incidental purchase evoked a tremendous labor. And it went on daily.

It would be presumptuous for a pupil to attempt to assay fully the character and qualities of his master, and praise would be an impertinence. We who have benefited so greatly from his teachings and his example can only be happy that the privilege was ours to be near him. I am one of those who will always feel that here was a man who lived completely for the medicine of his day. Everything he touched he made better. His opening up of the field of neurosurgery was but a small part of the man, for this accomplishment, just as his amassing a great library, his knowledge of medical history, his exquisite ability as a writer and his splendid laboratory contributions all flowed from the basic desire to do the best he could for suffering humanity. Of no other has it ever been more correctly said that he "lived this life up to the hilt."

And what will the patients say? Miss Ida Cannon has told me of the reaction of a patient with Raynaud's disease at the Massachusetts General Hospital when Harvey Cushing was a house pupil (1895). The patient, a bandage on her foot, had viewed with alarm the abrupt approach of the young man in white with a large pair of scissors which she anticipated meant amputation then and there. She related how the first dressing and all others which followed were accomplished with exquisite gentleness and care. She remained a worshipful patient at this same shrine all her life. How could it be otherwise? Never was there a better doctor in the real sense of the word. Everything that had to do with a patient was vitally important, the position in bed, the pillows, the daily bowel movement, the removal of the sutures all assumed equal importance with the surgical operation itself. Here was what sickness needed—complete understanding, great patience and exquisite gentleness.

As I try to look back over a quarter of a century and view not only the immense works but also his effects as a teacher, the latter seems very simple. Harvey Cushing taught by example. He never asked any assistant to work as hard as he did. It was the age-old method of apprenticeship. He hated class exercises and disliked lectures. If there was a patient, it was all right and he would let the class draw their own conclusions. His house staff learned chiefly from his example, certainly the internes did. When one had climbed further up the ladder, either in his clinic or in the laboratory, it was different. The master and pupil met there more or less as equals trying to settle matters. It was natural that Dr. Cushing's curiosity, when coupled with a primitive desire for perfection, should sprout problems daily and many a casual conversation with a member of the house staff ended with the beginning of a new series of investigations.

Little wonder that such an ardent and serious person was impatient with incompetence and slovenliness. It has been said that Harvey Cushing was a severe taskmaster. He was when it was necessary. There is no place for half-heartedness and mediocrity when one deals with life. No effort can be too great if it can be of assistance. Those who worked longest with Dr. Cushing came to admire and love him best, for they knew the depth of feeling and vision behind the critical remarks. Moreover, criticisms were always accompanied by the vision of a better way the next time. And it was not all stern and cold. There were many sympathetic and generous moments. His little kindnesses were not only to the old and devoted pupil, they came often to total strangers in his path. A distinguished surgeon of to-day has recently related to me his early contacts wih Dr. Cushing. He as a young surgeon had spent a month watching from the operating room seats or on ward rounds. But practically no contact had been made. Suddenly, one Saturday morning, Harvey Cushing summoned him: "Here, take this seat to the Harvard-Yale football game!" A moment later, as our friend stood abashed by this sudden offer, "Have you rubbers?" "No." "A raincoat?" "No." "Go down and tell my secretary to give you mine." It was that rainy day of 1923 when "Ducky" Pond derived his pseudonym, acquired a fumbled ball and waddled down a marshy field for a touchdown! And this story had its counterpart many times.

There is no doubt in my mind that Dr. Cushing disliked elaborate functions, and was happiest when at work. Moreover, he wanted to become acquainted with all the people about him and therefore rather frowned on big institutions feeling that there the effect of the master would be either lost or so attenuated there would be little productivity. His devotion to the apprentice system (Hippocratic, he called it) of teaching medicine was well recognized in the Harvard Faculty, where he opposed any movement in medical education that in any way robbed the student of opportunities to meet a teacher at the bedside of a patient.

This method of teaching was the only one Harvey Cushing ever concerned himself with. The author was secretary of the Department of Surgery during an early part of this period and recalls the impossibility of interesting Harvey Cushing in any part of the surgical curriculum which had to do with class efforts. On the contrary, he fought hard in his department and on the floor of the Faculty Room for any change that brought the student and the teacher together at the bedside of sick people. Nor is it difficult to understand this attitude of Harvey Cushing's toward education. He had previously experienced the value of study and independent work, and at the Johns Hopkins Hospital and Medical School this personal experience had been intensified by the methods of teaching so brilliantly successful in that school. Halsted had demonstrated to him the experimental method and had allowed him great latitude in acquiring experience in technical surgery. As a result Cushing would trust his own five senses above laboratory methods and the teaching of others. Moreover, his natural scepticism encouraged the accumulation of personal experience as a chief road to education. Thus he insisted on others acquiring their information through a similar system and method.

Other than this emphasis on education through self-experience, Cushing's influence as a teacher was essentially that of teaching through example. He utilized fully the stimulus which comes through personal contacts and emulation. As a rule, a man of few words, he produced his effect on his pupils by virtue of his example. He lived for and by work, and to those privileged to associate themselves with him he was as stimulating and instructive a master as there could be. This influence, by the very reason of its method, was a restricted one and produced its chief results among his immediate assistants in the Brigham Hospital and in the Laboratory of Surgical Research of the Harvard Medical School. Such an influence could not permeate the entire student body and though his amphitheater clinics were well attended, there were many students who failed to appreciate his historical embellishments and even avoided his exercises except when they covered the nervous system or the ductless glands, in which fields he was so obviously a leader. But within the hospital walls it was different. Here the young assistant saw and recognized at once two great attributes worthy of constant emulation. First, the perfection of his technical methods. Nowhere else could he see such exquisite handling of tissues; in no other clinics did wounds heal so kindly, nor such dangerous procedures go forward with such little difficulty, moribidity and mortality. Secondly, the pupil envisaged the perfect care of the patient; the unsparing efforts to provoke confidence and comfort; the value of thorough records and their proper use. He was taught that no detail which added either to the information about the patient or to the comfort of the patient could be neglected.

Harvey Cushing's life is ended. His great accomplishments are known wherever civilization flourishes and will pass down the ages to benefit the generations to come. He became a chief decoration of every institution he served, brought great merit to them and assisted many young men to assume a way of life certain to bring comfort and happiness to humanity. He himself would like most to be remembered as one who upheld the first tradition of our profession—let nothing be neglected that can benefit a patient! This was his "vade mecum" and made him stand out as a chief physician of his time.

# THE PRESENT STATE OF SOLAR ACTIVITY AND ASSOCIATED PHENOMENA

By Dr. HARLAN T. STETSON

MASSACHUSETTS INSTITUTE OF TECHNOLOGY

THE rise in solar activity recently reported in SCIENCE[1] has been accompanied by changes in the electrical state of the earth's atmosphere made evident by numerous displays of aurorae and ionospheric disturbances affecting radio transmission. While many sunspots have been conspicuous during the last few months, a study of the sunspot numbers during the last few years shows that the actual maximum occurred in 1937. The graph of sunspot numbers from the minimum of 1933 to date printed herewith (Fig. 1) shows the present state of solar activity with respect to the maximum so recently passed.

The curve has been drawn through individual monthly values derived by taking the moving averages of three months at a time. Inspection will show that the highest three months average occurred in July, 1937, with a Wolfer index of 137. It will be noted that this high was followed by an abrupt drop to the end of the year, with a recovery in 1938 to a three-months high of 131.6 centering in June of last year. The subsequent rise during the early part of this year yielded an index of 111 centered about May, 1939. The maximum passed in 1937 was the highest since the maximum of 1870, when the corresponding Wolfer solar index stood at 165.

The rapid decline in the sunspot numbers during the early part of October indicates a decreasing activity for the next six months and that the major trend will be definitely downward for the next four or five years. The next minimum may be expected to fall in 1943 or 1944.

In reviewing the activity of the sun in recent years, it is interesting to note that the interval between the last two maxima—that of 1928 and that of 1937—has been but nine years, as compared with the mean interval between maxima usually taken as 11.2 years. This is the shortest interval between maxima for over a century. Had we attempted to predict the present maximum by adding the 11.2—year average interval to the last maximum, we should not have expected the present period of heavy solar activity until 1940.

At a meeting of the American Association held at St. Louis in 1935, I ventured to predict on the basis of sunspot activity at that time that the next maximum would occur at the end of 1937 or the very early part of 1938. On the basis of the sun's performance during the subsequent four years, it would appear that the sun anticipated even this prophecy by possibly six

[1] SCIENCE (Supplement), 90: 2337, 9, October 13, 1939.
[2] John Q. Stewart and H. A. A. Panofsky, *Astrophysical Journal*, 88: 4, 385–407, November, 1938.
[3] Newbern Smith, Theodore R. Gilliland and Samuel S. Kirby, National Bureau of Standards Research Paper RP1159, Vol. 21, December, 1938.

months. However, if the top of the curve is smoothed to eliminate the secondary fluctuations, it would appear that the mid-maximum falls very near this predicted time.

The irregularities in the so-called sunspot cycle have presented many difficulties from the point of view of prediction. Attempts to forecast solar behavior on the basis of harmonic analyses of many years of sunspot data have frequently brought disappointing results when projected into the future. Astrophysicists acquainted with the irregular variations in many stars of unpredictable performance have come to believe that no combination of fixed periods can ever safely be used for predicting the future of solar behavior.

in extraordinarily close agreement with the subsequently observed data. In making his forecast, Mr. Clayton purposely avoided using any observed data subsequent to 1910 to test the validity of his prediction. The desirability of even short-range prediction of solar activity is coming to be of increasing importance, due to the many now recognized ionospheric changes that parallel so closely the solar cycle.

Among the generally recognized phenomena of a terrestrial nature that show changes with the sunspot cycle, the most obvious are the auroral displays such as have been unusually active during the last two years. Through the courtesy of Director C. H. Brooks, I have examined the records of the Blue Hill Observa-

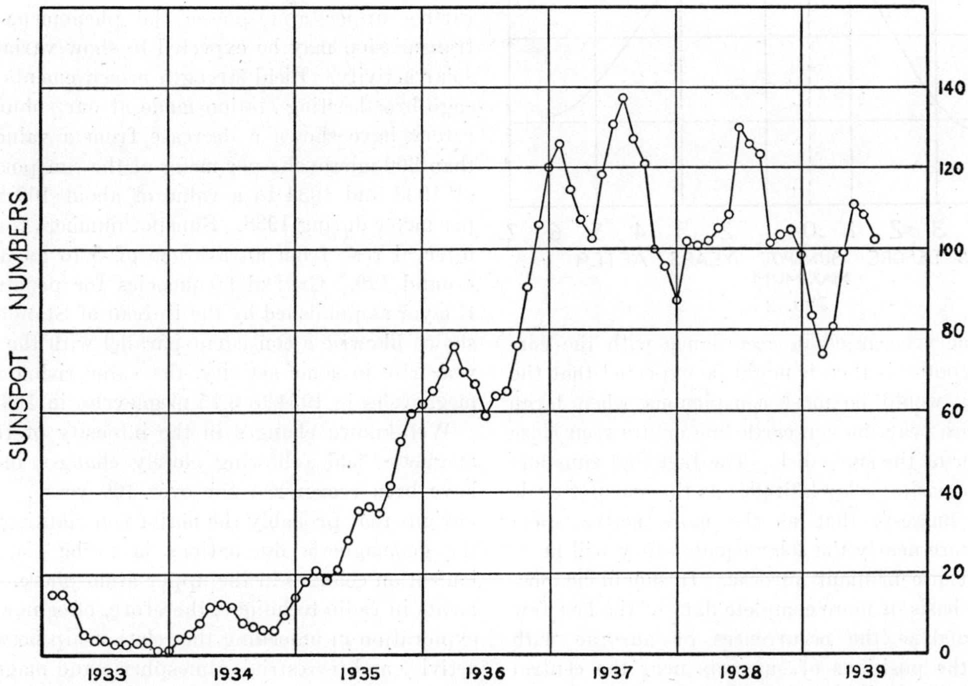


FIG. 1

Abandoning Newcomb's conclusion "that an underlying regularity of period governs the sunspot cycle," J. Q. Stewart and Panofsky[2] have recently made a mathematical analysis of 16 solar cycles from the point of view of the "outburst" hypothesis of Halm and Waldmeier and have derived an expression for the sunspot number $R$ for each given year after an observed minimum. Their quantity $R$ depends upon the general form of the family of curves that appears to be typical of the rise and subsidence of sunspots once a new period of solar activity has started. On the basis of such short-range prediction they have derived an average sunspot number for 1937 as 114.4 agreeing closely with the actual observed value of 115.1.

Still holding to the principle of underlying periods, H. H. Clayton three years ago predicted the date of the coming maximum of sunspots to be 1937.5, a value

tory, which have been kept since its inauguration in 1885, and find a very marked tendency for the maximum frequency of brighter aurorae to occur on the average about a year after sunspot maximum (Fig. 2). In treating the data the number of aurorae for a given year was weighted with the observed intensity and the moving averages of three consecutive yearly values taken in plotting the curve.

The delay in the maximum of auroral frequencies with respect to the sunspot maximum calls for some explanation. Differences of opinion exist as to the exact mechanism connecting solar activity with auroral phenomena. Some investigators believe that the ionization responsible for the displays of the polar lights is produced by bursts of ultra-violet light from the sun accompanying the period of maximum solar activity. Dr. Carl Störmer, on the other hand, favors, the hypothesis that corpuscular emission of some sort emanates from sunspot centers and has been remarkably successful in computing the actual forms of auroral streamers on the basis of the behavior of charged particles coming from the sun and entering the upper atmosphere along paths distorted by the magnetic field of the earth.

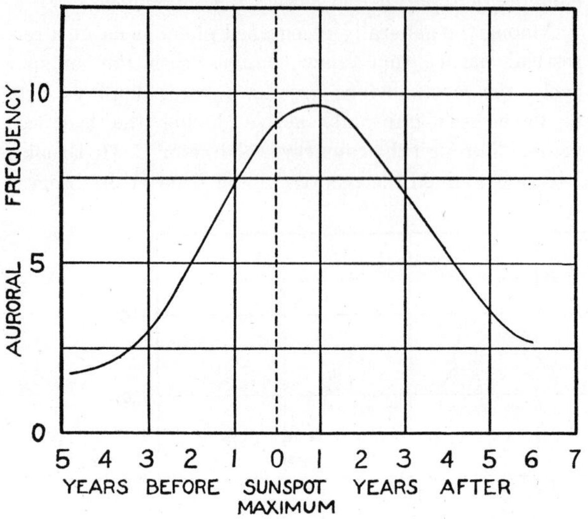


FIG. 2

If aurorae are caused in accordance with the corpuscular hypothesis then it might be expected that the polar lights would be most conspicuous when large sunspots pass near the sun-earth line or are seen close to the center of the sun's disk. The fact that sunspots occur at decreasing solar latitudes as the sunspot cycle progresses suggests that as the more active spots approach more nearly the solar equator they will more frequently cause brilliant aurorae. It should be possible on the basis of more complete data of the last few years to analyze the occurrences of aurorae with respect to the positions of sunspots near the central zone.

By the time spots begin to appear within 5° of the sun's equator, the numbers of sunspots have so appreciably waned as to diminish very considerably the presumable cause for auroral phenomena. Even on the hypothesis of flares of ultra-violet associated with chromospheric eruptions in the vicinity of sunspots, one would expect the latitude effect to be important in the production of aurorae. In either case, therefore, we have a possible qualitative explanation for the maximum in auroral frequency occurring after the actual maximum of sunspot numbers has been passed.

Since it is evident that an increased emission of ultra-violet radiation from the sun and possibly also the emission of particles in the vicinity of sunspots are directly associated with increased ionization of the earth's upper atmosphere, the phenomena of radio transmission may be expected to show variations with solar activity. Field strength measurements of a Chicago broadcasting station made at our suburban laboratory have shown a decrease from a value of more than 300 microvolts per meter at the sunspot minimum of 1933 and 1934 to a value of about 100 microvolts per meter during 1938. Sunspot numbers for the same interval rose from an average of 5 to an average of around 120. Critical frequencies for penetrating the E layer as published by the Bureau of Standards[3] have shown likewise a consistent parallel with the last four-year rise in solar activity, the value rising from 3.05 megacycles in 1934 to 3.75 megacycles in 1938.

Well-known changes in the intensity of the earth's magnetic field following closely changes in sunspots have been recognized for over 100 years. It is now obvious that probably the major contributing factor in the geomagnetic fluctuations is to be found in the ionization changes in the upper atmosphere. Developments in radio technique, therefore, offer new tools for exploration in unlocking the relationship between solar activity and terrestrial, atmospheric and magnetic phenomena.

# SCIENTIFIC EVENTS

## A DISCUSSION OF FRANKLIN AND HIS TIMES

A DISCUSSION of Franklin and his times entitled "Meet Doctor Franklin" is being held under the auspices of the Franklin Institute with the cooperation of the American Philosophical Society and the Historical Society of Pennsylvania.

The conferences are being held on Fridays at 5:15 P.M., beginning on October 20 and ending on April 19. The program follows:

Opening address, Dr. Carl Van Doren, author and editor, New York City.

''The Philosophical Revolutionist,'' Bernhard Knollenberg, librarian, Yale University.

''Dr. Franklin: Friend of the Indians,'' Dr. Julian P. Boyd, librarian and editor, Historical Society of Pennsylvania.

''The Colonies and the Mother Country,'' Dr. Verner W. Crane, professor of American history, University of Michigan.

''The Diplomat,'' Dr. Frank, Monaghan, assistant professor of American history, Yale University.

''Self-Portraiture: The Autobiography,'' Dr. Max Farrand, director, Huntington Library, San Marino, Calif.

''Looking Westward,'' Professor Gilbert Chinard, professor of French, Princeton University.

''Molding the Constitution,'' George Wharton Pepper, member of the Franklin Institute, Philadelphia.

''The Printer at Work,'' Dr. Lawrence C. Wroth, librarian, John Carter Brown Library, Providence, R. I.

"The Student of Life," Dr. Robert E. Spiller, professor of English, Swarthmore College.

"Adventure in Agriculture," Dr. Carl R. Woodward, secretary of Rutgers University.

"Dr. Franklin as the English Saw Him," Dr. Conyers Read, professor of English history, University of Pennsylvania.

"Dr. Franklin and Science," Dr. R. A. Millikan, physicist, California Institute of Technology.

Closing address, Dr. Carl Van Doren.

## THE EIGHTH AMERICAN SCIENTIFIC CONGRESS

THE eighth American Scientific Congress will be held in Washington, D. C., from May 10 to 18, 1940, under the auspices of the government of the United States of America.

Pursuant to a special act of the Congress of the United States, invitations on behalf of the President have been extended to the governments of the American Republics who are members of the Pan American Union to participate in the forthcoming meeting. Scientific institutions and organizations are also cordially invited to send representatives.

On April 14, 1940, the Pan American Union will celebrate the fiftieth anniversary of its founding. Although the eighth American Scientific Congress will convene a few weeks subsequent to the anniversary date, the congress will be one of the important phases of that celebration. It is hoped that the presence in Washington of many distinguished investigators from all the American republics as participants in this congress will serve as one of the many tributes to the Pan American Union on the occasion of celebrating the completion of a half century of invaluable service in the fostering of good-will and better understanding among the republics of the Western Hemisphere.

This series of inter-American meetings, serving as a medium for the exchange of scientific information of particular interest and importance to the governments and peoples of the Americas, has enjoyed a long and distinguished history, dating from the first Latin American Scientific Congress held at Buenos Aires in April, 1898.

The Honorable Cordell Hull, Secretary of State of the United States, has requested the following government officials and scientific men to serve upon an organizing committee, which is collaborating with the Department of State in formulating definite plans for the congress:

The Honorable Sumner Welles, Under Secretary of State, *chairman.*

Dr. Warren Kelchner, acting chief, Division of International Conferences, Department of State, *vice-chairman.*

Dr. Alexander Wetmore, assistant secretary of the Smithsonian Institution, *secretary.*

Dr. C. G. Abbot, secretary of the Smithsonian Institution.

Dr. Isaiah Bowman, president, The Johns Hopkins University.

Dr. Vannevar Bush, president, Carnegie Institution of Washington.

Dr. Ben M. Cherrington, chief, Division of Cultural Relations, Department of State.

Laurence Duggan, chief, Division of the American Republics, Department of State.

Dr. Ross G. Harrison, chairman, National Research Council.

Dr. Waldo G. Leland, secretary, American Council of Learned Societies.

Archibald MacLeish, librarian of Congress.

Dr. Thomas Parran, Jr., surgeon general, United States Public Health Service.

Dr. Stuart A. Rice, chairman of the Central Statistical Board.

Dr. Leo S. Rowe, director general, Pan American Union.

Dr. James Brown Scott, trustee and secretary, Carnegie Endowment for International Peace.

Dr. Wetmore has been designated also as secretary general of the congress.

The congress will be divided into the following sections, each to be in charge of a chairman, assisted by a vice-chairman, secretary and section committee:

I. Anthropological Sciences.
II. Biological Sciences.
III. Geological Sciences.
IV. Agriculture and Conservation.
V. Public Health and Medicine.
VI. Physical and Chemical Sciences.
VII. Statistics.
VIII. History and Geography.
IX. International Law, Public Law and Jurisprudence.
X. Economics and Sociology.
XI. Education.

The chairman of the respective sections will be selected at an early date, after which the detailed agenda of each section will be announced. The official languages of the congress will be English, Spanish, Portuguese and French.

The Department of State and the organizing committee are preparing an entertainment program which will include visits to places of scientific and general interest in Washington and its environs.

## AWARDS OF THE AMERICAN SOCIETY OF MECHANICAL ENGINEERS

THE American Society of Mechanical Engineers will hold its fifty-ninth annual meeting at the Hotel Bellevue-Stratford, Philadelphia, from December 4 to 8. A list of the 1939 honors and awards to be presented on December 6 to members and junior members of the society has been made public. They are:

The Melville Medal, presented annually for an original paper or thesis of exceptional merit presented before the society, to L. M. Goldsmith.

The medal of the American Society of Mechanical Engineers to James E. Gleason, president, the Gleason Works, Rochester, N. Y., "for service to the cause of safer and better transportation."

The Holley Medal to Dr. Carl Edvard Johannson, Eskilstuna, Sweden, "in recognition of his pioneer work in the development of basic measuring gages," which are used throughout the world by machine and engine manufacturers.

The Worcester Reed Warner Medal to Dr. Rupen Eksergian, Edw. G. Budd Mfg. Co., Philadelphia, Pa., "for influential engineering papers of permanent value published in the *Transactions* of the American Society of Mechanical Engineers.

The Pi Tau Sigma Medal to John I. Yellott, assistant professor at Stevens Institute of Technology, Hoboken, N. J., with the citation, "outstanding young mechanical engineer of 1939."

The Charles T. Main Award of $150 to James R. Bright, Swampscott, Mass., graduate of Lehigh University, and now a student engineer, General Electric Co., for his paper, "The Economics of Investment in New Manufacturing Equipment—With Concrete Cases."

The Undergraduate Student Award of $25 to David T. James, Modeltown, N. Y., graduate of Michigan State College and now cadet engineer, E. I. du Pont de Nemours and Co., Niagara Falls, N. Y., for his paper, "Bells—Concerning Their Tones."

## AWARD OF THE WILLARD GIBBS MEDAL

Dr. Vladimir N. Ipatieff, who came to this country from Russia in 1931, has been awarded the Willard Gibbs Medal of the Chicago Section of the American Chemical Society for 1940. The citation referred to him as "occupying a place of the first order in modern chemistry."

Dr. Ipatieff is internationally known for chemical discoveries basic to petroleum refining and to the organic synthesis of artificial rubber and of many other industrial products. He is now professor emeritus of Northwestern University, where he directs research in catalytic high pressure syntheses, and director of chemical research in the Riverside, Ill., laboratories of the Universal Oil Products Company.

In announcing the award Dr. Cary R. Wagner, chairman of the Chicago Section and of the Medal Jury, gave the following account of Dr. Ipatieff's work:

Dr. Ipatieff's chemical achievements in the field of catalysis and high pressure synthesis date from 1897. During the World War, Dr. Ipatieff was in charge of all chemical work for the Russian Government, with the rank of general and after the revolution he became president of the Central Chemical Bureau and founder of the High Pressure Research Institute. For this work he received the Lenin prize.

Dr. Ipatieff's work is of the same high order as that of the other European Willard Gibbs Medalists, who have included Mme. Marie Curie, of France; Svante Arrhenius, of Sweden; Sir James Irvine, of Scotland, and Dr. Richard Willstaetter, of Munich.

His discoveries of catalytic dehydration, hydrogenation, dehydrogenation and polymerization have placed his work in a commanding position for the past four decades and are the basis for many industrial processes, particularly in the refining of petroleum and synthesis of hydrocarbons.

Between 1900 and 1933 his researches were published almost entirely in Russian and German publications. In the last eight years he has been able to start research afresh in a new land with results that have been very far-reaching. His newer researches have extended the chemistry of the hydrocarbons greatly. He has developed a polymerization process to make high octane gasoline.

In 1897 in the laboratory of Professor Adolf von Bayer, Ipatieff synthesized for the first time isoprene, building stone of the complex rubber molecule, thus making possible the later synthesis of artificial rubber. In 1901 he began research in catalytic reactions under high pressures while working in the laboratory of the Academy of Artillery in St. Petersburg. He noticed, in 1901, the effect of catalysts on the decomposition of compounds, especially alcohols under high pressures and elevated temperatures. Simultaneously he discovered a method of making olefins from alcohols by passing the latter over alumina, a catalyst. Olefins have become the "raw" material for many organic compounds. The discovery was of very great industrial importance.

Dr. Ipatieff in 1903 and 1904 experimented extensively with the use of high pressures in the hydrogenation of various organic compounds, and these experiments were the forerunner of the Bergius process by which motor fuel is produced from coal. In 1905 he first introduced high pressures in polymerization of ethylene and other olefins. Continuing studies of polymerization in the presence of various catalytic agents, he found a catalyst which allows the transformation of a portion of the olefin-containing gases from cracking operations into an excellent high octane gasoline.

The work of Dr. Ipatieff in catalysis during the last thirty-five years enriched science by several major discoveries. He discovered several new catalytic agents, such as iron, zinc, manganese and their dioxides, important in the manufacture of dyes and fuels. He also first indicated the action of promoters, substances which aid catalysts, on the accelerated activity of catalytic agents. He has developed the chemistry of the paraffin hydrocarbons, compounds from which motor fuels and lubricants are made.

## RECENT DEATHS

Dr. Wilfred Thomas Dawson, professor of pharmacology in the School of Medicine of the University of Texas, died on September 19. He was forty-four years of age and had been connected with the School of Medicine since 1925. He was appointed to the professorship of pharmacology in 1927.

Dr. Nelson Fithian Davis, professor of biology and head of the department of biology of Bucknell University from 1907 to 1937, died on November 11 at the age of sixty-seven years.

DR. WILLIAM REGINALD MORSE, co-founder and dean for fifteen years of West China Union University Medical School at Chengtu, died in Boston on November 11 at the age of sixty-three years. For the last two years he had been working at Harvard University. Dr. Morse spent thirty years in West China, where he had been engaged in medical work and anthropological research.

DR. ROBERT MARSHALL, chief of the Division of Recreation and Lands of the U. S. Forest Service, died suddenly on November 11. He was thirty-eight years old.

WENDELL PHILLIPS HOGE, laboratory assistant and computer at the Mount Wilson Observatory, died on November 14 at the age of seventy-two years.

SIR WILLIAM J. POPE, for thirty-one years professor of chemistry at the University of Cambridge, died on October 17 at the age of sixty-nine years.

VASILY ROBERTOVICH WILLIAMS, of Moscow, a specialist in agronomy, died on November 11 at the age of seventy-six years.

DR. ARTHUR JOHN HOPKINS, professor of chemistry emeritus of Amherst College, died on November 10 at the age of seventy-five years. A correspondent writes: "Professor Hopkins was born September 20, 1864, in Bridgewater, Mass., graduated from Amherst College in 1885, and took his Ph.D. under Morse at Johns Hopkins University in 1893. In 1894 he came back to Amherst, becoming full professor in 1907, in which position he served until his retirement in 1934. In 1895 he married Margaret Sutton Briscoe. He is survived by his wife and his daughter, Mrs. Cornelia Allen. Although he is credited with a number of contributions to the field of inorganic and analytic chemistry, in which he was always interested, Professor Hopkins was best known for his life-long study of the early history of the science. His 'color theory' of early alchemy has done much to clarify the obscurity of the Greek alchemical writings. In a series of articles in *Isis* and in his book, "Alchemy, the Child of Greek Philosophy," published by the Columbia University Press in 1934, he showed that the Alexandrian alchemists, believing that color was the chief property of metals, were trying to put into practice the philosophical ideas of Plato and the Gnostics. They were trying to push the baser metals along the road to 'improvement,' through a series of color changes which can be recognized as actual chemical processes, carried out with ingenious if primitive chemical apparatus."

# SCIENTIFIC NOTES AND NEWS

PROFESSOR P. DEBYE, director of the Kaiser Wilhelm Institute of Physics at Berlin-Dahlem, will be the George F. Baker non-resident lecturer in chemistry at Cornell University for four months, beginning with the second term of the academic year. He will discuss the determination of molecular structure by the method of interferences. The German Government has granted Dr. Debye leave of absence to accept the lectureship.

PROFESSOR THEODOR VON KÁRMÁN, director of the Daniel Guggenheim Aeronautical Laboratory of the California Institute of Technology, will give the fifteenth Josiah Willard Gibbs Lecture of the American Mathematical Society. The title of the lecture is "The Engineer Grappling with Non-linear Problems." It will be given at the annual meeting of the society, which will be held at Columbus on December 28, 29 and 30 in conjunction with the American Association for the Advancement of Science.

THOMAS H. CHILTON, director of the Technical Division of the engineering department of the E. I. du Pont de Nemours and Company, Wilmington, Del., was presented with the Charles Frederick Chandler Medal at a ceremony held at Columbia University on November 7. The presentation was made by Dean Joseph Barker, of the Columbia School of Engineering, which is celebrating the seventy-fifth anniversary of its founding as the first School of Mines in the United States by Dr. Chandler and his associates in 1864. Following the presentation Mr. Chilton gave the annual Chandler lecture entitled "Engineering in the Service of Chemistry." Mr. Chilton is the seventeenth Chandler medalist. The medal was awarded to him for "the discovery and formulation of principles underlying the unit operations of chemical engineering, and in the application of these principles to process development, equipment design and chemical plant construction and operation."

THE medal of the Society of Chemical Industry was presented on November 10 to Dr. Robert E. Wilson, president of the Pan American Petroleum and Transport Company, at a meeting at New York City of the Chemists Club, sponsored by the American Section of the Society of Chemical Industry and the New York Section of the American Chemical Society and the New York Section of the American Institute of Chemical Engineers.

DR. ARTHUR H. COMPTON, Charles H. Swift distinguished service professor at the University of Chicago, on November 8 was the guest of honor at a dinner at St. Louis sponsored by several scientific and religious groups. Dean Alexander S. Langsdorf, of the Washington University School of Engineering and Architecture, presided. Following the dinner, Dr. Compton spoke at the Centenary Church.

DR. HUGH S. TAYLOR, David B. Jones professor of chemistry and chairman of the department of chemistry of Princeton University, was the guest of his associates and former graduate students at a dinner held on the evening of October 21, given in honor of "twenty-five years of distinguished service to chemistry at Princeton." Following the dinner he was presented in the name of former graduate students with a silver smoking set by Dr. W. N. Henderson, of the Allied Chemical and Dye Corporation, New York. Dr. Taylor, in his response, surveyed the development of chemistry at Princeton in the last quarter century.

A MEETING was held at the St. Louis Medical Society on October 24 in honor of Dr. William Washington Graves, professor of neuropsychiatry at the St. Louis University School of Medicine. At this meeting Dr. Graves was awarded the certificate of merit and a gold medal for scientific accomplishment. The certificate reads: "In consideration of the usefulness of his classification of scapulae and other inherited characters, and of his discovery of 'The Age-Incidence Principle of Investigation,' both of which resulted in new approaches to the qualitative evaluation of inherited variations in relation to the inherited qualities of human constitution, expressed in inherited predisposition to health or disease, and in inherited capacity for education, for adaptability and for longevity." On only two occasions before this the St. Louis Medical Society has awarded this certificate of merit for scientific accomplishment. The first was given to Dr. Evarts A. Graham and his associates in 1927 for their work in cholecystography; the second to Dr. Edward A. Doisy in 1935, for his achievements in hormone chemistry and physiology.

DR. JOSEPH B. DE LEE, professor emeritus of obstetrics and gynecology of the School of Medicine of the Division of Biological Sciences, University of Chicago, observed his seventieth birthday on October 29 at a party planned to benefit the Chicago Maternity Center, which he founded. He was presented with cuff links forged from a pair of forceps that he used in his early days of practice.

THE Soviet Government has awarded the Order of Lenin to Dr. Vladimir Leontievitch Komarov, president of the Academy of Sciences of the U.S.S.R., in honor of his seventieth birthday and "in appreciation of his great services to science."

DR. SETON PRINGLE, surgeon to the Hospital of the Royal City of Dublin and lately president of the Royal College of Surgeons of Ireland, has been elected president of the Irish Royal Academy of Medicine.

AT the autumn meeting of the Virginia Chapter of Sigma Xi, the following officers were elected: *President,* Gordon T. Whyburn; *Vice-president,* James E. Kindred; *Secretary,* Joseph K. Roberts, and *Treasurer,* Lawrence R. Quarles. Dr. Jesse W. Beams, professor of physics at the University of Virginia, will be one of the lecturers this year. His subject will be "High Speed Centrifuging."

DR. DARIEL E. HOWELL has been appointed assistant professor of entomology at Oklahoma Agricultural and Mechanical College to take the place of Dr. L. E. Rozeboom, who resigned to become a member of the department of medical entomology at the Johns Hopkins University. Dr. Howell will have charge of investigations dealing with insect and tick transmission of bovine anaplasmosis, and will teach courses in medical entomology and pest control.

DR. JOHN C. HAFF, of the petrographic laboratory of the Bureau of Reclamation in Denver, has been appointed assistant professor of geology at the Colorado School of Mines.

AT the meeting of the Board of Scientific Directors of the Rockefeller Institute for Medical Research, New York, held on October 28, Professor Warfield T. Longcope, of the Johns Hopkins Hospital, was elected president of the board to succeed Dr. Charles R. Stockard, who died on April 7 of the present year. Professor Ross G. Harrison, of the Osborn Zoological Laboratory, Yale University, was elected a member of the Board of Scientific Directors of the Institute.

PROFESSOR EDMUND W. SINNOTT, professor of botany at Barnard College, Columbia University, has been elected a member of the Board of Trustees of *Biological Abstracts.* Members of the editorial board have been elected as follows: Dr. Robert S. Breed, Agricultural Experiment Station, Geneva, N. Y., "Dairy Bacteriology"; Professor Adriance S. Foster, University of California, "Morphology and Anatomy of Vascular Plants"; Dr. A. G. Karlson, University of Minnesota, associate editor, "Infectious and Other Diseases of Lower Animals"; Dr. Josef N. Knull, the Ohio State University, "Coleoptera"; Professor Gilbert M. Smith, Stanford University, "Algae"; and Robert G. Stone, Blue Hill Observatory of Harvard University, "Biometeorology and Bioclimatology."

DR. LOUIS B. BISHOP, of Pasadena, Calif., has been given an honorary appointment on the staff of Field Museum of Natural History as research associate in the division of birds. Dr. Bishop was responsible for the assemblage of one of the largest and most important collections of North American birds. It is known as "the Bishop collection" and was recently acquired for addition to the department of zoology. More than 50,000 specimens, representing nearly every known form of bird found in North America, are included.

THE Committee on Scientific Research of the American Medical Association has made a grant to Robert R. Sealock, of the Univeristy of Rochester, to continue his investigations on the relationship of ascorbic acid to the metabolism of the melanin pigment precursors.

DR. HUGH S. CUMMING, formerly surgeon-general of the U. S. Public Health Service, sailed for Europe on November 11. He will attend a meeting of the Health Committee of the League of Nations.

DR. OSCAR RIDDLE, of the Research Staff of Carnegie Institution Station for Experimental Evolution at Cold Spring Harbor, N. Y., gave an address before the Massachusetts State Chapter of Sigma Xi at Amherst on the evening of November 15 on "Our Uncontrollable Governor—the Pituitary Gland."

DR. ROBERT MEYER, formerly director of the Pathological Institute (Gynecological Clinic) and honorary professor of the Friedrich-Wilhelms University, Berlin, will give on December 6 and 7 the Charles Sumner Bacon lectures of the University of Illinois for 1939–1940 in the Medical and Dental College Laboratories Building at Chicago. The titles of the lectures are: "The Basis of the Histological Diagnosis of Carcinoma" and "Diagnosis of Early Carcinoma of the Cervix."

PROFESSOR K. K. LANDES, chairman of the department of geology of the University of Kansas, recently presented a series of three exchange lectures at the University of Cincinnati. The titles of the lectures were: "Pegmatites," "Igneous Rocks of the Mississippi Valley" and "Volcanic Ash in the Western United States." A fourth lecture, on a geologic exploring trip in Alaska, was given before the Cincinnati chapter of Sigma Xi. Professor N. M. Fenneman, of Cincinnati, had previously given a series of lectures on physiographic topics at the University of Kansas.

AT the twenty-fourth annual meeting of the Institute of Medicine of Chicago at the Congress Hotel on December 5, Dr. Arthur H. Curtis, professor and chairman of the department of obstetrics and gynecology at Northwestern University Medical School, will deliver the presidential address on "Some New Features of Gynecological Anatomy and Related Clinical Problems."

THE two hundred and thirtieth regular meeting of the American Physical Society will be held in Chicago on Friday and Saturday, December 1 and 2.

THE University of North Carolina on Monday, December 4, will celebrate the opening of the new Medical Laboratories Building as part of its general Sesqui-Centennial Celebration. The exercises will consist in the morning of an address by Professor E. K. Marshall, Jr., of the Johns Hopkins Medical School, on "Medical Research: the Story of Sulfanilamide." In the afternoon Dr. David Riesman, professor emeritus of clinical medicine and professor of the history of medicine, the Medical School of the University of Pennsylvania, will make an address entitled "The Making of a Clinician," and Dr. G. Canby Robinson, lecturer in medicine and director of the Medical Clinic of the Johns Hopkins University Medical School, will speak on "The Application of Medical Science to the Individual." An informal tea in conjunction with the inspection of the medical laboratories and the medical dormitory will be held in the Charles E. Kistler Memorial Library of the Medical School. In the evening Dr. Frank G. Boudreau, executive director of the Milbank Memorial Foundation, will speak at a dinner gathering on "New Health Frontiers." Greetings will be brought to the university and to the Medical School by various alumni and friends.

IT is announced that requests to the National Research Council Committee for Research in Endocrinology for aid during the fiscal period from September 1, 1940, to June 30, 1941, will be received until February 29. Application blanks may be obtained by addressing the Division of Medical Sciences, National Research Council, 2101 Constitution Avenue, Washington, D. C. In addition to a statement of the problem and research plan or program, the committee desires information regarding the proposed method of attack, the institutional support of the investigation and the uses to be made of the sum requested. No part of any grant may be used by the recipient institution for administrative expenses. Applications for aid of endocrine research on problems of sex in the narrower sense can not be given favorable consideration, but the committee will consider the support of studies on the effects of sex hormones on non-sexual functions—*e.g.*, on metabolism.

DR. STEPHEN DUGGAN, director of the Institute of International Education, has been forced to cancel for the duration of the war all student exchanges between the United States and Europe. The institute had expected to send four hundred American students abroad on fellowships. Three hundred of these have been cancelled, since they were for European universities, but the remainder, involving Latin America, Canada and the Far East, have not been affected.

OVER two hundred courses in clinical medicine for practicing physicians are being given by the Columbia University School of Medicine at metropolitan hospitals affiliated with the school during the academic year 1939–40. These are designed for continuation training and advanced experience in the clinical fields of medicine, and are divided into separate sections for general practitioners and for specialists. The hospitals affiliated with the School of Medicine are as follows: Bellevue; Hospital for Joint Diseases; Institute of Ophthalmology; Lenox Hill; Montefiore; Mount Sinai; Margaret Hague Maternity Hospital; Neurological Institute; New York Post-Graduate Medical School; New York State Psychiatric Institute and Hospital; Presbyterian Hospital; St. Luke's; Welfare Hospital for Chronic Diseases, and Woman's Hospital.

# DISCUSSION

## THE FOUNDING OF A DEPARTMENT OF FISHES IN THE MUSEO POEY OF THE UNIVERSITY OF HAVANA

FELIPE POEY (1799–1891) was Cuba's greatest naturalist. He was made professor of natural history in the University of Havana in 1830, and in 1839 he was appointed director of the museum in the university. He published rather widely on Cuban natural history, but he is best known by reason of his excellent work on Cuban fishes. His first ichthyological contribution appeared in 1851 and his last in 1883. In the space of these thirty-two years his publications on fishes number nineteen, and of these five were stout volumes. These volumes were issued in fascicules or parts as they were finished and were then gathered into volumes with inclusive titles. If these individual parts could be counted, they would probably treble the number of Poey's separate contributions. Only by thumbing through his works could the total number of fishes described by him be ascertained. But it is said that he described *de novo* more than 230 species.

Since Poey's day the study of Cuban fishes has been carried on intermittently by various investigators from various countries. These studies have consisted mainly of descriptions of one or a few species or at best of small collections. Now, however, plans are on foot for extensive and far-reaching studies, which will recall the days of Felipe Poey. His work is to be taken up and continued by a man who has already written extensively on Cuban fishes and who bids fair to be a worthy successor of Poey.

The Museum of Zoology (Museo Poey) of the University of Havana has recently established a department of fishes for the study and preservation of the fishes of the West Indian fauna, and particularly those of the Cuban waters.

The organization and establishment of this department are due to the initiative and activities of Dr. Luis Howell Rivero, professor in the faculty of science. Dr. Rivero was for two years (1934–1936) a fellow of the Guggenheim Foundation doing research work on West Indian fishes at the Museum of Comparative Zoology at Harvard College and at the Museum of Zoology of the University of Michigan. He has had the cooperation of his colleague, Dr. Carlos G. Aguayo (also a former Guggenheim fellow), and of Dr. José M. Cadenas, rector of the University of Havana, who has provided the necessary appropriation for the maintenance of the department.

The first great collections for the establishment of this department are the following accessions:

Fishes obtained by the "Tomas Barrera Expedition" in 1914, under the direction of Dr. Carlos de la Torre, from the University of Havana and of Dr. Paul Bartsch, of the U. S. National Museum.

Fishes obtained by Dr. Rivero in Jamaica in the spring of 1937, during a survey of the fishes of Jamaica done under the auspices of the Museum of Comparative Zoology at Cambridge, Mass., the Department of Science and Agriculture of Jamaica and the University of Havana.

Fishes obtained by the "Harvard-Havana Expedition" in the spring of 1938, and by the second expedition, March to May, 1939, under the auspices of Harvard University and the University of Havana, undertaken on board the research vessel *Atlantis*.

Besides, there are several small local collections made by Dr. Rivero, Dr. Aguayo and others, as well as many donations which have been made to the museum.

At the present moment and taking into consideration its very early stage, the department of fishes has over 50 per cent. of the species of the known Cuban fauna represented in its collections, and now that this department is prepared adequately to care for specimens, it is confidently expected that much valuable material will be presented to the Museo.

In this new department of the university, courses of lectures and laboratory work will be given by Dr. Rivero, its founder. In addition opportunities will be afforded graduate students to do research work on fishes under Dr. Rivero's immediate direction. Thus the Museo Poey of the University of Havana may be expected to become the center of work on the West Indian ichthyological fauna.

CORRESPONDENT

## A NOTEWORTHY AURORA

ON the night of August 1, 1937, there occurred an extremely spectacular display of the aurora borealis, visible, no doubt, in many of our northern states and in Canada. I watched it from the Musselshell Valley of central Montana, where I write this, and was so impressed by its many unusual aspects that I felt a brief account of it might be of interest for permanent record. Before I could find opportunity to work up my notes for this purpose, a very fine and detailed description of what was doubtless the same phenomenon was published in SCIENCE by Ernest H. Cherrington, Jr., and my own contribution was allowed to lapse.

The aurora of the night of August 11 of this year, also witnessed by me from this spot, ranked with the foregoing as one of the three most magnificent I have had the good fortune to witness,[1] but in some particulars it was altogether unique. When first observed at about 9:20 P.M. it comprised a single sweeping auroral arch in the northern heavens, but one reared so high that it included almost half the horizon between its termini, while its vertex nearly attained the zenith. At this time it appeared from my window as a simple broad band of strong whitish light, not without a serene majesty of its own. This was little prophetic of the glory to come, yet I roused a friend, Harold M. Hill, who had never witnessed an aurora, and it was consequently our good fortune to be in the open with an unimpeded view of the entire firmament when the climax came.

The first evidence of breaking was a narrow beam or ray which appeared to the northwest just under the span. The arch then rapidly broke up, with strong cloud-like patches of light appearing to east and west, while the portion between evolved into an array of luminous shafts or streamers so grouped as to seem to radiate from a roughly stellate centrum just south of the zenith in the general neighborhood of Vega. The best of the display occurred from about 9:45 to 10:00 o'clock, when the fast-changing beams and rays covered more than half the heavens, and rapidly shifting lesser flickerings were flashing all over and through the whole. At its peak nearly three fourths of the sky was illuminated, although the radiating streamers to the south of the centrum were very short, in contrast to those extending far down the northern sky and the still longer ones to east and west. Also on the south there was more of a tendency for the beams to give way to scattered, irregular spots and clouds of light than in other parts of the heavens. By this time considerable color had developed, mostly reddish, orange and pinkish brown tones which again were much more in evidence to the extreme east and west than elsewhere. After 10:00 o'clock the illumination lost its active motion and most of its color, retreating more and more into the northern sky, where it finally resolved itself into a simple diffused arch of the more usual type. This endured until we retired, and was still in evidence when I arose to look, around 1:00 A.M. and again just before dawn, though meanwhile considerable cloudiness had developed to obscure its details. I was unable to note any recurrence of the more lively pyrotechnics. As long as the first arch persisted, the northern sky remained quite dark under it, but at no time did I observe the intense contrasting *blackness* there which was so conspicuous an accompaniment of the arch of August, 1937.

It occurred to me at the time that the centering of the major display so definitely *south* of the zenith might well entail a visibility in much lower latitudes than is ordinarily the case for such phenomena. This has since received confirmation through newspaper reports, from one of which[2] it transpires that on this night the aurora was seen at least as far south as Summit Lookout in Cajon Pass and Lake Arrowhead in the San Bernardino Mountains of southern California, where some observers are reported to have interpreted it as the glow of a distant forest fire.

S. STILLMAN BERRY

WINNECOOK, MONTANA

## OZONE IN THE '38 HURRICANE

DURING the hurricane on September 21, 1938, the smell of ozone was strong during the latter part of the storm. The peak of the storm was shortly after 6 P.M. (D.S.T.); the lowest barometer 28.41 (corrected) at Amherst, Mass., being at 6:05, and the highest wind velocity, 80 miles, at 6:17. During the heavy rain, about 6 to 6:30, the ozone was strong, and later, when the rain stopped, the ozone was so strong I was uncomfortable. At this time my watch said 7 o'clock. No odor of ozone was noticed in the first part of the storm nor was any noticeable in the house. My colleague in chemistry, in the Massachusetts State College, Dr. Walter S. Ritchie, independently reports similar observations.

CHARLES A. PETERS

AMHERST, MASS.

## THE INTERNATIONAL UNION OF CHEMISTRY

COMMUNICATIONS have been received from individuals and organizations of many lands requesting advice as to whether or not they should endeavor to continue the work of the Union and its various commissions during the present chaotic condition of the world, or suspend operations until the return of peace and the general resumption of friendly international relations.

The answer to this question in the judgment of the writer should be unequivocally that the work is to go on, if possible still more actively than heretofore, not only in its local national field, but particularly in its international aspects. The Union, as its name signifies,

[1] For the third of these see SCIENCE, 44: 496, 568, 678, October and November, 1916.

[2] *Redlands* (Calif.) *Daily Facts*, August 12, 1939.

is an organization of scientists banded together for the good, not of any one country, but of all. Its aims are the welfare and happiness of all mankind, through the advancement of civilization by the triumphs of chemistry. No science offers greater opportunities for service and beneficent achievement. When the Union and its affiliated congress meet, as at Rome last year, where about 3,000 attended, representing some 30 nations, national boundaries and misunderstandings are forgotten, and mutual appreciation, esteem and good fellowship prevail. This spirit of friendship and regard, carried back home by all the delegates, is often like a breath of fresh air in dispersing the fogs of a murky local atmosphere of misapprehension and suspicion. Nor does it cease upon their arrival in the homeland, but in many cases is continued through correspondence. Individually the bonds of friendship so established may seem relatively unimportant, but collectively their Lilliputian character becomes a force not to be ignored.

The usefulness of the International Union of Chemistry and of its various commissions and committees will be determined primarily by the wholeheartedness with which the associated nations cooperate, and the fact that certain nations are now at war is no reason why the other nations concerned should not continue to cooperate and, to the best of their ability, take advantage of those opportunities for important useful service which the International Union offers, so that when the world finally returns to normal we shall be that much further along on the road to our goal. Even in the warring nations, it is to be hoped that they will still "carry on," as conditions permit, for their own ultimate benefit and that of the rest of the world. Their chemical societies are still active. Why should their international chemical problems be either dropped or forgotten?

To suspend activities now might give the impression of a malingering and pessimistic attitude, totally at variance with the inspiring vision and courage of chemists the world over.

MARSTON TAYLOR BOGERT,
*President, International Union of Chemistry*

COLUMBIA UNIVERSITY,
NEW YORK

# SCIENTIFIC BOOKS

## RECENT BOOKS IN GEOLOGY

*Geology: Principles and Processes.* By W. H. EMMONS, G. H. THIEL, C. R. STAUFFER and I. S. ALLISON. 2nd edition. 451 pp. 468 figs. New York: McGraw-Hill Book Company. 1939. $3.50.

*Elements of Geology* (with Reference to North America). By WILLIAM J. MILLER, professor of geology, University of California at Los Angeles. 2nd edition. viii + 524 pp. 367 figs. New York: D. Van Nostrand Company. 1939. $3.50.

*Textbook of Geology, Part I—Physical Geology.* By CHESTER R. LONGWELL, ADOLPH KNOPF and RICHARD F. FLINT. 2nd edition. ix + 543 pp. 340 figs. New York: John Wiley and Sons. 1939. $3.75.

THE second edition of the book by Emmons, Thiel, Stauffer and Allison, members of the department of geology in the University of Minnesota, originally published under the short title "Geology," has been considerably revised and completely reset. It is intended for use in a one-semester introductory course for college students, dealing with the physical phases of the science. The chapter on the atmosphere and the work of the wind has been enlarged and includes a brief consideration of certain meteorological principles as well as the discussion of weathering. The treatment of varved glacial lake sediments and their importance in glacial and post-glacial chronology has been expanded. The chapter on diastrophism has been enlarged to include structure of rocks. A new chapter on sediments and sedimentation has been added. The chapter on earth history is omitted. The volume is well organized, and its subject-matter is presented in an interesting manner. It contains an unusually large number of excellent photographs, sketches and maps. The numerous block diagrams are a valuable feature. The layman as well as the student will benefit from reading it.

First published in 1931, Professor Miller's textbook is one of the few designed to serve a one-semester course in general geology, covering both the physical and historical phases of the science. The principal changes made in this new edition are outlined by the author in his preface. Distinct and important improvements are the enlarged, more attractive format, superior quality paper and especially the greatly improved reproduction of the photographs. More photographs and block diagrams are used, and these have been brought up to date. Several chapters have been rewritten to coincide with modern data and concepts. A unique feature is the discussion of the instability of the earth's crust immediately after the introduction before the materials of the earth are considered. The chapter is understandable even at this early stage in the development of the subject and serves to stimulate interest at the beginning of the course. The text may seem to be rather long for a one-semester course, but this characteristic is shared by most other texts intended to serve such a purpose without becoming too "popular" in character. A relatively large number of technical terms and stratigraphic names are used.

The well-known text-book by Longwell, Knopf and Flint has likewise been thoroughly revised to include much new material from laboratory and field studies of recent years. Although the general plan of the book remains unchanged, two new chapters have been added. One of these considers such movements of surficial material as those resulting from creep and landsliding, all of which are included in the suggested term "mass-wasting." The other is devoted to the sculpturing of the lands and follows the development of the principles of weathering, mass-wasting and stream erosion. This gives opportunity for the consideration of the erosion cycle under diverse climatic conditions and leaves room in the preceding chapter for a brief but effective treatment of the problems of soil erosion and destructive floods. In contrast to certain other comparable text-books, technical terms have been avoided as much as possible, and some of the newly added references are to popular or semi-popular books. Many of the new illustrations are also in keeping with this highly commendable tendency to put vitality into a subject which ought to have a wide appeal to everybody.

*Physiography of Eastern United States.* By Nevin M. Fenneman. 691 pp., maps, photographs and diagrams, index. New York: McGraw-Hill Book Company. 1938. $6.00.

This excellent reference work summarizing the physiographic features of Eastern United States is a companion volume to the author's "Physiography of Western United States" and follows the same general plan. The portion of the United States east of the Great Plains is divided into provinces and sections similar, but not precisely equivalent, to those shown on the map of the "Physical Divisions of the United States" which accompanies the earlier volume. The boundaries of each province and section are traced in detail, and the reasons for the choice of boundaries are discussed. Each province and section is systematically treated by means of a brief résumé of the lithology and structure, a general description of the topography, an account of the origin of the topography and finally the history of its development. The space given each province corresponds roughly to its size and importance. The book is well indexed and so systematically divided that the description of any particular region can easily be found.

In discussing the origin and history of the topography the views of many workers are carefully considered and appraised, the conservative view being finally accepted in most instances of conflict. Frequent references to important physiographic problems and their proper interpretation enhance the interest in the subject-matter and the value of the book for the student.

The enormous amount of descriptive material packed into the volume places a severe strain upon the memory of the reader, and unfortunately many of the illustrations do not aid him in understanding the text as much as might be desired. But the very difficult task of assembling such a vast amount of uncoordinated data and reconciling the conflicting opinions of so many workers has been accomplished with remarkable success. The book is a valuable reference work for any natural scientist who may have occasion to be interested in the land surface of the eastern states and its genesis.

*A Textbook of Geomorphology.* By Philip G. Worcester. 565 pp. 375 illustrations. New York: D. Van Nostrand Company. 1939. $4.00.

Geomorphology is the interpretative description of the relief features of the earth. So runs the definition preferred by the author of this handsome volume, who for many years has been professor of geology in the University of Colorado. The term is therefore practically synonymous with physiography, the designation more commonly used in America for the science of land forms. Probably there is an advantage in using a term that by derivation implies study or interpretation rather than one that implies merely description.

The book has been planned for an introductory course in the geological sciences, and its table of contents differs only slightly from that ordinarily found in an elementary text for a course in dynamic geology. From it one may learn to distinguish orthoclase from plagioclase, as well as eskers from drumlins. More space is given to the causes of vulcanism than to the topographic forms resulting from the deposition of wind-blown sand. Professor Worcester approaches the subject from the point of view of the geologist rather than from that of the geographer.

There is still need for a treatise on geomorphology of a more advanced nature, designed for use by those who are already fairly well acquainted with the principles of dynamic geology and who need a thorough-going critique of the resultant land forms and their interpretation. Neither the volume now in hand nor the recently published book by Dr. A. K. Lobeck is adequate for the professional geomorphologist; both are intended for the beginning student and for the layman interested in the landscape. As a matter of fact, Professor Worcester appropriately stresses in his preface the cultural value of geomorphology and the responsibility of the teacher for the "thousands [who] may become interested in the subject and gain enduring pleasure from continued studies of their physical environment, wherever they may be."

The wealth of illustrations deserves high commendation and contributes much to the value of the book, especially for the audience which Professor Worcester has in mind. Most, though not all of the photographs, are superb both from the point of view of photography and of reproduction. All are well chosen to illustrate the ideas ably presented in the text. The line drawings, including many block diagrams, are uniformly excellent and for the most part were originally prepared for this book by Julian W. Low. Many of the contour maps are reproduced in two colors, with the drainage features in blue. Both author and publisher are to be congratulated for producing so excellent a volume.

*Geology and Engineering.* By ROBERT F. LEGGET. xviii + 650 pp. 223 illustrations. New York: McGraw-Hill Book Company. 1939. $4.50.

DURING the last few years the application of the science of geology to the art of civil engineering has become a matter of prime importance. Whereas a generation ago the geologist was frequently called for a post-mortem examination of a leaking dam, collapsed bridge or faulty tunnel, he is to-day even more frequently requested to cooperate in the preliminary investigations of the materials on which or in which the engineer is to build his structure or do his work. The results in the saving of human lives and the reduction in the cost of engineering works are beyond estimate. Such cooperation has also contributed much valuable information to geological lore. Professor Legget's up-to-date treatise is a veritable milestone on the highway of human progress toward accurate synthesis of the diverse problems encountered in the arena of interplay between man and his environment.

As stated by Professor P. G. H. Boswell, of the Imperial College of Science and Technology, London, in his foreword, the several text-books of engineering geology previously available have been written by geologists. "Where engineering applications are discussed, in particular, they indicate what the geologist from his rather different viewpoint, imagines that the engineer should know." In contrast, "this book is the work of an engineer with the additional training of a geologist" and has a background that would scarcely be possessed even by a geologist of wide experience as a consultant on engineering problems. It therefore fills a long-felt want and will be widely used in engineering schools and as a valuable tool of the professional geologist and civil engineer. Many a college teacher of geology will use to good advantage in his classroom the accounts of the practical application of geological principles with which Professor Legget has pointed his precepts.

The first four chapters introduce the engineering student to those phases of geological science with which he is most likely to be later concerned. The remaining sixteen chapters deal lucidly and succinctly with the application of geology in civil engineering. Tunnels, open cuts, road construction, bridge foundation, dam sites, silting up of reservoirs, wells and boreholes, landslides and soil mechanics, these and many other topics are ably handled. Especially commendable is the wealth of illuminating experiences drawn from engineering practice the world over and including such current projects as those of the T.V.A. and Boulder Dam. There are four appendices, which include a glossary of geological terms, an annotated list of the geological surveys of the English-speaking world and a list of geological societies and periodicals.

KIRTLEY F. MATHER

HARVARD UNIVERSITY

# SOCIETIES AND MEETINGS

## THE SEMI-CENTENNIAL CELEBRATION OF THE MEDICAL SCHOOL OF THE UNIVERSITY OF MINNESOTA

THE University of Minnesota celebrated from October 12 to 14 the fiftieth anniversary of the founding of its Medical School. The occasion was used as an opportunity to bring together a number of contributors to scientific medical progress in several fields, who presented accounts of recent advances with particular emphasis upon the unsolved problems which have been exposed and appear to be amenable to solution.

Progress in the application of physical chemistry to medicine was discussed by Professors Herbert M. Freundlich and Maurice B. Visscher, of the University of Minnesota, and John P. Peters, of Yale University. These investigators described living organisms as systems at steady states frequently, if not usually, at some distance from true equilibrium. The importance of the structure and properties of the colloidal systems in cells and of the metabolic energy-yielding reactions in maintaining these steady states was discussed.

Some recent investigations in metabolism were detailed by Professors Lee I. Smith and George O. Burr, of the University of Minnesota, who discussed organic chemical problems in relation to Vitamin E, and the metabolism of the fatty acids, respectively, by Professor George H. Whipple, of the University of Rochester, who treated the problem of production, utilization, and significance of the blood proteins, and by Professor Charles H. Best, of the University of Toronto, who summarized the present state of knowledge concerning the chemistry and physiology of heparin and concerning the clinical physiology of thrombosis.

Chemical problems in immunity were discussed by Professor Michael Heidelberger, of Columbia University. Professor Robert G. Green, of the University of Minnesota, described experimental modification of pathogenic viruses in relation to the general problem of the nature of viruses. Professors Perrin H. Long, of Johns Hopkins University, and Henry F. Helmholz, of the Mayo Foundation of the University of Minnesota, discussed modern chemotherapy, the first with particular reference to the sulfanilamide group, and the latter with reference to the specific problem of urinary antisepsis.

Several approaches to the problems of the nervous control of the organism were discussed. Professor Irvine McQuarrie, of the University of Minnesota, described experiments showing important chemical factors in the production and control of convulsions in man and in animals. Professor Herbert S. Gasser, of the Rockefeller Institute for Medical Research, presented a general treatment of methods of analysis of nervous action which are being and can be extended in the investigation of the more intimate character of nervous conduction. Professor Detlev W. Bronk, of the University of Pennsylvania, described the results of observations upon nervous control of such visceral processes as circulation and respiration. He dealt with the problem of chemically sensitive receptors in reflex regulation of body activities, showing the interdependence of chemical and physical mechanisms in such control. Professor Walter B. Cannon considered the problem of chemical mediation of excitation at synapses. He marshalled the existing evidence for chemical mediation, particularly at cholinergic structures.

Public meetings were addressed by Dr. Thomas Parran, Jr., surgeon-general of the U. S. Public Health Service, on "Medical Education, Research and the Public Health"; by Professor Anton J. Carlson, of the University of Chicago, on "The Role of the Fundamental Sciences in Medical Progress"; by President Guy Stanton Ford, of the University of Minnesota, upon "The Place of Medicine in a University," and by Governor Harold E. Stassen, on "Medicine in the Commonwealth." These speakers emphasized the peculiar importance of public support for medical education and research on a high plane in the interests of the community itself, the necessity of research in the basic sciences for sound progress in the applied science of medicine, and the importance of broader and better cultural training for physicians themselves so that they may play a larger and more enlightened role in the social and political changes which are going on at a rapidly accelerating pace. The relatively more important part that American science must play on the world scene in view of the catastrophies of war and authoritarianism in Europe and Asia was stressed as an additional reason for intensification and improvement in our scientific and cultural institutions. The scientific and general lectures presented at the semi-centennial celebration will shortly be published in two separate volumes by the University of Minnesota Press.

Since the State of Minnesota undertook responsibility for the guidance and support of medical education and research fifty years ago, the aims and needs for such service have changed greatly. Initially, the undergraduate training of physicians was viewed as its main task. About twenty-five years ago the university undertook the problems of graduate training and research in a serious way. At the present time the graduate teaching program is a larger undertaking than the undergraduate teaching. In comparison with some four hundred undergraduates in medicine there are over six hundred graduate students working toward advanced degrees in the several fundamental and clinical medical fields in this university. The larger share of those working in the latter fields are doing their work at the Mayo Foundation of the university at Rochester. With the extension in medical knowledge and the rise of specialization this work has acquired increased importance.

Relative to the wealth of the state, Minnesota has given large support to higher education, including medicine. Smaller support, which in the aggregate amounts to five millions of dollars, has come to the university for medical work from private sources, mainly from individual donors, but in smaller part from the large foundations.

The State of Minnesota has in the past accepted the principle that each generation should pay its debt to society for the scientific and cultural heritage which it enjoys by adding to the stock of knowledge which is the real groundwork of human wealth. In celebrating the completion of a half century of service to the community in medical education and research, the dominant note was the necessity for sound planning of a program for the future. President Ford expressed the conviction of many when he said, "If ever this nation, this state, this university had a responsibility for supporting science and research in the name of the common welfare, that responsibility is a measure now full and running over by reason of the tragic days just behind and just before the nations who fling from dying hands the torch to us to-day."

M. B. VISSCHER

THE MEDICAL SCHOOL,
UNIVERSITY OF MINNESOTA

# SPECIAL ARTICLES

## TOXIC EFFECTS OF DESOXYCORTICO-STERONE ESTERS IN DOGS[1]

IN the spring of 1939, a number of our patients with Addison's disease who were undergoing treatment with synthetic desoxycorticosterone acetate developed cardiac insufficiency. This varied considerably in degree but was severe in three instances. Furthermore, two patients complained of rapidly progressing weakness and died at home at a time when the blood pressure had been normal and no signs of adrenal insufficiency were recognized.

In view of the implication of these observations, it seemed imperative to study the effect of the protracted administration of synthetic desoxycorticosterone esters in animals. To this end, in July, 1939, two female dogs with carotid loops were selected for the experiment. One of these, S.E., was a normal animal, the other, N., one year before had had a unilateral nephrectomy, and the renal artery to the remaining kidney was slightly constricted by a Goldblatt clamp. The dogs were given the regular maintenance diet, containing some meat, and were injected subcutaneously with 20 mg of desoxycorticosterone acetate[2] in peanut oil daily for 70 days. In addition, two normal male dogs, maintained on a low potassium diet, have also been treated with daily injections of 25 mg of synthetic hormone. After 10 days of treatment in one instance and after 20 days of treatment in the other, both animals have developed changes similar to those shown by the other animals. The results may be summarized as follows:

(1) The changes in the blood constituents are shown in Table 1 and demonstrate a striking decrease in serum potassium, a slight increase in serum sodium, a slight decrease in serum protein and non-protein nitrogen and no definite change in blood sugar or serum calcium.

TABLE 1

| Dog | Date | Na m.eq. per l. | K m.eq. per l. | Non-protein nitrogen mgm per 100 cc | Serum protein per cent. | Blood sugar mgm per 100 cc | Blood pressure mm Hg | Body weight Kgm |
|---|---|---|---|---|---|---|---|---|
| S.E. | Control 7/11 | 145.0 | 4.1 | 27 | . . | 86 | 185 | 17.0 |
| | Maximal effect | 152.1 | 2.2 | 22 | 5.9 | 74 | 205 | 13.1 |
| N. | Control 7/11 | 147.5 | 4.5 | 34 | 6.5 | 80 | 170 | 14.4 |
| | Maximal effect | 158.4 | 2.3 | 25 | 5.8 | 74 | 215 | 10.6 |
| B. | Control 10/20 | 143.9 | 4.3 | 20 | 6.1 | 82 | . . . | 13.0 |
| | Maximal effect | 147.0 | 2.4 | 20 | 5.6 | 93 | . . . | 13.1 |
| P. | Control 10/20 | 146.4 | 4.8 | 23 | 7.3 | 73 | . . . | 16.5 |
| | Maximal effect | 147.6 | 2.5 | 19 | 6.4 | 74 | . . . | 15.1 |

(2) All the dogs have shown curious periodic weakness with inability to stand or raise the head. The tendon reflexes have been active, and when the animals have been able to get on their feet they have held their limbs in marked hyperextension, but have usually been unable to raise their heads, apparently because of flaccidity of the neck muscles. These bouts of paralysis, except for persistence of reflexes, have closely resembled familial periodic paralysis in man, which is also associated with marked decrease in serum potassium. A number of the attacks of paralysis have remitted spontaneously in the course of one to three days, but others have been markedly alleviated in one half to eight hours apparently by the intravenous or oral administration of potassium chloride. (Intravenous dosage up to 1 gram in 2 per cent. solution and oral dosage up to 15 grams in one day). The administration of large doses of KCl appears to protect the animal from paralysis for one to three weeks.

(3) After several weeks of administration of synthetic hormone the ingestion and excretion of water have been definitely augmented. This "diabetes insipidus" has been most apparent at those times when varying degrees of paralysis have been present. The administration of KCl has further emphasized the disturbance of water regulation. The daily urine volume has frequently been in excess of 2.5 liters and has even exceeded 4,000 cc.

(4) X-ray studies of the heart before and at the conclusion of hormone administration showed no increase in cardiac contour. The dogs did not receive large amounts of salt in their diet in addition to hormone in contrast to the patients who developed cardiac dilatation.

(5) Electrocardiographic studies made by Dr. N. Williams showed irregular changes in the T waves, which were perhaps most apparent when the serum potassium content was strikingly decreased.

(6) In the dogs with carotid loops there was a maximal increase in arterial pressure of 45 mm and 20 mm Hg, respectively.

(7) Following the withdrawal of hormone all the abnormalities recorded disappeared in the course of

[1] From the Departments of Medicine and Neurology, College of Physicians and Surgeons, Columbia University, and the Presbyterian Hospital, New York.

[2] Supplied by Roche-Organon, Inc., Nutley, N. J.

three to four days and no manifestations of adrenal insufficiency appeared.

DANIEL KUHLMANN
ROCKEFELLER FOUNDATION FELLOW FROM
UNIVERSITY OF STRASBOURG, FRANCE
CHARLES RAGAN
JOSEPH W. FERREBEE
DANA W. ATCHLEY
ROBERT F. LOEB

## THE ENCEPHALITOGENIC PROPERTY OF HERPES VIRUS[1]

MODIFICATIONS have recently been reported in the virulence of the viruses of human influenza,[2] vaccinia,[3,4] infectious bronchitis of fowls[5] and pseudorabies,[6,7] following cultivation on the chorio-allantois of chick embryos. This communication is to describe an increase in virulence for chick embryos and a reduction in virulence for rabbits which have occurred in a neurotropic strain of herpes simplex (HF, Rockefeller Institute) during 70 serial passages on the chorio-allantois of chick embryos. The technique of establishing and maintaining membranal strains of viruses has been described elsewhere.[8]

The original HF virus on membranes metastasized rarely to the heart and brain. After the twentieth passage it regularly induced metastatic lesions in the heart, liver, lungs, spleen and kidneys of embryos. Lesions in the heart, liver and spleen are grossly visible areas of necrosis. By subinoculation of membranes, embryonic blood was shown to contain virus at 24, 48, 72 and 96 hours. There was no localization of virus in the brain from the blood stream. The lethal effect of infection has increased so that at the 75th passage embryos rarely survived 96 hours, whereas at the tenth, most embryos survived infection 6 or 7 days.

As virulence for chick embryos has increased, it has diminished for the rabbit. After the 25th passage the membranal strain no longer induced a typical keratitis in rabbits. Fifteen rabbits scarified and inoculated on the cornea at intervals between the 25th and 65th membranal generations have shown only slight lacrimation, mild inflammation of conjunctiva without suppuration, no elevation of temperature and no symptoms of encephalitis. This is in contrast to an invariably fatal encephalitis which follows a suppurative keratitis induced by the original strain.

To determine whether or not this modified virus traveled along the fifth nerve from the cornea to the brain without causing encephalitis, two rabbits were inoculated on their right corneas: one with the 50th membranal generation, the other with HF. Corneal reactions typical of each strain developed. The rabbits were killed at 96 hours. The right Gasserian ganglion and brain at the entrance of the fifth nerve were removed from each animal and inoculated onto membranes. Herpes virus transmissible in series was recovered from both the Gasserian ganglion and the brain of the HF control rabbit. Virus could not be demonstrated grossly or microscopically on membranes inoculated with material from the rabbit with the modified virus. This experiment was repeated with the same result using rabbits inoculated with the 53rd generation virus and sacrificed at 96 hours and at 7 days. Material from the medulla of one of these rabbits inoculated intracerebrally into another rabbit induced no symptom.

These experiments led to the conclusion that the HF strain of herpes virus had lost its ability to invade the central nervous system following corneal inoculation in rabbits. A second series of passages through 30 generations over a period of 6 months has not induced a similar modification. Modification of the first strain was observed at the 25th generation 11 months after initiation of the chick strain. Whether the already established modification is a repeatable *Dauermodification* induced by prolonged passage of the virus on chick embryos or a suddenly appearing mutation remains to be determined.

To test the virulence of the modified strain following intracerebral inoculation, suspensions of HF virus (1st membranal generation) and the 62nd membranal generation in dilutions of $10^{-3}$, $10^{-4}$ and $10^{-5}$ were inoculated intracerebrally into rabbits. All 3 rabbits receiving HF virus died within 5 days of herpetic encephalitis. Each rabbit receiving the modified virus had a remarkably delayed elevation of temperature. One ($10^{-4}$) is alive 60 days after inoculation; one ($10^{-3}$) died on the 20th day, and the other ($10^{-5}$) died on the 26th day.

Preliminary experiments indicate that corneal inoculation with the modified strain induces a stable degree of immunity to HF inoculated on the cornea.

KATHERINE ANDERSON
VANDERBILT UNIVERSITY MEDICAL SCHOOL

[1] Aided by a grant from the John and Mary R. Markle Foundation.

[2] F. M. Burnet, *Brit. Jour. Exp. Path.*, 17: 283, 1936.

[3] C. Levaditi, *et al.*, *Revue d'Immunologie*, 4: 481, 1938.

[4] L. Molina, *Zbl. f. Bakt., I. Orig.*, 139: 493, 1937.

[5] F. R. Beaudette (personal communication).

[6] F. M. Burnet, Dora Lush and A. V. Jackson, *Aust. Jour. Exp. Biol. and Med. Sc.*, 17: 35, 1939.

[7] R. E. Glover, *Brit. Jour. Exp. Path. and Med.*, 20: 150, 1939.

[8] E. W. Goodpasture and G. J. Buddingh, *Am. Jour. Hyg.*, 21: 319, 1935.

## THE CHEMICAL COMPOSITION OF SUCKLEYA SUCKLEYANA

FOLLOWING the discovery of hydrocyanic acid in *Suckleya suckleyana* during 1937, together with the experimental work which proved its toxicity to cattle, sheep, rabbits and guinea pigs, the etiology of many of the heretofore unexplained losses in cattle and sheep in eastern Colorado was explained.[1]

[1] Frank Thorp, Jr., A. W. Deem, H. D. Harrington and J. W. Tobiska, *Colo. Exp. Sta. Tech. Bul.*, 22: 1–19, 1937.

This seemed a desirable plant in which to study the factors influencing HCN formation. The chemical composition of *Suckleya suckleyana* and its relation to the toxic properties of the plant is an important physiological problem.[2]

Preliminary studies of the carbohydrate and nitrogen content of poison Suckleya showed the soluble carbohydrates to be chiefly reducing sugars which varied from one per cent. in seedlings to 2.5 per cent. in three-months-old plants. The sucrose content never exceeded 0.25 per cent. at any stage of development studied.

The starch content showed only moderate variation from early June to August.

Close relationship was found between the HCN and reducing sugar content. The HCN varied from a minimum of 0.018 per cent. at the time of minimum sugar content to a maximum of 0.240 per cent. when the sugar was highest.

Young plants contained a higher percentage of protein or colloidal nitrogen than old plants, but the older plants were higher in soluble nitrogen.

The marked reduction of protein nitrogen with advance of the season, accompanied by an equally rapid formation of HCN, is a behavior worthy of further investigation which may help to clarify some of the problems of nitrogen metabolism in plants. It is probable that following the exhaustion of available nitrates from the soil, synthesized proteins may be digested and the nitrogen constituent of the molecule then used in the formation of glucosides which yield HCN upon hydrolysis.

The data showed no accumulation of starch during the period of protein nitrogen diminution but rapid increase of reducing sugars. This relationship between the hexose sugars, colloidal nitrogen, soluble nitrogen and HCN suggests that the presence of available carbohydrates may stimulate the synthesis of the HCN—containing glucoside. The above relationship also suggests that this synthesis probably is not checked by limited nitrates, providing factors have been favorable for liberal protein formation in the early part of the season.

C. G. BARR
H. W. REUSZER
FRANK THORP, JR.
COLORADO AGRICULTURAL EXPERIMENT STATION

## EXPERIMENTAL CHRONIC CADMIUM POISONING[1]

CONTINUED feeding of albino rats with an adequate diet to which cadmium as the chloride had been added has been conducted in this laboratory for the purpose of studying the toxicity of chronically ingested cadmium. The details of this study will be reported elsewhere, but three symptoms of toxicity are so striking and of such importance as to justify a preliminary announcement in addition to the report presented at the twenty-third annual meeting of the Pacific Division of the American Association for the Advancement of Science.

The concentrations of cadmium added to the basic diet were 0.0031, 0.0062, 0.0125, 0.025 and 0.05 per cent. The symptoms of toxicity observed were bleaching of the enamel of the incisor teeth, anemia, and cardiac hypertrophy. The bleaching of the teeth is similar to, if not identical with, that produced by fluorides, and occurred on all dosage levels of cadmium. The degree of bleaching was proportional to the dosage. The anemia was likewise present on all dosage levels of cadmium, the severity increasing with the percentage of cadmium added to the diet. The cardiac hypertrophy was most evident on cadmium concentrations of 0.0062, 0.0125, and 0.025, and less evident on a concentration of 0.05 because the rats died before the hypertrophy could fully develop. Since the cardiac hypertrophy was not limited to the left ventricle, it is believed that the anemia rather than hypertension resulting from kidney damage was the causative factor.

ROBERT H. WILSON
FLOYD DEEDS
BUREAU OF AGRICULTURAL CHEMISTRY AND ENGINEERING, U. S. DEPARTMENT OF AGRICULTURE, AT THE DEPARTMENT OF PHARMACOLOGY, STANFORD UNIVERSITY SCHOOL OF MEDICINE

[1] Food Research Division Contribution No. 455.

[2] A paper presented at the Virginia meeting of the American Society of Plant Physiologists.

## BOOKS RECEIVED

HENDRICK, IVES. *Facts and Theories of Psychoanalysis.* Second edition, revised. Pp. xiv + 369 + xv. Knopf. $3.00.

HERZBERG, GERHARD. *Molecular Spectra and Molecular Structure; I, Diatomic Molecules.* Pp. xxviii + 592. 181 figures. Prentice-Hall. $6.50.

*Palao Tropical Biological Station Studies, No. 4; A List of the Fishes of the Palao Islands, and Other Papers.* Pp. 523–694. Illustrated. Japan Society for the Promotion of Scientific Research, Tokyo.

*Texas Agricultural Experiment Station: Fifty-first Annual Report, 1938.* Pp. 281. Agricultural and Mechanical College of Texas.

*University of Illinois Bulletin; Papers Presented at the Fifth Short Course in Coal Utilization, Held at the University of Illinois, May, 1939.* Pp. 173. Illustrated. The University. $0.50.

*Vitamin E.* A Symposium Held Under the Auspices of the Food Group (Nutrition Panel) of the Society of Chemical Industry, April, 1939, at the School of Hygiene and Tropical Medicine, London. Pp. viii + 88. The Society. 5/–.

*Zoologica; Scientific Contributions of the New York Zoological Society.* Pp. 265–384. Illustrated. The Society.

SCIENCE

Vol. 90 | Friday, December 1, 1939 | No. 2344

*The American Association for the Advancement of Science:*
*Preliminary Announcement of the Columbus, Ohio, Meeting:* Edited by Dr. F. R. Moulton ... 499

*Scientific Events:*
*The Platform of the American Medical Association; Inter-American Society of Microbiology; Activities of the U. S. Geological Survey; Award of the Egleston Medals of the School of Engineering of Columbia University; Recent Deaths and Memorials* ... 507

*Scientific Notes and News* ... 510

*Discussion:*
*A Dozen Mathematical Errors in the "Encyclopaedia Britannica":* Professor G. A. Miller. *A Remarkable Example of Polar Mirage:* Professor William H. Hobbs. *Index to Schoolcraft's "Indian Tribes":* M. W. Stirling. *Available Lectures in Geology and Geography:* Professor Chester R. Longwell ... 512

*Scientific Books:*
*Developments in Physics:* Dr. C. G. Montgomery. *Physiological Phenomena:* Dr. Walter B. Cannon 514

*Special Articles:*
*Sperm Agglutination in the Keyhole Limpet and the Sea-urchin:* Professor Albert Tyler and Sidney W. Fox. *The Control of Experimental Alcaptonuria by Means of Vitamin C:* Dr. Robert R. Sealock and Hannah E. Silberstein. *Some Crystalline Constituents of the Non-saponifiable Fraction of Bone Marrow:* Professor Harry N. Holmes and Ruth E. Corbet ... 516

*Scientific Apparatus and Laboratory Methods:*
*Latex Emulsions in Human Vascular Preparations:* Professor Oscar V. Batson. *Liquid Latex as an Injection Mass for Blood-vessels:* Dr. D. L. Gamble 518

*Science News* ... 10

SCIENCE: A Weekly Journal devoted to the Advancement of Science, edited by J. McKeen Cattell and published every Friday by

THE SCIENCE PRESS
New York City: Grand Central Terminal
Lancaster, Pa. Garrison, N. Y.

Annual Subscription, $6.00 Single Copies, 15 Cts.

SCIENCE is the official organ of the American Association for the Advancement of Science. Information regarding membership in the Association may be secured from the office of the permanent secretary in the Smithsonian Institution Building, Washington, D. C.

# THE AMERICAN ASSOCIATION FOR THE ADVANCEMENT OF SCIENCE

## PRELIMINARY ANNOUNCEMENT OF THE COLUMBUS, OHIO, MEETING

**Edited by Dr. F. R. MOULTON**
PERMANENT SECRETARY

From next December 27 to January 2 the association and about 30 of its affiliated and associated societies will meet in Columbus, Ohio. This will be the one hundred fifth meeting of the association.

Columbus, the capital of Ohio, is a city of approximately 500,000 inhabitants situated near the center of the state and the center of population of the country. It is the seat of the Ohio State University, which has more than 17,000 students. Although the university has a campus of nearly 400 acres, most of its fifty buildings are within three miles of the business and hotel district of the city. A number of other state institutions and the Ohio Wesleyan University, located at Delaware only twenty-three miles distant, add to the large scientific population of the region. Moreover, Ohio is noted for having perhaps more colleges than any other equal area in the world.

### Registration

Registration will be in the Civic Auditorium, which is only a few blocks from the Deshler-Wallick Hotel, the headquarters of the meeting. The Annual Science Exhibition and social center of the meeting will also be in the same building.

Each person registering will receive a General Program of the meeting and a badge of admission to the address of the retiring president and to other general sessions. The General Program contains the programs of all sections and societies and their places and times of meeting, a schedule of all general sessions, a list of all symposia, a catalogue of exhibits in the annual science exhibition, a schedule of all dinners, luncheons, social functions and excursions, and an alphabetical list of all persons who present addresses, papers or exhibitions during the meeting. Since about 200 scientific sessions will be held, before which at least 1,600 addresses and papers will be presented, a well-organized general program is necessary for a person to make best use of the precious hours he will be among his fellow scientists in Columbus.

Although the registration fee is only $1, there has been a tendency for the members of some affiliated societies to neglect to register at the meetings. With the growing complexity of science and the increasing importance of the inter-relations of science, scientists owe it to themselves, even from the most selfish point of view, to mingle widely with their fellow scientists. And quite apart from their own direct interests, they owe a heavier responsibility to our civilization than ever before. The British Association for the Advancement of Science requires a person to register before he may attend any sessions whatever of the meeting, and the registration fee is about $10!

### Hotels and Headquarters

*General Headquarters:* Deshler-Wallick Hotel.

Headquarters of the sections of the association and of the affiliated and associated societies meeting with the association in Columbus are as follows:

*Deshler-Wallick:* All sections of the association except G and O, American Physical Society, American Association of Physics Teachers, Sigma Pi Sigma, American Society of Zoologists, American Association of Economic Entomologists, Entomological Society of America, American Society of Parasitologists, American Society of Naturalists, American Microscopical Society, Metric Association, American Science Teachers Association, Society of the Sigma Xi, United Chapters of Phi Beta Kappa, Honor Society of Phi Kappa Phi and Pi Gamma Mu. Rates: with bath—single, $3–$7; double, $5–$10.

*Neil House:* Section on Botanical Sciences (G), Botanical Society of America, American Phytopathological Society, American Society of Plant Physiologists, Mycological Society of America, Sullivant Moss Society, American Fern Society, Genetics Society of America, National Association of Biology Teachers. Rates: with bath—single, $3–$5; double, $4.50–$7.

*Fort Hayes:* Section on Agriculture (O), Ecological Society of America, Limnological Society of America, Phi Sigma Society, American Society of Agronomy, Potato Association of America, Gamma Alpha Graduate Scientific Fraternity. Rates: with bath—single, $2 and up; double, $3.50 and up.

*Chittenden:* American Meteorological Society, Society for Research on Meteorites, American Nature Study Society, History of Science Society, American Mathematical Society, Mathematical Association of America, National Council of Teachers of Mathematics. Rates: with bath—single, $2.50–$3; double, $3.50–$4.50; without bath—single, $1.50–$2.50; double, $2.50–$3.50.

### Other Hotels in Columbus

*Seneca:* Rates: with bath—single, $2; double, $3.50–$6.

*Southern:* Rates: with bath—single, $2.50–$3; double, $3.50–$4.50; without bath—single, $1.50–$1.75; double, $2.50–$2.75.

*Virginia:* Rates: with bath—single, $2 and up; double, $3–$4; without bath—single, $1.50; double, $2.50.

*Broad-Lincoln:* Rates: with bath—single, $2 and up; double, $3–$4.50.

*Note:* The Deshler-Wallick Hotel has available large-capacity rooms with combination tub and shower and single beds; three persons in a room, $2.50 per person per day; for four persons in a room, $2 per person per day.

The mathematical societies, the American Society for Horticultural Science and Sigma Delta Epsilon Graduate Women's Scientific Fraternity have arranged for rooms in dormitory buildings on the campus of the Ohio State University. Information about these rooms will be contained in announcements from the societies named.

### Transportation

Columbus is at the almost exact geographical center of Ohio, and it is about 200 miles east of the center of population of the United States. Columbus may be reached conveniently by railroad, by airplane or by bus. Forty highways pass through Columbus, 15 divisions of five trunk-line railways serve the city, and there is airplane service on two lines.

Railway fares have been substantially reduced this year, both for one-way tickets and for round-trip tickets. Special fares will be in effect during the period of the meeting, information respecting which and time schedules may be obtained from local agents of transportation companies. At the present fares, round-trip railroad tickets to Columbus, exclusive of Pullman fares, from representative cities are as follows: Baltimore, $28.25; Boston, $44.70; Chicago, $18.30; New York, $35.40; Philadelphia, $30.70; Washington, $28.25; Atlanta, $28.50; New Orleans, $44.80; San Francisco, $109.20.

### Official Meetings

*The Executive Committee* of the association, to which matters for the council are first submitted, will meet at 10:00 A.M. on Wednesday, December 27, in the permanent secretary's rooms in the Deshler-Wallick Hotel, and thereafter as may be arranged. The council of the association will meet at 2:00 P.M. on Wednesday, December 27, in the Wallick Suite of the Deshler-Wallick Hotel and thereafter as may be arranged. The council will elect a president and other officers of the association at a meeting that will be held in the Wallick Suite at 9:00 A.M. on Saturday, December 30.

*The Academy Conference* will be held at 3:00 P.M. on Wednesday in the Wallick Suite of the Deshler-Wallick Hotel. The conference will be followed by a complimentary dinner to one representative of each affiliated academy and to designated representatives of the association.

*The Secretaries Conference* will be held at 9:15 on Friday evening in the Wallick Suite of the Deshler-Wallick Hotel. The secretaries of the sections of the association and of all affiliated and associated societies are invited to attend.

### ANNUAL SCIENCE EXHIBITION

The annual science exhibition, which will be housed in the Civic Auditorium within five minutes' walk of the principal hotels, will include exhibits both of research laboratories and of manufacturers of scientific apparatus, equipment and supplies. In addition, the outstanding books on science published during 1939 will be on display and available for examination. Interesting and important scientific motion-picture films will be exhibited adjacent to the science exhibition.

### SYMPOSIA AND JOINT SESSIONS

Recent meetings of the association have been distinguished by comprehensive symposia organized by the sections and cooperating societies. The Columbus meeting will maintain the high level of previous meetings. Among the symposia that promise to be of importance and wide interest are those on "Isotopes" and "Photosynthesis," organized by the Section on Chemistry; "Speciation," organized by the American Society of Zoologists, in cooperation with the Genetics Society of America; "The Relation of Ecology to Human Welfare," organized by the Ecological Society of America; "Defense Mechanisms in Plants and Animals," organized by the American Society of Naturalists; "The Internal Environment and Behavior," organized by the Section on Psychology; "Effects of Science upon Human Beings," organized by Alan Gregg for the Section on the Social and Economic Sciences; and "Blood, Heart and Circulation," organized by the Section on Medical Sciences. For a complete list of symposia and joint sessions consult the programs of the sections and societies which follow.

The association is publishing symposia that are "of such high order of scientific merit that it can not afford not to publish them." It has published several in the field of public health on such subjects as "The Cancer Problem," "Tuberculosis and Leprosy," "Syphilis" and "Mental Health," with "The Gonococcus and Gonococcal Infection" now in press. Each of these symposia has added to the value and prestige of the previous ones, and the officers of the association look with satisfaction on others to follow on such subjects as "Blood, Heart and Circulation" (the Columbus Meeting) and "Malaria" (the Philadelphia Meeting). It is desired that other sections and societies, especially those in the broad fields of biology, will even more vigorously than in the past formulate plans for series of symposia of the highest character in respect to organization, participants, character of contributed papers and comprehensiveness with the hope that they will be published by the association. The success of the symposium on "Problems of Lake Biology" (now in press), organized by the Limnological Society of America, is a promise of the welcome that they will receive. In organizing, presenting and publishing such symposia, the societies concerned and the association will fulfil their primary purposes.

### GENERAL SESSIONS

All evening general sessions will be held at 8:15 in Memorial Hall, which has a seating capacity of 3,500 persons. The places at which other general sessions will be held are stated in connection with their announcement.

*Wednesday evening, December 27.* Dr. Wesley C. Mitchell, of Columbia University, will deliver an address as retiring president of the association on "The Public Relations of Science."

*Thursday evening, December 28.* The annual address under the joint sponsorship of the association and the Society of the Sigma Xi will be delivered by Dr. Kirtley F. Mather, of Harvard University, on "The Future of Man as an Inhabitant of the Earth."

*Friday, December 29.* At 4:30 P.M. Dr. Julian Huxley, of London, England, will deliver the first address in America under the arrangement with the British Association for the Advancement of Science for exchange lectures on alternate years. His address, on "Science, War and Reconstruction," will be delivered in the Chapel in University Hall.

*Friday evening, December 29.* The annual address under the auspices of the United Chapters of Phi Beta Kappa will be delivered by Dean Marjorie Nicolson, of Smith College, on "Science and Literature."

### BREAKFASTS, LUNCHEONS AND DINNERS

*Wednesday, December 27*

*Luncheon:* American Meteorological Society.

*Dinners:* Section on Chemistry. Ecological Society of America.

*Thursday, December 28*

*Luncheons:* Gamma Alpha. Sigma Delta Epsilon.

*Dinners:* American Mathematical Society and The Mathematical Association of America. Section on Chemistry. American Association of Economic Entomologists and The Entomological Society of America. The American Phytopathological Society. American Society of Plant Physiologists. Joint dinner by Section on Psychology and Section on Education. Biologists' Smoker.

*Friday, December 29*

*Breakfasts:* Phi Kappa Phi. Sigma Delta Epsilon.

*Luncheons:* American Astronomical Society. American Society of Parasitologists. Genetics Society of America. American Nature Study Society. Pi Gamma Mu. Sigma Pi Sigma.

*Dinners:* American Astronomical Society. American Society of Zoologists. Section on Teaching of American Association of Economic Entomologists. The Botanical Society of America and all botanists. National Association of Biology Teachers. American Society for Horticultural Science.

*Saturday, December 30*

*Luncheon:* Subsection on Dentistry.

*Dinners:* American Society of Naturalists. Phi Sigma Society.

## SECTION AND SOCIETY PROGRAMS

*Section on Mathematics and Affiliated Societies.* On Thursday morning the section will hold a joint session with the American Mathematical Society, at which J. R. Kline, retiring chairman of the section and vice-president of the association, will deliver an address on "The Jordan Curve Theorem." On Thursday evening the Section on Mathematics, the American Mathematical Society and The Mathematical Association of America will hold a joint dinner. On Friday morning the Section on Mathematics, the Section on Geology and Geography and the American Mathematical Society will hold a joint session on "Applications of Mathematics to Geological and Geophysical Problems."

The American Mathematical Society will hold a session on Thursday afternoon, before which D. H. Lehmer will deliver an invited address on "The Applications of Bernoulli Polynomials to Some Problems in Diophantine Analysis."

On Wednesday afternoon at 4:30 the J. Willard Gibbs annual lecture will be delivered by Theodor von Kármán on "Grappling with Non-linear Problems."

The Mathematical Association of America will hold sessions on Friday afternoon and Saturday morning, with addresses by W. B. Carver and T. C. Frye on "The New Mathematical Reviews." Papers will also be presented by Henry Blumberg, Saunders MacLane, G. T. Whyburn and E. F. Beckenbach. On Friday afternoon the Mathematical Association of America and the National Council of Teachers of Mathematics will hold a joint session for discussing subjects of common interest.

*Section on Physics and Affiliated Societies.* On Friday afternoon the section will hold a joint session with the American Physical Society and the American Association of Physics Teachers at which Herbert E. Ives, retiring chairman of the association, and John T. Tate, president of the American Physical Society, will deliver addresses.

The American Physical Society will hold its forty-first annual meeting (its 232d regular meeting) from Thursday to Saturday, inclusive. The society and the American Association of Physics Teachers will hold a joint dinner on Friday evening.

The American Association of Physics Teachers will hold sessions from Wednesday to Friday, inclusive. The American Meteorological Society will hold sessions on Wednesday and Thursday, the principal feature of which will be a program on "Rainfall and Evaporation in Relation to Run-off and Floods." A luncheon of the society will be held on Wednesday. The honorary society in physics, Sigma Pi Sigma, will hold a luncheon on Friday.

*The Section on Chemistry.* The section will hold sessions all day Wednesday and Thursday and on Friday morning, and will have its annual dinner on Wednesday evening in honor of the retiring vice-president of the section, Harold C. Urey, to which all friends of Dr. Urey are invited. On Thursday evening there will be a dinner especially for those interested in the symposium on "Photosynthesis," following which there will be a round-table discussion of the papers presented at the symposium. It is requested that those planning to attend either or both of these dinners notify, previous to the meeting, Dr. A. B. Garrett, Ohio State University, Columbus. The program of the symposium on "Isotopes," which will be held on Wednesday, beginning at 9 A.M., is as follows:

### ISOTOPES

1. The Dependence of Physical and Chemical Properties on Mass, and the Separation of Isotopes. H. C. UREY.
2. The Nitrogen and Carbon Heavy Isotopes in Kinetic Research. H. S. TAYLOR.
3. The Electrical Separation of Isotopes in Quantity. LLOYD P. SMITH.
4. Measurement of Isotopic Abundances in the Heavy Elements. A. J. DEMPSTER.
5. Methods of Increasing the Efficiency in Thermal Separation of Isotopes. A. KEITH BREWER.
6. Thermal Separation of Isotopes. W. W. WATSON.
7. The Atomic Masses of the Lighter Isotopes. K. T. BAINBRIDGE.
8. Accurate Determinations of the Relative Abundances of Isotopes. A. O. C. NIER.

The program of the symposium on "Photosynthesis," which will be held on Thursday at 9 A.M., is as follows:

PHOTOSYNTHESIS

1. Introductory remarks. CHARLES FRANKLIN KETTERING.

2. Induction and Related Phenomena. E. D. MCALISTER.

3. The Efficiency of Photosynthesis. FARRINGTON DANIELS.

4. The Absorption of Radiant Energy by Leaves. W. E. LOOMIS.

5. Relation of Photo-Oxidation to Solarization. J. E. MEYERS and G. O. BURR.

6. A brief review of Certain Investigations on Chlorophyll and Photosynthesis at the C. F. Kettering Laboratories. O. L. INMAN.

7. Factors Influencing the Apparent Efficiency of Photosynthesis. ROBERT EMERSON.

8. The Growth of Plants under Artificial Light. JOHN M. ARTHUR.

9. On the Purification of the Chlorophyll Components. F. P. ZSCHEILE.

10. Relative Amounts of Photosynthesis in the Yellow, Green, and Blue Mercury Lines. G. RICHARD BURNS.

11. Variations in the Daily Rate of Photosynthesis in Mature Apple Trees during Four Successive Seasons. A. J. HEINICKE.

12. A Contribution to the Theory of Photosynthesis. JAMES FRANCK.

13. Chlorophyll as the Prosthetic Group of a Protein in the Green Leaf. EMIL L. SMITH.

14. The Physico-Chemical Properties of Chlorophyll in their Relation to Photosynthesis. EUGEN RABINOWITCH.

On Friday at 9 A.M. a session will be held at which 12 papers on a variety of subjects will be presented.

*Section on Astronomy and Affiliated Societies.* The section and its affiliated societies will meet from Wednesday to Saturday, inclusive. The sessions on Wednesday will be held at the Ohio State University and those on Thursday and on Friday morning at the Ohio Wesleyan University, at Delaware. On Friday afternoon, at the Ohio State University, R. M. Stewart will deliver an address at a joint meeting of the section and the American Astronomical Society as retiring chairman of the section and vice-president of the association. On Saturday morning the section will hold a joint session with the Society for Research on Meteorites. On Saturday and Sunday the Observatory of the Ohio Wesleyan University will be host to members and guests of the A. A. A. S. irrespective of their section affiliations.

*Section on Geology and Geography and Affiliated Societies.* The section and the Geological Society of America, in collaboration with the Section on Geology of the Ohio Academy of Science, will hold eight sessions, before which approximately 50 papers will be presented, including two joint sessions, one with the Section on Mathematics and one with the Section on Astronomy and The Society for Research on Meteorites. The general topic of the papers which will be presented on Wednesday morning is "Geomorphic and Glacial Problems on the Appalachian West Slope." On Wednesday afternoon Walter H. Bucher will deliver his address as retiring chairman of the section and vice-president of the association on "Problems of the North Atlantic Ocean." Dr. Bucher's address will be followed by a session for the presentation of papers on "The Non-Metallic Mineral Industry." The topic which will be discussed on Thursday morning is "Methods and Problems in the Teaching of Elementary Geology." On Thursday afternoon the subject for discussion is "Current Research in the Paleozoic Stratigraphy of the Ohio Basin." On Friday morning the section will hold a joint session with the Section on Mathematics and The Mathematical Society of America on "Applications of Mathematics in the Earth's Sciences." At the same time a joint session will be held with the Society for Research on Meteorites on "Meteorite Falls and the Rate of Accretion." The subject for discussion on Friday afternoon is "Hydrologic Problems in the Ohio and Michigan Basins." Among the speakers representing the section in the joint sessions are Walter D. Lambert, Lachlan Gilchrist, M. M. Slotnick, Archie Blake and Fletcher Watson.

*Section on Zoological Sciences and Affiliated Societies.* No section has stronger or more active affiliated societies than has Section F. Consequently, in order to serve most effectively the interests of zoology, the section gives way to the American Society of Zoologists, the Entomological Society of America, the American Association of Economic Entomologists and the American Society of Parasitologists in organizing programs in the field of the zoological sciences.

The American Society of Zoologists will hold sessions on Thursday, Friday and Saturday, at which approximately 300 papers will be presented. On Thursday afternoon the society will join with the Genetics Society of America in the presentation of a symposium on "Speciation," organized by Th. Dobzhansky, at which papers will be presented by Sewall Wright, E. M. Mayr, L. R. Dice, Warren P. Spencer and Th. Dobzhansky. On Friday morning the society will present a symposium on "Experimental Study of Cellular Organization," at which Robert Chambers, L. V. Heilbrunn, Daniel Mazia, M. H. Jacobs and Francis O. Schmitt will present papers. On Saturday afternoon the society will join with the American Society of Naturalists in sponsoring a symposium, organized by W. H. Taliaferro, on "Defense Mechanisms in Plants and Animals," at which papers will be presented by F. W. Went, W. C. Price and William Bloom. On Thursday evening, at 9 o'clock, the society will join with the American Society of

Naturalists and the members of other biological societies in the Biologists' Smoker. The annual dinner of the society, to which all zoologists and friends are invited, will be held on Friday evening, at which Wesley R. Coe, retiring chairman of the section and vice-president of the association, will deliver an address on "Divergent Pathways in Functional Development."

The Entomological Society of America will hold its thirty-fourth annual meeting on Wednesday, Thursday and Friday. On Wednesday afternoon the society will join with the American Association of Economic Entomologists in a symposium on "Fifty Years of Entomological Progress." On Thursday morning the society will hold a joint session with the Ecological Society of America, at which the papers will be devoted to insect ecology. The annual public address of the society will be delivered by A. Avinoff on "Adventures of a Lepidopterist in Jamaica," which will be illustrated by colored motion pictures and Kodachrome slides. On Thursday evening the society will join with the American Association of Economic Entomologists in the Entomologists' dinner. The other sessions of the society on Wednesday morning, Thursday afternoon and Friday will be devoted to papers by members of the society in the general field of entomology.

The American Association of Economic Entomologists will hold sessions from Wednesday to Saturday, inclusive, at which a total of 112 papers will be presented. In celebration of the fiftieth anniversary of the founding of the society, a symposium will be held jointly with the Entomological Society of America on "Fifty Years of Entomological Progress," with Herbert Osborn presiding. Papers will be presented on this program, each devoted to a period of ten years, by C. L. Marlatt, Lawson Caesar, C. L. Metcalf, E. O. Essig and S. A. Rohwer. The presidential address of the society will be delivered by E. R. Sasscer on "Undesirable Insect Aliens." The banquet of the society will be held on Thursday evening. On Friday morning the society will hold a joint symposium with the Section on Plant Quarantine and Inspection of the American Association of Economic Entomologists and the American Phytopathological Society on "Viruses and Plant Quarantine." On Friday evening the society's Section on Teaching will hold a dinner at the Southern Hotel, followed by a session at the Deshler-Wallick Hotel.

The American Society of Parasitologists will hold sessions on Thursday, Friday and Saturday, at which 77 papers and demonstrations will be presented, this being the largest program in the history of the society. At the sessions on Friday afternoon 33 papers will be presented on a demonstration program representing all fields of parasitology. On Thursday afternoon Cornelius B. Philip, United States Public Health Service, will show a thirty-minute colored motion-picture film on "How Rocky Mountain Spotted Fever Vaccine Is Prepared and Used." On Friday morning Horace W. Stunkard, president of the society, will deliver an address on "Life History Studies and the Development of Parasitology." On Friday at 12 o'clock a parasitologist luncheon will be held in Pomerene Hall of the Ohio State University, following which the society will hold its annual business meeting.

*Section on Botanical Sciences and its Affiliated Societies.* The section and its affiliated societies will meet from Thursday to Saturday, inclusive. On Thursday at 2 P.M. Raymond J. Pool, retiring chairman of the section and vice-president of the association, will deliver an address on "White Man versus the Prairie." This address will be followed by a paper on "Problems in Breeding for Disease Resistance," by Donald Reddick, another on "Recent Investigations in the Cytogenetics of Maize," by Barbara McClintock, and one on "The Communal Nature of the Fruiting Process in the Acrasieae," by Kenneth B. Raper.

The Botanical Society of America will hold meetings of its General, Paleobotanical, Systematic and Physiological sections on Thursday, Friday and Saturday mornings. On Thursday afternoon the society will hold a joint session with the other botanical societies. On Friday afternoon the Physiological Section of the society will hold a joint session with the American Society for Horticultural Science and the American Society of Plant Physiologists. Also on Friday afternoon, the General Section of the society will hold a joint session with the Ecological Society of America. On Friday evening the society will join in its annual dinner for all botanists, at which Arthur J. Eames, retiring president of the society, will deliver an address. On Saturday afternoon the society will join in the symposium on "Defense Mechanisms in Plants and Animals" organized by the American Society of Naturalists.

The American Phytopathological Society will hold its thirty-first annual meeting from Wednesday to Saturday, inclusive, at which approximately 120 papers will be presented. The first session of the society will be held on Wednesday afternoon. Among the papers presented at this session will be one on "The Influence of Ultraviolet Irradiation on the Pathogenicity of *Phytomonas tumefaciens*" by B. M. Duggar and A. J. Riker. On Wednesday evening at 7:15 the society will hold a "Plant Disease Survey," and at 8:15 P.M. a second conference on "The Resistance of Plants to Diseases," the latter under the chairmanship of E. C. Stakman. On Thursday morning three sectional meetings of the society will be held, one on "Diseases of Fruits," another on "Diseases of Small Grain Crops," and the third on "Diseases of Southern and Miscellaneous Crops." On Thursday afternoon the society will hold a joint session with the

Section on Botanical Sciences and its other affiliated societies. Also on Thursday afternoon the Extension Plant Pathologists will hold a conference on "Fire Blight of Apple and Pear." On Thursday evening the society will hold its annual dinner at 6:30 o'clock in the Neil House. On Friday morning the society will hold a joint session with the American Association of Economic Entomologists. Also on Friday morning the society will hold three sectional meetings, one on "Virus and Tobacco Diseases," the second on "Diseases of Vegetables," and the third on "Fungicides and Diseases of Cherries." On Friday afternoon the society will hold a round-table conference on "Laboratory Testing of Fungicides," during which such subjects as standardization of the fungus and factors involved in deposition of sprays will be considered. On Friday evening a conference will be held on "Eradicant Fungicides," with reports on old and new eradicant fungicides by G. W. Keitt, H. W. Anderson, R. C. Baines and E. E. Wilson. On Saturday morning the society will hold a joint session with the Potato Association of America. Also on Saturday morning the society will hold a joint session with the Floriculture Section of the American Society for Horticultural Science on "The Diseases of Ornamental Plants." A third joint session will be held on Saturday morning with the Mycological Society of America. A fourth joint session will be held on Saturday morning with the Society of American Foresters on "The Diseases of Trees." On Saturday afternoon the society will hold a joint session with the Physiological Section of the Botanical Society of America and the American Society of Plant Physiologists on "Cotton Diseases and the Relation of Physiology to Disease." Two distinguished foreign scientists will appear on the program of the society, Dr. Jean Dufrenoy, of Corrèze, France, and Dr. A. A. Bitancourt, of São Paulo, Brazil. Special attention is called to the fact that the society has made arrangements for a display of phytopathological exhibit material during the meetings. Pathologists who desire to exhibit material are requested to communicate with Dr. A. L. Pierstorff, Ohio State University.

The American Society of Plant Physiologists will hold sessions from Thursday to Saturday, inclusive. On Thursday afternoon the society will hold a joint session with the Section on Botanical Sciences, the Botanical Society of America and the American Phytopathological Society. On Thursday evening the society will hold its annual dinner at which the presidential address will be delivered by W. F. Loehwing and the Charles Reid Barnes life membership award will be announced. On Friday morning the society will hold a session for the presentation of papers and on Friday afternoon a joint symposium with the American Society for Horticultural Science on "Physiological Processes of Plants in Relation to Temperature." On Friday evening the society will join in the dinner for all botanists. Following the dinner a symposium will be held under the chairmanship of O. F. Curtis on "The Teaching of Plant Physiology." On Saturday morning a session will be held for the presentation of general papers. On Saturday afternoon the session will be held in two sections, the second of which will be a joint symposium with the American Phytopathological Society and the Physiological Section of the Botanical Society of America on "Cotton."

The Mycological Society of America will meet from Thursday to Saturday, inclusive. On Thursday morning the address of the retiring president of the society will be delivered, following which will be a regular program, including papers on new fungi from the northwest and Bermuda, fungi parasitic on man, fungi parasitic on plants, and several papers on morphology, physiology and genetics of fungi. On Thursday afternoon the society will hold a joint meeting with the Section on Botanical Sciences, and on Saturday morning it will present a joint program with the American Phytopathological Society.

The American Fern Society will hold its annual meeting on Saturday morning, at which Robert T. Clausen, president of the society, will deliver an address.

*Societies Affiliated with the Sections on Zoological Sciences and Botanical Sciences.* The American Society of Naturalists will hold its fifty-seventh annual meeting on Thursday afternoon, at which, in cooperation with the American Society of Zoologists, the Botanical Society of America and the Genetics Society of America, it will present a symposium on "Defense Mechanisms in Plants and Animals." The program consists of three formal papers; "Local Reactions in Plants," by F. W. Went; "Generalized Reactions in Plants," by W. C. Price; and "Local and Generalized Reactions in Animals," by William Bloom. The annual business meeting will follow the symposium, and the Naturalists' Dinner will be held at 6:30 in the evening, at which the presidential address will be delivered by Ivey F. Lewis on "Cell Reactions."

*The Ecological Society of America* will meet from Wednesday to Saturday, inclusive. The program for Wednesday morning consists of a business meeting and a general session for animal ecologists. On Wednesday afternoon the society will present a symposium on "The Relation of Ecology to Human Welfare," Charles C. Adams presiding. The participants in the symposium are Homer L. Shantz, C. W. Thornthwaite, Benton MacKaye, Robert E. Park, A. B. Hollingshead and E. C. Lindeman. The society will hold a banquet on Wednesday evening, at which the retiring president, Charles T. Vorhies, and A. H. Wright will speak. On Thursday morning the society will hold a joint session with the Entomological Society of America and also a general session for animal ecologists. On Thursday afternoon, in addition to a session on animal ecology, there will be a meeting, at 4 o'clock, of the Committee on the Preservation of Natural Conditions. On Friday morning the society will hold a general session, a joint session with the Botanical Society of America and a joint session with the Limnological Society of America.

The American Microscopical Society will hold its fifty-eighth annual meeting on Thursday afternoon. The formal session will consist of a meeting of the executive committee, followed by the annual meeting of the society.

The Genetics Society of America will meet from Thursday to Saturday, inclusive. On Thursday it will join the American Society of Zoologists in a symposium on "Speciation," and on Saturday it will join the American Society of Naturalists and other societies in a symposium on "Defense Mechanisms in Plants and Animals." On Friday the society will present an invitation program at which the speakers will be Karl Sax, L. C. Dunn, M. R. Irwin, M. Gordon and B. P. Kaufman.

The Limnological Society of America will hold its fifth annual meeting on Thursday to Saturday, inclusive. It is planned to have at least three half-day sessions for the presentation of papers. On Friday forenoon the society will hold a joint meeting with the Ecological Society of America and will provide about one half the program.

Phi Sigma Society will hold sessions on Friday and Saturday. The speakers on the scientific programs will be student members of the society. A banquet will be held on Saturday evening, at which Paul B. Sears will deliver an address on "The Scientist as a Citizen."

The National Association of Biology Teachers will meet on Friday, both morning and afternoon, and will hold a dinner in the evening.

*The Section on Anthropology* will hold a one-day session on Wednesday at the Museum of the Ohio State Archaeological and Historical Society. Papers will center on the theme of the North American Indians and their archeological cultures. The address of the retiring chairman of the section, Diamond Jenness, will be on "Canada's Indian Problems." Section members will be shown the Museum by Director H. C. Shetrone and will inspect the recently established Lithic Laboratory. At the conclusion of the sessions adjournment will be to the Chicago meeting of the American Anthropological Association.

*The Section on Psychology* will hold sessions from Wednesday to Friday, inclusive. Besides several sessions for the presentation of general papers, there will be a symposium on Thursday morning on "The Internal Environment and Behavior," under the chairmanship of Ross A. McFarland. In this symposium, the effect of changes in the blood stream on the brain and consequent alterations in behavior will be discussed. Special emphasis will be given to the effect of alterations in temperature, oxygen, blood sugar and the endocrines. Also on Thursday, there will be a joint session with the Section on Education and a joint dinner with the same section, at which J. F. Dashiell will speak on "A Neglected Fourth Dimension to Psychological Research."

*The Program of the Section on the Social and Economic Sciences* will consist of three parts, a session on Friday under the chairmanship of Alan Gregg, a conference under the sponsorship of the American Association of Scientific Workers on "Science and the Public," and a luncheon by Pi Gamma Mu on Wednesday, at which officers of the association will speak.

*The Program of the Section on Engineering* will consist in part of a session by the Institute of Radio Engineers.

*The Section on Medical Sciences* will present a program, consisting of six sessions for the presentation of a symposium, on "Blood, Heart and Circulation," and a joint session with the biological societies sponsoring the symposium on "Defense Mechanisms in Plants and Animals." The subjects of the six divisions of the symposium on "Blood, Heart and Circulation" are: "Blood"; "The Physiology of Coronary Blood Flow"; "Pathology of the Coronary Circulation"; "Cardiac Failure"; "Hypertension," and "Heart and Circulation in Special Territories." On Thursday morning the address of Carl J. Wiggers, retiring chairman of the section and vice-president of the association, will be delivered on "Pathways of Natural Progress." On Thursday afternoon the Theobald Smith Award in Medicine will be presented to Albert B. Sabin by Walter B. Cannon, president of the association, following which Dr. Sabin will deliver an address entitled "Constitutional Barriers to Involvement of the Nervous System by Certain Viruses."

*The Subsection on Pharmacy of the Section on Medical Sciences* will hold a session on Wednesday morning at which five papers will be presented, and another on Wednesday afternoon at which four papers will be presented. The papers for the morning program are: "The Chemistry of the Viburnums," by Justin L. Powers; "Methenamine Mandelate: Preparation, Toxicity, and Antiseptic Value," by Glenn L. Jenkins; "The Bioassay of Aconite," by B. V. Christensen and J. W. Nelson; "The Use of Oral Vaccine in the Prophylaxis of the Common Cold," by Leonard J. Piccoli; and "Solanum Carolinense," by R. L. Murray. The papers for the afternoon session are: "A Method for the Determination of Peptic Activity," by Carl J. Klemme and Lee F. Worrell; "Employee Predictive Tests," by C. M. Brown; "The Pharmacology of Soaps," by Leroy D. Edwards; and "A Criterion for Distinguishing between Virgin and Parous Animals," by Richard A. Deno.

*The Subsection on Dentistry of the Section on Medical Sciences* will hold a session on Thursday, at which papers will be presented on "Definite Oral Manifestations in Systemic Disease," by Lester Cahn, T. J. Cook, T. R. Blayney, Norman Topping, George Stein, W. N. Taylor and Bruce Wiseman.

*The American Society for Horticultural Science* will hold its meetings from Thursday to Saturday, inclusive. On Thursday afternoon the Vegetable Crop Section of the society will hold a joint session with the Potato Association of America. On Friday afternoon the society will hold a joint session with the American Society of Plant Physiologists, the Physiology Section of the Botanical Society of America, and the American Society for Horticultural Science on "Effects of Temperature on Absorption, Growth and Reproduction in Plants." On Saturday morning the Floriculture and Ornamental Horticulture Section of the society will hold a joint session with the American Phytopathological Society. On Saturday afternoon the society will hold a joint session with the Section on Agriculture and the Society of American Foresters, at which R. M. Salter, retiring chairman of the Section on Agriculture and vice-president of the association, will deliver an address on "Some Soil Factors Affecting Free Growth," following which there will be a symposium on "Problems of Fruit, Shade and Forest Trees." In addition to the program of 294 papers, the largest number in the history of the society, there will be four round-table discussions on Thursday evening on the following subjects: "Fruit Varieties and Nomenclature," "Extension Work," "Educational Methods" and "Vegetable Variety Types." At the banquet and social evening on Friday the retiring president, V. R. Boswell, will deliver an address on "Performance and Attitude of the Individual in Relation to Research Accomplishment."

The Potato Association of America will hold sessions on Thursday, Friday and Saturday. On Thursday afternoon the program will consist of a joint discussion with the American Society for Horticultural Science. On Saturday morning a joint session with the American Phytopathological Society will consider such topics as irrigation, grading and packaging, internal quality, crop reporting, bacterial ring rot and breeding for disease resistance.

### OTHER PROGRAMS

*The Society of the Sigma Xi* will hold its fortieth annual convention at 4 P.M. on Thursday afternoon. The eighteenth annual lecture, given under the joint auspices of the association and the society, will be delivered by Kirtley F. Mather, of Harvard University, on "The Future of Man as an Inhabitant of the Earth."

*The United Chapters of Phi Beta Kappa* on Friday evening will present the fifth of its series of lectures at annual meetings of the association. Dean Marjorie Nicolson, of Smith College, will deliver an address on "Science and Literature."

*The Graduate Scientific Fraternity, Gamma Alpha,* will hold its annual meeting on Thursday, including a luncheon at the Hotel Fort Hayes.

*The Honor Society of Phi Kappa Phi* will hold business meetings on Thursday and Friday mornings, present a lecture open to the public on Thursday afternoon, and unite at a breakfast on Friday morning.

*The Graduate Women's Scientific Fraternity, Sigma Delta Epsilon,* will meet on Wednesday, Thursday and and Friday. On Wednesday afternoon the society will hold a business meeting. On Thursday a luncheon will be held for all women in science, at which Dr. Marie J. Weiss will deliver an address on "Genius and Youth in Mathematics." The annual breakfast of the society will be held on Friday morning, following which the annual convention of the society will be held.

*The American Nature Study Society* will hold meetings on Thursday, Friday and Saturday. On Thursday the society will meet jointly with the American Science Teachers Association; on Friday it will be host to the American Science Teachers Association in a program which will emphasize the place of nature study in the community, children's museums, teacher's colleges, the public press, conservation and the wildlife program. A broadcast will be demonstrated. The society will hold a luncheon on Friday noon. The Saturday program will be devoted to specific school problems, nature study work in state parks and a discussion of the contributions of affiliated chapters.

*The American Science Teachers Association* will meet on Thursday and jointly with the American Nature Study Society on Friday.

# SCIENTIFIC EVENTS

## THE PLATFORM OF THE AMERICAN MEDICAL ASSOCIATION

IN the various actions of the House of Delegates during the special session held in Chicago in September last year, and again at the meeting in St. Louis, according to the *Journal* of the association, certain constructive proposals were made which had the full approval of the House of Delegates. Now the Board of Trustees has formulated these concepts into a constructive platform. This platform is set up as a guide to indicate the trend which the American Medical Association believes should be followed in the development of health activities and medical care for the people of the United States. It is as follows:

1. The establishment of an agency of the federal government under which shall be coordinated and administered all medical and health functions of the federal government exclusive of those of the Army and Navy.

2. The allotment of such funds as the Congress may make available to any state in actual need, for the prevention of disease, the promotion of health and the care of the sick on proof of such need.

3. The principle that the care of the public health and the provision of medical service to the sick is primarily a local responsibility.

4. The development of a mechanism for meeting the needs of expansion of preventive medical services with local determination of needs and local control of administration.

5. The extension of medical care for the indigent and the medically indigent with local determination of needs and local control of administration.

6. In the extension of medical services to all the people, the utmost utilization of qualified medical and hospital facilities already established.

7. The continued development of the private practice of medicine, subject to such changes as may be necessary to maintain the quality of medical services and to increase their availability.

8. Expansion of public health and medical services consistent with the American system of democracy.

## INTER-AMERICAN SOCIETY OF MICROBIOLOGY

At the close of the third International Congress of Microbiology held in New York on September 9 and 10, steps were taken toward the establishment of an Inter-American Society of Microbiology.

The preliminary discussion clearly showed that inter-American cooperation in the field of microbiology presents opportunity for the solution of two major problems, both concerned with the advancement of the science of microbiology and making such accumulating knowledge more readily available to all scientific men in the Western Hemisphere.

The first of these problems consists in devising means for effecting a better exchange of the results of important studies in microbiology now being carried out in Latin America and in North America to the mutual advantage of all.

The second problem, directed toward essentially the same end, and of equal if not greater importance, comprehends the use of all present resources and the establishment of new ones to effect a more intimate affiliation between the workers of all countries in the study of those diseases which are common to all. This contemplates not only an exchange of the results of work done, but of workers as well, thus fostering through intimate association a better understanding of microbiological questions in the broader sense supplemented by a knowledge of the peculiar conditions which different geographic areas may bring to bear on such questions.

The basis for the first of these problems is the unfortunate fact that investigators in Canada and in the United States gain but fragmentary knowledge of the increasingly numerous important original contributions emanating from Latin America. This is due largely to the fact that comparatively few scientific men in North America are familiar with the Spanish and Portuguese languages.

It is the purpose of the Inter-American Society to approach a solution of this problem; first, through assuming editorial responsibility for one or more journals devoted to microbiology and allied subjects, and second, through organizing periodic inter-American congresses of microbiology.

The initial step in the problem involves the establishment of an *Inter-American Journal of Microbiology,* this to serve as the official organ of the society. It is proposed to make its pages available to contributors from both Latin America and North America, the necessary editorial work, including translations into English of the Spanish and Portuguese papers being done in the United States.

The Inter-American Society proposes to hold, within the next three years, the first Inter-American Congress on Microbiology at Rio de Janeiro in order to carry out that part of its program which can not be undertaken immediately. Dr. J. C. N. Penido, of Rio de Janeiro, was chosen to organize a committee to prepare for the congress. The presiding officer at this congress will be Dr. A. Fontes.

Dr. A. Sordelli, director of the Bacteriological Institute for the Department of Hygiene of Buenos Aires, was elected first president of the society. Dr. F. Duran-Reynals, of Yale University, was chosen executive secretary, charged with the duty of organizing within each of the American Republics a local committee to foster the interests of the society.

## ACTIVITIES OF THE U. S. GEOLOGICAL SURVEY

Dr. W. C. Mendenhall, director of the U. S. Geological Survey, has sent to Science the following particulars in regard to the work of the survey.

The following members of the Geologic Branch have recently returned to Washington after completing their season's field work on the projects indicated: G. F. Loughlin, chief geologist, made an inspection trip of geologic field parties in the West. He spent two weeks examining the underground workings of gold mines in the Little Rocky Mountains, Montana, and conferred with field parties in the San Juan and Cripple Creek districts, Colorado, and in Death Valley, and also with officials in Denver and Salt Lake City; G. R. Mansfield attended the meetings of the Industrial Minerals Division of the American Institute of Mining and Metallurgical Engineers in Tuscaloosa, Ala., conferred with W. H. Monroe, of the Geological Survey, regarding investigations of the geology around Livingston, Ala., and Jackson, Miss., and inspected bentonite deposits in Monroe County, Miss.

For the fifteenth consecutive field season, geologic work was conducted by the Federal Survey in Colorado in cooperation with the Colorado Geological Survey and the Colorado Metal Mining Fund. The following projects were in progress this season: Geologic mapping, commenced in 1938 in the Alta and Palmyra Basins, was continued by John S. Vhay; field work on the geology and ore deposits of the Red Mountain area, Colo., has been concluded by W. S. Burbank; A. H. Koschmann continued his study of structure and ore deposits in the Cripple Creek mining district, and E. N. Goddard completed a study of gold deposits at Gold Hill.

Field work connected with the remapping of the Eureka mining district, central Nevada, has been terminated for this season by T. B. Nolan. During the summer, Mr. Nolan devoted approximately a month to study of tungsten districts in Nevada, California and Arizona; E. N. Goddard completed field work on the manganese deposits of the Philipsburg district, Montana; Charles F. Park continued field work on manganese deposits of the Olympic Peninsula, Washington. Mr. Park, assisted by Russell G. Wayland, also examined manganese deposits in the Butte district, Montana; F. G. Wells mapped chromium deposits in the Grants Pass and Kerby quadrangles, Oregon. He also studied the Pilliken chromium mine, in Eldorado County, Calif.; field work on the geology and mineral deposits of the Seven Devils mining district, western Idaho, conducted in cooperation with the Idaho Bureau of Mines and Geology, has been concluded by R. S. Cannon.

On the evening of November 6, Dr. J. B. Mertie, Jr., of the Alaskan Branch of the Geological Survey, delivered a lecture before the New York Academy of Sciences in the American Museum in New York City. Dr. Mertie, who has a background of many field seasons in Alaska, took for his title the ''Geological Features of Alaska.''

Glenn L. Parker, district engineer of the Tacoma, Washington, district since May 31, 1913, has recently been appointed chief hydraulic engineer of the Water Resources Branch.

S. K. Love, of the Water Resources Branch, has returned from Idaho, where he has been determining run-off and silt removal from areas believed to be representative of different types of vegetative and timber cover and of various grazing practices. The investigation is being conducted by the Geological Survey in cooperation with the Flood Coordinating Committee of the U. S. Department of Agriculture.

A comprehensive study of the surface- and ground-water resources of southeastern Florida was recently begun by the Geological Survey in cooperation with the cities of Miami, Miami Beach and Coral Gables, and Dade County. A field office has been established at Miami with William P. Cross in general charge. The surface-water investigations are under the general supervision of Donald S. Wallace, district engineer, Ocala, Florida, and the ground-water investigations under the general supervision of V. T. Stringfield.

## AWARD OF THE EGLESTON MEDALS OF THE SCHOOL OF ENGINEERING OF COLUMBIA UNIVERSITY

TWELVE distinguished graduates of the School of Engineering of Columbia University were presented at a special convocation on November 27 with the medals for "distinguished engineering achievement" established this year by alumni in memory of Professor Thomas Egleston, who played the chief role in founding the school as the first School of Mines in the United States seventy-five years ago.

The medalists are:

Walter H. Aldridge, a member of the class of 1887, president of the Texas Gulf Sulphur Company.

Major Edwin H. Armstrong, '13, professor of electrical engineering at Columbia.

Marston T. Bogert, '94, professor emeritus of organic chemistry at Columbia.

Gano Dunn, '91, president of Cooper Union.

Arthur S. Dwight, '85, president of the Dwight and Lloyd Metallurgical Company, New York.

Henry Krumb, '98, New York, consulting engineer.

Irving Langmuir, '03, associate director of the General Electric Research Laboratory, Schenectady, N. Y.

Leon S. Moisseiff, '95, New York consulting engineer.

Robert Peele, '83, professor emeritus of mining at Columbia.

Sir Stephen J. Pigott, '03, managing director of the John Brown Company, Clydebank, Scotland.

Robert C. Stanley, '01, president of the International Nickel Company.

Arthur L. Walker, '83, New York consulting metallurgist.

The presentations were made by Dr. Nicholas Murray Butler, president of the university, in the rotunda of the Low Memorial Library, in connection with the anniversary celebration of the School of Engineering. Dr. William O. Hotchkiss, president of the Rensselaer Polytechnic Institute, spoke on "Seventy-five Years of Progress; Empirical Art to Technological Science," and Dr. Harvey N. Davis, president of the Stevens Institute of Technology, made an address entitled "Seventy-Five Years of Engineering Education."

In the future the Egleston Medal will be awarded annually to a single alumnus who has "distinguished himself either in the furtherance of his branch or the profession, in the development of processes or of technique, or in the application of engineering principles."

## RECENT DEATHS AND MEMORIALS

PROFESSOR GEORGE ERLE BEGGS, chairman of the department of civil engineering at Princeton University and a member of the faculty for twenty-five years, died on November 23. He was fifty-six years old.

LOUIS B. MARKS, illuminating engineer of New York City, died on November 22 at the age of seventy years.

DR. EARLE KENNETH STRACHAN, associate professor of chemistry at Brown University, died on November 21 at the age of fifty-three years.

DR. E. E. FREE, consulting chemist and physicist, editor of "The Week's Science," died on November 24 at the age of fifty-six years.

DR. HENRY CLINTON FALL, of Tyngsboro, Mass., the entomologist, died on November 14 in his seventy-seventh year.

DR. EDWARD PALMER POULTON, physician at Guy's Hospital, London; the elder son of Sir Edward Poulton, Hope professor of zoology at the University of Oxford from 1893 to 1933, died on October 18 at the age of fifty-six years.

MEMORIAL services for Dr. Jacob Goodale Lipman, dean of the College of Agriculture of Rutgers University and director of the New Jersey Agricultural Experiment Station, who died on April 19, were held on November 23 at Temple Emanu-El, New York. The services were sponsored by institutions, including Columbia and Rutgers Universities and the U. S. Department of Agriculture. The speakers included Dr. Henry G. Knight, head of the Bureau of Chemistry and Soils of the Department of Agriculture; Dr. Gabriel Davidson, general manager of the Jewish Agricultural Society; Professor O. S. Morgan, of the department of agriculture of Columbia University; Dr. Carl R. Woodward, secretary of Rutgers University; Dr. Harold B. Allen, of the National Farm School, and Dr. Arthur D. Goldhaft, of the Baron de Hirsch Agricultural School Alumni Association.

# SCIENTIFIC NOTES AND NEWS

ROYAL Medals of the Royal Society, London, which is at present conducting its work at Trinity College, Cambridge, have been awarded for the current year as follows: To Dr. P. A. M. Dirac, professor of mathematics at the University of Cambridge, for the leading part he has taken in the development of the new quantum mechanics, and to Professor David Keilin, Quick professor of biology at the University of Cambridge, for his contributions to biochemistry and entomology; in particular for his demonstration of the part played by cytochrome in the oxidation reduction mechanisms of the living cell; and for his studies of the higher Diptera.

SIR ARTHUR SMITH WOODWARD, until his retirement in 1924 keeper of the Geological Department of the British Museum of Natural History, has been awarded the Hayden Memorial Geological Medal of the Academy of Natural Sciences of Philadelphia. The medal, which is awarded every three years, was given in recognition of "notable contributions in the field of vertebrate and invertebrate paleontology."

THE Anthony F. Lucas Gold Medal for 1940 of the American Institute of Mining and Metallurgical Engineers has been awarded to Dr. Everette Lee DeGolyer, consulting petroleum geologist of Dallas, Texas, in recognition of "distinguished achievement in improving the technique and practice of finding and producing petroleum" and as "one of the first to visualize the possibilities of the application of geophysics to oil prospecting."

THE German Goethe Medal for art and science has been awarded to Dr. Franz Fischer, director of the Kaiser Wilhelm Institute for Research on Coal, situated at Mülheim in the Ruhr.

AT the recent meeting of the Acoustical Society of America at Iowa City, a luncheon was given in honor of Dr. Carl E. Seashore, research professor of psychology at the State University of Iowa, and of Dr. George W. Stewart, professor of physics and head of the department, in recognition of their contributions to acoustics. On the same evening former students and friends of Professor Seashore gave a musical soirée in recognition of his contributions to the science of music, and presented a bronze bust, which was accepted by President Gilmore as a gift to the university.

A LUNCHEON was given in New York on November 22 by the American Association of University Women in honor of Dr. Katharine B. Blodgett, research physicist in the laboratories of the General Electric Company at Schenectady, N. Y.; Dean Virginia Gildersleeve, of Barnard College; Dr. Harry David Gideonse, president of Brooklyn College, and William E. Haskell, Jr., assistant to the president of *The New York Herald-Tribune*.

DR. CHARLES F. BOLDUAN, director of the Bureau of Health Education of the Health Department, New York City, was the guest of more than a hundred co-workers on November 22 at a surprise party in the Health Building to celebrate the thirty-fifth anniversary of his work for public health.

THE degree of doctor of science has been conferred by the University of London on Dr. Niels Bohr, director of the Institute of Theoretical Physics at the University of Copenhagen, and on Sir Robert Robinson, professor of chemistry at the University of Oxford. Because of the war and the absence of the university from London, it will not be possible this year to confer honorary degrees at the Senate House on Foundation Day. By the authority of the Senate the chancellor has therefore conferred the degrees, *honoris causa, in absentia*.

DR. ROBERT DOERR, professor of hygiene in the faculty of medicine of the University of Basle, has been made a doctor *honoris causa* in natural science in recognition of his work on ultra-virus diseases, especially psittacosis, and the relations between herpetic virus and encephalitis.

DR. WILLIAM B. PORTER, professor of medicine at the Medical College of Virginia, Richmond, has been elected president of the American Clinical and Climatological Association.

PROFESSOR ALPHEUS W. SMITH, chairman of the department of physics of the Ohio State University, has been appointed dean of the Graduate School. Dr. Smith succeeds Dr. George F. Arps, who died on September 16. He will act as dean of the school until a permanent appointment is made.

DR. LAWRENCE F. MARTIN, associate chemist in the Bureau of Chemistry and Soils of the U. S. Department of Agriculture, has been appointed senior chemical engineer in the Chemical Engineering and Development Division of the Southern Regional Research Laboratory at New Orleans.

DR. C. LALOR BURDICK, since 1928 assistant chemical director in the Ammonia Department and technical investigator in the Development Department of the E. I. du Pont de Nemours and Company, has been appointed assistant to the president, succeeding Henry B. du Pont, who was recently advanced to the position of vice-president and member of the executive committee. In 1935 Dr. Burdick organized the Lalor Foundation for the support of purely scientific research.

THE University of Michigan has granted leave of absence for the second semester to Dr. Bradley M. Davis, professor of botany; to Dr. George Y. Rainich, professor of mathematics; to Dr. Ralph A. Sawyer, professor of physics, and to Dr. William P. Wood, professor of chemical and metallurgical engineering.

THE Council of the Royal Horticultural Society, London, has appointed Sir Daniel Hall, from 1902 to 1912 director of the Rothamsted Experimental Station, editor of the society's journal and publications and keeper of the library, in place of the late E. A. Bunyard.

DR. K. K. DARROW, of the Bell Telephone Laboratories, addressed the Ohio Physics Club on November 4 at Findlay College, Ohio. He spoke on "The Fission of Uranium."

DR. E. M. K. GEILING, professor of pharmacology at the University of Chicago, gave the third annual Rockwood lecture of the College of Medicine of the State University of Iowa on November 14. His subject was "The Comparative Anatomy and Pharmacology of the Pituitary Gland."

DR. S. ALFRED MITCHELL, director of the Leander McCormick Observatory of the University of Virginia, recently gave an illustrated lecture before the West Virginia chapter of Sigma Xi, entitled "With an Astronomer to the South Seas."

DR. FREDERICK S. GOUCHER, of the Bell Telephone Laboratories, will give a lecture demonstration entitled "The Microphone and Research," in the Auditorium of the Museum of Science and Industry, Chicago, on the evening of December 1 before a joint meeting of the American Physical Society and the Physics Club of Chicago.

DR. B. HOLLY BROADBENT, director of the Bolton Foundation, affiliated with the School of Medicine of Western Reserve University, delivered the fourth Frank Billings lecture of the Thomas Lewis Gilmer Foundation of the Institute of Medicine of Chicago, on November 24. His subject was "Clinical Significance of a Roentgenographic Method of Measurement of Disturbances of Facial Growth."

BY the will of the late Murry Guggenheim, who died on November 15, the sum of $5,000,000 is bequeathed to the Murry and Leonie Guggenheim Foundation. The foundation, which Mr. and Mrs. Guggenheim incorporated in 1929, built and maintains a dental clinic. It has for its purpose "the promotion, through charitable and benevolent activities, of the well-being of mankind throughout the world." By the will funds are provided for the Dental Clinic to enable it to erect and operate "a fully equipped dental clinic which affords charitable and benevolent assistance to the children of Greater New York through the practical application of dentistry and oral hygiene." Mr. Guggenheim named the Guaranty Trust Company of New York a trustee of the fund. He expressed the wish that Dr. S. S. Goldwater, Commissioner of Hospitals, whose "outstanding ability contributed in such large measure to the establishment of the Murry and Leonie Guggenheim Clinic," would consent to act in a consulting capacity in connection with the construction and equipment of any clinics that may be established.

AMONG recent gifts to Columbia University amounting to $87,760, the largest contribution, $29,100, came from an anonymous donor for a study of respiratory physiology to be carried on for three years. The William J. Matheson Foundation gave $12,450 for research in the departments of bacteriology and neurology; the W. K. Kellogg Foundation contributed $10,000 for the study of rheumatic fever, and Philip

Morris and Company presented $7,000 for research in the department of pharmacology. The department of psychology received from anonymous donors the sum of $4,000 for a salary.

ACCORDING to *The British Medical Journal*, Professor H. C. Souja-Aranjo, member of the Brazilian Academy of Medicine and vice-president of the International Leprosy Commission, has founded two prizes at the academy, each of the value of $2,000—namely, the Kadrowsky Prize for the best work on the bacteriology of leprosy, and the Lieras Acosta Prize for the best work on the immunology of leprosy.

THE trustees of Western Reserve University and of the Brush Foundation have entered into an agreement by which the work on human growth, development and sex initiated by the late Dr. T. Wingate Todd for the Brush Foundation and other foundations as well as future studies sponsored by the Brush Foundation will be conducted through the School of Medicine. Dr. William W. Greulich, research associate in anatomy and physical anthropology at Yale University School of Medicine, has been appointed director of the foundation and professor of physical anthropology and anatomy in the department of anatomy in the medical school.

AT the third International Congress of Neurology held at Copenhagen from August 21 to 25, which was attended by about five hundred neurologists from all countries, it was decided that the next congress should be held in Paris in 1942 or 1943.

THE autumn meeting of the American Society of Agricultural Engineers will be held from December 4 to 8 at the Stevens Hotel, Chicago, under the presidency of K. J. T. Ekblaw.

THE annual dinner of the New York Academy of Sciences and affiliated societies will be given on Wednesday, December 13, at the Hotel Astor at 7:00 P.M.

MORE than sixty professional psychologists and psychiatrists from eastern Massachusetts recently attended a discussion meeting at the President's House, Tufts College, as guests of the following psychologists and psychiatrists connected with the college: Douglas A. Thom, professor of psychiatry; Abraham Myerson, professor of neurology; A. Warren Stearns, professor of psychiatry; Herbert Barry, lecturer in psychology; Leonard Carmichael, president of the college; John L. Kennedy, assistant professor of psychology; Leonard C. Mead, instructor in psychology; Edwin A. Shaw, professor of education; John P. Tilton, assistant professor of education; Nils Y. Wessell, assistant professor of psychology; and Robert A. Young, instructor in education. Among those who spoke briefly on the topic of the relationship between psychiatry and psychology were: C. Macfie Campbell, professor of psychiatry at the Harvard Medical School; Truman Lee Kelley, professor in the Graduate School of Education at Harvard; Edwin G. Boring, professor of psychology at Harvard; Gordon Allport, professor of psychology at Harvard; Ross A. McFarland, of the Fatigue Laboratory of the Harvard Business School; Edna Heidbreder, professor of psychology at Wellesley College; David Shakow, clinical psychologist at the Worcester State Hospital; Vernon Jones, head of the department of psychology at Clark University; Hudson Hoagland, head of the department of biology at Clark University; and E. Stanley Abbott, psychiatrist and psychologist of Boston.

# DISCUSSION

## A DOZEN MATHEMATICAL ERRORS IN THE "ENCYCLOPAEDIA BRITANNICA"

IN the preface to the "Encyclopaedia Britannica" (1938) it is stated that "three thousand five hundred scholars, scientists, experts, and men of affairs" co-operated in the production of this work. It is to be expected that some errors appear in a work which had so many contributors and which covers such a wide field of knowledge, notwithstanding the emphasis on accuracy and the great claims made along this line. Some of these errors relate to details which interest only the specialists, but there are others which are of wider interest and affect adversely the users of this highly respected and widely distributed work of reference. The latter include the fundamental laws known as the associative law and the commutative law of mathematics. Contrary to common usage these appear in the plural in the articles devoted thereto in the encyclopedia in question. While this is somewhat striking it is not the worst feature thereof, even if it is at first disconcerting.

Under the entry "associative laws," for instance, it is stated that they are "two laws relating to numbers, one with respect to addition and the other with respect to multiplication." The same sentence appears under the entry "commutative laws." In fact, there is only one law in each of the two cited cases. It is the same law when it is used in addition as when it is used in the multiplication of numbers, and it has a large number of other applications. For instance, in the second edition of Webster's "New International Dicitonary" under the entry "associative law," it is said to be a fundamental law of group theory when the elements are combined, but these elements are usually not numbers, as is now commonly known.

The groups whose elements obey the commutative law when they are combined are known as Abelian groups, and under the entry of "groups" in this encyclopedia it is stated (volume 10, page 914) that a set of independent generators of such a group can be so selected that their orders are powers of distinct prime numbers. This is clearly only possible in the special case when the Abelian group is a cyclic group. Among the other errors which appear under the same entry is the assertion that the group of the cube is the same as the group of the regular tetrahedron, while the latter group contains only one half as many elements as the former, and is a subgroup of the former. The regular solids have received considerable attention in mathematics since the times of the ancient Greeks, and hence it may be assumed that their groups of movements are of general interest.

Under the entry "algebra" in this encyclopedia it is stated that "the earliest known treatise containing problems which would at present be called algebraic is the Ahmes Papyrus (also called, from the name of its former owner, the Rhind Papyrus) now in the British Museum and written 1700–1600 B.C. It is now known that the work along the line of algebra by the ancient Sumerians and the ancient Babylonians is more advanced and probably older than that of the ancient Egyptians. On the following page it is said that the biquadratic equation was solved by Ferrari (1540). As Ferrari was born in 1522 he would have been only about eighteen years old when he first solved this equation. The solution was first published in the *Ars Magna* by H. Cardan in 1545, and there is no evidence to support the statement that Ferrari had obtained it long before the time of its publication and at such an early age as about eighteen years.

Several very elementary errors appear under the entry "arithmetic." On page 356 of volume 2 there appears the following statement: "The fact that twelve is scientifically a more convenient radix than ten (having its half, third and fourth easily expressible), seems to have led to the use of eleven and twelve instead of oneteen and twoteen, after which the denary scale was followed." Since eleven means etymologically one left and twelve means two left, these terms relate to the base ten and have no connection with the base twelve. On the same page it is stated that "the distinction between *abstract numbers,* like 4, and *concrete numbers,* like 4 ft., is an inheritance that serves no important purpose." On the contrary, the concept of abstract mathematics is of fundamental importance and it appears in the earliest extant mathematical developments. The early appearance of abstract mathematics is one of the primary facts of history.

Under the entry "Euler, Leonard" it is said that a complete edition of his works was begun in 1926. As a matter of fact, the first volume of this edition was published in 1911 and edited by H. Weber. As this was an international undertaking which was greatly delayed by the World War, the given date is somewhat striking, especially in view of the publicity given to the vast project of publishing Euler's complete works after several failures along this line. Under the entry "Descartes, René" it is stated in volume 7, page 252, that his lines of reference were preferable at right angles to one another. On the contrary, both he and Fermat commonly used lines of reference which are not at right angles to one another. Unfortunately, it is stated in many other places that the lines of reference used by Descartes were preferably at right angles to each other, and hence this error deserves emphasis. In view of the fact that Descartes's Collected Works are widely available this error can easily be verified.

Under the entry "coordinates" it is stated in volume 6, page 391, that the polar coordinates are attributed to Gregorio Fontana (1725–1803). In fact, these coordinates were used much earlier by Jakob Bernoulli (1694) but were not widely used before the appearance of the *Introductio* by L. Euler. On page 75 of volume 15 there appears the following sentence: "The number of mathematical societies, clubs, and circles organized since the early one at Hamburg in 1690 is exceedingly large, but the number of mathematical periodicals since the seventeenth century is very much larger." Since no one knows the number of mathematical organizations which were formed since 1690 it is misleading to imply the contrary. Many of these organizations lasted only a short time and did not publish any of their discussions. In fact, the number of mathematical periodicals since the seventeenth century is not definitely known.

G. A. MILLER

UNIVERSITY OF ILLINOIS

## A REMARKABLE EXAMPLE OF POLAR MIRAGE

IN midsummer of the present year those on board the schooner *Effie M. Morrissey,* while midway between the tip of South Greenland and Iceland, were favored by a remarkable example of superior or polar mirage. Captain Robert A. Bartlett, master of the *Morrissey,* who has reported the occurrence to me with a view to its publication in SCIENCE, has during an experience of more than forty years in the Arctic seen many polar mirages, but, as he says, none so remarkable as this and certainly none so well checked for position and distance.

On July 17, the schooner was from its noon observation in sunshine found to be in latitude 63° 38′ N and longitude 33° 42′ W. The ship's three chronometers had been checked daily by the Naval Observatory signal, and the air was calm and the sea smooth. At 4 P.M. with sun in the southwest the remarkable mirage appeared in the direction of southwestern Iceland. The Snaefells Jökull (4,715 feet) and other landmarks well known to the captain and the mate were seen as though at a distance of twenty-five or thirty nautical miles, though the position of the schooner showed that these features were actually at a distance of 335 to 350 statute miles. A checking observation of the sun made at 6 P.M. gave the latitude at that time as 63° 42′ N and longitude 33° 32′ W. It was warm and rainy; the air had throughout been calm and the sea smooth. Captain Bartlett writes: "If I hadn't been sure of my position and had been bound for Rejkjavik, I would have expected to arrive within a few hours. The contours of the land and the snow-covered summit of the Snaefells Jökull showed up almost unbelievably near."

It should be pointed out that superior or polar mirage is always a phenomenon concerned with great distances and, further, is visible for any given features only within a comparatively limited area. This is because the rays from the object must be directed upward into the warmer air layers of an *inversion,* and these inversions are generally at elevations in excess of a thousand meters where the differences in temperature are represented by a few degrees only. The refraction of the rays necessary to bring them down to the surface of the sea where they would be visible thus represents very flat curvatures and correspondingly great distances. The writer has drawn attention to examples where distances of 100 to 300 miles are involved. The example furnished by Captain Bartlett is somewhat in excess of the examples already described.[1]

WILLIAM H. HOBBS

## INDEX TO SCHOOLCRAFT'S "INDIAN TRIBES"

THE monumental six-volume work by Henry R. Schoolcraft entitled "Historical and Statistical Information Respecting the History, Condition and Prospects of the Indian Tribes of the United States." which was published in 1851–1857, represents the first systematic attempt on the part of the Federal Government to study the ethnology and archeology of the North American Indians. Because of this fact and because of the early date at which the information was collected, it will always remain a most valuable source of information on American ethnology.

While this report has proved an important reference work on American Indians for nearly ninety years, its usefulness has been greatly hampered because of the fact that heretofore no index has been available. Mrs. F. S. Nichols, of the editor's office of the Bureau of American Ethnology, has now completed an index consisting of about 22,000 entries on cards, which is available in its present form to ethnologists, librarians and other workers who may wish to make use of it.

Those who can not consult it in person may write to the Editor's Office, Bureau of American Ethnology, Smithsonian Institution, and information requested will gladly be furnished by mail.

M. W. STIRLING

BUREAU OF AMERICAN ETHNOLOGY

## AVAILABLE LECTURERS IN GEOLOGY AND GEOGRAPHY

SEVERAL months ago a note in SCIENCE announced a tentative plan to furnish university departments with information regarding distinguished foreign geologists and geographers who may be available for lectures. During the summer and early fall, the names of five scholars who wish to make lecture tours were registered with the Division of Geology and Geography. Some of these men have already arranged to give lectures at several universities, and will be glad to make other appointments. Departments that are interested may secure detailed information by writing to the office of the division.

In this connection, attention is called to the Institute of International Education, which acts as a clearing house of information on available lecturers in all fields of learning. This institute publishes a "News Bulletin," issued monthly from October to May, giving specific information about individual lecturers. The bulletin is published at 2 West 45th St., New York.

CHESTER R. LONGWELL,
*Chairman, Division of Geology and Geography, National Research Council, 2101 Constitution Ave., Washington, D. C.*

# SCIENTIFIC BOOKS

## DEVELOPMENTS IN PHYSICS

*Atomes, radioactivité, transmutations.* By MAURICE DE BROGLIE. 269 pp. Bibliothèque de Philosophie scientifique, Flammarion, Paris, 1939. Paper covers, 22 francs.

WITH the distinctive clarity so characteristic of French authors, M. de Broglie gives an account of the developments in physics during the last thirty years culminating in a discussion of the modern concepts of the atomic nuclei and the transmutation of one element into another. Apart from the more profound philosophical aspects of the recent work in this field, and

[1] W. H. Hobbs, *Ann. Assoc. Amer. Geog.*, 27: 229–240, December, 1937.

its fundamental importance to physics, the new science of nuclear chemistry has already demonstrated its usefulness in its applications to medicine and physiology. The promises it holds for the future are nearly unlimited. It is particularly valuable to have at hand a volume which is so up to date and readable as the present one. The book does not require a specialist to understand it, but it will not appeal to the large class of readers of "popular" scientific works who desire more to be mystified than to be informed. Physics is essentially a simple discipline. It becomes abstruse only when it strives for the necessary preciseness by employing the language of mathematics. The text of M. de Broglie approaches closely to this ideal by the written word alone. It is a pity that this quality is so difficult to translate into English, or that we do not have more authors of such lucid style. All of us might well profit, if there were more books of this kind.

*Measurement of Radiant Energy.* Edited by W. E. FORSYTHE. xiv + 452 pp. Prepared under the direction of a Committee on Methods of Measurement of Radiation of the Division of Physical Sciences of the National Research Council. McGraw-Hill Book Company, Inc., New York and London, 1937. $5.00.

THIS volume consists of a series of contributions by twenty-one authors, each an authority in his field. It describes in detail the methods of measuring radiation in the ultra-violet, visible and infra-red regions. There are four phases of the problem presented: the fundamental concepts of radiation, the sources of radiation, the determination of frequency and the determination of intensity. Each phase is competently presented, and all the necessary precautions are discussed. There are numerous references to the original papers listed at the end of each chapter. The completeness and quality of the material presented are noteworthy, and the detail is carried so far as to include, for example, a chapter on galvanometers and their characteristics in relation to the measurements. The book is an extremely useful addition to the literature of physics, and will become, no doubt, indispensable to a large number of workers.

*Atomic Structure.* By LEONARD B. LOEB. xiv + 446 pp. John Wiley and Sons, Inc., New York, 1938. $4.50.

TO provide a text for a course of lectures to third-year students at the University of California, Professor Loeb has written this volume. He has gathered together from many sources much useful and important material which is generally available only in the more advanced and more specialized treatises in the field of atomic structure. The subject is developed in more or less the chronological order. The first part of the book consists of four chapters dealing with the discovery and elementary properties of x-rays and electrons leading up to a discussion of the scattering experiments of Rutherford which are the basis of the nuclear atomic model. The fifth chapter deviates from the historical order and gives an account of the discovery of the positive electron and the neutron and presents some of the present-day ideas of the structure of the nucleus. The chapter is somewhat of a digression, but it in no way interferes with the logical arrangement. The second part of the book consists of a presentation of the classical quantum theory of Bohr which is outlined in sufficient detail to enable the breakdown of the theory, as shown by the necessity for half integral quantum numbers, to be indicated. The third portion consists of descriptions of the various kinds of impacts among atoms, electrons and photons, and is summarized by a chapter in which all the processes are written in the form of chemical reaction equations.

Professor Loeb states in the preface that "it is his firm conviction that it is impossible to introduce the student properly to the subject directly from the rather abstract and modern wave mechanical view-point. In order that a student really understand and be able to use the modern developments, he must grow into these, much in the same way as the physicists who developed the field have done." Younger physicists who do not regard wave mechanics as so "abstract and modern" will perhaps read this statement with suspicion, and wonder whether Professor Loeb is prejudiced in his text against the newer ideas. Although a criticism of this nature may be partially justified, the reviewer feels that Professor Loeb does not regard wave mechanics as any more abstract than the concept of electrons moving in Bohr orbits, but simply as being mathematically more complex. As a result the text is well balanced and fitted to the abilities of the students for whom the book is intended. It may be remarked that, in common with most other authors, Professor Loeb omits all reference to the fact that J. W. Nicholson derived the stationary orbits of hydrogen a year before Bohr's publications on the subject.

The volume closes with a short chapter on the kinetic theory of gases and two excellent chapters on the electron theory of metals, including a discussion of Fermi-Dirac statistics. This extremely important field is generally not presented to students until they are more advanced. Its inclusion in this work seems an excellent idea.

C. G. MONTGOMERY

THE BARTOL RESEARCH FOUNDATION
OF THE FRANKLIN INSTITUTE,
SWARTHMORE, PA.

## PHYSIOLOGICAL PHENOMENA

*Analisis Experimental de los Fenomenos Fisiologicos Fundamentales.* By JOSÉ J. IZQUIERDO. xxii + 334 pp. Mexico, 1939.

DR. IZQUIERDO presents in this volume, which has been prepared for serious students of biology, a well-selected series of illuminating experiments accompanied by explanations and by stimulating questions. The procedure is that of letting the experiments lead the student from observations on physical and physico-chemical states and processes to observations on the properties and responses of living structures as affected by these conditioning agencies. Thus, diffusion, osmotic pressure and the characteristics of solutions are first considered, and then these phenomena are applied to an understanding of changes induced in simple biological units. Similarly, hydrogen-ion concentration, colloidal solutions and properties of interfaces, the polarization of membranes, chemical equilibria and the processes of oxidation and reduction are dealt with in such manner as to yield insight into an understanding of biological events. The final sections of the book are devoted to the phenomena of excitability and the contractions of cilia and muscles. Throughout, the student learns not only the important facts of general physiology but the application of the physical and chemical methods which are employed in examining biological responses to experimental tests. An introduction to the use of mathematics in evaluating data obtained by experimentation is a feature of the discipline imposed by the book. Frequent references to the original investigators whose experiments the student repeats bring him in touch with the masters of the subject.

In a preface Dr. Merkel H. Jacobs has characterized Dr. Izquierdo's book as "an admirable introduction to the fundamental principles of physiology." This judgment is well warranted. Spanish-speaking students who follow Dr. Izquierdo's excellent experimental course in the basic aspects of biological reactions should not only be very soundly instructed but should be stimulated to further studies.

WALTER B. CANNON

# SPECIAL ARTICLES

## SPERM AGGLUTINATION IN THE KEYHOLE LIMPET AND THE SEA-URCHIN

THE spermatozoa of the giant keyhole limpet, *Megathura crenulata,* show a striking agglutination reaction upon addition of egg water. The reaction differs from that described by Lillie[1] and Just[2] in the sea-urchin and other animals in that it does not spontaneously reverse. Instead of the clumps breaking up they continue to enlarge by fusion with one another and, in a sufficiently high concentration of the agglutinin, one large agglutinate forms containing most of the sperm. The spermatozoa agglutinate by the tips of their tails as well as by their heads. The agglutinates are spherical in shape with a thin shell of sperm heads at the surface separated from the central mass of sperm by a distance roughly equal to the length of the tail. In small agglutinates, the tips of the tails occupy the center. The reaction resembles that described by Sampson[3] for chiton sperm and by Henle, Henle and Chambers[4] for bull sperm in anti-sera. The head agglutination is, however, not due to a separate head agglutinin present in the egg water but represents an aggregation reaction.

The limpet agglutinin precipitates in nearly saturated ammonium sulfate, and it is retained by a collodion membrane. By these means active concentrates have been prepared. The preparations give definite xanthoproteic, Millon's and biuret tests. The agglutinin is inactivated by solutions of crystalline trypsin or chymotrypsin (supplied by the courtesy of Dr. J. H. Northrop). Complete inactivation is obtained in 6 days with 1 per cent. chymotrypsin at pH 8 and 22° C.; in 7 days with 1 per cent. trypsin. The controls retain practically their full activity during this period. During the first 3 to 4 days of digestion there is no appreciable loss of activity. After complete inactivation of an agglutinin solution of such titer as to give, when mixed with an equal volume of 1 per cent. sperm, a 10 second macroscopic reaction, the formol titration showed $8 \times 10^{-6}$ equivalents of $-COOH$ per ml. of solution for the trypsin digests and $13 \times 10^{-6}$ for the chymotrypsin.

In the sea-urchin, *Arbacia punctulata,* Glaser[5] reported obtaining no definite protein tests except for a faint xanthoproteic reaction. In *Strongylocentrotus purpuratus* we obtain, with material prepared by $(NH_4)_2SO_4$ precipitation and dialysis of concentrated egg water (care being taken to avoid injury to the eggs), the same protein tests as with the limpet. Also, the sea-urchin agglutinin is rapidly inactivated by one of the crystallized proteinases, namely, chymotrypsin.

1 F. R. Lillie, "Problems of Fertilization," The University of Chicago Press. 1919.

2 E. E. Just, *Protoplasma,* 10: 300, 1930.

3 M. M. Sampson, *Biol. Bull.,* 50: 301, 1926.

4 W. Henle, G. Henle and L. A. Chambers, *Jour. Exp. Med.,* 68: 335, 1938.

5 O. Glaser, *Biol. Bull.,* 26: 367, 1914.

Lillie[1] showed that the activity of sea-urchin sperm is increased upon the addition of egg water. The preparations of limpet and of sea-urchin agglutinins also have this effect, as shown by direct observation and by measurements of the respiratory rate of the spermatozoa. In Arbacia it has been reported[7] recently that echinochrome causes the increased activity of the spermatozoa. The eggs of Strongylocentrotus do not contain echinochrome and attempts[8] to increase the activity of the spermatozoa with this substance have proven unsuccessful.

In both the limpet and the sea-urchin, the agglutinin is obtained in highest titer when the jelly surrounding the eggs is dissolved by means of acid. Other evidence points to the agglutinin being either identical with the jelly or located in it, but not continuously produced by the eggs. The limpet agglutinin is extremely heat-stable, being half-inactivated only after 24 hours boiling at pH 3. The sea-urchin agglutinin is half-inactivated after 5 minutes boiling. Both sea-urchin and limpet agglutinins are stable in isotonic NaCl but not in distilled water. At alkaline pH in sea water the agglutinins are absorbed by the precipitate of calcium and magnesium carbonates and hydroxides that forms. In isotonic NaCl the agglutinins are rapidly inactivated above pH 11 and below pH 2.

ALBERT TYLER
SIDNEY W. FOX
CALIFORNIA INSTITUTE OF TECHNOLOGY

## THE CONTROL OF EXPERIMENTAL ALCAPTONURIA BY MEANS OF VITAMIN C[1]

IN a study of the relation of vitamin C to the metabolism of the melanin pigment precursors tyrosine and dihydroxyphenylalanine in the guinea pig[2] it was observed that the animals receiving tyrosine excreted in the urine a substance of melanin-like properties. Upon examination this proved to be not melanin but homogentisic acid. The production of experimental alcaptonuria in the white rat by phenylalanine feeding has been recently reported by Papageorge and Lewis[3] and by Butts, Dunn and Hallman.[4] Our results may be considered as a further example of artificial alcaptonuria although arising from tyrosine feeding and in another species, the guinea pig. In our experiments it appeared that the animals receiving the smaller doses of ascorbic acid excreted the greater amount of homogentisic acid. Experiments were then designed to test this possibility. The guinea pigs were housed in metabolism cages and the urine collected for quantitative analysis. The feeding of 0.5 gm of l-tyrosine with an amount of basal diet containing 0.5 mg of ascorbic acid per day resulted in the excretion of 20–50 per cent. of the theoretical amount of homogentisic acid when determined by the method of Briggs.[5] With the addition of 5 mg of ascorbic acid per day all but a trace of the homogentisic acid disappeared from the urine within one or two days. Subsequent withdrawal of the extra vitamin C resulted in the reappearance of the homogentisic acid to the same extent as before within one to three days. This process could be repeated at will. In order to confirm the results of the quantitative procedure the homogentisic acid was identified by means of the usual qualitative tests, by the characteristic behavior of the lead salt and finally by isolation and identification of the dibenzoyl homogentisamide by the method of Papageorge and Lewis.[3]

The effectiveness of ascorbic acid in controlling this artificial alcaptonuria in the guinea pig led us to perform experiments on two normal human subjects. On a diet practically free of ascorbic acid the daily ingestion of l-tyrosine resulted in the excretion of significant amounts of homogentisic acid which could be completely prevented by the ingestion of reasonably large doses of crystalline ascorbic acid. The lack of alcaptonuric patients in this vicinity has made it impossible to test the effect of extra amounts of the vitamin on an individual who normally excretes homogentisic acid, but we hope that such experiments can be carried out elsewhere in the very near future.

In a further study of this relation of ascorbic acid we have utilized the unnatural d-tyrosine and find that it also causes the excretion of homogentisic acid by the guinea pig although not to the same extent as does the natural isomer. More striking is the fact that we as yet have been unable to prevent the excretion of homogentisic acid arising from d-tyrosine by the administration of the amount of ascorbic acid which completely checks its production from l-tyrosine. This latter point is being further investigated.

The effectiveness of ascorbic acid in influencing the metabolism of tyrosine so as to prevent the excretion of homogentisic acid not only throws new light upon the physiology of this vitamin but furnishes an extremely useful tool in further studies on the intermediary metabolism of the amino acids phenylalanine and tyrosine.

ROBERT R. SEALOCK
HANNAH E. SILBERSTEIN
UNIVERSITY OF ROCHESTER

7 M. Hartmann, O. Schartau, R. Kuhn and K. Wallenfels, *Naturwissenschaften*, 25: 433, 1939.; R. Kuhn and K. Wallenfels, *Ber. des deutsch. Chem. Ges.*, 72: 1409, 1939.

8 A. Tyler, *Proc. Nat. Acad. Sci.*, 25: 523, 1939.

1 Aided by a grant from the Committee on Scientific Research of the American Medical Association.

2 R. R. Sealock, B. Ziegler and R. L. Driver, *Jour. Biol. Chem.*, 128: lxxxix, 1939.

3 E. Papageorge and H. B. Lewis, *Jour. Biol. Chem.*, 123: 211, 1938.

4 J. S. Butts, M. S. Dunn and L. F. Hallman, *Jour. Biol. Chem.*, 123: 711, 1938.

5 A. P. Briggs, *Jour. Biol. Chem.*, 51: 453, 1922.

### SOME CRYSTALLINE CONSTITUENTS OF THE NON-SAPONIFIABLE FRACTION OF BONE MARROW

WE were interested in the isolation of pure substances from yellow bone marrow in the hope that we might find one or more especially effective in the formation, maturing and release of white blood cells, especially the granulocytes. Others have reported that it is the non-saponifiable fraction of bone marrow fat which is effective in the treatment of agranulocytosis. Consequently, we centered our efforts on this fraction, amounting to a few tenths of one per cent. of the entire marrow.

Since the greater part of the marrow in the large bones of beef is fat, we first had this fat extracted by suitable solvents and then saponified it, extracting the valuable non-saponifiable portion from the soap. Our second method called for direct saponification of the entire marrow, a process that probably broke down certain protein structures in the aqueous fraction of the marrow with release of more fat or lipid than is possible with solvents alone. There are advantages in both methods.

By careful fractional crystallization of the non-saponifiable fraction from suitable solvents we isolated four crystalline substances of high purity and a few others which, if not quite pure, are mixtures of closely related compounds not readily separated by solvent fractionation. All these substances were obtained by the second method mentioned above, that is, saponification of the entire bone marrow. Of course, the proteins and water solubles of the aqueous-type fraction were eliminated by the solvents used in extraction.

In addition to the four colorless crystalline products reported below we secured a number of highly colored oily or semi-solid fractions set aside for further study. The four listed below contained oxygen and were carbinols.

CRYSTALLINE PRODUCTS

(1) Carbon 73.6 per cent., hydrogen 13.4 per cent.; melting point 66°–67° C. The benzoate melted at 35°–36° and the acetate at 34°–35°. Molecular weight by Rieche micro method (usually found 5–10 per cent. low on known pure substances) was 296.

(2) Carbon 83.8 per cent., hydrogen 12.2 per cent.; melting point 147°. Benzoate melted at 144°–144.5°, acetate at 113.5°–114°. The sterol recovered by saponification of the benzoate melted at 147°. Gave good Liebermann-Burchard test for sterols. Mixed melting point test with cholesterol confirmed identity of this substance with cholesterol.

(3) Carbon 76.9 per cent., hydrogen 13.0 per cent.; melting point 61°–63°. The benzoate melted at 137°–138° with preliminary softening and the acetate at 37°–38°. Molecular weight by Rieche method, 268.

(4) Carbon 82.2 per cent., hydrogen 12.1 per cent., for substance contaminated with cholesterol. Melting point after removal of cholesterol was 124°, not sharp. The benzoate of the purified substance melted at 123°–125°. A sterol, forming a digitonide.

This report is wholly preliminary. Further separations and purifications of marrow substances, in addition to biological testing, are in process and will be reported later in greater detail.

We are greatly indebted to the Abbott Laboratories of North Chicago for preliminary processing of the bone marrow which was generously supplied by Swift and Company, and to Dr. H. K. Alber, of the Biochemical Research Foundation of Philadelphia, for his micro determinations of carbon, hydrogen and molecular weights.

HARRY N. HOLMES
RUTH E. CORBET
OBERLIN COLLEGE

## SCIENTIFIC APPARATUS AND LABORATORY METHODS

### LATEX EMULSIONS IN HUMAN VASCULAR PREPARATIONS

FOR generations vessels and ducts have been filled with materials to make them stand out in anatomic preparations. Many different substances and combinations have been used. The older anatomists introduced many masses which are still useful. For example, in Paris one sees the preparateur injecting melted tallow colored with vermilion. In this country in human anatomy the use of a starch paste prepared by mixing lump starch and color, either red lead or a red lead substitute, with cold water is a common practice. Teichmann's mass was preferred for many years and is still used occasionally. This mass is essentially a heavy oil paint. The late Professor C. R. Bardeen, at the University of Wisconsin, used a shellac which was colored with Prussian blue pigment, in the arteries of human cadavera. This violation of the classic color for arteries resulted in giving the students an opportunity to see small arterioles in beautiful contrast to the surrounding reddish tissues. For many years I have used, both here and formerly at the University of Cincinnati, a variation of this mass, a material prepared for the electrical industry. This material (Ajax—insulating varnish, black air drying No. 26, Sherwin-Williams) I demonstrated at the meetings of the American Association of Anatomists at Cleveland. It has been equally as satisfactory as the mass that I learned to use in Dr. Bardeen's laboratories. It has the advantage of being ready prepared and cheap.

For corrosion preparations the completely satisfactory mass has not yet been found. Substances satisfactory for smaller structures are unsatisfactory for large cavities and vessels. Some of the newer materials produced by synthetic chemistry partially bridge this.[1]

With the continuing chemical advances new substances will be available; one of these seems to be latex emulsion. In 1936 I first became acquainted with the properties of latex emulsion through Dr. George P. Phillips, of Boston. Dr. Phillips told me something of the working properties of the material and advised me as to where it might be obtained and also stated that the firm was very cooperative in supplying small amounts of the material to the dental and to the medical profession. Since that time I have used the material in its various forms, colored and uncolored, in the preparation of prostheses and in various laboratory procedures.

Latex emulsion (Vultex[2] is the preparation that I have used) is a slightly ammoniated water emulsion of rubber. When freshly received, the clear material has a milk-white appearance and is of the consistency of cream. In my experience the emulsion may be "cracked" in three ways; simple drying reduces the emulsion to the consistency of rubber found in latex rubber gloves. The emulsion is cracked by acidulating it with any weak acid. It retains its milk-white color until the water has thoroughly dried out. The emulsion can be made into rubber by pouring it into plaster of Paris moulds. These moulds should not be previously treated in any way which would destroy their porosity. The porosity of the mould absorbs the water from the emulsion, leaving the rubber behind. It takes several days or even a week or two for this remaining material to assume its final character.

Considering my interest in the injection of vessels and in corrosion preparations I am surprised that I did not try latex until this present year. We have now in the laboratory several human cadavera in which the arteries and the veins have been injected with colored latex emulsion. We have also used this material for three color injections of the kidney. Our work on the nasolacrimal apparatus has not been satisfactory because of the difficulty in causing the material to flow through small caliber cannulae. The elasticity of the material makes it seem ideal for the routine injection of human cadaveric material. It is not suitable for corrosion preparations where one expects to retain the size of the vessel. Corrosion is accomplished as usual with concentrated hydrochloric acid. In my work with latex in plaster moulds I have found a shrinkage of about one in six, so that when sizes must be duplicated one has to expand the mould to allow for this shrinkage.

Our procedure for human material is as follows. We use air pressure and an injecting bottle for the latex emulsion much as one would use for the injection of a gun-cotton mass. We rinse the system with weak ammonia water before adding the latex emulsion. We make all connections between the bottle and the structure being injected as short as possible to simplify cleaning. If the material has become somewhat thickened from standing we dilute it slightly with weak ammonia water. We find that about one liter suffices for the arterial injection of the average cadaver. This amount compares with what is used with the other colored masses in the human cadaver. The amount is increased to advantage in many instances. The material is injected from 12 to 24 hours after the intra-arterial embalming is completed. For special venous injections we sometimes make the latex injection before embalming, so that the vessels are not filled with the blood from the capillaries. In work with the human cadavera we have not found it satisfactory to routinely practice the washing out of the venous system. Occasionally we open a vein to allow for some lessening of blood on the venous side.

In working with latex and in preparing to describe its use I made inquiry concerning a material used by a biologic supply firm.[3] The nature of this material was not disclosed, but its description by letter seemed to fit the material that I was using. A reply to a direct question confirmed the fact that this material was indeed a latex emulsion. Examination of a purchased specimen also showed this. There has recently appeared in the house organ[4] of another firm an account of the use of latex emulsions. I can not agree with the statement there made about the expansion of the material. This expansion, if it occurs at all, is very transient and is immediately followed by shrinkage.

The material in question can be obtained from the Vultex Chemical Company, 666 Main Street, Cambridge, Massachusetts. The specific materials that I am at present using for colored injections are as follows: F-934 Red No. 244, F-934 Blue No. 9B, and F-934 Yellow No. 154. Previously the material was furnished in glass or in tin screw-top containers and now for two or three years in iron buckets. In the course of time, especially after opening the material, it begins to rust the bucket, therefore, we transfer the material to glass containers in the laboratory.

Using Abernathy's[5] classification this material would have to be a coarse mass. It will never be suitable for such fine vessels as one may inject with preparations of vermilion nor will it be suitable for formal museum corrosion preparations. I believe it will be invaluable

1 O. V. Batson, SCIENCE, 81: 2108, 519–20, March 24, 1935.

2 Trade name used by the Vultex Chemical Company for their material prepared under the Schidrowitz patents.

3 Ward's Natural Science Establishment, Rochester, N. Y.

4 *Turtox News*, General Biological Supply Company, Chicago, Ill.

5 Abernathy: *Phil. Trans. Roy. Soc.*, London (for 1798), 18: 287, 1809.

for routine preparation of human cadaveric material and will lead to a better concept of structures in many parts of the body. We have adopted it as our routine mass.

It's a pleasure to again acknowledge my indebtedness to Dr. Phillips for having first introduced me to this material, and I should also like to express my thanks for the great consideration given numerous queries and small orders by the various members of the firm of the Vultex Chemical Company.

OSCAR V. BATSON
GRADUATE SCHOOL OF MEDICINE,
UNIVERSITY OF PENNSYLVANIA

## LIQUID LATEX AS AN INJECTION MASS FOR BLOOD-VESSELS

NUMEROUS substances have been used in injecting the circulatory systems of laboratory specimens to enable students to trace the course of blood-vessels with greater ease. Gelatin and corn-starch masses in various colors have been used for many years, but both of these have serious faults. Gelatin tends to stain tissue by "jumping" the capillaries and has the added disadvantage of becoming excessively brittle in formaldehyde. Starch mass does not set well if used too thin, and when made thick enough to prevent the running of the mass when a blood-vessel is accidentally cut by the student, it will not fill the smaller vessels.

Recently, plastics have been used with some degree of success, but the polymerization to the solid substance after injection presents such formidable obstacles that it is not yet practical to use for laboratory specimens.

Mr. William Kruse, of Ward's Natural Science Establishment, first suggested the use of latex as an injection mass in March, 1939. Since that time experiments have proven that latex is the perfect substance for this purpose. It will enter the smallest vessels without staining tissue; it may be diluted with water to give the proper consistency; it is used cold, and solidifies to form a tough, flexible solid which forms a perfect cast of the circulatory system. Latex will replace all other substances previously used for filling blood-vessels, and in addition has untold possibilities for use in research on the circulatory, respiratory and excretory systems.

Latex solution of heavy consistency and high pH value, colored with fast, soluble dyes, has proven most practical in this work. The latex may be thinned to any desired consistency by adding distilled $H_2O$. In larger vessels and ducts the mass should be thicker than for use in smaller cavities and thinner when it is desired to fill blood-vessels to their smallest branches. Syringes with glass cylinders and rubber pistons must be used since it was found that contact with the lubricants used for smooth operation of an all-metal syringe set the mass around the piston, causing it to stick. All-glass syringes were unsatisfactory because rubber solution filled the tiny cavities in the ground-glass piston and set under pressure, making the piston immovable.

The material is injected in the ordinary way through metal hypodermic needles inserted into the cavity it is desired to fill. It sets into a tough, flexible solid almost immediately in animals that have been previously embalmed with solutions of phenol or phenol derivatives or preserved in formaldehyde. When injected into larger spaces in freshly killed animals it is difficult to set. When freshly killed animals are used they must be fixed immediately either in alcohol, embalming fluids containing phenol or phenol compounds or in solutions of 5 to 8 per cent. formalin containing 1 or 2 per cent. glacial acetic acid. If the latter fixative is used it must be injected internally so that it will come into close contact with injected vessels and organs and the animals should also be immersed in the fixative. To prevent the latex from escaping when the needle is withdrawn, a drop of 1 per cent. glacial acetic acid or 95 per cent. alcohol may be applied at the spot where the needle was inserted. A clamp or tie should be used on larger vessels.

Dr. Oscar V. Batson, in the current issue of SCIENCE, describes the use of an emulsion of latex sold under the trade name Vultex. He states that he has experienced difficulty in causing the material to flow into the very finest vessels and further expresses the opinion that latex emulsion will never be suitable for the injection of fine vessels.

Dr. Batson undoubtedly refers to vessels of almost capillary size. We have found that our material, which is a rubber solution in contrast to an emulsion, will pass through capillaries if diluted sufficiently and can be used with the finest of cannulae.

D. L. GAMBLE
WARD'S NATURAL SCIENCE ESTABLISHMENT, INC.
THE FRANK A. WARD FOUNDATION OF NATURAL SCIENCE OF THE UNIVERSITY OF ROCHESTER

## BOOKS RECEIVED

ARMSTRONG, HARRY G. *Principles and Practice of Aviation Medicine.* Pp. xii + 496. 86 figures. Williams and Wilkins. $6.50.

MAIN, ROLLAND J. *The Care of a Small Rat Colony.* Pp. 101. 12 figures. Mosby.

PONTRJAGIN, L. *Topological Groups.* Translated from the Russian by EMMA LEHMER. Pp. ix + 299. Princeton University Press. $4.00.

*Report of the British Association for the Advancement of Science.* New Quarterly Series, No. 1, October, 1939. The Association, London. 5/–.

VITRAY, LAURA, JOHN MILLS, JR. and ROSCOE ELLARD. *Pictorial Journalism.* Pp. xvi + 437. 43 figures. McGraw-Hill. $4.00.

WENDT, GERALD. *Science for the World of Tomorrow.* Pp. 316. Illustrated. Norton.

# SCIENCE

VOL. 90 FRIDAY, DECEMBER 8, 1939 No. 2345

*The Argument for Chemical Mediation of Nerve Impulses:* DR. WALTER B. CANNON ..... 521

*The Basic Needs of American Archeology:* DR. CARL E. GUTHE ..... 528

*Obituary:*
*Floyd Karker Richtmyer:* PROFESSOR EARLE H. KENNARD. *William Henry Brown:* PROFESSOR E. D. MERRILL. *Recent Deaths and Memorials* ..... 530

*Scientific Events:*
*Engineering Education; The Alaska Fisheries Experimental Commission; The Biological Research Division of the Edmund Niles Huyck Preserve; Awards of the Royal Geographical Society; Survey of Research in Industry* ..... 533

*Scientific Notes and News* ..... 536

*Discussion:*
*Heavy Water and Longevity:* DR. H. G. BARBOUR and DR. F. S. HAMMETT. *Heparin and Blood Clotting:* DR. K. M. BRINKHOUS and OTHERS. *Mastodon Remains Found in West Virginia:* PROFESSOR W. J. SUMPSTINE and PROFESSOR B. R. WEIMER. *Borgmeier's Revista de Entomologia:* DR. J. BEQUAERT ..... 538

*Scientific Books:*
*Medical Climatology:* PROFESSOR ELLSWORTH HUNTINGTON ..... 540

*Special Articles:*
*The Bacteriostatic Action of Sulfanilamide under Anaerobic Conditions:* DR. R. H. BROH-KAHN. *Effect of Nicotinamide on Respiration of Dysentery Bacilli:* DR. ALBERT DORFMAN, STEWART A. KOSER and DR. FELIX SAUNDERS. *Somatoplastic Sterility in Medicago sativa:* PROFESSOR R. A. BRINK and D. C. COOPER ..... 543

*Science News* ..... 8

SCIENCE: A Weekly Journal devoted to the Advancement of Science, edited by J. MCKEEN CATTELL and published every Friday by

THE SCIENCE PRESS
New York City: Grand Central Terminal
Lancaster, Pa. Garrison, N. Y.

Annual Subscription, $6.00 Single Copies, 15 Cts.

SCIENCE is the official organ of the American Association for the Advancement of Science. Information regarding membership in the Association may be secured from the office of the permanent secretary in the Smithsonian Institution Building, Washington, D. C.

# THE ARGUMENT FOR CHEMICAL MEDIATION OF NERVE IMPULSES[1]

By Dr. WALTER B. CANNON

GEORGE HIGGINSON PROFESSOR OF PHYSIOLOGY, HARVARD MEDICAL SCHOOL

WHEN an impulse travels along a nerve it is attended by a quick rise of negative electrical potential, followed by a quick fall. The duration of this "spike potential" includes the absolutely refractory and the relatively refractory periods of nerve function. The fall is not immediately to zero, but is checked by a slower, negative after-potential. And that in turn is followed by a longer, positive after-potential. The changes are more rapid in fibers of large diameter than in small fibers; the spike lasts only 0.4 msec. in the fastest fibers (*e.g.,* those supplying skeletal muscles) and thereupon the nerve can be stimulated again.[2] As elsewhere in the body, such electrical phenomena are signs of physicochemical or chemical processes which accompany functional activity. In nerve there must be to a large extent a restoration of the resting state, when an impulse has passed, before another impulse can traverse the same course. Associated with the electrical phenomena of nervous activity is a use of oxygen, an output of carbon dioxide and a display of heat. Since a nerve soon ceases to transmit impulses in the absence of oxygen, it is reasonable to assume that the increased metabolism, demonstrable when a nerve functions, indicates that chemical work is involved. According to evi-

[1] The annual Alpha Omega Alpha address, given on October 13, 1939, at the celebration of the fiftieth anniversary of the founding of the Medical School of the University of Minnesota.

[2] H. S. Gasser, Harvey Lectures (Baltimore), 32: 169–174, 1937.

dence furnished by Schmitt and Gasser,[3] the negative after-potential depends on active oxidation. It is depressed by asphyxia, and after asphyxia it is much augmented by conditions which favor oxidation. And when this potential is augmented the rate of recovery is hastened. It is highly probable, therefore, that even in the subsidence of the spike potential—for in fibers of fast conduction the negative wave "is first seen at its maximal value"[4]—an oxidative restorative process occurs, essential for returning to the nerve the ability to act again.

*The electrical theory.* The spike potential, sweeping along a nerve which has been effectively stimulated, causes an electric current to run, in a conductor external to the nerve, from inactive points to the active region, the "action current." It is assumed that a polarized state exists in the surface membrane of each nerve fiber (the outer charges positive); that a stimulus decreases or abolishes the potential difference across the membrane at a node of Ranvier, thus making it permeable and depolarizing it; and that thereupon adjacent nodes of the fiber discharge through the node already discharged so that new nodes in turn become permeable, depolarized and activated, and cause next proximal nodes to do the same. That the circulating local currents resulting from this traveling negative electrical wave can cause stimulation of successive portions of a nerve has been proved by Hodgkin,[5] who has demonstrated that, when an impulse reaches a region blocked by cold or compression, the local currents extend beyond the block and set up there a change of potential with an accompanying change of excitability. Blair and Erlanger[6] have brought supporting evidence by showing that an action current will pass an inert polarized region of the nerve and stimulate the responsive segment beyond. According to the traditional theory of transmission of influence from neurones to other neurones (as in a sympathetic ganglion) or from neurones to the cells of an effector organ (a muscle or gland), that is the sort of process which occurs—it is supposed that the local circuits reach beyond the limits of the active nerve and excite, electrically, the next element in the series.

At the synapse between neurones and effectors there is evidence of a protoplasmic discontinuity. As Bronk and Brink[7] and also Forbes[8] have pointed out, this introduces a physical condition not found in Hodgkin's experiments. As Forbes has remarked, "The structural and presumably the electrical conditions are quite different in an unbroken but inactive axon from those at the synapse. Here, at the termination of the neurone, histology seems to reveal a transverse membrane, which may well act as a short circuit to the action potential. . . . If the membrane theory of nerve conduction holds good, there is every reason to expect such a short-circuiting effect at the termination of the axon." Furthermore, Rosenblueth and I[9, 10] have shown that smooth muscle—that of the nictitating membrane—though readily responsive to a single nerve volley, is, after being deprived of its nerves, quite unresponsive to a single electric shock. Similarly, the cells of a gland (the adrenal medulla in our tests), easily activated by impulses delivered by their nerve supply, are, after denervation, affected to only a very slight degree, even when electric shocks are applied so powerful and prolonged as to injure the tissue. Obviously, there are synapses at which the possibility of stimulation by the action current appears to be highly improbable.

*The chemical theory.* In recent years evidence has accumulated that when an impulse arrives at a nerve ending it sets free a chemical substance—adrenaline at sympathetic synapses, acetylcholine at parasympathetic synapses and at synapses in motor end plates and in sympathetic ganglia—and that these substances rouse in the next distal element its typical reaction—secretion, contraction, relaxation or nervous conduction. Two theories of synaptic transmission have been proposed—the traditional electrical theory and the newer chemical theory. Each theory has its ardent advocates, and a vigorous controversy prevails between them. For purposes of the present discussion these advocates may be called the "electragonists" and the "chemagonists"—"agonist" meaning contestant or combatant!

There is agreement of the agonists on certain points. In order to simplify the consideration of these points, and also the points of difference, I propose to limit the present discussion to synapses in which there is evidence that acetylcholine is involved. The liberation of this substance at parasympathetic synapses and at the synapses of sympathetic ganglia and motor end plates, on the arrival of nerve impulses, is frankly admitted by the electragonists. They also admit that tissues where acetylcholine appears contain a cholinesterase which quickly destroys that highly unstable combination of choline and acetic acid. They admit, further, that acetylcholine, when perfused in very minute amounts through organs in which it is dis-

[3] F. O. Schmitt and H. S. Gasser, *Am. Jour. Physiol.*, 104: 320, 1933.

[4] H. S. Gasser, *loc. cit.*

[5] A. L. Hodgkin, *Jour. Physiol.*, 90: 193, 211, 1937.

[6] E. A. Blair and J. Erlanger, *Am. Jour. Physiol.*, 126: 97, 1939.

[7] D. W. Bronk and F. Brink, *Ann. Rev. Physiol.*, 1: 398, 1939.

[8] A. Forbes, *Jour. Neurophysiol.*, 2: 465, 1939.

[9] A. Rosenblueth and W. B. Cannon, *Am. Jour. Physiol.*, 108: 384, 1934.

[10] W. B. Cannon and A. Rosenblueth, *Am. Jour. Physiol.*, 119: 221, 1937a; *C. r. Soc. de Biol.*, 124: 1262, 1937b.

charged by nerve impulses, will influence these organs as do the impulses themselves. They admit, likewise, that when present in excess acetylcholine has not a stimulating but a paralyzing action. And, finally, they admit that the acetylcholine naturally set free at parasympathetic endings in slowly reacting structures —*e.g.*, in the heart, smooth muscle and glands—is the agent which affects these structures. The main difference now concerns the rôle of this mediator in the transmission of influence from nerves to skeletal muscle cells and from nerves to nerve cells at ganglionic synapses. Electrical stimulation will, indeed, excite both muscle cells and nerve cells; and therefore the action current, if it reaches with effective intensity beyond the junctions, would act as a stimulus. But, if that is the mode of transmission, why the discharge of acetylcholine by the nerve impulse? This is where theories begin to conflict.

In evaluating two antagonistic theories, nothing is to be gained by a recital of the phenomena which both can explain. Deeper insight into the processes concerned in the theories is likely to result from a survey of the phenomena which only one, or neither, can account for. On that basis we may proceed to compare the two theories—electrical and chemical—as explanations of observed facts.

*A comparison of the electrical and the chemical theories.* First, the analogy between evidence for chemical mediation in the slowly responsive heart and evidence for it in rapidly responsive striate muscle and sympathetic ganglia. In all three structures a perfusate obtained while they are not stimulated contains no demonstrable acetylcholine. In all three, nerve-stimulation causes the appearance of acetylcholine, though eserine may have to be used to prevent its sudden destruction by cholinesterase. In all three, perfusion with acetylcholine induces the typical effects of nerve impulses—inhibition of the heart beat, contraction of skeletal muscle and discharge of ganglion cells. And in all three the effect of acetylcholine can be blocked by drugs, without preventing its liberation at nerve endings—in the heart by atropine, in striate muscle by curare and in the ganglion by nicotine. Under these conditions, with nerve impulses delivered to the tips of the active nerve fibers, as shown by the discharge of acetylcholine there, and with the recipient elements still sensitive to electrical stimulation, the action current is without influence.

The practical identity of evidence for chemical mediation in the three regions raises pertinent questions. If the action current is the true transjunctional stimulus, what is the use of acetylcholine, regularly produced during stimulation? How is the efficacy of minute amounts of acetylcholine, as a stimulus to ganglion cells and muscle fibers, to be accounted for? Why should there be a concentration of cholinesterase in sympathetic ganglia and at the motor end plate (*cf.* Marnay and Nachmansohn, 1937;[11] Feng and Ting, 1938?[12] The electragonists surely face difficulties in answering these questions, difficulties not encountered in the chemical explanation. The orthodox electragonists, moreover, are inconsistent; they agree that acetylcholine is a deputy of nerve impulses at vago-cardiac synapses, but deny it that function for neuromyal synapses. Furthermore, they confront a dilemma—on the one hand, agreement that acetylcholine is a chemical mediator of nerve impulses, and on the other, admission that the wide-spread arrangements for its routine production and prompt destruction at synapses, where it can stimulate, are merely a false and futile show. In attempted avoidance of this dilemma hypothetical suggestions of imaginary functions have been offered, *e.g.*, that acetylcholine may serve to increase excitability at synapses, or to delay the onset of fatigue, or to dilate blood vessels locally, or to exert vague "trophic influences."[13] Perhaps it "may"; but it can demonstrably do things to muscle cells and to sympathetic neurones; it can excite in them their peculiar functions. Confessedly, the argument implied in emphasizing the presence and capacity for action of acetylcholine at synapses is based on the reasonableness of means being adapted to ends. In biology, however, that argument is so generally valid as to be, in special cases, quite respectable.

The electragonists have set up what they regard as a serious obstacle to the chemical theory in stressing the brevity of the latent period of the postsynaptic elements before action occurs. In supporting this criticism Fulton[14] has expressed the judgment that "synaptic transmission is probably brought about directly by the action currents of the axon terminal rather than by a specific humoral agent such as acetylcholine," which, in his opinion, "appears to be a by-product of nerve metabolism." It is true that the synaptic events are very brief. In the neurones of the superior cervical ganglion the latent period of the most rapid responses ranges from 2 to 4 msec.,[15] and in the fibers of some skeletal muscles it can be shorter, 1 to 2 msec. (Eccles, footnote 13). If acetylcholine is the transmitter it must flash forth and excite in that brief time; and since a single nerve volley induces a single response the acetylcholine must be quickly rendered ineffective during the refractory phase of the responding elements (which lasts in neurones and muscle fibers about as long as the latent period) be-

[11] A. Marnay and D. Nachmansohn, *C. r. Soc. de Biol.*, 125: 41, 1937.
[12] T. P. Feng and Y. C. Ting, *Chinese Jour. Physiol.*, 13: 141, 1938.
[13] J. C. Eccles, *Physiol. Rev.*, 17: 538, 1937.
[14] J. F. Fulton, "Physiology of the Nervous System." New York, 1938.
[15] G. L. Brown, *Physiol. Rev.*, 17: 485, 1937.

fore another nerve volley can act again. The time is too short, the electragonists assert, for these chemical changes to occur. It is pertinent to point out that this is an assumption. Too little is known of the speed of chemical processes at synapses to justify categorical limitations. Furthermore, the electragonists neglect the fact that the nerve fiber itself, when it transmits an impulse, must recover before it can transmit another. Evidence indicates, as we have noted, that this recovery is an oxidative chemical process, and in fast mammalian fibers it lasts less than 1.0 msec., *i.e.,* it may be much more rapid than the transmission at ganglionic and muscular synapses, which the electragonists assume to be too rapid to be chemical. Until they can offer better evidence for their assumption they have a frail basis for belittling the speed of intimate molecular changes.

The argument that the delay at synapses is too short for the processes required by the chemical theory can be turned against the electragonists. When an electric current is applied to a nerve, the interval between the instant of shock and the discharge of the nerve impulses ranges between 0.2 and 0.4 msec. The delay between the arrival of the impulse at the superior cervical sympathetic ganglion and the discharge of the ganglion cells is at least 5 times as long as that for the quickest cells and at least 11 times as long for the next quickest.[16] If a weak electric current can activate the nerve fibers almost instantly, and the electric action current activates the ganglionic neurones, as the electragonists argue, why this protracted latent period? The relatively long delay in the ganglion is matched by a similar delay in the motor end plate. Here the electragonists have a real problem. The chemagonists, on the other hand, can readily account for the extra time as due to the requirements of an interposed chemical mediation.

At this point may be mentioned an attempt to bring electrical events in the ganglion into relation to electrical events in the nerve trunk. As shown by Gasser and Erlanger[17] and Graham and Gasser,[18] nerves have a heightened electrical excitability during the negative after-potential and a decreased excitability during the subsequent positive after-potential. These two phases, negative and positive, following the spike potential, can also be recorded from the ganglion after it has been stimulated; and Eccles[19] has claimed that submaximal volleys of nerve impulses delivered to the ganglion during its negative after-potential evoke smaller spikes than the original. These observations, if confirmed, might bring support to the electrical theory. In the present discussion a detailed review of the evidence and arguments against Eccles's contentions is impossible. Suffice it to remark that Rosenblueth and Simeone[20] have recorded variations of the spike potentials of the ganglion, responding to maximal and submaximal stimulation, that were precisely opposite to what the inferences of Eccles would predict—maximal spikes when the ganglion was maximally positive, and noteworthy decrease of the spikes at the peak of the negative phase. Furthermore, they noted that by altering conditions the synaptic delay could be shortened to less than 1 msec. or increased to twice its usual length. Because of the lack of correlation between after-potentials and the responsiveness of the ganglion cells and also because of the large variations in synaptic delay, as well as for other reasons, Rosenblueth and Simeone concluded that the electrical theory, instead of being in agreement with observed facts, is definitely opposed by them.

*Evidence for the chemical theory from experiments with curare.* The action of curare confronts the electragonists with a perplexing question. As is well known, this drug is capable of paralyzing muscles by interrupting the nervous influence at the neuromuscular junctions. It does not, however, prevent the discharge of acetylcholine at the nerve endings; the nervous action currents, therefore, run their full course. And with small doses of curare the inherent irritability of the paralyzed muscle is not altered.[21] Yet the muscle does not respond to the nerve impulse. The paralyzing effect of curare at the motor end plate offers no difficulty for the chemical theory. What curare does is to reduce the sensitiveness of the responsive element in the plate. In studies on denervated skeletal muscle Rosenblueth and Luco[22] demonstrated that even with doses too small to stop action of the respiratory muscles curare markedly lessens the contractions resulting from uniform injections of acetylcholine. And the same phenomenon is seen in normally innervated skeletal muscle.[23] In short, curare acts as if it raised the threshold to acetylcholine. Then the normal amount of the mediator which is released by the nerve impulse is incapable of causing the muscle to contract. Thus, while a curare paralysis displays a phenomenon hard for the electragonists to explain, it forms a part of the factual support for chemical transmission.

16 J. C. Eccles, *Jour. Physiol.,* 85: 179, 1935.

17 H. S. Gasser and J. Erlanger, *Am. Jour. Physiol.,* 94: 247, 1930.

18 H. T. Graham and H. S. Gasser, *Proc. Soc. Exp. Biol. Med.,* 32: 553, 1934.

19 J. C. Eccles, *Jour. Physiol.,* 85: 464, 1935; 88: 1, 1936.

20 A. Rosenblueth and F. A. Simeone, *Am. Jour. Physiol.,* 122: 688, 1938.

21 H. Grundfest, *Jour. Physiol.,* 76: 95, 1932.

22 A. Rosenblueth and J. V. Luco, *Am. Jour. Physiol.,* 120: 781, 1937.

23 G. L. Brown, H. H. Dale and W. Feldberg, *Jour. Physiol.,* 87: 394, 1936.

Recent studies on curarized end plates present the electragonists another hard problem to solve. In experiments performed by Luco and Rosenblueth[24] two symmetrical muscles (*e.g.*, the soleus of each side) were arranged to record simultaneously. After a paralyzing dose of curare had been injected the motor nerve of one of the muscles was stimulated continuously at the rate of 60 shocks per sec. When the control muscle was periodically tested through its nerve, and by its response proved that complete recovery from curarization had occurred, the continuously stimulated muscle was usually not contracting at all. If given a brief rest and then again subjected to the stimulation, it contracted momentarily and thereupon promptly became inert; *i.e.*, it manifested extreme fatigue. Clearly, this was not a fatigue of the muscle, for the curare throughout the whole period of stimulation had protected the muscle from being forced into activity. And it was not a fatigue of the nerve, for that remarkable structure can carry impulses at the rate of 60 per sec. during an indefinitely long time. Furthermore, records of the spike potentials proved that the nerve impulses might be full-sized when they were having no effect. The fatigue occurred at the point of transmission. Even if curare should somehow block the nerve action current, the electragonists would have trouble solving this riddle, because the curare block disappeared while the continuous stimulation of the nerve was evoking no muscular contraction. In other words, at a time when both the electrical excitability of the muscle and the spike potentials of the nerve were quite normal, the nerve impulses failed to stimulate. Before this situation the electrical theory breaks down. The chemical theory, on the other hand, has no trouble in explaining it. Prolonged rapid stimulation results, after an initial large outburst of acetylcholine, in a gradually reduced discharge until the concentration falls below the effective range.[25] In these circumstances, according to the chemical theory, a muscular response would not occur. And it does not.

*Evidence from experiments with eserine.* In order to introduce another important series of facts supporting the theory of chemical transmission at muscular and ganglionic synapses, I wish to present evidence regarding the action of eserine. (That term will be used as equivalent to physostigmine and prostigmin). It will be recalled that eserine is able to protect acetylcholine against destruction by a cholinesterase. It will be recalled, also, that if acetylcholine is present in excess it is not a stimulating agent but a depressant.

As Rosenblueth and Morison[26] demonstrated, eserine has quite opposite effects on two symmetrical muscles, one recording responses to slowly repeated nerve impulses, the other responding to similar but rapid stimulation. A small intravenous injection of eserine causes the less frequently stimulated muscle to contract more strongly, and simultaneously it causes the corresponding, more frequently stimulated muscle to contract less strongly. This very striking difference of effect is not due to altered action currents, for the intensity of the nerve spike potential is not affected by eserine. Eccles (*Ergebn. d. Physiol.*, 38: 339, 1936) has suggested that eserine exerts its influence by increasing the sensitiveness of the responding structures. Obviously that suggestion does not apply to the depressant effect on the rapidly stimulated muscle. That effect has its explanation in the change produced in the functioning of such a muscle when acetylcholine is injected so that it is present in excess; the contractions are depressed as they are depressed by eserine. The action of eserine, therefore, can reasonably be accounted for, in these circumstances, by its shielding of the acetylcholine as it is set free by the nerve impulses, against attack by cholinesterase. Since the impulses are quickly recurring, the time for destruction is abbreviated, and with protective eserine at hand, the acetylcholine accumulates until it reaches a concentration which paralyzes some of the end plates. Thus would the chemagonists clear up the phenomenon.

But how account for the opposite effect in the slowly stimulated muscle? That, again, finds an explanation in the shielding of acetylcholine by eserine. Under normal conditions a single volley of nerve impulses evokes a single response in a muscle, as registered by the spike potential of the muscle fibers. If eserine is administered, however, a single volley from the nerve induces a repetitive response and hence a greater muscular shortening. As Brown, Dale and Feldberg[27] have pointed out, this sort of response to single volleys after eserine may reasonably be attributed to the persistence of the acetylcholine released by the motor impulse at the neuromuscular junctions.

The only difficulty which the chemagonists meet in clarifying the remarkably opposed effects of eserine on slowly and on rapidly stimulated muscles is that of understanding why these effects are prolonged. It is known that potassium ions are liberated simultaneously with acetylcholine, and they, as persistent agents, may play a rôle not yet evident. Whatever may be the final chapter of this story it is clear now that the results of injecting eserine are such as to

[24] J. V. Luco and A. Rosenblueth, *Am. Jour. Physiol.*, 126: 58, 1939.

[25] G. L. Brown and W. Feldberg, *Jour. Physiol.*, 88: 265, 1936.

[26] A. Rosenblueth and R. S. Morison, *Am. Jour. Physiol.*, 119: 236, 1937.

[27] *Loc. cit.*

place still unsurmounted obstacles in the path of the electragonists, while presenting the chemagonists additional support for their views.

*Evidence for the chemical theory from experiments with different rates and periods of stimulation.* Thus far the discussion has been concerned mainly with transmission at neuromuscular synapses. Many years ago Elliott[28] called attention to striking resemblances between characteristics of motor end plates and of cell bodies in sympathetic ganglia. For example, nicotine in small doses stimulates at both places, and in larger doses it paralyzes both; curare blocks transmission to skeletal muscle, and in greater concentration it has a similar influence in the ganglion; and, whereas the postganglionic axons can not replace motor fibers, the preganglionic axons, effective on the ganglionic cells, can be cross-sutured and will grow out and make good functional union with striated muscle cells. To these resemblances we can now add the following: acetylcholine in small doses excites at both synapses; and when present in excess acetylcholine, like nicotine, has a depressant or paralyzing influence. We have learned recently that there are still other remarkable similarities between these two transmission points. It will be convenient, therefore, to consider them together.

As shown by Rosenblueth and Morison,[29] if a muscle is stimulated through its nerve at a rapid rate—*e.g.*, 240 shocks per sec.—the muscle first shortens in a sharp strong contraction, then changes promptly to a low contraction or fails to contract at all, and thereupon it shortens in a strong contraction again. Thus with recurring impulses of a constant high frequency the muscular response manifests three distinct stages—a sequence of plus, minus, plus. Now if the stimulation is continued the muscle enters a well-known fourth stage, that of lessened efficiency or fatigue. If the stimulation is at a slow rate from the start, stages 2 and 3 drop out; then stage 1 merges directly with stage 4. Curiously enough, as revealed in the experiments of Rosenblueth and Luco,[30] continuance of the stimulation at a slow fatiguing rate (60 per sec.) causes the muscle to enter gradually a fifth stage in which its performance progressively improves; the contractions increase in strength—displaying a tension as great as 60 per cent. of the highest tension developed at the beginning—and this betterment may last for several hours.

By use of the nictitating membrane of the cat as an indicator of the discharge from the superior cervical sympathetic ganglion the effect of stimulation of preganglionic fibers on the ganglion cells can be examined. In experiments which Rosenblueth and I[31] performed we were able to duplicate, with rapidly repeated stimuli, the first four stages—plus, minus, plus, minus—seen in skeletal muscle. The only difference was a preliminary dose of eserine in experiments on the ganglion. And a few months ago Lanari[32] and Rosenblueth succeeded in recording in the ganglion performance the fifth stage, that of partial recovery of the original efficiency, if only the fatiguing stimulation is patiently continued.

Here is a challenging sequence of events. Why do muscle cells and ganglion cells, when continuously stimulated, respond well at first, then poorly; well again, then poorly again; and finally well for a long period? As proved by Rosenblueth and Luco,[33] who took records of the nerve action potentials periodically during four or five hours of stimulation, there may be a slow diminution in the height of the spikes or there may be no diminution, but in no case is there any correlation between the electrical phenomena of the nerve and the various stages of muscular activity. These conditions at motor end plates and at ganglionic synapses—and with normal blood supply, let it be noted—disclose a puzzle which the philosophy of the electragonists has not dreamed of. What clue to its solution can the chemagonists present?

As previously remarked, when a nerve is continuously stimulated there is at first a flush discharge of acetylcholine at the nerve endings, and then the discharge gradually diminishes. Now if the stimuli are repeated at very high frequency time will be lacking for destruction of the relatively abundant acetylcholine by cholinesterase; thereby the initial great outburst becomes accentuated and the acetylcholine accumulates until it is present in a paralyzing concentration. Thus, the primary contraction of the muscle (stage 1) is quickly followed by less contraction or an actual failure to contract (stage 2). In the ganglion a small dose of eserine, protective against the destructive cholinesterase, allows the acetylcholine to act in the same manner, so that it has the same paralyzing effect. As the primary outburst quickly subsides, the depressant concentration of acetylcholine ebbs away, to be replaced by an optimal lower concentration which is highly stimulative; hence the rise of the muscular tension into stage 3. That this is the correct explanation is proved by the injection of a small amount of acetylcholine during stage 2, whereupon the depressed condition is prolonged; or during stages 1 or 3, whereupon, not stimulation, but, instead, depression is induced. The fourth stage, the stage of fatigue, can be explained by so great a reduction in the output of

[28] T. R. Elliott, *Jour. Physiol.*, 35: 367, 1907.
[29] *Loc. cit.*
[30] *Loc. cit.*
[31] See footnote 10.
[32] A. Lanari and A. Rosenblueth, *Am. Jour. Physiol.*, 127: 347, 1939.
[33] *Loc. cit.*

acetylcholine that it fails to stimulate some of the cells; hence the lessened degree of response—*i.e.*, the appearance of "fatigue." That this interpretation is correct is proved by injecting at this stage the same dose of acetylcholine as that which caused depression in stages 1 and 3 and finding that it now causes an improvement of the response. This, of course, is strictly in accord with the theory of chemical transmission.

The astonishing recovery of function in the fifth stage has been investigated by Rosenblueth, Lissák and Lanari.[34] They have assayed the acetylcholine content of nerves, quickly frozen *in situ* by carbon-dioxide snow, or instantly excised and dropped into liquid air (in order to prevent any change), after continuous, rapid stimulation for various lengths of time. They found a progressive decrease in the content during the first ten minutes—a decrease which turned to an increase when there was a brief period of rest. In the fifth stage the concentration of acetylcholine had gradually increased over that in the fourth stage. If, now, it is assumed that depolarization of the surface membrane of the nerve fibers is attended by a greater permeability for the acetylcholine contained within them, the output per impulse would vary directly with the concentration. In the fifth stage, when the fibers have more acetylcholine, they give forth more, and the result is a larger response. This is the view presented by Rosenblueth, Lissák and Lanari. It is substantially based on the agreement between the evidence of acetylcholine liberation from nerves at the different stages of stimulation and the evidence of concentration of acetylcholine in nerve fibers.

I have described a group of events in the transmission of nerve impulses from neurone to neurone and from neurone to muscle cell. I can find no adequate explanation for these perplexing events in terms of the electrical theory. On the contrary, I can see that supporters of the theory of chemical transmission need only use demonstrated facts in order to give a reasonable answer to the whole intricate riddle.

*Evidence for the chemical theory from degenerating nerves and muscles.* The main assumption in the foregoing account of the five stages of transmission at peripheral synapses was that the output of acetylcholine per nerve impulse would vary with its concentration in the nerve fiber. The recent research by Rosenblueth, Lissák and Lanari, *loc. cit.*,[34] already noted, has furnished evidence that when a nerve has been cut and is undergoing degeneration there is a gradual reduction of the acetylcholine content after the first twenty-four hours. A highly significant fact is that during these first twenty-four hours no functional change is observable. As the concentration of acetylcholine diminishes in the second twenty-four hours, however, the possibility of evoking stage 5 is regularly lost, and stages 2 and 3 may largely disappear or be wholly absent. *At the same time the nerve spike potentials are of normal intensity.* The results are quite in accord with the assumption mentioned above, for, as will be recalled, tests revealed that stages 2 and 3 were due to an excess of acetylcholine and stage 5 to an improved production of it. In the degenerative process, with the acetylcholine of the nerve gradually becoming less, these periods of excessive production fade out and as they do so the attendant variations of activity likewise fade out. And, as might have been anticipated, the fourth stage, that of fatigue, becomes unduly emphasized—the transmission from degenerating nerves "fatigues" much sooner than normally. Now the further important fact emerges that while nerves in the late steps of degeneration can still conduct, as revealed by a definite, though reduced, spike potential, they may not stimulate across the synapse. All these observations harmonize perfectly with the chemical theory of transmission and find no illumination whatever in the electrical theory.

Perhaps no further testimony is needed to justify the claims of the chemagonists. There is one other observation, however, which is demonstrative and well worth presenting. As is now generally recognized, autonomic nerves do not end on striated muscle. They do end on blood vessels—vessels intimately distributed throughout striated muscle fibers. Among the autonomic nerves which give off acetylcholine is the lingual, supplied to the vessels of the tongue. In 1937 Rosenblueth and Luco recorded the action potentials of the tongue muscles which had been deprived of motor nerves for about a week. Stimulation of the lingual nerve induced the appearance of typical action currents in the completely denervated muscle fibers. Here is a stimulation of muscular units clearly not due to electrical transmission, for the nerve stimulated was not distributed to the muscle which responded, and, furthermore, the latent period (60 msec.) was too long for that occurrence. It was a clear instance of a contractile response to acetylcholine, liberated by nerve impulses, to be sure, but not nerve impulses delivered to the contracting fibers. Electrical transmission was definitely excluded. Until the electragonists can display an instance of electrical transmission without acetylcholine at neuromuscular and neuroneuronal synapses their argument can not be on the same footing as that of the chemagonists.

Meanwhile they have arduous tasks in explaining away the evidence which has repeatedly proved the adequacy of the chemical theory of nervous transmission.

[34] A. Rosenblueth, K. Lissák and A. Lanari, *Am. Jour. Physiol.* In press.

# THE BASIC NEEDS OF AMERICAN ARCHEOLOGY

By Dr. CARL E. GUTHE

CHAIRMAN OF THE DIVISION OF SOCIAL SCIENCES, NATIONAL RESEARCH COUNCIL

LATE in April of this year there was appointed in the Division of Anthropology and Psychology of the National Research Council a committee to study the basic needs of American archeology. This committee is composed of W. D. Strong, *chairman,* Clark Wissler, A. V. Kidder, Fay-Cooper Cole, W. C. McKern, J. O. Brew and W. S. Webb. Before undertaking a detailed examination of the archeological problems, the committee felt that it was best to limit its sphere of interests by an analysis of the principles which govern the methods and procedures of American archeological research. At a meeting late in June a preliminary statement of these principles was prepared, upon which this article is based. This first report of the committee constitutes a declaration of the field of interest of the committee and indicates the nature of the basic needs of American archeology which will be studied in its future deliberations. Mimeographed copies of this preliminary report may be obtained from the Division of Anthropology and Psychology, National Research Council, 2101 Constitution Avenue, Washington, D. C.

The aim of American archeology is "to make the past live again," to preserve for posterity the story of the rise and spread of early cultures on this continent and their influence on white settlement. From such studies much can be learned, not only in the field of human history, but also of such significant subjects as long-continued land utilization, cycles of climatic change and the history of important agricultural crops. It is obvious that the competent archeologist must be completely trained in all aspects of anthropology and historical method, in order to be able to interpret these data adequately.

In every part of this country a great deal of excavation and collecting has been carried on, often by untrained persons and without well-defined aims. These activities have irrevocably destroyed many pages of unwritten American history.

More recently state and federal projects have been inaugurated, in some cases to afford employment, in others to rescue prehistoric records in districts about to be flooded. Out of these latter efforts, and through excavations carried on by universities and other scientific organizations, much experience and knowledge have been gained. These projects are being continued, and others are contemplated. It therefore seems urgent that this committee of the National Research Council set forth in brief form what it believes to be the minimum requirements for any future work, whether under public or private auspices.

In initiating an archeological research project, a definite need should be shown for the solution of a well-defined archeological problem or for the conservation of prehistoric material placed in jeopardy by public works or other agencies, whether natural or human. The program of the work should propose a comprehensive archeological investigation. The sponsoring scientific institution or learned society should be able to guarantee adequate supervision and field management, laboratory restoration and study of material, permanent conservation of all materials and records and the publication of a final report. The committee suggests it is essential in the case of all archeological projects sponsored by federal funds that the representative of the sponsoring agent should be approved by the Smithsonian Institution, whose national character and scientific attainments make it the most satisfactory qualifying agent in the country.

Field operations should be conducted by trained field men with academic training as well as field experience. The general supervision of the field work should insure that adequate records be kept and that the work be done with a clear comprehension of the problem under attack. Naturally a balanced supply of surveying instruments, cameras, tools, supplies and storage and transportation facilities must be available. The supervisory staff must be given time for experimentation, rechecking of records and data, and careful completion of operations begun, as well as for the preparation of a full and complete field report. Time limitations should never be permitted to induce rush tactics which might promote carelessness or curtail efficiency.

The laboratory phase of the project should be conducted by trained laboratory technicians and a sufficiently large staff to care for field material as rapidly as it is acquired. The general supervision of the work should insure close cooperation between laboratory and field work in order that each may aid the other in the solution of the problem. As many allied sciences as may be necessary should be brought to bear upon the laboratory investigation.

The methods and techniques used in an archeological project are different, of course, in the field and in the laboratory. Both phases of the project should be under the general direction of a director. The active field director should possess a comparative knowledge of methods of work and the ability to adjust or revise these to suit the particular conditions under which he is working. In organizing a field party, specific types of work should be placed in the hands of capable men under the immediate direction of competent supervisors. In order to secure most efficient service on the part of all concerned, it is essential that responsibility be vested with corresponding authority.

In survey work the preparation of maps and charts is one of the primary objectives. An accurate map should show the relationship of a site to the natural and significant cultural environment. The more detailed working plan, whether based upon the grid system or other arrangements of reference points and lines, should insure accuracy both for the initial surface charts and for the vertical and horizontal records. In so far as possible the site nomenclature should be in accordance with a statewide plan.

The methods employed in excavation should be selected to facilitate the clearest perception of the archeological phenomena. The soil may be removed by peeling, by vertical sectioning, by horizontal stripping in arbitrary levels or by combining these several procedures as dictated by the specific nature of the problems involved and the peculiarities of the site. In all cases, work must be conducted in a manner which promises to disclose all available evidence on formation and structure, and to preserve all data on stratigraphy, age, time succession, cultural and historical activities and cultural processes.

In all field work, whether it be a survey or an excavation, complete documentation is essential. The progress of the work must be fully documented by charts and texts. There must be full recording of finds and associations, preferably by filling out a standard form to insure complete and comparable information. Finally, there must be well-organized and integrated identifications, including good and complete photographic records.

The satisfactory application of laboratory methods presupposes the existence of a well-equipped laboratory for the storage of materials and for their analysis in order to facilitate definition of types, cultural synthesis and broad cultural comparisons.

The many and varied activities of the laboratory consist of: the recording, preservation and technical analysis and study of all tangible materials, including physical anthropological data; the integration and filing of all documentary records; the coordination of material data with other data to determine culture complexes and relationships, as well as the origin and development of these cultures; and finally, the preparation of the manuscript report for publication.

All the foregoing activities are nullified unless followed by prompt publication. There are several essential steps in the realization of this final scientific objective. Firstly, the daily notes on excavations, plans of trenches, lists of finds and photographs should be typed and otherwise recorded from day to day. This is so essential that the appropriation for each project should provide for the necessary clerical assistance in the field.

Secondly, when the record is approved by the archeologist in charge, three complete copies should be made. Where projects are under government auspices, one of these should be deposited in the Smithsonian Institution. If the sponsoring institution possesses an adequate library, the second copy should remain there; otherwise, it should be placed in the library of the state university. The third may be used as the working copy of the archeologist in charge, but ultimately should be deposited in some important library.

Thirdly, adequate arrangements should be made to supply the archeologist in charge with time and clerical and technical assistance for the preparation of an adequate final report of the work. It must be remembered, in this connection, that the study of materials and the preparation of a final report normally requires at least as much time as is devoted to field work.

A satisfactory final report should contain at a minimum a statement of the problem attacked, a description of the methods employed, an adequate descriptive and illustrative review of the data and a final section containing such interpretations and conclusions as are justified by the data.

Finally, in establishing any archeological program, whether for purely scientific purposes or in conjunction with problems of state or federal employment, the basic need for national conservation must be given primary consideration. Not only should each site opened be excavated with the greatest care, the material completely studied, and the results fully published, but also certain sites in every area should be carefully preserved for research in the future as new techniques are developed. The fencing, restoration, marking and guarding of important prehistoric sites is particularly applicable at the present time, permitting as it does the use of local labor and the advancement of historical interest.

Such forward-looking activities should extend from the National Park Service on the one hand to State Historical Societies and municipalities on the other. They will advance the growth of national consciousness as well as scientific progress, and should receive every encouragement.

It should always be remembered that the number of archeological sites in the United States is strictly limited, and that once a site has been carelessly excavated its value is totally destroyed. These ancient ruins are really material documents that comprise the very stuff of American history. From them we may learn not only the manner in which the New World was originally settled and how its strongly individualized and truly remarkable civilizations arose, but also determine the history and nature of various important American agricultural crops. In addition, the practical problem of the sequence and duration of postulated post-glacial climatic cycles may only be solved when the archeological record is clear.

For these and similar reasons, it is the fundamental belief of the Committee on Basic Needs in American Archeology of the National Research Council that unless the foregoing minimum requirements of scientific archeology can be fully met by any federal, state or local institution, it should not undertake archeological research.

# OBITUARY

## FLOYD KARKER RICHTMYER

ON November 7 death came without warning to Dean Richtmyer of Cornell University. He collapsed while preparing to go to a concert with his family, and before the doctor arrived he was dead from coronary thrombosis. Thus was struck down, in the full tide of amazing activity, a prominent figure of the Cornell campus and one of the most influential members of several learned societies and institutions.

Floyd Karker Richtmyer was born on October 12, 1881, in the rural community of Cobleskill, New York. He showed an early interest in scientific research as an undergraduate at Cornell University. After graduation in 1904 he married and taught for two years at Drexel Institute, Philadelphia; then he returned to Cornell as instructor in physics, and in 1910 was awarded the degree of Ph.D.

In his activities as a graduate student, the main lines and characteristics of Richtmyer's life work are already visible. Stimulated by E. L. Nichols to an interest in photometry, he presented a paper before the Illuminating Engineering Society in which he advocated more instruction in the subject of illumination for engineers and described a new laboratory course in the subject. Thus he showed an early interest both in educational problems and in the applied side of physics. For the subject of his Ph.D. research, however, he chose the photoelectric properties of the alkali metals. In this investigation he did the careful, clean-cut experimental work for which he possessed an unusual talent; and he also revealed his outstanding characteristics of looking at a set of data from all angles and extracting from them every possible conclusion. He was preeminently a man with a passion for doing things well; and he saw many things to do.

From this point, Richtmyer's career falls naturally into three periods. During the first, he taught physics for students of engineering and pursued his interests in applied optics. In the Illuminating Engineering Society we find him on the council and on several committees, acting as chairman of a committee on education. Furthermore, in 1916 he assisted in the organization of the Optical Society of America, and throughout his life he contributed greatly to the work of that society; he was president in 1920, and for 22 years he participated in the conduct of the *Journal,* becoming editor in 1933.

About 1918, however, when he became full professor of physics, Richtmyer began to turn toward other fields. After a brief interlude in the study of thin films he developed an interest in x-rays which was destined to be permanent and to establish him as an authority in the field. After spending a sabbatic year as "investigator" in the laboratories of the General Electric Company, he undertook at Cornell a series of well-planned and precisely executed measurements on topics related to x-ray absorption, the principal result of which was to establish the law that absorption due to ionization in a given shell in an atom is proportional to the cube of the wave-length of the x-rays and to the fourth power of the atomic number. Then, in 1927, as a result of several months in Siegbahn's laboratory in Uppsala, Sweden, he became interested in the faint x-ray lines known as "satellites." He proposed a new theory concerning the origin of these lines, ascribing them to jumps made simultaneously by two electrons in an ionized atom; and he made a series of experimental studies in an endeavor to support the theory. Later he himself recognized, in the light of further developments, that most of the observed satellites are probably due to a mechanism proposed earlier by others, namely, to a one-electron jump in a doubly ionized atom; but it is still possible that some of the faintest lines are of his double-jump type.

Richtmyer's interest in x-ray research continued to the end. He inspired and supervised a number of investigations which did much to clear up the subject of x-ray line widths and shapes; after 1930, however, the actual work was done by others. His enthusiasm and obvious mastery of fact and technique attracted many graduate students into his field, and during many years he had the help of an assistant. His attainments as a scientist were given recognition by his election as president of the American Physical Society in 1936, and as vice-president in charge of section B of the American Association for the Advancement of Science in 1930; and in 1932 he was elected to the National Academy of Sciences (councilor in 1938).

About 1931 began the third period of Richtmyer's activities, during which most of his time was devoted to administrative work of wide variety. In that year he became dean of the graduate school at Cornell. In this capacity he strove, with tact and infinite patience, for the maintenance of high standards, hampered by the circumstance that he had neither a budget nor direct control over students' work. In 1931, also, he participated in the organization of the American Institute of Physics, and thereafter he contributed greatly to its management, as a member of the executive committee of the governing board and of several other committees. Finally, in the same year he participated in the founding of the American Association of Physics Teachers, of which he remained a member of the executive committee and served several years as vice-president (1935, 1936), president (1937, 1938) or associate editor of the *Journal*.

In spite of these new responsibilities he continued to be active in the American Association of University Professors, of which he was vice-president in 1932 and 1933; serving on various committees, he took the leading part as chairman of a committee which studied the effects of the depression on higher education. As dean of the graduate school he was also brought actively into the work of the Association of American Universities; besides membership on several committees, he acted as chairman of one on foreign student problems which did a great deal to improve the lot of foreign students in America. In 1938 he was chosen to be the first personal permanent secretary of the association. And, finally, he continued until 1937 to share in the work of the National Research Council, of which he became a member in 1923; he was chairman of the division of physical sciences from 1930 to 1935 and on the fellowship board from 1930 to 1937.

During later years Richtmyer's teaching was restricted to an occasional graduate course and a senior course of his own devising. The subject-matter of the latter he published in 1928 as a book, "Introduction to Modern Physics," in which he surveyed from the experimental standpoint the advances of the present century. In this book, as on the lecture platform, he showed himself a master of clear and forceful exposition. He was often invited to lecture on scientific or educational topics; during the last two years he gave at least 15 lectures on his experiences as a physicist accompanying the National Geographic Society-U. S. Navy expedition to the South Pacific to observe the solar eclipse of 1937.

Richtmyer was a member of many scientific societies. In Sigma Xi he headed a committee on revision of the constitution, and from 1924 to 1926 he was president. He also took a warm interest in the Cosmopolitan Club of Ithaca, doing a great deal to establish this club on a sound basis. He seemed to feel surest that here he had, beyond all possibility of dispute, accomplished something to benefit mankind. It was characteristic of him in general that he was always willing to lend a helping hand to others; there are many, within the university and without, who feel a deep personal sense of gratitude toward him for such assistance. This trait and his graciousness as friend and host won him many friends, both on and off the campus. His closest friends speak of his frankness, sincerity and modesty. His going leaves many with a sense of irreparable loss.

He is survived by his widow, Bernice Davis Richtmyer, and three children: Robert D., now instructor in physics at Stanford University, Sarah (Mrs. Mann) and Lawson E.

EARLE H. KENNARD

CORNELL UNIVERSITY

## WILLIAM HENRY BROWN

WHEN an active and productive man, experienced and successful in research, in teaching, in the preparation of important texts and in administration, altogether too rare an association of talents, suddenly and unexpectedly dies at the relatively young age of fifty-five years, not only his colleagues and associates keenly feel his loss but science itself suffers. This statement applies preeminently to Dr. William Henry Brown of the department of botany, Johns Hopkins University, whose death occurred in Baltimore on the morning of November 9, 1939.

Dr. Brown's active and productive career centered in the Philippines, for with the exception of one short vacation trip to the United States in 1925, he resided there continuously for twenty-seven years, a very long term of tropical service. Yet his investigations and his publications have given him a distinctly wide and favorable clientele not only in the Philippines and in the United States, but in all parts of the world where botany is an established and recognized field of instruction and research.

Dr. Brown was born in Richmond, Va., on October 6, 1884, receiving his bachelor's degree from Richmond College in 1906. In the fall of 1906 he entered Johns Hopkins University, taking advanced work in botany under the late Dr. Duncan S. Johnson. In 1909, after Dr. Burton E. Livingston joined the Johns Hopkins staff, he became more and more interested in plant physiology, and in this year accompanied the latter as research assistant to the Desert Laboratory of the Carnegie Institution, Tucson, Ariz. As an interim appointment he also served as scientific assistant in 1908 at the United States Fisheries Laboratory at Beaufort, N. C. While a graduate student at Johns Hopkins University he served as graduate assistant in botany, was appointed a fellow in 1909, and, after receiving his Ph.D. degree in 1910, was appointed a Bruce fellow, a post-Ph.D. fellowship for studies planned to be carried on at the Desert Laboratory. In the fall of that year, however, he resigned the Bruce fellowship to accept an instructorship in plant physiology at Michigan State College. These brief data suffice to cover his formative years, but in whatever field he worked, technical publications resulted.

At about this time it was decided to initiate work in plant physiology in the Bureau of Science at Manila, and the undersigned made a survey of available candidates, the result being the selection of Dr. Brown for appointment in the Philippine service. It was in Manila, in a decidedly stimulating, even although a tropical environment, that Dr. Brown established himself as a productive scientist, for his work there added distinctly to the prestige of the small group of individuals on whose shoulders fell the responsibility of developing and maintaining the scientific work fostered and supported by the Philippine Government.

It soon became apparent that Dr. Brown's interests were by no means confined to plant physiology, and gradually he entered the field of ecology, the result being the publication in 1919 of his monographic "Vegetation of Philippine Mountains," based on a long, arduous and critical series of field studies in the primary forests of Mount Maquiling. He retained his Bureau of Science appointment from 1911 to 1923, but in this period acted as associate (later professor) of botany, in the University of the Philippines from 1919 to 1924, and as chief of the Division of Investigations in the Philippine Bureau of Forestry from 1919 to 1920.

His teaching experience led him into the text-book field, for he soon found that there were no properly balanced botanical text-books available for instruction in the subject for students resident in the tropics. Most texts had previously been prepared by individuals familiar from long residence with the vegetation of the temperate zone, but with little or no tropical experience. The result of Dr. Brown's efforts here was his very excellent "Textbook of General Botany," published in 1925, a text characterized by its balance, remarkable for its excellent illustrations and for its adaptability to the actual teaching of the subject in any climate. Ten years later this was followed by his equally excellent and authoritative "Plant Kingdom."

With an active and inquiring mind, fully at home in several diverse fields of botanical science, including plant physiology, ecology, morphology and economic botany, for in the latter field Dr. Brown was also a productive worker, his actual botanical output was limited for the next nine years, from 1924 to 1933, for in the former year he was selected to succeed the undersigned in the distinctly exacting position as director of the Bureau of Science in Manila. Here he proved himself as an administrator, his work involving the general supervision of an enormously wide range of subject-matter as well as the editorship of the *Philippine Journal of Science*. In this position Dr. Brown's period of service was longer than that of any of his three predecessors, except that of the first incumbent, Dr. Paul C. Freer.

Retirement from administrative work and from the Philippine service in 1933 gave Dr. Brown the opportunity of devoting practically full time to the advancement of research in the field that now claimed his attention, that of general morphology, with special reference to the significance of the floral nectaries as indicators of broad relationships of the major groups of plants. He elected to remain in Manila after his retirement from the government service, where he had access to a wealth of fresh material essential to the proper prosecution of his special studies. As the work developed he commenced to feel the need of access to other than tropical types, and in the latter part of 1936 correspondence was initiated between himself and the late Dr. Duncan S. Johnson, tentative plans being then made for him to locate in or near Baltimore or Washington, where he could have access to ample herbarium and library facilities. At the time of Dr. Johnson's death in February, 1937, laboratory space had been made available to Dr. Brown in Johns Hopkins University. It was then learned that Dr. Brown was about ready to transfer his botanical activities from the Philippines to the United States, whereupon he was offered a lectureship in botany at Johns Hopkins University. He took up his residence in Baltimore in February, 1938, having charge of the botanical laboratory and of the botanical garden at the university.

Here in addition to his teaching duties he concentrated on his studies of the significance of the floral nectaries, having in mind the ultimate production of a major work, planned to cover all possible groups (families) of flowering plants. His untimely death leaves this culminating task incomplete, although it is hoped that ways and means may be devised to continue the work.

Dr. Brown's botanical interests were unusually wide, and he fortunately had exceptional opportunities available to him through a very long period of service in a tropical environment. Taking advantage of these opportunities, his published results were uniformly excellent, no matter in what field he worked. He was a member of numerous organizations, including the American Ecological, Meteorological and Botanical Societies, a fellow of the American Association for the Advancement of Science and a member of Phi Beta Kappa. He married Mary Angus Blythe in Manila, on June 3, 1927, who with two sons survive him. His loss is a serious one to America and to world botany.

E. D. Merrill

## RECENT DEATHS AND MEMORIALS

Dr. Charles Skeele Palmer, consulting chemical engineer, inventor of a gasoline-cracking process that separated mineral oil into gasoline, fuel oil and gas, previously professor of chemistry at the University of Colorado, died on November 30 at the age of eighty-one years.

PROFESSOR FREDERICK NEWTON WILLSON, emeritus professor of descriptive geometry, stereotomy and technical drawing at Princeton University, died on November 15. He was eighty-three years old.

PROFESSOR R. V. WHEELER, professor of fuel technology in the University of Sheffield, died on October 28 at the age of fifty-three years.

DR. WILFRED TROTTER, professor of surgery at the University College Hospital Medical School and surgeon to the University College Hospital, London, died on November 25 at the age of sixty-seven years.

A PORTRAIT of the late Professor Henry Smith, formerly dean of the School of Mines of Columbia University, painted by H. E. Ogden Campbell, was unveiled in the Low Memorial Library on November 27.

A MEETING dedicated to the memory of Dr. William Hallock Park, emeritus professor of medicine in the New York University College of Medicine until his retirement in 1936 and director of the Bureau of Laboratories of the New York City Department of Health, was held on November 28 at the New York Academy of Medicine. The speakers included: Mayor La Guardia; Dr. Harry Woodburn Chase, chancellor of New York University; Dr. Malcolm Goodridge, president of the academy; Dr. Anna W. Williams, formerly assistant director of the Health Department Bacteriology Laboratories under Dr. Park, and Dr. Augustus B. Wadsworth, director of laboratories and research for the New York State Department of Health.

# SCIENTIFIC EVENTS

## ENGINEERING EDUCATION

A REPORT on "Present Status and Trends of Engineering Education in the United States," by Dr. Dugald C. Jackson, emeritus professor of engineering at the Massachusetts Institute of Technology, has been issued by the Engineers' Council for Professional Development, with the aid of funds supplied by the Carnegie Foundation for the Advancement of Teaching. The report is one of the valuable by-products of the task of accrediting curricula in engineering undertaken by the Committee on Engineering Schools of the Engineers' Council for Professional Development.

Dr. Jackson's report may be divided roughly into four parts. An appendix has been provided by Allen W. Horton, Jr., who acted as secretary to the committee during the period in which the accrediting procedure was developed and put to the test, and the data collected. In the early chapters of the report Dr. Jackson traces the history of developments that led up to the accrediting program, summarizes the well-known Mann, Wickenden and Potter reports that have played important roles in that development, and sketches briefly the status of engineering education in America in 1939. He next turns his attention to the Committee on Engineering Schools of the Engineers' Council for Professional Development, to the procedure it adopted in its task of accrediting curricula and to comments on some of the perplexing problems it had to face and the progress of the committee's own thinking and methods that resulted from actually coming to grips with these problems.

The data themselves, which cover 679 curricula in 139 institutions, assembled, coordinated and analyzed in the form of tables and charts, with Dr. Jackson's comments, occupy the third portion of the report. These data were gathered for the purpose of the accrediting program, which they usefully served, but they constituted a store of information of value to engineers and educators, and were so fruitful for the improvement of engineering education that the committee was able to secure from the Carnegie Foundation for the Advancement of Teaching the funds necessary to put them in shape for public use.

As to the present status, Dr. Jackson provides a convenient summary in the following passages quoted from the report:

> It is reasonable to say that the majority of the substantially one hundred and sixty engineering schools in the United States are now in a sound status and are wide-awake to improve their effectiveness. The principal defects in the quality of faculties are perhaps a lack of recognition of the unity of learning in science and in political economy as applied in engineering, an inadequate espousal of professional ideals as distinguished from either craftsmanship or speculative philosophy, a failure to impress on all students that a successful engineer's life demands continuous study throughout its length, and a failure to dovetail the curricula into political economy on one side as thoroughly as they are dovetailed into physical science on the other. . . . Part of the onus for the defects named may be appropriately laid at the doors of administrative officers. . . . There is an additional fault . . . which is the failure to recognize that the proper use of research vitalizes all levels of engineering education, from the sophomore undergraduate level to the most advanced levels, which makes it a requisite and important factor in such education.

## THE ALASKA FISHERIES EXPERIMENTAL COMMISSION

AN Alaska Fisheries Experimental Commission has

been organized with an appropriation from the Legislature of $20,000 for cooperation in the establishment of a fishery products laboratory in Alaska.

The members of the commission are the governor of Alaska, Dr. Ernest Gruening; J. W. Mendenhall, of Ketchikan, member for industry, and Seton H. Thompson, member for the bureau. At a meeting on August 20 Governor Troy, who has since resigned, was elected chairman and Mr. Mendenhall, secretary. It was then decided to enter into a cooperative agreement with the U. S. Bureau of Fisheries for the operation of the laboratory.

At this meeting it was also decided to establish the office of the commission at the laboratory building in Ketchikan, when constructed, and Mr. Mendenhall was designated as liaison officer with authority to consult appropriate officials of the Bureau of Fisheries regarding construction, maintenance and operation.

A site has been selected on which to construct the laboratory, and the sum of $50,000 has been allocated for this purpose by the Public Works Administration. The building will be approximately 60,000 cubic feet in size.

The laboratory will serve as headquarters for the Alaska technical and economic research staff, who will conduct studies on the capture, preservation and marketing of Alaska fishery products.

In general, it is proposed to conduct research along the following lines:

Improvement of processes and methods of capture, handling and preserving of species now utilized.

Development of new methods for processing species now utilized.

Preparation of useful commodities from species not utilized.

The purpose of this work will be to extend the processing or fishing season over a longer period of the year. At present most of the fishing and packing business is done in the summer.

## THE BIOLOGICAL RESEARCH DIVISION OF THE EDMUND NILES HUYCK PRESERVE

THE Edmund Niles Huyck Preserve at Rensselaerville, Albany County, New York, was incorporated in 1931. The purpose of the preserve, as outlined in the certificate of incorporation, is to

preserve the natural beauty of Rensselaerville Falls, Lake Myosotis, Lincoln Pond and the lands around them in the town of Rensselaerville; to increase the general knowledge and love of nature, particularly that of trees and wildlife, by maintaining a demonstration of reforesting and forest culture, and by providing means for increasing and protecting the birds, wild animals and fish within the boundaries of said land.

The preserve covers nearly a square mile of diversified habitats. Two lakes, one of eighty acres, numerous streams, dense beech-hemlock stands and arable fields provide a diverse attraction for the naturalist. The elevation is 1,650 feet above sea. As a preliminary step to the possible establishment of a biological station on the preserve a study of the biota was made during the summers of 1937 and 1938.

Three fellowships (two of three months each and one for the entire year) have been provided, the recipients to conduct basic zoological investigations in the field of animal behavior or ecology. Donald Griffin, of Harvard University, and Dr. E. C. Raney, of Cornell University, were awarded the 1939 summer fellowships. Dr. Eugene P. Odum, a graduate of the University of Illinois, has accepted the post of resident naturalist for 1940.

Members of the Scientific Advisory Committee are Dr. W. J. Hamilton, Jr., *chairman;* Dr. Lewis A. Eldridge; Dr. John R. Greeley; Dr. G. Kingsley Noble; Dr. Thomas Ordway and William Vogt. Inquiries regarding the Biological Research Division should be addressed to W. J. Hamilton, Jr., Cornell University, Ithaca, New York.

## AWARDS OF THE ROYAL GEOGRAPHICAL SOCIETY

THERE have already been given in SCIENCE the names of those who received the awards of the Royal Geographical Society at the annual meeting in London on June 26. The citations made by Field Marshal Sir Philip Chetwode, president of the society, follow:

With the approval of His Majesty, the Founder's Medal has been awarded to Mr. Arthur M. Champion. Mr. Champion has spent thirty years in East Africa, largely in the administrative service of Kenya. For some years he was in administrative charge of the Turkana Province. On his appointment, Mr. Champion made it his duty to carry out the first systematic survey of the Province on a trigonometrical framework, producing a valuable map in six sheets on the scale of 1/250,000. In addition to this he investigated the physical geography and geology of the area, and more particularly of Teleki's Volcano and the lava fields south of Lake Rudolf. He has communicated the results of his work in valuable papers to the society, and has recently shown to us the film which he made on a motor journey across Africa from Cape Verde to Nairobi, carried out after he had retired from the Colonial Service. Mr. Champion has now made his home in Kenya, and we look forward to further contributions from him on the geography of East Africa.

His Majesty the King has approved of the award of the Patron's Medal to Professor Hans Ahlmann, of the University of Stockholm, for his exploration and glaciological studies in the Arctic. He has specialized in studying the work of ice and snow and for this purpose he organized and led the two Swedish-Norwegian expeditions to Spitsbergen in 1931 and 1934, and the Swedish-Icelandic expedition to Vatnajökull in 1936–37. The many important scientific monographs resulting from these expeditions have been noticed from time to time in the *Geographical Journal,* and we have had the pleasure on a former occasion of hearing a paper by him upon the physical characteristics of glaciers. Professor Ahlmann's work has stimulated much interest in this important branch of our science, and younger explorers and students owe a great deal to his encouragement and assistance. He is leaving in a few weeks' time to continue his researches in northeast Greenland.

The Murchison Grant has been awarded by the council to Mr. Robert Bentham for his surveys and geological investigations in Ellesmere Land. Mr. Bentham first went to the Arctic with the Oxford University Exploration Club's Ellesmere Land Expedition in 1934. In 1936 he returned by himself to the police post at Craig Harbour, Jones Sound, where he spent two years making a plane-table survey of southeast Ellesmere Land and in geological and archeological work. He also made an extended journey to the northwest.

The Back Grant has been awarded by the council to Lieutenant-Commander R. E. D. Ryder, R.N., for his captaincy of the *Penola* and his marine surveys on the British Graham Land Expedition. Commander Ryder's achievement in navigating the *Penola* in high latitudes and often in uncharted waters, with a crew which had little nautical experience before leaving England, was a fine feat of resourceful seamanship. He also took every opportunity of extending our hydrographical knowledge of the island-strewn waters and coasts of western Graham Land, and his surveys have been incorporated in the official charts. Commander Ryder being absent on duty, I shall ask his father, Colonel Ryder, to accept the award on his behalf.

The Cuthbert Peek Grant has been awarded by the council to Mr. W. V. Lewis for his physiographical studies in Great Britain and Iceland. Mr. Lewis, who is university demonstrator in geography at Cambridge, has taken part in one expedition and led another to Iceland. His interests are chiefly in the evolution of glacial features and of shorelines and he had also pursued these studies in Great Britain. At various times he has imparted to us the results of his observations on Dungeness Foreland, the Chesil Beach and elsewhere on the English coast, as well as upon the coast of southeast Iceland.

The council has awarded the Gill Memorial to Mr. J. V. Harrison for many years' exploration in Central and South America and southern Iran. Mr. Harrison, who is a geologist by training, saw active service during the war with the Royal Engineers in Mesopotamia. Since then he has been engaged on topographical and geological surveys in Iran, Mexico, Venezuela, Colombia, Honduras and the West Indies. In particular he has described to the society his journeys and surveys of the mountainous and inhospitable Bakhtiari and Kuhgalu country in southwestern Iran, formerly difficult of access to travelers and unsurveyed, the homes of restless tribes. Mr. Harrison's work has not only provided us with our first precise knowledge of the topography of these regions, but has also contributed to the elucidation of some major problems of the earth's structure. He is now at work in the Central Andes of Peru, and I shall ask Dr. G. M. Lees to accept this award on his behalf.

## SURVEY OF RESEARCH IN INDUSTRY

THE appointment of Raymond Stevens, vice-president of Arthur D. Little, Inc., of Cambridge, Mass., as director of a nation-wide survey of research in industry which is to be started at once, has been announced by Dr. Ross G. Harrison, chairman of the National Research Council. The announcement followed the first meeting of a special committee held at the Engineers' Club in New York City to formulate initial plans. Mr. Stevens has obtained leave of absence that will permit him to devote a principal portion of his time to the survey, the headquarters of which will be in the National Research Council Building in Washington. He is known as an authority on the organization of large-scale research programs, as well as the application of research for the solution of specific problems in industry.

In announcing the appointment, Dr. Harrison stated that while funds for the work had been made available by the National Resources Planning Board, of which Frederic A. Delano is chairman, the survey would be conducted and the report prepared by the National Research Council. This is in accordance with plans approved by an advisory committee of leading scientific men, industrial research directors and executives, of which F. W. Willard, president of the Nassau Smelting and Refining Company, New York, is president. The report will be submitted in printed form by the council next year and will present "an objective study of industrial research as a national resource, as a means of aiding in its further development and utilization."

The National Research Council is composed largely of the accredited representatives of about eighty-five national scientific and technical societies. It was established in 1916 at the request of President Woodrow Wilson, by the National Academy of Sciences, to coordinate the research facilities of the country for work on war problems involving scientific knowledge. An executive order by President Wilson in May, 1918, complimented the National Academy and the National Research Council on war services and requested that the academy perpetuate the National Research Council with six peace-time objectives: to stimulate research in natural sciences for national defense and public welfare; to survey larger possibilities and formulate comprehensive research projects; to promote cooperation in research at home and abroad; to promote active cooperation with War and Navy Departments and civil branches of the government; to direct attention of scientific workers to war problems and to make available scientific information at home and abroad in cooperation with other agencies.

# SCIENTIFIC NOTES AND NEWS

DR. JULIAN HUXLEY, secretary of the Zoological Society, London, was the guest of honor on December 2 at a dinner arranged by the Smithsonian Institution, the American Association for the Advancement of Science and *The Scientific Monthly.* Dr. Forest Ray Moulton, permanent secretary of the association, presided. Remarks were made by a representative of the Marquis of Lothian, the British Ambassador, who was unable to be present, and by Dr. Charles G. Abbot, secretary of the Smithsonian Institution. Dr. Isaiah Bowman, president of the Johns Hopkins University, introduced Dr. Huxley, whose address was entitled "Science, Social and Unsocial."

DONALD WILLS DOUGLAS, president of the Douglas Aircraft Company, Santa Monica, Calif., has been awarded by the Institute of the Aeronautical Sciences the Daniel Guggenheim Medal for 1939 "for outstanding contributions to the design and construction of transport airplanes."

THE Lamme Medal of the Ohio State University was presented to Thomas Alvin Boyd, since 1923 head of the fuel department of General Motors Research Laboratories, who was the codiscoverer of anti-knock effects of liquid lead compounds, at a dinner of the fourth annual Industrial Research Conference.

FREDERICK SKENE, who for eighteen years has been dean of the School of Technology of the College of the City of New York, was the guest of honor at a reception by the Engineering Alumni on November 29 at the City College Club.

FRANCIS P. GARVAN, JR., has been elected *president* of the Chemical Foundation, an office held by his father, the late Francis P. Garvan, from the formation of the foundation until his death in 1937. George J. Corbett was elected *vice-president;* William M. Buffum, *treasurer,* and Edward J. Muhs, *secretary.*

CERTIFICATES of honorary membership in the American Society of Mechanical Engineers were presented at the sixtieth annual meeting, which opened in Philadelphia on December 4, to Dexter Simpson Kimball, dean-emeritus of the College of Engineering, Cornell University; to Edwin Jay Prindle, retired patent attorney and mechanical engineer, East Orange, N. J.; to Charles T. Main, industrial engineer and expert on power and textile plants, Boston, Mass., and to Henry Hague Vaughan, consulting engineer and president of the Canadian Foreign Investment Corporation, Montreal, Canada.

DR. WILDER PENFIELD, director of the Montreal Neurological Institute and professor of neurology at McGill University, has been elected president of the Royal College of Physicians and Surgeons of Canada.

THE degree of doctor, *honoris causa,* has been conferred by the faculty of medicine of the University of Bordeaux on Dr. Constantin Daniel, professor of obstetrics and gynecology at the University of Bucharest. The diploma and the insignia were handed to him in the presence of the deans of the university and of prominent citizens.

DR. NAGAMICHI KURODA, an authority on the birds of Japan and eastern Asia, has succeeded to the title of Marquis Kuroda previously held by his father, who died last August at the age of seventy-two years.

ACCORDING to the *Australian Journal of Science,* the title of emeritus professor has been conferred by the senate of the University of Sydney on Dr. J. Douglas Stewart, who recently retired from the chair of veterinary science at the university. Professor Stewart was the first professor of veterinary science at Sydney, and served for thirty years as dean of the faculty.

DR. W. ALBERT NOYES, JR., has been appointed head of the department of chemistry of the University of Rochester. He succeeds Professor Victor J. Chambers, who has become professor emeritus.

DR. HARRY STACK SULLIVAN, chairman of the faculty of the Washington School of Psychiatry, has been appointed professor of psychiatry and director of the department of psychiatry and neurology at the Georgetown University School of Medicine. He succeeds the late Dr. Daniel Percy Hickling, who was a member of the faculty for more than forty years.

*Industrial and Engineering Chemistry* reports that Jules Bebie, for a number of years director of research at the Monsanto Chemical Company, has been appointed lecturer in chemical engineering at Washington University, St. Louis.

ERWIN H. AMICK has resigned his position with the Standard Oil Development Company to become an assistant professor in chemical engineering at the University of Pennsylvania.

SIR ROBERT KELLY, from 1922 to 1939 professor of surgery at the University of Liverpool, has retired with the title emeritus.

DR. RICHARD VAN DER RIET WOOLLEY has been appointed director of the Commonwealth Solar Observatory at Mount Stromlo, Australia. Dr. Woolley was chief assistant at the Royal Observatory, Greenwich, from 1933 to 1937, and since then has been John Couch Adams astronomer in the University of Cambridge. He has been editor of *The Observatory* since 1933.

DR. ELMER O. KRAEMER, formerly connected with the Experimental Station of E. I. du Pont de Nemours and Company, has recently returned from Europe, where he spent a year as fellow of the Lalor Foundation, continuing his researches on the sizes and shapes of giant molecules with Professor The Svedberg at the University of Upsala, Sweden. Dr. Kraemer is now associated with the Biochemical Research Foundation of the Franklin Institute in Philadelphia.

Dr. Charles O. Warren, Jr., instructor in physiology at Cornell University Medical College, has been awarded a grant from the Committee on Scientific Research of the American Medical Association for the continuation of studies on the metabolism of bone marrow. A renewal has been made of the grant of last year to Dr. Joseph H. Roe, professor of biochemistry in the School of Medicine of the George Washington University, in support of the continuance of his work on methods for the determination of ascorbic acid and of a study of the effect of vitamin C upon gastric function.

Dr. Irvine McQuarrie, head of the department of pediatrics at the Medical School of the University of Minnesota, has leave of absence. He plans to spend six months as visiting professor of pediatrics at the Peiping Union Medical College. He will leave for China early in January.

According to *The Harvard Alumni Bulletin,* Dr. Lewis W. Hackett, who represents the International Health Division of the Rockefeller Foundation in the Mediterranean region, has moved from Rome to Egypt. His address after January 30 will be the Public Health Laboratories, Cairo.

Harlan B. Holmes returned to the service of the Bureau of Fisheries in October after a four-year period of detail to the War Department, during which time he designed the fishways at Bonneville Dam and supervised the initial period of their operation. Mr. Holmes now assumes charge of the recently established Hydraulics Section of the Division of Scientific Inquiry. Associated with Mr. Holmes in the Hydraulics Section is O. W. Lindgren, associate hydraulic engineer, who has recently been engaged in directing the installation of screens at various federal irrigation projects in the Northwest.

Dr. William M. Mann, director of the National Zoological Park, Washington, D. C., lectured on November 30 to an audience numbering over eight hundred before the Lancaster Branch of the American Association for the Advancement of Science. He described the work accomplished by the National Geographic Society-Smithsonian Expedition of 1937 in the Dutch East Indies.

Professor Douglas Johnson, of Columbia University, gave an illustrated lecture on "The Physical History of the Grand Canyon District" before the students and faculty of the Connecticut College on October 31. On December 7 he addressed the Geology Society of the College of the City of New York on "The Supposed Meteorite Craters of the Carolina Coast."

Dr. F. F. Nord, of Fordham University, editor of *Ergebnisse der Enzymforschung,* lectured under the auspices of the Research Council at the Iowa State College on November 27 and 28, on "Low Temperature and Its Relation to Colloid Chemistry" and on "The Enzyme System of Fusaria and Its Action." At a meeting of Sigma Xi he spoke on "The Modern Concepts of the Mechanism of Alcoholic Fermentation."

Dr. George Jobberns, head of the department of geography of the Canterbury University College, Christchurch, New Zealand, is a visiting scholar in geomorphology at Columbia University during the current semester. In November he delivered a course of four illustrated lectures on "The Geology of New Zealand," under the auspices of the department of geology. On November 28 he gave an illustrated lecture on New Zealand Landscapes, under the auspices of the Columbia Institute of Arts and Sciences.

The Croonian lecture of the Royal Society was delivered by Professor J. Gray at the department of zoology of the University of Cambridge on November 16. His subject was "The Aspects of Animal Locomotion."

According to *The Fisheries Service Bulletin,* Leo D. Sturgeon, Foreign Service Officer of the Department of State on detail in the department, has been assigned to serve as assistant to Counselor R. Walton Moore. The primary duty of Mr. Sturgeon is to assist in the formulation of policy and in the coordination of action in the State Department on international aspects of fishery matters. This will involve the study and handling of problems concerning methods of regulating the fisheries and the formulation of arrangements for the conservation of international fisheries of concern to American interests. Mr. Sturgeon will act as liaison officer between the Department of State and other government agencies.

The *Journal* of the American Medical Association reports that members of the state board of examiners in the basic sciences for Florida include the following recently appointed by the governor: Dr. Mark Wirth Emmel, professor of veterinary science, University of Florida, *chairman;* Dr. John Ferguson Conn, professor of chemistry, the John B. Stetson University, *secretary;* Dr. Ezda May Deviney, professor of zoology, Florida State College for Women; Dr. Jay F. W. Pearson, professor of zoology, University of Miami, and Dr. Donald D. Bodé, professor of chemistry, Tampa University.

Dr. A. O. Weese, professor of zoology in the University of Oklahoma, was elected president of the board of directors of the newly incorporated Grassland Research Foundation at a meeting held in Norman, Okla., on November 7. Other officers are G. W. Goldsmith, professor of botany at the University of Texas, and V. E. Shelford, professor of zoology at the University of Illinois, *vice-presidents;* J. M. Aikman, professor of botany at Iowa State College, *secretary;* and Mrs. M. W. Shackleford, professor of biology at the Oklahoma College for Women, *treasurer.* Incorporation of the group has been completed under the laws of Oklahoma. Membership, however, includes those living in the grassland area as far distant from Oklahoma as Saskatchewan, Oregon, Arizona, Texas and Illinois. A meeting of the corporation will be held in Columbus, Ohio, during the Christmas vacation, as part of the meeting of the American Association for the Advancement of Science. The Grassland Research Foundation is the outcome of the work of the committee on ecology of the grasslands of the National Research Council.

FOR the positions in the Bureau of Animal Industry, Department of Agriculture, of protozoologist at a salary of $3,800 a year, of associate protozoologist at a salary of $3,200 a year and assistant protozoologist at a salary of $2,600 a year, applications must be on file with the U. S. Civil Service Commission at Washington, D. C., not later than January 2. Vacancies in positions requiring similar qualifications will be filled from these examinations, unless it is found in the interest of the service to fill any vacancy by reinstatement, transfer or promotion. The salaries named above are subject to a deduction of 3½ per cent. toward a retirement annuity. Separate lists of eligibles will be established in each of the above grades in: (1) Coccidiosis; (2) parasitic protozoa of the blood; (3) general parasitic protozoa. Permanent employees in the classified service will, upon earning a passing mark in these examinations, have their names placed upon a separate list of eligible government employees, which list may be certified separately to fill appropriate vacancies in accordance with the civil-service rules.

DR. ERNEST CARROLL FAUST, secretary of the American Academy of Tropical Medicine, reports that the sixth annual session of the academy was held in conjunction with the American Society of Tropical Medicine meeting with the Southern Medical Association at Memphis, Tenn., on November 23. The presidential address was delivered by Dr. W. W. Cort, of the Johns Hopkins University, on the subject "Research on Helminth Diseases and Public Health Progress." The second presentation of the Theobald Smith Gold Medal of the George Washington University for distinguished work in tropical medicine was presented by Dr. Alfred C. Reed, of the University of California, for the academy, to Dr. Richard P. Strong, of the Harvard Medical School. At the business session of the academy, the officers elected were: Admiral Charles S. Butler, *president;* Dr. Marshall A. Barber, *vice-president;* Dr. Ernest Carroll Faust, *secretary;* Dr. Thomas T. Mackie, *treasurer;* Colonel George R. Callender, *councillor.* Five new members were elected, and Dr. L. O. Howard, member, was elected to honorary membership. It was voted to hold the seventh annual session of the academy with the American Society of Tropical Medicine at Louisville, Ky., in November, 1940.

ACCORDING to the *Journal* of the American Medical Association, the Milwaukee Academy of Medicine and the Marquette University School of Medicine have consolidated their medical libraries, forming a collection of 34,000 volumes. Dr. Irving S. Cutter, dean of Northwestern University Medical School, Chicago, was the speaker at the ceremony inaugurating the new library on October 17. Facilities have been enlarged at the university to receive the academy's library, the most important part of which is the collection of the late Dr. Horace Manchester Brown.

# DISCUSSION

## HEAVY WATER AND LONGEVITY

THE suggestion by Barnes[1] that deuterium oxide would be found to retard life processes, thus favoring longevity, was predicated upon the lower energy content of deuterium as compared with hydrogen.

The undersigned[2] have shown, during the past summer, that heavy water retards four chief growth activities of *obelia geniculata.* This is a sessile marine animal living in colonies of a few millimeters length. Forty-six experiments on 27,000 animals were made with concentrations up to 10 per cent. $D_2O$. The results accord with the general trend of observations by others on the growth of various low forms of life[3] and can best be interpreted on the assumption that deuterium oxide blocks anabolism. Since the evidence concerning regressive and senile stages of obelia also favors retardation rather than acceleration by $D_2O$, the prolongation of individual existence in these animals appears established.

While our results, as far as they go, fulfill the prediction of Barnes, they do not contribute convincingly

[1] T. C. Barnes, *Jour. Am. Chem. Soc.,* 55: 4332–4333, 1933.

[2] F. S. Hammett and H. G. Barbour, *Growth,* 3: 4, 1939.

[3] See reviews: S. L. Meyer, *Jour. Tenn. Acad. Sci.,* 10: 111–115, 1935; H. G. Barbour, *Yale Jour. Biol. Med.,* 9: 551–565, 1937; C. B. Davenport, *Ann. Rev. Physiol.,* I: 81–108, 1939.

to the question of mammalian longevity. The retarding effects of $D_2O$ on the growth of mice bearing tumor transplants were demonstrated by Barbour and Allen.[4] One fifth saturation with deuterium oxide retarded the growth of both tumors and hosts, the latter showing shorter survival periods than the $H_2O$ controls. A number of other mice have for several months tolerated one fifth saturation with $D_2O$, without evidence for enhanced longevity.

More significant is the fact that while the obelia offers evidence for decreased catabolism in low forms of animal life, mammals respond to one fifth saturation of deuterium oxide by catabolic stimulation persisting for many days.[5] Such difference in mammals may be attributable to checks and balances acquired in their phylogenetic development, as are, for example, provided by the elaboration of hormones. Now, deuterium oxide, presumably by providing a slow-acting form of hydrogen, protects and "prolongs the life" of at least two of these unstable hormones, namely, epinephrine[6] and acetylcholine.[7] The first of these has been found responsible for the metabolic increases, up to +20 per cent., which tend to make the mice "live faster" rather than slower.

Therefore, although deuterium oxide retards growth and anabolism and in toxic concentrations even delays catabolism in all forms of life so far examined, it is not to be expected that mammals enjoying the luxury of partial saturation with this substance will exhibit enhanced longevity.

H. G. BARBOUR

YALE UNIVERSITY
SCHOOL OF MEDICINE

F. S. HAMMETT

LANKENAU HOSPITAL
RESEARCH INSTITUTE,
NORTH TRURO, MASS.

## HEPARIN AND BLOOD CLOTTING

THERE recently appeared an article in which Astrup[1] confirmed our observation[2] that normal plasma contains an unknown factor, which, in conjunction with heparin, blocks the transformation of prothrombin into thrombin. Both his work and ours showed that heparin alone has little or no effect in blocking this reaction—a finding which conforms to the earlier experiments of Mellanby[3] and Quick.[4] However, in mixtures containing both the plasma factor and heparin, our work and that of Astrup showed that marked inhibition of thrombin formation results.

In a recent note in this column, Ferguson[5] discussed these results, and indicated, erroneously, we believe, that Howell and Holt's[6] original work had brought out all these same facts. It is true that they did find that the *destruction* of thrombin by heparin requires a plasma factor ("pro-antithrombin"), but they believed that heparin interfered *directly* with the conversion of prothrombin into thrombin (antiprothrombic action of heparin). Our work and that of Astrup has brought out the new concept that a plasma factor is needed for this inhibitory action of heparin.

Although we have suggested that this new plasma factor and the pro-antithrombin of Howell may be identical chemically, as yet no data are available on this point and the question must be left for future work.

K. M. BRINKHOUS
H. P. SMITH, JR.
E. D. WARNER
W. H. SEEGERS

DEPARTMENT OF PATHOLOGY,
STATE UNIVERSITY OF IOWA

## MASTODON REMAINS FOUND IN WEST VIRGINIA

ON Monday, October 9, there was brought to the biological laboratories of Bethany College the proximal portion of a long bone, too large to be that of any local domesticated animal. This bone fragment had been uncovered and picked up by a Mr. Funk, the operator of a steam shovel engaged in stripping coal about two miles west of Bethany, W. Va., in Brooke County, on a tract of land known as the Pendleton Farm and owned by a Mr. Petzol, of Hollidays Cove, W. Va.

The undersigned went immediately to the stripping operation and there found a number of other fossilized bones, as well as a portion of a tooth. These materials were removed to the biological laboratories of Bethany College. Dr. Leroy Kaye, paleontologist of the Carnegie Museum, Pittsburgh, Pa., was called into consultation and it was agreed that these were parts of a skeleton of the American mastodon.

The skeleton remains were found in a deposit of blue clay about 18 feet below the surface. This layer of clay was 6′ 3″ in thickness. It was probably a Pleistocene deposit. This layer contained an abundance of Gasteropod and Pelecypod fossils, as well as numerous pieces of fossilized wood. Overlying this was another layer of yellow clay of a gravelly nature,

[4] H. G. Barbour and E. Allen, *Am. Jour. Cancer*, 32: 440–446, 1938.

[5] H. G. Barbour and L. E. Rice, *Jour. Pharm. Exp. Therap.*, 62: 292–300, 1938.

[6] H. G. Barbour, Internat. Physiologen-Kongr., 16, Zurich, 1938, *Kongressber.*, pt. 2, 34–35.

[7] H. G. Barbour and V. C. Dickerson. *Jour. Pharm. Exp. Therap.*, 65: 281–286, 1939.

[1] T. Astrup, SCIENCE, 90: 36, 1939.

[2] K. M. Brinkhous, H. P. Smith, E. D. Warner and W. H. Seegers, *Am. Jour. Physiol.*, 125: 683, 1939.

[3] J. Mellanby, *Proc. Roy. Soc. B.*, 116: 1, 1934.

[4] A. J. Quick, *Proc. Soc. Exp. Biol. and Med.*, 35: 391, 1936.

[5] J. H. Ferguson, SCIENCE, 90: 272, 1939.

[6] W. H. Howell and E. Holt, *Am. Jour. Physiol.*, 47: 328, 1918.

approximately 11′ 6″ in thickness; both overlay a thick stratum of shale above a vein of Pittsburgh coal.

A study of the geology of the region revealed that in the geological past the bed of clay formed the bottom of an ancient stream bed. Fortunately the mining operations cut across the strata, thus revealing the geological history quite definitely.

The portions of the skeleton recovered thus far consist of the heads of both femurs, the proximal end of the humerus, a practically complete right scapula, a number of foot and toe bones, together with portions of the vertebra. A number of other bony fragments are in the laboratories and will be assembled later.

Two large fragments of a molar were found and these have been fitted together. The figuration of the tooth and the marks established the identity of this animal definitely as a mastodon.

To the best of our knowledge this is the first report of the finding of mastodon remains in this section of the State of West Virginia. Thirty-seven years ago a portion of a tusk was found in a gravel pit near Brilliant, Ohio, eight miles west of Bethany, W. Va., on the west bank of the Ohio River.

It is planned to continue the search in the region of the original find and make a more detailed report at a later date.

W. J. SUMPSTINE
B. R. WEIMER

BETHANY COLLEGE (W. VA.)

## BORGMEIER'S REVISTA DE ENTOMOLOGIA. AN APPEAL TO ENTOMOLOGISTS

IN the field of entomology, many of us have depended for years on foreign journals, the channels for publication being wholly inadequate in this country. I notice, in my case, that in 1938 nearly half of my papers were published abroad. In the near future, some of the European periodicals will be completely closed to us, while others plan to carry on on a modest scale or even to suspend for the duration of hostilities. It seems most opportune to call the entomologists' attention to a New World publication, which, with the proper support of American workers, may well prove the ideal solution to our present difficulties. Started in 1931, the *Revista de Entomologia,* of Rio de Janeiro, is now running through the tenth volume, and has kept up an unequaled standard of excellence. Each of the nine completed volumes covers some 500 pages, adequately illustrated with text-figures and half-tone plates. The papers are cosmopolitan in authorship (being written in English, German, French, Spanish and Portuguese) and cover practically every phase of entomology, theoretical as well as practical. Each issue, of which there are now three to a yearly volume, concludes with an extremely valuable critical bibliography of neotropical entomology. This feature alone makes the *Revista* indispensable to all students of Central and South American insects. From the start, the *Revista* has been conducted as a labor of love by Father Thomaz Borgmeier, O.F.M., an entomologist of repute in his own field. As most European subscribers are likely to drop out at present, it is to be feared that the editor will run into some unexpected difficulties. All American entomologists are urged to rally to his support. Beginning next year, Father Borgmeier plans to accept for publication papers dealing with North American insects also. The editor's address is Convento S. Antonio, Largo da Carioca, Rio de Janeiro, Brazil.

J. BEQUAERT

HARVARD MEDICAL SCHOOL,
BOSTON, MASS.

# SCIENTIFIC BOOKS

## MEDICAL CLIMATOLOGY

*Medical Climatology.* By CLARENCE A. MILLS. 296 pp. Baltimore, Md.: Charles C Thomas. 1939.

MILLS's "Medical Climatology" is symptomatic of a movement which may become a mighty tide a generation hence. For two generations or more biological investigation has centered upon the organism itself far more than upon its environment. The structure of the cell, the mechanism of inheritance, the chemical composition of glandular secretions and the influence of bacteria and other internal parasites have engrossed attention. As a result not only have the ravages of infectious diseases diminished greatly, but new and valuable varieties of domestic plants and animals have been produced in great numbers. This progress, however, has gone hand in hand with comparative neglect of the other side of the shield. Our knowledge of how the organism is influenced by the external environment represented by climate, soil and so forth is still pitifully small. The botanists, to be sure, have recently made good progress in ecology, but only the merest beginning has been made in studying the ecology of animals and man. The significance of "Medical Climatology" lies in the fact that it opens up many new lines of approach to the fruitful field of human ecology.

The thesis of the book is that two main types of disease—infectious and degenerative—display opposite relations to climate. The basic reason for this, as Mills sees it, is that human metabolism varies greatly in response to weather and climate. Warm and monotonous climates lower the rate of metabolism; thus diminishing people's power to resist all sorts of infections. Cold and variable climates increase metabolism, thus making people active, energetic and able to resist infection. Unfortunately, however, this metabolic activity places too great a strain upon the vital organs, thus leading to degenerative diseases of the heart, kidneys, nervous system, and so forth. Hence in warm, mild, enervating climates, infectious, parasitic diseases are especially common, whereas in cool, variable and stimulating climates degenerative diseases are dominant. Recent medical progress has greatly diminished the danger from infectious diseases, such as tuberculosis, diphtheria, measles, yellow fever and malaria. It has had little effect, however, upon the degenerative diseases, and these are increasing as the elimination of the infectious diseases lengthens the span of life.

Mills's thesis is that we fail to conquer the degenerative diseases because we do not recognize that their major cause is the incessant drive of cool, stormy and variable climates, which reach their greatest extreme in the north central United States. The most valuable part of his book is a series of maps showing that the death rate from a considerable series of diseases increases from south to north in the United States, and varies in corresponding fashion according to the climate of other parts of the world. The diseases include diabetes, goiter, pernicious anemia, leukemia, pneumonia, tuberculosis, appendicitis, arteriosclerosis and heart failure. Suicides and homicides behave in much the same way. Most of the diseases show a maximum death rate in winter and a minimum in summer. Mills shows that in general the geographical distribution of mortality from these diseases is the same for whites and Negroes, and also for both rural and urban populations. The Negro death rate, to be sure, always exceeds that of the whites, and the urban and rural rates may differ. In all cases, however, the variations from region to region are similar.

Mills takes issue with Winslow, Herrington and others who claim that such diseases owe their distribution mainly to urban conditions and to the intensity of modern industrial life. To the reviewer it seems that Mills does not pay enough attention to the fact that even in villages our modern urban and industrial life is quite highly developed, and that it surely has an effect upon health in general and upon metabolism in particular. On the other hand, Winslow and his coadjutors fail to pay enough attention to the fact that this kind of life is found only in climates that are highly stimulating, and that it would not be there to any such degree if the climate were different.

Another important point made by Mills is that in many infectious diseases the number of *cases* is especially high in the more stimulating climates, but the *deaths* in proportion to the cases are few. In warmer climates, on the contrary, the number of cases is small, but the death rate in proportion to the cases is high. His interpretation of this is that although the overstimulation of the cool stormy type of climate leads to degeneration of certain organs, its general effect on the body is so good that people are often able to overcome disease. In warm monotonous climates, on the contrary, if people become ill for any cause whatsoever, they have relatively little power of resistance. There the number of deaths is high in proportion to the cases, although absolutely low. In this connection Mills finds that China and, to a less degree, Japan behave like tropical countries. Western Europe is more like the eastern United States, while the north central part of this country is peculiarly subject to the stimulus and the diseases induced by low temperature and great storminess.

Here is Mills's own way of putting his main conclusion: "Atmospheric turbulence, with sudden changes in temperature and barometric pressure, is a factor largely responsible for the initiation of infectious attacks, particularly in the respiratory and enteric systems. But ability to successfully resist the invasion seems to depend closely on the energy level engendered in the population mass by the stimulation of the climatic habitat. People living at low levels of energy and bodily vigor in regions of moist heat show little ability to throw off infections that once gain a foothold. Fortunately, in most tropical regions of moist heat, atmospheric stability is the rule. Only in the somewhat limited areas of tropical typhoons is man doubly handicapped in his struggle for survival. In these regions such infectious (?) diseases as tuberculosis, leprosy, acute nephritis and acute appendicitis take heavy toll. In the cooler portions of the stormy temperate regions ability to fight infectious invasions rises to much higher levels. There it is that most remarkable advances have been made in the fight to lessen the infectious disease death rates. But while these advances are being recorded, energetic inhabitants of these stimulating regions are exhibiting an increasing rate of exhaustion and bodily breakdown that provides an evil foreboding of what may eventually result from the too intensive climatic drive (pp. 161–2)."

In spite of much that is convincing, "Medical Climatology" needs greater precision. For example, "in Greenland the Norse colonies died out around 1000 A.D. (page 278)." That is the time when they went there. They disappeared four centuries later. Again page 256 mentions "a time when Pittsburgh has just become adapted to heat more severe than that of Texas." The reader understands that Pittsburgh, where the average July temperature is 75°, has a hotter season than Texas, where the July average at altitudes under 3,500 feet is 80° to 88°. Mills fails to explain that he refers to a particular instance when a brief heat wave made Pittsburgh hotter than Texas.

Much more important is the author's uncertain attitude toward changes in barometric pressure, an attitude which is prevalent among many others. For instance, "Tropical typhoon storms sweeping eastward over the West Indies and Caribbean region bring added instability during the winter months. These latter storms cause little temperature change, but their sharp pressure fluctuations seem to bring many of the same body disturbances that are associated with temperate zone storm changes [page 222]. . . . There is a strong suggestion that the sudden change of barometric pressure which accompanies tropical hurricanes may be just as important a factor in promoting many types of infectious diseases as are similar changes accompanying temperate zone storms [page 216]. Nevertheless, ". . . our knowledge of the physiologic effects induced by pressure changes is still far too incomplete even to be called evidence. There are hints, however, that fluctuations in atmospheric pressure do result in marked alterations in certain body functions, particularly those of the nervous system, reflex acts and glandular activity [page 258]. . . . The only significant experimental results so far published," however, "are those of Smith, showing a positive water balance in the body with pressure reduction and a negative balance with pressure increase. Body tissues in this respect act as a sponge [page 54]." In spite of the scarcity of evidence, ". . . Sudden changes in air temperature and barometric pressure, as major storm disturbances sweep across the continent, seem to be the most potent factors predisposing to acute infectious attacks [page 123]."

In many other places changes in atmospheric pressure from day to day are mentioned as if on a par with changes in temperature. Smith's conclusions, to which Mills refers, are based on differences less than the probable observational error in one of his two experiments, and only a little larger in the other. Most writers on this subject take no account of the fact that whenever we drive among hills which cause our altitude to vary as much as three or four hundred feet, we subject ourselves to changes of pressure like those in an ordinary storm, but much more sudden. Nevertheless, no one is conscious of any effect. Mills tells us, however, that "tropical populations living in typhoon regions exhibit the world's most severe tuberculosis problems, . . . particularly . . . in such typhoon-afflicted regions as the Philippines . . . the West Indies, and parts of Mexico . . . that are battered by this type of storm disturbance [page 138]." The obvious implication of this last statement and of those previously quoted is that the changes in pressure accompanying typhoons or hurricanes, especially in winter, are a main cause of tuberculosis. This ascribes far too much to these tropical disturbances. In the West Indies as a whole, for example, there are only about four hurricanes per year on an average. In any one region there are far less. Jamaica, for example, near the center of the hurricane belt, had only 14 in 36 years. Moreover, there are few hurricanes in winter, as appears from the following data as to their total number in the entire West Indies from 1876 to 1911:

| | | | | | | | |
|---|---|---|---|---|---|---|---|
| Jan. | 0 | Apr. | 0 | July | 5 | Oct. | 44 |
| Feb. | 0 | May | 1 | Aug. | 35 | Nov. | 3 |
| Mar. | 0 | June | 8 | Sept. | 45 | Dec. | 2 |

Another feature of "Medical Climatology" which will at least arouse discussion is the map of climatic stimulation on page 82. It is based on (1) the difference between the maximum and minimum temperature of each day, (2) the difference between the maxima of successive days, (3) the difference between the minima of successive days, and (4) the number of days having temperatures above 64° and below 38°. From the standpoint of ordinary climatology and geography the resultant map seems inconclusive. It brings together regions which have little unity from the standpoints of vegetation, health or human activity. The greatest climatic stimulation is indicated in places as diverse as (1) the high Andean plateau within the tropics, (2) the plateau of Tibet, 25° farther north, (3) the plains of North America from Nebraska to the Arctic Circle, and (4) New Zealand. The northeastern United States, the North Sea region of Europe and a vast area in central Siberia, although reckoned by Mills as highly stimulating, are placed in a lower category. It must be clearly understood, however, that Mills distinguishes sharply between climatic stimulation and climatic efficiency. His whole book centers around the idea that the climate of some regions is so stimulating that its beneficial effect is in part counteracted.

In spite of these criticisms Mills's book is of high value. It blazes a pioneer trail in its suggestion that the study of climate may be the clue which will lead ultimately to a reduction in metabolic or degenerative diseases comparable to that which has taken place in infectious diseases. It also contains a number of interesting minor suggestions. For example, the place for sanitaria is not where a given disease is most common, but where it is rarest because that is where the climate helps to eliminate the disease. If all lepers were taken to Switzerland, the disease would presumably disappear. Again, dental caries increases not only from south to north in the United States, but as one goes downward in river valleys. In a book where so many new ideas are set forth, the chance for error is necessarily great. On the other hand, the searcher for fruitful research problems in the rich new field of the influence of physical environment will find in this book a perfect mine of valuable suggestions.

ELLSWORTH HUNTINGTON
YALE UNIVERSITY

# SPECIAL ARTICLES

## THE BACTERIOSTATIC ACTION OF SULFANILAMIDE UNDER ANAEROBIC CONDITIONS

ALTHOUGH the therapeutic use of sulfanilamide and allied compounds has been attended with much clinical success, the mechanism of their action in overcoming various infections is still in dispute. The *in vitro* studies of Locke,[1] Fox and coworkers[2] and the theoretical deductions of Shaffer[3] have led many investigators to assume that sulfanilamide is bacteriostatic only in the presence of oxygen. Contrary to such claims are the important findings of Bliss and Long[4] who reported bacteriostasis of streptococci and pneumococci under anaerobic conditions. However, Fox[5] claimed that Bliss and Long had been unable to obtain complete anaerobiosis in their experiments and attributed these results to small amounts of oxygen still remaining in their media.

We wish to report some data which completely substantiate the claim of Bliss and Long that sulfanilamide may be bacteriostatic under anaerobic conditions. During the course of some experiments designed to test the validity of the reduction potential theory of Shaffer and of the anti-catalase hypothesis of Locke, we have had occasion to examine the effects of sulfanilamide on the growth of *E. coli*. This was done primarily because the respiratory mechanisms and nutritional requirements of this organism are better understood than are those of the coccus group and because it has been pointed out[6] that *E. coli* is an excellent test organism for the accumulation of hydrogen peroxide.

Sulfanilamide produces, under given circumstances, marked bacteriostasis in cultures of *E. coli*. Thus, in ordinary meat extract broth, bacteriostasis is observed under aerobic but not under anaerobic conditions. On the other hand, in broth containing 1 per cent. glucose, sulfanilamide produces but little effect. It might be claimed that this protective action of glucose is attributable to its powerful reducing properties. Such does not appear to be the case, however. Both cysteine and ascorbic acid, powerful reducing agents themselves, fail to protect against the sulfanilamide bacteriostasis. Furthermore, as will be reported in another paper, glucose does not protect against the activity of sulfanilamide towards *E. coli* in certain other media.

It appears more probable that the protective action of glucose is based on its ability to supply to the cell a source of food and energy that is unaffected by the presence of sulfanilamide. *E. coli,* when growing in nutrient broth, depends on the various constituents of this medium for its supply of food materials, and if sulfanilamide, for any reason whatsoever, prevents the assimilation of various of these the growth of the cells will be adversely affected. On the other hand, if another substance (glucose) assimilable in nutrient broth even in the presence of sulfanilamide is added to the basal medium, growth will not be affected to any noticeable degree provided that such a substance can supply energy sufficient to permit growth to the same degree as do the constituents of the basal medium.

The proposition that sulfanilamide inhibits the mechanisms which enable the organism to grow aerobically at the expense of the constituents of nutrient broth finds some support in the following facts (Table I). *E. coli* grows well aerobically in nutrient broth

TABLE I

THE EFFECT OF SULFANILAMIDE ON GROWTH OF *E. coli* IN NUTRIENT BROTHS

| Oxygen tension | Nutrient broth enriched with | | | |
|---|---|---|---|---|
| | 1 per cent. glucose | | ——— | |
| | Sulfanilamide 10 mg per cent. | ——— | Sulfanilamide 10 mg per cent. | ——— |
| Aerobic .......... | ++++ | ++++ | + | +++ |
| Anaerobic ........ | ++++ | ++++ | + | + |

but only poorly under anaerobic conditions. In the presence of oxygen, the energy required for the multiplication of such a facultative anaerobe as *E. coli* is obtained simultaneously from two different sources—the one, an aerobic, the other an anaerobic mechanism. If sulfanilamide inhibits only the aerobic mechanism, the degree of growth in the presence of this chemical and oxygen should approximate that obtained in the absence of oxygen, and sulfanilamide should have no effect under conditions which induce anaerobiosis. Such is actually the case.

Moreover, since the addition of glucose enables the organisms to grow luxuriantly both in the presence and absence of oxygen, neither type of growth in glucose broths should be affected by sulfanilamide if the latter does not inhibit the assimilation of glucose. The results in Table I demonstrate that both aerobic and anaerobic growth in glucose broth are the same in the presence as in the absence of sulfanilamide.

[1] A. Locke, E. R. Main and R. R. Mellon, SCIENCE, 88: 620, 1938.
[2] C. L. Fox, B. German and C. A. Janeway, *Proc. Soc. Exp. Biol. Med.*, 40: 184, 1939.
[3] P. A. Shaffer, SCIENCE, 89: 547, 1939.
[4] E. Bliss and P. Long, *Proc. Third Internat. Microbiol. Cong.*, New York, 1939.
[5] C. L. Fox, *Proc. Third Internat. Microbiol. Cong.*, New York, 1939.
[6] R. H. Broh-Kahn and I. A. Mirsky, *Jour. Bact.*, 35: 455, 1938.

The type of bacteriostasis that has just been described is quite similar to that observed in the case of the hemolytic streptococci, since there is in both cases the same lag period before the bacteriostatic action becomes evident.

Quite different results were observed when the organism was grown in a synthetic medium of the following composition:

| | |
|---|---|
| 4.0 g. $(NH_4)_2HPO_4$ | 0.7 g. $MgSO_4$ |
| 1.0 g. NaCl | Trace $FeSO_4$ |
| 1.0 g. $KH_2PO_4$ | 1000 cc. distilled water |

Adjust to pH 7

As has been demonstrated by Quastel *et al.*,[7] *E. coli* grows well aerobically in such a medium when 1 per cent. lactate is added, but not at all under anaerobic conditions. On the other hand, the addition of both 1 per cent. lactate and 1 per cent. nitrate enables the organisms to grow anaerobically as well as aerobically, since the cells can utilize the energy obtained from the oxidation of lactate by nitrate to multiply in the absence of oxygen.

When sulfanilamide is added to cultures growing aerobically in the lactate medium, very little bacteriostasis is evident. The same is true for aerobic cultures growing in the lactate-nitrate medium. However, anaerobic cultures in the latter medium are markedly inhibited by the action of sulfanilamide. This, then, is an example of a case in which sulfanilamide is bacteriostatic in anaerobic but not in aerobic environment.

It is apparent that sulfanilamide prevents the oxidation of lactate by nitrate and so exerts its effect in anaerobic cultures. In this respect its action is similar to that of the cyanides (Table II).

THE EFFECT OF SULFANILAMIDE AND CYANIDES ON THE GROWTH OF *E. coli* IN A SYNTHETIC MEDIUM

| Oxygen tension | Synthetic medium + 1 per cent. Lactate enriched with | | | | | |
|---|---|---|---|---|---|---|
| | —— | | | 1 per cent. nitrate | | |
| | Sulfanilamide 10 mg per cent. | KCN M/400 | —— | Sulfanilamide 10 mg per cent. | KCN M/400 | —— |
| Aerobic .. | ++ | ++ | ++ | +++ | ++ | +++ |
| Anaerobic . | — | — | — | — | — | +++ |

These results are not affected by the various methods employed to obtain anaerobiosis, and they have been observed under conditions in which the oxygen content is so low that it will not affect electrode potentials or reoxidize leuco dyes. The following biological criteria of anaerobiosis could be obtained under the conditions employed. It is known[8] that *E. coli* is extremely sensitive to oxygen when grown in media containing cyanides and certain reversible oxidation-reduction systems. Furthermore, the growth of *H. influenzae* in the absence of hemin is inhibited by the slightest traces of oxygen in the medium[9] and our methods of securing anaerobiosis were sufficient to permit the growth of both organisms under the conditions mentioned. Certainly, the few molecules of oxygen that remain in the medium are insufficient to produce enough peroxide, "blue substance"[10] or oxidized sulfanilamide to cause bacteriostasis.

These observations of the differences between the effects of sulfanilamide in the nutrient broths and in synthetic media suggest that sulfanilamide selectively inhibits only certain mechanism. It follows that if, perchance, such mechanisms are either essential or beneficial to multiplication, the growth of the organism will be inhibited to a greater or less extent.

The above results should not necessarily be construed to indicate that the theories of Locke, Shaffer and Fox may not explain the bacteriostasis observed *in vitro* under special conditions, but they appear to demonstrate that such mechanisms can not be the sole ones concerned. Experiments in this laboratory have led us to believe that the bacteriostasis produced by sulfanilamide and allied compounds can not be attributed to any general, non-specific mechanism and that all efforts to derive knowledge concerning its mode of action will be futile unless its effects are examined in a variety of media under different conditions.

This work has been carried on with the technical assistance of Dan Perry.

R. H. BROH-KAHN

COLLEGE OF MEDICINE,
UNIVERSITY OF CINCINNATI,
AND THE CINCINNATI GENERAL HOSPITAL

## EFFECT OF NICOTINAMIDE ON RESPIRATION OF DYSENTERY BACILLI

NICOTINIC acid has been shown to be essential for the growth of the dysentery organism on a synthetic medium composed of amino acids, glucose and salts.[1] Derivatives of nicotinic acid such as the amide, coenzyme I and coenzyme II, and other closely related compounds will also function as growth factors in a synthetic medium.[2] On the other hand, Lwoff and Lwoff have shown[3] that *Hemophilus parainfluenzae*

[7] J. H. Quastel, M. Stephenson and M. Whetham, *Biochem. Jour.*, 19: 304, 1925.

[8] R. H. Broh-Kahn and I. A. Mirsky, *op. cit.*

[9] T. L. Snyder and R. H. Broh-Kahn, *Nature*, 142: 153, 1938.

[10] C. L. Fox, B. German and C. A. Janeway, *op. cit.*

[1] Koser, Dorfman and Saunders, *Proc. Soc. Exp. Biol. Med.*, 38: 311–13, 1938.

[2] Dorfman, Koser, Reames, Swingle and Saunders, *Jour. Infectious Diseases*, 65: 163–82, 1939.

[3] *Proc. Roy. Soc., London*, B122: 352–9, 1937.

needs the entire molecule of coenzyme I or coenzyme II and can not synthesize it from nicotinamide. The dysentery organism when grown on a synthetic medium with nicotinamide can synthesize a compound (or compounds) identical with or an adequate substitute for one or more of the coenzymes needed by *H. influenzae*.[2]

By means of the Thünberg technique, Lwoff and Lwoff have shown[4] that *H. parainfluenzae* cells grown in a medium which is deficient in the "V" factor (presumably coenzyme I or coenzyme II) have their respiration markedly stimulated by the addition of coenzyme I or coenzyme II to the Thünberg tubes. A similar stimulation of oxygen uptake could be demonstrated by means of the Warburg technique. This stimulation disappears when the cells are grown in a medium containing larger amounts of "V" factor, *i.e.*, the addition of coenzymes to the Thünberg tubes does not increase the respiration.

We have performed similar experiments in which we used dysentery bacilli grown on a medium containing suboptimum amounts of nicotinamide. We found that the rate of reduction of methylene blue is greatly increased not only by the addition of coenzyme I, but also by the addition of nicotinamide or nicotinic acid to the Thünberg tube, as shown by the following protocol. This effect of nicotinamide and nicotinic acid has not previously been reported for any system. The cells (Strain D76) were grown 24 hours in synthetic medium containing 0.005γ nicotinamide. The cells from 100 cc of medium were collected in the centrifuge and suspended in M/20 buffer (pH 7.4). The cells were again centrifuged and suspended in 34 cc of buffer. Two cc of this suspension was added to each tube. Each tube also contained 0.30 cc of a 2 per cent. solution of glucose and 0.50 cc of a solution of methylene blue containing 100γ of methylene blue per cc. The nicotinamide and nicotinic acid solutions contained 100γ per cc. The cozymase solution contained 300γ per cc and was 40 per cent. pure. Smaller quantities of a pure cozymase preparation from Euler's laboratory showed the same effect. Water was added to the controls to make the dilution the same in all cases. The tubes were equilibrated 10 minutes at 37° before tipping.

TABLE 1

| Tube | Control | 1 | 2 | 3 |
|---|---|---|---|---|
| Nicotinamide | 0 | 0.15 cc | 0 | 0 |
| Nicotinic acid | 0 | 0 | 0.15 cc | 0 |
| Cozymase | 0 | 0 | 0 | 0.15 cc |
| Time (in sec.) | 460 | 170 | 170 | 200 |

If we consider the ratio of the time of reduction control/nicotinamide, we find that the ratio decreases as the amount of nicotinamide in the *medium* is increased until with cells grown in a medium containing 0.020γ per cc it is about one. Thus at 0.003γ, the ratio is 3.8; at 0.005γ, 2.6; at 0.007γ, 1.8; at 0.010γ, 1.5; and at 0.020γ, 1.1. In controls containing nicotinamide, etc., but not glucose, reduction was much slower, 600 seconds or more. In controls which contained cells alone the methylene blue was reduced even more slowly or not at all. Nicotinamide, nicotinic acid or cozymase and glucose gave no reduction of methylene blue in the absence of cells.

The same stimulation of respiration by nicotinamide, etc., was found when oxygen uptake was measured by the direct Warburg method. It should be emphasized that various strains of the dysentery organism differ in their nicotinamide requirements. Further work in an attempt to elucidate the mechanism of this codehydrogenase action of nicotinamide is in progress in this laboratory.

ALBERT DORFMAN
STEWART A. KOSER
FELIX SAUNDERS

UNIVERSITY OF CHICAGO

[4] *Ibid.*, 360–73.

## SOMATOPLASTIC STERILITY IN MEDICAGO SATIVA[1]

THE collapse of ovules during the early stages of post-fertilization development frequently occurs in alfalfa, particularly after self-pollination.[2] Histological study shows that the collapse follows abnormal growth of the somatic tissue adjacent to the embryo sac. Since local hyperplasia of the maternal structures appears to be the essential feature of the developmental course leading to collapse, the term somatoplastic sterility is here proposed for a type of seed failure believed to occur in many plants.

The reproductive process in angiosperms may fail at any stage between fertilization and maturity of the seed. The early stages are of critical importance for survival of the ovule in alfalfa. Although somatoplastic sterility is not necessarily limited to this period, it is in young ovules that one would expect it to be manifested in simplest form. The case is of interest, therefore, as affording a point of departure in defining the significant histological features and in discovering the cause of a rather obscure, although probably widespread, form of sterility in plants.

The embryo sac in the mature ovule of alfalfa is surrounded by two integuments. The inner integument, which is composed of two layers of cells, lies in direct contact with the embryo sac except at the chalazal end where a few disintegrating cells, remnants of

[1] Papers from the Department of Genetics, Agricultural Experiment Station, University of Wisconsin No. 248. The authors desire to express their appreciation for financial aid from the University Research Committee and for assistance from WPA project in the Natural Sciences No. 8649.

[2] Brink and Cooper, *Proc. Nat. Acad. Sci.*, 24: 497–499, 1938.

the nucellus, are found. Shortly after fertilization active cell division is initiated in the integuments as well as in the endosperm mother cell and the zygote. The cells of the inner integument divide longitudinally so that this tissue normally continues to have two layers of cells at the later stages of development. The cells adjacent to the endosperm are tapetal-like in appearance.

In material collected 48 to 72 hours after pollination in which the collapse of fertile ovules is frequent the cytoplasm of the cells immediately adjacent to the endosperm becomes finely vacuolate and densely staining, and the resemblance to tapetal cells is gradually lost. This condition, which makes its first appearance on the funicular side of the ovule in the region of the vascular bundle, is often seen before any impairment of the embryo sac becomes evident. Breakdown of the endosperm follows, beginning in the chalazal region and progressing toward the embryo. At this stage there is extensive meristematic activity in the chalazal portion of the inner integument. Through transverse division of the cells this tissue may come to be three to five layers in thickness. The ovule may continue to enlarge for several hours, even after the endosperm has broken down, but its growth soon ceases.

The frequency of collapse of fertile ovules in alfalfa is much higher following self-pollination than after outcrossing to unrelated plants. In a representative experiment involving seven individuals on which the two types of matings were made under strictly comparable conditions the average values were 34.4 per cent. and 7.1 per cent., respectively, in the interval up to 144 hours after pollination.[2] The relatively high survival of ovules containing hybrid, as compared with inbred, embryos and endosperms affords a clue to the cause of somatoplastic sterility.

Fertilization initiates development of the embryo and the endosperm and stimulates mitosis in the surrounding somatic tissue. The ovule, quiescent prior to gametic union, suddenly springs into active growth. Further development of these structures is largely dependent upon food moved in from other parts of the plant, the visible reserves immediately at hand in alfalfa being very limited in amount and quickly disappearing after fertilization. The critical factor for survival at this stage seems to be the manner in which the translocated food is shared between the endosperm, on the one hand, and the inner integument, on the other. The partition of nutrients appears to depend upon the rate of growth inside and outside the embryo sac. It may be assumed that the synthetic processes are essentially alike in the different tissues concerned, and hence, that the same raw materials are in concurrent demand. Under these conditions of parallel growth the available foods will be shared between the inner integument and the structures within the embryo sac in proportion to the velocity with which growth is occurring in the respective tissues. Continued development of the ovule following fertilization demands a balance in rate of growth between the endosperm, which is the dominant tissue within the embryo sac, and the adjacent maternal tissue which will insure the nourishment of both. If, during early development, the balance is upset by failure of the endosperm to keep pace with growth in the extensive surrounding tissue the endosperm starves and, eventually, the ovule collapses.

Following hybridization in alfalfa, the rate of growth of the endosperm, as measured by the number of nuclei, is found to be significantly higher than after selfing. The two classes of embryos, on the other hand, grow at only slightly different, and much lower, rates. As mentioned above, only about one fifth as many fertile ovules collapse after crossbreeding as after selfing. The initial conditions in the ovule outside the embryo sac being alike in the two cases, it seems clear that the higher survival following crossing is the result of the more active growth of the hybrid endosperm. Conversely, following self-fertilization, the rate of growth of the endosperm is frequently so low that the balance soon shifts in favor of the integument. The hyperplasia we have described then arises, causing collapse of the endosperm and, eventually, terminating development of the ovule.

R. A. BRINK
D. C. COOPER
UNIVERSITY OF WISCONSIN

## BOOKS RECEIVED

ADAMSTONE, F. B. and WALDO SHUMWAY. *A Laboratory Manual of Vertebrate Embryology; Anatomy of Selected Embryos of the Frog, Chick and Pig.* Pp. vii + 87. 38 figures. Wiley. $1.25.

American Geophysical Union. *Transactions of 1939. Part I, Reports and Papers, Regional Meetings, Los Angeles and Spokane, December, 1938. Part II, Twentieth Annual Meeting, Washington, D. C., April, 1939; Symposium on Floods. Part III, Twentieth Annual Meeting, Reports and Papers, General Assembly and Sections of Geodesy, Seismology, Meteorology, Terrestrial Magnetism and Electricity, Oceanography and Volcanology. Part IV, Twentieth Annual Meeting; Reports and Papers, Section of Hydrology.* National Research Council of the National Academy of Sciences, Washington.

CLARKSON, ROSETTA E. *Magic Gardens; a Modern Chronicle of Herbs and Savory Seeds.* Pp. xviii + 369. Illustrated. Macmillan. $3.00.

Cooper Union for the Advancement of Science and Art. *Eightieth Annual Report, July, 1939.* Pp. 121. Cooper Union, New York.

EDDINGTON, SIR ARTHUR. *The Philosophy of Physical Science.* Pp. ix + 230. Macmillan. $2.50.

JOHANNSEN, ALBERT. *A Descriptive Petrography of the Igneous Rocks. Vol. I, Introduction; Textures, Classifications and Glossary.* Revised edition. Pp. xxiv + 318. 145 figures. University of Chicago Press. $4.50.

MABY, J. CECIL and T. BEDFORD FRANKLIN. *The Physics of the Divining Rod.* Pp. xv + 452. 51 figures. Bell & Sons, London. 21s.

# SCIENCE

Vol. 90 — Friday, December 15, 1939 — No. 2346

*Dr. Robert Henry Thurston's Eighteen Years at Cornell:* Dr. William F. Durand ..... 547
*Photoperiodic Aspects of Phasic Development:* Professor W. F. Loehwing ..... 552
*Obituary:*
*Margaret Floy Washburn:* Dr. Karl M. Dallenbach. *Oscar Henry Plant:* Dr. E. G. Gross and Dr. I. H. Pierce. *Recent Deaths and Memorials* ..... 555
*Scientific Events:*
*Mining Education in England; Lectures to the Laity of the New York Academy of Medicine; Statement of the Board of Trustees of Biological Abstracts; The Annual Meeting of the Council of the Union of American Biological Societies; Award of the Penrose Medal of the Geological Society of America* ..... 558
*Scientific Notes and News* ..... 561
*Discussion:*
*Grassland as a Site for Basic Research on Terrestrial Animals:* Dr. V. E. Shelford. *Oxygen Requirements for Germination of Seeds of Nyssa aquatica—Tupelo Gum:* Dr. Ivan V. Shunk. *On "A New Color Reaction for Vitamin $B_1$ (Thiamin aneurin)":* Dr. Guy E. Youngburg. *Chronica Botanica:* Dr. D. T. MacDougal, Professor F. E. Lloyd and Professor H. S. Reed ..... 564
*Scientific Books:*
*Physics:* Dr. F. C. Brown ..... 566
*Reports:*
*Grants of the American Philosophical Society* ..... 568
*Special Articles:*
*Photosynthesis with Radio-carbon:* Dr. S. Ruben and Others. *The Preparation and Purification of Brucella antiserum:* Dr. I. Forest Huddleson and R. B. Pennell. *Selenium and Duck Sickness:* Dr. Arthur C. Twomey, Sarah J. Twomey and Loring R. Williams ..... 570
*Scientific Apparatus and Laboratory Methods:*
*A Simple Method for the Filing of Microfilm Records in Short Length Strips:* Dr. Harold P. Brown and James A. Austin ..... 573
*Science News* ..... 8

SCIENCE: A Weekly Journal devoted to the Advancement of Science, edited by J. McKeen Cattell and published every Friday by

THE SCIENCE PRESS
New York City: Grand Central Terminal
Lancaster, Pa. Garrison, N. Y.

Annual Subscription, $6.00 Single Copies, 15 Cts.

SCIENCE is the official organ of the American Association for the Advancement of Science. Information regarding membership in the Association may be secured from the office of the permanent secretary in the Smithsonian Institution Building, Washington, D. C.

## DR. ROBERT HENRY THURSTON'S EIGHTEEN YEARS AT CORNELL[1]

By Dr. WILLIAM F. DURAND
LELAND STANFORD UNIVERSITY

To me has been allotted the pleasant task of giving you some account of the life and work of Dr. Thurston during his eighteen years as director of the Sibley College of Cornell University. To compress into a period of some twenty-five or thirty minutes' time any adequate account of the activities over a period of eighteen years of a man such as was Dr. Robert Henry Thurston will be, I am sure you will agree, quite out of the question; and I can only hope to give some account of what appear to be the more important features of this story.

The initial point in the sequence of events which led to Dr. Thurston's call to Cornell appears to have been a gradually growing conviction in the minds of the then president, Dr. Andrew D. White, and members of his board of trustees, that the Sibley College, as representing the School of Mechanic Arts of Cornell, was hardly realizing, in its condition during the middle eighties of the last century, the full measure of its potential standing in the domain of higher technical education.

This is evidenced by the appointment by the trustees, on June 18, 1884, of a special committee known as the "Committee on Revision of Sibley College." This committee comprised the president of the university, Dr. Andrew D. White, Honorable Hiram Sibley (the founder of Sibley College), the chairman of the Board of Trustees, and one graduate of the Department of Mechanic Arts to be selected by the trustees. The resolution calling for the appointment of this committee prescribed its duty as that of considering "all

[1] Address at the celebration at Cornell University of the hundredth anniversary of the birth of Robert Henry Thurston, October 25, 1939.

questions relating to the Mechanic Arts Department," and the resolution itself was accompanied by a declaration of purpose reading as follows:

*Resolved:* that it is the wish and purpose of the Trustees of Cornell University to establish and maintain an Engineering and Mechanical Department either by union under one head or by division into two departments—a complete system of instruction in all that belongs to this important branch of a thorough university education.

The members of this committee approached their study with a sense of its serious importance. They early reached the conclusion that in order to realize the purposes in view some new form of organization was needed, with a new directive head with enlarged authority and responsibility. The crux of the situation was obviously the man to be called as head of the reorganized college. The field was surveyed with care and several eminent engineers were considered and their qualifications passed in review. Finally, almost exactly a year later, on June 17, 1885, this committee submitted a written report from which some extracts may be given:

. . . They have met various gentlemen eminent in the profession, and several of these gentlemen on the invitation of the president of the University, and the chairman of the board of trustees, have visited the University, looked carefully into the affairs of Sibley College, and discussed them freely with resident members of the committee. After such full consideration, the committee unanimously report in favor of establishing a professorship of mechanical engineering to be called the Sibley professorship, . . . and that there be attached to the same the directorship of Sibley College, in the duties of which shall be included the chairmanship of the faculty of mechanical engineering or mechanic arts with large powers as to the laying out of the course or courses in the department, the assignment of duties to the various professors especially connected with it, the decision as to the character and amount of various kinds of instruction, including drafting and shop work, subject to this board, the executive committee, and the president of the University so far as their spheres include his own, and having the special faculty of Sibley College as his advisory council. . . . They also recommend that the professor be immediately called and asked at once during the summer vacation to begin a careful study of the various questions involved and to prepare and have ready for this board at the coming annual meeting in October a full report on these subjects and all others which he deems best to bring before the board, and especially to include any plan that occurs to him in regard to any possible consolidation of instruction in his own and kindred departments.

Your committee, in looking about among candidates, have found various distinguished gentlemen, many of whom would do high honor to their profession and to the University. But they have unanimously concluded to recommend Professor Robert H. Thurston, LL.D., a graduate of Brown University, at present professor of mechanical engineering in the Stevens Institute at Hoboken, N. J. Professor Thurston is a gentleman of about forty-four years of age, has taken the highest rank in his profession, has published reports and various documents showing a wide range of knowledge and great depth of thought, has built up a high reputation as a teacher, has held the position of president of the American Association of Mechanical Engineers, as well as consulting engineer of the United States Navy, has been intrusted with some of the most important theoretical and practical tests by the Government of the United States and by large private corporations, and has thus gained an experience and a knowledge which cannot fail to enure to the benefit and the reputation of the Sibley College of our University. He has also proved his teaching ability by sending forth for several years past a number of graduates from the Stevens Institute who have taken high positions. And as to his standing among his associates in his profession, your committee would submit herewith certain letters from eminent mechanical engineers and others, sent directly to the members of the committee, which show that Professor Thurston is all that we could desire him to be.

The hope and belief of your committee is that if this nomination be ratified by the board, we shall have a professor and director of the fullest competence and of the highest standing, one who will at once by his counsels, his teachings, his influence upon the students, and the weight of his opinion on the country at large give to Sibley College a standing among the foremost institutions of the kind in existence.

The board of trustees lost no time in acting on this report with approval and among the minutes of this meeting it is recorded that:

Upon ballot duly had, Robert H. Thurston was unanimously elected Professor of Mechanical Engineering and Director of Sibley College.

There is also extant an account written by President White, thirty years later in 1915, and giving his recollection of the circumstances which led to the selection of Dr. Thurston out of the field of possible choice of presumably available material. Only a small part of this account can be quoted here. Speaking of conditions in Sibley College at that earlier period, he says:

. . . There were differences of opinion, some of them very acute, in the Sibley faculty, and, to the great regret and even dismay of those interested in the department, Professor Sweet left it. It was clear that a thorough reorganization was needed, and it fell to my lot to seek a professor who should take the post of director of the College, who could speak as one having authority, and who should have both theoretical and practical acquaintance with all the departments and, at the same time, a position among mechanical engineers throughout the whole country which would command respect and justify authority. But the question was where to find him.

Then, further speaking of Dr. Thurston, he says:

. . . His position was one of great eminence. He had certainly, in an astonishing degree, the qualities I sought, but his reputation as a professor at Hoboken and his distinction as a consulting engineer at New York City were such that it seemed impossible to dislodge him. All I had hoped to do was to secure from him information regarding various candidates throughout the country. A whole morning was spent by me in obtaining from him opinions regarding the work of different men who seemed promising, and at last I departed, more than ever impressed with the difficulties of the situation. Taking leave of Professor Thurston, I walked slowly down the pathway from his door, when it suddenly occurred to me to make one more attempt, such as, thus far, I had not dared. It was a sudden thought, and returning to the door, I asked Professor Thurston one more question, simply whether, under any circumstances, he could come to Cornell. He answered that he had no desire to change his surroundings at Hoboken, but he gradually confided to me that he and Mrs. Thurston had sometimes agreed that, for their children's sake and, indeed, for their own tastes, they would have preferred a life more remote from a great city and with more rural surroundings. A new hope sprang up within me. I presented the attractions of Cornell and its neighborhood, dwelt upon the possibilities of a great work under his direction, and, before leaving the house, had secured his promise to come to us.

It is well known that the qualifications of other engineers of high standing in those days were also canvassed carefully by this committee on the "Revision of Sibley College." Among these was the late William Kent, between whom and Dr. Thurston there had existed for many years a warm personal friendship. Correspondence between these two men shows that they discussed the situation frankly regarding Cornell. Up to the very last, it was generally assumed, certainly by Dr. Thurston himself, that his role was that of an adviser rather than an active candidate himself. Finally, however, in a letter from Thurston to Kent under date of June 16, 1885, he refers to a telegram from Dr. White accepting the conditions which he, Thurston, had proposed as essential to his consideration of their offer to himself of the position; he then expressed to Kent the feeling that, "had I not been in the way, you would, perhaps have gone there, and that causes me regret."

Between the accounts given in copies of Dr. Thurston's letters to Kent and Dr. White's account written some thirty years after the event, there is some uncertainty as to just when and where Thurston first received the suggestion of considering the appointment for himself. It is clear, however, that he did not give his final acceptance of the offer until certain conditions had been met, conditions which he considered essential to the proper realization of the major purposes in view.

Thus there is extant a letter written by Dr. Thurston to President White under date of May 26, 1885, setting forth his views and understanding regarding the authority and responsibility to be vested in the position to which he had been invited. This letter apparently served as the basis of a final and definite understanding regarding these matters, as evidenced by the telegram from White to Thurston, referred to in the letter from Thurston to Kent, noted above.

The attitude of the committee regarding the choice of Dr. Thurston for the position is clear from correspondence between the late Walter C. Kerr, the alumnus member of the committee, and Dr. White, showing clearly that Thurston was the choice of the committee from the start, and if there was delay in making a direct approach to him regarding the matter, it was doubtless due to a fear that with his connections in and about New York City, it would not be easy to interest him in taking up the work at Ithaca.

So in 1885 began the new era for Sibley College. In the article by Dr. White previously quoted from, and speaking of the period immediately following 1885, he says:

So began a new era for Sibley College, for Cornell University, and indeed, for the country. . . . Professor Thurston's coming put an end to all divided counsels and began a new and better order of things.

The picture which Dr. Thurston had formed in his own mind of a college of mechanical engineering was far removed from the relatively simple plan which had so far been followed. As set forth in his first annual report, he visualized a comprehensive system of schools of engineering and of the underlying mechanic arts. In the lower or fundamental departments, these schools would offer instruction in the principal departments of industry, and then, built upon these, schools of the industries in which, to quote his own words, "the use of the apparatus of the several industries as well as the scientific and statistical facts and principles underlying them should be exhibited and illustrated by learned and expert teachers." And then, finally, schools of the constructive professions of engineering, architecture and industrial art, conducted by men distinguished in their respective professions; and then, in immediate contact with all of this splendid picture, he visualized a department of experimental research in which, again to quote his words:

. . . men who have earned their spurs in the earlier struggles of previous years, and who have acquired a right to liberty to continue their work of solution of the great problems of the unknown, shall give themselves wholly, with all their time, talent, strength and genius, to the work which attracts them. . . .

And then he closes with the words: "All this is now and here a possibility—given capital."

As we know, not all of this splendid picture was realized. Limitations arose in time, in funds and in human effort. Graduate schools in naval architecture and marine engineering and in railway engineering were organized and carried on for some years, but the experience with these schools showed that the idea as expressed wholly in terms of *graduate* study was somewhat ahead of the temper and demands of the time.

Just as Dr. Thurston was transferring to Cornell, the newly organizing field of electrical engineering was beginning clearly to show its importance, though few of its foremost protagonists could, at that time, have imagined the brilliant future which lay just ahead of this newly developing domain of engineering work.

A few years earlier, in 1883, a course of instruction in electrical engineering at Cornell had been organized and announced. The work was wholly in the department of physics under Professor Anthony. Dr. Thurston in 1886 took steps, through a cooperative arrangement with the department of physics, to supplement and round out the work in the department of physics with courses of instruction and training in the more directly professional phases of the subject.

Thus in the late years of the decade 1880–90, Sibley College became a college of mechanical and electrical engineering, with courses substantially the same for the first three years, but diverging each along its special line for the senior and graduate years.

Another cardinal feature in Dr. Thurston's picture of a great school of engineering—the Department of Experimental Research—was promptly organized and carried along vigorously in the lines of both mechanical and electrical engineering.

The growth of Sibley College both in numbers and in prestige was continuous and notable throughout the period of his work at Cornell. In 1885, there were seven members on the teaching staff and about sixty students. At the time of his death in 1903, the respective numbers were forty-three and nine hundred and sixty.

If the attempt be made to sum up in a single sentence the results of Dr. Thurston's work at Cornell, it may be said that they were manifest in a broadening and strengthening of the courses of instruction, and in an infusion into the work, especially of the junior, senior and graduate years, of a more distinctly professional atmosphere; in giving to the college front rank prestige and standing among the engineering schools of the country and of the world, and finally in putting the imprint of his spirit and fine idealism on some sixteen hundred graduates who passed into and through the college during the years of his life as its directing head.

In the paper by President White previously quoted from, he says further, in speaking of Dr. Thurston's work as a whole:

He brought the institution immediately into touch with the leading men in the profession, not only in this country but in other lands. It became my duty later, at various places and institutions, in company with him, to perfect our relations with leading establishments for mechanical engineering, at home and abroad, and everywhere he was received as an authority and treated as a full equal among the leaders in the profession. At home, in his class room, in his business office, in his study, he was a center toward which students in ever increasing numbers were attracted; his books, his lectures, his talks were an inspiration. Various men prepared by him, who were destined to carry on his work, will, everyone of them, testify to his influence upon his students, upon the institution at large and upon the whole field of its activity. How Sibley College, in those days, was increased in its numbers, improved in its work, and altogether, how a new epoch began, not only for itself, but for the University, is known especially by all those who had the great privilege and honor of graduating under him.

Again in a different connection but referring to these same years, President White says:

Few days in the history of Cornell University have been so fraught with good as that on which Thurston accepted my call to the headship of Sibley College. At the very outset he gained the confidence and gratitude of trustees, professors, students, and indeed, of his profession throughout the country, by his amazing success as professor, as author, as an organizer and administrator of that department, which he made not only one of the largest, but one of the best of its kind in the world. The rapidity and wisdom of his decisions, the extent and excellence of his work, his skill in attracting the best men, his ability in quieting rivalries and animosities, and the kindly firmness of his whole policy were a source of wonder to all who knew him.

As a writer, during these years, Dr. Thurston maintained a steady pace, both in the production of books and of papers on technical subjects.

At Stevens Institute he had outlined, in mind, a great series of engineering texts. Of these, his treatise on "Friction and Lost Work in Machinery and Millwork" was completed at Stevens Institute in 1885, just as he was transferring to Cornell. He had projected two great works, one on the steam boiler and another on the steam engine. Some work had been done on these books, but they were unfinished, and to their completion and publication he gave much time and energy during his earlier years at Cornell. The "Manual of Steam Boilers" was published in 1888 and that on the steam engine in 1891–92. In addition to this, there was, during the entire period of his life at Cornell, continued work on revision of books already published as well as a continued output of papers on technical and more general subjects, astonishing in their number and in the wide variety of topics treated.

In addition to the work of organization, administration and instruction in Sibley College and to his tremendous output of technical writing, Dr. Thurston found time for much service of a public character. Only a few illustrations need be given. Thus: service as a member of the New York State Commission on Voting Machines; service as a member of a New York State Commission to report on a Modern Rifle for the National Guard; service on the United States Industrial Commission on Improvements in Manufacturing Methods and on the United States Commission on Safe and Vault Construction for the U. S. Treasury.

In 1889 he attended the French Exposition in Paris and took a prominent part as vice-president of one of the juries. Again in 1893 he served as a member of the Jury of Awards at the World's Columbian Exposition in Chicago. Again and in widely different lines Dr. Thurston served for six years as a member of the board of aldermen for the city of Ithaca, for most of the time as chairman of the finance committee and at a later time as a member of its board of water commissioners.

Dr. Thurston was always ready and willing, within the limits of his obligations otherwise, to undertake service for the public good or where he believed that his training and experience might be of specific and definite value. He was, furthermore, sufficiently human to distinctly enjoy public service of an important character and where the work was such as to bring him into contact with other men of note.

The family life of Dr. Thurston was most fortunate and happy. His family comprised his wife, three daughters and, for portions of the time, Mrs. Thurston's mother and sister, Mrs. and Miss Boughton.

Soon after coming to Cornell he built a comfortable house on East Avenue, and I can not refrain from adding here the source of the funds for the construction of this house. In connection with the capture of the blockage runner *Princess Royal* during the Civil War, and to which reference has been made by Admiral Brown, Thurston received as prize money the sum of $2,291.99. This was first invested in government bonds and later in real estate, first in Providence, R. I., and later in Hoboken. As a result of the advances in value realized in these various transactions, he was able, selling out these holdings, to build his house at Cornell; and it was always a matter of much satisfaction to him that, through the judicious use of this prize money, he had been able to furnish the major part of the funds necessary for the provision of comfortable housing for himself and his family for the remainder of his days.

I have spoken thus far chiefly of Dr. Thurston as an educator; somewhat incidentally as an engineer, as a public servant and as a writer. I can not bear to close my tribute, however, without a word regarding him as a man among men, as a friend and neighbor, as a social unit in the delightful atmosphere of the Cornell campus. If I were to attempt the briefest possible specification of the character of Dr. Thurston, I would say that the controlling elements in this complex were an abiding faith in himself, unwavering persistence toward his objectives and a steadfast optimism, all combined with generous and kindly human impulses toward those about him, with a serene, cheerful and confident outlook regarding both present and future. He was always ready to accept responsibility and to undertake any task which seemed to fall in the line of his duty, which seemed worth while and for which the means were at hand. These characteristics are illustrated throughout his entire life.

I would not imply, however, that his faith in himself was such as to lead to reckless and ill-considered measures. It was tempered with a wise restraint. In the face of important steps his strategy included not only a most careful survey and analysis of the matter by himself, but the taking of counsel with those in whose opinion he had confidence. In the end he might or might not follow advice given, but if not, it was always after a careful and generous weighing of such counsel given. He was ready at the last to accept responsibility for the final judgment and to make it in the light of all the assembled evidence which he could bring to bear on the problem.

No characteristic was perhaps more marked than his persistence in following through in the face of discouraging obstacles. Repeated return to the attack, again and again, always with the same cherry optimism, gives the secret of the successful outcome of some of his undertakings carried forward against obstacles which might well have discouraged a soul less persistent, less hopeful and less assured of the righteousness of the ends for which he was working.

Members of the board of trustees of those days have told in later years of the cheerful and unruffled manner in which he would accept unfavorable action with regard to the grant of funds or regarding some other measure which they might not find themselves in a position to forward as rapidly as he might wish. With no exhibition of impatience or disappointment, he would bid them a cheery and courteous good day, with the assurance that in due time he would venture to present the matter again in the hope that it might then commend itself to their more favorable consideration. One of the trustees of that period, speaking of these matters, once remarked that "it was no wonder that a man like that got what he wanted in the end."

Not many in this room have, perhaps, seen Dr. Thurston in the flesh. I wish that I might give some adequate picture of him, for example, in his daily walk across the campus from his home to the Sibley buildings. The late Dr. W. A. Hammond, of the department of philosophy at Cornell, who will be remembered by many in this audience, once told me that in going to classes in the morning, his path often crossed that of Dr. Thurston and that he grew to look forward to these meetings with anticipation; that Dr. Thurston's manner of saying "Good morning" would always make the day seem brighter and fairer for him.

In physical frame, Dr. Thurston was moderate in stature, rather spare of build, erect in carriage and mien. His hair with full beard and moustache were in early and middle life black, becoming gray with the passing years. His eyes were dark and piercing, often with something kind and quizzical shining through. His gait was rapid and firm, with figure trim and erect, a characteristic tracing back, perhaps, to his naval training, but none the less a natural expression of his personal energy and normal outlook on the world about him. This daily walk between his house and office, with black portfolio of lecture notes under his arm, body erect, shoulders back, head up and eyes to the front, formed a picture of personal dignity and of purpose toward an intended goal which will surely long be remembered by those who saw this as a familiar sight during the years of his life at Cornell.

I wish that there were time for some of the anecdotes which illustrate his kindly nature, his intense human sympathy, his resourcefulness in adapting himself to the unexpected, all combined with his optimistic outlook on his environment, his abiding faith in the ultimate working out of the great enterprise in which he was embarked, but time presses and I must close.

The fall of 1903 found Dr. Thurston in seeming good health, in the midst of interesting and important work and apparently with many years of fruitful activity before him. On the occasion of his birthday, thirty-six years ago to-day, Mrs. Thurston had arranged for a small dinner party of intimate friends. Sitting quietly in his home waiting for the arrival of these friends, the final summons came—apparently through an aneurism of the heart. Peacefully and with hardly a movement he passed on, and so out of the busy life in which he had wrought so long, so courageously and so well.

In the shuffling of human characteristics by the Fates, only too rarely do the combinations give us a man such as was Dr. Robert Henry Thurston. We shall not soon look upon his like again.

# PHOTOPERIODIC ASPECTS OF PHASIC DEVELOPMENT

By Professor W. F. LOEHWING

THE STATE UNIVERSITY OF IOWA

THE concept of phasic development of plants has, in less than a decade, profoundly influenced the fundamental philosophy of plant growth as well as theory and practice in plant physiology, ecology, agronomy and genetics. This theory emphasizes especially the differences between the thermo- and photo-phases of plant growth. In view of the fact that recent advances in our knowledge of photoperiodism show variable effects of a given light period upon the different processes involved in sexual reproduction, it now seems desirable to evaluate this evidence to determine the possible desirability of subdividing the photophase of plant development into (*a*) an initial flowering phase as distinguished from a subsequent (*b*) gametogenic phase concerned with the formation of viable gametes.

When the photoperiodic concept was first clearly enunciated by Garner and Allard (1920), formation of macroscopic flowers in known periods of diurnal illumination was taken as a criterion of photoperiodic response. It was soon learned, however, that plants receiving minimal periods of photo-induction frequently produce flowers of anomalous shape and marked sterility. *Xanthium* of one short photoperiod, for example, exhibits marked pollen sterility (Hamner and Bonner, 1938; Neidle, 1939). Kirichenko and his associates (1934–36) had also previously observed that though flowers developed in *Triticum erythrospermum* when exposed for several weeks to a daily two-hour photoperiod, pollen when present was invariably sterile. The data of Kirichenko and other investigators indicate that the development of viable pollen requires (*a*) a longer period (6 hours or over) of photo-induction, consisting both of more days and longer daily light periods than necessary for the differentiation of pistil and ear. In conformity with other light-induced, formative processes, once the requisite period of photo-induction has been supplied, *Triticum erythrospermum* then continues to produce viable pollen indefinitely in all ranges of illumination from continuous day to continuous night. Oleson (1938) observed similar conditions in *Fuchsia* and *Begonia*.

The work of Rosenbaum (1937) on 18 varieties of soybean indicates that not only stamen but also perianth and ovule development can be suppressed by extremely short day length (8 hours or less), thus reducing the fruits to parthenocarpic, seedless pods. A 13-hour day, on the other hand, results in normal flowers producing pods with the usual complement of viable seeds (Hamner, 1938). Earlier still, Schaffner (1927–30), Richey and Sprague (1932) noted the absence of tassels in corn grown during very short photoperiods, especially in low intensities of light, and that ears formed normally, or sometimes apically in place of tassels. Short day thus rendered corn dioecious. In cucumbers, it has been known for many years that short day of low intensity results in a preponderance of pistillate flowers (Edmond, 1930; McCollum, 1934; Miller, 1938; Zukova, 1938). The production of staminate flowers requires longer days and higher light intensity. Allard (1938) found that the flower habit of the hog peanut changed from hypogeic to cleistogamous and finally to anthesitic as the photoperiod increased. Aerial flowers required a 13½ hour day for their formation, but hypogeic forms developed in as little as a five-hour light period.

It is evident from the foregoing data that the photoperiod exerts a variable effect on the different parts of the flower, just as it does upon different vegetative structures. Thus, if flower fertility is to be made the criterion of photoperiodicity, the conditions will be somewhat different from those necessary to cause the inception of primordia alone.

The contrast in the photoperiodic demands of staminate and pistillate tissues is a manifestation of sex, and it is to be expected that these organs will differ as much in metabolism and composition as in mode of origin. In fact, as the evidence on flower physiology accumulates, it shows increasingly that the most profound compositional and developmental changes in the plant's entire existence occur in the brief period of floral differentiation, a condition as yet inadequately appreciated, probably due to the rapidity, extreme localization and inconspicuousness of the changes involved. The technical and analytical difficulties in physiological studies of this sort are obvious, and they constitute a further reason for the meagerness of quantitative data on reproduction. Once the importance of such information is generally recognized, it is to be expected that adequate techniques and increased investigation will follow. It would be helpful, however, if some consensus could be reached as to precisely what constitutes flowering. If inception of floral primordia is to be the criterion, then there is definite need of distinguishing gametogenesis from the origin of the other floral parts, since inception of primordia and perianth development are no absolute guarantee of the production of viable gametes.

The common denominators of flowering, in both long- and short-day species, such as the non-specific character of the florigenic hormone, suggested by the researches of Cailachian, Murneek, Loehwing, Hamner and Bonner and many others, as well as similarity in stem anatomy of all flowering types as worked out by Roberts and his associates, are all valuable inventories of the various attributes of normal flowering. They still leave much unanswered, however, as to the physiological nature of sporogenesis and the differentiation of the sex organs. In addition to those features which are common to all plants in the flowering phase, we must identify the physiological stimuli responsible for differences between pistils and stamens.

More than a decade of research by the writer and his students upon dioecious species suggests that, among the most important physiological differences of the sexes, are the oxidation-reduction enzymes, marked quantitative if not qualitative differences in soluble carbohydrates and qualitative contrasts in proteins. Mild hydrolysis of proteins in sexually differentiated hemp plants discloses arginine and lysine but no proline or histidine in staminate individuals, while pistillate plants are the exact converse. Tests for these amino acids in foliar tissues of vegetative plants without flower primordia enable one to forecast the eventual sex of the mature plant (Kiesel and Pachewitsch, 1938; Loehwing, 1939). Inception of staminate organs seems to be characterized by a preponderance of soluble sugars and presence of oxidase. Pistillate loci have a preponderance of nitrogen and marked reducase activity (Loehwing, 1937; Stanfield, 1937). Though the foregoing appear to be significant physico-chemical differences between the sexes, we have not as yet successfully distinguished cause and effect, nor have we the desired degree of voluntary control over carpo- and andro-genesis.

Not only are the photoperiodic requirements for development of pollen and embryo sac different from one another, but they in turn also differ from the post-fertilization processes of fruit enlargement. Fertilization marks the inception of the new sporophyte phase and as such, essentially the recommencement of vegetative activity, temporarily of a parasitic sort with a high food demand. In many plants, it seems that the photoperiodic conditions favorable for fruit development are more similar to those for vegetative growth than for flowering. In brief, the optimal photoperiodic conditions change as the plant progresses from inception of primordia to differentiation of floral parts and finally to fruiting.

This fact has been recognized in varying degrees by many investigators, but has recently been well formulated by Eguchi (1937), who suggests a double photoperiodic classification for plants. Eguchi's system not only recognizes but definitely emphasizes the difference in the light optima of flowering and fruiting. Following Garner and Allard's classification, he postulates three fundamental types of plants, namely, long day, short day and photoperiodically indifferent. With respect to flowering, the plant may have a short optimal period but a long or indifferent light requirement with respect to fruiting. There are, then, nine possible permutations of these three classes as given in Table 1:

This synoptic classification is perhaps a bit extreme

TABLE I

| Optimal photoperiods for: Flowering | Fruiting | Representative species |
|---|---|---|
| Short | Long | Strawberry, Cineraria |
| Long | Long | Oxeye Daisy, Spring Barley |
| Long | Short | *Physostegia virginiana*, *Boltonia latisquama* |
| Short | Short | Soybeans, *Cosmos bipinnatus* |
| Long | Indifferent | *Phlox paniculata* |
| Short | Indifferent | Late rice varieties |
| Indifferent | Short | *Chrysanthemum articum* |
| Indifferent | Long | Spinach, Many wheats |
| Indifferent | Indifferent | Pepper, Early rices, *Stellaria media*, *Poa annua* (Tincker, 1924) Buckwheat (Arthur, 1930) |

and as a result not wholly clear. A plant may be long day with reference both to flowering and fruiting, yet nevertheless have a shorter optimum by several hours for fruiting than for flowering. It will be noted that this classification of Eguchi controverts the original suggestion of Lysenko that long-day species are at their optimum in continuous-day and short-day species in continuous-night. Even with reference to flowering alone, we already have abundant evidence that this interpretation by Lysenko is too extreme (Singh, 1937; Allard, 1938; Borthwick and Parker, 1938; Murneek, 1937; Celjadinova, 1937).

The fact that the optimal photoperiod for fruiting is different than for flowering in some species, often causes delay in the enlargement and even abscission of the earliest fruits. Oleson (1938) noted that after the first crop of *Begonia* and *Fuchsia* fruits appeared in early spring, about four to six weeks elapsed before these began to enlarge under conditions of normal day-length. Many fruits abscissed during the period from late February to late April. Neither pollination with viable pollen nor stimulation with indole acetic, indole butyric or phenyl acetic acids was capable of inducing ovary growth until late April or early May. These earliest successful fruits, both natural and parthenocarpic, were seedless. As the days became longer, ovules filled out in both naturally and artificially stimulated fruits. In cucumbers, a similar favorable effect of long day was noted in setting of natural and parthenocarpic fruits by Miller (1938). Whyte (1939) has recently suggested that in fruit growth, temperature plays a somewhat more important role, along with the photoperiod, than it does in the pre-fertilization processes.

The period of embryo development is preceded by extensive mobilization of food reserves, so profound that the entire plant is involved. Renewed root growth and absorption is a concomitant of this phase, making the applications of soil nutrients peculiarly effective at this time (Polster, 1938; Kraus and Kraybill, 1918; Hamner, 1938; Borodin, 1931; Auchter, 1924; Combes, 1935; Howlett, 1934–36; Murneek, 1937; Dobrunov, 1938).

If we consider photoperiodic responses as one stage of phasic development in the sense of Lysenko's concept, a number of open questions still remain. Though Lysenko originally considered the thermal and light phases qualitatively distinct, there is now evidence of overlap between them as shown by the ability to complete a portion or all the essential photoperiodic induction in swollen seeds and seedlings undergoing low temperature vernalization (Wöber, 1936). Harder (1937) has shown this to be true in *Sinapsis*, *Agrostemma* and winter rye. If the thermo- and photophases are wholly separate, we as yet possess neither readily recognizable criteria of the completion of the former nor inception of the latter. Though the transitions are functional rather than structural, they should be identifiable nevertheless. Changes in permeability, oxidase enzymes and protein iso-electric point have been suggested, but the data are thus far too meager to be conclusive (Bassaraskoja, 1936; Richter, 1936). There also remains the question as to why morning light is more effective than evening light in a long-day species as shown by Fabian (1938) for *Ullucus* and contrariwise for short-day forms as shown by Bünning (1936) for *Phaseolus*.

Lysenko and Whyte (1939) have also postulated the irreversibility of phases. Yet it is possible to rejuvenate a reproductive plant photoperiodically, making it again vegetative. While in some cases a shift from reproductive to vegetative photoperiod leads to the death of the apical meristem and initiation of subsequent vegetative growth from previously dormant lateral buds well down on the stem, as in hemp, there are, however, also cases of vegetative proliferation of the apical meristem of flowering plants, as in the *Compositae*. Whether such rejuvenation is possible only in plants on the threshold of reproduction but not in those which have been exposed for a considerable length of time to an optimal reproductive photoperiod is not yet definitely settled. It seems likely, however, that the rigidity of Lysenko's concept as to irreversibility in the light phase may, on the basis of recent data, undergo modification as already has the previous belief in irreversibility of the vernalization phase. Instances of devernalization with age and unduly prolonged low temperature treatment appear to be well established (Gregory and Purvis, 1937–38).

When a rejuvenated plant is shifted from a vegetative to a slightly reproductive photoperiod, certain anomalous yet progressive transitional intergrades from vegetative to reproductive structures are often obtained. Older portions of the stem produce green and leafy perianth segments devoid of stamens and pistils. Younger regions near the tip of the main axis produce increasingly perfect flowers until normal, functional flowers appear at the apex. This response often occurs in ornamentals of the *Solanaceae*, such as *Petunia*. Another aspect of reversion is the effect of change in temperature by means of which a short-day type such as *Xanthium* can be induced to exhibit long-day response (Gilbert, 1926, 1934).

The recent observation by Melchers (1939) that a vegetative scion of tobacco is able to induce flowering in a vegetative stock in the first year of the biennial species, *Hyoscyamus niger,* presages an early and profound revision of the current form of the florigen concept. Melchers' painstaking experiments were conclusive and clearly significant statistically. With reference to the normal flowering of biennials, Melchers postulates the formation of a new hormone, tentatively designated "vernalin," at low temperatures at the end of the first season. Upon this "vernalin" in turn depends the ability to produce florigen in the reproductive photoperiod of the second year. Melchers points out that our knowledge of the reproductive physiology of biennials, such as *Hyoscyamus niger* with which he worked, is almost as nebulous as our understanding of the day-neutral group of plants. Melchers' results also contradict the suggestion previously made by Cailachian that the photoperiodic effect is proportional to the area of foliage. Melchers noted no such quantitative relationships. Recent temperature studies suggest that radical revisions are also imminent in regard to the supposed indispensability of light for inception of flowering in the so-called photophase (Roberts, 1936–37–38–39; Thompson, 1933–36; Chroboczek, 1934).

In conclusion, it would seem, on the basis of recent evidence, that the thermo- and photo-phases are not as rigidly set apart nor as irreversible as originally suggested by Lsyenko. Further, it may prove desirable and conducive to a better understanding of reproduction if the photophase is subdivided into a flowering and gametogenic stage. If the profound and rapid transformations occurring between inception of flower primordia and fertilization, namely, the phenomena of sex, are studied as intensively as vernalization and photoperiodism, they promise to contribute fully as much as the former to our understanding of reproduction. If speed and magnitude of transformation be criteria of vital significance, the gametogenic or sexual phase *per se* represents the stage of most profound alterations in the ontogeny of the higher plants.

# OBITUARY

## MARGARET FLOY WASHBURN
### 1871–1939

MARGARET FLOY WASHBURN, emeritus professor of psychology at Vassar College since June, 1937, and a member of the Vassar faculty for thirty-six years, died after a long illness at Poughkeepsie, N. Y., on the afternoon of October 29, 1939. Her illness dated from a cerebral hemorrhage suffered on March 18, 1937—on the eve of the meeting of the Eastern Psychological Association, which was held at Vassar College in observance of her approaching retirement. She was at the time of her death in her sixty-ninth year, having been born in Harlem, New York City, on July 25, 1871, the only child of Rev. Francis and Elizabeth Floy (Davis) Washburn.

Professor Washburn was one of the foremost women in American science and was long recognized as a leader in her field. Her services and contributions to psychology were many and outstanding, and she received in recognition of them the highest honors and awards at the disposal of her confrères.

In 1919–1920, when the Division of Psychology and Anthropology of the National Research Council was formed, she acted as a representative of psychology, and again in 1925–1928. In 1921, she was president of the American Psychological Association. That same year she was awarded the prize of $500 by the Edison Phonograph Company for the best research on the effects of music, an investigation, done in collaboration with a colleague in the Vassar Department of Music, on "The Emotional Effects of Instrumental Music." In 1927, she was vice-president of Section I (Psychology) of the American Association for the Advancement of Science and was the recipient of a *Festschrift* and of an honorary degree of D.Sc. The *Festschrift,* volume 39 of *The American Journal of Psychology,* was dedicated to her by its authors, thirty-two colleagues from the various editorial boards upon which she had served, "in recognition of thirty-three years of distinguished service to psychology." The degree, *honoris causa,* was conferred upon her by Wittenberg College during the International Symposium on Feeling and Emotion that was held there at the dedication of the new psychological laboratory. She was elected, in 1929, to the International Committee on Psychology (the governing body of the International Congresses) and to the Society of Experimental Psychologists; and, in 1931, to fellowship in the National Academy of Sciences (the second woman to receive that honor, Dr. Florence Sabin having been elected before her in 1925). She was president, in 1931, of the New York Branch of the American Psychological Association (now the Eastern Psychological Association) and chairman of the Society of Experimental Psychologists. In 1932, she was the U. S. delegate to the International Congress of Psychology in Copenhagen. Professor Washburn was also a member of the National Institute of Psychology, the American Philosophical Society, the New York Academy of Sciences, the American Association of University Professors and Sigma Xi.

Besides publishing nearly 200 scientific articles and

reviews, Professor Washburn translated Wundt's "Ethical Systems," 1897, and wrote two books: "The Animal Mind," 1908, and "Movement and Mental Imagery," 1916. "Animal Mind" went through three more editions, every one thoroughly rewritten and enlarged (1917, 1926 and 1936). The first edition was translated into Japanese in 1918. "Movement and Mental Imagery," a development of her article in G. Stanley Hall's *"Festschrift"* in 1903, marked her break with Titchener's doctrine and her espousal of a motor theory of consciousness for which she was thereafter widely known. Between 1905 and 1938, she published in *The American Journal of Psychology* sixty-eight studies from the Vassar Psychological Laboratory. During this period she also gave unsparingly of her time to editorial work. She was cooperating editor of *The American Journal of Psychology,* 1903–1925 and co-editor since 1926; cooperating editor of the *Psychological Bulletin,* 1909–1915; associate editor of the *Journal of Animal Behavior,* 1911–1917; advisory editor of the *Psychological Review,* 1916–1930, and associate editor of the *Journal of Comparative Psychology,* 1921–1935.

Professor Washburn was an able and accomplished woman, the product of a good inheritance and a good environment. In her autobiography, published in 1932 in Volume II of the "History of Psychology in Autobiography"—a series of biographies to which the foremost psychologists in the world were invited to contribute—she tells that her ancestry was Dutch and English: Long Island and Westchester County Quakers and Maryland Cavaliers, with a dash of Connecticut Yankee. Most of her ancestors were in America before 1720. She was a precocious child. Though she did not enter school until she was seven years old, she had learned to read and write long before then. As a child, as throughout her life, she was an omnivorous reader. Her first school was one conducted in the home of a retired Presbyterian minister by his accomplished daughters. From them she learned the rudiments of mathematics and acquired a good foundation in French and German. When she was eleven years old, her father was called to the rectorship of the Episcopal Church in Kingston, N. Y. There she attended the public schools. Her progress was rapid, and she was graduated from the Kingston High School at fifteen years of age, in 1886. That fall she entered Vassar College. Due to a lack of Latin, which was required for college entrance at that time, her first year was spent in the preparatory department. In 1891, she was graduated from Vassar with the acquisition of an abiding interest in science and philosophy.

Hearing of the psychological laboratory that had just been opened by Cattell in Columbia University, she determined to become his pupil—though the graduate school at Columbia was then closed to women. Characteristically she persevered in her determination to be admitted to his classes and finally succeeded, as a result of special permission by the trustees of the university, in registering as a "hearer." Thus she was a pioneer in the struggle for equal educational opportunities for women. Cattell treated her as a regular student and permanently fixed her interest in psychology. As no fellowship was available to her at Columbia, she applied for and was granted a fellowship in the newly established Sage School of Philosophy at Cornell University. In 1892, she became Titchener's first doctoral student. After a year at Cornell, Vassar College awarded her an M.A. degree *in absentia* for work done under Titchener. A year later, in June, 1894, she obtained the Ph.D. degree from Cornell University. Her doctoral dissertation, "The Influence of Visual Associations on the Spatial Perceptions of the Skin," was published by Wundt in German in his *Philosophische Studien*—the first foreign study printed in that journal. Miss Washburn's doctoral minors were ethics with Schurman and philosophy with Albee, Hammond and Thilly.

In the fall of 1894 she went to Wells College as professor of psychology, philosophy and ethics. She remained there for six years. Then followed two years at Cornell as warden of Sage College—that is, head resident of the women's dormitory—and, during the second year, as lecturer in psychology. She gave two courses: social psychology, based on Wundt's "Völkerpsychologie," and animal psychology, which was to remain a life-long interest. Finding the duties of warden ("concerning oneself with the behavior of other people") uncongenial, she accepted at the end of two years the offer of an assistant professorship with full charge of the department of psychology at the University of Cincinnati. Though conditions there were to her liking, she could not resist the call of her *alma mater* and so went to Vassar College in the fall of 1903 as associate professor of philosophy. Her duties were at first divided between philosophy and psychology, but in 1908, psychology and philosophy having been divorced, she became professor of psychology and head of the newly created department.

Professor Washburn was an indefatigable and persistent worker. Except for the summers of 1913–1917, when she taught in the summer school of Columbia University; the spring of 1928, when, on sabbatical leave, she took a Mediterranean cruise; and the summers of 1929 and 1932, during which she took short trips to England and Copenhagen—she never was far nor long away from her work in her laboratory and study at Poughkeepsie. That she was also an inspiring teacher is attested by the growth of her department, by the many studies that came from her laboratory and by the number of her students who continued in psychology.

Hers was strictly an undergraduate department. As far as graduate study was concerned she was a proponent of coeducation. She wrote in her autobiography, "I deprecate graduate study for women at any but coeducational universities." True to her convictions, she encouraged her students to go to such universities for their final training. Many did, and wherever they went—to California, Columbia, Cornell, Harvard (Radcliffe), Illinois, Indiana, Iowa, Michigan, Ohio State, Yale—they made splendid records.

Professor Washburn's life and work should be an inspiration to women as it is a testimonial to the value of the equality of educational opportunity for which she determinedly strove.

KARL M. DALLENBACH

CORNELL UNIVERSITY

## OSCAR HENRY PLANT

ON October 1, 1939, Dr. Oscar Henry Plant, professor of pharmacology in the College of Medicine of the University of Iowa, apparently in good health and at the height of his career, passed away suddenly, following an attack of coronary insufficiency. He is mourned as a teacher, a scientist and a man.

Dr. Plant was born at Lawrence, Kansas, on September 30, 1875, the only son of Thomas Henry and Anna Stewart Plant. Early in his boyhood his family moved to East Texas. As educational facilities there were limited, he spent his winters with his grandparents in Topeka, Kansas, where he attended the public schools.

Dr. Plant joined his father when the latter removed to Galveston, and his high-school work was completed in that city. At the age of fourteen he determined to enter the field of medicine. With this object in view, he spent all his spare time and vacations working as an assistant to a Galveston pharmacist. This experience was a factor in directing his interest toward the field of pharmacology, to which he contributed so much in his later years. He entered the Medical School of the University of Texas in 1897 and graduated with the class of 1902, being compelled to drop out for one year to replenish his finances.

When a senior in medicine, Dr. Plant was selected by Dr. W. S. Carter, then professor of physiology, as an instructor in that department. To Dr. Carter's help and influence may be attributed his choice of a teaching career and the inspiration for his great success.

After graduation, Dr. Plant entered upon a five-year period of active practice in Galveston, retaining, however, his instructorship in physiology. In 1907 he decided to follow teaching as a career and became assistant professor of physiology.

Prior to this time instruction in pharmacodynamics had been carried on by the lecture and text-book method. Realizing a deficiency in this method, Dr. Plant undertook, on his own initiative, to conduct experimental demonstrations of the action of drugs on animals. His resourcefulness and ingenuity in this important field were always a source of wonder to his associates. His experiments were always worked out to the minutest detail, so that students never had any difficulty in properly performing the laboratory work. His most noteworthy contribution to research while at Texas was a study of fat absorption from Thiry-Vella loops, published in the *American Journal of Physiology.*

In 1911 Dr. Plant was called to the University of Pennsylvania as instructor in pharmacology under Dr. A. N. Richards. He was advanced to an assistant professorship in 1914 and to the rank of professor in 1918. He was associated with Dr. Richards in the well-known research on kidney function carried on by Dr. Richards and his colleagues.

In 1920 Dr. Plant was appointed professor and head of the department of pharmacology at the University of Iowa, in which position he continued until his death. The facilities for the laboratory teaching in pharmacology were very meager, so with characteristic energy he set about organizing the courses and building up what became in a comparatively short time one of the outstanding teaching laboratories of the United States. At the same time he developed an extensive research program. His outstanding contributions were studies of the action of morphine on the alimentary tract and his fundamental work on the problem of morphine addiction. Other contributions were studies on the cardiac action of camphor and a series of papers on the effects of carminatives.

Dr. Plant was a member of the American Physiological Society and the American Society for Pharmacology and Experimental Therapeutics. He was treasurer of the latter society from 1929 to 1934, vice-president from 1935 to 1936 and was elected president in 1939. He was also a member of the Society for Experimental Biology and Medicine and the American Association for the Advancement of Science. He was intensely interested in all organized scientific activities and gave his unstinted time and devotion to their welfare. His election to the presidency of the American Pharmacological Society is best proof of the high esteem in which he was held by his colleagues in the society. For the past few years he served on the Board of Editors of the *Journal of Pharmacology and Experimental Therapeutics* and the *Proceedings* of the Society for Experimental Biology and Medicine. Papers submitted to him for criticism always received the most careful attention. In addition to his many other duties, he devoted much time during the past year in directing the preparation of a Formulary for the University Hospital, copy of which was distributed to the various departments the day before he died.

In spite of all his many official duties, Dr. Plant found time for many outside interests. He was keenly interested in bird life, wood carving, fishing and stamp collecting. He was always immensely thrilled by the sight of the first migrant birds in the spring and spent many hours in the City Park with his field glasses.

In 1904, Dr. Plant was married to Ella Mary Beissner, of Galveston. She and their son William are the only direct relatives to survive him. Although he had only one son of his own, he often said that there were former students all over the United States who were like sons to him.

Dr. W. S. Carter, under whom Dr. Plant began his career, testifies to his character and personality in these words:

> His relations with the students were always most pleasant. He understood their difficulties and was most patient and sympathetic in helping them. He endeared himself to his students and to his colleagues, so that he commanded at all times the highest respect and admiration of those who knew him.
>
> His delightful personality, unusual ability, faithful and enthusiastic devotion to duty, and his loyalty to his friends, all contributed to a warm friendship which I prized very highly and which lasted throughout his lifetime. His death is a great loss to his many friends, as well as to his family and to the university which he served so well.

Those who were associated with Dr. Plant at the University of Iowa feel that Dr. Carter's tribute expresses the feeling of all his colleagues, friends and students. His loss will be keenly felt in the university and the community, and he and his work will not soon be forgotten.

E. G. GROSS
I. H. PIERCE
THE STATE UNIVERSITY OF IOWA

## RECENT DEATHS AND MEMORIALS

DR. ROYAL N. CHAPMAN, dean of the Graduate School of the University of Minnesota since July, died on December 2. He was fifty years old. Dr. Chapman resigned last year as director of the experiment station at the Pineapple Producers Cooperative Association, of Honolulu, to return to Minnesota, where he was formerly chief of the division of entomology and economic zoology of the School of Agriculture of the university.

DR. SENECA EGBERT, emeritus professor of hygiene at the Medical School of the University of Pennsylvania, known especially for his work in public health, died on December 6. He was seventy-six years old.

BENJAMIN WALLACE DOUGLASS, formerly state entomologist of Indiana, died on December 6 at the age of fifty-seven years.

THE death is announced of Dr. Arthur P. Beddard, chairman of the British Pharmacopoeia Commission, formerly lecturer in medicine in Guy's Hospital, London.

DR. VIGGO CHRISTIANSEN, formerly professor of neurology at Copenhagen and president of the Third International Neurological Congress, died suddenly on November 3.

CHARLES VALLIANT, of Paris, known for his work as a radiologist, died on December 4 at the age of sixty-seven years.

PROFESSOR UGO MONDELLO, of Florence, Italy, seismologist, formerly director of Ardenza Observatory, died on December 3 at the age of sixty-one years.

THE Louisiana Iris Conservation Society held a memorial meeting at Tulane University on September 29 as a tribute to the work of Dr. John K. Small, who until his death on January 20, 1938, was chief research associate and curator at the New York Botanical Garden and who was responsible for the discovery and preservation of many of the native irises of the southern states.

IN a note in SCIENCE, page 533, in regard to a portrait of the late Henry Smith Munroe, formerly dean of the School of Mines of Columbia University, his surname was unfortunately omitted.

# SCIENTIFIC EVENTS

## MINING EDUCATION IN ENGLAND

IN the annual report of the governing body of the Imperial College of Science and Technology, South Kensington, as summarized in the London *Times,* it is stated that mining as a career does not appear to make a great appeal to boys in the English public secondary schools. It is hoped that the provision of certain scholarships may help to spread at schools knowledge of the interest and advantages of this career, while making it possible for the necessary training to be given to a number of boys who might otherwise be prevented from obtaining it for financial reasons.

The governing body expresses its thanks to mining companies that have contributed £2,700 a year, in the first instance for seven years, to provide scholarships to be awarded to suitable candidates desiring to enter the Royal School of Mines. Provision has also been made for two, and possibly for more, scholarships for students taking an honors course in oil technology.

The Appointments Board of the Imperial College, in an appendix to the report, states that the year was a record one for the employment of college-trained graduates. Of the 247 on the register of the board only 11 were unemployed at the end of the year, and unemployment had never been so low. A remarkable feature was the persistently small number of candidates from the Royal School of Mines during the past few years; as was the case last year, there had been very many more demands for men trained in mining, metallurgy, oil, etc., than could be met.

The total number of students during the year was 1,143, made up of 530 at the Royal College of Science, 123 at the Royal School of Mines, and 490 at the City and Guilds College.

In a review of research development during the year it is reported that the Rockefeller Foundation has made an appropriation of a sum not exceeding £12,000 for researches on vitamins, sterols and related compounds, under the direction of the professor of organic chemistry, during the seven years to September 30, 1945. New subjects of research being investigated with the assistance of outside bodies included infestation of stored grain and grain products by insects, wear problems, investigation of thin carcinogenic films, combustion characteristics of coal dust and diseases of spring lettuce.

## LECTURES TO THE LAITY OF THE NEW YORK ACADEMY OF MEDICINE

THE Fifth Series of Lectures to the Laity sponsored by the New York Academy of Medicine opened on Thursday, November 30, with an address entitled "The Inheritance of Mental Disease" by Dr. Abraham Myerson, clinical professor of psychiatry at the Harvard Medical School. The presiding chairman was Dr. Malcolm Goodridge, president of the academy.

The lectures are given on Thursdays at 8:15 P.M. in the building of the academy at 2 East 103rd Street. Subsequent lectures will be as follows:

*December 28.* The Ascent from Bedlam, Richard H. Hutchings, M.D., professor of clinical psychiatry, emeritus, Syracuse University Medical College. "The remarkable growth of the mental hospital. Is mental disease increasing? New standards for mental health." *Presiding chairman,* A. A. Brill, M.D.

*January 25.* The Story of our Knowledge of the Blood, Paul Reznikoff, M.D., assistant professor of clinical medicine, Cornell University Medical College. "Blood has had a fascinating importance for humans since ancient times. The invention of the microscope, and modern knowledge of blood. The great medical significance of the recent hematological discoveries." *Presiding chairman,* Lloyd F. Craver, M.D.

*February 29.* The Romance of Bronchoscopy. Chevalier Jackson, M.D., and Chevalier L. Jackson, M.D., professors of broncho-esophagology, Temple University School of Medicine, Philadelphia. "The bronchoscope, what it is, how it is used and what is seen through it will be demonstrated by lantern slides and motion pictures." *Presiding chairman,* Charles F. Tenney, M.D.

*March 28.* The Story of the Viruses, Thomas M. Rivers, M.D., director, the Hospital of the Rockefeller Institute for Medical Research. "The development of knowledge of viruses; an historical review, and an evaluation of that knowledge in relation to certain other biological facts." *Presiding chairman,* Wilbur A. Sawyer, M.D.

*April 25.* Chemical Warfare against Disease, Perrin H. Long, M.D., associate professor of medicine, the Johns Hopkins University, Baltimore. "It has been the hope of physicians for many years that chemical compounds would be available which would cure bacterial infections. Since the introduction of Prontosil, remarkable strides have been made in the treatment of bacterial infections with sulfanilamide or its derivatives. It now appears as though within time the majority of infectious diseases may be conquered by chemical products." *Presiding chairman,* William S. Ladd, M.D.

## STATEMENT OF THE BOARD OF TRUSTEES OF BIOLOGICAL ABSTRACTS

THE Board of Trustees of *Biological Abstracts* is conscious of their great responsibility in maintaining an abstracting service available to all biologists, and it has been a matter of great concern that the cost has been so high that the benefits of this service have been largely lost to those who feel that they can not afford to subscribe. Unfortunately the editorial costs of preparing such a service are great, and it is apparent that the only possibility of decreasing the cost to the individual lies in securing a great increase in subscriptions.

For a long time it has been felt that some plan should be formulated that would more actively stimulate the interest and support of members of the several biological societies. In the hope that this plan will provide a greater service to biologists generally the trustees have approved the following: A reduction of $1.00 in the subscription price to any section, or sections, of *Biological Abstracts* will be granted the membership of any society *provided* that:

(1) They receive subscription pledges from at least 30 per cent. of their membership.

(2) It is understood that section subscriptions will be non-duplicating, *i.e.*, in cases where individuals are members of several societies, they will have the right to designate the society to which their section subscriptions will be credited.

(3) It is also understood that, in the case of an individual subscribing to *more than one section,* he may designate the appropriate societies to which each section subscription will be credited.

It is further understood that this plan does not supersede existing plans for support, such as direct subsidy of $2.00 a member by the American Society of Zoologists, but that it may be supplementary to such plans. As a further aid to individual biologists the costs of sectional subscriptions have been reduced in some cases.

It is hoped that many societies will take advantage of the opportunity to render this greater service to their membership. It is requested that a committee of interested members be appointed by each biological society to handle the matter. Further information on this plan, or a sample copy of a section, may be secured by addressing the Business Manager, *Biological Abstracts,* University of Pennsylvania, Philadelphia.

## THE ANNUAL MEETING OF THE COUNCIL OF THE UNION OF AMERICAN BIOLOGICAL SOCIETIES

The annual meeting of the Council of the Union of American Biological Societies will be held in the Colonial Room of the Neil House, Columbus, at 4:00 P.M. on the afternoon of Thursday, December 28, 1939. It is hoped that all representatives to the council will make a special effort to attend this meeting, since matters of more than ordinary interest will come up for consideration.

There will be a brief report by the editor-in-chief of *Biological Abstracts,* Dr. John E. Flynn. This will include a summary of the financial situation, the effect of the war and plans for Volume 14 (1940).

Dr. Riddle, as chairman of the Union's Committee on Biological Science Teaching, reports that the committee has continued its efforts to enroll greater numbers of high-school teachers in the National Association of Biology Teachers, which this committee sponsored and founded last year. In various ways individual members of the committee, as well as Dr. D. V. Miller, committee representative, have supported the new journal—*The American Biology Teacher.* Professor E. W. Sinnott became a member of this committee in July of this year, other members being Drs. E. V. Cowdry, F. L. Fitzpatrick, H. B. Glass and B. C. Gruenberg. During recent months the committee has given much care to the preparation of a questionnaire dealing with conditions affecting the teaching of biology in our secondary schools. This questionnaire was mailed in late November and early December to nearly 15,000 high-school teachers in 48 states. The results of this inquiry will guide and determine the committee's future efforts. The work of this year, like that of 1938, was financed through funds made available by the Carnegie Foundation for the Advancement of Teaching.

It is also planned to consider an amendment to the constitution of the union which will make possible a second type of membership, namely, "individual membership." It is hoped that the representatives of the various member societies will be prepared to consider this matter carefully.

George W. Hunter, III,
*Secretary*

## AWARD OF THE PENROSE MEDAL OF THE GEOLOGICAL SOCIETY OF AMERICA

Professor William Berryman Scott, of Princeton University, has been named by the Council of The Geological Society of America as the Penrose Medalist for 1939. The gold medal will be presented on December 29 at the fifty-second annual meeting of the society at Minneapolis.

The Penrose Medal was established in 1927 for the Geological Society by the late Dr. R. A. F. Penrose, to be awarded, under the terms of the deed of gift, "in recognition of eminent research in pure geology" and "of outstanding original contribution or achievements which mark a decided advance in the science of geology."

Professor Scott is the eleventh geologist to receive this medal. Born in Cincinnati, Ohio, in 1855 and now retired from active teaching, he was for fifty years Blair professor of geology and vertebrate paleontology at Princeton University. In the words of the Committee on Penrose Medal Award of the Geological Society,

> he is generally regarded as the leading American student of the Tertiary mammal faunas of the western hemisphere, with particular reference to their historical development and migrations. A familiarity with these problems led him also to a fruitful study of the principles of evolution. His many years of exploration of the Tertiary deposits in western United States and collaboration with Hatcher and others in Patagonia have resulted in more than fifty monographs as well as several comprehensive books. His wide range of interests is also indicated by his authorship of an excellent general text-book of geology.
>
> The importance and quality of his scientific attainments have been recognized by the award of honorary degrees from the Universities of Pennsylvania, Harvard, Oxford and Princeton, by medals from the Geographical Society of Philadelphia, the Geological Society of London, the National Academy of Sciences, the Academy of Natural Sciences, and by his election to the presidencies of the Paleontological Society, the American Philosophical Society and the Geological Society of America.

In nominating Professor Scott as Penrose Medalist for 1939 the committee on the Penrose Medal Award stated that "The award of the Penrose Medal to Professor Scott at this time is recommended because of the distinguished place he has won for himself in the science of paleontology and its related fields of organic evolution and historical geology." The committee included Professors Eliot Blackwelder, Stanford University, *chairman;* E. L. Bruce, Queen's University, Kingston, Ontario; John P. Buwalda, California Institute of Technology; James Gilluly, University of California at Los Angeles; Adolph Knopf, Yale University; Donald H. McLaughlin, Harvard University, and Dr. W. P. Woodring, United States Geological Survey.

Previous recipients of the Penrose Medal are: 1927, Professor Thomas Chrowder Chamberlin, University of Chicago; 1928, Dr. Jakob Johannes Sederholm, director of the Geological Survey of Finland; 1930, Professor François Alfred Antoine Lacroix, director of the Mineralogical Laboratory of the Museum of Natural History of Paris; 1931, Professor William Morris Davis, Harvard University; 1932, Dr. Edward Oscar Ulrich, United States Geological Survey; 1933, Professor Waldemar Lindgren, the Massachusetts Institute of Technology; 1934, Professor Charles Schuchert, Yale University; 1935, Professor Reginald Aldworth Daly, Harvard University; 1936, Dr. Arthur Philemon Coleman, University of Toronto, and 1938, Professor Andrew Cowper Lawson, University of California.

# SCIENTIFIC NOTES AND NEWS

THE Hughes Medal of the Royal Society, London, has been awarded to Dr. G. P. Thomson, professor of physics at the Imperial College of Science, London, for his "important discoveries in connection with the diffraction of electrons by matter." Professor Thomson is the son of Sir J. J. Thomson.

THE Sigma Xi lecture at the Columbus meeting of the American Association for the Advancement of Science will be given by Dr. Kirtley F. Mather, professor of geology at Harvard University, on Thursday, December 28. He will speak on "The Future of Man as an Inhabitant of the Earth." In honor of Dr. Mather, the society has arranged a dinner preceding the lecture. Dr. George A. Baitsell, president of the society, will preside.

IN honor of Robert J. Moore, development manager of the Varnish and Resin Division of the Bakelite Corporation, a dinner was given at a recent meeting of the American Institute of Chemists. The speakers were Dr. Marston T. Bogert, Dr. Robert Calvert, Dr. W. T. Read, Dr. F. D. Snell and Dr. Maximilian Toch.

DR. OLIVER E. BUCKLEY, executive vice-president of the Bell Telephone Laboratories, New York City, with which he has been associated since 1925, has been elected president to the Engineering Foundation to succeed the late Professor George E. Beggs. F. F. Colcord, vice-president of the United States Smelting Company, has been made vice-chairman of the foundation; Kenneth H. Condit has become chairman of the research procedure committee, and E. M. T. Ryder a member of that committee. Professor Walter I. Slichter, of Columbia University, has been elected a member of the executive committee.

DR. W. H. PIERRE, head of the department of agronomy at the Iowa State College, was elected president of the Soil Science Society of America at the New Orleans meeting. During the past year he was secretary of the society.

OFFICERS for 1940 of the Mineralogical Society, London, have been elected as follows: *President,* Arthur Russell; *Vice-presidents,* Professor C. E. Tilley, Dr. W. Campbell Smith; *Treasurer,* F. N. Ashcroft; *General Secretary,* Dr. G. F. Claringbull; *Foreign Secretary,* Sir Thomas H. Holland; *Editor of the Journal,* Dr. L. J. Spencer.

DR. HENRY W. HOLMES has retired as dean of the Harvard Graduate School of Education. He will continue his work as professor of education and has become chairman of the newly established University Committee on Educational Relations. Dr. Francis T. Spaulding succeeds him as dean of the school.

FREDERICK M. FEIKER, executive secretary of the American Engineering Council and a former director of the United States Bureau of Foreign and Domestic Commerce, has been named dean of the School of Engineering of the George Washington University.

D. W. MACCORQUODALE, formerly assistant professor of biochemistry at the School of Medicine of St. Louis University, has joined the research staff of the Abbott Laboratories, North Chicago, Ill., where he is in charge of hormone research.

RAYMOND P. SLOAN, vice-president of the Modern Hospital Publishing Company, Inc., associate editor of *Modern Hospital* and managing editor of *The Nation's Schools,* has been elected a member of the Board of Trustees of the Long Island College of Medicine.

DR. WILLIAM F. TALBOT, who in June joined the staff of Arthur D. Little, Inc., chemists and engineers of Cambridge, Mass., for the purpose of carrying out studies for the General Printing Ink Corporation, has recently been made research director of this company.

PROFESSOR EDWARD L. MORELAND, dean of engineering at the Massachusetts Institute of Technology, a member of the engineering firm of Jackson and Moreland, has been elected a member of the corporation of the Babson Institute, Wellesley Hills, Mass.

DR. DONALD WYMAN, of the Arnold Arboretum, Harvard University, has been appointed chairman of the newly constituted committee on arboretums and botanic gardens of the American Institute of Park Executives.

DR. C. MONTAGUE COOKE, JR., of the Bishop Museum, Honolulu, was made chairman of the standing committee on the distribution of terrestrial faunas in the inner Pacific of the Pacific Science Congress, which was held in San Francisco last summer.

DR. COLIN BARNARD, of the Council for Scientific and Industrial Research, Canberra, has been appointed local honorary secretary for the Australian and New Zealand Association for the Advancement of Science in the Australian Capital Territory, to fill the vacancy caused by the resignation of Professor G. A. Currie.

A COMMITTEE of members of the faculty of the School of Medicine of Yale University has been appointed to make a survey of the plan of instruction of the school in the light of the primary educational objective of giving broad training to qualified men and women for medical work. Members of the committee are as follows: Dr. Hebbel E. Hoff, associate professor of physiology, *chairman;* Drs. Warren T. Brown, assistant professor of psychiatry and mental hygiene; Philip B. Cowles, assistant professor of immunology; Daniel C. Darrow, associate professor of pediatrics; Alfred Gilman, assistant professor of pharmacology and toxicology; John C. Leonard, instructor in medicine; Gustaf E. Lindskog, assistant professor of surgery; Leon S. Stone, associate professor of anatomy; Herbert Thoms, associate professor of obstetrics and gynecology; John H. Watkins, assistant professor of public health; Abraham White, assistant professor of physiological chemistry; Harry M. Zimmerman, associate professor of pathology, and Dean Bayne-Jones, *ex officio.*

GRANTS recommended by the National Advisory Cancer Council, of which Professor Ludvig Hektoen is executive director, at its meeting on December 4 include Dr. Albert Tannenbaum, Michael Reese Tumor Clinic, Chicago, $3,600, for work on factors in the initiation of induced and spontaneous tumors; Dr. Wm. Ray Bryan, Duke University, $1,000, toward work on the papilloma virus protein and related material; Dr. Herbert M. Evans, University of California, $1,800, for study of nature and amount of urinary gonadotropic hormone coincident with various testicular neoplasms; Dr. Mont R. Reid, University of Cincinnati, $2,400, toward the improvement of present methods of diagnosis and treatment of cancer, and National Research Council, Washington, D. C., $3,000, in support of the American Registry of Pathology.

DR. ROBERT A. MILLIKAN, chairman of the Executive Council of the California Institute of Technology, who is engaged in a study of cosmic rays on a trip around the world, was in India when last heard from. He will continue his trip to Egypt and plans to return to the United States in February.

KARL P. SCHMIDT, a member of the Magellanic Expedition of the Field Museum of Natural History, has returned to Chicago and to his work as curator of amphibians and reptiles. Other members of the expedition, the leader, Dr. Wilfred H. Osgood, chief curator of zoology; Colin C. Sanborn, curator of mammals, and John Schmidt, assistant, will remain in the field for at least four months more. At present they are collecting in Chile, and soon will move on to the extreme southern tip of South America, along the Straits of Magellan, and to the island of Tierra del Fuego, where they will continue the research begun in 1834 by Charles Darwin on the cruise of the *Beagle.* Mr. Schmidt brought back approximately 500 specimens of mammals, 250 birds, 1,200 reptiles and amphibians, 400 fishes and a number of insects and invertebrates. The great majority are of species entirely new to the collections of Field Museum, and therefore of great importance to zoological research.

D. F. HEWETT, of the U. S. Geological Survey, has returned after ten weeks' absence in the West, where he visited most of the mining districts in which geologists of the survey are engaged in studies of strategic mineral deposits. He also conferred with numerous cooperating state officials. J. T. Pardee returned at the close of the field season, during which he supervised an examination of manganese deposits at Philipsburg, Mont., as a part of the strategic minerals program, and examined a dam site on Carbon River, near Tacoma, Wash., for the Water Resources Branch of the Geological Survey. H. E. Gregory spent about three weeks in the Washington offices of the Survey completing his report on the geology of the Zion National Park. He has returned to Honolulu.

DR. KARL F. MEYER, professor of bacteriology at the University of California and director of the Hooper Foundation for Medical Research, will deliver on December 21 the third Harvey Society Lecture of the current series at the New York Academy of Medicine. He will speak on "The Host-Parasite Relationship, with Particular Reference to Heterogeneous Infection Chains."

DR. M. L. CROSSLEY, director of research of the Calco Chemical Company, Bound Brook, N. J., recently gave an address on "The Sulfanilamides as Chemotherapeutic Agents" before the New York Section of the American Chemical Society at the Chemists' Club. Professor Louis P. Hammett, of Columbia University, chairman of the section, presided at the meeting, which was preceded by a dinner at the club.

THE annual Huxley Memorial Lecture of the Royal Anthropological Institute, London, was delivered on November 28 by Dr. R. R. Marett, rector of Exeter College, Oxford. The title of the lecture was "Charity and the Struggle for Existence."

DR. EARNEST A. HOOTON, of Harvard University, gave an illustrated lecture, entitled "Anthropology and the Belligerents," on December 11 and 12 at the Smith College Club at Cambridge.

DR. PHILIP FOX, director of the Museum of Science and Industry of Chicago, was one of the speakers at a conference on vocational problems held at Northwestern University on December 6.

PROFEESSOR DONALD E. CUMMINGS, of the University of Colorado School of Medicine, was the guest speaker at a meeting on November 25 of the Colorado Alpha chapter of Alpha Epsilon Delta, the national honorary pre-medical fraternity. The subject of his address was "Silicosis." Dr. C. E. Burford, head of the department of urology in the St. Louis University Medical School and president-elect of the Missouri Medical Association, was the guest speaker at the annual initiatory banquet of the Missouri chapter. His subject was "Some Shallow Excursions into the Fringes of Medicine."

THE seventh annual meeting of the American Science Teachers Association will be held on December 27 and 28 in conjunction with the American Association for the Advancement of Science under the presidency of W. L. Eckenberry, of the New Jersey State Teachers College at Trenton. On Wednesday morning, Thomas Midgley, Jr., Worthington, Ohio, chairman of the Board of Directors of the American Chemical Society, will make an address on synthetic rubber, in connection with which there will be an exhibit by the du Pont Company and an address on the anti-scorbutic vitamins by Dr. Charles Glen King, professor of chemistry at the University of Pittsburgh. "A History of Science in Mural Painting," by Elmer E. Taflinger, will be presented and briefly explained by Robert Lovell Black, instructor of biology at the Emmerich Manual Training High School, Indianapolis. At the luncheon meeting on Thursday Dr. Walter B. Cannon, president of the association, will make an address entitled "The Rôle of Chance in Discovery."

THE Geological Society of Philadelphia will hold one meeting each year at which a symposium will be presented on a major problem in the science of geology. Authorities on the subject will be invited to present their views, and other speakers will be welcomed. One problem, preferably of a controversial nature, will be fully considered. The subject of the first symposium will be the origin of anorthosites of the Adirondack type. Professor Robert Balk, of Holyoke College, and Professor A. F. Buddington, of Princeton University will speak on the Adirondack anorthosite. Katharine Fowler-Billings will discuss the Laramie (Wyoming) anorthosite and Dr. T. F. W. Barth, authority on certain Norwegian anorthosites, will take part. The opening session will be held at the Academy of Natural Sciences in Philadelphia at 8 P.M. on December 21, and the meetings will be continued next morning at Bryn Mawr College. Officers of the society are H. H. Hess, *president;* E. H. Watson, *past-president,* and A. E. Meier, Swarthmore College, *secretary.*

THE American Society of Tropical Medicine held its thirty-fifth annual meeting in Memphis, Tenn., from November 21 to 24. Special features of the meeting included the fourth Charles Franklin Craig lecture on tropical medicine, on "The Mechanism of Acquired Immunity to Metazoal Parasites," by Dr. W. H. Taliaferro, of the University of Chicago. The presentation of the Walter Reed Medal to Dr. William B. Castle, of Harvard University, was made by Dr. Richard P. Strong. Dr. Alfred C. Reed delivered his presidential address on "The Future of Tropical Medicine" at the annual luncheon of the society on November 23. On Thursday afternoon a joint session was held with the National Malaria Committee.

THE Geological Society of London announces that the eighteenth session of the International Geological Congress, which was to have been held in London from July 31 to August 8 next year, is indefinitely postponed. The London *Times* states that the invitation to hold the congress was accepted by the bureau of the seventeenth congress in Moscow, 1937, and was the outcome of a strong desire on the part of the fellows of the Geological Society of London and of British geologists in general to reciprocate the hospitality received by them on so many occasions in other countries, and to fulfil the wish that the congress, which last met in Great Britain in 1888, should meet there again. Sir William Bragg, president of the Royal Society, had been elected honorary president of the general organizing committee.

THE School of Mathematics of the Institute for Advanced Study each year allocates a small number of stipends to gifted young mathematicians and mathematical physicists to enable them to study and to do research work at Princeton. Candidates must have given evidence of ability in research comparable at least with that expected for the degree of doctor of philosophy. Blanks for application may be obtained from the School of Mathematics of the institute, Fuld Hall, Princeton, N. J., and are returnable by February 15, 1940.

THE Rumford Committee owns a perfect diamond slab 9 × 9 × 3 millimeters. The large surface and that at one end are flat to 0.1 wave-length of sodium light and are set at 90 degrees, the edge appearing perfectly sharp under a 300-fold magnification. The other surfaces are all rough cleaned. If any person would like to borrow this slab for experimental purposes, application should be made to the chairman of the committee, Norton A. Kent, the American Academy of Arts and Sciences, 28 Newbury Street, Boston, Massachusetts.

THE Galton Laboratory, of University College, London, is carrying on its work at the Rothamsted Experimental Station, Harpenden, Hertfordshire. It is announced in *Nature* that in view of the importance of chemical engineering at the present juncture, the Ramsay Laboratory of Chemical Engineering at University College, London, has reopened, and students will be accepted for training in chemical engineering and research.

AT the State Serum Institute, Copenhagen, Dr. Th. Madsen has established an International Salmonella Center, financed by the Commonwealth Fund. This laboratory supplies to Salmonella Centers in the various countries the sera and cultures necessary for serological diagnosis, *i.e.,* 50 sera and 100 cultures. So far, thirty-seven Salmonella Centers have been established. Those in the United States are: New York City, Dr. F. Schiff, Beth Israel Hospital; Albany, N. Y., Dr. A. Wadsworth, Department of Health, and Lexington, Ky., Dr. P. R. Edwards, department of animal pathology, University of Kentucky. The centers will receive and investigate doubtful cultures without charge.

# DISCUSSION

## GRASSLAND AS A SITE FOR BASIC RESEARCH ON TERRESTRIAL ANIMALS

THE greater part of a century has passed since Darwin published his famous work on the origin of species, and as yet no lands nor combined *natural* outdoor and laboratory facilities have been provided to study competition and the interchange of forces, which made up the basis of his theory. With the development of modern ecology and ecological processes, methods have come into use whereby studies of biotic interaction may profitably be carried on alone or in combination with laboratory studies. Various scientists have long hoped for lands and a laboratory where the interactions of land plants and animals and their physiological relations to climate can be studied just as the marine plants and animals are investigated in seaside biological stations. Pure science studies of terrestrial animals may well have much more intimate relations to human needs than marine inquiries. The sea has attracted the efforts of scientific men and the funds of granting bodies and philanthropists perhaps to an extent disproportionate to its human value. It has been demonstrated at the State University of Iowa that grassland grasshopper eggs may be used as a material for basic physico-chemical research, rivaling the sea urchin egg. The investigators at the University of Chicago have made use of striped ground squirrels taken from their native grassland haunts, for fundamental studies in hormones and for studies of the environmental factors that influence the important function of reproduction.

A grassland laboratory possesses facilities for research not available in some other types of land, such as forest or agricultural land. The great complication of forest vegetation makes many types of shelter and many niches affording protection from the elements to animals and smaller plants, which renders observations difficult. Tundra shares the advantages of grassland for researches involving field observations. These barren lands, however, are in a climate forbidding to continued scientific research and are remote from academic centers. Grassland, however, affords unrivaled opportunities for scientific biological study for the following reasons:

(1) Grassland allows full visibility of the more important larger animals and plants.

(2) Niches and hiding places for animals, such as tree tops, fallen and hollow trees and dense thickets do not occur in Great Plains areas to retard observation.

(3) The life histories and life span of the principal plants are about one tenth that of forest trees, and this greatly facilitates long-time observation because of the more rapid turnover and hence, the quicker response to climatic fluctuations.

(4) The grassland flora and fauna have intimate relations to the general problems of agriculture and human welfare on the Great Plains.

(5) Grassland constitutes about 40 per cent. of the original vegetation of the earth's land surface and is of great importance to mankind in general.

(6) It has been much less studied than forest.

(7) Stable primeval areas or semi-primeval areas of large size are rapidly disappearing. In another generation the program proposed by biological scientists may perhaps be impracticable.

(8) The field is unencumbered by organized pure science research projects.

(9) It is a vegetation type in which ecological interest is great and much important plant ecological work has been done on the moist eastern portion of the grassland, but all animal relations and their interactions with plants have been neglected.

(10) The problems of wind and water erosion of soil and the attendant dust movement are essentially biological problems.

(11) Suitable lands are of *low* economic value.

(12) Its climate is suitable for the work of investigators.

The plans of interested scientists have called for an undisturbed check area which could be under observation for a sufficiently long period to permit an analysis of drouths and dust storms, and rodent, predator and grasshopper outbreaks that occur separated by rather long intervals such as 30 to 50 years or more.

Agricultural lands are subject to such erratic overturn that causes of cyclic phenomena can not ordinarily be followed in a scientific manner. Game preserves and other small areas are, necessarily or unnecessarily, so managed as to obscure natural phenomena and render scientific conclusions unavailable or uncertain. Students of grasshopper outbreaks and, to a lesser extent, infestations of rodents desire large areas to follow the normal population of these pest animals. The need of a large area has been voiced by many, including grasshopper specialists, whose scientific results require freedom from *marginal effects* in this migratory group. For example, a tract of a few dozen sections of land surrounded by cultivated and overgrazed areas is so completely sprinkled with wind-borne organisms as to render conclusion as to natural trends uncertain.

The hope is that in the not too distant future scientific men can interest government agencies and granting bodies, which have helped with such projects in the past, to cooperate in providing land and facilities for basic terrestrial biological research. For example, an endowed laboratory could be set up on land of its own for the purpose of carrying on observations continuously. Such research would include analyzing the physiology of the animals in their relation to weather and climate, studies of competition, natural selection, reproduction, hormones, etc. For example, the National Park Service is interested in setting up a Great Plains National Monument large enough to prevent domestication of plains animals and to be managed on a hands-off basis. A laboratory adjacent to such an area would have many advantages.

V. E. SHELFORD

UNIVERSITY OF ILLINOIS

## OXYGEN REQUIREMENTS FOR GERMINATION OF SEEDS OF NYSSA AQUATICA—TUPELO GUM

IN the swamp forests of the southeastern United States frequently two species of trees are found to be dominants, *Nyssa aquatica* and *Taxodium distichum*. These trees have often been considered as very similar in their ecological requirements. Some time ago, 1932,[1] it was shown that *Taxodium* seeds can not be made to germinate under water, although after the seedling has attained a certain growth the roots and lower parts of the stem may be submerged indefinitely without harm. This is of interest ecologically, since it prevents the coming in of *Taxodium* in marshes that are continuously covered with water unless a dry season reduces the water to the point that the upper layers of soil become fairly dry.

So far as the writer has been able to learn, little has been known regarding the capability of seeds of *Nyssa aquatica* to germinate under water, although the trees may stand in water for indefinite periods.

The drupaceous fruits of *Nyssa aquatica* were collected in eastern North Carolina in September, 1938. They were allowed to dry and the fleshy exocarp and mesocarp tissue was removed, leaving the very hard endocarp enclosing the seed. On October 25 some of these "seeds" (endocarp plus seed) were placed in a metal cylinder containing sand, covered with water and placed out of doors at Raleigh, N. C. Similarly, a number of "seeds" were placed in a cylinder in moist sand out of doors at the same time.

On May 9, 1939, the cylinders were brought into the laboratory, and on the following day the sand containing the "seeds" was removed from the cylinders and placed in moist chambers kept in the laboratory. Those "seeds" kept moist but not flooded during the winter were kept in moist sand, and those that had been flooded were kept flooded under 3 to 4 cm of water.

When brought into the laboratory on May 9, three of the "seeds" from moist sand had already germinated. Subsequently, up to May 27 six additional "seeds" sprouted, giving a total germination in moist well-aerated sand of nine out of 21 "seeds." Up to the latter date none of the "seeds" kept flooded showed any signs of germination. Of 32 "seeds" kept flooded until May 27, sixteen were taken out on that date and placed in moist but well-aerated sand, the others kept flooded. From May 27 to June 16, eight of the "seeds" taken from the flooded container and given oxygen in moist sand germinated. None of the seeds kept flooded germinated up till the present, late July.

Since lack of aeration apparently prevents sprout-

[1] Delzie Demaree, *Ecology*, 13: 258–262, 1932.

ing of the "seeds" of *Nyssa aquatica*, it, like *Taxodium*, can not come in on an area kept constantly flooded.

IVAN V. SHUNK

N. C. STATE COLLEGE OF THE
UNIVERSITY OF NORTH CAROLINA

## ON "A NEW COLOR REACTION FOR VITAMIN B₁ (THIAMIN, ANEURIN)"

VILLELA and Leal[1] report that pure synthetic Vitamin $B_1$ produces an intense blue color by the use of ammonium molybdate in sulfuric acid solution and aminonaphthosulfonic acid solution, and prescribe the quantitative method of Fiske and Subbarow, which is primarily used for phosphorus determinations.

The author was interested to ascertain if the blue color would be produced likewise when using stannous chloride as the reducing agent instead of aminonaphthosulfonic acid. Both reagents are used in phosphorus determinations by the blue color methods, and if thiamin interfered in one or both, it should be taken into account. Also since there is a distinct need for an efficient thiamin method, reports should be considered and evaluated.

By employing the stannous chloride reduction method,[2] it has now been found that thiamin (Vitamin $B_1$ Hydrochlor. Cryst. Merck) gives no blue color. Neither does thiamin give any blue by the Fiske and Subbarow method. Presumably, Villela and Leal[3] used thiamin chloride or hydrochloride, since no report of the isolation of the pure base has yet been made. However, by first treating thiamin chloride hydrochloride with NaOH (to produce the strong base),[4] neutralizing and immediately following with the procedure prescribed by Villela and Leal, no blue resulted. Reagents and procedure were, of course, thoroughly checked.

It is concluded that thiamin, or Vitamin $B_1$, does not give a blue color by the Fiske and Subbarow method nor by the stannous chloride reduction method. Thus thiamin does not interfere in phosphorus determinations. It is suggested that the blue color indicated by Villela and Leal was probably due to impurities.

GUY E. YOUNGBURG

UNIVERSITY OF BUFFALO MEDICAL SCHOOL

## CHRONICA BOTANICA

COMMUNICATIONS from Dr. Fr. Verdoorn in November convey the information that the difficulties arising from the war situation in Europe which threatened the existence of *Chronica Botanica* have been solved.[1] It is announced that this important periodical will be published as a weekly beginning January, 1940, with the number of pages increased to 850 annually, with about 150 illustrations. Publications of all planned volumes of the "New Series of Plant Science Books," including numbers by Lloyd and Reed and H. I. Baldwin, together with the production of Volume 1, "Tree Growth" by MacDougal, will be carried out. The editor advises that urgent letters be sent by air mail and that all other mail be designated via "Holland America Line."

D. T. MACDOUGAL
F. E. LLOYD
H. S. REED

DECEMBER 5, 1939

# SCIENTIFIC BOOKS

## PHYSICS

*Physical Science in Modern Life*. By E. G. RICHARDSON. 256 pp. 16 plates. D. Van Nostrand Company, Inc. $3.00. The English Universities Press, Ltd. 8/6d.

THE publisher's blurb on the jacket is: "If you have wondered how an aeroplane flies—what constitutes a quicksand—why it is usually necessary to shake an embrocation, but not a mayonnaise—how a man can glide for four hours in an engineless aircraft—what limits clarity on a television screen and power in broadcasting stations—how a fish swims—whether we shall ever have trips to the moon—here is the book for you."

Certainly there can not be too many works that excite wonder or clarify the problems born in wonderment. The author claims to have set his back to the atom and the molecule and to have faced those recent advances which make contact with everyday existence. Perhaps his incentive came from his aunt, who was fond of lauding the advances in psychic science at the expense of those in the material world. When she asked him what physics had done for her, he replied that the tram had brought her up the hill that day. Thus he says the book might be called "tramway physics."

Perhaps beginning students and others do display glassy eyes when the conversationalist or lecturer begins by mentioning atoms, molecules, electrons, neu-

---

[1] Gilberto G. Villela and Aluiso M. Leal, SCIENCE, 90: 179, 1939.

[2] Guy E. Youngburg and Mamie V. Youngburg, *Jour. Lab. Clin. Med.*, 16: 158, 1930.

[3] It is to be noted that Villela and Leal use twice as much Molybdate II as Fiske and Subbarow. It made no difference, however, in this application.

[4] R. R. Williams, *Ind. Eng. Chem.*, 29: 980, 1937.

[1] Robert F. Griggs, SCIENCE, 90: 4418, November 3, 1939.

trons, cosmic rays, etc. Possibly it is wise to disarm the 'aunties' by promising them that words or ideas that hurt or produce drowsiness will not be used. It is certainly a worthy objective, to fill the great human void of understanding about the physical world without using logic or ideas against which many people are mentally allergic. There are millions who love birds but know them only by sight, sound and habitat. It seems reasonable that millions should have a vibrant alertness for the discernment of natural phenomena commensurate with the alertness of the man in the grand stand waiting for a home run.

Mechanics is covered in the chapter "Streams and Eddies," with the idea that motion is a more attractive starting point than statics. No equations are given and the reader may not even discern that mathematics was necessary in the formulation of the knowledge. Generally the ideas are developed using the word "particle" instead of "molecule," but in a few places he uses "molecule" without apology.

In the subject of heat, molecules are mentioned, but it seems to the reviewer it would have been better to have recognized heat as molecular energy. It would have been easier to explain the hot wire anemometer and the hot wire vacuum gauge. In this connection it would have fitted the objective to have explained the dark streaks on the plastered ceiling of the usual farm house or the patches of dust collection on the plastered wall back of the radiators.

Physicists and mathematicians generally should read this book, partly to learn facts, but more especially to appreciate how good an understanding of the subject can be given without using equations and formulae. The author's presentations and scope, with trifling exceptions, are sound. Recently an editor desired to correct a writing to read that an ellipse was a flattened circle. There is not an instance where the author has been guilty of describing an "ellipse as a flattened circle."

Without decrying the need for physicists capable of super-mathematical analysis, one can not help feeling the need of more physicists who can reach out to the other men of common clay and thereby bring greater benefits to all. In general, such men will use formulae and complicated analysis for personal achievement rather than to dazzle and daze the audience.

F. C. BROWN

MUSEUM OF SCIENCE AND INDUSTRY,
CHICAGO

*Demonstration Experiments in Physics.* By RICHARD MANLIFFE SUTTON. viii + 545 pp. New York: McGraw-Hill Book Company. 1938. $4.50.

THIS is a compilation of lecture demonstrations in physics originated by the American Association of Physics Teachers, as suggested by Professor C. J. Lapp. Upon recommendation of a committee composed of Professors John Zeleny, C. T. Knipp and H. W. Farwell, the editor was appointed in 1935. More than 200 members of the association contributed.

The work is designated as a "cook-book" for teachers of physics to illustrate the principles of physics in a manner to develop a fascination and an understanding of the physical world about us. A "cook-book" is rarely read by others than cooks. The designation is rather modest, for this book should be used wherever there is need or latent desire to understand the simple elements of the physical world.

In general, the demonstrations are simple and require the minimum equipment for performance and are well designed to clarify fundamental principles rather than to daze the student or "show off" the instructor. There is, however, full recognition of the incentive for a student to think if he is amazed or intrigued. Thus brilliant brass trimmings are not specified, as garnishings may be recommended in a "cook-book." It is pointed out that every mathematical formulation of a principle can be translated into an experiment and that the skilful teacher will constantly resort to simple demonstrations to emphasize the relationships involved.

Most of the 1,200 demonstrations described are familiar to the experienced instructor. Nevertheless, every one will find unfamiliar and delightful new ones. For example, the "Falling Chimney—Free-Fall Paradox" was new to the reviewer. In this a ball is rested on the upper end of a meter bar, pivoted at an angle of 30°. A paper cup is attached to the meter bar 15 cm from the upper end of the bar. When the meter bar is released, the ball falls in the cup. This shows that the upper end of a pivoted bar travels faster than a freely falling body. This was recently shown to two most eminent teachers to whom it was new, both as to the principle and technique involved. Many demonstrations of this character are included. The reviewer would have welcomed two others in similar category—one is the free fall of a calling card, with edges turned up, in a stairwell. In this case the card falls with amazing steadiness perpendicular to direction of motion. The other is the "Robeval Enigma" involving the same explanation in balances as in M-41 (a).

The reviewer would praise this compilation of demonstrations by expressing the wish that two companion volumes might be published. One, "Automatic Demonstrations in Physics," would comprise descriptions with diagrams and illustrations that would be useful in the construction of equipment designed for students and others to operate, view and study without the necessity of an attendant instructor. Such demonstrations, like books in a library, would be available for study and pleasure at least forty hours a week instead of a meager ten minutes that might be possible in a class period. The art of construction of such demonstrations is an extension of the automatic principles developed for manufacture and merchandizing.

The other desirable volume might be called "Showing off the Physical World." The demonstrations in this book should be designed for stage production for the fascination and education of the general public. In this connection one thinks of such performances as given by the Bell Telephone Laboratories, the General Electric Company, the Westinghouse Electric and Manufacturing Company and the General Motors Corporation.

F. C. BROWN

CHICAGO, ILLINOIS

# REPORTS

## GRANTS OF THE AMERICAN PHILOSOPHICAL SOCIETY

THE following grants in the natural and exact sciences were awarded by the committee on research of the American Philosophical Society in December, 1938, and in April, June and October, 1939. Grants in renewal of previous grants are not included, as these have already been published in SCIENCE.

Reginald D. Manwell, Syracuse University, for experimental animals in connection with the study of the exoerythrocyte cycle in avian malaria, and its relation to the development of immunity; the study to be centered about *Plasmodium circumflexum*. $300.

John Ernst Weaver, University of Nebraska, for technical assistance, travel in connection with studies on the damage done by drought, the adjustment of grassland to these injuries, and the method and rate by which prairie is being reestablished. $450.

University Museum, University of Pennsylvania, for excavations at Piedras Negras, Guatemala. $3,000.

Simon Freed, University of Chicago, for part payment of a research assistant in the study of the symmetries of the electrical fields about ions in solution and their relation to chemical thermodynamics. $750.

Francis Harper, John Bartram Association, for the preparation for publication, with annotations, of John Bartram's manuscript diary of his journey through the Carolinas, Georgia and Florida in 1765–66; of William Bartram's manuscript report to Dr. John Fothergill on his travels in the Carolinas, Georgia and Florida in 1773–74; and of a new edition of William Bartram's "Travels" (1791). $1,000.

H. H. Hess, Princeton University, and M. Ewing, Lehigh University, for traveling expenses in the continuation of a gravity survey of the Caribbean area and the correlation of the gravity field with the geologic structure. $1,000.

J. Percy Moore and Olin Nelsen, University of Pennsylvania, for the purchase of a micro-manipulator with a warm chamber to be used in connection with experimental studies on the free uterine eggs and blastocysts of the opossum to test the existence of embryonic organizers and the mutual interrelation of parts and related problems. $300.

Harvey Harlow Nininger, American Meteorite Laboratory, for field work in the search for and laboratory investigations of meteorites. $500.

Emil W. Haury, University of Arizona, for a part of the expenses of the excavation of a prehistoric village on Forestdale Creek, Fort Apache Indian Reservation, Arizona, occupying the area of direct contact between the Mogollon and Anasazi cultures. $500.

Research Council on Problems of Alcohol, for technical assistance, chemicals, animals and apparatus, to be used in connection with the study of the toxic factors in alcoholism. $1,500.

L. S. Cressman, University of Oregon, for field work in connection with the archeological exploration and excavation in southeastern Oregon. $600.

Samuel King Allison, University of Chicago, for part payment of a research assistant in making a precise measurement of the energies of short-range particles produced in nuclear disintegrations. $500.

James A. Shannon, New York University, for part payment for technical assistance in the study of the relationship between the renal tubular reabsorption of water and the role of the antidiuretic principle of the posterior pituitary; the effect of the composition of the body fluids upon the latter variable. $600.

Francis Owen Rice, Catholic University of America, for technical assistants in connection with his studies on the synthesis of polynuclear ring systems by a method of thermal polymerization. $1,000.

Merritt L. Fernald, Harvard University, for traveling expenses for himself and two assistants, equipment, etc., in connection with the collection of plants in eastern Virginia and the Carolinas. $1,500.

Carl C. Speidel, University of Virginia, for photographic equipment to be used in investigations of the histological changes exhibited by cells and tissues as these are subjected to various experimental procedures, and to record the changes by cinephotomicrography. $400.

Margaret Lantis, University of California, for travel and other expenses in Alaska involved in making an ethnographic study, through the complete seasonal round of the year, of the Eskimos of Nunivak Island, Alaska, as the culturally best preserved group of the important but little known Alaskan Eskimos south of Bering Strait. $950.

Robert W. Pennak, University of Colorado, for apparatus to be used in making a study of the comparative limnology of north central Colorado. $350.

Rodney H. True, University of Pennsylvania, for traveling expenses and assistance in making investigations of materials and personalities of significance alluded to in Thomas Jefferson's manuscript book on his garden operations at Shadwell and Monticello, Va. $750.

Louis W. Chappell, West Virginia University, for traveling expenses and equipment for the collection and preservation of folklore in West Virginia; folk-songs, folk-tales, legends, riddles, proverbs, superstitions, animal and plant lore, etc. $500.

Karl Sax, Harvard University, for a technical assistant in studying the effect of radiation on chromosome structure. $600.

Arthur C. Cope, Bryn Mawr College, for a technical assistant in the study of three carbon tautomerism between 1-alkenyl and alkylidene malonic and cyanoacetic esters. $600.

Adam G. Böving, Bureau of Entomology and Plant Quarantine, U. S. Department of Agriculture, for traveling expenses in making an anatomical investigation of the taxonomically important structures of the larvae of the beetles of the genus *Phyllophaga*. $800.

Paul Weiss, University of Chicago, for apparatus, technical assistance, etc., in connection with his study of the "resonance" principle of neuromuscular coordination in mammals, studied by nerve crossing and muscle transplantation, using motion pictures and electrical action potentials as indicators. $350.

Charles B. Davenport, Department of Genetics, Carnegie Institution of Washington, for a statistical assistant in the study of postnatal development of the extremities in *Homo*. $500.

Richard H. Shryock, University of Pennsylvania, for traveling expenses in connection with the study of the modern history of irregular medical practice in Europe (medical sects, folk medicine and quackery) with particular reference to Great Britain, France and Germany and the influence exerted by developments therein upon the United States since the eighteenth cntury. $250.

B. Edwin Blaisdell, Massachusetts Institute of Technology, to hire a computer for the numerical integration of Laplace's differential equation for the equilibrium meridian of a fluid drop of axial symmetry. $250.

Herbert S. Harned and Gosta C. Akerlof, Yale University, for construction of apparatus for making vapor pressure measurements of high precision for solutions with one volatile component. $1,000.

Horace W. Babcock, Astrophysical Observatory, California Institute of Technology, for supplies, travel, etc., in connection with the systematic measurement of the spectrum of the night sky and of its integrated intensity, to discover the most favorable spectral region and the type of photographic emulsion to reduce the effect of this light to a minimum. $1,000.

Harry B. Friedgood, Harvard Medical School, for technical assistance, chemicals, etc., for the biochemical study of hirsutism and virilism in women. $500.

Roy Winfield Jones, Central State College, Oklahoma, for technical assistance, purchase of fish and equipment in determining the effect of growth-promoting substances, such as auxilin (indolebutyric acid), on the early differentiation of fish embryos, as expressed by the rates of cell division in such embryos. $275.

M. Bruce Fisher, R. I. State College, for equipment and machinist's labor in connection with the determination of the relation between the critical fusion frequency of flicker at the fovea of the human eye and the size, brightness and position of the surrounding field. $125.

Lloyd P. Smith, Cornell University, for a technical assistant and apparatus in connection with the electrical separation of the isotopes of calcium, phosphorus and boron in sufficient quantities for biological, medical and nuclear investigations, respectively. $1,500.

Dwight L. Hopkins, Mundelein College, for laboratory space, chemicals and supplies for further studies of the adaptation of amoebae to changing concentration and the regulation of the water content of the protoplasm. $250.

Frederick A. Saunders, Harvard University, to purchase a camera to be used in the investigation of the mechanical action of old and new violins. $500.

Benjamin R. Coonfield, Brooklyn College, for laboratory fees, supplies and traveling expenses in connection with an investigation on the problems of regeneration in the ctenophores and color change in embryo fishes. $300.

Paul R. Stewart and B. K. Stewart, Waynesburg College, for excavation, travel, slides, etc., in connection with a paleontological survey of the 1,100 ± ft. above the Monongahela formation in southwestern Pennsylvania. $500.

E. G. Anderson, California Institute of Technology, for a cytological technician to assist in the genetic and cytological analysis of the chromosomes of maize. $300.

Irvin M. Korr, New York University College of Medicine, for part payment of apparatus to be used in the study of the relation between cellular activity and cellular respiration in mammalian tissues, with particular attention to changes in rate, foodstuffs burned, and catalysts involved as the tissues are made to pass from the resting to the active state. $400.

Dorothy M. Spencer, University of Pennsylvania, for traveling expenses, equipment, informants, etc., in connection with an intensive study of one group among the Munda-speaking peoples of Central India. $1,500.

Richard C. de Bodo, New York University, for animals, chemicals, materials, etc., for the study of the cause and mechanism of the loss of hypersensitivity to insulin and the return of gluconeogenesis to a normal level. $850.

Leslie Lyle Campbell, Washington and Lee University, for apparatus, etc., for the continuation of investigations into the Hall and allied effects in metals. $350.

Morris H. Harnly and Ruth B. Howland, Washington Square College, New York University, for care of stocks, preparation of slides and technical assistance, in the analysis of the effect of the vestigial locus during the embryological and larval periods. $500.

Serge A. Korff, Bartol Research Foundation, to purchase a ten milligram radium-beryllium neutron source for the investigation of the disruption of the nuclei in the upper atmosphere by cosmic radiation. $325.

Isaac Starr, University of Pennsylvania Hospital, for an assistant in ascertaining and defining the clinical utility of the ballistocardiogram, an instrument which records the heart's recoil and the blood's impact in man. $480.

Eugene Pacsu, Princeton University, for technical assistance, chemicals and apparatus for the physico-chemical investigation of polypeptides and proteins produced synthetically. $1,500.

Willis L. Tressler, University of Buffalo, for apparatus to be used in the limnological study of New York Lakes. $250.

Peter van de Kamp, Swarthmore College, for a technical assistant in making an accurate measurement of relative positions of close double star components by interferometer methods with special reference to close binaries with rapid orbital motion. $500.

Frances G. Wick, Vassar College, for a technical assistant, in making an investigation of the effect of neutrons as source of luminescence excitation and a study of the relation of luminescence to changes in physical state and changes in crystal structure. $500.

Carl A. Hoppert and Harrison R. Hunt, Michigan State College, for food for rats, laborer, etc., in connection with the determination whether there are inherited differences in rats with respect to susceptibility to dental caries, and if so to discover (if possible) the number of genes involved. $425.

Hudson Hoagland, Clark University, for an assistant in the investigation of the controlling chemical pacemakers (master reactions) involved in respiration of different brain centers. $600.

GRANTS AWARDED FROM THE ELDRIDGE REEVES JOHNSON FUND

*Academy of Natural Sciences of Philadelphia:*

James A. G. Rehn and John W. H. Rehn, for travel expenses in connection with field investigations of the *Orthoptera* of the Southern Alleghanies, Cumberland Plateau, Ozark and Ouachita Mountain Areas. $420.

# SPECIAL ARTICLES

## PHOTOSYNTHESIS WITH RADIO-CARBON

ANTICIPATING the appearance of a complete report now in preparation, we wish to summarize very briefly the results obtained in the past year using unicellular green algae (*Chlorella pyrenoidosa*)[1] and radioactive carbon dioxide ($\overset{*}{C}O_2$). In some respects the $\overset{*}{C}O_2$ reduction is similar to that found in barley and sunflower plants previously reported.[2]

The rate of photosynthesis was measured simultaneously by the Warburg manometer method and the radioactive technique. The two methods agreed within the experimental error. The $\overset{*}{C}O_2$ reduction was found to be markedly affected by such poisons as hydrogen cyanide and phenyl urethane. The light and dark reduction was enormously decreased by $10^{-2}$–$10^{-3}$ M. HCN. It was observed, manometrically,[3] that at these concentrations of HCN photosynthesis was strongly inhibited, whereas respiration remained unchanged. We feel certain, therefore, that the radioactive indicator method as applied to *Chlorella* is not complicated by possible reversible steps in the respiratory process.

As in the case of the higher plants,[4] *Chlorella* cells reduce $\overset{*}{C}O_2$ in the dark. We have found this to be a reversible reaction; 85 to 95 per cent. of the *dark* reduced radioactive carbon could be extracted by boiling approximately one minute with water; 70 to 80 per cent. of the C* in this extract was precipitated[5] by barium or lead ion in 80 per cent. ethanol. The barium precipitate from the *light* reduction extract contained a smaller fraction of the C*. Prolonged boiling with 1 N. HCl did not decrease the barium-insoluble radioactivity. These and other experiments indicate the presence of a carboxyl group in the radioactive molecule(s). Decarboxylation (dry distillation of barium salts) carried out on the dark water soluble material showed that most, if not all, of the labeled carbon was in the carboxyl group. To a far lesser extent this was also true of the light extract. A considerable number of naturally occurring carboxylic acids (*i.e.*, formic, acetic, propionic, oxalic, tartaric, malic, maleic, fumaric, citric, succinic, ascorbic) have been found inactive. Water-soluble proteins as well as a large number of molecules (aldehydes, ketones, ketoacids, carbohydrates, hydrolyzable polysaccharides) containing a free carbonyl group were also inactive. Benzoylation experiments indicated the presence of at least one alcoholic hydroxyl group in the radioactive molecule(s).

Preliminary experiments with glass diffusion discs (method of Northrop and Anson[6]) yield values for the diffusion coefficient of the radioactive substance in the water-soluble extract from *Chlorella* exposed to $\overset{*}{C}O_2$ for short times in light or dark which suggest the molecular weight to be large. A lower limit may be set at 200 although all indications are that the molecular weight is considerably greater.[7] Precautions were taken to ensure the diffusion measurements were made with a

[1] Sterile cultures were used. We are indebted to Dr. W. Arnold and Dr. H. A. Barker for much help and advice in this connection.

[2] S. Ruben, W. Z. Hassid, M. D. Kamen, *Jour. Am. Chem. Soc.*, 61: 661, 1939.

[3] O. Warburg, *Biochem. Zeits.*, 100: 230, 1919.

[4] E. D. McAlister, *Jour. Gen. Physiol.*, 22: 613, 1939, using a different method, has also found a dark uptake of $CO_2$ by wheat.

[5] A mixture of different carrier substances was added in all the chemical analyses.

[6] J. H. Northrop and M. L. Anson, *Jour. Gen. Physiol.*, 12: 543, 1929.

[7] Lack of information about the shape of the molecule(s) prevents a reliable estimation of the molecular weight. Experiments with Professor McBain using the ultracentrifuge are in progress and it is hoped these will make an accurate molecular weight evaluation possible.

true, non-colloidal solution. Within the experimental accuracy, the molecular weight was independent of the extraction method employed as well as time of exposure to $\overset{*}{C}O_2$.

The reversible uptake of $CO_2$ in the dark may be written as follows:

$$\text{(I)} \qquad CO_2 + RH \rightleftarrows R{-}\overset{\overset{\displaystyle O}{\|}}{C}{-}OH.$$

The formation of carboxyl is a probable reaction energetically and structurally and is suggested by the presence of radioactivity in the carboxyl group. According to thermal data for similar reactions, this process may be exothermic by 1–2 K. cal. The experimental data accumulated thus far indicate $\triangle$ F can be unfavorable by 1–2 K. cal. Free energy values for a reaction such as I, involving large molecules, are not available, however. For small molecules, the free energy change is +5–10 K. cal. Conjugation in the "R" to the carboxyl group may furnish resonance energy to help the reaction. A more favorable free energy balance may be gained by the occurrence simultaneously of processes involving other molecules or taking place within R itself. This reaction is undoubtedly catalyzed by an enzyme system. Evidence bearing on the nature of RCOOH (at least after extraction) is its molecular weight of 3,000 or more, solubility in water, insolubility in ether, absence of free carbonyl groups, presence of alcoholic groups and absence of pigments (chlorophyll, etc.).

At present the dark reversible uptake of $CO_2$ may reasonably be considered a part of the photosynthetic process,[8] since (1) it is found to be similarly poisoned by HCN, (2) the molecular weight of R is the same as that of the photosynthetic products (whether ultimate or not) formed in the light. That $CO_2$ does not combine with chlorophyll but with some other substance present in the cell has been suggested by many workers.[9]

Since the net reaction for photosynthesis is

$$nh\nu + H_2O + CO_2 \longrightarrow 1/x(C \cdot H_2O)_x + O_2$$

one may, without specifying the various steps[10] involved, represent the photochemical process by the following schematic equation:

$$\text{(II)} \qquad RCOOH + H_2O + nh\nu \longrightarrow RCH_2OH + O_2.$$

The CO–$O_2$ balance in photosynthesis, together with the absence of carbonyl groups in the observed products, infers reduction to hydroxyl. The similarity between the molecular weights and other properties of the molecules in the light and dark reactions suggests strongly that R in I and II are identical. The energy required for II is about 110 K. cal per mole of $CO_2$ reduced.

We may add that formaldehyde formation, sometimes postulated, would require about 135 K. cal per mole. In addition the above picture avoids the necessity of polymerization steps. The $RCH_2OH$ may add another $CO_2$ and repeat the cycle to build up long carbohydrate-like chains. Indeed, R itself may be such a chain. Processes in which carbohydrates are formed by interaction of accumulated reduction products, are of course, not excluded.

We wish to acknowledge our indebtedness to our many associates, and especially to Professors W. M. Latimer, W. F. Libby, W. C. Bray and T. D. Stewart, for their interest and many valuable discussions and suggestions. The continued cooperation of Professor E. O. Lawrence and his colleagues in the Radiation Laboratory has made this work possible. Our thanks are also due to the Rockefeller Foundation for financial support to the Radiation Laboratory.

S. RUBEN
M. D. KAMEN
W. Z. HASSID
D. C. DEVAULT
UNIVERSITY OF CALIFORNIA, BERKELEY

[8] We wish to thank Professor G. Mackinney and Dr. H. A. Barker for friendly criticism.

[9] R. Emerson, *Ergeb. Enzymforsch.*, 5: 305, 1936; H. Gaffron and K. Wohl, *Naturwissenschaften*, 24: 81, 103, 1936; K. V. Thimann, SCIENCE, 88: 50c, 1938.

[10] These may be part of a process involving either a photosynthetic unit (Emerson and Arnold, *Jour. Gen. Phys.*, 16: 191, 1932) or a sequence of reactions as suggested by Franck and Herzfeld, *Jour. Chem. Phys.*, 5: 231, 1937.

## THE PREPARATION AND PURIFICATION OF BRUCELLA ANTISERUM[1]

THE constituent of *Brucella* cells responsible for the clinical manifestations of brucellosis in man and animals appears from our studies to be a toxic soluble fraction.[2] Its toxicity may be demonstrated by any route of parental injection.

Preliminary studies have shown that the toxic action of the soluble fraction for experimental animals can be neutralized *in vitro* before injection by the precipitating action of a specific antiserum or by injecting a sufficient amount of antiserum shortly before the toxic antigen.

In order to obtain an antiserum of high precipitin titer or neutralizing power, and as free as possible of non-specific substance for therapeutic application in certain forms of human brucellosis, several procedures were examined.

The serum used was obtained from the cow. The fresh untreated serum precipitated the antigenic frac-

[1] Journal Article No. 396 n.s. from the Michigan Agricultural Experiment Station. This study was supported by a grant from the Horace H. and Mary A. Rackham Fund.

[2] R. B. Pennell and I. F. Huddleson, *Technical Bulletin* 156, Michigan Agricultural Experiment Station, 1937.

tion up to a dilution of 1:32,000. When the serum was diluted progressively, and the dilution of the antigen kept constant, precipitation ceased above a 1:40 dilution.

The procedures examined for the concentration and purification of the antiserum were: (1) dissociation of specific precipitates; (2) precipitation of immune globulin by dilution of serum with distilled water; (3) precipitation of immune globulin with alcohol; (4) purification by the use of salts of heavy metals; (5) disaggregation of serum proteins by means of pepsin and removal of non-specific protein by heat coagulation; (6) dissociation of serum proteins by sodium-chloride.

A combination of procedures (4) and (5) was the only one that proved to be of any value. Procedure (5) used by us is a modification of the ones described by Parfentjev (2) and Pope (1), (2), (3).

An outline of the procedure found adaptable to the purification of *Brucella* antiserum from the cow is as follows: To 500 cc of fresh serum was added 446 cc of 0.5 per cent. $AlCl_3$. The precipitate was centrifuged out and the excess of $AlCl_3$ removed from the supernatant by neutralization. The volume of supernatant recovered was 700 cc. Following this step, purified pepsin (Difco) was added to the serum to a final concentration of 0.5 per cent., the pH adjusted to 4 with citric acid, and the mixture digested for 1 hour at 37° C. Following digestion, the mixture was adjusted to a pH of 5.5, heated for 30 minutes at 60° C., and then centrifuged to remove heat-coagulated protein. The supernatant was recovered and precipitated with $(NH_4)_2SO_4$ at half saturation. The precipitate formed was removed and dialyzed in a Cellophane casing under pressure against distilled water until free from $(NH_4)_2SO_4$. The volume of the dialysate was now 300 cc.

Methiolate was added as a preservative and sufficient sodium chloride added to make the final concentration 0.85 per cent. The purified serum was sterilized by passing through a Seitz filter.

Table I shows the precipitation valves of the serum at different steps in its preparation.

The results of one of several experiments which demonstrate the high neutralizing ability of the purified antiserum *in vivo* are illustrated in Table II. In order to obtain complete neutralization of the toxic antigen *in vivo,* it is necessary to inject the antiserum at least ten minutes before the antigen. If a toxic dose of the antigen is injected before the antiserum or the two are injected simultaneously, no neutralization is obtained.

In order to determine whether the purified antiserum had any therapeutic action on the course of certain forms of human brucellosis, five patients were given daily subcutaneous injections of the purified serum

TABLE I

| | Maximum precipitation of antigen | Maximum precipitin titer |
|---|---|---|
| Untreated serum ....... | 1:32,000 | 1:40 |
| After $AlCl_3$ treatment... | 1:256,000 | 1:128 |
| After pepsin treatment.. | 1:4,000,000 | 1:2048 |

TABLE II

NEUTRALIZING ACTION OF PURIFIED *Brucella* ANTISERUM ON *Brucella* ENDOANTIGEN *in vivo*

| G. Pig No. | Amount of anti-serum cc | Amount of endo-antigen mg | Temperature reaction | Result |
|---|---|---|---|---|
| 1 .... | 1 | 10 | Normal | Lived |
| 2 .... | 0.5 | " | " | " |
| 3 .... | 0.1 | " | " | " |
| 4 .... | 0.05 | " | " | " |
| 5 .... | 0.01 | " | " | " |
| 6 .... | 0.005 | " | " | " |
| 7 .... | 0.0025 | " | " | " |
| 8 .... | 0.00125 | " | " | " |
| 9 .... | 0.000625 | " | −5 degrees | Dead 6 hours |
| 10 .... | 0.000312 | " | Normal | Lived |
| 11 .... | 0.000156 | " | " | " |
| 12 .... | None | " | −5 degrees | Dead 6 hours |
| 13 .... | " | " | −5 degrees | " |

All injections intradermally.
Antiserum given one hour before endoantigen.

in amounts varying from 0.1 cc to 5 cc. Two of the patients failed to respond to treatment with the antiserum. The temperatures of two returned to normal and remained so after two injections. The temperature of the remaining one returned to normal following one injection, but again became elevated after a lapse of seven days. Three more daily injections were then given following the rise in temperature. The temperature again returned to normal and remained so.

I. FOREST HUDDLESON
R. B. PENNELL
MICHIGAN STATE COLLEGE

## SELENIUM AND DUCK SICKNESS

A PREVIOUS communication[1] indicated that low concentrations of selenium produced poisoning in ducks in which the syndrome was identical with that described as produced by *Clostridium botulinum* type C.[2] Since the original work it has been possible to secure field material which would indicate that selenium is an important factor in western duck sickness in the areas studied. These results appear sufficiently significant to warrant recording.

Analyses of the livers of ducks and shore birds found dying of duck sickness in the Great Bear Marsh area, Utah Lake and the Lake Front Project, fifteen miles northwest of Salt Lake City, showed definite traces of selenium. Black ducks and mallards collected in the vicinity of Pymatuning Swamp, Pennsylvania (a non-seleniferous area), exhibited negative tests when

[1] A. C. Twomey and S. J. Twomey, SCIENCE, 83: 470, 1936.
[2] U. S. Dept. Agr., *Bull.* 411, May, 1934.

treated in like manner. In the chemical analyses of these tissues, a modification of the Robinson, Williams,

TABLE 1

LIVER ANALYSES

| No. | Species | Dry wt. liver | Ppm selenium |
|---|---|---|---|
| A*1 | American pintail | 5.197 gms | 7 |
| 2 | " " | 4.201 | 16 |
| 3 | Common mallard | 3.667 | 19 |
| 4 | " " | 6.776 | 16 |
| 5 | " " | 4.716 | 40 |
| 6 | Green-winged teal | 1.669 | 44 |
| 7 | " " | 1.426 | 52 |
| 8 | " " | 1.307 | 76 |
| 9 | " " | 2.311 | 43 |
| 10 | White-faced glossy ibis | 4.075 | 25 |
| 11 | Avocet | 2.971 | 25 |
| B†1 | American pintail | 3.196 | 11 |
| 2 | " " | 3.268 | 18 |
| 3 | " " | 2.065 | 39 |
| 4 | " " | 3.358 | 24 |
| 5 | " " | 1.519 | 40 |
| 6 | Common mallard | 2.369 | 34 |
| 7 | Green-winged teal | 1.635 | 148 |
| 8 | " " | 1.629 | 49 |
| 9 | " " | 2.522 | 32 |
| 10 | " " | 1.300 | 92 |
| 11 | Shoveller | 3.105 | 19 |
| 12 | American coot | 2.434 | 49 |
| C‡1 | Green-winged teal | 2.335 | none |
| 2 | Redhead | 5.065 | none |
| 3 | American pintail | 5.380 | none |
| 4 | " " | 4.635 | none |
| 5 | Common mallard | 6.015 | 10 |
| 6 | Redhead | 5.910 | 10 |
| 7 | Common mallard (juv.) | 4.545 | 10 |
| D§1 | Common mallard | 6.737 | none |
| 2 | " " | 6.091 | none |
| 3 | " " | 12.477 | none |
| 4 | " " | 7.976 | none |
| 5 | " " | 6.537 | none |
| 6 | Common black duck | 7.326 | none |
| 7 | " " " | 8.626 | none |

* A Samples from Utah Lake (dead ducks).
† B Samples from Lake Front Project, 15 miles northwest of Salt Lake City (dead ducks).
‡ C Samples from supposedly healthy birds collected on shooting grounds near Brigham, Utah, prior to an outbreak.
§ D Samples from healthy birds obtained from Pymatuning Swamp area, Pennsylvania.

Dudley and Byer[3, 4] method of determining selenium was used. Blank tests were run on all reagents. (See Table 1.)

A marked decrease in the size and weight of livers was noted in the specimens obtained from waterfowl dying of the duck sickness. This supports the experimental finding that ducks, which were poisoned on low concentrations of selenium as sodium selenite (up to 18 ppm.), fed in the drinking water, showed a reduction in the size and weight of the livers. The experimental birds also showed all the symptoms of western duck sickness in successive stages. Higher concentrations of selenium produced death within ten to twenty-four hours, and the birds died without perceptible shrinkage of livers.

Vegetation, including *Potamogeton pectinatus, Salicornia rubra, Chara* and *Ruppia maritima,* taken from Willard Spur and Unit 3 of the Great Bear Marsh area on August 29, 1939, showed no evidence for the presence of selenium. Soil and water samples taken from the same places contained no selenium.

Although large numbers of birds die during major outbreaks of duck sickness, they represent but a small percentage of the actual birds present in the areas.

The waterfowl poisoned with selenium probably ingest it in either an organic or inorganic form from small, restricted areas.

These results would indicate that selenium is a factor in western duck sickness.

ARTHUR C. TWOMEY
SARAH J. TWOMEY
CARNEGIE MUSEUM
LORING R. WILLIAMS
UNIVERSITY OF NEVADA

# SCIENTIFIC APPARATUS AND LABORATORY METHODS

## A SIMPLE METHOD FOR THE FILING OF MICROFILM RECORDS IN SHORT LENGTH STRIPS

RECENTLY L. R. Dice[1] described a simple method of filing microfilm records. For the past three years, we have employed a different method which we believe has advantages commending its description. We have found the method applicable to an industrial laboratory library, a school library and to private libraries.

Much attention has been given to the filing of 25-, 50- and 100-foot lengths of microfilm copies of documentary material. Little attention has been given to lengths of film of not over 3 feet, and often under 18 inches in length. As it is customary to photograph 16 pages of the ordinary magazine, journal or similar material on a 1-foot length of 35-millimeter film, it often happens, particularly in the fields of science, that an entire article can be copied on one foot or less of film. We have found it more convenient to use such copies in their short-strip form rather than splice them together into long film lengths.

The film strips are conveniently stored in an ordinary 10 × 12-inch filing cabinet drawer by making use of specially prepared filing cards of this size. These cards are prepared by taking a 10 × 12-inch piece of 1/16-inch cardboard and sewing onto one or both surfaces of the card layers of cloth, so that pockets are formed. A convenient type of card, which we have employed extensively, consists of four pieces of cloth sewn on one side of the cardboard. This results in six rows of three pockets each or a total of eighteen pockets. Each pocket is capable of holding a one-foot film strip, or 16 pages; thus, on one card, it is possible to file 288 pages of microfilm copies of documentary material.

[1] SCIENCE, 89: 39–40, 1939.

[3] Robinson, *et al., Ind. Eng. Chem. Anal. Ed.,* 6: 274, 1934.

[4] *South Dakota Exp. Sta. Bull.,* No. 311, 1937.

We have used many different cloths in preparing these cards. If no attention is paid to the expense, a most excellent material is tracing cloth. However, we have found equally suitable and much cheaper ordinary book-binding fabrics. Another inexpensive material which we have used successfully is oiled silk. We have noted no injury to our films as a result of the use of the latter material. Any cloth which does not ravel along its cut edges and presents a smooth, non-scratching surface can be used. In sewing the cloth to the board, care must be taken that it is not pulled tight across the board but rather caused to cup slightly between rows of stitching to provide space for the insertion of the film strips. This may be accomplished by putting a small piece of cardboard, slightly greater in thickness than the film strips, underneath all the pieces of cloth when sewing the material to the cardboard. In order to have pockets accommodating 16 pages, the seams are run lengthwise of the card. In some cases, it is convenient to prepare cards to hold shorter strips, running the seams crosswise. It is also advantageous to indent each successive cloth layer one quarter of an inch further from the right-hand edge of the card than the cloth layer immediately beneath it. This affords easy access to the various pockets in a given row and reduces the number of pages which can be stored in the top pocket of a three-pocket card by only one page. Each pocket is 40 millimeters wide, thus giving ample clearance for the 35-millimeter film.

In filing the film, it is convenient to record the identifying data concerning the film and the source of the material which has been copied on a strip of gummed paper which can be pasted onto the cloth surface. There is ample room on the top surface of each row of pockets to record full information concerning each of the three films filed in the three pockets beneath. The films themselves may be given identifying numbers or notches on the leader of the film indicating pocket and card numbers, readily facilitating the return of the film to the card and pocket in which it belongs.

The use of such a system of cards makes possible the assembling of material pertaining to a given topic from widely divergent sources. On the other hand, we have used the cards as a means of assembling copies of several items from the same volume of a journal. The system is quite flexible and, as peculiar needs for variation in the filing scheme arise, can readily be adjusted to meet the immediate needs. For libraries, the issuance of an entire film card to the patrons can at least partially combat the drawback of the inability to scan shelf titles in a library of film, since the scanning of related titles on the card may serve to suggest further readings of interest.

Another use which we have made of these filing cards is to file copies of complete books and volumes of bound magazines in short strip lengths rather than in long reels. An advantage which we have found in this procedure is that, particularly in the case of reference works, it is more convenient to examine a short strip length containing the desired page rather than going through the majority of a 50- or 100-page reel to obtain a desired page reference. One other advantage of this scheme is that more than one person may make use of a book at the same time, provided that they wish to consult different pages. It is particularly convenient to file indices in this fashion.

The majority of books which are copied on microfilm do not exceed 550 pages. It will be noted that it is possible to file such a book on two cards prepared as described above to hold 288 pages each. However, if 18 pockets are prepared on each side of the cardboard, the entire book may be filed on one card. Probably most material on film lengths of 25 feet or more can best be filed in roll form. But it has been our experience in acquiring research material on microfilm during the last five years that a large majority of the items which we have required in connection with chemical research have been articles of 16 pages or less. Frequently the items do not exceed five pages.

We have found that this method of filing enables us to put a maximum number of films into a given space when short film lengths are involved. Thus it is possible to file, in a 28-inch filing drawer, 65,000 pages of material. If cloth is sewn on both sides of the cardboard and if more numerous pockets seem advisable, this number may be increased. Certainly such a system of filing makes possible the assembling of the research material required by individuals and small industrial research laboratories in an ordinary 4-drawer filing case.

A catalogue notation on $3 \times 5$-inch filing cards recording, in addition to the ordinary information found on library catalogue cards, the file card and pocket number in which the film is kept serves to locate the film. We have found an author and a journal listing of items received useful.

HAROLD P. BROWN
UNIVERSITY OF KANSAS CITY

JAMES A. AUSTIN
JENSEN-SALSBERY LABORATORY

## BOOKS RECEIVED

BENNETT, H., Editor. *The Chemical Formulary.* Vol. IV. Pp. 638. Chemical Publishing Co. of N. Y. $6.00.

National Resources Committee. *Consumer Expenditures in the United States; Estimates for 1935–36.* Pp. iii + 195. Illustrated. Superintendent of Documents, Washington. $0.50.

SEDGWICK, W. T. and H. W. TYLER. *A Short History of Science.* Revised by H. W. TYLER and R. P. BIGELOW. Pp. xxi + 512. 61 figures. Macmillan. $3.75.

SOKOLNIKOFF, IVAN S. *Advanced Calculus.* Pp. v + 446. McGraw-Hill. $4.00.

# SCIENCE

VOL. 90 — FRIDAY, DECEMBER 22, 1939 — No. 2347

*Summary Statement of the Activities of the National Research Council, 1938–39:* DR. ROSS G. HARRISON and DR. ALBERT L. BARROWS ... 575
*Medals of the Royal Society:* SIR WILLIAM BRAGG ... 580
*Obituary:*
*Livingston Farrand:* SURGEON-GENERAL THOMAS PARRAN. *Waldemar Lindgren:* DR. W. H. NEWHOUSE. *Recent Deaths* ... 583
*Scientific Events:*
*The School of Tropical Medicine of the University of Puerto Rico; Research Grants of the Virginia Academy of Science; The Carnegie Institution of Washington; Grants of the Carnegie Corporation of New York* ... 585
*Scientific Notes and News* ... 587
*Discussion:*
*Non-Technical Books on Science:* DR. F. R. MOULTON. *The Large Mammals of the Great Plains:* DR. V. E. SHELFORD; *Zoology for Pre-Medical Students:* DR. WALTER C. KRAATZ; *Scientific Invention and Social Consciousness:* PROFESSOR M. F. ASHLEY-MONTAGU ... 590
*Scientific Books:*
*Miller's Collected Works:* PROFESSOR W. A. MANNING. *A Guide in Entomology:* PROFESSOR I. E. GRAY ... 593
*Societies and Meetings:*
*Indiana Academy of Science:* WILL E. EDINGTON. *The New England Intercollegiate Field Geologists Conference:* DR. LLOYD W. FISHER ... 593
*Special Articles:*
*The Mechanism of the Biological Citric Acid Synthesis:* DRS. NIILO HALLMAN and P. E. SIMOLA. *Loss of Biologically Fixed Nitrogen from Soils and Its Bearing on Crop Production:* DR. T. R. BHASKARAN and DR. S. C. PILLAI. *The Availability of the Iron in Dried Peas and Beans:* DR. LEAH ASCHAM, DR. MARY SPEIRS and DOROTHY MADDOX 594
*Scientific Apparatus and Laboratory Methods:*
*Culture Technic for Quantitative Growth Studies with Myxophyceae:* DR. LEE WALP. *An Inexpensive Small Air Compressor:* PROFESSOR G. J. RALEIGH. *A Convenient Method for Obtaining Blood Serum:* DR. E. M. ABRAHAMSON ... 597
*Science News* ... 14

SCIENCE: A Weekly Journal devoted to the Advancement of Science, edited by J. MCKEEN CATTELL and published every Friday by

THE SCIENCE PRESS

New York City: Grand Central Terminal

Lancaster, Pa. — Garrison, N. Y.

Annual Subscription, $6.00 — Single Copies, 15 Cts.

SCIENCE is the official organ of the American Association for the Advancement of Science. Information regarding membership in the Association may be secured from the office of the permanent secretary in the Smithsonian Institution Building, Washington, D. C.

# SUMMARY STATEMENT OF THE ACTIVITIES OF THE NATIONAL RESEARCH COUNCIL, 1938–39

By Dr. ROSS G. HARRISON
CHAIRMAN

and

Dr. ALBERT L. BARROWS
EXECUTIVE SECRETARY

## INDUSTRIAL RESEARCH

MUCH of the attention of the National Research Council has been directed during the past year, based upon the culmination of previous interests, to various aspects of the function of research in industry. Large as are the expenditures for research in scientific institutions and in universities, the traditional seat of the quest of knowledge, and for research by the agencies of government, necessary in connection with their administrative and regulatory functions and service to the public, probably both of these together are now nearly equaled by the expenditures for research by industry. Moreover, if the amounts appropriated by the government for research in agricultural and engineering fields were added to the amounts directed to research in private industry, by far the greater amount of money expended at present for scientific work in this country would be found to be devoted to the applied sciences. Although mere expenditures of money are an imperfect criterion for real values, they are nevertheless indicative in these cases of the avidity with which knowledge is being sought after and increased for man's direct profit and advantage.

These trends are reflected in some of the activities of the Council. During the past year the Division of Engineering and Industrial Research of the Council has been reorganized with particular view to bringing the resources of industrial research into more effective touch with emergency needs of the Government. An Industrial Research Institute has also been organized under auspices of this division of the Council to study problems relating to the organization of research for industrial uses, mainly in manufacturing. The Council published last winter the sixth edition of a directory of industrial research laboratories of the United States, listing some 1,769 such laboratories. A study of the physiological, psychological and social effects of working conditions upon employees in industry has also been carried on for the past two years.

Last spring the National Resources Committee requested the National Research Council to undertake a study of research in industry in the nature of an appraisal of the scientific resources and interests represented. This is for the purpose of knowing more clearly than we do now how extensively industry has come to depend on the rational application and development of scientific knowledge, the trends of progress of the scientific industries, the range and capacity of industrial laboratories for scientific work and the ways in which science and technology are influencing or affecting human welfare through the utilization of human labor in industry and through the manufacture of useful products and the rendering of convenient services.

### FELLOWSHIPS

The post-doctorate fellowships of the Council, supported by funds provided by the Rockefeller Foundation, are now administered by two boards, one for the medical sciences and one for the natural sciences. The Medical Board at its meeting early last spring made nine new appointments and three reappointments out of a total of 77 applications considered. These appointments are for twelve months at stipends ranging from $1,600 to $2,300 for the year. In the natural sciences 155 applications were considered by the Board and 24 appointments were made, including one reappointment. These are at annual stipends ranging from $1,600 to $2,000.

In reviewing recently the course of the administration of these fellowships during the past twenty years, the National Research Fellowships Board in the Natural Sciences has felt that distinct changes have occurred in the educational situation, in conditions of professional employment and in the progress of research during this period, and that changes should accordingly be made in the administration of these fellowships as a stimulus and aid to the advancement of science. Among changes adopted in its policies, the most significant perhaps are the intention of the board to make its future appointments, as a rule, from applicants who have taken the doctor's degree a year or more before applying for a fellowship and to reappoint fellows for a second year less frequently than heretofore. The basic annual stipend for fellowships in the natural sciences will be increased from $1,600 to $2,000 (effective for 1940–41). The Board has also advanced the date of announcement of fellowship appointments to about March 15 instead of May 1, beginning with 1940, and correspondingly the closing date for the receipt of applications has been changed from February 1 to December 15.

During the past year the Board offered a plan for participating fellowships in cooperation with universities. This plan received some expressions of interest, but in the particular cases considered it was not possible to put the plan into operation. Under this plan the Board will contribute one half of an annual compensation of $2,000, to be matched by a similar contribution from the university. The fellow, jointly appointed, will have approximately one half of his time free for research, but will be expected to devote the other half of his time to university duties. For the coming year the Board intends to repeat its offer of cooperation with universities in this way.

### SCIENTIFIC AIDS TO LEARNING

For the past two years a committee of the Council on scientific aids to learning has been engaged in directing studies upon the utilization of recent technological achievements in motion pictures, radio, photography, sound recording and reproduction, and other devices for aid in the process of learning in the schools. These studies have been supported generously by the Carnegie Corporation of New York. The program of the committee includes over forty projects of investigation which have been undertaken with the assistance of specially engaged investigators in some cases or with the cooperation of institutions and individuals interested in the matter. Several of these projects are concerned with the utilization of sound recording in public school teaching, as, for instance, in courses in speech, in English drama and in general science; with the possible classroom usefulness of sound slide films; and with the selection and improvement of instruments for the reproduction of visual and auditory material. The committee has been instrumental in arranging assistance to scholars requiring the development of instruments for the handling of large masses of data. Its interest in promoting the scholarly uses of microfilm has led to the setting up of a study of the whole problem of visual fatigue.

Results of the visual fatigue study should have an important bearing upon the use of the eyes in many occupations and skills and in general reading as well as in the narrower field of microfilm. For its orientation in the matter of visual fatigue, the Council arranged for a conference (on May 20 and 21, 1939) to consider the several aspects of the problem and to develop information essential to a program of investigations leading to a clearer recognition of the conditions which bring on excessive fatigue of the eyes. An advisory committee, the personnel of which includes physicists, psychologists, ophthalmologists and physiologists, is setting up a program of study for this purpose.

Several reports have been published for the Committee, which maintains offices in its own name (Committee on Scientific Aids to Learning) at 41 East 42d Street, New York City. These include:

Reports on the Reading of Microfilm.

The Present Status of Equipment and Supplies for Microphotography.

Auditory Aids in the Classroom.

The Possibility of Improving Documentation in Research Centers by Microfilming.

Eye Fatigue in the Reading of Microfilm.

Local Broadcasts to Schools.

Broadcast Receivers and Phonographs for Classroom Use.

### AMERICAN GEOPHYSICAL UNION

The twentieth annual meeting of the American Geophysical Union was held in Washington, D. C., from April 26 to 29, 1939. Regional meetings of the Section of Hydrology were held in Los Angeles on December 16 and 17, 1938, and in Spokane on December 28, 1938. The *Transactions* of these meetings have recently been published in four parts, totalling 740 pages.

The American Geophysical Union was also engaged during the past year in preparations for the seventh triennial general assembly of the International Union of Geodesy and Geophysics, which was held in Washington, D. C., during the period from September 4 to 15, 1939. The invitations for this assembly had been extended through the National Research Council to the Union at its meeting in Edinburgh in 1936. The funds to cover necessary expenses were contributed in approximately equal shares by (1) the Federal Government, (2) the Carnegie Corporation of New York, (3) the Geological Society of America, (4) the National Research Council and (5) the members and friends of the American Geophysical Union.

The registered attendance at this general assembly of the International Union was 546, including delegates and guests from 23 of the 34 countries adhering to and from three countries not adhering to the Union. Over 300 papers were presented and discussed at this meeting, and a large number of national reports on earth physics and of additional papers were recorded in the program, to be published later in the *Transactions* of the assembly and of the seven individual associations of the Union. Although the increasing tenseness of the international situation in Europe during the weeks just before the meeting and the eventual outbreak of war prevented many delegates from attending from abroad or from remaining for the assembly after reaching the United States, the program was carried through in its entirety.

### SIXTH PACIFIC SCIENCE CONGRESS

Much of the attention of the Council during the past year has been devoted to the preparations for the sixth Pacific Science Congress, with assistance from a Pacific Coast committee on arrangements. The congress was held between the dates July 24 and August 12, 1939, with sessions on the campus of the University of California and of Stanford University, and at Pacific House on the grounds of the Golden Gate International Exposition. The registered attendance was about five hundred, and over 700 papers were included in the program. These papers will be published during the coming year in the *Proceedings* of the congress. While most of the attendants at the congress were from the United States, representatives were included from some thirty countries of the Pacific region and of European countries having colonies in the Pacific.

In the absence in the Orient of international congresses in special fields which occur so frequently in Europe, this series of Pacific Science Congresses, of which the first was held in Honolulu in 1920, represents the coordinated interests of scientific men in all parts of the Pacific area in problems of that region in a number of the major fields of science. These include, for example, the relationships of land masses, the lines of volcanic and seismic activity, the courses of the ocean currents, the meteorology of the region as a whole, its plant and animal migrations, the movements of its peoples, its biological and mineral resources and the distribution of disease. Vast as the region is, the scientific problems of its various parts can be seen as closely related, and those of one field of science as bearing significantly upon those of another. For these reasons this series of congresses with their wide range of discussion has been found to be of great value. The seventh congress of this series has been announced to be held in Manila in 1943.

### WASHINGTON BIOPHYSICAL INSTITUTE

For the purpose of stimulating the adaptation of the methods of physics to biological research, and also for the encouragement of quantitative studies of the physical aspects of the functioning of the plant and animal organisms, the Rockefeller Foundation has given to the Council a generous appropriation to be available over the five-year period ending June 30, 1942. The use of this fund is in charge of an agency organized in 1934 and termed the Washington Biophysical Institute, which operates as a committee of the Council.

The value of this institute lies in the fact that it provides a means through which the interests of university physicists and biologists implemented by the appropriation of special funds can be coordinated with the interests and facilities of governmental agencies in this field. The work is conducted in the laboratories of the National Institute of Health in Bethesda, Maryland. The facilities of the National Bureau of Standards are available for the construction and testing of apparatus. A staff of several investigators and instrument makers is maintained responsible directly to the Biophysical Institute, but having access to the large facilities of these two government laboratories.

The main program of the institute is the investigation of biological substances by photochemical methods. Sterol and bile acid derivatives have been selected for these studies because they afford a rich source through body processes for derivative substances of great biological importance. The work, it is hoped, will throw light upon the origin in the animal body of such substances as antirachitic vitamins, hormones and muscle stimulants as well as the possible formation of carcinogenic substances.

In connection with this research a large number of pieces of special apparatus have been designed and constructed by the staff of the institute in collaboration with the associated government bureaus, including monochromators to produce light of known and controllable quality, self-recording spectrographs in visible, infra-red and ultra-violet light, as well as photocell detectors and integrators for specific regions of the spectrum.

The Washington Biophysical Institute has initiated a number of lines of work which have already found a continuing place in government research, including studies of genetic and lethal action of ultra-violet, photosensitized action of visible radiation, isotopic tracing and the development of spectrocytology by means of the ultra-violet microscope. The institute looks forward to the development of services which it is hoped will be of general value in biophysical research.

### NARCOTICS RESEARCH

The program of research on the chemistry and pharmacology of narcotic drugs which the Council undertook in 1929, through its Committee on Drug Addiction, has undergone a transition during the past year. The chemical and pharmacological studies, which have been pursued at the University of Virginia and at the University of Michigan since the beginning of the committee's work, are now being carried on as a major part of the program of chemotherapy investigations of the United States Public Health Service at the National Institute of Health. The Committee on Drug Addiction is acting as an advisory committee to the Public Health Service in the continuation of this work. It is also pushing ahead the clinical program which was undertaken as the necessary corollary to the chemical and pharmacological studies. A publication of the Public Health Service issued last fall[1] summarizes the results obtained during the course of the committee's work, "with special reference to the chemical structure of opium derivatives and allied synthetic substances and their physiologic action."

The problem of the committee has been to produce a substance of high analgesic properties with a minimum of euphoric characteristics, which on this account would be a more nearly ideal drug than the present derivatives of opium. Although the ideal drug has not been found, nor as yet a substance which can be unqualifiedly recommended as a substitute for morphine, much has been learned fundamentally concerning the chemistry of alkaloids and methods for testing their physiologic effects. Through the cooperation of hospitals not only for the treatment of drug addiction itself but also for the treatment of tuberculosis and cancer as well, certain of the substances, numbering over 400, which have been produced by the chemists have been or are being tested therapeutically, and there is some indication that a better drug than morphine may result from this work.

Whereas, when this work was initiated, only one or two American chemists were interested in alkaloid chemistry, now a corps of highly competent investigators has been developed in this field. Also, a procedure for patenting new narcotic substances and for providing the necessary control over them has been devised for the benefit of the public, and a pattern for successful cooperation among university groups, industrial laboratories and governmental scientific and control agencies.

### RESEARCH IN PROBLEMS OF SEX

For the current academic year the Committee for Research in Problems of Sex has made eighteen research grants, totalling $57,080, to collaborators located at fifteen institutions, continuing in the main investigations which it has been supporting for some years with funds furnished by the Rockefeller Foundation for the purpose. The Committee "was appointed eighteen years ago because of our ignorance concerning phenomena of sex and reproduction and the prevalence of prejudice against inquiry into sexual phenomena. The primary purpose, as originally conceived and recognized in policy, was the furtherance of the study of fundamental phenomena of sex. In the last two decades progress in the field of interest of the committee has been rapid, and the current

[1] Supplement No. 138 to the Public Health Reports.

research situation is radically different from that which it originally faced. Inquiry has become much more varied; endocrinology has developed remarkably; psychobiology has discovered new ways of investigating, and of using investigatively, aspects of sexual behavior." The committee has, accordingly, changed the direction of the support which it has been giving, and five years ago decided that the fields of endocrinology and of hormonal reactions needed but little further assistance on its part. In the less well-developed fields of research relating to sexual phenomena to which the committee has since turned its principal attention are the neurological and psychobiological problems of sex, and among the grants made by the committee for the current year about as many grants have been made in these fields as for general physiological problems. A second edition of the volume "Sex and Internal Secretions," edited by Dr. Edgar Allen, of Yale University, was published last spring.

### ENDOCRINOLOGY

The Committee on Research in Endocrinology has continued the program of coordinated research in this field which it inaugurated in 1937. Its program is adjusted with that of the Committee for Research in Problems of Sex by including the operation of gonadal factors on bodily processes in the general range of endocrinology, but omitting problems dealing directly with sex and reproduction, and the procedure followed by this committee is similar to that of the Committee for Research in Problems of Sex. For the current year (1939–40) twenty-nine grants have been made, totalling $54,300, from funds provided by the John and Mary R. Markle Foundation, carrying forward most of the investigations which were supported last year. These covered problems concerning neoplasia and internal secretions, the relation of endocrines to old age, carbohydrate metabolism and diabetes, the pituitary or "master-gland" of the body, endocrine control of gastro-intestinal functions, lactation, water and salt metabolism, changes in organs with diet and growth and methods of testing for endocrine secretions.

### RADIATION

With the termination of funds this summer the program of investigations which the Committee on Radiation has been conducting for the past eleven years upon the biological effects of various forms of physical emanations has been brought to a close. The resources of the committee, generously furnished in funds by the General Education Board, the Commonwealth Fund, the Rockefeller Foundation and through the contribution or loan of apparatus and supplies by a considerable number of manufacturers, have been devoted during this period to the application of new techniques to the old biological problems of modifiability and inheritance. These new methods have opened up large new fields of experimentation in genetics and its relation to evolution, and there are now many agencies and many investigators engaged upon these problems.

The trend of present work in this field includes the mechanism by which radiations influence the development, the morphology, the cytology and the genetics of organisms, and especially the effects of different wavelengths of emanation, the photosynthesis of hormone reactions in plants, radiosensitivity of tissues, photodynamic reactions and more recently the action of neutrons on living cells, the use of artificially radioactive substances in tracing the metabolism of minerals in the animal body and the mechanism of the process of the recovery of cells after injury by various forms of radiation. This committee has thus been supporting by means of grants and the loan of apparatus to collaborators in a large number of institutions work which is similar to that which the Washington Biophysical Institute is conducting directly in a portion of this field in cooperation with government laboratories.

### OTHER ACTIVITIES OF THE COUNCIL

It is not possible to refer in this brief report to all the current activities of the Council. These will be covered in the regular annual report to be published later. A word, however, may be said here about some of these developments, as follows:

Two monographs have recently been issued (through a commercial publisher), VII. "Internal Constitution of the Earth" and VIII. "Terrestrial Magnetism and Electricity," in the series of monographs on "The Physics of the Earth," which have been published by the Council since 1931.

In addition to the *Proceedings* of the eighteenth annual meeting of the Highway Research Board last fall, the Board has issued this year: (1) A discussion of rural traffic problems (mimeographed); (2) a résumé of contributions at the annual meeting concerning roadside improvement; (3) a census of highway research in progress (mimeographed); (4) a volume on "Soil Mechanics and Soil Stabilization."

Annual meetings of a committee on electrical insulation held some years ago have expanded to the proportions of two-day conferences for the presentation and discussion of technical papers, the eleventh having been held in Pittsburgh last November with an attendance of over one hundred electrical engineers and university physicists.

The Third Report of the Council's Committee on Catalysis, reviewing advances in this field since 1930, was issued last summer. Arrangements have also been made for the publication (commercially) of a catalogue of ring systems used in organic chemistry, which has been under compilation for a number of years and now presents diagrams and formulae for some four thousand organic substances.

A symposium of contributions on processes of geologic sedimentation prepared under auspices of a committee of the Council has been published by the American Association of Petroleum Geologists. Arrangements are also being made for the commercial publication of a "Symposium on Some Relations of Structural Features to Ore Deposition."

The Council has subscribed for a table at the Naples Zoological Station, which is at the disposal of American zoologists on request. Committees of the Council have prepared programs of investigation on the biological processes of aging and for studies of inheritance in man.

A committee of the Council's Division of Anthropology and Psychology has advised in recent years in the conduct of archeological excavations made in the Tennessee Valley in areas to be inundated by the building of power dams, and the division has also been requested to advise the Work Projects Administration in regard to basic problems of American archeology. A second edition of an international directory of anthropologists is now in preparation.

Among other new undertakings of the Council, as represented by the appointment of committees during the year, are the following:

The application of x-rays to physics and chemistry, and the use of spectroscopy in analytical chemistry.
The compilation of thermochemical data for the chemical industries.
The technology of organic plastics.
The organization of basic geographic data and the development of new techniques for geographical research.
The construction of a Pleistocene glacial map for North America.
The importance of breeding pure-line strains of animals for scientific purposes.

### International Scientific Meetings

The Council has been represented at international scientific congresses abroad as follows:

15th International Geographical Congress and General Assembly of the International Geographical Union, Amsterdam, July 18–28, 1938 (at which cartography in the United States was represented by an extensive exhibit); 4 representatives.
6th General Assembly of the International Astronomical Union, Stockholm, August 3–10, 1938; 6 representatives.
6th General Assembly of the International Scientific Radio Union, Venice, September 5–15, 1938; 5 representatives.
7th International Congress of Genetics, Edinburgh, August 23–30, 1939; 5 representatives.

# AWARD OF THE MEDALS OF THE ROYAL SOCIETY[1]

By Sir WILLIAM BRAGG

THE Copley Medal has been awarded to Professor Thomas Hunt Morgan.

In those branches of biology which are called botany and zoology the most important advance during the present century has been the development of genetics. The establishment of definite laws of heredity, and the discovery of the mechanism, the gene, by which hereditary qualities are carried on from generation to generation, has revolutionized our outlook on the function of the nucleus of the cell and of the chromosomes it contains; it has enabled us to understand the significance of the maturation of the germ cells and of fertilization as they occur in higher animals and plants, and thus led to a very rapid development of nuclear cytology. The theory of the gene has given us a new outlook on the determination of the development of an animal or plant. But nowhere has genetics produced greater changes than in our attitude to evolution. The observation that mutations arise *de novo* at a definite rate, that the number of different mutations occurring in a single species may be very large and that the mutations in allied species are essentially identical, have shown us for the first time the materials which are available as a basis for evolutionary change. The quantitative nature of genetics has made it possible to examine the effects which result after many generations from the establishment of a community by a few individuals of different hereditary composition, and to estimate the effect of a definite advantage attaching to one particular quality on the ultimate composition of a population. It has thus put the theory of natural selection on a sound theoretical basis. Furthermore, it has enabled us to observe indirectly the effects of natural selection in wild populations, and to plan experiments to determine its effects.

The practical applications of genetics are as important as its influence on theory. The whole of the breeding of many cultivated plants, including maize, is now firmly based, and the process of improvement immensely hastened by cytological examination. Genetics is already influencing animal breeding, and in its modern developments is throwing much light on the possi-

[1] From the address of the president at the anniversary meeting, November 30, 1939.

bility of controlling hereditary diseases in man. Thus the influence of genetics is already very wide-spread, and it will become important even in fields in which it is now little appreciated.

In the development of genetics the work of the Morgan school has been paramount. It is to Morgan that we owe that exploitation of *Drosophila melanogaster* which is the basis of most modern developments. To him we owe the theory of the gene, which is fundamental, and the explanation of "crossing over" which forms the basis of the conception of the linear arrangement of the genes and the chromosomes. From these starting points all other work springs, and much of this work comes from Morgan himself, his associates and his students. Thus, although in the case of a man working for many years in the closest association with very able men, it is impossible to isolate his individual contributions, it is evident that Morgan has done more than any other man to establish genetics and thus to revolutionize our ideas in many different fields of work, in practical affairs as in pure theory.

A Royal Medal has been awarded to Professor Paul Adrien Maurice Dirac.

Dirac's chief work has centered around the fundamental principles of modern theoretical physics. The new quantum mechanics was discovered by Heisenberg in 1925. Dirac at once realized the great importance of this discovery, started to work out its fuller implications and by a remarkable combination of originality, mathematical skill and uncanny instinct rapidly established himself as a great leader in this field. His earliest efforts were directed towards tidying up the intermediate field between that of the new quantum mechanics and the Newtonian. In this connection he established the importance of the Poisson bracket expressions of the old mechanics. An early and very important paper was on the fundamental equations of quantum mechanics. This was a generalization of any earlier work in this field, and for the purpose he introduced a new algebra, that of non-commutative numbers.

Probably his greatest achievement was that of ending the conflict between quantum mechanics and relativity mechanics by showing how to make the fundamental equations of quantum mechanics invariant under a Lorenz transformation, at any rate to a first approximation which has not yet been improved on. This led to a revision of the theory of the hydrogen atom which confirmed Sommerfeld's formula for the fine structures of spectrum lines and x-ray levels. This formula had been derived hitherto from a mixture of empirical results and theoretical guidance, but had not been deduced from general fundamental principles. The idea of a quantized electron spin also fitted naturally into the new theory. The harmonization of the quantum and relativity mechanics also required the introduction of the strange conception of negative energy states (holes) and this is generally regarded as a prediction of the existence of the positive electron (positron) since discovered by Anderson.

His book, "The Principles of Quantum Mechanics," is an important and original work, a comprehensive account of the subject by an acknowledged master in this field.

A Royal Medal has been awarded to Professor David Keilin.

Professor Keilin's contributions to entomology extend over nearly thirty years. In the main they concern the higher Diptera: with critical ability and a great capacity for detailed observation he has demonstrated the very close correlation that exists between larval structure and habits in these insects. As the result of Keilin's work it has become possible to determine the habits of almost all such larvae from an examination of their mouthparts and pharyngeal ridges. Among his many papers those on carnivorous Anthomyidae and on the remarkable life-cycle of the parasite of *Pollenia rudis* deserve especial mention.

Professor Keilin's main contributions to biochemistry have been his studies on cytochrome, published in a series of papers from 1925 onwards. These have filled an important gap in our knowledge of cell respiration and, in particular, have shown how various mechanisms, the existence of which was already known, are related to one another through the linking mechanisms which Keilin himself has discovered. He has shown that cells contain a respiratory pigment, cytochrome, composed of at least four components related to haematin. One of these is in all probability the enzyme previously known as indophenoloxidase. The catalytic activity of this enzyme depends entirely on cooperation with the other three components of cytochrome. The complete cytochrome system forms within the cell a highly active catalytic mechanism which by utilizing molecular oxygen can easily oxidize hydrogen atoms of certain substrate molecules which have been activated by dehydrogenase systems. This shows that the enzyme component of cytochrome may be identified with the previously undiscovered oxygen-transporting enzyme of Warburg and his coworkers.

Other work of Professor Keilin in this field has included the characterization of certain oxidizing enzymes which make use of molecular oxygen, and the preparation in a pure condition of the polyphenol oxidase of mushrooms. The latter has been shown to be a copper protein compound. Recently he has also isolated in a pure state copper protein compounds from blood corpuscles and liver (haemocuprein and hepatocuprein) which may be of biological importance, though they are not apparently concerned in oxidase reactions. Keilin has thus provided us with an integrated picture of cellular respiration which, though it does not cover all respiratory mechanisms, is an enormous advance on the much less systematized knowledge that we had before his work was published.

The Davy Medal has been awarded to Professor James William McBain.

McBain's claim to special recognition rests essentially on the circumstance that he created, and has led the development of, a new and important chapter of physical chemistry—the study of colloidal electrolytes. It was as the result of a long series of precision measurements on the electrical and thermodynamic properties of soap solutions that McBain originally defined this new class of materials, which combined in a special way the properties of colloids and electrolytes. The definition and constitutional theory proved to be the key to the orderly exploration, which thenceforth proceeded with continually growing impetus, of a large and fruitful field—incidentally one of considerable technical importance. The materials include soaps, nearly all modern synthetic detergents, a number of inorganic substances, such as silicates and tellurates, as well as many dyes, proteins and biocolloids. The value from a physical point of view of their classification as colloidal electrolytes and the general correctness of the micellar description of the thermodynamic and electrical properties which distinguish these materials are to-day universally recognized.

In the continued investigation, in which numerous workers have contributed to the general development of the subject, McBain has been a leader, and his work has thrown much light not only on the special properties of the ionic micell, but also on the physical properties of colloidal particles as a whole. In the course of this work a great variety of experimental methods have been developed—chemical, electrical, optical and mechanical methods—which are novel in their application and are in some cases novel in themselves. Reference may be made to the quantitative study of "solubilization" and the elaboration of the air-borne ultra-centrifuge in illustration of McBain's versatility of technique.

In addition to the composition and organization of a colloidal particle, its interface with the continuum has a decisive influence on its properties, and this gives special importance to the section of McBain's work which deals with the structure, composition and depth of macroscopic interfaces, especially of the surfaces of colloidal electrolyte solutions. Here also he has devised many methods of study, one of the most striking being the "microtome" method whereby the outermost layer of a solution can be peeled off with a rapidly moving knife blade so that the surface concentration of solute can be directly determined.

The Hughes Medal has been awarded to Professor George Paget Thomson.

Thomson's researches have been spread over a wide range of experimental and theoretical physics.

Most of his earlier experiments were connected in some way or another with positive rays, and in this field he obtained a number of valuable results. Probably the most important of these is his discovery that the small angle scattering of protons in hydrogen could not be accounted for by treating the protons and electrons as point charges obeying the inverse square law of force, but that there must be some other law of force operating at the small distances of approach during the very close encounters involved.

The scope of his work in pure physics is indicated by the titles of three books he has written or, in one case, helped to write. These are: "The Atom," "Wave Mechanics of the Free Electron" and the third edition of "Conduction of Electricity through Gases." The last is a joint effort with his father and is the most important work there is on the subject. Within this range his work is both experimental and theoretical, but the experimental part predominates both in quantity and in importance.

Thomson has also made notable contributions to aeronautics. They include research work for the fighting air services during the Great War of 1914–18, a book entitled "Applied Aeronautics," 1919, and various contributions to government publications.

Thomson's most distinguished work is based on Davisson's discovery—finally established in 1927—that electrons were reflected by single crystals as if they were possessed of the characteristics of waves. By brilliant experiments and able reasonings thereon, Thomson has opened out a new field of research which has been singularly fruitful and is still full of promise. He has been able to prove by direct experiment the correctness of Louis de Broglie's ideas of wave mechanics, not merely qualitatively but also quantitatively. In fact electrons of mass $m$ and velocity $v$ on passing through a crystal give a diffraction pattern identical with that given by a beam of x-rays of wave-length $\lambda = h/mv$, where $h$ is Planck's constant, when passed in the same direction through the same crystal. In this way the lattice constants of the crystal can be measured instead of with x-rays, and in his first paper Thomson showed that the values he found using electron diffraction agreed to within one per cent. with the values previously got by the use of x-rays.

# OBITUARY

## LIVINGSTON FARRAND

IN Livingston Farrand, who died on November 8, public health lost a great leader; education, a most able administrator; science, a distinguished contributor; the underprivileged of the nation, a valiant friend.

Rarely is it given to one man to contribute so largely to so many and such diverse fields. Even more rarely is such a contribution rich in the human values which give the scientific implications force and power.

Born in Newark, N. J., on June 14, 1867, Livingston Farrand received his undergraduate education at Princeton, where he was a member of the class of '88. He received his degree in medicine at the College of Physicians and Surgeons in 1891 and afterward took postgraduate work for a year at Cambridge and the succeeding year at Berlin. He returned to this country to teach in the department of psychology of Columbia University until 1903, when he was advanced to the chair of anthropology, a position which he held until 1914. In 1901, Dr. Farrand was married to Margaret K. Carleton, of New York. Five children, three daughters and two sons, were born of this union.

Among Dr. Farrand's many unusual capacities was that of being able to carry on active creative work simultaneously in widely separated fields. He became secretary of the National Association for the Study and Prevention of Tuberculosis and devoted much time to the strengthening of its organization during the same year in which he assumed the professorship of anthropology at Columbia and interspersed both duties with expeditions to study the primitive populations of the northwest coast and in British Columbia. His conclusions were stated in several authoritative monographs on anthropology.

From 1914 until 1919 Dr. Farrand served as president of the University of Colorado. During that period, in addition to conventional academic tasks which he executed with unconventional vigor and efficiency, he devoted himself to effecting a complete reorganization of the medical school of that institution; at the same time giving generously of his time to act upon a series of conciliation boards during a period of bitter labor disputes in the great industries of Colorado.

By 1917 Europe had been at war for three long years. Health conditions had become distressing among the civilian populations behind the lines of each nation involved. In France, especially, tuberculosis was doing vast damage. Accordingly, Dr. Farrand was asked to take leave of absence from the University of Colorado in order to organize the fight against this disease among the French people; a difficult task, for they were unfamiliar with the modern methods of searching out early and incipient cases and isolating active cases for treatment. Also, they were bitterly antagonistic to the interference in their daily lives which this involved and were distinctly suspicious of the intruding Americans. Dr. Farrand handled the problem with distinction, however. In recognition of his services, he was made an Officer in the Legion of Honor. Because of his excellent relations with the French and his familiarity with the work of the American Red Cross overseas, he was suggested by their War Council as the proper person to direct the work of the organization after the war. He had almost completed the process of transition, in which the war activities of the Red Cross were transmuted into useful labors for a nation at peace, when he was chosen for the presidency of Cornell University.

From his installation at Ithaca, N. Y., in 1921 until his retirement at the age of 70 in 1937, Dr. Farrand was not only a great university president, as measured by the growth in size, prestige and support of the institution during that period, but he found time to contribute to many causes, especially in the interest of medicine, public health and education. He was first treasurer, then president of the American Public Health Association, and an editor of the *American Journal of Public Health.* From 1930 to 1932 he headed the State Health Commission appointed by Governor Roosevelt which drew up a 20-year plan to conserve the vital resources of the State of New York. He was among the first to place himself publicly on record against the Prohibition Amendment. He headed the emergency committee of American educators for the assistance of German scholars exiled by Hitler. In 1932 he succeeded Dr. William Allan Neilson of Smith College as chairman of the board of trustees of the Carnegie Foundation for the Advancement of Teaching. He was a member of the board of the Milbank Fund and other foundations for the promotion of human welfare. In 1937 he was elected a member of the board of governors of New York Hospital and a trustee of the American Museum of Natural History. He devoted much time during his latter years to study of the needs and the development of sound policies for better medical care for the masses of American people.

Dr. Farrand was continually besought to assume executive responsibilities, because of his great capacity to see the best in men and get the best out of them, particularly in inducing them to work loyally alongside those with whom they differed. He was the great moderator, the composer of factions, the friend of freedom of thought and unity of action. He knew how to implement an idea without regimenting the men who marched under its aegis. A great tribute was offered him on June 9, 1937, upon the conclusion of sixteen years as president of Cornell University and becoming president emeritus. In a volume engrossed on parchment and signed by nearly 500 members of the Cornell faculty, there are among other glowing words of praise, these lines which summarize the deep significance of Dr. Farrand's life and work:

> We wish to dwell upon that warm fellow-feeling which has characterized your daily association with members of the faculty.
>
> Few there are among us who have not upon some occasion sought your advice or practical assistance. We have always left your office with gratitude for the helpfulness and sympathy which you have invariably manifested.
>
> Coming to the headship of the university in the full maturity of your mind and with rich experience in education and in public affairs, you have not thought it necessary to seek innovation for the sake of innovation.
>
> You have, on the other hand, missed no opportunity to reaffirm those fundamental principles of education which as members of the faculty we treasure most highly.
>
> During your presidency there has been in this university no question involving freedom of speech, no question as to the authority of the faculty in strictly educational matters, no question as to academic security. The years of your presidency have been free from factional strife. We have enjoyed the academic peace which must prevail in an educational institution if it is to be worthy of the name.

Men come, they serve, and they move forward to their greater to-morrow. Never for the cause of humanity which he loved, have we needed so much as now the skill and strength, the human kindliness and salty wisdom of Livingston Farrand.

THOMAS PARRAN

## WALDEMAR LINDGREN
### 1860–1939

WALDEMAR LINDGREN died on November 3 after an illness of eleven months. His influence will long be present with those who work in his beloved geology, but they will miss his friendly greeting and counsel.

His interest in geology began in early boyhood with walks in the pleasant countryside near Kalmar in southern Sweden. Soon he was making trips farther afield to the famous mineral localities and mines of Central Sweden which have stimulated the curiosity and imagination of so many Swedish scientists. By this time he had decided to make geology his life work. Until the closing year of his life he labored in this chosen field with a sustained enthusiasm and singleness of purpose that resulted in a remarkable unity of man and vocation.

At the age of eighteen Lindgren entered the Royal Mining Academy at Freiberg, Saxony, was graduated four years later, and remained for an extra year of graduate work. While at the Academy he studied under the leading workers in geology and mineralogy of that time. Typical of Lindgren was his remark that one of the most valuable lessons he learned at Freiberg came from a reproof by one of his teachers, Weisbach, that the student should rely on himself and not on the professor. This wholesome philosophy Lindgren later passed on to generations of field assistants and students.

In 1883 he came to the United States, and a year later began work with the U. S. Geological Survey. A long succession of reports on the geology of important mining districts came from his pen during the next three decades. Among these were the classical descriptions of portions of the Mother Lode and other districts in California; Silver City and De Lamar, Idaho; Clifton-Morenci, Arizona; Cripple Creek, Colorado; National, Nevada; and Republic, Washington. The long intensive field studies of these and other ore deposits provided the data for the theories and generalizations with which he so greatly enriched the science of mineral genesis.

In 1911 he was appointed chief geologist of the Survey, a testimonial to his broad grasp of all fields in geology. He resigned this position in 1912 to become the William Barton Rogers professor of geology and head of the department of geology at the Massachusetts Institute of Technology. In 1933 he was appointed professor emeritus.

The first edition of "Mineral Deposits" appeared in 1913. It became the leading reference and text-book of this subject the world over. The later editions have maintained this position to the present time.

Lindgren was a stimulating teacher. The generations of students who came from many lands to work with him have been lavish in praise of the man and the mentor. The respect with which students came to him as a teacher soon was tempered by respect and admiration for him as a friend. Those who came to know him well treasure the memories of the man, and the friend, beyond those of the teacher. The even temperament, the ability to infuse life into a geological discussion, the disarming kindness with which he presented forceful objections to some theory were characteristic of the man.

For decades Lindgren has been recognized as the world's leading student and interpreter of ore deposits. He made important contributions to our knowledge and theory of alterations or changes in the rocks adjacent to fissure veins and igneous intrusions; the process of replacement; the influence of physical conditions on ore deposition; the rôle of igneous processes in the formation of ores; the conception of ore deposition within certain geological periods and provinces; and the importance of colloids in the formation of certain ore deposits. Transcending all these in importance, however, was his comprehensive philosophy of mineral genesis and the far-reaching effect this has had on a host of other workers.

Lindgren's achievements can not be regarded as due to a golden age of opportunity during the exploration of virgin mining camps in the rapidly growing West; rather he achieved because of a remarkably keen and analytical mind, an inordinate love for his subject, and a great capacity for work. In addition to his own investigations and those of others to which he gave stimulus, he was always keenly interested in the interchange of geological knowledge. With a reading knowledge of at least eight languages he kept abreast of the events in his field in amazing degree. He helped to establish the *Journal of Economic Geology,* and also the "Annotated Bibliography of Economic Geology."

Lindgren received the highest honors that his appreciative fellow workers could bestow on him. Formal honors included election to many American and foreign scientific societies. The honorary degree of doctor of science was awarded him by Princeton and later by Harvard. In the citation made by President Conant of Harvard when he was conferring the degree he described Lindgren as ". . . a geologist to whom all men turn for knowledge of the metallic secrets hidden within the rock." A leading German geologist has spoken of him as "Teacher and Master"—a phrase which has often been echoed in other parts of the world. The widespread recognition of the position he held in his science is indicated by the remark of an old prospector in a western mining camp who said, with something like awe in his voice, that he had eaten breakfast the day before in a restaurant next to Lindgren, and that Lindgren had sat at the counter and eaten pancakes just like any ordinary man.

Lindgren built an impressive edifice which future work will probably change, but the blocks which he hewed out for the building will be used again and again.

W. H. NEWHOUSE

## RECENT DEATHS

DR. FREDERIC SCHILLER LEE, until his retirement in 1938 professor of physiology at Columbia University, died on December 14 at the age of eighty years.

DR. STANLEY SYLVESTER SEYFERT, head of the department of electrical engineering at Lehigh University, died on December 11. He was fifty-eight years old.

DR. JOHN BLACK JOHNSTON, from 1914 until his retirement in 1937 dean of the College of Science, Literature and the Arts in the University of Minnesota, died on November 19 at the age of seventy-one years.

DR. JOHN JACOB PIEPER, professor of crop production in the University of Illinois, died on November 26, while *en route* home from the annual meeting of the American Society of Agronomy at New Orleans. He was fifty-three years old and had been a member of the staff of the University of Illinois for twenty-two years.

# SCIENTIFIC EVENTS

## THE SCHOOL OF TROPICAL MEDICINE OF THE UNIVERSITY OF PUERTO RICO

THE report of Dr. George W. Bachman, director of the School of Tropical Medicine of the University of Puerto Rico, which is under the auspices of Columbia University, has been made public.

Nearly a dozen scientific, educational and governmental institutions collaborated with the school in researches during the past year. More than forty investigations are in progress.

An extensive building program begun in 1935 will be completed by the end of next year. Two three-story wings have been added for offices and laboratories, the university hospital plan has been reconditioned, an extra story has been put on each wing and a modern animal house for research purposes has been constructed with funds made available by such Federal agencies as the Department of the Interior and the Puerto Rico Reconstruction Administration. A new library and a building for physiology are now being erected on land transferred to the school by the United States War Department.

Researches in progress include:

An analysis of the physical measurements of certain groups of agricultural workers; studies on the nutritional values of Puerto Rican forage crops; research into the chemistry of plants; ultra-violet solar radiation preliminary to work on climate and health; vital statistics and maternal health and the prevalence of syphilis. Streptococcus infections in the tropics, the tropical disease sprue, the biological characteristics of pneumococci isolated in Puerto Rico, the rôle of experimental tuberculosis and diet with vitamin $B_1$-free rats, gland tuberculosis, cattle disease, infections from intestinal bacteria and intestinal parasites. The American Leprosy Association is collaborating in an epidemiological survey of St. Thomas and neighboring islands.

In the Department of Clinical Medicine, studies are in progress or have been completed on mucositis of the gastrointestinal tract and the effect of sulfanilamide on recurrent tropical lymphangitis.

The Department of Medical Mycology and Dermatology has completed a study of the organism causing black "piedra."

The Department of Pathology has made studies of

filterable viruses, acute rheumatic fever and skin reactions to bacilli causing abortion diseases in cattle and on the effect of vitamin A-deficient diets, as compared with normal diets, in experimental schistosomiasis, or blood fluke disease.

The Division of Parasitology of the Agricultural Experiment Station, in cooperation with the department of medical zoology, has carried on the study of the tropical diseases of calves and horses, on fluke diseases of domestic pigeons, and has made a survey of the active parasites of the island from the standpoint of both human and animal diseases.

Fourteen gibbons and 439 rhesus monkeys were added during the year to the primate colonies on the island of Santiago in order to make available conditioned animals free from disease with known histories.

A program of weekly conferences and lectures for the medical profession has been successfully developed. Dr. Bachman recommends that plans be made for the creation and maintenance of a department of tropical physiology. The importance of this work in relation to the investigations that are now being conducted can not be overemphasized.

The school has collaborated during the past year with scientific men associated with the University of Chicago, the University of Wisconsin, Duke University, the Columbia School of Medicine, the University of Puerto Rico, the Presbyterian Hospital, the Agricultural Experiment Station at Rio Piedras, the Puerto Rico Reconstruction Administration, the American Leprosy Association and the National Committee on Maternal Health.

## RESEARCH GRANTS OF THE VIRGINIA ACADEMY OF SCIENCE

THE Research Committee of the Virginia Academy of Science met on November 18 to make the regular awards for the encouragement of scientific research in Virginia. It had available for distribution $650.15, which included the sum of $125 from the American Association for the Advancement of Science. It had in hand eleven applications for grants amounting to $960. After careful consideration of each request the following awards were made:

To Miss M. Katharine Cary, of the Medical College of Virginia, $75 for a study of the relation of alkalemia and acidemia to resistance to infection.

To Dr. E. Ray Casto, of Emory and Henry College, $50 for student assistance in the tabulation and graphing of data on the influence of climate on agriculture and manufacturing.

To F. F. Ferguson and Dr. E. R. Jones, Jr., of the College of William and Mary, Norfolk, $25 for aid in the collection of Turbellaria in the Norfolk area.

To Professor F. H. Fish, of the Virginia Polytechnic Institute, $50 for the purchase of a colorimeter for use in the study of organic analytical reagents.

To C. C. Flora and W. C. Thacker, of the Virginia Polytechnic Institute, $25 for aid in the construction of a thermostatically controlled water bath for use in a study of the digestibility of the fat in various forms of milk.

To Dr. Allan T. Gwathmey, of the University of Virginia, $105 for the purchase of a special camera for the photomicrography of the various surfaces of single crystals of various metals.

To Dr. J. Frank Hall and Dr. R. L. Simpson, Jr., of the Medical College of Virginia, $50 for the purchase of materials to be used in the construction of dental bridges in a study of the effects of such structures on the teeth and other tissues concerned.

To King A. Jamison, of the Virginia Polytechnic Institute, $50 for the purchase of canaries to be used in a survey of the incidence of malarial parasites in the wild birds of Virginia.

To A. F. Meyer, Jr., of the Virginia Military Institute, $35 for the purchase of supplies and materials for use in a study of the sterilization of dishes and equipment used in public eating places.

E. C. L. MILLER,
*Secretary*

## THE CARNEGIE INSTITUTION OF WASHINGTON

THE annual meeting of the Board of Trustees of the Carnegie Institution of Washington was held on December 15, in the Administration Building of the institution at Sixteenth and P Streets. The Honorable W. Cameron Forbes, chairman of the board, presided. The following trustees were present: Thomas Barbour, James F. Bell, Robert Woods Bliss, Frederic A. Delano, Homer L. Ferguson, W. Cameron Forbes, Walter S. Gifford, Walter A. Jessup, Frank B. Jewett, Charles A. Lindbergh, Roswell Miller, Stewart Paton, Elihu Root, Jr., Henry R. Shepley, William Benson Storey, Richard P. Strong, Charles P. Taft, James W. Wadsworth, Lewis H. Weed.

The president of the institution, Dr. Vannevar Bush, submitted his annual report on the work of the institution during the past year, and the board authorized appropriations totaling $1,316,500 for conduct of research activities of the institution for the year 1940.

Governor Forbes was reelected chairman of the board for the next three years. Walter S. Gifford was reelected vice-chairman and Frederic A. Delano secretary for the same period.

The Honorable Robert Woods Bliss, Dr. Walter A. Jessup and Dr. Lewis H. Weed were reelected as members of the executive committee for the ensuing three years.

Standing committees of the Board of Trustees were appointed by the chairman for the year 1940 as follows:

Committee on Astronomy: Herbert Hoover, *chairman*, Walter S. Gifford, Roswell Miller, Elihu Root, Jr., William Benson Storey.

Committee on Terrestrial Sciences: Frank B. Jewett, *chairman,* Frederic A. Delano, Homer L. Ferguson, Henry S. Morgan, James W. Wadsworth.

Committee on Biological Sciences: Lewis H. Weed, *chairman,* Thomas Barbour, James F. Bell, Alfred L. Loomis, Stewart Paton.

Committee on Historical Research: Henry R. Shepley, *chairman,* Robert Woods Bliss, Charles A. Lindbergh, Richard P. Strong, Charles P. Taft.

## GRANTS OF THE CARNEGIE CORPORATION OF NEW YORK

THE annual report of Dr. Frederick P. Keppel, president of the Carnegie Corporation of New York, has been issued. Grants amounting to $4,846,126 were made during the fiscal year 1938–39 by the corporation to organizations and individuals in the United States and in the British Dominions and Colonies. Of this sum, $697,200 was given for library interests, $1,157,325 for the arts, $1,253,650 for research, studies and publications, $204,921 for adult education and $1,533,030 for the general program of the corporation. The largest grant made during the year was $250,000, given to complete the sum necessary to establish joint academic library services for Vanderbilt University, Peabody College and Scarritt College at Nashville, Tennessee.

Grants for scientific research amounted to $137,500, and those for educational investigation, $233,550. Grants were made to the amount of $432,500 for the purpose of carrying forward the work of the Institute of International Education, with headquarters in New York, and of the New Zealand Council for Educational Research. The American Association for Adult Education, the National Occupational Conference, the Committee on Scientific Aids to Learning and the American Law Institute received the sum of $295,400 for work in their respective fields; $177,000 was voted to the Association of American Colleges, the American Council of Learned Societies and the National Bureau of Economic Research.

Grants of $500,436 were made for the British Dominions and Colonies. In South Africa these funds have been used chiefly for scientific inquiry; in New Zealand and Australia emphasis has been on educational research, libraries and social services. In Canada grants have been made primarily to continue research programs in colleges and universities and to forward library extension.

Appropriations for scientific work authorized and payable during the fiscal year 1938–1939 included:

University of Puerto Rico, School of Tropical Medicine, development of library. $13,500.
University of Michigan, experiments in microphotography. $8,000.
New York Museum of Science and Industry. $52,625.
American Museum of Health, studies in field of health education. $30,000.
American Museum of Natural History. $25,000.
American Association of Museums. $12,000.
Research in genetics as it relates to intelligence, University of Iowa. $2,000.
The Carnegie Institution of Washington. $79,000.
School of Medicine, Yale University clinic of child development. $30,000.
Harvard University. $57,500.
National Research Council. $106,300.
American Mathematical Society, to establish in the United States an international journal of mathematics. $60,000.
Research Council on the Problems of Alcohol, preliminary survey. $25,000.
Marine Biological Laboratory, Woods Hole, Mass., emergency support. $20,000.
National Academy of Sciences, survey regarding a national science fund. $15,000.
Zoological Society of London, publication of *Nomenclator Zoologicus.* $6,000.
American Neurological Association, research on heredity of mental diseases. $3,000.
Long Island Biological Association. $3,000.
Dental research, various institutions. $53,500.
In aid for research on insulin. $5,000.
Comprehensive study of the Negro in America. $55,000.
Brown University, development of work in mathematics. $6,000.
American Mathematical Society, support of International Congress of Mathematics, 1940. $4,500.
American Association for the Advancement of Science, support of educational program. $4,000.
American Geophysical Union, Seventh Triennial Assembly of International Union of Geodesy and Geophysics, 1939. $3,000.

# SCIENTIFIC NOTES AND NEWS

DR. HENRY NORRIS RUSSELL, director of the observatory at Princeton University, was elected to honorary membership in the New York Academy of Sciences at the recent annual meeting.

THE decoration of "Officer of the Order of Leopold" has been conferred by the King of the Belgians on Dr. James B. Murphy, member of the Rockefeller Institute, New York, in recognition of his work in the field of cancer research.

THE President of the Republic of Cuba has awarded decorations of the Order of Carlos J. Finlay to several public health workers from the United States and Mexico. The recipients, who were decorated at a recent meeting of the Florida Public Health Association at Jacksonville by Dr. Domingo F. Ramos, director of Public Health in Cuba and Minister of National Defense, included Dr. Angel de la Garza Brito, dean of the School of Hygiene, Mexico City; Dr. G. T. Dunnahoo, past assistant surgeon of the United States Public Health Service, Miami; Dr. George MacDonnell, city health officer, Miami, each of whom received the officer's medal, and Dr. Reginald M. Atwater, executive secretary of the American Public Health Association, New York, who received the Commander's medal.

AT a testimonial meeting at the Bohemian Club of San Francisco, Dr. Karl F. Meyer, director of the Hooper Foundation of Medical Research of the University of California, and Dr. J. C. Geiger, director of public health of San Francisco, were presented with special embossed scrolls "in recognition of their service in the conquering of botulism and of the appreciation of the nation's canners." Representatives of the University of California, Stanford University, the State of California, the City of San Francisco and of the canning industry were present. The work on botulism was initiated by the late Dr. E. C. Dickson, who was later joined by Dr. Meyer and Dr. Geiger.

DR. MARY SWARTZ ROSE, professor of nutrition at Teachers College, Columbia University, received the annual award of the Associated Grocery Manufacturers of America at the recent annual convention in New York, "in recognition of her contributions to the science of nutrition, the part she has played in the dissemination of scientific information concerning foods, her authorship in this field and her outstanding career as a teacher of others who teach nutrition."

MARY C. BUEHNE, administrative assistant in the office of the secretary of the American Chemical Society, completed twenty-five years of service on November 17. Her associates gave her a testimonial luncheon to express their appreciation and esteem on November 18. Miss Buehne was presented with a silver coffee service.

DR. GOTTLIEB HABERLANDT, professor emeritus of plant physiology at the University of Berlin, celebrated his eighty-fifth birthday on November 12.

OFFICERS elected at the recent Pittsburgh meeting of the American Public Health Association were: *President,* Dr. Edward S. Godfrey, Jr., Albany, N. Y.; *President-elect,* Dr. W. S. Leathers, Nashville, Tenn.; *First Vice-president,* Elisabeth L. Smellie, R.N., Ottawa, Canada; *Second Vice-president,* Dr. Domingo F. Ramos, Havana, Cuba; *Third Vice-president,* Dr. Wilton L. Halverson, Pasadena, Calif.; *Treasurer,* Dr. Louis I. Dublin, New York, N. Y.; *Executive Secretary,* Dr. Reginald M. Atwater, New York, N. Y.; *Chairman of Executive Board,* Dr. Abel Wolman, Baltimore, Md.

DR. THOMAS T. MACKIE, New York, was named president-elect at the recent annual meeting in Memphis of the American Society of Tropical Medicine. Dr. Malcolm H. Soule, professor of bacteriology at the University of Michigan, was elected vice-president, and Dr. E. Harold Hinman, senior biologist of the health section of the Tennessee Valley Authority, was elected secretary. Dr. Louis L. Williams, Jr., Washington, D. C., became president.

AT the annual dinner meeting on December 12 of the New York Academy of Sciences, Dr. Roy Waldo Miner, curator of living invertebrates at the American Museum of Natural History, was elected president to succeed A. Cressy Morrison. Vice-presidents elected were: Leslie E. Spock, Anne Anastasi, Horace E. Wood, 2d, Ralph Linton and Victor K. LaMer. Other officers elected were: *Recording Secretary,* Duncan A. MacInnes; *Corresponding Secretary,* C. Stuart Gager; *Treasurer,* Wyllys Rosseter Betts, Jr.; *Librarian,* John Hendley Barnhart; *Editor,* Erich M. Schlaikjer; *Councilors,* W. J. V. Osterhout and Douglas W. Johnson; *Members of the Finance Committee,* Herbert F. Schwarz, John D. Sherman, Jr., and Wayne M. Faunce. The address of Mr. Morrison, the retiring president, was entitled "The Practical Benefactions of Pure Science." Richard Archbold gave an account of his third expedition to New Guinea illustrated by motion pictures.

THE following officers and members of the Council of the Royal Society, London, were elected at the anniversary meeting on November 30: *President,* Sir William Bragg; *Treasurer,* Professor T. R. Merton; *Secretaries,* Professor A. V. Hill, Professor A. C. G. Egerton; *Foreign Secretary,* Sir Albert Seward; *Other Members of Council,* Professor F. C. Bartlett, Professor P. G. H. Boswell, Professor F. T. Brooks, Dr. C. G. Darwin, Professor H. M. Fox, Dr. H. J. Gough, Dr. A. D. Imms, Professor C. K. Ingold, Professor G. B. Jeffery, Professor R. T. Leiper, Professor H. S. Raper, Sir Owen Richardson, Professor E. K. Rideal, Dr. F. J. W. Roughton, Professor W. W. C. Topley, Professor R. Whiddington.

DR. F. G. DONNAN, formerly professor of chemistry at the University of London, has been elected president of the British Association of Chemists.

AT a meeting of the British General Medical Council on November 28 Dr. H. L. Eason, principal of the University of London, was elected president to succeed Sir Norman Walker, who has served since 1931.

DR. HARRY STACK SULLIVAN, president of the William Alanson White Psychiatric Foundation, has resigned as professor of psychiatry at Georgetown University School of Medicine.

PROFESSOR B. S. MONROE has been made acting dean

of the Graduate School of Cornell University. He succeeds Dr. Floyd K. Richtmyer, who died on November 7. Professor Monroe has been secretary of the Graduate School since 1917.

Professor Harry Dexter Watson, who is directing the civilian aviation program, has been appointed acting head of the department of mechanical engineering at the College of Technology of the University of Maine. His appointment, which is for the remainder of the academic year, is to fill the vacancy created by the recent death of Professor William Jordan Sweetser, who had been head of the department since 1915.

Dr. Stanislas Francis Snieszko, of the University of Krakow, a former Rockefeller Foundation scholar at the University of Wisconsin, has been appointed research assistant in the department of bacteriology at the University of Maine for the remainder of the academic year. The appointment has been made possible through the cooperation of the Maine Canners' Association.

Recent appointments in the Division of Plant Pathology and Physiology of the Texas Agricultural Experiment Station include: Dr. Charles E. Minarik, plant physiologist in rice investigations at Beaumont, and Dr. Glenn KenKnight, plant pathologist, who will conduct investigations of peanut, watermelon and cantaloupe diseases at Stockdale.

Major General Charles Ransom Reynolds, who retired last June as Surgeon-General of the United States Army, has been appointed chief of the Division of Tuberculosis Control of the Pennsylvania State Department of Health.

Dr. J. Alfred Hall, formerly associate director of the California Forest and Range Experiment Station, U. S. Forest Service, has been named director of the Central States Forest Experiment Station, with headquarters at Columbus, Ohio, to succeed Willis M. Baker, who has resigned to become chief forester for the Tennessee Valley Authority. Dr. Hardy L. Shirley, formerly in charge of silviculture investigations at the Lake States Forest Experiment Station, has been made director of the Allegheny Forest Experiment Station, with headquarters at Philadelphia. He succeeds R. D. Forbes, who will devote his full time to special assignments.

Dr. William Bowie, who retired in 1937 as chief of the Division of Geodesy of the U. S. Coast and Geodetic Survey, has been appointed executive secretary of the Society of American Military Engineers and editor of *The Military Engineer,* the journal of the society. He took over his work at the national headquarters in Washington on December 1.

Dr. Max Cutler, from 1931 to 1937 director of the Tumor Clinic of the Michael Reese Hospital, Chicago, and Dr. George M. Smith, research associate in anatomy, Yale University School of Medicine, have been appointed members of the National Advisory Cancer Council to succeed Dr. Ludvig Hegtoen, and Dr. Clarence C. Little, director of the Roscoe B. Jackson Memorial Laboratory of Bar Harbor, Me., whose terms have expired. Members include Dr. James B. Conant, president of Harvard University; Dr. Arthur H. Compton, professor of physics at the University of Chicago; Dr. Mont R. Reid, professor of surgery at the University of Cincinnati, and James B. Murphy, of the Rockefeller Institute for Medical Research.

Dr. E. D. Adrian, professor of physiology in the University of Cambridge, has been appointed to succeed the late Professor John Mellanby as a member of the British Medical Research Council.

Dr. John N. Couch, of the department of botany of the University of North Carolina, has been granted leave of absence for the winter quarter. He will leave Chapel Hill on January 1 for special work in Mexico. He will work in conjunction with the Mexican Department of Forestry, which will furnish guides in return for duplicate specimens of all that is collected.

Dr. Wladyslaw Gorcynski, from 1919 to 1928 chief of the Polish Weather Bureau, is now working at the Scripps Institution of Oceanography of the University of California. He is gathering data for a comparative study of the sunshine in Southern California and the Mediterranean region. Dr. Gorcynski was attending a meeting of the International Union of Geodesy and Geophysics in Washington, D. C., when Germany invaded Poland.

Dr. Isaiah Bowman, president of the Johns Hopkins University, and Dr. Perrin Long, associate professor of medicine in the Medical School, spoke at the annual meeting on December 12 of the Johns Hopkins Alumni Association of New York, New Jersey and Connecticut. Dr. Bowman's address was entitled, "Who is Responsible for Peace?" Dr. Long spoke on "Sulphanilamide."

The History of Science Society will meet with the American Association for the Advancement of Science at Columbus on December 29. The morning session will be devoted to the history of agriculture, with Drs. H. G. Good and C. A. Browne as speakers. At the afternoon session on medical history, the speakers will be Drs. L. T. Moore and E. R. Lang. At the annual dinner Dr. Louis Karpinski, professor of mathematics at the University of Michigan, will give an address on "Organic Unity of the Contributions to the Progress of Mathematical Science."

THE Society of American Bacteriologists will hold its forty-first general meeting at New Haven on December 28, 29 and 30, under the presidency of Professor Arthur T. Henrici, of the University of Minnesota. The occasion will mark the fortieth anniversary of the founding of the society at New Haven on December 29. Professor C.-E. A. Winslow, a charter member, will review "The First Forty Years" of the society's development at the annual banquet, at which the living charter members will be introduced by the toastmaster, Dr. Karl F. Meyer, and presented with testimonials. The annual presentation of the Eli Lilly and Company Research Award in Bacteriology and Immunology will be made at this time. The scitific program will emphasize bacterial chemotherapy, immunity, filterable viruses and fermentation. Other sessions will consider bacterial physiology, dissociation, taxonomy and various aspects of agricultural and industrial microbiology. Round-table discussions will be held on the History of Bacteriology, Bacterial Chemotherapy, the Teaching of Bacteriology and Fermentation.

THE Emergency Executive Committee of the International Congress of Mathematicians has decided definitely to postpone until some more favorable date the congress which was to have been held in Cambridge in September, 1940. Notice to that effect is being sent to the invited speakers and to others interested.

INDEFINITE postponement of the eighteenth session of the International Geological Congress fixed for July 31 to August 8, 1940, in London has been announced. An invitation from the Geological Society of London for the eighteenth session to meet in Great Britain during 1940 had been accepted by the bureau of the seventeenth congress in Moscow in August, 1937. The last previous meeting of the congress in Great Britain was held in 1888, and geologists throughout America had been formulating plans to attend. At date of taking action to postpone the meeting the officers of the congress had anticipated an attendance of the order of fifteen hundred. The prospective program for the congress had included a wide range of subjects of international interest and importance. Sixteen excursions before and after the session had been arranged to conduct visiting geologists throughout England, Scotland and Wales. Twenty-two individual geological and mining societies and societies concerned with related sciences had supported the Geological Society of London in organizing the session.

FERENCE VON TOMPA, president of the International Congress of Prehistoric and Protohistoric Sciences, announces that the third session of the congress, which was to have been held in Budapest during the summer of 1940, has been postponed pending the establishment of peace in Europe. The American members of the permanent council of the congress are: A. L. Kroeber, University of California; George Grant MacCurdy, Yale University; Harriett M. Allyn, Mount Holyoke College, and Carl E. Guthe, University of Michigan.

THE American League against Epilepsy, composed of physicians, has sponsored an organization called the "Laymen's League against Epilepsy," formed for the purpose of educating the public concerning the various aspects of epilepsy and for stimulating contributions towards research. Officers elected at the first annual meeting on December 4 are as follows: *President,* Mrs. Francis B. Riggs; *Vice-presidents,* Clinton H. Crane and Dr. William G. Lennox; *Secretary-Treasurer,* Mrs. Mary L. Fleming. *Medical sponsors,* Dr. Stanley Cobb, Dr. Irvine McQuarrie, Dr. Adolf Meyer, Dr. Wilder Penfield, Dr. Tracy Putnam and Dr. William Kerr. The office of the society is at the Harvard Medical School, Boston.

# DISCUSSION

## NON-TECHNICAL BOOKS ON SCIENCE

Two years ago the American Association for the Advancement of Science began the publication of those symposia presented at its meetings that are judged to be "so comprehensive and of such high order of merit that it can not afford not to publish them." Six of these symposia have been published—"Tuberculosis and Leprosy," "Syphilis," "Applications of Surface Chemistry in Biology," "Recent Advances in Chemical Physics," "Mental Health" and "The Migration and Conservation of Salmon." Two more—"Problems of Lake Biology" and "The Gonococcus and Gonococcal Infection"—are about to appear from the press. The manuscripts of two additional symposia—"The Cell and Protoplasm" and "Blood, Heart and Circulation"—will soon be ready for the printer.

Experience has already proved that in publishing distinguished symposia the association is making an important contribution to the progress of science. For one thing, it is exercising its function as a synthesizing agency. For another, it is making available important scientific material which, at least in the field of public health, is having a profound influence on the country. The inauguration of the publishing of these symposia constitutes the beginning of a new period in the history of the association.

The association is now entering on a new undertaking that promises to be equally important in a different field. It has entered into a contract with Doubleday, Doran and Company, Inc., for the publication of a series of non-technical books on science to be known as American Association for the Advancement of Science Series. The books of this series will be on important subjects of wide public interest and will be written by competent and distinguished authorities. They will be for the intelligent general public—every scientist is an amateur except in his own field—for, in the final analysis, science and all the other avenues of progress depend upon society as a whole. Consequently, from the narrow view of the defense of science the association is justified in entering on this new undertaking.

There are, however, broader considerations, for it would not profit science even though it were worshipped if civilization should die. Science is no longer regarded as something quite apart from the strong currents of life. It is, on the contrary, the principal force that is hurrying mankind forward, whether toward a precipice or into serene waters of a finer and nobler civilization is not yet generally accepted as certain. Although theologians and philosophers and politicians are often despairing of civilization, scientists are haunted by no such misgivings. They have as a background the long history of the evolution of life on the earth. They know of the slow rise of man, with his many ups and downs, from the level of the lower animals. They are well aware of his physical, mental and moral imperfections and the ease with which he can stumble. Yet on the whole they regard his prospects with steady eyes, for they are developing methods of learning the realities of the inorganic and the organic worlds, and are confident that the continued pursuit of these realities and the organizing of both individual lives and society in harmony with them will lead inevitably to a better future.

There are no complexities in the arrangement the association has made for the publication of this series of non-technical books on science. Any person planning to write such a book may offer it to the association as one of its series. If it is accepted by the committee appointed to represent the association, and if the publishers approve of the book, the author will make a direct contract with the publishers for its publication under the usual terms and royalties for such works. The publishers assume all the financial risks.

Upon the appearance of a book of this series from the press, the association will buy from the publisher from time to time, at a substantial discount, as many copies as it may require and will offer them to its members at a substantial discount from the publisher's retail price. The publisher will also sell the book through the usual channels. The association will advertise each book published under this contract in both SCIENCE and *The Scientific Monthly*. And in all advertisements of each of these books the publisher will state that it is one of the American Association for the Advancement of Science Series.

All that remains is to secure manuscripts that have the desired qualities—soundness, timeliness, importance and literary excellence. It is expected that only a few books will be published each year, at least at first. The development of the plan will be guided by experience, as in the publication of the symposia. If the books in this new series are kept on a correspondingly high plane of excellence, they will set the general pattern for non-technical science and exert in time a profound influence on science and society. Inquiries respecting the project are invited.

F. R. MOULTON,
*Permanent Secretary*

## THE LARGE MAMMALS OF THE GREAT PLAINS

IT is cogent to ask if the larger game animals of the Great Plains are not rapidly undergoing domestication. One who makes a brief study of the Great Plains big game reserves is likely to be impressed that the bison and antelope are rapidly being domesticated in all of them, due to (1) winter feeding on hay, and (2) various schemes for regulating breeding and care of young in close quarters.

The reserves are at the same time overgrazed to a considerable degree. One of the largest of these, at Wainwright, Alberta, is very badly overgrazed (1939). Here the smaller animals are, accordingly, deprived of shelter and are wanting or deficient as to numbers. Some of them, such as the badger, small vertebrates and various invertebrates, are threatened with extirpation.

This brings us to the consideration of the size of area necessary to prevent domestication of these animals and their associates. Taking the minimum daily range from home and normal wandering of a community of plains animals, for example, in Nebraska, 1,250,000 acres is found to be near the minimum. Men with large experience regard 1,000,000 acres as the ideal area at which to aim in the case of plains animals. Animals which roam the national forests and connected national parks have very much larger areas available. Boerker's list of national forests as of 1917 shows more than half of them with 800,000 acres of actual Forest Service-owned land. The Kaibab Forest contained 1,072,375 acres, giving ample range to the deer, the Kaibab squirrel, etc.; probably not over one fourth of the area is grazed by cattle, leaving 800,000 acres for the wild animals, recreation, etc.

Future generations have a right to see these animals

in a wild state. There would be many distressing appeals from botanists if redwoods, beech and giant cedars and other trees with their associated shrubs and herbs were rapidly coming under cultivation as nursery stock.

This need has been realized by animal ecologists and students of wild life for some time. It was brought to more general attention at about the same time by the National Park Service and a committee of the Ecological Society. This resulted in the investigation of thirteen areas, four or five of which were considered suitable for a Great Plains National Monument.

V. E. SHELFORD
UNIVERSITY OF ILLINOIS

## ZOOLOGY FOR PRE-MEDICAL STUDENTS

UNDER the above title, Dr. H. S. Diehl[1] advised less zoology and criticized the alleged arts college advice to pre-medics "to take as much zoology as they can possibly get in."

Zoologists in charge of pre-medics are really not advising "all they can possibly get in," but urging all such zoology courses (as well as those chemistry courses) which will give the pre-medics a sufficiently thorough preparation to do well in the medical aptitude tests, and get in and stay in medical school. To "take only those courses which are required for entrance to medical school," as we are told some medical deans advise, is ambiguous. It probably means the well-known minimum, as given in all medical catalogues, including one year of zoology or biology, one of physics and three semesters of chemistry. It is ambiguous, because experience shows such zoology (and chemistry) inadequate, and considerably more zoology advantageous, as we are assured in reading the aptitude tests and in heeding all that is related by our graduate pre-medics who visit after a year or two in medical school.

Moreover, and most important here, medical school catalogues when studied more, as I studied over 40 of them, show many cases of various other required zoology courses and other courses that are recommended. I summarized in detail these courses for half a dozen medical schools, nearer our institution or to which most of our pre-medics have gone. This summary was found to be too extensive to appear in these columns, however. To prepare our students advantageously in this larger scope and different pattern of zoology requirements, we have in our four-year pre-medic curriculum three times as much zoology as the one-year minimum, plus a course in bacteriology. Only the latter would not be necessary according to the various requirements and recommendations.

Dr. Diehl criticized taking arts college courses of the same type as medical school courses, to which we agree, as most likely such courses in arts college would be dilute and poor. A course in human physiology should be displaced by a foundational laboratory course in general physiology. Following advice of medical school men, we give that type of course. Genetics is an essential course. Human embryology (which our critic cites) is not to my knowledge given in arts colleges, but a basic laboratory course in general vertebrate embryology, on frog and chick mostly, is and should be given. Finally, comparative vertebrate anatomy is an entirely different course in the arts college from human anatomy in the medical school. The comparative may not cause students to make an appreciably higher grade in mastery of details of regional gross anatomy when working on the cadaver, but it will give the beginning medical students a far broader and wiser outlook upon human anatomy.

WALTER C. KRAATZ
UNIVERSITY OF AKRON

[1] SCIENCE, 89: 604, June 30, 1939.

## SCIENTIFIC INVENTION AND SOCIAL CONSCIOUSNESS

SOME months ago, in the pages of this journal,[1] before aerial frightfulness broke out in Europe, I drew attention to the remarks made in 1670 by the inventor of the first airship, Francesco Lana. Lana conceived the greatest objection to his invention to be the inhuman and unconscionable uses to which it might be put by unscrupulous men.[2] Now that submarine frightfulness has for some time been under way in Europe, it may not be without some interest to hear what the inventor of the first submarine, who wrote 170 years before Lana, thought of his work. He writes (about the year 1500):

> How by an appliance many are able to remain for some time under water. How and why I do not describe my method of remaining under water for as long a time as I can remain without food; and this I do not publish or divulge on account of the evil nature of men who would practice assassination at the bottom of the seas, by breaking the ships in their lowest parts and sinking them together with the crews who are in them; and although I will furnish particulars of others they are such as are not dangerous, for above the surface of the water emerges the mouth of the tube by which they draw in breath, supported upon wine-skins or pieces of cork.

The writer of these words was Leonardo da Vinci.[3]

M. F. ASHLEY-MONTAGU
HAHNEMANN MEDICAL COLLEGE
AND HOSPITAL,
PHILADELPHIA

[1] SCIENCE, 90: 180, 1939.
[2] F. Lana, Prodromo, Brescia, 1670.
[3] Leicester Mss., 22 v. See Edward MacCurdy, "The Notebooks of Leonardo da Vinci," 850–51, New York, 1939.

# SCIENTIFIC BOOKS

## MILLER'S COLLECTED WORKS

WITH the publication by the University of Illinois Press of the second volume of the Collected Works of George Abram Miller this set begins to take on the appearance of an imposing monument to a long and well-spent life. The large body of mathematicians who are interested in the advancement of group theory realize with gratitude the great convenience to them of this collection of so many scattered papers, long and short, into a readily accessible form.

The papers of Volume II date mostly from the years Miller spent in California. He was then much interested in groups generated by operators with given relations between them, in groups of isomorphisms, in extensions of Sylow's theorem and in groups of prime power order. Of the many topics discussed in this volume, probably the most important is that of the groups of order $p^m$ which contain cyclic subgroups of order $p^{m-2}$. This is well covered by three papers, on pages 89, 165 and 271. Certainly the most brilliant results are to be found in the paper, written in collaboration with H. C. Moreno, on non-Abelian groups in which every proper subgroup is Abelian. The most extensively studied and the most baffling problem of finite group theory is that of the existence of simple groups of odd composite order. In one of these papers (see page 83) Miller showed that if such a group does exist there must be more than 50 members in any complete set of conjugate operators or subgroups. The statement on page 13 that Turkin has announced the solution of the problem seems to be a mistake.

What with book reviews, short expository articles, reports on the progress of group theory prepared for the American Mathematical Society and historical essays at the beginning and end of this volume, it, like the first, has much to interest the general reader.

STANFORD UNIVERSITY W. A. MANNING

## A GUIDE IN ENTOMOLOGY

*A Laboratory Guide in Entomology.* By ROBERT MATHESON. vii + 135 pp. 48 plates. Ithaca, N. Y.: Comstock Publishing Company. $2.00. 1939.

FOR many years there has been need for a satisfactory laboratory manual for the study of insects. Consequently, those entomologists and zoologists who are called upon to teach beginning courses in entomology will welcome Matheson's new laboratory guide. The manual seems to be well done, and, in as much as it presents a general view, it should be serviceable in giving a fundamental knowledge of insects to those who will branch out into other fields of biology as well as furnishing preparation for advanced studies in entomology.

The manual is based on the work offered in the beginning course in entomology at Cornell University. It begins with a brief study of a crayfish to refresh students' minds as to the fundamental structure of the arthropods. The essentials of insect anatomy, both external and internal, are gained from a thorough study of a grasshopper. This is followed by a comparative study of mouth-parts; metamorphosis and growth; structure and classification of principal orders, with keys for identification of families; and some work on adaptation, social life, insect pollinators, relation of insects to animal and plant diseases and insect control. Of practical value is the appendix on how to collect, prepare, mount, preserve and rear insects. Brief lists of references are given in connection with some of the exercises. There are forty-eight well-executed plates, most of which are for the student to interpret and label. The pages are perforated and punched so that the plates may be removed and inserted in a loose-leaf notebook. A glossary of technical terms used in the manual is included.

I. E. GRAY

# SOCIETIES AND MEETINGS

## INDIANA ACADEMY OF SCIENCE

THE fifty-fifth annual meeting of the Indiana Academy of Science was held on November 9, 10 and 11, in Terre Haute, Ind., with Indiana State Teachers College as host. Some 350 scientists from Indiana and adjoining states were in attendance. The general meetings were presided over by Dr. L. A. Test, vice-president, Purdue University, in the absence of the president, Dr. T. G. Yuncker, DePauw University, who is on a botanical research expedition in the South Seas. Dr. Willis S. Blatchley, one of the charter members of the academy and now eighty years of age, gave the principal address on "The Days of a Naturalist."

Some eighty-six research papers were read at the nine divisional meetings, and a panel discussion on "Teaching Bacteriology" was also carried out in the Bacteriology Division. The following divisional chairmen were chosen for 1940: archeology, Paul Weer, Indianapolis; bacteriology, Dona G. Graam, Indiana State Teachers College; botany, Ralph M. Kriebel, Soil Conservation Service, Bedford; chemistry, Karl Means, Butler University; geography and geology, W. D. Thornbury, Indiana University; mathematics, Cora B. Hennel, Indiana University; physics, James F. Mackell, Indiana State Teachers College; psychology, R. A. Acher, Indiana State Teachers College; zoology, W. H. Hiestand, Purdue University.

The dinner meeting was held on Friday evening with 150 in attendance, after which President

Yuncker's address on "Parasitism as a Way of Life" was read by Dr. Winona Welch, DePauw University.

The officers chosen for the year 1940 are: *President,* Frank Wallace, state entomologist, Indianapolis; *Vice-president,* S. S. Visher, Indiana University; *Secretary,* W. P. Allyn, Indiana State Teachers College; *Treasurer,* W. P. Morgan, Indiana Central College; *Editor of the Proceedings,* Paul Weatherwax, Indiana University; *Press Secretary,* Will E. Edington, DePauw University.

The Junior Academy of Science held its meetings on Saturday with an attendance of 200. A number of papers were read by the young scientists, and the various high-school clubs had very interesting exhibits on display. The principal address was given by Dr. W. P. Allyn, Indiana State Teachers College, on "Indiana Fauna." Miss Ruth Downey, George Washington High School, Indianapolis, and Robert Bennett, Mishawaka High School, were chosen as the two outstanding junior scientists and were recommended for the honorary memberships in the American Association for the Advancement of Science. The officers of the Junior Academy for 1940 are: *President,* Jack Wilkie, Elmhurst High School, Fort Wayne; *Vice-president,* Dorothy Smitha, George Washington High School, Indianapolis; *Secretary-Treasurer,* Robert Karler, Mishawaka High School.

The state societies of taxonomists and entomologists, which are affiliated with the academy, held their meetings on Saturday.

The annual meeting of the academy for 1940 will be held in Muncie, Ind., with Ball State Teachers College as the host institution.

WILL E. EDINGTON,
*Press Secretary*

### THE NEW ENGLAND INTERCOLLEGIATE FIELD GEOLOGISTS CONFERENCE

THE thirty-fifth annual conference of the New England Field Geologists was held in Hartford, Conn., on October 20, 21 and 22. Dr. Edward L. Troxell, of Trinity College, was in charge of local arrangements, and was assisted by geologists from Wesleyan and Yale Universities. More than 150 geologists attended the field trips and the discussion meetings at the College Lounge. Dr. Remsen Ogilby, president of Trinity College, welcomed the visitors.

The Friday afternoon field trip was led by Dr. Troxell. This trip included the relations between the lava flows and Triassic sandstones on the Trinity Campus, the pillow structure and mineral content of the flows near New Britain, and a spatter cone in a trap rock quarry near Farmington.

Dr. Chester R. Longwell, of Yale University, conducted a trip on Saturday to the eastern border of the Triassic Lowland. The geologists studied the evidence of the great eastern boundary fault, as recorded in sediments and structure of Triassic strata, in features of Triassic igneous rocks and in structure of pre-Triassic rocks. The distribution of fan-glomerate and increase of grain size away from the fault were emphasized.

The glacial geology of the Hartford-Middletown region was studied under the direction of Dr. Richard F. Flint, of Yale University. The features of the dissected clay plain, red gravel knolls, continuous knolls of "kame" type, ice-contacts, varved silt and clay, kettle complex in kame terraces and parallel-bedded dunes were discussed.

Dr. Joe Webb Peoples and Dr. Dave Keppel, of Wesleyan University, conducted an excursion on Sunday to show the lithology and structures of some of the crystalline rocks bordering the Triassic on the east between East Hartford and Portland. Parallelism between the structural lines of the crystalline Glastonbury gneiss, Bolton schist, Maromas gneiss and pegmatites with the Triassic was illustrated at numerous places. The trip was concluded at the Strickland quarry.

An excursion for glacial geologists was made to the Quinnipiac-Farmington lowland on Sunday under the leadership of Dr. Richard J. Lougee, of Colby College. A glacial delta with an attached esker was studied.

It was voted at the annual business meeting to meet at Dartmouth College, Hanover, N. H., in 1940, under the leadership of Dr. J. W. Goldthwait.

LLOYD W. FISHER,
*Permanent Secretary*

BATES COLLEGE

# SPECIAL ARTICLES

### THE MECHANISM OF THE BIOLOGICAL CITRIC ACID SYNTHESIS

THE role of pyruvic acid in the synthesis of citric acid in the animal organism has been studied earlier by Simola,[1] who found that administration of pyruvic acid to rats induces a comparatively powerful excretion of citric acid, and also by Simola and Alapeuso,[2] who demonstrated a synthesis of citric acid *in vitro* by adding pyruvic acid to finely ground tissue pulp. Continued research by Simola, Hallman and Alapeuso[3] showed that, under definite experimental conditions, addition of pyruvic acid together with fumaric or oxalacetic acid to the tissue pulp produced effects which were more pronounced than those caused by any

[1] P. E. Simola, *Skand. Arch. f. Physiol.,* 80: 375, 1938.

[2] P. E. Simola and H. Alapeuso, *Suomen Kemistilehti* (*Acta chemica fennica*) B, 11: 17, 1939.

[3] P. E. Simola, N. Hallman and H. Alapeuso, *Suomen Kemistilehti* (*Acta chemica fennica*) B, 12: 10, 1939.

of these acids alone. This combined effect is illustrated particularly clearly by Hallman's[4] work with the heart muscle.

Detailed investigations have now convincingly shown that pyruvic acid and the 4-carbon acids act in the animal organism as primary sources of the enzymic citric acid synthesis. In these investigations it was possible, under suitable conditions, to produce in the heart muscle enzymically about 0.2 per cent. of citric acid within a short period of time. The most pronounced effect was noted when pyruvic acid together with malic acid was used as substrate under aerobic conditions. Table 1 shows the results of one of such combination experiments.

TABLE 1

20 g MINCED HEART MUSCLE; 50 ml BICARBONATE BUFFER. INCUBATED AEROBICALLY; 30 MINS. AT 37°.

| Substances added | Na pyruvate 15.0 mg | Na malate 39.0 mg | Na pyruvate 15.0 mg Na malate 39.0 mg |
|---|---|---|---|
| Citric acid produced | 1.2 mg | 3.1 mg | 25.0 mg |

When larger quantities of malic and pyruvic acid were employed, under the above conditions, the amount of citric acid could be substantially increased. For instance, in an experiment with 325 mg Na pyruvate and 510 mg Na malate, 20 g heart muscle produced in 30 minutes 151 mg citric acid.

In the synthesis of citric acid, malic acid is obviously first dehydrated enzymically to oxalacetic acid, which then immediately reacts with the excess pyruvic acid to form an intermediate compound of citric acid. (That citric acid can be synthesized by purely chemical methods from pyruvic acid and oxalacetic acid, has been shown earlier by Knoop and Martius.[5])

To our surprise we found, however, that the effect of oxalacetic acid in the heart muscle was distinctly less pronounced than that of malic acid. The effect of fumaric acid was approximately equal to that of oxalacetic acid. In the other tissues examined, oxalacetic acid produced the best effects.

When boiled tissue was used, synthesis of citric acid could not be demonstrated—even in the presence of oxalacetic acid. Hence it can be concluded that under the conditions of our experiments, the citric acid formation is ascribable to enzymic processes.

It should also be observed that in the combination experiments the effect of *phospho-pyruvic* acid was definitely less than that of pyruvic acid alone.

Our experiments indicate that at least in the heart muscle—which, according to unpublished work of Hallman, effects a very powerful decomposition of citric acid—pyruvic acid is transformed to a large extent via citric acid. From the citric acid stage the decomposition follows the course discovered by Martius and Knoop,[6] to α-keto-glutaric acid and then further to succinic, fumaric, malic and oxalacetic acid. Following the union of the 4-carbon skeleton with pyruvic acid, to form the primary stage of citric acid, the cycle proceeds further. (It is probable that the vitamin $B_1$ plays an important role in the decarboxylation of this precursor of citric acid, formed from pyruvic and oxalacetic acids.) As a result of successive dehydrations and additions of water molecules, pyruvic acid is in this process ultimately burned to carbon dioxide and water, whereby each molecule of pyruvic acid requires 5 atoms of oxygen and produces 3 molecules of carbon dioxide.

NIILO HALLMAN
P. E. SIMOLA
DEPARTMENT OF MEDICAL CHEMISTRY,
UNIVERSITY OF HELSINKI, FINLAND

## LOSS OF BIOLOGICALLY FIXED NITROGEN FROM SOILS AND ITS BEARING ON CROP PRODUCTION

IT is well known that application of readily fermentable carbohydrates to soil leads to increased microbial activity, resulting in the fixation of considerable quantities of atmospheric nitrogen. With a view to finding out how far the nitrogen thus fixed is available for plant nutrition, a number of pot and field trials were carried out with different crops. Using molasses (a waste product obtained from the local sugar factory which is rich in sugars, having a total percentage of from 50 to 60 per cent. of sugars), it was found that although useful amounts of nitrogen are fixed in the soil, the major part of it was somehow not available for plant growth. Thus, in a typical field experiment using Ragi (*Eleusine coracana*) the results given in Table 1 were obtained:

TABLE 1

| Treatment | Yield of grain in gms. |
|---|---|
| Control (untreated) | 3,560 |
| Hongay cake | 5,704 |
| Sugars* (as molasses) | 4,810 |

* The sugar (as molasses) was applied in quantities such that it fixes the same amount of nitrogen in the soil as supplied in the form of Hongay cake.

From the foregoing table, it is evident that only a part of the fixed nitrogen is rendered available to the crop; probably the rest is being lost from the soil system. Mirchandani[1] has reported a similar type of nitrogen loss.

[4] N. Hallman, *Suomen Kemistilehti* (*Acta chemica fennica*) B, 12: 11, 1939.

[5] F. Knoop and C. Martius, *Zeits. f. Physiol. Chem.*, 242: I, 1936.

[6] C. Martius and F. Knoop, *Zeits. f. physiol. Chem.*, 246: I, 1937.

[1] T. J. Mirchandani, *Proc. Nat. Inst. Sci.*, Vol. III, 185, 1937.

The results of the laboratory studies relating to the fate of the nitrogen fixed in the soil are represented in Fig. 1.

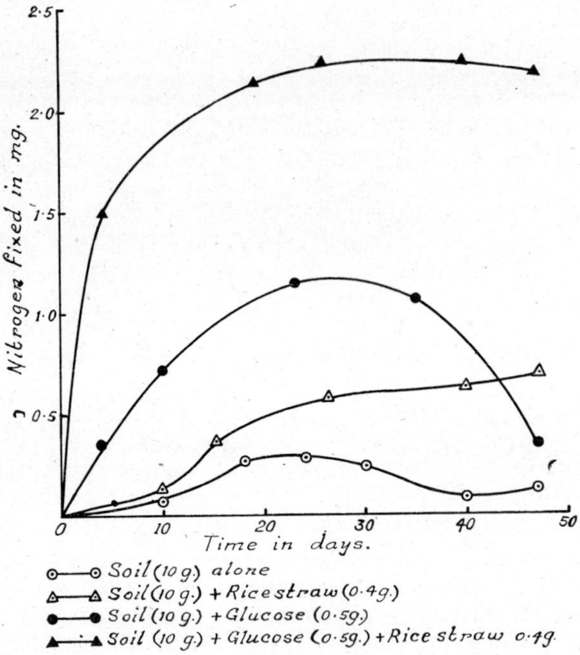


FIG. 1

These results show that the fixation of nitrogen under these conditions is almost immediately followed by its loss, so that both the processes proceed simultaneously till about three weeks, when the period of maximum fixation is reached, and during this period the rate of fixation is obviously greater. The loss continues steadily even after this period so that, within the following three to four weeks, more than 60 per cent. of the fixed nitrogen disappears from the soil system. This, combined with the fact that a period of rest extending up to four weeks is necessary between fertilizer application and sowing or transplanting, would indeed show that the crop can not fully utilize the nitrogen fixed by these materials. In presence of straw in the medium, however, the loss is prevented and the fixed nitrogen is retained in the system for a longer time.

The same type of loss is also observed when nitrogen in the form of dried Azotobacter cells is added to the soil (Table 2).

TABLE 2

| Time in days: | 5 | 7 | 12 | 17 |
|---|---|---|---|---|
| Nitrogen lost in mg from 10 g of soil | 0.74 | 0.80 | 1.08 | 1.62 |

It has also been observed that this loss of biologically fixed nitrogen can be prevented to an appreciable extent by the addition of cellulosic materials like straw.

Probably this loss of fixed nitrogen is of a general character in the soil even under natural conditions, more especially in tropical climes; and this same loss which is going on to a lesser extent to which natural fixation is also taking place, may have been magnified under the above experimental conditions. Full details of the experiments will be published elsewhere.

Experiments with a view to finding out the exact mechanism of this loss and methods of preventing it in actual field operations are in progress.

Our thanks are due to Dr. V. Subrahmanyan and Mr. B. N. Banerjee for their kind interest in the progress of the work.

T. R. BHASKARAN
S. C. PILLAI

INDIAN INSTITUTE OF SCIENCE,
BANGALORE, INDIA

## THE AVAILABILITY OF THE IRON IN DRIED PEAS AND BEANS

SINCE dried peas and beans have been considered important sources of dietary iron on the basis of their relatively high content of this element, an investigation has been made of the actual availability of the iron in blackeyed peas, green and yellow split peas, navy beans, pinto beans and butter beans. Blackeyed peas, which had been cooked preliminary to drying and grinding, were found to have all the iron available.[1] The details of the biological technic used may be found in a previous report upon the availability of iron.[1] In general the method consists of measuring the rise of hemoglobin in rats rendered anemic by an exclusive milk diet in response to the addition of the test food.

The process used in preparing the dried peas and beans for feeding consisted of drying them at 60° to 65° C., breaking in a mortar and grinding in a ball mill until the particles were fine enough to pass through a 40-mesh sieve. Analyses of the dried products for total iron by Farrar's method showed the following values expressed in mg per gm: blackeyed peas, 0.087; green split peas, 0.053; yellow split peas, 0.053; navy beans, 0.077; pinto beans, 0.077; butter beans, 0.78.

The experimental animals were weaned at 21 days of age and placed on a diet of fresh whole milk. When the level of hemoglobin had fallen below 3.0 gm per 100 cc of blood, the test foods were added to the diet at levels providing 0.2 mg of iron per day throughout the 6-week experimental period. Positive controls were fed 0.2 mg of iron, as ferric chloride. Negative controls were kept on the milk diet alone as a check on its freedom from contamination. Each animal receiving an iron-containing supplement was given daily 0.05 mg of copper, as copper sulfate, to insure that hemoglobin synthesis might be as complete as possible.

[1] Ascham L. M. Speirs and D. Maddox, *Jour. Nutrition*, 16: 425, 1938.

The animals were distributed to the various supplements as evenly as possible in respect to age, weight and litter mates.

The gains in hemoglobin during the experimental period in response to the various food supplements are shown in Table 1. As is evident from the figures for the standard deviation of the mean (S. D.), small differences may not be considered significant for these values. The hemoglobin of the animals receiving the test foods and of those receiving completely available iron, in the form of ferric chloride, rose to approximately the same levels. It appears, therefore, that the iron in the dried foods tested, namely, blackeyed peas, green and yellow split peas, navy beans, pinto beans and butter beans, is completely available to the nutritionally anemic rat for the regeneration of hemoglobin.

TABLE 1

THE REGENERATION OF HEMOGLOBIN IN ANEMIC RATS RECEIVING EITHER FERRIC CHLORIDE OR FOOD SUPPLEMENTS CONTAINING 0.2 MG OF IRON PER DAY DURING AN EXPERIMENTAL PERIOD OF 6 WEEKS

| Supplement | Number of rats | Gain in hemoglobin | ± S. D.* |
|---|---|---|---|
| | | gm/100 cc | |
| $FeCl_3$ | 25 | 9.3 | 0.26 |
| Blackeyed peas | 8 | 8.9 | 0.33 |
| Navy beans | 8 | 8.8 | 0.46 |
| Pinto beans | 9 | 8.9 | 0.42 |
| Butter beans | 9 | 9.3 | 0.31 |
| Green split peas | 7 | 10.1 | 0.54 |
| Yellow split peas | 6 | 10.3 | 0.20 |

* Standard deviation of the mean.

LEAH ASCHAM
MARY SPEIRS
DOROTHY MADDOX

GEORGIA EXPERIMENT STATION,
EXPERIMENT, GA.

# SCIENTIFIC APPARATUS AND LABORATORY METHODS

## CULTURE TECHNIC FOR QUANTITATIVE GROWTH STUDIES WITH MYXOPHYCEAE

THE procedure whereby aliquots are taken for cell counts from liquid or other large volume culture media is inaccurate because of unequal distribution. And the hanging-drop method of slide culture is difficult to manage for long periods when frequent changes of solution must be had. Therefore when studies of cell increase in number are to be made of small organisms somewhat larger than bacteria, other methods must be devised. Two such methods are here reported.

Chroococcus was grown in tiny paraffin boxes fixed to glass slides. The boxes were made from the sprocket holes of 16 mm uncoated movie film kindly donated by the Eastman Kodak Company of Rochester, New York. Short strips of the film were washed overnight in distilled water, dried, roughened by fine sandpaper and coated with hard (62°) paraffin. Pieces containing a single rectangular hole were affixed to cover-slips by warming. Into the little receptacle so produced the blue-green algae cells were transferred by micropipette from a Bristol solution culture. Accurate counts were made of the cells so introduced at the beginning and after any desired period up to 72 hours. Evaporation was controlled by keeping the preparation in large petri dishes containing wet filter paper and by adding distilled water when necessary.

The second method was found useful for microorganisms which have a gelatinous sheath, such as Anabaena and diatoms. Thoroughly clean cover-slips were broken into tiny pieces, washed and placed in small petri dishes in such manner that each little piece of glass remained free from the others. The preparation was sterilized while wet so that the glass fragments became attached and but one surface was available for algae growth. Over this preparation was then poured about 10 cc of a Bristol solution culture of the organism and the whole was allowed to stand for from 24 to 48 hours. By that time algae were attached and growing on the fragments. Single pieces were then transferred to hollow ground culture slides, one to each, and the number of cells counted. Anabaena was kept healthy and increasing in cell number under such conditions for as long as 120 hours with many changes of solution, while the accompanying growth was quantitatively determinable at will.

Although most of the blue-green algae grow nicely on agar and such colonies serve adequately as stock material, it is next to impossible to obtain a quantitative sample therefrom. Consequently, the procedure of first transferring from agar to Bristol solution was adopted. Cell increase in this medium takes place readily, and clumps can be so broken by mild shaking that samples for quantitative study can be obtained as described above.

LEE WALP

THE LANKENAU HOSPITAL RESEARCH
INSTITUTE AND MARIETTA COLLEGE

## AN INEXPENSIVE SMALL AIR COMPRESSOR

HOAGLAND[1] and others have stressed the desirability of adequate aeration of solutions if reliable experimental data are to be obtained from plants grown in culture solutions. Those working in greenhouses far removed from a source of compressed air are forced to choose between several rather unsatisfactory procedures. Small rotary pumps may not give sufficient pressure to assure air for all cultures. Conventional

[1] D. R. Hoagland, *Bot. Rev.*, 3: 307–334, 1937.

air compressors of smaller sizes pump so little air that they are likely to be inadequate for future requirements. Compressors of sufficient capacity to meet probable future needs are expensive. With the thought that it will later be replaced by a large compressor or by one such as that described in this journal,[2] an aerating system made as follows has been found very satisfactory. Its chief appeal is its very low cost. Most of the necessary equipment may be found in the laboratory and in the junk yard.

A Kellogg pump which was regular equipment on an old model Cadillac car (SJ series) was mounted on a heavy wooden frame. A twelve-inch V belt pulley was substituted for the gear on the pump. This together with the standard size three-inch pulley on a ¼ H.P. electric motor gave the pump a speed of about 400 r.p.m. A three-gallon spray tank was mounted on the same frame immediately above the motor. In order to reduce friction and avoid breakage of a metal tube, a heavy cloth-reinforced rubber hose was used to carry the air from the pump to the tank. The outlet from the tank connected with suitable reducers to a two-inch pipe twelve inches long filled with cotton—as a precaution against oil getting into the solutions.

This compressor,[3] which was assembled without expenditure for technically skilled labor and at no cash outlay except for the belt and the twelve-inch pulley, has supplied for three months continuous aeration for 120 containers (ranging in size from three quarts to three gallons) with pin-punctured rubber tube aerators. When fewer solutions are aerated the air pressure is regulated by the simple expedient of by-passing air through a rubber tube partially closed with a screw clamp.

Because the pressure in the entire system is dependent on all the lines remaining intact, it has been found desirable to use five-sixteenths-inch glass T tubes with grooved ends for one-quarter-inch rubber tubing used in the air lines.

G. J. RALEIGH

CORNELL UNIVERSITY

## A CONVENIENT METHOD FOR OBTAINING BLOOD SERUM

SERUM is used for a number of chemical analyses and is usually obtained by permitting a tube of blood to clot. The serum is obtained after freeing the clot from the walls of the tube by a thin knife or fine glass rod, which is insinuated between the clot and the walls of the tube and then passed around the clot. The tube is then centrifuged or allowed to stand until the clot shrinks sufficiently to liberate enough serum.

In carrying out these manipulations, the clot is frequently injured and the serum is often contaminated with cells, either intact or hemolyzed. The following method avoids all trauma to the clot.

A test-tube or centrifuge tube of suitable size is waxed on its inner surface by filling it with molten wax and pouring out the excess. The tube is allowed to cool while rotating it so as to spread the wax uniformly on its walls. After the wax has solidified, a small pledget of dry cotton is placed at the bottom of the tube by means of a glass rod. The tip of the tube is then placed in the Bunsen flame momentarily. The wax melts and secures the cotton to the bottom of the tube.

The tube is filled in the usual way. The cotton serves to initiate clotting and to fix the clot to the bottom of the tube. Then, as the clot shrinks, it will be well away from the surface of the blood, since it does not stick to the waxed walls. The serum can be pipetted away from the clot or poured into a suitable vessel, the clot remaining in the tube.

E. M. ABRAHAMSON

THE JEWISH HOSPITAL,
BROOKLYN, N. Y.

[2] H. W. Beams, A. T. Casteel, R. L. King, SCIENCE, 86: 428, 1937.

[3] The pump was furnished by F. W. Barrett, and the assembly was made by C. J. VanEtten.

## BOOKS RECEIVED

BENNETT, H. *Standard Chemical and Technical Dictionary.* Pp. xlii + 638. Chemical Publishing Co. $10.00.

Carnegie Corporation of New York. *Report of the President and of the Treasurer, 1939.* Pp. 167. The Corporation.

CLAPP, ELSIE R. *Community Schools in Action.* Pp. xviii + 429. Illustrated. Viking Press. $3.75.

GERSHENFELD, LOUIS. *Biological Products.* Pp. xliv + 236. Illustrated. Romaine Pierson Publishers, New York. $4.00.

HOU, H. C., and others. *Chinese Medical Association, Report Series No. 12: Nutritional Studies in Shanghai.* Pp. 92. The Association, Shanghai. $1.00.

LAMB, FRANK H. *Book of the Broadleaf Trees.* Pp. 367. Illustrated. Norton. $3.75.

MATLIN, D. R. *Growing Plants without Soil.* Pp. 137. Illustrated. Chemical Publishing Co. $2.00.

MILLIKAN, R. A. *Cosmic Rays.* Pp. 134. 42 figures. Macmillan. $2.50.

SCHNEITER, CARL. *Die Skelette aus den Alamannengräbern des Zürichsee-, Limmat- und Glattales (inklusive Greifensee- und Pfäffikerseegebietes).* Pp. 148. 8 plates. Anthropologischen Institut der Universitat, Zurich.

SHEPPARD, W. F. *British Association for the Advancement of Science Mathematical Tables, Volume VII: The Probability Integral.* Pp. 34. Cambridge University Press, Macmillan. $2.50.

*Svenska Linné-Sällskapets Årsskrift. Årg. XXII, 1939.* Pp. 148. Illustrated. Almqvist and Wiksells, Uppsala.

TURNER, WAYNE I. and VICTOR M. HENRY. *Growing Plants in Nutrient Solutions; or Scientifically Controlled Growth.* Pp. xiii + 154. 29 figures. 3 plates. Wiley. $3.00.

WRIGHT, W. D. *The Perception of Light: An Analysis of Visual Phenomena in Relation to Technical Problems of Vision and Illumination.* Pp. 100. 49 figures. Chemical Publishing Co. $2.50.

# SCIENCE

VOL. 90 — FRIDAY, DECEMBER 29, 1939 — No. 2348

*The American Association for the Advancement of Science:*
*The Public Relations of Science:* DR. WESLEY C. MITCHELL ... 599
*Obituary:*
*Frederick Adams Woods:* DR. CHARLES B. DAVENPORT. *Fred William Tinney:* CORRESPONDENT. *Henry Clinton Fall:* PROFESSOR T. D. A. COCKERELL. *Recent Deaths and Memorials* ... 607
*Scientific Events:*
*The Status of the Engineering Profession; The Francis Amory Septennial Prize of the American Academy of Arts and Sciences; A Zoological Expedition of the Field Museum; Soil Conservation; The Minneapolis Meeting of the Geological Society of America and Associated Societies; Officers of the American Chemical Society* ... 609
*Scientific Notes and News* ... 612
*Discussion:*
*Radioactivity in Biological Experiments:* PROFESSOR S. GOUDSMIT. *Pseudomethemoglobin and Its Reaction with Carbon Monoxide after Reduction:* DR. GEORG BARKAN and OTTO SCHALES. *An Experiment on Retinal After-image and Judgment of Size:* PROFESSOR RICHARD M. SUTTON. *The Occurrence of the Two Rare Genera, Protohydra and Protodrilus, on the East Coast of North America:* DR. T. K. RUEBUSH ... 615
*Scientific Books:*
*The Teachers of Physics:* DR. NIEL F. BEARDSLEY 618
*Special Articles:*
*A Defect in the Metabolism of Aromatic Amino Acids in Premature Infants: The Role of Vitamin C:* PROFESSOR S. Z. LEVINE, ELEANOR MARPLES and H. H. GORDON. *Reaction of Variola Vaccine Virus to Roentgen Rays:* PROFESSOR JOHN W. GOWEN and PROFESSOR ALFRED M. LUCAS. *Electrophoretic Study of Pituitary Lactogenic Hormone:* DR. CHOH HAO LI, DR. WILLIAM R. LYONS and DR. HERBERT M. EVANS ... 620
*Scientific Apparatus and Laboratory Methods:*
*The Determination of Carotene:* GEORGE KERNOHAN. *Protection of Herbarium Specimens:* C. S. SEMMENS. *Marking Rocks, Minerals and Fossils:* PROFESSOR GEORGE D. HUBBARD ... 623
*Science News* ... 6

SCIENCE: A Weekly Journal devoted to the Advancement of Science, edited by J. MCKEEN CATTELL and published every Friday by

THE SCIENCE PRESS
New York City: Grand Central Terminal
Lancaster, Pa. — Garrison, N. Y.

Annual Subscription, $6.00 — Single Copies, 15 Cts.

SCIENCE is the official organ of the American Association for the Advancement of Science. Information regarding membership in the Association may be secured from the office of the permanent secretary in the Smithsonian Institution Building, Washington, D. C.

# THE PUBLIC RELATIONS OF SCIENCE[1]

By Dr. WESLEY C. MITCHELL
PROFESSOR OF ECONOMICS, COLUMBIA UNIVERSITY

UNTIL recently the attitude of the public toward science seemed to be growing more appreciative. There have always been folk who objected strenuously to the supposed implications of certain scientific hypotheses, but on the whole science was generally esteemed the most progressive factor in culture, man's best hope for bettering his lot upon earth. Of late this tide of approval has ebbed. There is a widespread disposition to hold science responsible for the ills men are bringing upon themselves—for technological unemployment, for the rise of autocracies, for the suppression of freedom, for the heightened horrors of war. For their part, scientific men are appalled at the hideous uses to which their discoveries are put. They feel an urge to combat the misuses of science, to protect the social values they cherish, but what they can do is not clear. The quandary is one that all who cherish science should face, however unwelcome and difficult the task. I offer no apology for asking your attention to a discourse of uncertain issue on an unpleasant theme thrust upon us by developments we deplore.

[1] Address of the retiring president of the American Association for the Advancement of Science, Columbus, Ohio, December 27, 1939.

## I

Let me start by recalling certain changes in the relations of science to society that may help us see our present problems in historical perspective.

The beginnings of scientific knowledge have been traced to man's dealings with the implements of his daily life—the sticks and stones, the skins, fibers and clay he shaped to his uses, and in the shaping learned to know. Human beings are born speculators; even the simplest cultures have their explanations of matters that puzzle us to-day—diseases, weather changes, animal behavior, the creation of the world, what happens after death. Without this speculative bent human intelligence could not have evolved far; but neither could it win much useful knowledge without subjecting speculative explanations to practical tests. As the nursery of scientific thinking, the humdrum work of making and using household equipment had this great advantage: it required frequent repetitions under roughly similar conditions, when there was no great emotional stress, and when attention was centered upon immediate material results. In such activities it was least difficult to find out what operations were followed by the desired consequences, and what operations were superfluous.

Whether or not we accept this speculation about the humble beginnings of science, we know that at a later stage of cultural advance thinking about natural phenomena, like thinking about religious observances, tended to break away from direct associations with daily work. The slowly improving techniques of tracing the motions of heavenly bodies, keeping track of the seasons, measuring lands, developing mathematical propositions and erecting large structures called for unusual intelligence and training. Possessors of special knowledge wished to guard their trade secrets, to make mysteries of them, to initiate merely a few of their own choosing, and so increase their prestige. Mathematics is the subject least dependent upon the use of material objects, and it led the development of systematic thought, closely followed by its cousin, logic. Dealing with a rational universe of concepts, its affiliations seemed to be with religion and philosophy rather than with industry. So far as knowledge dissociated itself from technology, it escaped from continual subjection to matter-of-fact tests. That left it free to pursue attractive lines of speculation, but took away its most vigilant corrective and its sharpest spur to self-criticism. Even mathematical inquiry lost its momentum when it soared aloft in mystical flights.

Such efforts to understand the world as the Middle Ages made were concerned chiefly with problems of a divine dispensation. Observation was not pertinent, and factual tests of conclusions were not possible. The highest authority upon all questions was Holy Writ, which nobody might question and which the church interpreted. This orientation made acceptable the later Greek preoccupation with formal logic and disdain of matter. Aristotle, that great investigator, was transmuted into an obstacle to further investigation of mundane phenomena. Intellectual acumen achieved triumphs in its chosen fields, but understanding of natural forces was not prominent among them.

The re-birth of science in the sixteenth and seventeenth centuries was brought about by turning from the study of concepts back to the study of nature. The new orientation was characterized by close observation, by the invention of devices to make observation more penetrating and accurate, by purposeful experimentation to simplify the processes observed, by close attention to quantity as well as to quality, by the practical application of mathematics to express the relations observed, by reformulation of concepts to fit the findings, by critical checking of one investigator's work by others, by the cumulation of tested conclusions in old fields of research and by the extension of this mode of inquiry to new fields. Inventing instruments for observing, setting up experiments, measuring and testing brought science again into intimate touch with the practical arts. Investigators took a keen interest in current affairs, sought to profit by the skill of craftsmen and to put what they learned to practical uses. Discoveries were applied not only to the production of goods, but also to navigation, fortification, ballistics and administration. By the close of the seventeenth century the dramatic achievements of "natural philosophy" were leading many to expect an almost limitless advance, and the promotion of science was recognized as a proper object of public policy. Kings lent their patronage to scientific societies. Philanthropists followed the royal precedents by offering prizes for improvements in the arts and later by endowing research.

Of course the public relations of science were not uniformly harmonious in this age of genius. But the celebrated clashes between scientific discoveries and beliefs held by churchmen did not affect many lines of inquiry and did not gravely retard the rising tide of investigation. Not less characteristic of the age than Galileo's troubles were Newton's services to churchly teachings and to the state. Scientific men have lamented that he devoted his later years to arguing the validity of biblical prophecies; they have paid less attention to his work as Master of the Mint. It was adjustments in the relative weight of the guinea and the shilling suggested by Newton that gave England a *de facto* gold standard in the eighteenth century, though Newton did not foresee this result.

An even more striking example of close relations between research and service to mankind is the life of Benjamin Franklin. The foremost American discoverer of his time, he was foremost also in applying and disseminating science to make life more comfortable, more secure, more interesting, more humane. These activities were incidents in the life of a busy printer, editor, politician, postmaster, legislator, colonial agent and diplomat. But while we wonder at the extraordinary versatility of a man who could become both a scientific discoverer and a great statesman under any conditions, we must remember that in Franklin's day science was still in its "natural philosophy" stage.

With the cumulation of results, science became a more exacting mistress, requiring of her votaries more exclusive attention. But science did not draw away from the material tasks of daily life as it did in Greece. On the contrary, these relations were becoming more intimate, while scientists were learning to speak symbolic dialects less and less intelligible to the public or even to one another. Let me illustrate the seeming paradox by the relations between science and industry.

To most of us the modern age is characterized by technological progress as markedly as by scientific discovery. We think of the two achievements as interdependent. This interdependence was less obvious to Franklin's contemporaries than to us. Theirs was a century of great inventions, but inventions made mostly by men not trained in science. The famous "agricultural improvers" worked by empirical methods. The great textile inventions came from handicraftsmen, one of them a barber. Metcalf, Telford and Macadam, the road builders, were "practical men"; so also was Brindley, the canal builder. Newcommen, "father of the steam-engine," was an ironmonger and blacksmith; his co-worker, Cawley, was a plumber and glazier. The Darbys, who found out how to smelt iron with coke, began as small ironmasters. A few inventors, it is true, tried methodically to discover scientific laws—Smeaton and Watt are eminent examples. Also, some scientists developed inventions out of their discoveries, as Franklin did with the lightning rod, and some set deliberately about the solving of industrial problems—Leblanc developed his process of making soda to win a prize offered by the Paris Academy of Sciences. But these instances were harbingers of a coming day rather than representative products of the eighteenth century.

This new day brought with it a division of labor in the conduct of industry matching the specialization evolving in science. The captains of industry who carried the Industrial Revolution through its youthful phases were often technical experts, business executives and capitalists united in one person. Men of this versatile type are still to be found even in "big business"; but they are becoming as rare as once they were common. For, as technology was elaborated, experts with special training were required to supervise its operations. Engineering became a learned profession—or rather a family of learned professions that multiplied by fission. It won a place in institutions of higher learning beside theology, law and medicine. Inventions continued to come from geniuses with little training, but more and more of them were made to order by experts. Business management meanwhile became so intricate, what with its problems of financing, selling, accounting, selecting personnel, planning investments, and the like, that a good-sized corporation required a staff of men with different skills to do part of the work that an old-fashioned captain of industry had performed for his small establishment. With a considerable lag behind engineering, business administration also raised claims to professional standing and developed schools of its own. As for capital, the requirements of business utilizing modern technology speedily outran the resources of the single enterpriser or partnership. By a series of inventions not less important than those of mechanics, methods were developed for bringing together the savings of countless individuals, rich and poor, by providing types of securities well enough adapted to their several needs to attract funds.

With this double division of labor, in science and industry, the scientist could stick closely to research and feel confident that whatever applications of his discoveries were feasible would be taken in hand by men who knew more about industry than he. The engineer could devote himself as sedulously to technological matters, putting research problems up to laboratory workers and leaving business worries to executives. The latter could get technical experts of many sorts from the schools, and could expect cumulative improvements in technology from the joint labors of scientists and engineers. Investors frequently knew little about the enterprises for which they provided capital; they inclined to rely upon the advice of professional financiers and to protect themselves by spreading risks.

The economic results produced by this unplanned organization of mutually stimulating activities astonished mankind. Industry after industry reorganized its processes time and again to take advantage of the latest engineering applications of scientific discoveries, and new industries kept cropping up. The efficiency of human labor increased greatly, per capita income rose, and hours of labor declined. Higher standards of living and applications of science to the prevention and cure of disease reduced death rates and prolonged the average duration of life. Population grew rapidly in the nations that led the scientific procession, and spread where it would over the earth, dominating, exploiting, sometimes exterminating the non-scientific peoples. Life became ampler if not easier for the beneficiaries of science.

What industry owed science is repaid in many ways. It provided in bewildering variety laboratory equipment more accurate and powerful than that made by hand. It stood ready to construct any new contrivance an investigator designed, and often improved upon the original plans. Fortunes accumulated in business were the source of many scientific endowments. Business corporations granted research funds to universities, and set up research staffs of their own, which were sometimes permitted to work upon fundamental problems.

Governments recognized the social importance of science by making place for an expanding array of scientific courses in public schools and universities, and by undertaking wide-ranging programs of research. In this country, the Federal Government became the largest employer of scientific men. At the time of the Civil War it chartered the Academy of Sciences, and in the World War the National Research Council to advise it upon scientific problems; in 1934 it set up the organization that has developed into the National Resources Planning Board with affiliations covering the full gamut of the sciences.

Finally, the public at large had a share in these great changes. It was the ultimate beneficiary of reductions in costs of production, of increasing per capita output, of new types of consumers' goods, of shorter working hours, of better protection against disease, of free education. And this share was not wholly passive. Wage-earners adapted themselves with less friction than might have been expected to the working conditions imposed by the new technology. If many disliked the impersonal regimentation of the factory and the monotony of machine tending, others delighted in their control over stupendous forces, in the precision of the work they turned out, in the efficiency of the organizations of which they were parts. It is a grave mistake to overlook the enthusiasms evoked by machines, big and little. As recent experience in Russia reminds us, a population that has not become mechanically minded in large measure can not effectively use modern technology. And at home the masses welcomed factory-made goods. In successive generations they thanked engineering and science for illuminating gas, sanitary plumbing, kerosene, telephones, electric wiring, inoculation against epidemic diseases, automobiles, motion pictures and radios. Almost every one participated in scientific discoveries to the modest degree necessary for using these contrivances with some skill. Besides material products, many folk enjoyed what Tennyson called "the fairy tale of science"; their thoughts were pleasurably enlarged by the telescope and microscope. Pasteur, Edison, Mendel, Mme. Curie, Einstein became romantic personalities to tens of thousands, rivaling in popular appeal politicians, business leaders, actors and athletes. Without this eager welcome from society at large, government, business and schools could not have fostered research as they did, and science could not have progressed so rapidly.

It can not be said that these eminently cordial relations between science and the public were consciously engendered by scientific men. Now and then when some scientific hypothesis or procedure was attacked, individual scientists rushed to the defense and sometimes organized protests by scientific bodies. The controversies over what the public called "Darwinism" and "vivisection" are examples. Also scientists answered calls for their services freely and took advantage of opportunities to make their livings on lecture platforms, in schools, governmental bureaus and business enterprises. On appropriate occasions they dilated eloquently upon the service of science to civilization, and investigators with skilful pens and need of royalties wrote popular books. But most of the men who made modern science what it is devoted themselves single-mindedly to research. Their deeds, not their words, won the esteem and raised the hopes of mankind.

In short, this policy of *laissez-faire* worked wonders. Science helped industry, and industry helped science. Even the backward art of agriculture, which faces so many difficulties and uncertainties, was benefiting by research. The dreaded "law of diminishing returns" seemed to be overbalanced by improvements in practice based upon the work of soil chemists, botanists and geneticists. The frightful prospect of overpopulation that Malthus had taught the thoughtful to fear seemed to be dissipated by scientific agriculture and scientific techniques of contra-conception. Best of all, science seemed to have found the secret of illimitable progress. What it had done was merely an earnest of the greater things it would soon do. One discovery led to another so continuously that men began to take for granted a cumulative rise in the standard of living. They moved the Garden of Eden from its traditional place at the beginning of human history into the calculable future, dreaming of a world from which poverty would be banished. If some souls felt oppressed by the materialism of the age, youthful sages arose from the non-scientific peoples to argue, in the words of Hu Shih, that there is more of the spiritual in the scientific effort to control natural forces than in passive resignation to poverty and disease.

## II

I doubt that any scientist ever accepted without qualification this idyllic version of the benefits science confers upon mankind. Certainly there were numerous protests from scientific quarters against misuses of the new technology. Geologists and economists warned against the rapid depletion of mineral deposits. Chemists feared for the nitrogen content of the soil. Geographers and meteorologists protested that wholesale cutting of forests and the plowing of grass lands produced deserts. Biologists lamented the extinction of animal species and anthropologists the callous stamping out of simpler cultures. Social scientists found much amiss within the countries that were most progressive. Urban and rural slums persisted as centers of disease and crime. The need of securing capital to utilize the new technology put control over it into the hands of the propertied classes. Labor was often grievously exploited. Huge fixed investments that could be used for only one purpose made competition destructive. The obvious escape from these hazards was to form monopolistic combinations. That was pleasant for the monopolists, but not for other business men or for consumers. Besides the obvious dangers of exploitation, many feared that the great combinations might purposely slow down technological advance because it threatened rapid obsolescence of their equipment. Business did not manage even its own interests properly, for every few years it generated a crisis and depression in which it suffered along with the whole community. And the international relations of the scientifically advanced peoples showed at his worst "the old savage in the new civilization." Demonstrations of the economic advantages of free trade no more stopped the imposition of protective tariffs than demonstrations of the horrors of war kept peace. Militant nationalism seemed to be spreading and growing more passionate. An appreciable fraction of scientific energy was devoted to contriving weapons of destruction. Thus against the glowing picture of science as a benefactor of mankind could be set a dark picture of science putting more power into the hands of certain individuals, classes, nations, generations, giving them a differential advantage over others which they exploited according to their several natures.

Though some of the Jeremiads I have been recalling belong to an earlier time, they did not produce a profound effect upon the public relations of science until recently. The ills complained of could be regarded as "growing pains." They were thought of as social "problems," which should be dealt with by arousing public opinion in a campaign of education that would lead to remedial legislation. Problems that could not be solved by this time-honored method would yield presumably to the slower processes of general enlightenment.

This optimistic attitude was particularly characteristic of democratic nations. It assumed tacitly that experts could devise whatever "reforms" were needed, and that the majority of voters were intelligent enough to understand and well disposed enough to support desirable changes. Science had a stellar role in this program for remedying the ills incidental to progress. It did not claim knowledge of good and evil; but it enabled men to make their value judgments more intelligent by tracing the consequences of actions. Many people were devoting their energies to the study of social problems; they spoke optimistically of their subjects as social "sciences." It seemed not too much to hope that science might presently begin to guide social practice in somewhat the same fashion as it guided practice in industry and medicine.

A man might be skeptical of the nascent social sciences; but he could scarcely deny that the leading scientific nations managed to readjust their economic, political and social institutions when the new technology produced results they deemed bad. True, the readjustments were usually made by attacking one evil at a time, without due consideration of indirect consequences, which were often unfortunate in good part, and sometimes canceled the gains. Also the processes of reform lagged so far behind the changes produced by applications of scientific discoveries that new troubles began and new social adjustments were needed before the preceding reforms had been perfected. Despite all this, the scientific nations believed themselves to be evolving a social order adapted to the times—one that enabled them to grasp ever more fully the ever larger benefits scientific progress was bestowing upon mankind. I question whether history can show another period in which human hopes soared so high as in the closing decades of the century between Waterloo and the first World War.

## III

That the public relations of science have recently become disturbing both to the public and to scientists is due, not to any change in the character of science or the behavior of scientists. but to changes in social conditions. While most people approved on the whole the applications of science before 1914, they have come to dislike many of the effects produced by later applications. To be specific: when scientific improvements in one industry after another threw men out of work in earlier decades, the victims might suffer in silence or protest riotously and perhaps smash machines. But the public at large was not deeply concerned over their sufferings; it repressed disorder, expected the displaced men to find new jobs for themselves, and blessed science for reducing costs of production. Now that a larger part of the public suffers from loss of work or obsolescence of investments, science is blamed for technological unemployment. When the modern arts of communication were used to facilitate the political processes of democratic nations, they were extolled on all sides. Now that these arts, further improved, are controlled in some countries by autocratic governments and used to suppress opposition, many good people treat science as the culprit. When the scientific nations used their superior arms against backward peoples, only a few sensitive souls were wrathful over the unfairness or iniquity of the procedure. Most people felt that science was good when it gave them a decisive advantage over those they wished to "civilize." Now that these same nations are threatened by still more terrible weapons in the hands of their peers, their moral horror is sincere, and they wish scientific warfare back to the pit from which it was digged.

This shift in attitude toward science as one happens to benefit or suffer from its applications is doubtless a mark of human frailty, but it is one at which scientists should not cavil without recalling a similar frailty of their own. Now that we are on the defensive, we discover that science is neither good nor bad in itself, but is merely an instrument that can be put to good or bad uses, and that the blame for bad uses should be visited upon those responsible for them. But when science was being lauded for good works, who among us argued that the credit belonged, not to science, but to those who used it for the benefit of mankind?

We made this discovery when difficulties forced us to think more carefully about the place of science in society. Well as the old policy of *laissez-faire* in public relations worked for a time, it had encouraged in us an indolent complacency foreign to the critical spirit of inquiry. We may not enjoy the shocks that have aroused us any more than an investigator rejoices over facts that disprove an elegant hypothesis; but we must face the situation and see what we can do to mend it. Every one concerned with the future of science or of mankind bears a share in the responsibility for trying to understand the present situation, and to decide what action, if any, is called for. It is not likely that a satisfactory solution can be produced in short order, for the problem is one of numerous variables in shifting combinations. But I venture to suggest an obvious proposition that seems to me of controlling importance, and to point out certain corollaries that should guide both our attempts to understand the public relations of science and our future policy concerning them.

## IV

The fundamental proposition is that scientific research is a social process as much as business, political or religious activities are, and as such is interwoven with all other social processes, influencing them and being influenced by them.

My historical sketch of the public relations of science supports this view. But let me borrow two illustrations from thoughtful physicists. David L. Watson has shown that social institutions impose their pattern upon research, putting a premium upon conventional inquiries and obstructing originality. Like other social activities requiring close cooperation, research gets organized, organizations become bureaucratic, bureaucrats may have routine efficiencies, but originality of thought and cordial welcome to originality in others are not conspicuous among them. Watson compiles a formidable list of instances in which scientific organizations have been slow to recognize fundamental discoveries, and he makes his point more uncomfortable by naming certain rather odd contemporaries who may be doing work more important than the men to whom we award medals.[2]

In a way that should come close home to every investigator, P. W. Bridgman has pictured the intellectual struggles a scientist must undergo if he strives seriously to live "an intelligently well-ordered life." Accustomed to subject his concepts in physics to operational tests, Bridgman tried to treat with similar rigor the concepts that count most in social intercourse. The results were disconcerting.

> Not one of our social institutions (he found) rests on the secure foundation that we so easily assume when we refute the skeptic or instruct our young. Never has any institution been justified in terms that anyone capable of close thinking could accept without stultification. Yet if ever the tragic need for close thinking and intelligent convictions on social questions was obvious it is at the present.

This loose thinking that characterizes social intercourse introduces confusion into the lives of all, though the confusion may be recognized only by those who try to live intelligently. For every one derives the words in which he thinks from society. They bring into mental processes all sorts of implications inherited from the past that will not bear analysis, and from which one can free oneself only by laborious analysis of the sort that has made the exact language of physics differ from the ambiguous language of everyday life.[3]

Scientific research, then, is one among many social activities carried on by the peoples of our culture. Like all such processes, it is carried on by men who learn in childhood languages ill suited to close thinking; by men who wish to eat, to make love, to win approval as well as to know; by men who are reared in an environment of emotional likes and dislikes; by men who become so absorbed in their technical tasks that they have little energy to criticize the non-scientific parts of their own make-up. And these scientific men form a tiny fraction of their communities. So far as they succeed in emancipating themselves from the misconceptions and prejudices pre-

[2] David L. Watson, "Scientists are Human," London, 1938.

[3] P. W. Bridgman, "The Intelligent Individual and Society," New York, 1938.

vailing in their social groups, they become by virtue of their partial emancipation queer creatures whose judgment most people mistrust outside of their specialties. Both the temperament that inclined them to research and the habits they form in research tend to make them awkward, ineffective, reluctant in appealing to the emotions that are so potent in influencing men. It is difficult to see how a few scattered individuals, each accusomed to think for himself and to be critical even of his fellow inquirers, can guide public opinion except by slow educational processes. In the long run their thinking may rule the world, just because it serves the purposes of mankind better than the traditional thinking it gradually replaces. But in the short run, others take of scientific discoveries only the parts that have an immediate application, and put these parts to such uses as they see fit—uses that serve whatever aims these others pursue. The prompt and potent influence of science upon society comes from these uses, good and bad, which scientists control only in small part.

Even in democratic countries, then, scientific men find it hard to bridge the gulf between their attitudes and those of the general public. In autocratic states the governments might give scientists fuller opportunities to direct public policies than they enjoy in democracies. But the autocratic states known to us are not built on that model. They are avid for science, to be sure, but only for science that is an uncritical servitor of ends the rulers determine. As between the difficult public relations confronting them in democracies and the shackling of free inquiry confronting them in autocracies, scientists can not hesitate. Theirs is a world of intellectual freedom, not perfect, alas, but the freest world the mind of man has yet created, and to let any authority under any pretense prescribe what conclusions they shall accept as scientific is to stultify the spirit of science.

## V

What, then, can scientists do to improve their public relations in communities where they are relatively free?

As I see the situation, they have two sets of opportunities and responsibilities: first, their opportunities and responsibilities as citizens; second, their opportunities and responsibilities as investigators.

It must be admitted that to many scientific men the performance of civic duties is an unwelcome interruption to their research work. Some brilliant investigators are temperamentally unfitted to share in the tumultuous processes by which a democracy reaches its decisions. Among the great discoverers of the past there have been cynics who despised the "common herd," recluses who could scarcely endure social contacts, geniuses so erratic that their judgments upon practical affairs seemed crazy, rationalizers who urged the insignificance of one citizen among millions as an excuse for shirking responsibilities. Presumably representatives of these types exist among our scientific contemporaries; but I know no ground for supposing that they form a larger proportion of the persons listed in Dr. Cattell's "American Men of Science" than of those listed in "Who's Who in America." A goodly majority of scientific men have normally balanced personalities and are competent citizens. They can be counted upon to take their civic responsibilities as conscientiously on the average as any other group, and to act with as much commonsense.

What scientific men can do as citizens is like what other intelligent men can do. If democracy is to work well, many people must form considered judgments upon a wide variety of problems. In forming a considered judgment on a given issue, what experts have to say should be taken into account. Who these experts are depends upon the character of the issue; more often than not contributions are needed from several kinds of specialists. All the many species of the genus scientist belong at one time or another in the list of desirable technical advisers; so also do lawyers, business organizers, labor leaders, social workers, educators, civil servants, politicians, and so on. When matters within the competence of some group of scientists are involved, they should contribute what they know, whether formally invited to do so or not. To make their advice effective they should welcome help from people more skilled than themselves in the arts of popular presentation. On matters concerning which a scientist has no special knowledge, he should listen to others and form the best judgment he can from what they advise. To an individual this task of sifting and weighing different opinions is time-consuming and difficult. On complicated issues organization is needed to bring into focus all the intelligence available in the community. Hence, one of the civic duties incumbent upon all scientific men in common with other citizens is to support vigorously but critically the nascent movement toward organizing all the intelligence we possess for constructive study of social problems before they become pressing emergencies that have to be dealt with in a hurry that allows no time for careful thinking.

The outside limits of what scientists can accomplish as citizens are set by their ignorance. Not merely does no individual have more than a tiny fraction of the knowledge that is needed; all the scientists of the country put together do not know enough to solve many of the problems that a democracy faces. In addition to the responsibilities they share with all other citizens, scientific men have the special duty of trying to increase the kind of knowledge required to deal intelligently with public problems. Their opportunities and responsibilities as citizens merge into their opportunities and responsibilities as investigators.

From the social view-point, the most urgent item in the unfinished business of science is to increase knowledge of human behavior. If we had keener insight into individual psychology, we might not be able to alter fundamental drives, but we might be able to direct them into beneficent channels. Preaching righteousness doubtless prevents men from being as bestial as they might otherwise become. Appeals to reason prevent them from making as many errors as they otherwise might. But the moralist and the rationalist admit that the results of their efforts are grievously disappointing. Scientific men with any gift of self-analysis realize that they have their own shares of selfishness and animosities. To subdue traits in oneself is hard enough to give an inkling of the difficulty of controlling them in society at large. Perhaps, and perhaps is all we can say, if we can come to a clearer understanding of how we behave, we can learn how to condition men so that their energies will go less into making one another miserable.

One of the things we have learned about individual behavior is that it is influenced greatly by social environment. In John Dewey's phrase, "all psychology is social psychology." Improving knowledge of social organization and its working is therefore part and parcel of the urgent task of learning how men behave. Though we may believe ourselves citizens of the most fortunate nation in the world, we have no more reason for complacency about the way in which our social organization works than for complacency about individual behavior. For example, our economic organization does not permit us to buy from one another as much wealth as our workers are able and eager to produce. Even in the best of years we fail to provide a national income large enough to give American families on the average what experts on household economics hold to be a standard of living adequate to maintain efficiency. In bad years this inadequate income falls off by a fifth or a sixth; in the very worst years by 40 per cent. or more. All this is true of our industrial equipment and practice as they stand. Proud as they are of our technological progress, engineers know that much of our equipment and many of our methods are far behind the times. We fail to make full use of knowledge that technological applications of scientific discoveries have put at our disposal. I might develop the shortcomings of our economic organization at great length, and then go on to exploit the weaknesses of our political and social institutions. It is needless to do so; for every candid and intelligent citizen can point out defects, however convinced he may be that, with all its faults, the American scheme of institutions is the best in the world. If scientists can do more than other intelligent citizens toward improving social organization, their contribution will consist in raising knowledge of social practice.

We all know that the social sciences lag far behind the natural sciences. That is because they deal with phenomena more complicated, more variable and less susceptible of experimental manipulation. Since investigators can not experiment at will upon social groups, they can not effectively apply to their problems the methods that have made the laboratory sciences strong. Max Planck once told J. M. Keynes that in early life he thought of studying economics, but found it too difficult.[4] Of course economic theory as we have it to-day is far easier to master than physical theory. But Planck was a true scientist, one who wished to gain knowledge that accounted for actual phenomena. He had learned enough to realize that it is far harder to get such knowledge of economic than of physical processes.

Yet the case of economics and its sister sciences is not hopeless. The rapid growth of statistics is providing mass observations upon social behavior of many kinds; the equally rapid growth of statistical technique enables us to learn more from a given array of data than our predecessors could. These materials and methods are making it possible to measure many social factors, some rather accurately, some roughly. Uniformities appear not only in averages but also in the way in which individual items are distributed about their means. Statements in terms of probability can be substituted for vague statements about the effect a certain cause "tends" to produce. True, work on this observational basis encounters many difficulties. It is limited by the variety, extent and accuracy of reliable data upon human behavior. It is laborious, slow and expensive. In presenting his work a realistic investigator begins with a critique of his data and methods, he ends by setting forth the probable errors and limitations of his results, and the road from the beginning to the end may be long. Instead of definitive conclusions he thinks others should accept, he presents tentative approximations he expects others to improve. The work has not even the advantage of calling for less hard thinking than speculative theorizing; for the relations among the variables in the problem are seldom manifest of themselves. All that can be claimed for this type of work is that it deals with actual experience, that its results stand or fall by the test of conformity to fact, and that it grows cumulatively after the fashion of the

[4] "Memorials of Alfred Marshall," edited by A. C. Pigou, London, 1925, p. 25, note.

observational sciences. But that is enough to give mankind strong reason for following this lead in seeking the knowledge required to improve social organization.

I do not imply that the social sciences can rapidly become such assured guides to social progress as the natural sciences are to technology. Because of difficulties inhering in their subject-matter, the social sciences will continue indefinitely to lag behind the natural sciences in precision and reliability. For a long time to come we shall have to form our opinions on many social issues in the light of common sense rather than of science. Knowledge of past experience should prove helpful in this uncertain process, and advice from specialists who have studied this experience should be sought. But wise technical advisers in these difficult matters will not pretend to certitude. As citizens we shall do well to suspect the intelligence, the candor or the disinterestedness of those who promise sure cures for social ills.

Scientific men are wont to face facts, whether these facts conform to their wishes or not. Most of them are sufficiently emancipated from conventional thinking to look critically upon social institutions. They contrast the society of to-day with its poverty in the midst of plenty, its class, racial and international animosities, its puerile aims and its destructive methods, to a society they can imagine living in security and comfort, using its increasing knowledge to provide a finer life for all mankind. This contrast should not be accepted in a spirit of resignation. It is a call to action. But scientific men will not be true to their own standards, they will not render to society the largest service of which they are capable, if they let their actions be guided by their feelings. No current discouragement should blind us to the great strides in human welfare made since science assumed its modern form; no fit of impatience over delays and relapses should make us forget that knowledge is won step by step, through the toilsome efforts of thousands of men. To jump this work with its numberless failures and its gradually cumulating successes, expecting to land in Utopia, is to give up faith in science for faith in magic. Men who take scientific methods seriously as the best hope of floundering mankind will seek to apply them just as critically and remorselessly in their social as in their physical thinking.

But science can not flourish in the future and yield the fruits for which we hope unless freedom of thought prevails. That is a condition we have been inclined to take for granted as part of the heritage our predecessors won. Now we realize that what they fought to win we must fight to maintain. The investigator's right to follow truth wherever it led was part of the common man's right to freedom of conscience and freedom of speech. These rights were established by political struggles and embodied in political institutions. The democratic way of life and the scientific way of thinking grew up together, each nourishing the other. If one now fails the other will falter. Where democracy is suppressed to-day science is fettered; for autocracy can not brook disinterested criticism of its dogmas or its practices. Freedom of scientific work in the years to come can be guaranteed only by preserving the institutions that secure freedom to all citizens. Perhaps scientific men have more at stake than any other social group in the struggle to maintain democracy.

To this struggle they can make a crucial contribution. The fate of free societies hangs upon the wisdom or folly of mass decisions. The gravest dangers to democracy come from within, not from without. They are ignorance and propaganda that turns ignorance to its uses. The best way of dispelling ignorance is by diffusing knowledge. The most effective defence against meretricious propaganda is critical inquiry. John Dewey is warranted in saying that "the future of democracy is allied with spread of the scientific attitude."[5] To foster this attitude among their fellow citizens by all means within their power is a duty incumbent upon us who cherish science. As teachers in schools and colleges we can help thousands to develop respect for evidence. As citizens we can be brave opponents of prejudice and hysteria. We can promote general understanding of the methods and results of science through our own writings or those of allies more skilled in popular exposition. These things we should do, not as high priests assured that they are always right, but as workers who have learned a method of treating problems that wins cumulative successes, and who would like to share that method with others.

# OBITUARY

## FREDERICK ADAMS WOODS

FREDERICK ADAMS WOODS was born at Boston, on January 29, 1873, and died on November 5, 1939, in Rome, Italy. His father was Solomon Adams Woods, who, born in Farmington, Maine, 1827, came to Boston about 1847 and became a successful manufacturer of wood-working machinery. Frederick Adams Woods's mother was Sarah C. Watts. She was fond of study. Her father was a seafaring man whose later life was spent in Boston devoted to study, especially of mathematics. Frederick's career was largely determined by

[5] "Freedom and Culture," New York, 1939, p. 148.

the heritage and environment into which he was born. He had a love of study and was especially interested in the application of mathematics to biology. He became, as Henry F. Osborn once called him, "the American Galton." He inherited a patrimony that left him relatively independent. He became one of the few scientific amateurs of his time in America.

Woods studied at the Massachusetts Institute of Technology from 1890 to 1894, graduating precociously. But his interest was man, so he studied at the Harvard Medical School (graduating in 1898) and remained there to teach histology and embryology for four years. He then became connected with M.I.T. as lecturer in biology and so remained for twenty years.

Woods was actively employed in study during these years of comparative freedom from the necessity of earning a living. His first book, "Mental and Moral Heredity in Royalty" (1906), was a contribution toward "the science of history"—a science based on statistical analysis. His book opens with a regret that "so little attention is paid to heredity in the biological sense." The work struck out on new lines. Seven years later (1913) was published his "The Influence of Monarchs; steps in a new science of history." This work correlated the qualities of the rulers (classified in three grades) with the condition (in three grades) of the countries over which they ruled. Here he concludes: "The true interpretation of history must hinge upon the gametes."

It was during the time between the publication of these two books that Woods sent to SCIENCE his paper, "Historiometry as an Exact Science," in which he analyzes at some length (as an illustration of method) the relative eminence of Euripides and Sophocles. Historiometry was the keynote of most of Woods's later work. In his researches he made much use of photographs of past monarchs and others, and this led to his discussion (1919) of evolutionary changes in type of face of the New England stock.

The World War aroused an especial interest in Woods. With Alexander Baltzby ("Adams Woods fellow in Harvard University"), he wrote a book on "Is War Diminishing? A study of the prevalence of war in Europe from 1450 to the present day" (1915). This study also is quantitative; it shows up Prussia as the most pacific of the European powers.

Woods was a man of rather striking personality, nearly six feet tall and slender—decidedly of the respiratory type. His intellectual interest was always in the biology of man, especially dynamical man. That is why teaching histology and embryology at the Medical School did not satisfy him. As early as 1899 he began to breed rabbits to test Galton's Law of Ancestral Inheritance and, in 1903, published in *Biometrika* a paper on "Mendel's Laws in Rabbit Breeding." He took very active interest in the American Breeders Association and its successor, the Genetic Association. During 1918–19 he was editor of the *Journal of Heredity* and contributed numerous articles on human heredity to it. He participated on committees of the Eugenic Congresses. The Galton Society was one of his main interests before he left this country to reside in Rome. He was elected president of the Eugenics Research Association, but his health did not permit him to serve. As a speaker and writer he was always clear and very serious. His life work was all a labor of love and a product of his rare personality.

CHARLES B. DAVENPORT
COLD SPRING HARBOR, L. I., N. Y.

## FRED WILLIAM TINNEY

FRED WILLIAM TINNEY was born at Saco, Montana, October 30, 1907. After graduation from the local high school, he entered the State Teachers College, Oshkosh, Wisconsin, where he received the degree of B.Ed. in 1929. He spent two years at the University of Oklahoma as assistant in botany, taking an M.S. degree in 1931. He then came to the University of Wisconsin as research assistant, which position he held until his appointment, in February, 1936, as assistant agronomist in the Bureau of Plant Industry of the U. S. Department of Agriculture, stationed at the University of Wisconsin, Madison, Wis. The degree of Ph.D. was received in 1933.

He married Madeline Morrissey on June 12, 1939. Both Dr. Tinney and his wife attended the International Congress of Genetics at Edinburgh. Both were passengers of the ill-fated *Athenia,* sunk off the coast of Scotland, on September 3, 1939. They were among those listed as missing since the disaster.

Dr. Tinney's research included a thoroughgoing study of heteropycnosis in two species of *Sphaerocarpos.* After this came an investigation of the cytology of an ornamental grass, *Agrostis nebulosa.* This led naturally to the study of the genetics and cytology of pasture grasses. After Dr. Tinney's appointment in the Bureau of Plant Industry, work in this field was carried on at Madison in cooperation with the department of agronomy of the University of Wisconsin. A paper embodying his extensive studies of blue grass (*Poa pratensis*) is in press. This grass has been the source of much confusion because of the multitude of races included within the species and of the variety of chromosomal conditions which these races manifest. Tinney's observations and studies of the peculiar methods of embryo-sac and embryo-development characterizing the species, go far toward explaining the peculiar genetic behavior of its varied forms. It promises, too, to supply a basis for the selection and breeding of improved strains of this and other grasses—a relatively new field of endeavor in America.

Deeply devoted to fundamental research in accordance with his training and inclinations, Dr. Tinney in his later work developed a keen insight into the applied aspects of his studies. Quiet and unassuming, he was highly respected by his fellow workers and many friends, who recognized in him the qualities of substantial leadership among the younger group of American scientists.

CORRESPONDENT

### HENRY CLINTON FALL

MOST people are not aware that the fauna of the United States is still very imperfectly known. Among the insects, in particular, new species can still be found in great numbers, and of most of those which have been described, little or nothing is known of their life history and habits. There is thus an immense task before us, to culminate eventually in a work of many volumes, describing the life of this continent in all its details. Such a work can never be really complete, but it might be as nearly so as existing treatments of the fauna of the British Islands or Central Europe. There is no organized effort to reach such ends, but many workers are dealing successfully with particular groups of animals, defining families, genera and species, arranging them according to their apparent natural affinities. During the past forty-five years, the name of Fall has been well known to all those concerned with American beetles. Henry Clinton Fall was born at Farmington, N. H., in 1862, and died at Tyngsboro, Mass., on November 14, 1939. He graduated from Dartmouth College with the degrees B.S. and Sc.D., the latter honorary. When I first knew him he was resident in Pasadena, Calif., happy in the extraordinary opportunities for the study of Coleoptera which he found in the arid southwest. He had been interested in the subject for fifteen years before he began to publish, but once he began to record his observations he soon became a prolific writer, especially known for his excellent revisions of various groups and important faunal papers, such as those dealing with Southern California, with New Mexico and Alaska. He described over 1,400 new species of beetles, and had one of the finest collections extant. All this was done in his so-called leisure time; he earned his living by high-school teaching. His entire collection goes to the Museum of Comparative Zoology, Harvard University.

T. D. A. COCKERELL

UNIVERSITY OF COLORADO

### RECENT DEATHS AND MEMORIALS

DR. CHARLES ZELENY, research professor of zoology, who had been a member of the faculty of the University of Illinois since 1909, died on December 21 at the age of sixty-one years.

FERDINAND AUGUSTUS SILCOX, chief of the U. S. Forestry Service, died on December 20. He was fifty-seven years old.

DR. HUGH KELSEA MOORE, for thirty years before his retirement in 1934 chief chemical engineer of the Brown Company, Berlin, N. H., died on December 18 at the age of sixty-seven years.

THE College of Medicine of the State University of Iowa has received a gift of $5,000 from Mrs. Edith Graham Mayo, of Rochester, Minn., in the name of herself and the late Dr. Charles H. Mayo for the establishment of a memorial to their son, the late Dr. Joseph Graham Mayo. The fund is for the support of a lectureship or research scholarship. Dr. Joseph Mayo was a graduate of the Iowa College of Medicine in 1927, who died in 1936.

## SCIENTIFIC EVENTS

### THE STATUS OF THE ENGINEERING PROFESSION

THE Engineers' Council for Professional Development, a joint cooperative body of seven engineering organizations, through its 1938–1939 Committee on Engineering Schools, of which Dr. Karl T. Compton, president of Massachusetts Institute of Technology, was chairman, has issued a list for 1939 containing 525 accredited undergraduate engineering curricula leading to degrees in 118 colleges and universities in the United States.

Since the inauguration of the accrediting program in 1935, the committee through its committees on inspection has appraised the various curricula in each school separately, considering such factors as qualifications of the faculty, standards of instruction, scholastic work of the students, records of the graduates, attitudes of the administration, as well as physical facilities, finances, requirements and size of staff and student body. According to Dr. Compton's report,

> while the committee has adhered rigidly to the policy that it should set no fixed standards for use as yardsticks in measuring the quality of engineering instruction, one principle however has been insisted upon, namely, that if any curriculum omits some portion of a subject in which the engineers in that field are expected by the public to have competence, then under such conditions the committee insists, as a necessary safeguard to the public, that the curriculum be not accredited. . . . However, it aims to preserve the independence of action of individual institutions and to promote thereby the general advancement of engineering education.

Besides Dr. Compton, other members of the Committee on Engineering Schools included: H. P. Hammond, dean of engineering, the Pennsylvania State College, *vice-chairman,* representing the Society for the Promotion of Engineering Education; G. M. Butler, dean of engineering, University of Arizona, representing American Institute of Mining and Metallurgical Engineers; Ivan C. Crawford, dean of engineering, University of Kansas, representing the American Society of Civil Engineers; P. H. Daggett, dean of engineering, Rutgers University, representing the National Council of State Boards of Engineering Examiners; A. B. Newman, College of the City of New York, representing the American Institute of Chemical Engineers; A. A. Potter, dean of engineering, Purdue University, representing the American Society of Mechanical Engineers; D. B. Prentice, president of the Rose Polytechnic Institute, and J. R. Killian, Jr. of the Massachusetts Institute of Technology. Dean Potter has been chosen chairman of the 1939–40 committee. J. W. Barker, dean of engineering, Columbia University, succeeds Dean Hammond on the committee and E. L. Moreland, dean of engineering, Massachusetts Institute of Technology, replaces Dr. Compton. President R. E. Doherty, of the Carnegie Institute of Technology, succeeds Dean Daggett on the committee.

## THE FRANCIS AMORY SEPTENNIAL PRIZE OF THE AMERICAN ACADEMY OF ARTS AND SCIENCES

IN compliance with the provisions of the will of the late Francis Amory, The American Academy of Arts and Sciences, as trustee of a fund given by the testator, announces a prize to be known as "The Francis Amory Septennial Prize" to be awarded for conspicuously meritorious work performed during the immediately preceding septennial period, "through experiment, study or otherwise, in the treatment and cure of diseases and derangement of the human sexual generative organs in general, and more especially for the cure, prevention or relief of the retention of urine, cystitis, prostatis, etc." While the donor wished especially to reward the discovery of any new method of treatment, he expressly authorized that the prize might be given to any author who might have contributed any theoretical or practical treatise of extraordinary or exceptional value and merit on the anatomy of said organs or the treatment of their diseases.

If there shall appear work of a quality to warrant it, the first award will be made in 1940. The total amount will exceed $10,000, which may be divided at the discretion of the academy among several nominees. While formal nominations are not expected and no essays or treatises in direct competition for the prize are desired, the committee invites suggestions looking toward the wise performance of their duty. Communications on this subject should reach the committee not later than May 15, 1940, and should be addressed in care of the American Academy of Arts and Sciences, 28 Newbury Street, Boston, Mass., U. S. A. The members of the committee on the Francis Amory Septennial Prize are: Dr. Roger I. Lee, *chairman;* Dr. Walter B. Cannon, Dr. David Cheever, Professor Leigh Hoadley, Dr. William C. Quinby, Dr. E. E. Tyzzer and Dr. Soma Weiss, secretary.

## A ZOOLOGICAL EXPEDITION OF THE FIELD MUSEUM

A ZOOLOGICAL expedition of the Field Museum of Natural History, sponsored and personally led by Leon Mandel, of Chicago, will sail from Havana in January on Mr. Mandel's yacht *Buccaneer* for a cruise to out-of-the-way cays, islands and rocks in the Caribbean Sea. Birds, mammals and reptiles will be collected, and fishes and other marine creatures will be sought in the surrounding waters. The scientific staff of the expedition plans also to make ecological studies of several species in the exotic fauna of the tropic American region to be visited. This is the fourth expedition Mr. Mandel has conducted for the museum. Rudyerd Boulton, curator of birds, and D. Dwight Davis, assistant curator of anatomy and osteology, who will accompany the expedition, have left for Havana. Mr. Mandel will also take an active part in the collecting, and another collector will be Captain William Gray, of Palm Beach. Mr. Boulton will concentrate his efforts chiefly on birds, and Mr. Davis will specialize in reptiles. Both will also seek desirable specimens of mammals and of oceanographic material, and will assist Mr. Mandel and Captain Gray in the collecting of fishes. Other members of the party include Mrs. Mandel and her mother, Senora Elvira Panerai.

Included in the itinerary are such places as Swan Island, a small possession of the United States; the Bay Islands, which belong to the republic of Honduras; Glover's Reef, Half Moon Cay, Turneffe Cay, Chinchorro Bank, Cozumel Island, Holbox Island and the Triangles—three large rocks in the Gulf of Mexico. The ship will also call at the Mexican port of Progreso, at which time a trip inland will be made to Yucatan's famous Maya archeological site at Chichen Itza. The expedition is expected to complete its work and return to Havana about the middle of February.

Among the objectives of the expedition is the collection of various specimens needed for a new hall of fishes in preparation at the museum. Efforts will be made to harpoon a large devilfish, a species of ray known as manta, which has a fin spread of twelve feet or more in fully developed individuals. An especially equipped fishing launch will be used for work in waters not navigable by the larger vessel. Two-way radio-telephone communication will be maintained between ship and launch. Specimens will be sought of large game fishes such as marlin, and attempts will be made to study their life history.

Many of the islands and cays to be visited have been incompletely explored biologically. Some of them are known to be inhabited by species and sub-species of birds and reptiles different from those of the adjacent mainland, and it is hoped that the expedition may be able to contribute to the further knowledge of an area which is of special interest to science.

## SOIL CONSERVATION

DR. W. C. LOWDERMILK, assistant chief of the Soil Conservation Service, has recently returned from an extended survey of the experience of older countries in the use of land as it relates to soil erosion, soil and water conservation and torrential flood control. His studies took him into Europe, including Great Britain, Holland, France, Italy, Algeria, Tunisia, Lybia, Egypt, Palestine, Trans-Jordan, Syria, Iraq and Lebanon. The war interrupted the course of the survey, which was to have continued through Turkey, Bulgaria, southern Germany and Switzerland and return.

The survey was made in overland travel by auto, including nearly 27,000 miles. It included conferences with more than 120 scientists, agriculturists and government officials, the examination and study of 124 areas of special interest, the collection of soil samples, particularly profiles dated by archeological evidence and the taking of some 3,500 illustrative photographs. Of special interest to American agriculture are evidences of an advanced degree of refinement in measures to control and conserve storm waters and to control erosion of a productive agriculture during the Roman epoch 2,000 years ago in Northern Africa and in ancient Syria. After the destruction of the Roman civilization and the traditions of agriculture by conquering nomad peoples, former measures of water and erosion control fell into disuse and were broken down. Soil erosion then began its damaging work and throughout this area has generally washed off soils from the slopes, sorting erosional débris and carrying the finer fractions out to the sea and spreading the coarser fractions over old alluvium on the valley floors. Increased torrential run-off from the bared slopes produces torrential streams, and is cutting gullies through the alluvium of the valley floors. This in short is the predominant process at work in the old lands south and east of the Mediterranean Sea, except in the broad alluvial plains of the Nile and Mesopotamia. Agricultural possibilities of to-day are restricted principally to the alluvium of lodged soils in the valley floors and outwash plains and in the improved management of vast grazing areas, where drought and famine have been the chief controls. It is possible to reforest the hill and mountain lands in Algeria, in Palestine and Syria, particularly where the country rock is limestone and to restore or to improve the productivity and prosperity of these wasted areas.

## THE MINNEAPOLIS MEETING OF THE GEOLOGICAL SOCIETY OF AMERICA AND ASSOCIATED SOCIETIES

THE Geological Society of America is meeting this week in Minneapolis. Many sections of the United States and Canada are represented, and the attendance was expected to reach five hundred. The principal universities, colleges, state and federal geological surveys of Canada and the United States planned to send delegates. Three associated societies—the Paleontological Society, the Mineralogical Society and the Society of Economic Geologists are meeting in conjunction with the Geological Society.

According to the preliminary program Dr. T. Wayland Vaughan, of Washington, D. C., president of the Geological Society, gave the address of the president on Thursday, December 28. His subject was "The Ecology of Modern Marine Organisms with Reference to Paleogeography." Earlier on Thursday Professor R. W. Chaney, of the University of California at Berkeley, retiring president of the Paleontological Society, addressed the several societies on "Tertiary Forests and Continental History." The title of the address of Professor E. S. Moore, of the University of Toronto, retiring president of the Society of Economic Geologists, was "Genetic Relations of Gold Deposits and Igneous Rocks in the Canadian Shield."

A general meeting of the four societies was held on Thursday morning. In the afternoon the sessions of the Geological Society were devoted to a discussion of structural geology; of the Paleontological Society to a discussion of new fossils; and of the Mineralogical Society to a discussion of crystal structure and textures. Papers read before the Economic Geologists were concerned with ground water supply and other applications of geology to the field of non-metallic resources. The technical sessions of the different societies were continued on Friday. On that day, in addition to the general session of the Geological Society, two joint sessions were held, one with the Paleontologists and one with the Mineralogists and Economic Geologists. Technical sessions were planned for Saturday morning, after which the meeting will close with an open house and tea at the Pillsbury Hall of the University of Minnesota.

## OFFICERS OF THE AMERICAN CHEMICAL SOCIETY

DR. WILLIAM LLOYD EVANS, head of the department of chemistry of the Ohio State University, has been elected president of the American Chemical Society for 1941. He will take office as president-elect on January

1, at which time Dr. Samuel Colville Lind, dean of the Institute of Technology of the University of Minnesota, becomes president, succeeding Professor Charles A. Kraus, of Brown University.

The president-elect was chosen by the council of the society from four nominees receiving the largest number of votes in a national poll by mail of the 24,000 members of the society. The council includes national officers, directors, editors of the publications of the society, past presidents, chairmen of eighteen professional divisions and councilors of the ninety-two local sections.

Other elections were:

*Directors:* Dr. Elmer K. Bolton, chemical director of E. I. du Pont de Nemours and Company, Wilmington, Del., *director-at-large.*

Leason H. Adams, director of the Geophysical Laboratory of the Carnegie Institution, for the fourth district of the society, comprising Alabama, Arkansas, District of Columbia, Florida, Georgia, Kentucky, Louisiana, Maryland, Mississippi, North Carolina, Oklahoma, South Carolina, Tennessee, Texas, Virginia and West Virginia.

Dr. Robert E. Swain, head of the department of chemistry at Stanford University, reelected for the sixth district, including Arizona, California, Colorado, Idaho, Iowa, Kansas, Minnesota, Missouri, Montana, Nebraska, Nevada, New Mexico, North Dakota, Oregon, South Dakota, Utah, Washington, Wyoming, Alaska and Hawaii.

*Councilors-at-large:* Dr. Per K. Frolich, director of the chemical laboratories of the Standard Oil Development Company, Elizabeth, N. J.; Dr. Edward Mack, Jr., of the Battelle Memorial Institute, Columbus; Dr. C. E. K. Mees, vice-president in charge of research and development of the Eastman Kodak Company; Professor William A. Noyes, Jr., of the University of Rochester, New York.

Professor Evans, who received the William H. Nichols Medal of the New York Section of the society in 1929 for his work on the chemistry of carbohydrates, has been a member of the faculty of the Ohio State University for thirty-five years and has been chairman of the department of chemistry since 1928. From 1892 to 1894 he was chemist of the American Encaustic Tile Company, Zanesville, Ohio. He served as assistant in the department of ceramics at the Ohio State University from 1896 to 1898, and instructor in the Colorado Springs High School from 1898 to 1902. He became assistant professor of chemistry at the Ohio State University in 1905, associate professor in 1908 and full professor in 1911.

# SCIENTIFIC NOTES AND NEWS

THE American Association for the Advancement of Science and some thirty of its associated and affiliated societies are meeting this week at Columbus. The address of the president, Professor Wesley C. Mitchell, is printed in the present issue of SCIENCE. This will be followed by other addresses of special interest. A general report of the meeting, edited by the permanent secretary, will be printed in the issue for February 2.

DR. ALEXANDER WETMORE, assistant secretary of the Smithsonian Institution, has been elected a corresponding member of the Royal Australasian Ornithologists' Union.

IT is stated in *Nature* that Dr. Gerhard Domagk, who was recently awarded the Nobel Prize for Physiology and Medicine for 1939, has been elected an honorary member of the Pharmaceutical Association of the Hindu University of Benares.

DECORATIONS of the Chinese Order of the Jade were presented on December 20 at a reception in New York City to Dr. John Dewey, professor emeritus of philosophy of Columbia University, in recognition of his work for Chinese students, and to Dr. Nicholas Murray Butler, president of Columbia University. The presentations were made by Dr. Tsune-chi Yu, Chinese Consul-General in New York.

PHILIP TORCHIO, who retired in 1938, at the age of seventy years, from the position of vice-president of the Consolidated Edison Company of New York, Inc., has been awarded the Edison Medal for 1939 of the American Institute of Electrical Engineers in recognition of "distinguished contributions to the art of central station engineering and for achievement in the production, distribution and utilization of electrical energy." The presentation will be made on the evening of January 24 during the winter convention of the institute, which will be held in the Engineering Societies Building, New York.

E. MEAD JOHNSON awards of $500 each were presented by the American Academy of Pediatrics at its annual meeting in Cincinnati to Dr. Frederic A. Gibbs, instructor in neurology, Harvard Medical School, and Dr. Dorothy H. Andersen, New York. The award was made to Dr. Gibbs in recognition of his work on epilepsy and to Dr. Andersen for her work on pancreatic disorders.

E. R. SQUIBB AND SONS have established an annual award of $1,000 to encourage investigation in endocrinology. The administration of this award has been intrusted to the Association for the Study of Internal Secretions, of which Dr. Philip E. Smith is president. Dr. Edward A. Doisy is chairman of the Committee on Awards. Nominations for the 1940 award must be received before March 1 by the secretary of the society, E. K. Shelton, 921 Westwood Boulevard, Los Angeles, Calif.

DR. T. L. ALTHAUSEN, associate professor of medicine in the Medical School of the University of California, has been awarded the Van Meter Prize of the American Association for the Study of Goiter in recognition of his work on the thyroid gland.

THE president of the University of Cincinnati and the faculty of the College of Medicine sponsored a dinner on December 6 at the Netherland Plaza Hotel, Cincinnati, in honor of Dr. Albert H. Freiberg, who recently retired as professor of orthopedic surgery. Dr. Martin H. Fischer was toastmaster, and the speakers were Dr. Raymond Walters, president of the university; Drs. Stanley E. Dorst, Mont R. Reid and David I. Wolfstein, and the Rev. Jesse Halsey, pastor of the Seventh Presbyterian Church. A portrait of Dr. Freiberg was presented to him.

DR. HORACE B. ENGLISH, professor of psychology of the Ohio State University, was elected president of the Association of Applied Psychologists at the recent Washington meeting of the association.

THE thirty-second annual meeting of the American Society of Agronomy and the fourth annual meeting of the Soil Science Society of America were held in the Roosevelt Hotel, New Orleans, on November 22, 23 and 24, with an attendance of approximately seven hundred. During the session a hundred and seventy-seven papers on various phases of soils and crops problems were presented. At a general meeting W. C. Lasseter, editor of the *Progressive Farmer,* spoke on "The Social and Economic Problems of Southern Agriculture" and Dean M. J. Funchess, dean of agriculture at the Alabama Polytechnic Institute, discussed "Agronomic Problems of the South." Officers of the American Society of Agronomy elected for 1940 are: *President,* Dr. F. J. Alway, University of Minnesota; *Vice-president,* Dr. L. E. Kirk, Central Experimental Farm, Ottawa; *Secretary-Treasurer,* Dr. G. G. Pohlman, West Virginia University; *Editor,* J. D. Luckett, New York Agricultural Experiment Station, Geneva; *Chairman of Soils Section,* Dr. W. H. Pierre, Iowa State College; *Chairman of Crops Section,* Dr. S. C. Salmon, Bureau of Plant Industry. Officers of the Soil Science Society of America for 1940 are: *President,* Dr. W. H. Pierre, Iowa State College; *Secretary,* Dr. C. E. Kellogg, Bureau of Plant Industry; *Treasurer,* Dr. G. G. Pohlman, West Virginia University.

PROFESSOR HENRI DARWIN HASKINS, for nearly fifty years a member of the faculty of the Massachusetts State College and more recently chief of the laboratory for fertilizer control, having reached the state retirement age of seventy years, the title of emeritus professor of agricultural chemistry has been conferred on him.

THE title emeritus has been conferred by the University of Missouri on Sidney Calvert, who retired in September as professor of organic chemistry and director of the chemical laboratory.

NEW appointments at the New York Medical College include: Dr. Ferdinand C. Lee, associate professor of surgery at the Johns Hopkins University, as professor and head of the department of surgery and dean of the college; Dr. Thomas I. Hoen, of Montreal, as professor of neuro-surgery and head of the department of neuro-surgery and neuropsychiatry; Dr. R. Townley Paton, surgeon of the Manhattan Eye, Ear and Throat Hospital, as professor and head of the department of ophthalmology, and Dr. William H. Everts, of the Neurological Institute of New York, as professor of neurology.

DR. ARTHUR SULLIVAN GALE has resigned as dean of the College for Men at the University of Rochester, effective on January 1. Dr. W. Edwin Van de Walle, professor of philosophy and chairman of the Committee on Advice, will succeed him. Dr. Gale will continue as Fayerweather professor and chairman of the department of mathematics, a post that he has held since 1906.

DR. JOSEPH MURDOCH has been appointed associate professor of geology at the University of California at Los Angeles, where he has taught since 1928.

DR. TZE-TUAN CHEN, a research fellow in the department of zoology of the Johns Hopkins University, has been appointed research associate in protozoology in the School of Hygiene and Public Health.

DR. BIENVENIDO M. GONZALEZ, who for the past twelve years has been dean and head of the department of animal husbandry of the College of Agriculture, University of the Philippines, was formally inaugurated as president of the university on October 19. President Gonzalez is succeeded by Dr. Leopoldo B. Uichanco as dean of the College of Agriculture. Dr. Uichanco continues to be head of the department of entomology.

DR. JUAN BACIGALUPO has been appointed professor of parasitology in the Faculty of Medicine at Buenos Aires to succeed Dr. D. Greenway, who has reached the age limit.

DR. R. Y. WINTERS has been appointed assistant director of research in the Department of Agriculture. He has been a staff member of the Office of Experiment Stations since 1937.

DR. K. A. C. ELLIOTT has been appointed research biochemist at the Institute of the Pennsylvania Hospital, Philadelphia, which is initiating a new program of research in mental and nervous diseases. Dr. Elliott will be in charge of the laboratory.

ALBERT C. CLINE, who has been on the staff of the

Harvard Forest in Petersham, Mass., since 1924, has been appointed director of the forest. He succeeds Ward Shepard, who was director for three years while on leave of absence from the Federal Government, but who has now returned to Washington.

A UNIVERSITY Committee on Pharmacotherapy has been formed at Harvard University. The function of the committee will be to coordinate the efforts of practising physicians and the members of the faculty in biology, chemistry and medicine and to develop research and improved graduate training in pharmacology and experimental therapeutics. In carrying out this program, the committee will bring together chemists and biologists from the Harvard Faculty of Arts and Sciences, pharmacologists, physiologists and biochemists from the Harvard Medical School, and physicians working with patients in hospitals. Dr. Soma Weiss, Hersey professor of the theory and practice of physic at the Medical School, is chairman of the new committee. The other members are: Dr. Fuller Albright, assistant professor of medicine; Dr. Henry K. Beecher, associate in anesthesia; Dean Burwell, *ex-officio;* Dr. Walter B. Cannon, George Higginson professor of physiology; Dr. William B. Castle, professor of medicine; President Conant, *ex-officio;* Dr. Louis F. Fieser, professor of chemistry; Dr. A. Baird Hastings, Hamilton Kuhn professor of biological chemistry; Dr. Frederick L. Hisaw, professor of zoology; Dr. Otto Krayer, associate professor of comparative pharmacology, and Dr. Reginald P. Linstead, professor of chemistry. Funds to support the work for the next five years have been donated by a group of corporations interested in medical and therapeutic research.

THE Wilson photoalidade, that was designed and built in the U. S. Geological Survey several years ago, will be used again this winter by T. W. Ranta in the office-mapping of part of the north slope of the rugged Wrangell Mountains, Alaska, from oblique airplane photographs. Mr. Ranta established the necessary ground control during the recent field season and will use photographs taken by Gerald Fitzgerald, of the Geological Survey, and Bradford Washburn, of the Harvard Institute of Geographical Exploration.

DR. JULIAN A. STEYERMARK, assistant curator of the herbarium of the Field Museum, Chicago, who is conducting an expedition in Guatemala, has during the first month collected specimens of more than a thousand varieties of plants. In the course of his exploration he climbed to the summit of the Sierra de las Minas, which rises above the Motagua River, a region probably never before visited by a botanist. He has also collected the flora of the Motagua Valley desert region of the Atlantic watershed. Dr. Francis Drouet, curator of cryptogamic botany, who with Donald Richards, of the University of Chicago, is collecting in the southwestern United States and northwestern Mexico, has forwarded to the museum a collection of 1,200 algae and other plants from the general region of Las Vegas. N. M.

DR. G. H. PARKER, of Harvard University, lectured on December 18 at an open meeting of the Brown University Chapter of Sigma Xi on the question, "Is Natural Selection a Brutal Process?"

A SERIES of eight lectures at Yale University on the history of science is planned by the Yale Chapter of the Gamma Alpha Graduate Scientific Fraternity. The first seven lectures will trace the history of the basic sciences. The last one will deal with the development of medicine in relation to the other sciences. The program includes lectures by the following members of the faculty of the university: January 16, *Astronomy,* by Dr. Frank Schlesinger; January 30, *Mathematics,* by Dr. Oystein Ore; February 13, *Geology,* by Dr. Chester R. Longwell; February 27, *Chemistry,* by Dr. John A. Timm; March 12, *Physics,* by Dr. Henry Margenau; April 2, *Biology,* by Dr. Lorande L. Woodruff; April 16, *Psychology,* by Dr. Walter R. Miles; April 30, *Medicine and the Sciences,* by Dr. John F. Fulton. Until the time of his death the late Dr. Harvey Cushing was collaborating with Dr. Fulton on the last lecture. In general the plan and scope of the series is similar to the series presented by the fraternity in 1920. Two new subjects, Psychology, and Medicine and the Sciences, have been added.

THE fifth International Congress of Pediatrics, which was to have been held in Boston in September, 1940, has been postponed to an indefinite date. Dr. Henry F. Helmholz, Rochester, Minn., is president of the congress; Dr. Kenneth D. Blackfan, Boston, general secretary, and Dr. Charles F. McKhann, Boston, assistant secretary.

THE new building of the New York Medical College, Flower and Fifth Avenue Hospitals, erected at a cost of $1,500,000, was dedicated on December 12. The speakers included Mayor La Guardia, President Harold Willis Dodds, of Princeton University; Dr. Lewis Hill Weed, director of the School of Medicine of the Johns Hopkins University, and Charles D. Halsey, chairman of the board of trustees. Dr. Claude A. Burrett, president of the college, presided.

BEQUESTS of about $1,500,000 to Northwestern University and $1,000,000 to the University of Chicago for medical and chemical research are provided in the will of Mrs. Clara A. Abbott, who died in 1924. She was the widow of Dr. Wallace C. Abbott, founder of the Abbott Laboratories of North Chicago. The gift to the University of Chicago makes the institution eligible for an additional $1,500,000 grant, given by the Rockefeller Foundation for Research in the biological sciences, with the proviso that the university raise an additional $500,000 for that purpose.

THE Ruth Lucie Stern Research Laboratory, the gift of Mrs. Louis Stern, built at the cost of about $97,000, has been opened at the School of Medicine of Stanford University at San Francisco. It is three stories high and has more than 6,000 feet of laboratory space. The second floor is occupied by research in pediatrics and the top floor by research in pathological gynecology, endocrinology and cancer.

ERNEST L. WOODWARD has made a gift of $45,000 to the University of Rochester to support the research in epilepsy of Dr. W. P. Van Wagenen, associate professor of neurological surgery at the School of Medicine and Dentistry. The facilities of the Craig Colony for Epileptics, at Sonyea, and of the Rochester State Hospital have been extended to him during the past year. Previous support of the work had come from the Markle Foundation.

THE will of Charles R. Walgreen, founder of the Walgreen drug store chain, who died on December 11, provides for the transfer of the balance of the 19,000 shares of the stock he had pledged previously to the University of Chicago.

LORD NUFFIELD has placed in the hands of trustees ordinary shares of Morris Motors, Limited, worth approximately £1,250,000, to be the nucleus of a fund for the provinces to finance a scheme of hospital regionalization.

THERE will be available on September 1, 1940, a research fellowship in the laboratory of pathology at the Collis P. Huntington Memorial Hospital and in the Department of Pathology at the Harvard Medical School. This carries a stipend of three thousand dollars and may be renewed for a second year. The fellow will be expected to devote most of his time to histologic and cytologic studies of the effects of radiation of different types on normal and pathological tissue. Application should be made to Dr. Shields Warren at the Collis P. Huntington Memorial Hospital, Boston.

# DISCUSSION

## RADIOACTIVITY IN BIOLOGICAL EXPERIMENTS

THE successful production of radioactive materials by a cyclotron has led to interesting biological experiments in which these substances are used as tracers. In this new field many results have already been obtained, some of which are in disagreement with previously held opinions. This has given rise to the fundamental question of whether a radioactive element has the same properties as the element in its normal form.

*Radioactivity.* This question is unfortunately sometimes the result of a misunderstanding of the nature of radioactivity. It is sometimes erroneously believed that radioactive atoms continually emit radiations. A radioactive atom does not emit any radiation at all until the very end of its existence, when it changes into another element. The tracer experiments involve only atoms which have not yet radiated. It is clear that future emission of such radiations can not have any influence upon the present atomic properties.

*Atomic Weight.* The radioactive atoms have an atomic weight slightly different from normal atoms. This can have an effect upon some of their properties such as the rate at which they diffuse through a membrane. However, effects of this kind are well known to be exceedingly small and barely observable even in specially designed physical experiments.

Normal elements also consist generally of a mixture of atoms of different atomic weights, called isotopes. There is some evidence[1] that the mixture has a slightly different composition when taken from different parts of the animal system. This difference is very small, showing clearly that living tissue does not possess a pronounced ability to distinguish between isotopes. It is obvious that such minute effects need only be considered after the quantitative accuracy of the tracer experiments has been very much improved.

*Presence of Radiation.* A fraction of the tracer atoms will emit radiations during the progress of the biological experiment. Though such atoms lose their rôle as tracer, one may ask whether the presence of this radiation does not alter the properties of the living organism and influences the result of the tracer experiment. In these experiments the radioactive element is so greatly diluted and the radiation so weak that such an effect seems very unlikely. The following simple observation can verify this in doubtful cases. If the result of the tracer experiment were due to the presence of the radiation, the yield of the experiment should be approximately proportional to the *square* of the amount of tracer administered instead of in direct proportion to it.

In this connection it is also interesting to examine Zwaardemaker's well-known hypothesis that the radioactivity of potassium is responsible for its physiologi-

[1] A. Keith Brewer (*Jour. Am. Chem. Soc.*, 58: 869, 1937) finds that the potassium in bone marrow consists for about 6.75 per cent. of the isotope of atomic weight 41; in other organic and inorganic sources the percentage is 6.58 per cent.

cal action. The basic experiment to support this idea is the beating of an isolated frog's heart when perfused with a certain solution of a mixture of salts, one of which has to be potassium chloride. The amount of potassium in this solution is so small that a simple calculation indicates that only about one potassium atom per hour radiates in the frog's heart. Since the whole experiment can be performed in a much shorter time, it is absurd to connect in this experiment the necessary presence of potassium with its radioactivity.[2]

*Conclusion.* The above remarks are meant to show that tracer experiments with radioactive elements, if carefully executed, give definitely reliable information about the behavior of the normal element. If unexpected results are found they should certainly not be ascribed to a difference in the properties of the radioactive isotope.

S. GOUDSMIT

UNIVERSITY OF MICHIGAN

## PSEUDOMETHEMOGLOBIN AND ITS REACTION WITH CARBON MONOXIDE AFTER REDUCTION

IN a discussion in this journal[1] recently, E. Ammundsen published her observations on the presence in the blood of "a kind of hemoglobin" combining with carbon monoxide only after reduction. With reference to that substance the author emphasizes that "for the present its composition and the cause of its appearance will have to be looked upon as unknown." In this connection the following facts may be of interest.

The normal presence of substances in human and animal blood not identical with hemoglobin but combining with carbon monoxide in a similar way was described by Barkan and Berger[2] in 1928. These authors pointed out that of the "easily split-off" blood iron ("leicht abspaltbares" Bluteisen) discovered by Barkan[3] (1925) one portion E combines with $O_2$ and CO following the distribution equation, while another portion E′ does not react with those gases. In 1937 we[4] demonstrated that both fractions of the "easily split off" blood iron are pseudohemoglobins which are intermediates in the formation of bilirubin from hemoglobin and accompany the hemoglobin within the red cells of the circulating blood. Pseudohemoglobins, according to our definition, are chromoproteins in which the protein is probably an unaltered globin, while the prosthetic group is an iron-containing heme or hemin derivative with an opened porphyrin ring, similar to that in Lemberg's[5] "verdohemochromogen." The two fractions E and E′ differ by the valency of the iron. The latter is bivalent in *E,* which combines with oxygen and carbon monoxide and hence was designated as a pseudohemoglobin *in sensu strictiori.* The iron is trivalent in E′, which does not combine with $O_2$ and CO and was designated as a "pseudomethemoglobin." By reduction with $Na_2S_2O_4$ we were able to transform the pseudomethemoglobin into pseudohemoglobin, which does combine with carbon monoxide.

Our work was published in different original articles[4, 6] and, in addition, some reviews[7] have been given. Taylor and Coryell[8] in an article (1938) dealing with the magnetic susceptibility of the iron in ferrohemoglobin confirmed our work. Using the same method as was later used by E. Ammundsen,[1] they found too that in normal blood and in oxyhemoglobin solutions there are present hemoglobin-like compounds which combine with carbon monoxide only after previous reduction.

GEORG BARKAN

BOSTON UNIVERSITY SCHOOL OF MEDICINE AND EVANS MEMORIAL, MASSACHUSETTS MEMORIAL HOSPITALS

OTTO SCHALES

HARVARD MEDICAL SCHOOL AND PETER BENT BRIGHAM HOSPITAL

## AN EXPERIMENT ON RETINAL AFTER-IMAGE AND JUDGMENT OF SIZE

BY an almost unconscious combination of elements, we judge the size of an object from the image it produces on the retina and from our judgment of its distance from the eye. If there is uncertainty in this latter judgment, there is corresponding uncertainty in judgment of size because we do not then know how far away to consider the object to be and do not know how to interpret the retinal image. It is common experience that we are incapable of estimating the

[2] A. J. Glazko and D. M. Greenberg (*Am. Jour. of Physiol.,* 125: 405, 1939) have shown that radioactive sodium can not replace the potassium in this experiment. Compare also a critical article by S. G. Zondek, *Biochem. Zeits.,* 121: 76, 1921.

[1] SCIENCE, 90: 2338, 372–373, October 20, 1939.

[2] G. Barkan and E. Berger, *Arch. exp. Pathol. u. Pharmakol.,* 136: 278–299, 1928; *Klin. Wochenschr.,* 7: 1868, 1929.

[3] G. Barkan, *Zeits. physiol. Chem.,* 148: 124–154, 1925; *ibid.,* 171: 179–193 and 194–221, 1927; *Biochem. Zeits.,* 224: 53–62, 1930; *Zeits. physiol. Chem.,* 216: 1–16 and 17–25, 1933; *ibid.,* 221: 241–251, 1933; *ibid.,* 236: 198–200, 1935. See also G. Barkan and O. Schales, *ibid.,* 244: 81–88, 1936; *ibid.,* 244: 257–265, 1936.

[4] G. Barkan and O. Schales, *Zeits. physiol. Chem.,* 248: 96–116, 1937.

[5] *Cf.* R. Lemberg, *Ann. Rev. Biochem.,* 7: 421–448, 1938; and original papers cited therein.

[6] G. Barkan and O. Schales, *Zeits. physiol. Chem.,* 253: 83–103, 1938.

[7] G. Barkan, Lecture in the Wiener Biologische Gesellschaft, June 14, 1937; *Klin. Wochenschr.,* 16: 1265–1268, 1937; *Dtsch. Mediz. Wochenschr.,* 64: 638–640, 1938; Kongressbericht II des XVI Internat. Physiol. Kongresses, Zürich (Schweiz), 1938, p. 250; G. Barkan and O. Schales, *Arch. Ital. di Sc. Farmacologiche,* Vol. Jubil. ad Benedicenti, 1937; O. Schales, Research Meeting of the Rockefeller Institute, Copenhagen, December 3, 1938.

[8] D. S. Taylor and Ch. D. Coryell, *Jour. Am. Chem. Soc.,* 60: 1177–1181, 1938.

size of the moon, for example, because, although we receive a clear image which subtends a certain angle, we receive no accompanying sense experience which might enable us to judge the distance of the object. (Astronomically determined distances are not, of course, perceived directly.) Elementary observations in optics show that whenever a real image is formed by a lens, as in the case of images formed on the retina by the lens of the eye, the size of the image decreases as the distance between lens and object increases. We learn in infancy to interpret this relationship between image size and distance of object. The following paragraphs describe a simple experiment which is, in a sense, the converse of our common experience with retinal images.

It is well known that exposure of the eye to bright light produces retinal fatigue and that after one has gazed intently for several seconds at a bright source, there may appear an after-image of the source soon after the eyes are shifted to some less brightly illuminated area. This after-image is commonly seen in a color complementary to that of the source, a fact which has heretofore played a part in hypotheses of color-vision, but which is, for the present, of secondary importance. It is the *size* of the after-image rather than its color to which the writer wishes to direct attention; for this persistent image may be used to produce the illusion of an external object whose apparent distance from the eye may be varied at will, with the result that the illusory "object" changes size, and its apparent size depends entirely upon the observer's judgment of its distance from the eye.

Let the observer, with one eye closed, look with the other eye steadily for ten seconds upon the bright filament of an unfrosted 60-watt lamp situated, say, two feet from the eye. If the gaze is then shifted to some less bright region, there soon appears a pronounced after-image of the lamp filament which may persist clearly for a minute or two because of the fatigue of that portion of the retina which has been so strongly exposed to light. If the observer has difficulty in discovering the after-image, it may be "developed" or made more apparent by blinking the exposed eye occasionally or by exposing it indirectly to intermittent flashing of a low-power lamp (15 or 25 watt). Once the image is seen, it may be followed from spot to spot about the room as the observer shifts his gaze; it may appear as a large object on a distant wall or as a small object on a piece of paper held close at hand. The change in apparent size of the illusory object is immediately evident; it is amusing, for example, to "fix" the object on a finger tip held not far from the eye and to observe the increase in its apparent size as the finger is moved farther away. By observing the after-image on a scale and by recording its apparent size as a function of the observer's distance from the scale, it is possible to check with reasonable accuracy that this apparent size of object is directly proportional to the distance between the eye and the scale on which the after-image appears to be situated.

Because of the well-known phenomenon of irradiation and because of involuntary movements of the eye during exposure to the light, the after-image on the retina is somewhat extended and looks larger than the lamp filament. However, the horseshoe-shaped filament of a 60-watt lamp gives an image which is readily recognized and is sufficiently definite in outline to serve for measurement. A frosted lamp may be used if it is obscured from view except for a small aperture of sharp outline and characteristic shape. The color of the after-image is not always the same but appears to depend upon length of exposure and upon external illumination. It may, at first, be dark blue (roughly complementary to the bright yellow of the source); but in many cases, especially under periodically changing illumination, it may change from dark blue to bright yellow, and by this reversal of color the after-image may be easily detected. In many cases it appears as a bright yellow object like the lamp filament, but with a blue border. When this experiment was tried with a group of twenty students at once, it was found that nearly all of them observed the effects described herein. The experiment may serve to demonstrate to students of physics and psychology certain fundamental facts of vision by the simple expedient of using a strong retinal after-image for purposes of measurement and observation. It is recognized that there may be danger to the eye in prolonged exposure to an intense source of light, but the writer has personally repeated the experiment a great many times without any observed harmful effects.

RICHARD M. SUTTON
HAVERFORD COLLEGE

## THE OCCURRENCE OF THE TWO RARE GENERA, PROTOHYDRA AND PROTODRILUS, ON THE EAST COAST OF NORTH AMERICA

THESE two genera, so far as can be ascertained, have never before been reported from the North American continent. The first form, *Protohydra leuckarti*, probably represents the most primitive coelenterate of the class Hydrozoa. It was found in a small brackish water creek formed at low tide on the mud flats in New Haven harbor together with numerous Protozoa, rotifers and Turbellaria. Only one specimen was found which after several hours' isolation divided by transverse fission. The two individuals thus formed lived for several weeks in the laboratory, when for some unaccountable reason they disintegrated over night. The animals, which lack tentacles, feed on small crustacea, rotifers and protozoa, which they capture by means of the expanded spoon-shaped peristome. Although discovered by Greeff in 1870 in Europe, the animal has been collected only occasionally since that time and consequently practically no experimental work has been done upon it. Recently, chiefly through the work of Westblad,[1] the sexual reproduction has been studied, and the extremely interesting observation made that the sex cells are of endodermal origin with the ovaries and testes projecting into the enteric cavity. Only two species are known, *P. leuckarti* Greeff and *P. caulleryi* Dawydoff.

The second animal, *Protodrilus leuckarti* Hatcheck, was collected by Mr. D. J. Zinn, of the Osborn Zoological Laboratory, from intertidae sand near Branford, Conn. Although some eleven species of this archiannelid genus have been reported from Europe, thus far none has been found in North America, chiefly, it is believed, because of failure to collect from its habitat. As is the case with *Protohydra,* little experimental work has been performed upon this form because of its comparative rarity. Very likely large numbers of European invertebrate genera are present here and will be discovered when our coasts are studied more intensively.

Both *Protohydra* and *Protodrilus,* it is believed, offer excellent possibilities for experimental work if they can be collected in more abundance and maintained in culture.

T. K. RUEBUSH

OSBORN ZOOLOGICAL LABORATORY,
YALE UNIVERSITY

# SCIENTIFIC BOOKS

## THE TEACHERS OF PHYSICS

WE have probably all listened to a teacher explain in glowing colors his way of teaching physics and have had the feeling that we should rush home and introduce his system into our classrooms. Closer thought, however, shows us that we have been listening to a happy, competent, enthusiastic teacher who has successfully fitted his teaching to his school, his students and his own personality. This same system forced on an overworked, less competent and unsympathetic teacher or a group of students of different training and point of view might well fail even worse than the system now being used. It seems that the same reasoning must be applied to text-books.

Probably most teachers are a bit dissatisfied with the text they are using. If only we could inject into the first-year student some of the enthusiasm of many graduate students, then our work would be made more easy. The advanced student is out on the front of new advances and new discoveries. Then should not these same "newest" ideas be made the theme of elementary texts? Some writers of text-books think so.

Smyth and Ufford (S & U)[1] is a text with this theme of "newness." The whole treatment is novel and new. The writers have not omitted the fundamental laws but rather have caused them to be brightened by the light of the advances of recent years. They are among the first writers of general texts to introduce and use the long recommended K.M.S. system of units with the Newton ($=10^7$ dynes) as the unit of force. This factor alone will doubtless influence some teachers in favor and some against this text. It would hardly be possible for the teacher to cling to the C.G.S. system and use this text.

In the hands of an experienced teacher who can keep in mind that good foundations are still necessary for safe construction and who nevertheless is willing to follow the spirit of the book S & U should be a real experience to the beginning college student. On the other hand, the inexperienced teacher who permits enthusiasm for the new to cause him to forget the necessary fundamentals or the teacher who puts this text into the hands of his student and then tries to teach in the conventional manner will produce neither good physicists nor clear thinkers.

Housman and Slack (H & S)[2] have avoided some of these dangers by writing a more conventional text with the material arranged as we are accustomed to find it, and yet they have included nearly every bit of new physics that S & U have used and some besides. A text which includes the "fission of uranium" and "non-reflecting glass," as does the H & S text, can hardly be called old-fashioned, yet these authors have kept their emphasis on teaching the fundamentals to the beginning student, to whom all physics is new. In their greater emphasis on fundamentals they have taken particular care to get the subject of units clear and straight in the student's minds. Also they have been careful to keep fundamental statements and definitions from becoming lost within long paragraphs of explanation.

There was some criticism on the part of teachers using H & S that the first edition showed a lack of care in the latter chapters compared to the earlier ones, as if the authors had been hurried to finish their task. This defect seems to have been eliminated completely in this second edition.

Both of these texts recognize that too many college students are poorly prepared in the art of working

[1] E. Westblad, *Arkiv för Zoologi,* 21A, No. 23.

[1] Smyth and Ufford, "Matter, Motion and Electricity." McGraw-Hill Book Co. $3.75.

[2] Housman and Slack, "Physics." Second edition. D. Van Nostrand Co. $4.00.

numerical problems and getting correct numerical answers. Hence they include a considerable number of carefully and completely worked-out numerical problems.

Both of these texts are of a difficulty which suggests their successful use only in the school where the students are rather above the average in ability and preparation. For the less capable students the older, well-tried and now rewritten Stewart[3] is in point of view much like H & S but with more qualitative description, less difficult mathematical discussion and, in general, of a lower level of difficulty but still a college text and not at all a glorified high-school text.

This reviewer feels at one disadvantage in writing of these texts. While these must be classed as among the best of the present texts, there are others which are completely comparable with these and which a teacher should also examine before deciding on the text for his classes.

Since the teaching of second-year electricity has escaped from the domination of Starling's "Electricity and Magnetism," whose red cover cast its controlling influence over this field for so many years, there have appeared a number of electrical texts. One of the newest is "Fundamentals of Electricity and Magnetism," by Loeb.[4]

This book was, according to the author, written to supply a text to accompany a course of twenty-six one-hour demonstration lectures. Hence the material was much influenced by the apparatus and conditions of those lectures. The students were to have had differential calculus before starting electricity and to be taking integral calculus concurrently with their electricity. Hence the first integral sign appears on page 87, following an unusually long historical introduction. The mathematical developments are rather less difficult than is common in such texts.

The author has followed the old convention of starting his development with the concept of a magnetic pole, which in spite of much criticism does seem to have its advantages. Similarly his treatment of B & H is quite conventional and no mention is made of the difficulties which have arisen in this field nor of the dicta of the International Electro-Technical Commission.

In his preface he states that he has found that "the greatest difficulty encountered by the student is the confusion in the definition and relation of the many electrical entities occurring in such a treatment." His definitions of field strength at a point as "the force exerted on a unit North pole at that point" (page 64) and potential difference as the "work to move unit quantity of electricity between those points," hardly agree with the criteria given by Worthing.[5]

There are a number of other minor criticisms which may be mentioned such as an unusual use of the expression "most efficient" on page 167 where it is used to mean "most current"; a strange diagram on page 328 where a damped sine function is plotted by straight lines: the failure to make clear the effect of line resistance in the self-induction experiment.

Where instructors wish a text which lies midway between the electricity of the conventional first year of college physics and the standard senior college course, Loeb's text will be found quite satisfactory and will fill a need in this field where few other texts are available.

A very different book is "The Fundamentals of Electro-Magnetism" by Cullwick.[6]

Professor Cullwick, recognizing that there has been a lack of clear thinking in many elementary texts, has attempted to put clarity and rigor into an elementary text. Mostly he has succeeded but some of his failures help to emphasize the difficulty of his undertaking. He has not produced a senior college text-book but he has produced a book which all teachers in this field should read both for its clarity and also for its confusion.

An elementary physics book[7] has been written by physicists and as nearly without mathematics as possible. No attempt has been made to "jazz up" the subject. Not at all a high-school text but, as the name implies, it is a survey for college students who can't or won't use simple mathematics.

"Mechanics for Engineering Students,"[8] is a textbook containing a very great number of carefully discussed mechanics problems, using only simple calculus. d'Alembert is mentioned, but not Lagrange nor Hamilton. Vectors are treated only by their components and no direct vector notation is used.

"Introduction to Laboratory Technique,"[9] is a book that will be found useful in any laboratory where work is being done. There are formulas and instructions for a great many things which a laboratory or shop man frequently needs to use. Aside from some English trade names and an occasional shop use of a word which will confuse a chemist or physicist, the instructions seem to be very clear and definite.

NIEL F. BEARDSLEY
RYERSON PHYSICAL LABORATORY,
UNIVERSITY OF CHICAGO

[3] O. M. Stewart, "Physics. A Text Book for Colleges." Third edition. Ginn and Company. $4.00. (First edition, 1924.)

[4] Loeb, "Fundamentals of Electricity and Magnetism." John Wiley and Sons. $4.00.

[5] A. G. Worthing, *American Physics Teacher*, 6: 50, 1938.

[6] Cullwick, "The Fundamentals of Electro-Magnetism." Macmillan, $4.50.

[7] Arthur E. Hass and Ira M. Freeman, "Elementary Survey of Physics." E. P. Dutton Company. $1.90.

[8] John E. Younger, "Mechanics for Engineering Students." International Textbook Company. $3.50.

[9] A. J. Ansley, "Introduction to Laboratory Technique." London: Macmillan and Company. $4.50.

# SPECIAL ARTICLES

## A DEFECT IN THE METABOLISM OF AROMATIC AMINO ACIDS IN PREMATURE INFANTS: THE ROLE OF VITAMIN C[1]

In the course of studies of the nitrogen metabolism of premature infants, a number of the infants were found to excrete substances in their urine which gave the Million reaction.[2] Further studies demonstrated the absence of appreciable amounts of tyrosine, dihydroxyphenylalanine, homogentisic acid and melanin, thus exempting them as the hydroxyphenyl compounds responsible for the reaction. Dr. Hans Clarke, professor of biochemistry at Columbia University, extracted from these urines crystals of l-p-hydroxyphenyllactic acid, identification being made by elementary analysis, melting point and optical rotation, the urinary substance conforming in all respects to the pure compound. Qualitative tests (a positive but transitory response to dilute ferric chloride, a precipitate with 2, 4-dinitrophenylhydrazine) also established the presence of a keto-acid, probably p-hydroxyphenylpyruvic acid in these urines, but it has not yet been isolated in a pure state. Reduction of phosphomolybdic acid by Medes' technique[3] has been employed for quantitative assay.

Since these substances were absent from the urine of premature infants receiving human milk and since their excretion was enhanced by the feeding of phenylalanine and tyrosine, it seemed reasonable to relate the defect to the higher content of these amino acids in cow's milk. The possibility that this defect in oxidation and decarboxylation of aromatic amino acids above a threshold level of intake might be related to an enzymatic deficiency remediable by administration of vitamins was suggested by the observation of Closs and Fölling[4] that the urinary excretion of phenylpyruvic acid following injection of phenylalanine was increased in rats by deficient intake of vitamin $B_1$. Such therapy with thiamin chloride in liberal dosage (20 mg daily) had no effect on the spontaneous excretion of hydroxyphenyl compounds in several of the infants. The effect of vitamin C therapy, however, was striking.

Shortly after birth five male premature infants were placed on diets of powdered cow's milk of adequate caloric, fluid and protein (5 gm per kg) content supplemented with vitamin A and D concentrates (20 drops of percomorph oil daily) but without added vitamins B and C. Complete 24-hour urines were quantitatively assayed for hydroxyphenyl derivatives.[5] The infants received from 50 to 200 mg of ascorbic acid parenterally at the ages indicated in Table 1, and in four of the five there resulted a prompt decline with virtual disappearance in excretion of hydroxyphenyl compounds within 48 to 72 hours. In the fifth infant (G. A.) 50 mg was ineffective, but the administration of 100 mg several days later was accompanied by a prompt response. In another infant (G. B.) the cycle of appearance of urinary hydroxyphenyl derivatives with omission of dietary vitamin C and disappearance with its resumption was demonstrated on two occasions. These results gain added interest in view of a recent report relating the production of experimental alcaptonuria to vitamin C deficiency[6] and the demonstration *in vitro* of the relation of dehydroascorbic acid to the breakdown of amino acids, including phenylalanine, to aldehydes.[7]

TABLE 1

The Effect of Vitamin C on the Excretion of Hydroxyphenyl Compounds

| Age days | Vitamin C supplement mg | Tyrosine* in urine mg | Age days | Vitamin C supplement mg | Tyrosine* in urine mg |
|---|---|---|---|---|---|
| | A. B. | | | G. A. | |
| 38 | | 953 | 20 | | 448 |
| 39 | 200 | 940 | 21 | | 477 |
| 40 | 200 | 67 | 22 | 50 | 524 |
| 41 | 100 | 33 | 23 | | 401 |
| 42 | 25 | 37 | 24 | | 436 |
| | | | 25 | 100 | 176 |
| | A. C. | | 26 | | 36 |
| 45 | | 1,079 | | | |
| 46 | | 1,067 | | G. B. | |
| 47 | 200 | 324 | 18 | | 606 |
| 48 | 200 | 38 | 19 | | 654 |
| 49 | 100 | 32 | 20 | | 534 |
| | | | 21 | 100 | 322 |
| | J. P. | | 22 | | 48 |
| 11 | | 525 | 23 | | 39 |
| 12 | | 627 | 28 | | 281 |
| 13 | 75 | 619 | 29 | | 469 |
| 14 | 75 | 251 | 30 | | 619 |
| 15 | | 30 | 31 | 200 | 494 |
| 16 | | 24 | 32 | | 340 |
| | | | 33 | 200 | 170 |
| | | | 34 | | 40 |

* Million reaction.[5] Figures represent hydroxyphenyl compounds expressed as tyrosine.

Analysis of the blood in three of the infants in the control periods showed no ascorbic acid.[8] After administration of vitamin C in amounts sufficient to suppress the excretion of hydroxyphenyl compounds, the blood ascorbic acid was still low, varying from 0.13 to 0.32 mg per ml, indicating that although a change in cellular oxidations had taken place, the blood had not reached normal levels. Roentgenograms of the long bones revealed no signs of manifest scurvy. The evidence suggests that the metabolic aberration in premature infants is an interrelated function of the level of intake of the aromatic amino acids, phenylalanine

1 Assistance in this work was given by the Children's Bureau, U. S. Department of Labor.

2 S. Z. Levine, *Am. Jour. Dis. Child.*, 58: 674, 1939.

3 G. Medes, *Biochem. Jour.*, 26: 917, 1932.

4 K. Closs and A. Fölling, *Ztschr. f. physiol. Chem.*, 254: 258, 1938.

5 O. Folin and V. Ciocalteu, *Jour. Biol. Chem.*, 73: 627, 1927.

6 R. R. Sealock and H. E. Silberstein, Science, 90: 517, 1939.

7 E. Alderhalden, *Fermentforschung*, 15: 522, 1938.

8 R. L. Mindlin and A. M. Butler, *Jour. Biol. Chem.*, 122: 673, 1938.

and tyrosine, and the degree of saturation of the tissues with vitamin C. Whether the same metabolic error is present in full-term infants under similar dietary conditions or in older infants with manifest scurvy is at present being investigated. Studies are also under way to determine the specificity of vitamin C in remedying the defect. The spontaneous occurrence of hydroxyphenyl compounds in the urine of premature infants fed cow's milk deficient in vitamin C affords the opportunity of studying the intermediary metabolism of aromatic amino acids in the growing human organism.

S. Z. LEVINE
ELEANOR MARPLES
H. H. GORDON

NEW YORK HOSPITAL AND THE
DEPARTMENT OF PEDIATRICS,
CORNELL UNIVERSITY MEDICAL COLLEGE

## REACTION OF VARIOLA VACCINE VIRUS TO ROENTGEN RAYS[1]

ROENTGEN ray irradiation of variola vaccine virus particles causes a reduction in number of active particles. The rate of inactivation proceeds exponentially.

Vaccinia virus[2] for irradiation was extracted from infected rabbit testis preserved in glycerine, by grinding the testis in sand and diluting it 1:10 with Locke's solution. After centrifuging, 0.75 cc of the supernatant solution which carried the virus was exposed to x-rays from a copper target tube.[3] The mean effective wave-length of this radiation was found to be 1.5 Å. The reduction in the velocity of virus inactivation was determined by titration experiments in which 0.1 cc of the irradiated and the control virus suspensions were inoculated intradermally into normal rabbits. Estimates of the infectious particles, remaining after irradiation, were made from those tests in the dilution series which gave both positive and negative takes.[4]

The inactivation curves of three experiments, in which vaccinia virus was irradiated with increasing dosages of x-rays, are plotted in Fig. 1. The logarithms of the numbers of infectious particles are the ordinates of the graph. The abscissae represent the Roentgen units of irradiation incident to the surface of the virus solution. Each curve is evidently linear

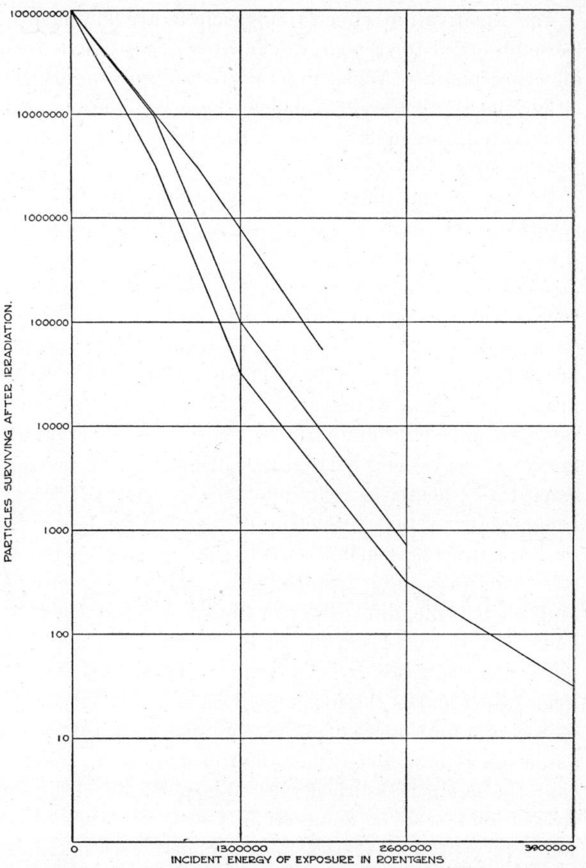


FIG. 1. Survival ratios of vaccinia virus treated with Roentgen rays of 1.5 Å.

in its trend; the inactivation of virus particles begins when irradiation commences. The small quantitative differences in the slope constants which do occur are partly accounted for by small variations in the Roentgen units in each experiment.

The linear nature of the raw data when plotted on the semi-logarithmic coordinates, and the absence of any initial lag during the inactivation of the virus is expected if we assume that one unit of radiant energy is sufficient to inactivate an infectious unit of the virus. The curve form would further postulate that the ultimate virus particles are held separate and distinct from each other in the water suspension when irradiation takes place—not in any conglomerate of particles —for if they were conglomerate the entities would require more than one unit of x-ray energy for inactivation and consequently lead to raw data having an initial lag period and a convex curvature instead of the straight lines observed.

The experimental observations are due to the inability of certain virus particles to reproduce after they have absorbed a unit of irradiation. The portion of the virus particle with which we are dealing is therefore only that which has to do with reproduction.

[1] Journal paper No. J-676 of the Iowa Agricultural Experiment Station, Ames, Iowa. Project No. 573. We are indebted to the Fuller Fund and the International Cancer Research Foundation for assistance in these researches.

[2] We are pleased to acknowledge our indebtedness to Dr. A. B. Sabin for the dried virus from which these experiments were started.

[3] L. E. Pinney, *Iowa State College Jour. Sci.*, 13: 269–273, 1939. We are indebted to Mr. Pinney for much other assistance.

[4] K. Iwaszkiewicz and J. Neyman, *Acta Biol. Exp.*, 6: 101–142, 1931.

The inactivation effects on vaccinia are similar to those observed for a widely separated group of viruses affecting plants. When exposed to radiant energy of either the x-ray[5] or ultra-violet[6] these viruses are also inactivated, the survival ratios following simple exponential curves of constant slope.

Curves of the linear type have been observed for several more highly organized forms of life when they are inactivated by Roentgen rays. The bacteria *Escherichia coli, Salmonella aertrycke* and *Staphylococcus aureus*[7] are all inactivated in this manner by various wave-lengths. *Drosophila melanogaster* sperm[8] are killed in like manner. These Drosophila results are of particular interest because of their analytical possibilities. Irradiation of Drosophila sperm by x-rays of wave-length from 2.29 Å–0.01 Å of radium caused (1) death in certain of the sperm, (2) rearrangements in the chromatin (either within the gene or linin thread) which expressed themselves as lethal effects in succeeding generations, crossing-over effects and phenotypic differences of the non-lethal type of gene mutations. Each of these effects of the radiant energy is described by exponential curves. Since the gene which makes these changes seems best interpreted as a single unit, and since the gene in some cases after radiation is modified rather than destroyed, it follows that the energy absorbed within it must be absorbed by different parts of the molecular structure, each dealing with different phases of the gene's several functions. Diverse expression of radiation effects are thus to be expected on irradiating viruses and may be expressed by loss of reproductive capacity (inactivation) and by mutation. Mutation effects and methods of converting the Roentgen dosages incident to the surface of the virus solution to those actually received by the virus will be discussed in the completed work.

JOHN W. GOWEN
ALFRED M. LUCAS

IOWA STATE COLLEGE

## ELECTROPHORETIC STUDY OF PITUITARY LACTOGENIC HORMONE[1]

AN electrophoretic study of White's crystalline lactogenic hormone has been reported by Shipley *et al.*[2] Using the Hellige apparatus developed by Tiselius,[3]

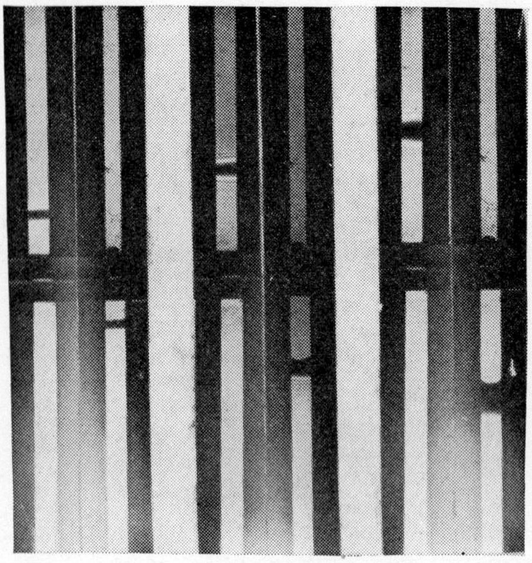

FIG. 1.

we have investigated the electrophoretic behavior and iso-electric point of our own lactogenic preparations.

The lactogenic hormone (L 269) was prepared in

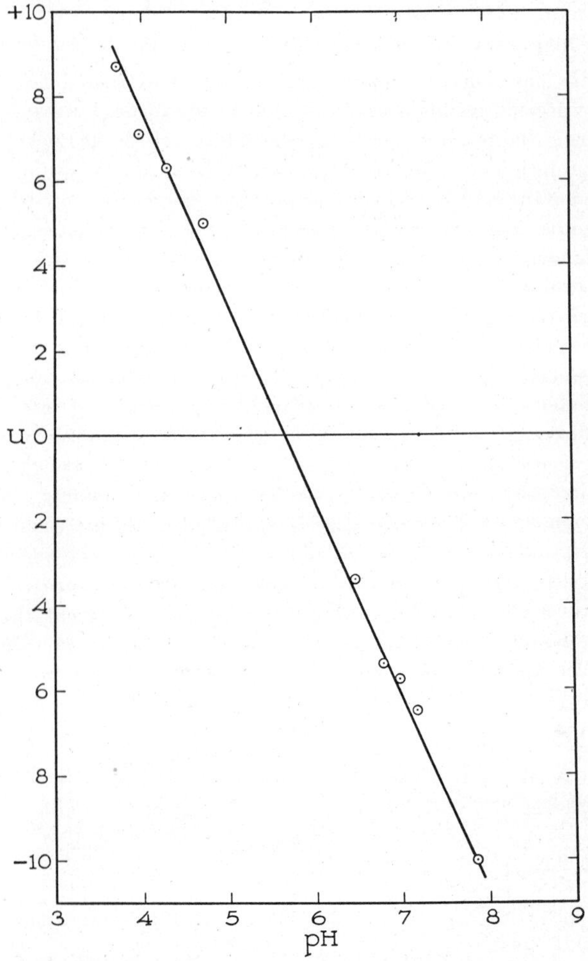


FIG. 2.

[5] John W. Gowen and W. C. Price, SCIENCE, 84: 536–537, 1936.

[6] W. D. Price and John W. Gowen, *Phytopath.*, 27: 267–282, 1937.

[7] R. W. G. Wyckoff, *Jour. Exp. Med.*, 52: 769–780, 1930; R. W. G. Wyckoff and T. M. Rivers, 51: 921–932, 1930; R. W. G. Wyckoff, 52: 435–446, 1930.

[8] J. W. Gowen and E. H. Gay, *Genetics*, 18: 1–31, 1933.

[1] Aided by grants from the National Research Council, the Rockefeller Foundation and the Board of Research of the University of California.

[2] R. A. Shipley, K. G. Stern and A. White, *Jour. Exp. Med.*, 69: 785, 1939.

[3] A. Tiselius, *Trans. Faraday Soc.*, 33: 524, 1937.

essentially the same manner as previously published[4,5] and contained approximately 20 Riddle-Bates units per mg. L 269 also caused lactation in normal, virgin, post-oestrus guinea pigs in a total dose of 4 mg or less. The hormone was dissolved with the help of a small amount of acid or alkali and dialyzed against the desired buffers for 24 hours or more until there was no difference in the pH and conductance between the dialysate and the buffer. The ionic strength of the phosphate or acetate buffer solutions was 0.055 in all experiments. The potential gradients were kept practically constant (*ca.* 9 volts/cm).

The schlieren photographs, taken at 15-minute intervals in a typical experiment with a 0.5 per cent. solution, are shown in Fig. 1. They show only one sharp boundary throughout the experiment. Since Tiselius[6] has demonstrated that 0.02 per cent. protein solution can be detected by electrophoresis, the single boundary shown by L 269 indicates that in all probability no great amount of contaminant, if any, is present.

The results of mobility studies made with 0.2–0.3 per cent. solutions of L 269 are recorded in Fig. 2. The + and − refer to charge on the protein, which is presumably the hormone. It will be seen that the iso-electric point of the preparation falls at pH 5.70. It is interesting to note that Shipley *et al.*[2] have reported an iso-electric point of approximately pH 5.6 for their preparation, although of the 4 electrophoresis experiments made with their crystalline prolactin, only 2 were made with "native" substance.

While it may be concluded that the single sharp boundary observed in these electrophoretic studies of our lactogenic preparation is suggestive of its purity, a more decisive conclusion may be reached from solubility studies now in progress.

CHOH HAO LI
WILLIAM R. LYONS
HERBERT M. EVANS

UNIVERSITY OF CALIFORNIA,
BERKELEY

4 W. R. Lyons, *Proc. Soc. Exp. Biol. and Med.*, 35: 645, 1937.

5 W. R. Lyons, *Cold Spring Harbor Symposia on Quantitative Biology*, 5: 198, 1937.

6 A. Tiselius, *Biochem. Jour.*, 31: 1464, 1937.

# SCIENTIFIC APPARATUS AND LABORATORY METHODS

## THE DETERMINATION OF CAROTENE

IN the study of plant pigments two methods were developed for the quantitative determination of carotene. Willstätter[1] used a two-phase solvent extraction method for separating carotene from xanthophyll and chlorophyll. Tswett[2] made use of an adsorbing column through which he passed a solution of plant pigments forming a chromatograph of the plant pigments with complete separation of carotene.

Many modifications of these two methods have been developed since Moore[3] discovered that carotene was converted into vitamin A. Schertz[4] modified Willstätter's method so that carotene, xanthophyll and chlorophyll could be determined quantitatively. Guilbert[5] modified Schertz method so that carotene determinations could be made more rapidly. Peterson, Hughes and Freeman[6] modified Guilbert's method by eliminating several unnecessary steps which further reduced the time required for making carotene determinations. Strain[7] used a modification of Tswett's method for obtaining carotene in crystalline form.

In the routine analysis of a large number of samples of dehydrated alfalfa for the quantitative determination of carotene any modification of the Willstätter method required considerable mechanical manipulation. Tswett's method, although requiring a longer time for the extraction of the plant pigments, is quite simple, rapid and accurate. For the past several years we have been using a modification of Tswett's method for the determination of carotene in dehydrated alfalfa.

Briefly, this method consists of placing a one-gram sample of alfalfa in a flask, to which is added 100 cc of petroleum ether. The flask is stoppered and set aside over night. The petroleum ether solution of plant pigments is poured on a column of finely divided soda ash and drawn through the column by the aid of suction. A chromatograph of the various plant pigments forms on the column with the separation of carotene, which passes through with the petroleum ether. Some of the petroleum ether is absorbed by the soda ash so that it is necessary to add fresh petroleum ether until it comes through clear in order to elute all the carotene from the column. The filtering column is made of a filter tube with a small plug of cotton in the bottom upon which is packed soda ash. Tswett recommended the use of $MgO$ or $CaCO_3$. We find, however, that soda ash is to be preferred to any other adsorbent which we have used.

GEORGE KERNOHAN
POULTRY PRODUCERS OF CENTRAL CALIFORNIA

1 "Carotinoids and Related Pigments," L. S. Palmer, pp. 202. The Chemical Catalog Co., Inc., 1922.

2 *Ibid.*, pp. 203.

3 Thomas Moore, *Biochem. Jour.*, 241: 692, 1930.

4 F. M. Schertz, *Plant Physiology*, 3: 211, 1928.

5 H. R. Guilbert, *Ind. Eng. Chem.*, Anal. Ed. 6: 452, 1934.

6 W. J. Peterson, J. S. Hughes and H. F. Freeman, *Ind. Eng. Chem.*, Anal. Ed. 9: 71, 1937.

7 H. H. Strain, *Jour. Biol. Chem.*, 3: 85, 1935.

## PROTECTION OF HERBARIUM SPECIMENS

THE use of Cellophane or any similar substance as a protective covering for herbarium sheets may not be an entirely new idea; the extent to which it is employed, however, may be readily determined by a visit to any one of the large Herbaria of this country. It would appear that some such method of covering would find greater application if a simple way of sealing the cover to the herbarium sheet were available. In schools and colleges where herbarium specimens are much used for teaching purposes it is often found that the friable nature of dried specimens is very much of a drawback to their full employment. It is possible that no satisfactory method of fixing a transparent cover over herbarium sheets has so far been introduced, so that the following particulars may prove of service to those concerned with the use or care of such specimens.

The actual covering material used by the writer has the trade name of "Flexiglass." It is a non-inflammable Cellophane-like synthetic substance, perfectly transparent and tough. It is obtainable in various thicknesses from most of the firms dealing with the usual laboratory supplies. From 1/20 mm to 1/10 mm is the range most suitable for the present purpose. If a standard size of mounting-sheet is used the Flexiglass may be purchased ready cut to the required dimensions or it may be bought in rolls for cutting to any odd sizes.

The firm of Offrex Ltd., 15 Newman Street, London, W.1., has placed on the market a very simple type of instrument called the Offrex Edge Binding Machine. This is easily operated and provides an excellent means of fixing the Flexiglass to the ordinary herbarium sheet. Particulars for operating the machine, a very simple process, are supplied with it.

A piece of the Flexiglass is cut to the size of the herbarium sheet in use and the dry specimen covered with this. The edges of the sheet and the cover, in register, are run through the machine and the edges thus bound together with tape. A range of colored tapes is available. An intelligent boy can bind up a sheet in about two minutes if supplied with ready-cut Flexiglass.

The initial cost of the machine with a supply of tape and Flexiglass amounts to about £4. The machine itself will, of course, serve many useful purposes, such as rebinding worn separates, strengthening wall diagrams, etc., and will last for years. The Flexiglass covering will be found to improve considerably the appearance of the specimens as well as protecting them from injury in handling or storage. The thicker material may be used for any valuable or delicate specimens that need to be stiffened as well as covered.

C. S. SEMMENS

DEPARTMENT OF BOTANY,
KING'S COLLEGE, LONDON

## MARKING ROCKS, MINERALS AND FOSSILS

CELLULOID dissolves in acetone in almost any proportion. Both substances are cheap and abundant. The celluloid, preferably clear, colorless, but discarded from other uses if need be, is chipped with scissors and dropped piece by piece into a wide-mouthed ground-glass-stoppered bottle until the solution attains the desired consistency (about that of thin mucilage). More of either can be added if, after trial, the consistency is not quite as desired.

Numbers or name labels are prepared by printing with india ink on good linen paper. Paper can be trimmed from waste letter heads of wealthy firms for economy's sake. When labels are made and ink is dry, use a small camel's-hair brush or even a toothpick to lay upon the specimen a small patch of the solution larger than the label. Before it dries press the label into the solution. As the acetone evaporates a celluloid film is left between the specimen and the paper. When the first application is about dry, spread a layer of the solution over the label and bordering solution and let all dry completely. There is then a "capsule" of celluloid firmly attached to the specimen with the label inside. It can be washed and handled with impunity. A series of specimens may be given the first step and allowed to dry before starting the second step.

Some of the more porous rocks as clays and infusorial earth sometimes release the celluloid unless a little shellac or varnish is first applied and dried.

This labeling material finds other uses in geologic laboratories. It has been used to make impressions of fossils and sections of surfaces by spreading it over a surface and, when dry, stripping it off, thus making a delicate, exact film of the fossil surface.

GEORGE D. HUBBARD

OBERLIN COLLEGE

## BOOKS RECEIVED

ARTHUR, PAUL. *Lecture Demonstrations in General Chemistry.* Pp. xvi + 455. 113 figures. McGraw-Hill. $4.00.

*Aspects of the Calculus of Variations.* Notes by J. W. GREEN after Lectures by HANS LEWY. Pp. vi + 96. University of California Press, Berkeley. $0.75.

BENNETT, HUGH H. *Soil Conservation.* Pp. xvii + 993. 358 figures. McGraw-Hill. $6.00.

BORGSTRÖM, GEORG. *The Transverse Reactions of Plants.* Pp. 230. 58 figures. Ejnar Munksgaard, Copenhagen. 6 kr.

*Cambridge Philosophical Society, Proceedings. Volume 35, Part 4.* Pp. 527–663. Cambridge University Press. 10/6.

CHENOWETH, LAURENCE B. *School Health Problems.* Second edition. Pp. xii + 419. 115 figures. Crofts. $3.00.

LAPAGE, GEOFFREY. *Nematodes Parasitic in Animals.* Pp. x + 172. Chemical Publishing Co. of N. Y. $1.75.

LOEB, LEONARD B. *Fundamental Processes of Electrical Discharge in Gases.* Pp. xviii + 717. 297 figures. Wiley. $7.00.

# SCIENCE NEWS

*Science Service, Washington, D. C.*

## THE SYMPOSIUM ON COSMIC RAYS

(*Copyright, 1939, by Science Service*)

COSMIC RAYS originate within the galaxy of stars which contains the sun and the earth, according to the report of Professor Arthur H. Compton, of the University of Chicago, at the symposium on cosmic rays at the University of Chicago.

Calculations show, Professor Compton indicated, that if the cosmic rays come from beyond the galaxy the northern hemisphere of the earth (the forward moving face of the earth) ought to receive one half per cent. more cosmic rays than does the southern hemisphere.

For three years Professor Compton's sensitive instruments for detecting cosmic rays have been aboard the *S.S. Aorangi* traveling back and forth between Vancouver, B. C., and Tasmania. The cosmic ray intensity received aboard the ship shows no such variation of one half per cent. The probable error of the readings is appreciably less than one half per cent. Professor Compton concludes that the evidence so far is most consistent with the view that cosmic rays rotate with our galaxy and do not come from outside.

Hesotrons—the newest kind of atomic particle found in cosmic rays and having a mass some 100 to 200 times as great as an electron—appear to be created by the bombardment of the upper atmosphere of the earth by the charged cores of hydrogen atoms (protons) coming in from outer space, according to Dr. Thomas H. Johnson, of the Bartol Research Foundation of the Franklin Institute. He explained that most of the mesotrons (extremely piercing component of cosmic rays on earth) appear to come from the westerly direction just as do positively charged particles found in the cosmic rays. He therefore concludes that impact of protons on the air in the stratosphere creates most of the mesotrons.

Dr. Victor F. Hess, who won the Nobel Prize in 1936 for first discovering cosmic rays twenty-four years earlier, described a small, almost undetectable 27-day cycle of cosmic-ray intensity which he explains as due to the magnetic field of the sun. The period of rotation of the sun is also 27 days.

## THE MESOTRON

(*Copyright, 1939, by Science Service*)

WHILE a hundred distinguished physicists gathered at the cosmic ray symposium at the University of Chicago, the meeting has been—in many ways—an honor for a Japanese 6,500 miles away.

Through the score and more of profound, prepared addresses, summarizing the known knowledge about cosmic rays, one word has appeared again and again. That word is mesotron and that is where Professor Hideki Yukawa, of Osaka University, comes in.

It was he who first suggested, in 1935, a kind of then-undiscovered particle which has since come to be called the mesotron. Two years later the mesotron was discovered by Drs. Carl Anderson and Seth Neddermeyer, of the California Institute of Technology, and almost simultaneously by Drs. J. C. Street and E. C. Stevenson, of Harvard University.

Professor Yukawa is not an expert in experimental cosmic ray investigations. He is a theoretical physicist with a fertile mind who had an excellent idea. What he started out to do, when he suggested mesotron particles—then unnamed—was to create a better explanation of the nuclear forces which bind atoms together. He conceived a kind of particle that would have the electrical charge of an electron, a mass about 100 to 200 times as great and—most important—the ability to disintegrate spontaneously. In the interchange of energy between two elemental particles the mesotron was conceived to help in the transfer and then die spontaneously by disintegration.

At this time the "Yukawa particle" passed unnoticed among most physicists. It came into prominence only when "heavy electrons" were found as a new and important constituent of cosmic radiation. Then it turned out that the "Yukons"—as they were sometimes called after Yukawa—were virtually a blue print supplied in advance to interpret the new discovery. For a year the terms Yukons, heavy electrons, X particles, and barytrons battled for acceptance in the scientific literature until finally Dr. Anderson suggested the present name mesotrons that has found general acceptance.

Mesotrons appear to give a reasonable explanation for the extremely piercing component of cosmic rays which are detected deep down in mines. They appear to be generated within the earth's own atmosphere by the impact of cosmic rays coming at the earth from outer space.

## ECONOMIC CONDITIONS IN THE STONE AGE

THERE is nothing new in our economic roller coaster with its ups and downs taken at top speed. Europeans in the Stone Age had to get used to quick economic changes and made the revolutionary change from a hunting life to agriculture abruptly, according to a paper read by Professor V. Gordon Childe, the archeologist of the University of Edinburgh, at the meeting of the Pacific Division of the American Association for the Advancement of Science.

The economics of the New Stone Age in northern Europe, over 4,000 years ago, are being emphasized in archeological studies. In the oldest Swiss lake dwellings of the New Stone Age, the people lived on meat of domestic animals mainly. Only thirty per cent. of their meat bones, left for archeologists to explain, are bones of wild game animals. But later on, nearly half the meat eaten by the lake dwellers was game, showing a back step in economic progress. The earliest pottery at these lake dwellings is pronounced "a magnificent product" by Professor Childe, while later people turned out coarse stuff.

Abruptness with which the New Stone Age developed in northern Europe, calling for a break with the hoary tradition of Old Stone Age hunting life, is seen by Professor Childe as evidence that the idea of farming economy was a foreign importation. This mode of life was worked out, he says, in the Fertile Crescent of the Near East, where

American excavators are now probing the origins of settled existence, beneath cities over 5,000 years old.

Professor Childe is convinced that trade and specialization of industry in Europe began no later than the dawn of the New Stone Age.

"Flint was systematically mined in Belgium and southern England," he said, "and the miners must have lived by bartering their products with neighboring groups. Axes were made from a specially suitable rock at Penmaenmawr in North Wales and exported as far as Wiltshire and Astrim. But the commodities thus traded were in fact luxuries; the consuming communities could have got along without them."

The village of Skara Brae in Orkney, Scotland, which Professor Childe unearthed, reveals to a modern world that New Stone Age people could be self-sufficing, but also the penalties of isolation. These remote villagers lacked timber, but they made their furniture, even to beds and dressers, out of stone, and built relatively large huts. They neither raised crops nor hunted or fished regularly, but lived mainly by breeding cattle and sheep. No trace of imported articles has been found in this exhibit village of a prehistoric adjustment to economic problems.

## VITAMIN CONTENT OF BREAD

A LOAF of white bread which has the vitamin $B_1$ content of a whole wheat loaf, some five times as much as ordinary white bread, was predicted to the food conference at the Massachusetts Institute of Technology by Charles Frey, Alfred Schultz and Lawrence Atkin, all of the Fleischmann Laboratories.

Vitamin $B_1$, or thiamin, is an important factor in nutrition, but it is not stored in the body to any significant extent and thus must be contained in basic foods. Cereal products, mainstay of the national diet, are suitable for this, but these products, especially bread, have been increasingly deprived of their natural vitamin content in recent years.

The problem of restoring this loss, sometimes as great as ninety-three per cent., has been tried along many lines, but the latest and most practical employs a new yeast. This yeast contains enough thiamin to produce a loaf of white bread with the vitamin content of a whole wheat loaf, but without any loss of palatableness. Although made by a new process, the yeast offers no new technical problems since its baking properties have not been altered. Possibility of such a loaf at a low cost increase would be a boon to low income groups.

Research aimed at irradiating yeast to convert its natural ergosterol to vitamin D and to include milk solids to supplement cereal protein and minerals in the "staff of life" were also described.

## RADIO SCIENTISTS FIND HOLES IN TROPICAL STATIC

*(Copyright, 1939, by Science Service)*

RADIO listeners plagued with the roar of summer static may find some encouragement in the results reported by Dr. G. W. Kenrick and Peter J. Sammon, of the University of Puerto Rico, to the meeting, in San Francisco, of the Institute of Radio Engineers.

Observations conducted in the tropics during the past few years have used radio direction finders of special design to locate static's origin much in the same way that we may trace the course of ships. Most of the static received in the United States in winter is found to come from Central and South America, while the instruments used are sensitive enough to detect some coming from Africa and other far-off continents.

Static fades just as the signals received on the same wave-lengths fade. Under some conditions these effects cause sudden drops in the static intensity usually at periods near sunrise and sunset. At the University of Puerto Rico, automatic recorders measure this static intensity day and night, and Dr. Kenrick showed examples indicating a sudden drop in static intensity persisting for minutes or even hours. Examples were also shown of use of static to study the path of hurricanes which may sometimes be traced by associated atmospherics. It was pointed out, however, that this static was usually feeble compared to that originating in thunderstorms in the tropical Americas and, during summer, in the United States.

Dr. Kenrick also showed results obtained in his studies of radio signal intensities and the upper atmospheric layers responsible for long distance radio. In the tropics these layers behave differently than in the North, but despite the small changes in temperature found in Puerto Rico, signal changes due to this radio roof seem even greater than in the rigorous climate of the northern United States.

## ITEMS

THE average person grows up a trifle lopsided, with a right arm bigger than his left. Comparatively few children or adults with equal-sized right and left arms were found, when Professor Clarence R. Van Dusen, of the Michigan State College, measured arms of nearly 100 small children and 77 grown-up college men. While the right is most likely to be longer, sometimes bigger left arms were found. So far as full length of arm goes, children are more apt to have longer right arms than adults, Professor Van Dusen says in a report to *Human Biology*. In adults the more frequent occurrence is a bigger right forearm, that is, longer, wider with the palm broader. The use that a right arm gets in every-day living may play some part in one-sided development. But Professor Van Dusen considers it probable that a tendency toward a mightier right may be a normal growth process attributable to heredity.

JAWBONE and shoulderblade of a small mammal that lived during the Age of Dinosaurs have recently been found in a coal mine in South Manchuria, and are described by H. Yabe and T. Shikama in a report to the Imperial Academy at Tokyo. The creature must have been quite small, no larger than a squirrel, for the jawbone is only a little more than an inch long. The teeth are primitive and simple in structure, from which circumstance the animal has been named *Manchurodon simplicidens*. The stratum in which the fossils were found belongs to the Jurassic geologic period, with an age estimated at between 120 and 150 million years.

# SCIENCE NEWS

*Science Service, Washington, D. C.*

## SUPER-HEAVY ELEMENTS AND COSMIC RAYS



THE astounding picture of cosmic rays generating in the dense white dwarf stars of the universe by the splitting of super-heavyweight elements, nearly 10,000 times as massive as any known on earth, is suggested by Dr. Felix Cernuschi, Argentine exchange scholar at the Massachusetts Institute of Technology.

To generate cosmic ray particles of 1,000,000,000,000 electron-volts, like those which have been observed, requires elements having atomic number 10,000 and atomic weight 26,000. (The heaviest element found on the earth is uranium of atomic number 92 and atomic weight 238.)

In a report to *The Physical Review,* Dr. Cernuschi suggests that the kind of splitting recently found to occur in uranium under neutron bombardment—which makes a single uranium atom liberate about 200,000,000 electron-volts of energy—is possibly going on in his hypothetical super-heavy elements too.

His X elements, or whatever name they may be given, would break down into two fission elements having atomic number 5,000 each. And then these would each in turn go into an element of 2,500 atomic number and so on; all the while liberating tremendous quantities of atomic energy that would appear both as light and as invisible atomic particles (the cosmic rays).

The new Cernuschi hypothesis is not only intriguing because it is the first application of the new uranium splitting phenomenon to cosmic ray theory, but also because the suggestion of super-heavyweight elements would account for the known dense white dwarf stars. These stars, like the small dwarf companion of the bright star Sirius, are known to have a density 50,000 times as great as water. A cubic inch of the material from this star would weigh tons. It has previously been suggested that such stars were ''collapsed'' stars consisting only of neutron particles. Dr. Cernuschi's suggestion gives an alternative explanation which possesses the additional virtue of providing a reasonable explanation of the origin of cosmic rays.

Professor M. S. Vallarta, well known for his work in astrophysics and cosmic rays, was the faculty adviser of Dr. Cernuschi.

Drs. W. Baade and Fritz Zwicky, of the California Institute of Technology, have suggested that super-novae stars (having a brightness of more than 630,000,000 times that of our sun) were exploding stars and the place of origin of super-high energy particles like those found in cosmic rays. Dr. Cernuschi says he is unable to agree with parts of their reasoning as to this origin of cosmic rays and adds that no known atomic transmutations appear sufficient to account for the tremendous energies cosmic rays possess. Hence he calls on his new hypothesis of the fission of super-heavyweight elements.

## THE NEW 60-INCH CYCLOTRON



THE world's most powerful beam of atomic ''bullets'' for bombarding atoms has been generated in the new 60-inch cyclotron of the University of California.

In its first official test the new instrument, whose magnets alone weigh 250 tons, generated deuterons of 16,000,000 electron-volts energy. When the nuclei of helium are used for the ''bullets'' it will be possible to produce a beam of alpha particles having an energy of 38,000,000 electron-volts.

In a report to *The Physical Review,* a research team of eight investigators, headed by Professor Ernest O. Lawrence, describes its success in the first test of the newest and most powerful atom-smasher in any physical laboratory. Nor is the present energy the limit, they say. ''We . . . see no difficulties in the way of producing with the present equipment 25 million volt deuterons and 50 million volt alpha-particles, and moreover we are convinced that much higher energies could be obtained from a cyclotron of larger dimensions.'' Professor Lawrence has already suggested that a 1,000-ton cyclotron could be constructed to go to even larger energies. The present test substantiates in real performance his previous hopes.

So potent is the beam from the new cyclotron that its particles can be observed emerging in air from the target window for a distance of over a meter and a half, or about five feet.

## CHEMICAL USED IN PHOTOSYNTHESIS

DISCOVERY of a chemical that allows the green plant to inhale waste carbon dioxide from air is announced by the Smithsonian Institution.

This hitherto unsuspected substance is a go-between for carbon dioxide and chlorophyll, the green coloring matter of plants. It seizes a molecule of carbon dioxide and delivers it to the chlorophyll. It is therefore one of the most important substances on earth, as without it sunshine energy could not be trapped in vegetation.

Dr. E. D. McAlister, biophysicist of the Smithsonian Institution, made the observation while making extremely delicate measurements of the amounts of carbon dioxide used by wheat seedlings. He found that plants continued to use carbon dioxide for a short interval after they had been plunged into darkness, which was contrary to conventional ideas about photosynthesis. He concluded that some intermediate chemical was playing an essential rôle.

The existence of the new chemical basic to life was thus demonstrated, but so fleeting is its existence that Dr. McAlister does not believe that it will ever be possible to isolate any of it.

Chlorophyll, by the process called photosyntheis, enables the plant to use sun energy to manufacture out of water from the soil and carbon dioxide from the air the various hydrocarbons, such as cellulose, starch, etc., used by men and animals for food and other purposes. Coal and oil contain the sunshine of past ages trapped in this way. Our breathing and the burning of fire use oxygen and pour out carbon dioxide into the air, while photosynthesis manufactures oxygen for the air. Thus the new chemical believed essential to photosynthesis is one of the important links in the energy cycle of life on earth.

## NEW FILM FROM CLAY

THE United States may soon be able to replace most of its imports of valuable sheet mica with an American-made substitute, it appears from chemical discoveries reported to the colloid symposium at the Stanford University meeting of the American Chemical Society.

The new mica substitute is Alsifilm, made from bentonite clays. Its development has been under way for some time and was first reported last year. The new advances and improvements were described in a paper presented by Professor E. A. Hauser, of the Massachusetts Institute of Technology, and Miss D. S. le Beau, of the Dewey and Almy Company, Cambridge, Mass.

The new film can be made thin and almost transparent (looking like celluloid or Cellophane) and has superior electrical insulation properties. It is composed of inorganic materials that make it fireproof. Mica sheet is at present on the War Department's list of strategic materials of which the United States lacks adequate sources.

The bentonite clays are remarkable materials most commonly known for their ability when wet to swell to many times their dry size. One common use of bentonite is for sealing leaks in earth dams or in ditches. Wet bentonite closes the cracks. As it dries it shrinks, a little water penetrates, then it becomes wet and swells up again. This process is repeated indefinitely.

In the form of thin films bentonite is compressed strongly into a permanently stable material which is virtually impervious to water and does not swell as does bentonite normally.

As a substitute for sheet mica the new film may be expected to replace, to some degree, existing imports of this strategic material. In 1938 sheet mica imports amounted to 4,646 tons of unsplit mica and 1,115 tons of split mica. The value of imports of sheet mica in 1938 was $664,419.

## VACCINE AGAINST HORSE PLAGUE

*(Copyright, 1939, by Science Service)*

TRAGEDIES such as the death from horse ''sleeping sickness'' of Dr. Charles E. Salsbery, of Kansas City, Mo., veterinary biologist who acquired the illness in the course of his scientific work, will probably be prevented in future.

A vaccine against the disease will be the means of preventing these tragedies. Such a vaccine already has been used successfully in protecting horses and a modified vaccine has been developed for human use. From 50 to 100 men and women who handle the dangerous virus in disease-fighting laboratories have already been vaccinated, according to information received by the U. S. Public Health Service.

The Federal Health Service, when asked, has advised firms manufacturing the horse-protective vaccine that they would be justified in using the horse vaccine to protect their employees so long as nothing better was available. Within the last month (June 9) the development of a vaccine suitable for human use was reported by Dr. Ralph W. G. Wyckoff, of the Lederle Laboratories at Pearl River, N. Y.

Dr. Salsbery was the fourth to be stricken with the disease in the course of the work. One other of the four, a girl laboratory technician, also died of it, the U. S. Public Health Service has learned. The name of the girl martyr and the laboratory where she was employed is withheld as being ''confidential information.''

Scientists and laymen alike were shocked at the announcement last fall of the first proved human cases of this horse ailment, which has the technical name of equine encephalomyelitis. There are two different viruses, one the Eastern and one the Western type. The Eastern type is more fatal among horses and according to present knowledge is apparently more fatal among humans also.

Thirty-eight human cases of the horse plague were reported in Massachusetts last year, of which 20 were fatal. There were six cases with one death reported from Minnesota and one fatal case in a child reported from California.

How the disease spreads is still a mystery. According to one theory, the virus is spread by mosquitoes or other insects, and some investigators believe that birds, rather than horses, constitute a reservoir of the disease. None of these theories has been proved as yet.—JANE STAFFORD.

## THE TEMPERATURE DURING JULY AND AUGUST

*(Copyright, 1939, by Science Service)*

JULY and August are going to be warmer than average, if this summer's weather follows the pattern determined by many years of observation, according to Charles D. Reed, senior meteorologist of the U. S. Weather Bureau. Mr. Reed bases his long-range forecast on the high-temperature record established for May and June.

May was an especially warm month over the country's great crop areas generally, with a ''plus departure'' of about six degrees for the month in Iowa. June has shown about two degrees in excess of normal. Statistical studies have shown that when May and June temperatures together are that much above normal they are practically invariably followed by a hot summer. Mr. Reed's figures and forecasts are based primarily on Iowa conditions, and apply with decreasing pertinence over widening zones away from that midland center.

Based on the general temperature forecast is a second forecast by Mr. Reed, that not more than five per cent. of Iowa's great corn crop will be caught by frost next fall. Over a fifteen-year period, the average amount of frosted corn comes to 15 per cent. of the total crop, so that the expected 95 per cent. of frost-free corn for this year will represent a considerable gain.

The most uncertain quantity involved in this crop forecast is the question whether the excess temperatures to come during the next two months will be high enough to harm the corn. A let-up in the rains is normally to be expected after the end of June, but shortage of moisture alone is less damaging to corn than too high temperatures even when there is a moderate amount of moisture remaining in the soil.

Fears aroused by a dry May that the summer of 1939 would be another disastrous drought season have been well dissipated by a June that brought abundant rainfall. By contrast with its arid predecessor, June has seemed an excessively wet month, but official figures show only a slight to moderate excess in precipitation for the month. However, soil moisture is mostly in normal condition, so that crops are in relatively good situation for the long pull through the hot-weather weeks ahead.—Frank Thone.

## THE PSYCHOLOGY OF CROWDING AND AIR TRANSPORT



The bad psychological effects of overcrowding of passengers will place a limitation on the size of long-range transport airplanes, it was reported at the San Francisco meeting of the American Society of Mechanical Engineers. A. F. Bonnalie, assistant to the director of flight operations for United Air Lines Transport Corporation, said, "One thing that seems to have definite limits, at least for any long-range aircraft, is the rapidly increasing crowding effect with increased numbers of passengers. . . . The problem becomes most acute when any more than a relatively small number of passengers are involved for more than a relatively short space of time."

The most crowded condition is represented by a trip of six people in a small motor car. About 114 cubic feet of space is available, or about 19 cubic feet per person. This is tolerable only for a group of friends or relatives with common interests and then only because the scenery is changing very rapidly near-by the car. High overhead in an airplane the scenery frequently is monotonous except on those particular flights which may traverse a mountainous region. Over-ocean flying is notoriously monotonous after the first few hours.

It is probable, according to experts, that 19 cubic feet of space for each passenger is the lower limit at which passengers can be attracted to aerial transport. Mr. Bonnalie pointed out that "As the number of passengers increases the difficulty of providing for the human pay load increases faster than the numbers involved. Even the development of airplanes large enough to have habitable wings may not be more than a minor relief. It is also going to be necessary to take these factors into consideration in the construction of terminal facilities, waiting rooms, and so on."

## ITEMS

The flash flood at Morehead, Ky., which brought death and heavy property damage to that little mountain community was caused by heavy rains of more than 2.6 inches in 48 hours, according to the report of the flood division of the U. S. Weather Bureau. The only rainfall station near Morehead is at Pikesville, Ky., where 0.58 inch of rain fell for the 24 hours ending July 4 at 7 A.M. For the next 24 hours rainfall was 2.02 inches, an almost unprecedented amount for this region. Louisville, Ky., and Cincinnati, Ohio, reported no precipitation and there is no flood danger on the major rivers and tributaries.

A huge cluster of sun-spots, so large that more than a dozen earths could be dropped into them, now sweeping across the face of the sun, is disclosed on photographs taken at the U. S. Naval Observatory. The current spots comprise the largest group seen in recent months. Three of the spots, with smaller satellite spots near-by, are lined up in an east-west direction across the sun. Not far away is a fourth group consisting of three small spots arranged in the form of a triangle. All passed the sun's meridian line about July 8 and should disappear off the western edge of the sun about July 15. If they keep their shape they should reappear again on the sun's eastern side near the end of July. The period of rotation of the sun, which determines the speed with which sun-spots appear to move, is about four weeks as seen from the earth.

American aviation hangs up another first with the establishment of the world's premier "windmill airplane" airline, which has started shuttling airmail between Camden airport, the Philadelphia flying field and the Philadelphia post office. Not only does Eastern Airlines' "land-on-a-dime" Kellett autogiro haul 400 pounds of mail in five minutes a distance a mail truck requires a half hour to negotiate, but it promises a solution to the big city airport problem as well. The autogiro can land on the post office building roof. With mail now successfully carried, passengers will be carried later just as quickly and easily.

Radio observations as to how the ionized layers in the earth's upper atmosphere reflect transmissions give a good index to the activity of the sun, according to W. M. Goodall, engineer of the Bell Telephone Laboratories. Comparing critical radio frequencies of what scientists call the F2 region of the ionosphere with astronomical observations of the calcium flocculi on the middle part of the sun, he finds both give measures of the sun's activity.

Special paints that change color when they are heated to definite temperatures are being used successfully in German airplane engine research. While temperature-indicating paints or "thermocolors" have been used previously, engineers of the I. G. Farbenindustrie at Oppau have developed a series of new paints that are reliable thermometers up to 825 degrees Fahrenheit. The exact compositions are not disclosed, although it is known that they are mostly metallic salts. Earlier thermocolor paints were effective only up to 150 degrees F. and the color change was not permanent. They consisted usually of double iodides of mercury and copper, or mercury and silver.

A new x-ray procedure which promises to help in the fight on tuberculosis was described by Drs. Israel Steinberg, George P. Robb and Ursula J. Roche, of New York City. The new method may enable doctors to determine the effect of lung collapse therapy, one of the new methods of treating tuberculosis, on the physiology of blood circulation in the lungs, and even to evaluate effectiveness of this treatment. "It seems certain," the inventors of the method said, "that many problems in pulmonary disease which previously have been studied only in animals or in autopsy material may now be investigated during life." The new procedure consists of injecting a concentrated solution of diodrast rapidly into the veins. This substance makes the veins opaque so they can be seen in the x-ray picture. Within a matter of seconds, the heart and the veins and arteries of lungs and chest of a normal person can be seen by this procedure. Striking decreases in the number of veins carrying blood away from the involved areas of the lungs were found to be characteristic of pulmonary tuberculosis. Other changes in the arteries of the lung were observed.

# SCIENCE NEWS

*Science Service, Washington, D. C.*

## PARIS ASTRONOMICAL CONFERENCE ON STELLAR EXPLOSIONS

LIFE histories of the heavens' most mysterious stars, gigantic and brilliant stellar explosions that are believed to end as almost unbelievably dense but very dim stars, are being explored at an international congress of astrophysics in Paris, July 17–23, that brings together fourteen of the world's leading astronomers, seven of them Americans.

Novae, or "new stars," and white dwarf stars are the special subjects of this congress. Those participating were this week in Paris as guests of the unique Singer-Polignac Foundation, sponsored and financed by the heiress of the Singer fortune, the American-born Princess Singer-Polignac, in memory of her late husband, Prince Polignac, who had been conducting research in astronomy before his death.

Professor Henry Norris Russell, of Princeton University, is presiding over the conference. The other Americans are: Dr. Gerard P. Kuiper and Dr. S. Chandrasekhar, of the Yerkes Observatory; Dr. Walter Baade, of the Mt. Wilson Observatory; Dr. Sergei Gaposchkin and Dr. Cecilia Payne Gaposchkin, of the Harvard Observatory; Dr. C. S. Beals, of the Dominion Astrophysical Observatory at Victoria, and Amos J. Shaler, of the Massachusetts Institute of Technology, who is secretary and interpreter.

Sir Arthur Eddington and Professor F. J. M. Stratton, of Cambridge, England, the Chanoine Georges Lemaître, the Belgian cosmologist; Dr. B. Strömgren, of Copenhagen; Professor K. Lundmark, of Lund, Sweden; Professor Bengt Edlen, of Uppsala, Sweden, and Professor N. Grotrian, of Potsdam, Germany, comprise the European delegation.

The conference is attempting to clarify the life history of a star. It is believed at present that an ordinary star, such as the sun, eventually reaches the point where it no longer can give forth its quota of heat and light. Its internal equilibrium becomes so disturbed that some change must occur. This change may take the form of a sudden explosion. Such violent explosions of stars and even entire galactic systems have not infrequently been observed by astronomers—the star becomes what is called a nova, or a "new" star. After the star has suffered an explosion of this sort, and it has settled down to a new equilibrium, its internal structure is radically different. It is thought that those white dwarfs—faint stars of a type characterized by densities so great that, volume or volume, they are millions of times heavier than lead—are the end products of the cataclysms observed as novae.

## THE SUPERNOVAE

DR. HENRY NORRIS RUSSELL, of Princeton University, in the address he expected to give at the opening of the Singer-Polignac Congress of Astrophysics on July 17, states that super-exploding stars, the supernovae, although they are the most tremendous phenomena known to man, constitute a mystery to astronomers.

There seems to be no escape, according to an advance copy of his address, from the conclusion that "a supernova may reach such amazing brilliance that it will shine for a few days with light comparable to that given off by a whole galaxy of stars. The fortunate recent discovery of two supernovae, one of the eighth magnitude, in time to permit detailed spectrographic observation, has greatly increased our information and also our puzzlement. The spectra, though similar from one supernova to another, are utterly unlike those of any other celestial bodies, so that despite careful study it has not yet been possible to identify a single feature with any radiation known in the laboratory."

Dr. Russell has not given up hope that the problem of the kind of light emitted by supernovae will be explained by known properties of atoms, perhaps atoms that are moderately ionized, that is, with not more than half-a-dozen electrons stripped from them. The energy emitted by a supernova is enormous, reaching as much as 50,000,000 times that of the sun. Two supernovae that occurred within the Milky Way, the galaxy in which the sun and earth are located, are authenticated. These are famous Tycho's star of 1572, the brightest ever observed visually, and one recorded in China and Japan in 1054, which survives as the nucleus of the Crab Nebula, which itself represents the material ejected during the cataclysm.

There are lesser exploding stars, the ordinary novae, which are now occurring with extraordinary frequency. Six very conspicuous novae have appeared during the first forty years of this century, an unequaled record. This happy accident—for astronomers—Dr. Russell attributes to the chance of our position in space because the actual dates of the outbursts differed by many centuries due to the differences in distance from the stars to the earth.

## MEASURING THE CURRENT IN LIGHTNING BOLTS

ATOP the 42-story tower of the University of Pittsburgh's Cathedral of Learning there is a spinning wheel that traps bolts of lightning, studies their electrical characteristics and then discharges them harmlessly through lightning arresters. The device spins at 3,400 revolutions a minute. In continuous operation since June 3, it turned over its 210,000,000th revolution on July 16. In a normal lightning season of 200 days it will come close to a billion revolutions.

The device that willingly and purposely awaits the direct hits of lightning is called the fulchronograph. Designed by Charles F. Wagner and Gilbert D. McCann, Westinghouse engineers, it is essentially a motor and a slotted aluminum wheel filled with laminated permanent magnet steel, projecting like fins from each side of the wheel and rotating through two coils which carry the total surge current from the lightning stroke being measured. As the small fins pass between the magnetic field of the coils they are magnetized in proportion to the amount of current that is carried by the lightning stroke in time intervals as brief as forty millionths of a second.

The fulchronograph gives a schematic picture of the wave shape and surges in a single lightning stroke. This

is compared with the wave shape and surges created by artificial lightning bolts in the laboratory, and can be used to improve the protection of exposed power circuits.

The first lightning stroke actually measured by the fulchronograph was found to last one sixtieth of a second and showed a maximum current of 21,000 amperes, or enough to light 40,000 ordinary light bulbs.

## CORRECT EATING

*(Copyright, 1939, by Science Service)*

VICTORIES over disease in the past have been won for us by others. Future victories will depend increasingly upon oureslves, our willingness to change our food habits and eat what is good for us, was pointed out by Dr. Victor G. Heiser, of New York City, in the eighth Maiben Lecture, delivered at Milwaukee before the recent meeting of the American Association for the Advancement of Science.

"In the past the extraordinary success in liberating man from the pestilential diseases has been achieved largely in the field of environmental sanitation. No great change has been required in man's personal habits. Typhoid fever and cholera have been controlled through the engineer providing man with safe water. He has been saved from plague by keeping rat fleas from him. Smallpox and diphtheria have been made puny enemies by vaccination, and malaria and yellow fever can also be prevented by community effort."

Now, however, man is confronted with the challenge of increasing his own welfare by his own efforts. Are we, Dr. Heiser asked, ready as whole peoples to wean ourselves away from tradition and custom and learn how to eat our own way to better health? Many of us voluntarily deny ourselves certain foods for religious reasons; we are conscientious vegetarians or we eat no pork or we abstain from meat on certain days. Will we do that kind of thing for the sake of our health?

The answer is not easy, the speaker admitted. He told of the dramatic demonstrations of the role of polished rice in producing the disabling disease, beriberi, among the millions of the Orient, of the equally dramatic disappearance of that plague from groups fed on the unpolished grain. Yet Orientals still blandly persist in their preference for polished rice—and still get sick with beriberi. And vast numbers of our own countrymen suffer needlessly from pellagra because of a similar dietary stubbornness.

A really enlightened diet will not only prevent the so-called deficiency diseases, it will ward off many of the conditions that now-a-days make surgical operations necessary. He told of large-scale experiments with colonies of white rats, which lived in perfect health as long as they were given a physiologically adequate diet, but which, when placed on rations of what might be called the "civilized poverty" level, proceeded to develop such surgical conditions as sinus trouble, infection of the middle ear, gastric ulcer, kidney and bladder stones, gangrene, heart diseases and bad teeth.

Correct eating need not be expensive eating, Dr. Heiser urged: "All too often we eat far too much of a substance that is not needed, and still suffer from hunger if a needed substance is not present in sufficient quantity."

FRANK THONE

## ITEMS

WHATEVER federal funds are allotted to tuberculosis control, a large proportion should go for training personnel, is the belief of Dr. Chesley Bush, of Livermore, Calif., as stated in his presidential address before the National Tuberculosis Association at Boston. Not the least of this training of personnel, he said, should be training in medical administration of institutions. In the fight against tuberculosis, prevention and treatment go hand in hand, he pointed out. For example, an operation to put the infected lung at rest may arrest the patient's disease but it also prevents the spread of infection. Similarly a family survey may detect a minimal case of tuberculosis and make this lung operation unnecessary.

NEUTRAL atomic fragments by the billions, 1,000 times more plentiful at thirteen miles overhead than at sea-level, give the first clue to a new kind of atom smashing, Dr. S. A. Korff, of the Bartol Research Foundation of the Franklin Institute, suggested to members of the American Physical Society. The fragments are neutrons, atomic particles without electrical charge that have amazing ability to pierce all atoms. Sending a new type of neutron detector 70,000 feet up in unmanned balloons, Dr. Korff found that while cosmic ray intensity was increasing 100 times over sea-level intensities the neutron intensity was increasing by 1,000 times. Explaining the origin of the stratosphere neutrons, Dr. Korff said: "If a cosmic ray collides with a nitrogen nucleus and completely disrupts it, seven neutrons will be liberated. The presence of neutrons may be an indication of some such explosion induced by cosmic rays in our atmosphere. Cosmic rays are the only agency with sufficient energy to produce such a disruption. Possibly these neutrons are the clue to an important new atom-smashing process."

A BILLION times a second, on the average, a molecule in a gas at ordinary pressure and temperature will collide with another, was reported by Dr. Eugene P. Wigner, of Princeton University, to the American Chemical Society symposium at Madison, Wis., on the kinetics of homogeneous gas reactions. Despite this large number of collisions all chemical reactions in gases are not instantaneous, because not every "bump" between molecules leads to a chemical change. A great many molecules are moving slowly and have too little energy. A certain threshold energy exists below which molecules will not react. This is known as the activation energy. Another reason for the lack of reaction when molecules collide, Dr. Wigner added, is that they may have too much energy. This excess energy may disrupt the newly-formed compound.

NOW adapted for household refrigerators are the new ultraviolet producing lamps which will kill bacteria and keep mold growth under control. The lamps developed by the Westinghouse Electric and Manufacturing Company for hospital operating rooms and the preservation of meats in stores are available as a 1939 refrigerator accessory. They burn only a fourth as much electricity as a small 25-watt bulb.

## NEW BOOK AND INSTRUMENT CATALOGUES

**APPLETON-CENTURY, D., COMPANY,** New York. *Fall Books, 1939.* Pp. 66.

**BAKELITE CORPORATION,** New York. *Bakelite Review; "Give Your Sales the Needle!" July, 1939.* Pp. 15. Illustrated.

**BAUSCH AND LOMB OPTICAL COMPANY,** Rochester. *Bausch and Lomb Microtomes and Accessories; Catalog D-16.* Pp. 15. Illustrated.

**BELL AND HOWELL COMPANY,** Chicago. *Filmo Topics; Vacation, 1939.* Pp. 12. Illustrated.

**DUTTON, E. P. AND COMPANY,** New York. *Dutton Books; Summer, June through September, 1939.* Pp. 24. *News of Books and Authors; July–August, 1939.* Pp. 8. Illustrated.

**GENERAL ELECTRIC COMPANY,** Cleveland. *Engineering Data on Fluorescent Mazda Lamps; June 1, 1939.* Pp. 16. Illustrated.

**GOLDSCHMIDT, E. P. AND COMPANY, LIMITED,** London. *Catalogue 52, Old Books; A Collection of Early Photographs and Books Commemorating the Centenary of Fox Talbot and Daguerre, 1839–1939.* Pp. 80. Illustrated.

**LEEDS AND NORTHRUP COMPANY,** Philadelphia. *Mueller Bridges for Highly Precise Measurements of Temperature; Catalog E-33C (1), 1939.* Pp. 16. Illustrated.

**LEITZ, E., INCORPORATED,** New York. *Leica Photography; June, 1939.* Pp. 26. Illustrated. Price, $0.10.

**MAICO, INCORPORATED,** Minneapolis. *Maico Model D-5 Audiometer; a Precision Instrument for the Measurement of Hearing Loss.* Pp. 8. Illustrated.

**OXFORD UNIVERSITY PRESS,** New York. *Bulletin of New Publications; April and May, 1939.* Pp. 16. Illustrated.

**QUARITCH, BERNARD, LIMITED,** London. *A Catalogue of Books on Botany; Agriculture, Forestry, Fruit-Culture, Gardens and Gardening, Tobacco; No. 563, 1939.* Pp. 100.

**WHITTLESEY HOUSE (McGRAW-HILL BOOK COMPANY),** New York. *1939 Fall Books.* Pp. 32. Illustrated.

**WILEY, JOHN AND SONS, INCORPORATED,** New York. *The New Wiley Engineering Handbook Series.* Pp. 12. Illustrated.

*Readers are requested to mention* SCIENCE *when they write for catalogues.*

# SCIENCE NEWS

*Science Service, Washington, D. C.*

## VITAMIN B

PROFESSOR C. A. ELVEHJEM, of the University of Wisconsin, discoverer of pellagra-curing nicotinic acid, the third B vitamin, reported to the chemical research conference, which was held at Gibson Island, Md., under the auspices of the American Association for the Advancement of Science, that Vitamin B has now been chemically sliced into ten different vitamins or factors and that the end is not yet in sight. He stated that the boundaries of the B complex are still unknown. The B complex is "the group of water-soluble vitamins found in yeast." Liver and whole grains are also richly supplied with this vitamin.

Oldest of the B vitamins is the chemical now known as thiamin, which prevents and cures the nerve disorder, beriberi. Next in line is riboflavin, recently discovered to be essential for human health, but known much longer as one of the B vitamins through discoveries of the dire effects on laboratory animals of a lack of this substance. Nicotinic acid, preventive and cure for pellagra, was the third B vitamin to be cut out of the group by chemical dissection.

The spectacled eye factor is the picturesque way Professor Elvehjem described one of the newest members of the B group. Rats lacking this vitamin develop the condition described as spectacled eyes. Pantothenic acid, acclaimed recently as a vitamin essential for all living forms, is the same vitamin that prevents a skin disorder in chicks. The anti-gray hair member of the B group is apparently a rat vitamin only. Another rat vitamin is $B_6$, also called Factor 1, and fortunately is now identified chemically and available in synthetic form. The chemical identification is fortunate because it helps to clear up some of the confusion about these vitamins. Factor W, for rats, and Factor U, for chicks, and another substance known at present as vitamin M, apparently complete the list of the 10 B vitamins so far known.

How many and which of them, outside of thiamin, riboflavin and nicotinic acid, are essential in the diet has not been entirely settled. The difficulties of chemical separation of the B vitamins from each other suggests that people eating plenty of the food sources, such as whole grains, liver and other fresh meat, and yeast, can not fail to get all the B vitamins.

The members of the group already available as chemical substances, thiamin and nicotinic acid, for example, are valuable for patients too sick to eat and assimilate the vitamin-containing foods.

## FROZEN SLEEP

FROZEN sleep may replace ether as anesthetic for surgical operations of the future. Instead of putting a smelly mask over the patient's face and telling him to "breathe deep" the surgeon of to-morrow may gently chill his patient to insensibility before getting to work with scalpel and needles. After the operation is over, the patient will be warmed back to consciousness without any unpleasant anesthetic after-effects.

Scientific evidence that this picture of future surgical operations is a distinct possibility appears in a report from Dr. G. H. Parker, emeritus professor of zoology of Harvard University. In an article in SCIENCE he states that frozen sleep has long been used in the Harvard laboratories for operations, even extensive ones, on fishes, amphibians and reptiles.

Use of the same method of inducing unconsciousness before operations on humans is suggested, Dr. Parker says, by "press reports of a kind of cold hibernation induced in human beings by a slight lowering of their bodily temperatures." This refers to the use of cold hibernation in treatment of inoperable cancer reported by Drs. Temple Fay and Lawrence W. Smith, of Temple University, Philadelphia, to the American Association for Cancer Research and the American Medical Association in April and May of this year. Without advocating the method as a cancer cure, but only as an aid in treatment, interest was aroused by the achievement of safe hibernation in humans through refrigeration methods which cooled the body three to four degrees below its normal temperature of 98.6 degrees Fahrenheit. Of the many investigators whose interest was aroused by reports of this use of frozen sleep, Dr. Parker is apparently the first to go on record with a practical suggestion for its use in fields other than cancer treatment.

The Harvard method of inducing frozen sleep, as Dr. Parker describes it, is similar to that used by cancer patients. At Harvard the fishes or reptiles are immersed for 10 to 15 minutes in water and cracked ice or cracked ice alone. They are then laid on cracked ice for the operation.

The Philadelphia doctors put their patients in a room cooled to about 50 degrees Fahrenheit, used an air-conditioning unit to keep the body temperature below 95 degrees Fahrenheit, and surrounded patients with ice bags and coils in which ice water circulates. The patients were kept in this frozen sleep for several days. Before turning on the cold, however, the patients were put to sleep with sleeping medicines.

The animals at Harvard, Dr. Parker says, recover quickly and satisfactorily from their frozen sleep at the ordinary temperature of the laboratory and "the animals so treated may be almost at once tested in a particular way without waiting for the gradual disappearance from their systems of an anesthetizing drug."

## SPECTROSCOPICAL ANALYSIS OF VIRUSES

THE first spectroscopic analysis of viruses, ultra-microscopic disease-producing entities, and their constituent proteins and nucleic acids, has been made by Dr. George I. Lavin, of the Rockefeller Institute for Medical Research.

Dr. Lavin investigated three plant viruses—the classic tobacco mosaic virus, the latent mosaic virus and the tobacco ringspot virus, all of them crystallized in the pioneer researches in this field by Dr. Wendell M. Stanley and Dr. Hubert S. Loring of Princeton.

The crux of his technique, as explained at the Conference on Spectroscopy at the Massachusetts Institute of Technology, was the use of a continuous light source, in preference to the more usual source, and fractionation or splitting of the complex biological substances with which he was dealing, a procedure which may well revolutionize accepted spectroscopic methods of attacking intricate medical and biological problems.

Nucleic acid is apparently a rather prominent constituent of some viruses at least, for Dr. Lavin found it in all three of the plant viruses with a particularly high concentration in the tobacco ringspot. The presence of indoleacetic acid was also indicated.

That the amino acids which go to make up a protein may at times be hitched together in a very peculiar way was indicated by Dr. Lavin's study of papain, a protein-splitting enzyme, in which he was unable to find the amino acid, tyrosine, until after the enzyme had been hydrolyzed by Dr. J. S. Fruton.

He has also used the spectrograph to analyze urine, photographing fractions prepared by Drs. K. Dobriner and C. P. Rhoads so precisely that he was able to identify a number of physiologically important materials. Two years ago he made the first spectroscopic analysis ever done of an enzyme, pepsin.

In all, Dr. Lavin has investigated proteins both containing and deficient in aromatic amino acids and with varying concentrations of nucleic acid, problems which are virtually hopeless chemically. He has also examined the protein fraction of pneumococci, the causative agents of pneumonia.

## SPECTROSCOPIC STUDIES OF HEMOGLOBIN

THE first studies ever made of hemoglobin, the red, oxygen-carrying material of the blood, within its natural environment of the red blood cells themselves, were reported to the Conference on Spectroscopy by Dr. David L. Drabkin, of the University of Pennsylvania.

Previous spectroscopic researches in this knotty but highly significant field have been limited to investigations of concentrated solutions of the pigment, prepared by actual destruction of the red cells themselves. Thus much of our knowledge has been drawn from studies not of the substances in their natural environment but of their solutions obtained by extraction, a procedure possibly risking chemical change.

Dr. Drabkin dealt with a rather complicated turbid suspension of the red blood cells which gave a distorted picture requiring interpretation. His results constitute the first accurate deductions ever made on biological material. Preliminary studies indicate that the spectra of hemoglobin and its derivatives are the same within the blood cells as those obtained extracellularly.

The method has already found an additional application, in facilitating accurate determination of hydrogen ion concentration within the red blood cells. This is done by intracellularly converting the hemoglobin to methemoglobin, its oxidized form, and using the well-known indicator properties of this latter compound. Dr. Drabkin said that this unique method of using the main cellular constituent to determine reactions within the cell appears "most promising." Heretofore such methods as puncturing the cell with a micro-needle, which injures the cell, have been used.

Dr. Drabkin also reported progress in a spectroscopic study of protein denaturation which may throw considerable light on the structure of the complex protein molecule. Urea, he found, may play an important role in the denaturation process, for whereas hemoglobin is denatured no more rapidly in alkali than in concentrated urea solution, the presence of both reagents speeds the process some sixty-fold.

## THE WING BEATS OF INSECTS

STUDIES of the almost incredibly fast beatings of insect wings, in some cases as high as 350 strokes per second, are in progress at Harvard's Biological Laboratories as the first step in a comprehensive research program aimed at understanding the physiological processes which sustain this exceptionally vigorous activity.

The investigation, directed by Dr. Leigh E. Chadwick, is aided by the high speed stroboscopic and photographic technique perfected by Professor Harold E. Edgerton, of the Massachusetts Institute of Technology. With exposures as fast as a 25,000th of a second, sharp, stop action photographs can be obtained of the whirring wings or the insects can be observed visually, either stopped altogether, at slow motion or even in reverse.

Outstanding among Dr. Chadwick's preliminary findings is the first conclusive answer to an old scientific argument, whether the speed of the wing beat varies among species, among individuals of the same species or even in the same individual under different external conditions. Dr. Chadwick finds there is considerable variation in all these cases.

Different individuals of his most useful subject, drosophila the fruit fly, for example, vary in wing speed from about 9,000 beats per minute to possibly 13,000 under normal conditions. Increasing temperatures skyrocket the rate from 6,000 at 50° Fahrenheit (10° Centigrade) to double that at 84° F. (29° C.) Fatigue naturally lowers the rate, even at high temperatures, but the fruit fly can usually manage two or three hundred thousand strokes before exhaustion.

Wing speeds of moths and butterflies also vary widely among different species. The common big yellow swallowtails, for example, average about six beats a second, while hawk moth speeds run as high as 90 per second. The honey bee averages between 160 and 220 per second, the bumblebee, 240, the common house fly about 160. Dragon flies, at 30 per second, have the peculiarity that the rear set of wings precedes the front set in the beating, in contrast to the case for other types of insects.

To appreciate these tremendous speeds, compare them with high-speed physical exercises of other animals: man can do a fast one-finger piano trill at about 10 beats per second; the leg of a scratching mouse does about 20 per second; the wings of a hummingbird, much too rapid to be seen, go about 50 beats per second.

Dr. Chadwick is also studying the effects of atmospheric pressure on wing-speeds and correlating his findings with oxygen consumption as a clue to internal physiological activity. Associated with him in the study are three research students, Carroll M. Williams, Darcy Gilmour and O. P. Pearson.

## THE NEW COURSE OF THE YELLOW RIVER

THE treacherous, silt-laden Yellow River, "China's Sorrow," will go on a flood rampage in a few weeks in the no man's land between contending Japanese armies and Chinese guerillas which will exceed the war in destructiveness, Norman D. Hanwell, of the American Council of the Institute of Pacific Relations, predicted. He stated that the river's new course, which it carved out for itself last year in one of its periodic shifts, is too small to take care of the flow of water from summer rains. Twelve million people in the province of Kiangsu, in one corner of which Shanghai is located, will eventually be dispossessed and forced to move because the land on which they live is below sea level and is also in the river's way.

"There is little hope that the river can be returned to the bed from which it so recently fled," according to Dr. Hanwell. "On former occasions efforts to force the river back to its 'proper' bed were under way long before it was able to form a definite new channel of its own. In addition, those charged with the responsibility of controlling the rampant river had certain facilities at hand which are no longer available. Access to transportation facilities and materials necessary for curbing the river are now cut off by the war. The most serious breach remains, it is reported, in the 'no man's land' between the Japanese and Chinese 'lines.' So long as hostilities continue . . . it appears unlikely that effective countermeasures can or will be taken to avert an otherwise almost inevitable catastrophe."

Last year the Yellow River caused enormous destruction when it changed its course, usurped the beds of two other rivers and ended up by flowing through the Grand Canal into the Yangtze River. The Yangtze, itself in flood due to melting western China snows and dykes cut by fighting armies, backed up and overflowed Lake Poyang as a result.

## ITEMS

ADMINISTRATOR CLINTON M. HESTER, of the Civil Aeronautics Authority, said in an address at St. Louis that airlines of the United States hung up an all-time year-round safety mark of 42,000,000 passenger miles per passenger fatality during the year ending June 30. While the nation's domestic lines were piling up 630,000,000 passenger miles, only 15 passengers lost their lives in four accidents. Mr. Hester's figures do not include American flag lines operating abroad. The best previous year-round record is about a third as good.

THE U. S. Antarctic Service, the newest government bureau, denied that its first project, the forthcoming Federal expedition to the Antarctic, is being made to claim South Polar region lands for the United States. It is stated by Roger Hawthorne, its press representative, that the expedition is being made for purposes of exploration and study. Land can be claimed only by formal proclamation of the State Department. The expedition will, however, make reports of its findings upon which the department may wish to act. The new Federal agency, of which Admiral Byrd is executive officer, has no definite plans beyond the expedition, although it is expected to be a semi-permanent government bureau. It may station men in the Antarctic for the next several years, if the expedition and the status of international claims for the region make it advisable.

A NEW highly purified diphtheria antitoxin, developed in England, is reported in the *Journal* of the American Medical Association. Animal experiments indicate that this refined antitoxin is more rapidly and completely absorbed from subcutaneous tissues than is the American antitoxin. The Wellcome Laboratories, England, have developed a method of large-scale purification of diphtheria antitoxin based on a fractional enzymic action. "The possibility that such enzyme purifications may be generally applicable to antiserums demands prompt investigation," according to an editorial appearing in the *Journal*.

BEES will fly in Russian greenhouses to pollinate flowers, just as they do out of doors, according to Tass, the Soviet telegraphic news agency. Experiments in the greenhouses of the Agricultural Exhibition of the Soviet Union showed that when bees were used for the pollination of hothouse cucumbers the crop was increased by forty per cent. over that obtained through the hand-pollination method.

THE first studies of remote interstellar "atmosphere" were announced at the meeting of the American Association for the Advancement of Science in Milwaukee by Dr. Otto Struve, director of Yerkes Observatory and of the new McDonald Observatory in Texas. It was at the latter institution that the studies were made, with a powerful new instrument known as the nebular spectrograph. Three-hour exposures were necessary, using specially sensitized photographic plates, to get "snapshots" of the faint glow of these gases of space, split up into the lines that tell of their chemical nature. Sixty-five such spectral photographs have been made. These gases, and indeed all kinds of drifting matter in the deeps between the stars, are of course very thinly spread out. Dr. Joel Stebbins, of Washburn Observatory, stated that light traveling through one mile of the earth's atmosphere loses more of its intensity than it would in passing through a quadrillion miles of interstellar space.

A STAR that periodically half hides itself behind a puff of smoke, like an automobile with a dirty, soot-choked muffler, was described by John A. O'Keefe, of the Yerkes Observatory, at the recent meeting of the American Association. This star, an inconspicuous member of the constellation Northern Crown, is a variable, that is, it undergoes periodic fluctuations in brightness. Five years ago another astronomer, E. Loreta, suggested that the star produced its own dimmings by puffing out clouds of obscuring matter. Mr. O'Keefe's studies indicate that these clouds are probably composed of carbon dust—in effect, smoke. The star apparently expels the carbon in the state of a vapor or gas, which speeds out to a distance of about four times the star's diameter and then condenses into solid particles.

# SCIENCE NEWS

*Science Service, Washington, D. C.*

## A VACUUM TUBE OF LONG LIFE

(*Copyright, 1939, by Science Service*)

A VACUUM tube that will give nearly eleven and a half years of continuous service, night and day, has been developed by Dr. A. W. Hull, of the General Electric Company. The tube, setting a new high in length of life for vacuum tube devices, is a mercury vapor thyratron which is used to convert alternating current into direct current. Tubes of this type carry very large electrical currents and can be used as commutators for direct current motors such as in elevators. They also are employed in experimental methods of power transmission by direct current.

The new tubes exceed by 100 per cent., in their probable length of life, the famous 50,000-hour tubes which early this year gained public notice by investigations of the Temporary National Economic Committee in Washington. Dr. Frank B. Jewett, president of the Bell Telephone Laboratories, was questioned by the committee about the vacuum tubes, giving 50,000 hours of useful service, which were employed by the telephone company as "repeaters" on its long-distance telephone lines.

High-cost precision construction explained the long-life of the telephone tubes. It was disclosed that while they were adaptable to the average radio set they would outlast the set several times and that the set would be obsolete long before its tubes were worn out. Their higher cost rendered them economically impracticable for ordinary radio use.

Dr. Hull's new vacuum tube owes its long life, in contrast, to a new type of cathode which emits the electrons within the tube. Ordinary cause of tube failure, he explains, comes because the electron-emitting material on the cathode (barium oxide) is gradually used up and finally fails. In the new Hull-type of thyratron there is built inside the tube a reservoir of the active electron-emitting material. Known as a "dispenser cathode" this reservoir serves the dual function of a heater (to make the electrons go off) and as a dispenser of the coating. Some of the new type tubes have been in experimental service for 30,000 hours, or nearly three and a half years.

One tube, accidentally broken at about 20,000 hours, was examined. It was found that less than half of the barium oxide supply had left its container at that time and that half of this half was still within the cathode enclosure doing its job of emitting electrons. This means that 20,000 hours is probably less than a quarter of the life of the tube. This is the reasoning behind the statement that the tubes may last 100,000 hours or nearly eleven and a half years of continuous service, 24 hours a day.

The thyratrons under test are carrying very high currents, 175 amperes, but have not yet shown any deterioration of their vacuum. The new tube is described in the current issue of the *Physical Review*.

## STAINLESS STEEL

THAT the Achilles heel of stainless steel—its inability to resist the corrosive action of sea water—may be protected by the addition of tiny traces of silver, has been discovered at the Massachusetts Institute of Technology.

The new discovery, which should have great importance in marine and naval construction, arose from observations that a salt of silver, silver chloride, is insoluble in sea water. Out of this knowledge Professor R. S. Williams and his associates have found that as little as 0.42 per cent. of silver will cut down stainless steel's salt water corrosion more than 80 per cent. Not only is corrosion resistance improved, but the heat conductivity of stainless steel—another weak point—is increased 26 per cent. by the addition of only .14 per cent. silver, according to the report of Arthur D. Little, Inc. Other advantages claimed for silver-steel is a greater ease of machining and an improved polish. A very uniform and highly polished surface in itself inhibits corrosion. The corrosion of stainless steel in sea water comes from tiny electrical batteries created on the surface of the steel plate by differences in oxygen concentration. A barnacle, on a ship's bottom, for example, might be the cause of this oxygen difference. In the myriad of tiny batteries created by this or a similar process, the formation of chloride compounds of the metals in the alloy is favored. These chlorides are soluble and wash away, leaving a pitted surface. As the pits deepen the difference in concentration of oxygen increases and the corrosion goes faster and faster until the entire plate of stainless steel becomes honeycombed. To the eye its surface may look unmarred but at the danger point it may suddenly collapse.

The function of the silver in the alloy is to make insoluble chlorides under the action of sea water which form a thin, guardian layer.

## THE MATERNAL DEATH RATE

THE death rate from childbirth in the United States is falling spectacularly. While there is much that can and should be done to improve American obstetrics, the situation is by no means as unfavorable as both the public and the medical profession have been led to believe.

The *Journal* of the American Medical Association recently published "an obstetric audit" made by Dr. Scott C. Runnels, of Cleveland, secretary of the Hospital Obstetric Society of Ohio.

The black picture of the maternal death rate in the United States, exceeded only by that of Chile and Scotland, has been much publicized. Dr. Runnels's audit shows that the charge that American hospitals are unsafe places in which to have a baby certainly does not apply to all hospitals. It further shows that the charge that preventable sepsis is rampant is, to say the least, "a flagrant misrepresentation." While deaths from all causes declined between 1929 and 1937 by 7 per cent., the puerperal death rate declined 30 per cent. Hospitals and obstetricians have, therefore, made tremendous strides.

Dr. Runnels makes a careful distinction between the puerperal death rate and the obstetric death rate. In the former are included abortions and ectopic (tube) preg-

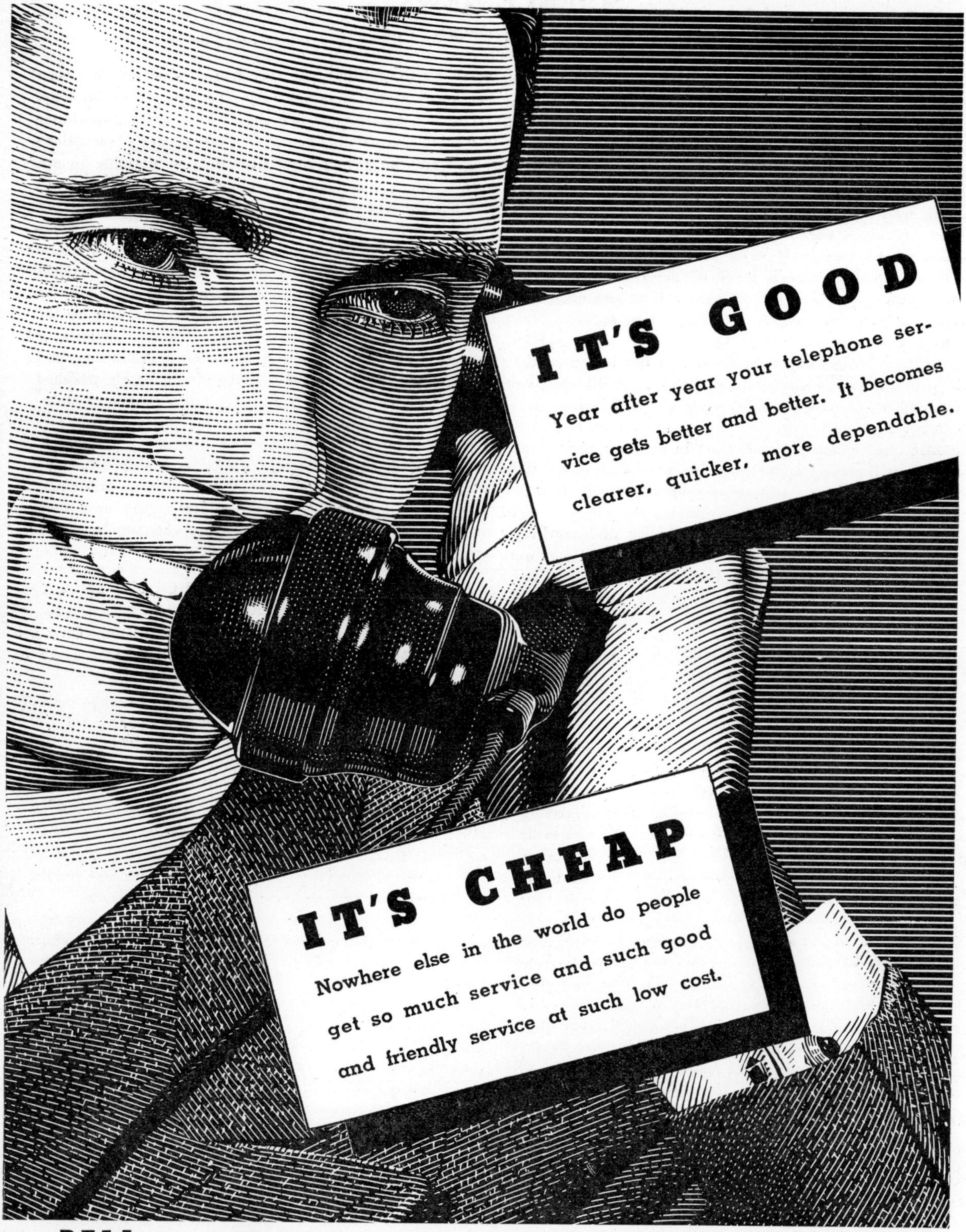
IT'S GOOD
Year after year your telephone service gets better and better. It becomes clearer, quicker, more dependable.
IT'S CHEAP
Nowhere else in the world do people get so much service and such good and friendly service at such low cost.

nancies. Neither of these situations can be charged against the obstetrician or the hospitals. Yet almost half of the deaths commonly classified as due to puerperal septicemia are due to abortion.

Localities show sharp variability in puerperal death rates. In 1938, for instance, the maternal mortality for the states ranged from a low of 25 per 10,000 births in Connecticut to a high of 92 in Nevada, a rate almost four times as great. Twelve states had a rate below 40; ten had a rate above 60. In cities the maternal death rate is higher than in rural areas. Dr. Runnels's audit attributes this fact to the influx of non-resident patients who are taken to city hospitals when serious conditions develop. The same explanation is given of the fact that the hospital puerperal death rate is higher than the home rate. When serious complications develop during labor at home, the patient is whisked off to the hospital.

In commenting on the decided and accelerated strides in the reduction of maternal mortality, Dr. Runnels concludes the following: "Supervision by the hospital of the character of obstetrics practiced within its walls and the enforcement of early consultation in the case of abnormal labor has become recognized as essential. As the births of the United States increasingly occur in well-organized hospitals and come increasingly under the supervision of trained obstetricians, maternal mortality and morbidity will continue to improve. If obstetric conditions were as favorable over the entire United States as are those existing to-day in a quarter of the country, there would be an annual saving of 2,500 lives."

## THYROID GLANDS KEPT ARTIFICIALLY ALIVE



A NEW lead for an attack on the kind of goiter known as Graves's disease has been obtained from human thyroid glands kept alive on artificial medium outside the body for the first time for from three weeks to two months in the Lindbergh-Carrel heart apparatus. The studies may revolutionize the treatment of this kind of goiter, characterized by popping eyes. They are reported by Drs. N. Chandler Foot, Lillian E. Baker and Alexis Carrel, of the Rockefeller Institute for Medical Research and Cornell University Medical College and New York Hospital, in the current issue of the *Journal of Experimental Medicine*.

The thyroid glands were taken from patients operated on for Graves's disease. The glands were immediately placed in fruit jars, the covers were clamped on, the jars wrapped in sterile cotton, and then whisked from the hospital to the neighboring Rockefeller Institute. There the glands, after preliminary treatment, were placed in the apparatus designed for Dr. Carrel by Colonel Charles E. Lindbergh. They were nourished on solutions or media instead of blood. Different kinds of solutions were tried, but the glands, it was found, could be kept alive and healthy for weeks on a completely artificial, synthetic solution which contained only a tiny amount of blood serum, just enough to act as a solvent for vitamin A.

A remarkable cancer-like change occurred in one of the glands during the six to eight weeks that it remained in the apparatus. The change was great enough to deceive a competent thyroid surgeon who examined sections of this gland into thinking the sections were from cancer tissue. No reason for this change was found, and after about one month, the gland became more normal looking.

A hint that the serious thyroid gland disorder, Graves's disease, may be due to some condition quite outside the gland was found in studies of the human glands in the Lindbergh-Carrel apparatus. The changes in the gland that appear in Graves's disease were increased and intensified when small amounts of extracts from the cortex of the adrenal glands and from the pituitary gland were added to the nourishing solution on which the glands lived in the Lindbergh-Carrel heart. Thyroid gland hormone itself, female sex hormone material, adrenalin and insulin were also tried, but produced changes only in connection with the adrenal cortex hormone and the pituitary hormone.

Dr. Baker, in response to a Science Service inquiry, said that "It is too early to say whether Graves's disease is a matter of something other than the thyroid gland." At present she is more concerned with the fact that human organs can be kept alive for long periods in the apparatus.

One of the great advantages of the method is that the organs can be kept alive on artificial media for long periods, during which the effect of the continuous action of small amounts of gland extracts and other chemicals can be studied. "Such experiments are probably of the utmost importance," Drs. Baker and Carrel state, "since this may be the way that certain profound changes are produced within the body."—JANE STAFFORD.

## A NEANDERTHAL SKULL FOUND IN CAVE NEAR ROME

FOLLOWING its discovery in a cave at Monte Circeo, a promontory on the Tyrrhenian Sea, fifty miles south of Rome, the world's most perfectly preserved specimen of a Neanderthal skull is being studied by Professor Sergio Sergi, head of the Institute of Anthropology at the Royal University of Rome, in an effort to uncover new racial characteristics of this early man.

Both Professor Sergi and Professor Alberto Carlo Blanc, who first identified the skull on the scene of discovery, say that it is in an almost perfect state of preservation except for a fracture in the right temporal area. This was caused by a series of blows on the head, probably during a battle with clubs, 70,000 or 80,000 years ago.

In addition to the anthropological importance of the skull, which is the third of its type found in Italy, fossilized bones of animals discovered in the cave give evidence of Neanderthal man's mode of life. The bones include fragments of those of prehistoric elephants, rhinoceri and giant horses, all showing evidence of fractures. The floor of the cave was literally paved with these bones.

Discovery of the cave was made by accident on the property of Antonio Guattari, owner of a small resort hotel at Monte Circeo. While digging foundations for enlarging the hotel, workmen found the entrance which had been sealed as the result of a landslip, believed to have occurred during the last glacial period, about 80,000 years ago. The skull was found in a large open space at the end of a passage in a crude circle of stones. It had lain there untouched for all these thousands of years. Guattari notified Professor Blanc, who completed the investigation, and brought the skull to Rome. Failure to find any bones of the skeleton leads to the belief that the skull may have been brought to the cave and possibly used in a sacrificial ritual. Other bones found on the floor have been identified as those of bears, deer, panthers, goats and hyenas.

According to Professor Blanc, scores of caves and grottoes in the Monte Circeo area were formed when the sea was thirty to forty feet above the present level, and its action scooped out hollows in the soft rock. At the beginning of the last glacial period the formation of ice fields caused the sea-level to drop. It was then prehistoric man found the dry grottoes and began living in them. Slowly a new change of climate took place causing sudden rises and drops in temperature. Alternating periods of freezing caused splitting of rocks and landslips, burying the caves under masses of stone and earth. In the post glacial period, melting of ice caused the sea to rise again, washing away the earth in many of the grottoes, but failing to reach the height of the cave of the Neanderthal skull, leaving it sealed until the accidental discovery.

Following the finding of the skull, the cave was closed by the Italian Paleontological Society, but exploration will be continued in the fall after assembling and cataloguing the bones taken out during first excavations. Two other Neanderthal skulls have been found in Italy, one in 1929 and the other in 1935, both in the Sacopastore region, near Rome, but neither is as well preserved as the new discovery. However, the occipital opening at the base of one of the skulls was particularly well preserved, enabling Professor Sergi, of the Royal University, to establish for the first time that Neanderthal man walked erect, and not with an ape-like posture with head thrust forward as previously believed. The horizontal plane of the opening in the skull shows that the bones of the neck fit perpendicularly into the opening, causing posture to be erect, as in present-day man.

## ITEMS

Discovery of a comet by an amateur French observer named Rigollet was bulletined to American observatories by Harvard Observatory on the receipt of data from the International Astronomical Bureau of Copenhagen. It is eighth magnitude and located near the horns of the constellation Taurus at right ascension 4 hours, 54 minutes; north declination, 26 degrees. It is moving about four degrees northeast daily and can be seen in the eastern sky just before dawn with a small telescope.

The Navy's study to determine if Anastasia Island, near St. Augustine off the Florida Coast, will be useful as a site for a new naval observatory has disclosed that it has already been used for astronomy on at least one previous historic occasion. On the top of old Fort Marion on the island is a plaque, showing that French army officers there observed a transit of Venus on December 6, 1882. Transits of Venus can occur only four times in 243 years, according to Captain J. F. Hellweg, superintendent of the U. S. Naval Observatory, who studied the old French marker.

Alaskan Eskimos have already been set to work by the Division of Arts and Crafts of the Office of Indian Affairs making mukluks—reindeer fur boots—and parkas or fur hoods for members of the forthcoming U. S. Antarctic Expedition. Sailmakers in Boston are also at work on clothing made of tight-woven cotton airplane fabric which is both wind-resistant and light in weight. The Antarctic Service, which is organizing the expedition, reports that the Eskimos are being paid for their work out of funds for the expedition. The Indian Office regularly employs them in making similar garments. Other clothing for the expedition will come from War Department stocks or will be bought from the open market. Leather ski boots are to be used for traveling. The men will wear long flannel underwear during the entire year they are in the Antarctic.

The Chinese Government is getting aid from the League of Nations in its fight against plague, cholera, malaria and other epidemic diseases, the League's Health Organization announces from Geneva. Experts in the fight against plague and cholera are now working in the northwest and center of China, according to Dr. M. D. Mackenzie, who has just returned from China where he has helped arrange for the assistance of the league to the Chinese Government. The league has established a transport service to provide these experts with the stores they need for the fight against plague and cholera. Health conditions on the road to Burma, China's life line at present, are under the supervision of a league expert who is serving as technical adviser to the Chinese Government. Malaria is particularly malignant in regions traversed by this road and constitutes a serious menace to the transport workers, the road menders and the regions to which the road leads. Much of the work of the medical and engineering experts has been concentrated on this road, at the request of the Chinese Government.

Specific chemical remedies, such as sulfanilamide, will be available in the future for practically all the common infections on germ diseases, was predicted by Dr. E. H. Northey, of the Calco Chemical Company, at a special research conference of chemists on Gibson Island, Md. Sulfanilamide itself and its derivatives have proved successful against a wide variety of diseases of bacterial origin, including blood poisoning, abscesses and sore throats where they are caused by streptococci; the venereal diseases, gonorrhea and chancroid; meningitis; erysipelas; and, most important from the viewpoint of mortality, pneumonia. Chemicals derived from sulfanilamide now under test show promise of value against tuberculosis and virus diseases, the latter being the group which includes infantile paralysis and influenza. Sulfanilamide derivatives reported by chemists working to produce new and better chemical remedies of this sort now number 778.

Identification of three previously undetected molecules of matter, which can probably soon be found in the sun, was announced to the conference on spectroscopy at the Massachusetts Institute of Technology by Dr. H. G. Howell, of University College, Southampton, England. They are the oxides of iron, nickel and cobalt, none of whose spectra has ever been reported heretofore. If found in the sun, these will bring to 30 the number of molecules known to exist there and in all probability in all stars of a similar type. Several other molecular combinations thought most likely to be present have not yet been found, partly due to lack of laboratory data concerning them and partly because the properties of these molecules make detection exceptionally difficult.

# SCIENCE NEWS

*Science Service, Washington, D. C.*

## THE ANTARCTIC CONTINENT

WHO discovered the Antarctic continent? In spite of centuries of exploration, extending back to the visit of Dirck Gherritz in 1599, this question remains unsettled, according to a paper presented to the Pacific Science Congress, meeting at Berkeley, by Dr. Bharne Aagaard, of Stavern, Norway. The paper gave a detailed account of the various claims, among which is included Bransfield's discovery of Trinity Land, January, 1820; Palmer's discovery of Palmer Land, November, 1820; Bellingshausen's discovery of Alexander Land, January, 1821; John Biscoe's discovery of Enderby Land, February, 1831.

Another question that remains to be settled is whether the Antarctic continent once formed part of a land bridge between South America and Australia. According to a paper presented by Dr. G. G. Simpson, geologist of the American Museum of Natural History, New York, students of zoogeography have supported such a theory as a result of fossil finds along such a speculative bridge, but there is little substantial evidence to bear this theory out from a geological standpoint.

While Dr. L. M. Gould, geologist of Carleton College and geologist with Admiral Bird in the Antarctic, advised the congress that Antarctica possessed a unity of climate, life and geographic conditions which are without parallel among the continental land masses of the earth, the surface of the great continent is not all snow and ice. The inland ice does not completely submerge the rocky sub-structure. In and around Palmer Land, mountain glaciers of great variety, island ice and shelf ice are the characteristic forms in which glaciation is manifested. But little is known of the ocean margins, where the ice meets the major waters of the Pacific Ocean. It is reasonable to assume that the inland ice moves directly into the sea over wide areas.

The former lofty mountains of Antarctica have been greatly lowered through erosion and glacial action, according to a paper presented by Dr. F. Alton Wade, geologist of Miami University, Oxford, Ohio. To-day some of those mountains are represented only by their igneous cores. Dr. Wade is also of the opinion that Palmer Land and related islands comprise a continuation of the Andean mountain chain of South America, while to the east in the Australian Quadrant is the great Antarctic Horst or depressed tract of the earth's crust, which is thought to be a continuation of the East Australian Horsts.

Climatically the continent of Antarctica exerts a tremendous influence over the whole south Pacific, according to Dr. Paul A. Siple, of Clark University. While present knowledge of climatic conditions is restricted to only five or six areas where meteorological stations are maintained, Antarctica appears to be under the control of a shallow, glacial anticyclone which periodically exchanges across the southern Pacific Ocean great masses of cold polar air for warmer masses.

## PAPERS BEFORE THE PACIFIC SCIENCE CONGRESS

IN certain regions earthquakes nearly always occur after a fall of atmospheric pressure, and in others after a rise in pressure, the fall being most common over the sea and the rise over the land. This is indicated by a report to the Sixth Pacific Science Congress, by Dr. R. C. Hayes, acting director of the Dominion Observatory, Wellington, New Zealand. He investigated the effects of atmospheric changes on the occurrence of 200 prominent earthquakes in the New Zealand region over the period 1931 to 1936, noting the pressure change during an interval from one to two days before the occurrence of the earthquake. The results, plotted on a map, indicated that sea earthquakes were preceded by a fall of pressure and land earthquakes by a rise. "As a fall of pressure indicates a removal of load," he said, "and a rise an increase of load, it is considered that the results give some indication of the general crustal movements at present taking place in the regions concerned."

TILTING of the ground near active volcanoes suggests the possibility of forecasting coming eruptive activities, was reported in a paper by Professor Takeshi Minakami, of the Earthquake Research Institute, Tokyo Imperial University. Tilting on a large scale preceded by about two months the explosive activity of the volcano Mount Asama, which began on April 20, 1935. The marked changes in the inclination of the ground during the active stage of the volcano clearly differ from the seasonal and other variations. Marked changes in the crater floor of Asama during eruptions were described by Professor Minakami. Two phenomena were noted, one wherein the floor rose as a whole, and the other in which explosions ejected a part of the floor from the crater in the form of volcanic bombs and ash. These two conditions differ greatly in character.

TRANSPACIFIC aviation, using coral atolls like Midway Island as "stepping stones" on the long over-water hops, would probably not yet be possible if the land had not been raised some five feet in recent times, according to Dr. Harold T. Stearns, of the U. S. Geological Survey. There is a "five-foot bench" in the Pacific, Dr. Stearns said. "So many coral atolls, as for example Midway Island, stand about five feet above sea-level that there can be little doubt that an emergence of approximately five feet has occurred in recent time." By "recent," geologists mean the epoch of time following the last Ice Age some 20,000 years ago.

THE Panama Canal may not have been the first Pacific-Atlantic water link between North and South America. Evidence presented to the Pacific Science Congress by Dr. Ralph W. Imlay, of the University of Michigan, indicates interoceanic connection across Mexico during the Jurassic and Cretaceous periods of millions of years ago. This connection may have been through the states of Oaxaca, Querrero and Colima, where it is described as the Balsas portal, and northern Sonora, where it is known as the Sonoran portal. Evidence of prehistoric animals indicates at least a temporary connection between the two oceans during the periods mentioned. The existence of the Balsas portal is substantiated by the occurrence of thick marine sediments

of Upper Jurassic and Lower Cretaceous times across southern Mexico nearly to the Pacific Ocean. The existence of the Sonoran portal is less certain, but seems most likely during the later Lower Cretaceous, when an arm of the Mexican Sea extended westward across Northern Sonora and Southern Arizona at least as far as the present Patagonia mountains.

DISCOVERY of ancient human bones in an Oregon cave, and the finding of man-made articles buried beneath pumice erupted when Crater Lake formed thousands of years ago, are clews to a new chapter in American prehistory, which will force a reconsideration of views now held in regard to the early Far West, is the opinion of Dr. L. S. Cressman, of the Oregon State Museum of Anthropology, who reported the latest finds of his expeditions to the Sixth Pacific Science Congress. Dr. Cressman told of finding skeletal remains of a human being in gravel of the late Pleistocene or early Recent times of geologic reckoning, and said that the bones were apparently deposited naturally, not buried. This ancient American was found in a cave in the Northern Basin in south-central Oregon. In another cave on Summer Lake, Oregon, articles used by man have been found beneath the pumice ejected at Crater Lake's formation, an eruption which by the most conservative estimate must have taken place 3,000 to 10,000 years ago.

## USE OF A CHEMICAL IN PLANT BREEDING

BIGGER and better cotton, tobacco, berries and fruits, with new chemical-created heredities, are about to result from research at the U. S. Department of Agriculture through use of a powerful and poisonous drug, colchicine. Fertile hybrids of economically important plants are being produced, successful plant crosses heretofore impossible are being achieved.

From pioneering experiments made several years ago by Dr. Albert F. Blakeslee, of the Carnegie Institution, the application of colchicine, extracted from seeds of the wild meadow saffron and used sometimes as a gout remedy, promises to give farmers better plants to grow in their fields. The drug causes rapidly growing young plants to double the number of chromosomes in their cells, juggling the heredity in such a way that the new plant created breeds true and is not sterile as are most hybrids. Chromosomes are the carriers of heredity within the cells and seeds.

Crossing of valuable Sea Island cotton of the Asiatic variety and American upland cotton is being undertaken by Dr. J. O. Beasley, of the Bureau of Plant Industry, working in North Carolina. For the first generation this cotton cross produces a form which gives the typical long fibers of Sea Island cotton with the early maturity of the American upland cotton. This hybrid, however, while fertile, goes to pieces after the first generation cross and loses its desirable qualities.

The drug colchicine, by doubling the number of chromosomes in the cells of the plant, allows the production of a fertile hybrid of the cotton that will breed true. To get a true-breeding strain depends on a freak of nature found commonly in Sea Island and at times in upland cotton. It is a twin embryo. Usually one of the embryos produces a shoot with only half the number of chromosomes in one set instead of the regular two sets required for fertility. By doubling the chromosome number of this shoot with colchicine, it is hoped to get a pure-line cotton with two sets of identical chromosomes which should breed true.

Dr. H. H. Smith, at the Arlington, Va., Experimental Farm of the U. S. Department of Agriculture, has obtained similar results with hybrid tobacco which, in some forms, has great value as an insecticide. This is especially true of wild tobacco of which one type contains nor-nicotine, an alkaloid related to nicotine but much more potent in killing insects.

Drs. Haig Dermen and G. M. Darrow, working at Beltsville, Md., have tried colchicine on berries and fruit trees and hope to produce a permanently reproducing cross between Loganberries and ordinary blackberries. Crossing of red raspberries with other berries is expected to yield a variety that will grow in warm southern climates. The work with peaches has only just been done. What its results will be can not yet be determined because it will take a year or two to obtain fruit from the trees.

## THE DEVELOPMENT OF ALASKA

By LEONARD H. ENGEL

*(Copyright, 1939, by Science Service)*

FORMATION of one or more private development corporations like the world-famous ''Hudson's Bay Company'' to people Alaska with American citizens and refugees and turn it into a prosperous ''Scandinavia of the West'' is to be suggested in a Department of Interior report slated for early publication.

A population of five million or more, the report will maintain, can easily be supported in the territory, which, one fifth the size of the United States, now has less than 60,000 inhabitants, including Eskimos and Indians.

It is urged that opening up the territory to large-scale colonization would provide a market for American capital goods equivalent to a heavy increase in the U. S. foreign market. At least half the settlers will be American citizens. Among the others would be carefully selected refugees from foreign lands. The plan would thus also be an American answer to European persecutions of minorities.

Private development corporations like the Hudson's Bay Company, which settled Canada, and the Plymouth Company, which sent the Pilgrims to the then unknown wilderness of the Atlantic coast, have been the most successful type of colonizing agency. One or more of them is therefore recommended for Alaska. Their dividends would be limited and their activities carefully delineated by law. Financing would be entirely private.

Providing that the plan secures support of Alaskans and others concerned, necessary legislation is expected to be introduced into the next session of Congress. Present immigration laws would be modified so as to permit aliens selected by the companies to settle in Alaska. Immigration quotas of the United States would not be altered. If the Alaskan settlers wished to become citizens or to enter the United States, they would have to apply for immigration quota numbers like other aliens. At least one large refugee-aid group is definitely interested.

Sponsors of the plan favor the establishment of more than one corporation. "Competition will be good for them," one declared. Besides, where diverse national and cultural groups are involved, they are likely to work better if each is allowed to work out its own problems instead of all being forced together into one company.

The society the colonists would build would be based primarily on manufactures exploiting Alaskan resources. The industries either would not duplicate those of the United States at all or would produce goods of a type now largely imported. Among the industries are paper manufacturing, lumbering, salting and pickling herring, woodworking, production of minerals such as tin, manganese and chrome ores, fur farming and leather working. Agriculture can supply a substantial part of the food supply of the new natives, although by no means all of it.

A National Resources Committee report quoted by sponsors of the plan indicates that Alaska is potentially richer than Sweden and Finland together. With an area two thirds larger and far better endowed by nature than the two Scandinavian countries, it now supports a population 1/165th as large. Half the population is Eskimo and Indian.

## SLIPPING OF METAL CRYSTALS

Slipping layers of material, such as produce ranges of high mountains in nature, are being used on a microscopic scale here to show how metals behave under severe pressures. In the metallic world, the slippage occurs along tiny crystal planes of the metal.

A research movie just completed at the research laboratories of the Westinghouse Electric and Manufacturing Company here under the direction of Dr. A. Nadai, consulting mechanical engineer, opens with a two-foot strip of steel, white and smooth. As a tremendous pull comes into play, the test specimen begins to elongate like a huge rubber band. While this stretch is within the elastic limit of the steel all goes well. But soon there appear the "villains"; first a tiny black line that runs diagonally across the specimen. Soon another, and another, each time about half an inch apart at an angle of approximately 45 degrees with the direction of pull. By the end of the film the whole test specimen is criss-crossed with a maze of these lines. These lines are the distinguishable marks of slip planes of the crystals of the metal.

Each of these microscopic crystals, containing about 27,000,000,000,000 (27 trillion) individual iron atoms will —if pulled strongly enough—start slipping and attempt to relieve the pressure in this way. Paradoxically the slipping does not occur uniformly throughout the steel bar, but in localized areas and the deformed part is stronger than the unaffected parts. Slip lines must be eliminated in the rolling of steel, for they might make their appearance through a paint finish on an automobile.

The stretching of a steel bar, says Dr. Nadai, parallels on a laboratory scale the large-scale effects of stresses in mountain building. An outstanding example is the Jura chain of mountains in Switzerland, which has been pushed together into a band some eighty miles north of the Alps.

## ITEMS

Dr. Robert A. Steinberg, of the U. S. Department of Agriculture, has discovered that traces of gallium are necessary for growth and reproduction of one of the common mold fungi, and he suggests that it may be proved necessary for other planets as well. Very little gallium was found sufficient for the needs of the fungus—10 to 30 parts per billion of water. No other element could be successfully substituted. Although gallium is one of the rarer elements, what there is of it is widely distributed in nature.

Shocking a patient by electrical means as a promising treatment for failing circulation of the blood is reported in the *Journal* of the American Medical Association. Many a surgeon has watched a patient sinking into traumatic shock and many a physician has observed a patient exhausted by illness, the editorial explains, only to find there is some element in the mechanics of blood circulation beyond medicine's control. Now Drs. G. G. Ornstein, Sidney Licht and Myron Herman, of Sea View Hospital, New York City, have reported a method of raising venous pressure in a case of shock, particularly applicable to circulation failure under spinal anesthesia. Towels soaked in salt solution are wrapped around the patient's body and legs. Electrodes are connected and an induced electric current is applied. This causes a distinct rise in pressure of blood in the veins. The original suggestion that low blood pressure arises from a failure in the tonus of the body's muscles which lowered the gentle pressure sending blood from the tissues into the veins and back to the heart came from Professor Yandell Henderson and his group of investigators at Yale University.

The "mummy" of a duckbill dinosaur that had old-age trouble with its back—ninety-five million years ago—is being studied at the Smithsonian Institution. The big creature had a stiff back due to ossified tendons, or the hardening of some muscles into bone, is the belated diagnosis of Charles W. Gilmore, Smithsonian paleontologist. Old turkeys sometimes have the same condition. "Mummy" dinosaurs, so-called because the print of the rough hide is preserved over the bones, are extremely rare, only about ten being known. The Smithsonian's specimen, from the dinosaur quarry in Alberta, Canada, shows the skin in fairly well distributed patches over the body. Mr. Gilmore infers that dinosaur hide would make excellent leather, if there were any left.

The use of safety plate glass on all the windows of motor vehicles will help to prevent many cases of "car sickness" and the headaches accompanying eye fatigue, according to Dr. A. H. Ryan, Chicago physician. Eye fatigue, he finds, is 62 per cent. greater when looking through safety sheet glass than it is when looking through safety plate glass. The tiny, almost imperceptible waviness of sheet glass, in contrast to the polished smooth surface of plate glass, distorts the vision, in laboratory as well as driving tests. The constant, automatic adjustment of the eye to this distortion causes fatigue. Most cars now have safety plate glass in the windshield, but the less smooth glass is often used in other windows. The tests were made for General Motors' Fisher Body division and the Libbey-Owens-Ford Glass Company.

# SCIENCE NEWS

*Science Service, Washington, D. C.*

## ISOTOPES, THE NEUTRINO AND URANIUM SPLITTING



A NEW way of separating isotopes quickly and effectively is suggested by Professor J. W. Beams and Dr. C. Skarstrom, of the University of Virginia, in the current issue of *Physical Review.* The new method would combine the whirling properties of high-speed centrifuges with the chemical fractionating column method employed by Professor Harold C. Urey, of Columbia University. Isotopes are the forms of chemical elements which have chemical properties so similar that ordinary chemical methods will not separate them. Yet they have slightly different atomic weights. Separating isotopes is one of the major tasks of physicists these days, for isotopes can be employed as "tracers" in studying the physiological happenings of the human and animal body and have already contributed much to knowledge of hitherto obscure body processes. To operate the new method would require a huge centrifuge, weighing tons, for the columns used at Columbia by Professor Urey are two stories high. An apparatus to whirl them around in a super-centrifuge would be very large.

In the same issue, Drs. H. R. Crane and J. Halpern, of the University of Michigan, describe their latest search for the elusive and never-found atomic particle, the neutrino, which is believed to have the mass of an electron, without electrical charge. By bombarding chlorine with deuteron particles from the huge Michigan cyclotron, the scientists have made it emit electrons, or beta rays. Studying the pictures of these beta rays in a Wilson cloud chamber has shown that the ordinary, every-day laws of classical momentum are not conserved unless one assumes that another particle (the neutrino) is liberated in the process. Because of the neutrino's neutral character actual pictures of its tracks have not been obtained, and probably they will never be found. But there are relationships showing definite directions in space in which the change of momentum occurs. This is interpreted as the line of direction of the neutrino.

The new attacks on the secrets of uranium splitting—the potential source of atomic power if scientists can ever find out how to create it efficiently and then control it after they have it—are also described. Professor Enrico Fermi and Drs. H. L. Anderson and Leo Szilard, of Columbia University, report that by bombarding uranium with slow neutrons they obtain a 20 per cent. gain in the number of neutrons emitted. This is evidence—slight but probably real—that the splitting of uranium, with its enormous release of atomic power, is probably accompanied by a chain reaction that creates more neutrons to produce more uranium fissions, and so on. The whole question of atomic power is still in the balance, for the experiments have yet to give a conclusive answer. The Columbia results are more conservative than reports which have come from France. Another new finding is the study by Drs. J. C. Mouzon and R. D. Park, of Duke University, on the delayed emission of piercing gamma rays from uranium excited by neutrons. Taking Wilson cloud chamber photographs of the bombardment out of a great number, one highly interesting picture was obtained. This may be the first evidence yet found of a multiple fission of uranium. Previously it has been shown that uranium can be split into two parts by neutron bombardment. The new pictures may reveal a splitting into three or more different products instead of into the usual two. More work will be needed to clear up this important point.

## ADVANCES IN THE MEDICAL SCIENCES



WARNING that the drug, salfapyridine, used successfully in treating pneumonia, can damage dangerously the white blood cells is contained in a report in the current issue of the *Journal* of the American Medical Association by Drs. Nathan Rosenthal and Peter Vogel, of New York City. They found granulocytopenia in three children treated with the drug. Sulfanilamide also causes the trouble, and cases caused by sulfapyridine have previously been reported in adults. Careful tests of blood for possible danger signs are advised when the drug is being used.

A unique case of a Japanese beetle feeding on the ear drum of a man is reported by Dr. Max Kimbrig, of Huntington, N. Y. The legs or biting equipment of the beetle were stuck fast in the ear drum when Dr. Kimbrig removed it, and a large part of the drum was perforated. Dr. Kimbrig writes: "Since the Japanese beetle is herbivorous, it is difficult to understand his appetite for human ear drums. I have been unable to find in the literature any report of the destruction of an ear drum by a beetle that lives on plants."

The recent report of Drs. Fritz Kogl and Hanni Erxleben, of Holland, that they had found unnatural forms of amino acids in malignant tissues, is given notice in the *Journal* of the American Medical Association, an editorial stating that if confirmed by other workers and if all types of cancer tissues contain them "a new and fertile field for study into the nature of cancer will be opened."

Stating that vitamin F has not been established as a vitamin although it has been commercialized by firms marketing cosmetics, a committee of the American Medical Association has endorsed the elimination of the term by the American Society of Biological Chemists and the American Institute of Nutrition. Reduction of the number of vitamin A and D preparations is recommended. Even since the committee on vitamins made its most recent report, the *Journal* observes that "vitamin $B_6$ has been synthesized, the chemistry of vitamin K has been clarified to a considerable extent, and evidence has accumulated concerning the significance of these factors and of riboflavin in human nutrition."

## THE CONGRESS OF AMERICANISTS IN MEXICO CITY

*(Copyright, 1939, by Science Service)*

NEWS of prehistoric America—its buildings concealed beneath buildings; its fortune-telling mothers; its first, all-but-wild corn crops—the latest scientific discoveries on these and several hundred more angles of ancient Americans are being reported in a barrage of papers read before the International Congress of Americanists in Mexico City.

Discovery of a temple which has been concealed for hundreds of years beneath the famous lofty Mayan temple "El Castillo," at Chichen Itza, was reported by José A. Erosa Peniche. The stairway, façade and chambers of this ancient building, which Mayan Indian architects covered over to raise a higher, more impressive temple on the lofty pyramid base, were found by tunneling beneath the present structure, to avoid damaging it. Other archeologists told of probing other Indian monumental buildings in similar fashion, as Mexico burrows deeper beneath the visible present.

Mayan Indians, greatest scholars of ancient America, knew exactly when to introduce inter-calendar days necessary to keep their year in step with the sun, according to Erwin P. Dieselforff, of Copan, Guatemala. He states that eclipses of the sun were of major interest to these ancient American astronomers, explaining the Mayan method of forecasting when eclipses would occur.

Mayan Indian mothers consulted astrologers in their anxiety to know what good fortune or bad might be the destiny of their babies. Four of the lists of days and their omens, found in the books of Chilam Balam, have been studied by Alfredo Barrera Vázquez, of the National Museum at Mexico City, and he has concluded that the custom of guarding babies' fortunes by giving them calendar names up to a certain age was used by Mayan mothers of Yucatan, as well as by those in Indian nations of Mexico proper.

Tackling the much-argued question of when the first corn was raised by the first New World farmers, Pablo Martínez del Rio advanced the theory that agriculture may have had a more rapid rise in America than in the Old World. Differences in methods of seed selection and cultivation, he believes, speeded up results for Indian farmers, so that it is not necessary to conclude, as some botanists have, that American Indians must have started on their road to higher civilization an extraordinarily long time back.

The newest excavations at Monte Alban, Mexico, scene of the discovery of a Treasure Tomb a few years ago, have demonstrated who built the mountain-top city. Indians of the same cultural heritage built both Monte Alban and the remarkable valley city of Milta not far away. Architectural ideas are the same in both cities, according to Dr. Alfonso Caso, director of Monte Alban excavations. Three stages of Monte Alban's ancient history have been traced, and can be linked in time with Mexico's cultural stages of the Archaic, older than the Christian era, then Teotihuacan or Toltec, and Aztec.

The effort to find out what was going on in different parts of Middle America, during its great Indian era, have led archeologists to explore pit tombs near Guatemala City. Dr. A. V. Kidder, of the Carnegie Institution of Washington, reported finding that these tomb-builders were living while Monte Alban in southern Mexico was in its middle stage, and the great Toltec Indian civilization in central Mexico was nearing its decline. Pottery from the Guatemalan tombs provides the key for linking the tomb builders with other tropical American cultures and drawing Central America more closely into the picture.

Success in finding one of the missing stone statues from Tiahuanaco, Bolivia, which a French traveler carried off to Europe a century ago, was reported by Henri Lehmann. Modern investigators have never seen these statues, he said, but one of them, a statue combining human and animal features, has been found and placed at the Gate of the Sun in Tiahuanaco.

## CORAL REEFS IN THE PACIFIC

CORAL reefs 1,200 miles long, extending as far as 150 miles from the coast line and sheltering huge clams four feet long and weighing more than a hundred pounds, were described by Professor C. M. Yonge, of the University of Bristol, England, speaking before the Sixth Pacific Science Congress meeting at Palo Alto on August 9.

"No ocean contains so rich a growth of coral reefs as does the Pacific," he told the congress. "Fringing reefs bound the land within the tropics especially along its western shores and atolls are scattered far and wide throughout the South Seas. But the greatest coral formation of all is the Great Barrier Reef of Australia. This immense series of reefs extends along the northeastern shores of Australia from the tropic of Capricorn in the south almost to the shores of New Guinea in the north, for a total distance of more than 1,200 miles. It is made up of thousands of individual reefs which extend in places as far as 150 miles from the coast."

The biology of the corals which form these reefs was examined by the Great Barrier Reef Expedition, which worked for more than a year in 1928–29 on a small coral island midway between the outer reef and the mainland.

"Corals are essentially sea anemones which have acquired the power of forming massive limey skeletons," Professor Yonge explained. Many grow to a great size, forming colonies which may be rounded and massive, branching and tree-like, or flat encrusting sheets, according to the region where they grow. Corals of the first type are found especially on the exposed outer surface of reefs, those of the second type in sheltered water in the lee of reefs, and of the third type on the summits of reefs where the surf sweeps over when the tide is out.

"Corals are all carnivorous. They feed, usually by means of delicate tentacles armed with batteries of stinging cells, on the minute animals which drift in the surface waters. Most corals only expand by night when alone; this animal life is abundant near the surface.

"Within their tissues are contained countless numbers of minute plants called zooxanthellae. It had been thought that these contribute to the food of corals, but this was found not to be the case. They do automatically remove the waste products formed by the corals and in this way probably aid in the remarkable rate of growth possessed by corals. These can frequently double the bulk of their skeletons in six to twelve months, and it is this rapid growth which has made possible the formation of reefs many miles in length, of great depth and thickness, which are capable not only of resisting the destructive action of the Pacific breakers, but of actually growing out against the full fury of the sea.

"Corals are among the most successful and most highly specialized of all marine animals and different kinds of corals are adapted for life in all regions of the reefs. On and in the reefs live an immense and diverse assemblage of animals and plants of all kinds and many, notably the fish, of great beauty. The most spectacular of all are the giant clams which may attain a length of more than four feet and which weigh more than a hundred-weight. These gigantic 'cockles' are the largest bivalve shellfish ever evolved."

## NEGROES AND INDIANS IN COLOMBIA

A racial struggle in America fought, not with guns, but in biological terms of the survival of the fittest, is being won in northern South America by African Negroes.

Losers in the struggle, Choco Indians of the Pacific coast of Colombia, are apparently doomed to extinction, according to the report of Dr. Robert Cushman Murphy, of the American Museum of Natural History, to the *Geographical Review,* the journal of the American Geographical Society. In one section of Choco country there is now one Indian to every 160 Negroes.

Calling the Negro "the fittest heir of the Choco," Dr. Murphy states: "Transplanted from Africa, the Negro has become, as regards survival, a 'native' superior to his predecessor, even over the obstacle of a greatly inferior sanitary code."

Dr. Murphy points out that the African is more resistant to white man's diseases than the Indian. Also, the African's traditional "million years" of selective evolution in the hot and humid Congo may help to explain why the Negro in Colombia's tropics thrives, while the Choco Indian with a mere 10,000 years of tropical heritage, at the most, is retreating farther into the interior and dwindling in numbers.

Psychological and psychic weapons of the struggle give the African another advantage. The Negro considers himself a Colombian, and the Indian a savage. This attitude stems from the Negro's association with white men, and his adoption of the Spaniard's language and attitudes. Magic power of the Negroes is held in universal awe by the Indians, who fear evil eye power that supposedly can kill fish by a glance or cause children to fall ill. Indians, on their side, arouse fear in the Negroes by their lore of poisons, and their handling and "planting" of deadly snakes to do harm. But the psychic advantage, Dr. Murphy concludes, is on the Negro's side. One of the most horrible demons in Choco Indian lore has taken on the guise of a Negro.

## ITEMS

The nation's infantile paralysis chart, closely watched by the U. S. Public Health Service, shows a rise for the week ending on August 5, when 208 new cases were reported. This figure, however, is well below the median of 250 cases, which might be expected in the height of summer for this disease. South Carolina reported 17 cases, California 57, Michigan 49, New York 13. Early September will see the disease start a downward curve, according to twenty years' observation of its summer course.

That the entire diameter of the sun is now covered with a band of sun-spots is disclosed by new photographs taken at the U. S. Naval Observatory. The band is about evenly distributed north and south of the sun's equator and consists of eight groups with two sun-spots to each group.

The Smithsonian Institution has acquired an implement that had more to do with the winning of the West even than Daniel Boone's famous long rifle. It is the first steel plow forged by John Deere at Grand Detour, Ill., in 1837. Made of an old sawmill saw because other suitable steel was lacking, it was able to shear through the tough roots of the prairie grasses that balked the relatively feeble Eastern-type plows which the pioneers had brought with them. The reputation of blacksmith John Deere's steel plows spread, and presently he and his partner gave up general blacksmithing altogether and became specialists in plow manufacturing. In 1846 they turned out 1,000 sod-breaking plows—a mass-production figure, for those days.

There's no metal from heaven in evidence inside the huge meteor crater in Arizona. All metal must have spattered outside when the meteorite crashed to earth, according to Samuel G. Gordon, Philadelphia Academy of Natural Sciences geologist, who has just returned from an expedition to study America's biggest "shell-hole." About 15 tons of fragments of the meteor, ranging from a few ounces in size to half a ton, have been found in a radius of several miles. Mr. Gordon found that the crater itself, several hundred feet deep, is filled with about 80 feet of sediment. Shells of existing types of water creatures in the sediment indicate that the meteor struck thousands of years ago, when the region was less dry. Mr. Gordon will supervise the making of a scale model of the crater for the exhibition of the academy.

A single determination of high lead content of blood or urine can not be considered a diagnostic sign of lead poisoning although it may be indication of it, according to Professor R. A. Sawyer, Dr. R. W. Waggoner and A. A. Erickson, of the University of Michigan, in a paper read before the conference on spectroscopy at the Massachusetts Institute of Technology. They reported spectroscopic analysis of about 1,000 samples, with every one showing measurable lead and typical random distribution. Seven apparently normal persons showed high content, while two definitely known cases of plumbism showed only average content. The findings were further complicated by day-to-day variations over wide ranges. There is, however, some correlation between average lead content and occupational exposure. The concentration in samples from painters, for example, was almost double that of white collar workers.

# SCIENCE NEWS

*Science Service, Washington, D. C.*

## PAPERS PRESENTED BEFORE THE GEOLOGICAL SOCIETY OF AMERICA



GREAT mud-laden "waterfalls" deep down in the ocean are pouring the sediment of California rivers into ocean bottom basins, Professor F. P. Shepard, of the University of Illinois, told the recent meeting at Berkeley of the Geological Society of America. About 150 miles west of San Diego and far under water is a submerged 10,000-foot mountain whose slopes have been found to be absolutely bare of the sediments which one might expect to find. Bare, too, are submarine canyons off the California coast out to depths of 5,000 feet. This raises the point of what happens to the tons upon tons of sediments borne to sea by California rivers. According to Professor Shepard: "A large amount of the sand poured in by rivers is brought back by the waves which distribute it on the beaches while the bottom currents carry the mud out over the (continental) sheaf into the deeper troughs and basins outside. The submarine canyons are kept clear of sediment largely by means of the great mud flows although currents are partly responsible."

The wide-spread sage-brush of the Great Basin area of the far west probably got its start because the Sierra Nevada-Cascade mountain range rose up and blocked off moisture-bringing winds from the Pacific, according to Dr. Daniel I. Axelrod, of the University of California. By a study of fossil plants he has been able to learn what plant life was like in the Late Pliocene era about 1,000,000 years ago. About this time, Dr. Axelrod reported, a great change in the weather occurred in the West. On the northwest coast, over what is now Oregon and Washington, rainfall dropped from 25 inches yearly to the 13 inches it is to-day. And in southeastern California it fell from 12 inches yearly to the three inches of rain which now falls on the land. The slow rise of the Sierra Nevada-Cascade Mountains probably was the basic cause of this. As they rose these ranges gradually intercepted more and more of the rain-bearing Pacific winds. Plants able to live in the increasingly drier climate prevailed. Sage-brush became king. A few of the Pliocene trees managed to survive—the pinyon pine, juniper, cottonwood and antelope brush—in Nevada. But generally they have continued to exist only in the mountains and on a few favorable sites bordering deserts.

Intensive studies of records of many California earthquakes have shown the "keel" of the southern Sierra Nevada mountain range, is stated in a paper by Professor Perry Byerly, of the University of California. One theory of geology, Professor Byerly recalled, is that mountain ranges are masses of heavy rock "floating" in weak rock not unlike ships floating on the ocean. The new discoveries indicate that the mountain ranges have a keel. Actually the keel seems to be a root of granitic rock penetrating much deeper into the weak rock under the range than does the range itself. Bottom of the Sierra Nevada range appears to be at a depth of 20 miles. The keel goes down still farther.

Fifty miles below the surface of the earth the ordinary crystalline structure of rocks gives way to a glassy condition, according to Professors B. Gutenberg and C. F. Richter, of California Institute of Technology. Studies of the records of earthquake vibrations have revealed this new knowledge. Highly important to geology is the discovery for it has long been suggested that the earth consists of many concentric shells of different materials packed, one around another, like the layers in an onion. "From all the evidence," Professor Gutenberg said, "it may be calculated that certain physical properties change at a depth of about 50 miles. From other clues we conclude that this depth is probably that at which the crystalline structure of the rocks is reflected by a glassy condition."

## PAPERS PRESENTED BEFORE THE AMERICAN PHARMACEUTICAL ASSOCIATION

A METHOD for detecting the presence of carbon monoxide in very minute quantities, as an impurity in oxygen intended for human inhalation, was described before the meeting in Atlanta of the American Pharmaceutical Association by Drs. Frederick K. Bell and John C. Krantz, Jr., of the School of Medicine of the University of Maryland. Oxygen is supplied compressed in cylinders for use by pneumonia patients and other critically sick persons, aviators at high altitudes, firemen, mine rescue workers, etc. The presence of even small quantities of poisonous carbon monoxide would of course be extremely dangerous, particularly in hospital use. The test is made with a reagent consisting of a dilute mixture of blood and pyrotannic acid. This is gray-brown in the presence of uncontaminated oxygen, but turns pinkish when it comes into contact with carbon monoxide in mixtures even as dilute as five parts per million.

EXPERIMENTS with an old-fashioned remedy which has long been discarded as of no particular value showed it to be capable of relaxing cramps in certain of the body organs was brought out in a report by Dean A. Richard Bliss, of the School of Pharmacy of Howard College, Birmingham, Ala. The drug is *Potentilla anserina.* It grows as a common weed everywhere, but Dr. Bliss had to send to Germany to get it in prepared drug form. Experiments on animals brought out its almost-forgotten value.

THE value of sodium hypochlorite solutions for treating athlete's foot was emphasized at the meeting of the American Pharmaceutical Association, by Drs. J. B. Vaughan and H. George DeKay, who reported the results of experiments carried on at Purdue University. Solutions of the chemical as weak as one tenth of one per cent. in available chlorine were found capable of inhibiting the growth of the fungus that causes athlete's foot, when permitted only 20 seconds' contact.

PECTIN, the stuff that makes jelly "jell," is the base of a new type of medicated paste that is having great success in the healing of bed sores and stubborn ulcers. Dr. Bernard Fantus and H. A. Dyniewicz, of the University of Illinois Medical College, stated that advantages claimed for the new paste are that it gives the healing tissue a more nearly natural medium in which to grow, that it needs to be changed less often than the dressings now used, and that its cost is much lower. To the base, which may be either pectin or gum tragacanth, Dr. Fantus and Mr. Dyniewicz add Ringer's solution, which is a synthetic approximation of the inorganic parts of the blood fluid. The paste is applied thickly, covered with a piece of waterproof transparent cellulose sheeting, and the dressing fastened down with adhesive tape. Different medicaments may be added for specific types of ulcers: sulfanilamide for streptococci, ethyl aminobenzoate for painful ulcers, urea when necrotic tissue is present, etc.

## "MELANOID," A SKIN PIGMENT



"MELANOID," a hitherto unknown kind of coloring matter, has been discovered in skins of all peoples, from pale blonds to Negroes, through the use of a new optical instrument, the recording spectrophotometer. This discovery, made in the course of researches by Dr. Edward A. Edwards, of the Harvard Medical School, and Dr. S. Quimby Duntley, of the Massachusetts Institute of Technology, raises the number of known skin pigments to five.

The researches of Drs. Edwards and Duntley constitute the first precise study ever made of the complex factors underlying variations in the color of human skin. The investigation, which may have significant bearing on many important and puzzling medical problems, is in progress at the Massachusetts Institute of Technology. Already the results are enabling doctors to diagnose anemia far more effectively than has been heretofore possible and to watch minutely the progress of attempts to stem its wasting tide. The experiments may also afford medicine a valuable diagnostic tool and method of observing treatment in circulatory disorders and various vascular and skin diseases, and may also contribute to studies of disturbances of the endocrine, or ductless, glands which produce those all-important chemical messengers of the body, the hormones. Disorders of these glands underlie a wide variety of far-reaching bodily ills.

Key instrument in the research is the recording spectrophotometer developed by Professor Arthur C. Hardy. With its aid it has been possible to make speedy and precise analyses of skin colors which are as objective as the temperature readings of a thermometer. Thus not only does it improve on previous methods, which have relied largely on the erratic human eye, but it also automatically analyzes the color of the skin by examining its capacity to reflect light at each separate wave-length, a task impossible for the human eye.

Melanoid is a diffuse form of melanin, long known as a skin pigment. Melanin is characteristic of brunets, and dominates the complexions of Negroes and other black races. A third pigment, carotene, which is responsible for the hue of carrots, has never previously been recognized as a color component of the human skin. The other two pigments involved in skin color, and the most important in producing its pinkish flesh tint, are the two forms of hemoglobin found in the blood, oxy-hemoglobin and reduced or oxygen-free hemoglobin. The turbidity of the deeper layers of the skin furnishes an added effect of light-scattering, which adds a bluish component to the general skin color. Without this scattering, a phenomenon probably best known for giving the sky its blue, the normal skin would appear much like a piece of Cellophane-wrapped, raw beefsteak.

All peoples have these five color pigments. Variations in skin color, from Nordic to Negro, are due entirely to the proportions in which they are blended. Melanin and melanoid are particularly important, for their abundance results in a dark skin and a lack of them gives a light skin. The bodily distribution of these pigments is identical for all races, but the amount is purely a matter of constitutional and racial factors. White men have the least melanin, they found, and it steadily increases in the Japanese, Hindu, Mulatto and Negro, in that order.

The research is reported in the current issue of *The American Journal of Anatomy.*

## SKIN RASH FROM SYNTHETIC INSECTICIDE

DISCOVERY that a new synthetic insecticide was causing a skin rash or dermatitis among the workers who handled it in the chemical manufacturing plant where it was being made for the market has resulted in suspension of operations for the time being. Drs. Louis Schwartz and Leon H. Warren, of the U. S. Public Health Service, who investigated the case, recommend that all insect sprays be given a cautionary label, for any of them is capable of injuring sensitive persons, with damage suits against manufacturers as a possible consequence.

The new chemical is known as alpha naphthyl isothiocyanate. Although not so poisonous to flies as pyrethrum and derris, vegetable poisons now commonly used in sprays, it is so much cheaper that it was intended to mix it with these ingredients in commercial liquid insecticides. Then it was discovered that some of the chemical workers who came into contact with it were getting a troublesome rash on their skins. Investigation by the U. S. Public Health Service followed.

It is not thought at present that manufacture of the chemical must be stopped permanently, especially since the ingredients already used in insect sprays are known to be poisonous to some persons. If manufacture is resumed, the compound is to be handled only in a closed system of containers, filters and pipes, by workers well protected with inhalers, goggles and special clothing.

Finally, Drs. Schwartz and Warren make the following recommendations for all spray insecticides, including those now on the market: "The directions on the cans should be worded in such a manner as to impress on the consumer the fact that the contents are toxic and irritating to the skin unless they are used according to directions. This would place the emphasis on their toxicity and tend to make people more careful in using them. Indeed, placing poison labels on all insecticides would better safeguard not only the health of the consumer but also the financial interests of the manufacturer by helping to protect him against lawsuits. The directions for use should state that in spraying these substances protective clothing should be worn, the face and other portions of the skin should be exposed as little as possible to their action, and that the containers should be kept away from articles of food and out of the reach of children.''

## CORN AND TEOSINTE

(*Copyright, 1939, by Science Service*)

Corn is not descended from the heavy-stalked Mexican grass called teosinte; more likely teosinte is descended from corn. Evidence pointing strongly in this direction was presented at the opening session of the seventh International Congress of Genetics, by Professor P. C. Mangelsdorf, of the Texas Agricultural Experiment Station.

It has long been contended that corn was derived, in some long-forgotten age, from teosinte, largely because teosinte grows abundantly in the wild state in Mexico and Central America, where corn, whose wild ancestor has never been found, was the staff of life of the great Indian civilizations.

Professor Mangelsdorf, suspecting that teosinte, not corn, might be the descendant, tried making hybrids of corn with a related wild grass, Tripsacum. He obtained intermediate forms, that suggested teosinte in some of their properties. A critical re-examination of teosinte disclosed the interesting fact that every character of teosinte is found in either corn or Tripsacum, or is intermediate between the two. Not only is this the case, but analysis of the heredity-bearing chromosomes within the cells of his hybrid plants showed that the germ-plasms of corn and Tripsacum are capable of the intimate mixtures and interchanges that are required for the origination of stable hybrid forms.

As more probable ancestor to corn, Professor Mangelsdorf pointed to pod corn, a strange type with each kernel covered in an individual husk, now grown only as a curiosity. He suggested that a wild pod corn may still be growing, somewhere in the lowlands ''back of the Andes,'' in whose valley and plateau lands corn was first extensively used by highly civilized Indian nations.

## ITEMS

The home of the world's weather—the zone of atmosphere just above the surface of the earth where warm and cold air masses intermingle to produce rain, clouds and hot and cool spells—has now been shown to act as a mirror for radio waves. Professor R. C. Colwell and A. W. Friend, of West Virginia University, describe their studies of radio reflections at the sharp boundaries between hot and cold air layers in *Nature.* The radio mirrors are not at extreme heights of scores of miles in the ionosphere at the place where radio reflections are commonly known to occur. Rather they appear to come in the troposphere at altitudes no greater than a mile and a half or about 9,000 feet. Some seem to occur as low as 6,000 feet. Three years ago such reflections were suggested from radio measurements alone. Now they give, side by side, a comparison of the radio reflections and the existing height of the layers of temperature inversion in the troposphere. Airplane flights directly over the experimental radio transmitter used in the tests during the times of the experiment furnished accurate, conclusive proof of the equal heights of the sharp temperature boundaries and the place of radio reflection.

A successful and cheap method for manufacturing colloidal fuel from coal is being sought, through an industrial research fellowship at Kansas State College. Although colloidal fuel is not now being used industrially anywhere in the United States, investigations to date have offered promise of finding a technique which would be cheap enough to make it an important possibility for railroad fuel and for use in power plants where either fuel oil or pulverized coal is now burned. Dean R. A. Seaton, of the Division of Engineering of the Kansas State College, explained that a satisfactory colloidal fuel would help to utilize effectively the petroleum supplies of the United States.

European sleeping sickness, a disease that has appeared during post-war years, may be growing weaker, or mankind may be growing stronger against it. These alternative hypotheses for its declining incidence are offered by the Matheson Commission which has been investigating the disease, under the chairmanship of Dean Willard C. Rappleye, of the School of Medicine of Columbia University. Epidemic encephalitis, as the disease is technically known, has been attacked with various medical weapons. Newest is benzedrine sulfate, the so-called ''pep pills'' of exam-cramming students. It is given either alone or in combination with atropine. The combination treatment is said to yield best results. However, a real cure seems still as remote as it did ten years ago.

A new type of organic resin material which can be made into artificial silk fibers has been patented at the U. S. Patent Office by the Canadian inventors, George O. Morrison and Aubrey F. Price, of the Province of Quebec. The new resins are of the vinyl-acetyl type. Fourteen different ways of preparing them are described in the patent, which has been assigned to Shawinigan Chemicals, Ltd., of Montreal. Three of the methods yield materials ''suitable for the manufacture of threads of artificial silk.'' Other forms also have wide use. Some are suitable for the interior lining of bottle caps and cans because of their insoluble properties. Others can be made into clear, colorless transparent sheeting suitable for wrapping materials.

Dr. Samuel F. Hildebrand, of the U. S. Bureau of Fisheries, has made a detailed study of the fish found in the Panama Canal when the locks are dewatered, and reports 159 species, ranging in size from anchovies to tarpon, as well as crabs, shrimp and several other kinds of invertebrates. Not all the 159 species are known to pass through the canal. The water changes from salt to brackish to fresh and back to salt again so that both freshwater and saltwater fishes have to be able to adapt themselves rapidly to changes in both salinity and temperature. Not many fish can do this; nevertheless a considerable number of Atlantic fish have been found in locks opening to the Pacific, and *vice versa.*

# SCIENCE NEWS

*Science Service, Washington, D. C.*

## PROTACTINIUM YIELDS TO ATOM SPLITTING

*(Copyright, 1939, by Science Service)*

RARE protactinium has now joined heavy uranium and thorium on the list of elements that undergo splitting into two parts under the bombardment with neutrons.

The cyclotron at Columbia University made possible the new discovery, according to an announcement in the *Physical Review* by Professor John R. Dunning and Dr. E. T. Booth, of Columbia University, and Dr. A. von Grosse, of the University of Chicago.

Protactinium has atomic number 91, midway between uranium No. 92 and thorium No. 90. Its atomic weight is 231. Dr. von Grosse was among the first to isolate protactinium and made available the small specimen that served as the target for the neutrons shot out by the cyclotron.

Chemical separation of the "splitter" products of protactinium's fission show that rubidium and caesium are created. At the same time enormous amounts of atomic energy are released of the order of 200,000,000 electron volts and about the same order of magnitude as the energy released in the fission of uranium and thorium.

The splitting of protactinium can only be accomplished with "fast" neutrons. In this the new discovery is similar to the findings already known for thorium's fission. In contrast uranium can be split by very weak "slow" neutrons.

One hope that lies, little mentioned, in scientific reports on atom splitting and the releasing of atomic energy is that by this process atomic power might somehow be made available in a useful form. It does not appear that protactinium can serve as a "fuel"—even potentially—for such use. Releasing atomic power is possible on an economical hypothetical basis only if each splitting can somehow set off a similar fission in near-by atoms and the whole matter perpetuated by a "chain reaction." For uranium, where weakly energetic neutrons appear to have the power to do this splitting, the idea of "power" from atoms is not beyond the realm of possibility. With protactinium, however, the need for fast neutrons to do the splitting probably means that a chain reaction would not be set up and that power (in any real economical sense) would not be forthcoming.

## PAPERS READ BEFORE THE INTERNATIONAL CONGRESS OF GENETICS

*(Copyright, 1939, by Science Service)*

GENES, the bearers of life, and viruses, that bring disease and death, may be very much alike. This suggestion was laid before the meeting of the seventh International Congress of Genetics at Edinburgh on August 28 by Professor John W. Gowen, of the Iowa State College. Professor Gowen also told of his use of x-rays as measuring tools, to get an estimate of the size of both these types of vitally important particles, which are too small to see with even the most powerful of microscopes. He found the virus particles to be super-sized molecules, with a molecular weight of approximately 16 million. This is in fairly close agreement with measurements obtained by other means. Regarding the possible essential similarity between genes and virus particles, the American scientist said: "Possibly the only difference between these small viruses and the gene is that the latter is attributed a place in the cell chromatin whereas the former is free to move, making its isolation in relatively pure form possible. But even this difference is likely to break down. With better techniques of recognizing gene effects, these substances may very possibly be found within the cell cytoplasm or even in the circulation of the animal or plant."

DEFINITE hereditary physiological traits go along with visible bodily character in different breeds of fowl, according to Professor F. B. Hutt, of Cornell University. Thus, White Leghorn hens lay thicker-shelled eggs than do heavier breeds like Plymouth Rocks or Rhode Island Reds, and they adjust more readily to changes in outside temperature. Inheritance of abnormalities in fowls, producing the seldom-seen "freak" breeds, such as Creeper and Dark Cornish, were reported by Professor Walter Landauer, of the Connecticut Agricultural Experiment Station. In these breeds there is a hereditary shortening of the leg and wing bones, producing a kind of Dachshund-in-feathers effect. In the purest-bred (homozygous) specimens this shortening extends to other bones, and the phenomenon may be so pronounced that the chick is unable to hatch at all, but dies within the shell.

SOME of the strangest cells ever seen through a microscope were described by Dr. Charles A. Berger, S.J., of Woodstock College. If twice or four times the normal number of the heredity-bearing chromosomes are found in the cells of an animal or plant, that is considered something worth mentioning at a scientific meeting. But Dr. Berger has found cells in the lining of the digestive tract of mosquito larvae that have 48, 96 and once in a while even 192 times the normal chromosome number. Ordinarily a doubling in chromosome number within a cell is the preface to division into two cells. But these strange cells in the mosquito "wigglers" just pile up their chromosome counts without dividing. Finally, when the larva is preparing to change into a winged adult, the divisions appear all at once, and the chromosome numbers go back to normal in the new cells.

IT is hard to think of an insect no bigger than a gnat being afflicted with tumors. Yet such is the case. Professor Mary B. Stark, of the New York Medical College, told of such growths which she has studied in the larval stage of Drosophila, the gnat-sized fly that is the favorite animal of geneticists. In certain strains of Drosophila these tumors appear generation after generation, in the digestive tract. They are sex-linked, appearing only in males—and they kill half of these. In another strain, the tumors appear in both sexes, but are not lethal.

FAILURE to grow a full set of teeth is a hereditary trait,

that "runs in families," and it is linked to hair color, according to Dr. Barbara S. Burks, of the Carnegie Institution of Washington. Tooth deficiency may manifest itself in any of the teeth: incisors, pre-molars, molars. Perhaps the commonest form is the failure to develop third molars or wisdom teeth. This is due to the same genetic factor that causes failure to grow teeth farther forward in the jaw. Sometimes, instead of a total absence of a tooth, the deficiency will be expressed by the growth of a very small, almost rudimentary tooth—a "peg" or "rice" tooth. Study of all available family histories, supplemented by examination of all brother-and-sister combinations exhibiting the deficiency that could be found, indicates that tooth deficiency and hair color are linked. That is, members of a family strain exhibiting tooth deficiency tend to have the same color of hair.

SUDDEN shocks of heat or cold speed the production of the abrupt evolutionary changes known as mutations, was reported by Dr. H. H. Plough, of Amherst College. With his colleagues, Drs. George P. Child and Philip T. Ives, Dr. Plough subjected the small insects, Drosophila, to quick jumps and drops in temperature. Mutations appeared at considerably higher rates than they did in control groups of the insects kept at ordinary temperature levels.

## ITEMS

SUN-SPOT groups so large they can be seen with the unaided eye behind smoked glasses are now visible according to photographs taken by the U. S. Naval Observatory. Eighty spots are seen in all, arranged in seven groups. The total area of the spots covers 41.5 square degrees on the sun's surface. Since a square degree on the sun amounts to 725,000,000 square miles, the total sun-spot area now visible is about 30,000,000,000 square miles. Over 600 "earths" could be dropped into the sun-spot area that may now be seen.

PERSIMMON wilt, the new and deadly enemy of persimmon trees, has crossed the Mississippi. It has been found as far west as Oklahoma, by Drs. K. Starr Chester and W. W. Ray, of Oklahoma Agricultural and Mechanical College. Persimmon trees have a threefold importance: their wood is ideal for golf club heads and similar small objects, their fruit is one of the most important wildlife foods, and their tough, ropelike roots made them favorites with soil conservation workers as plantings to check erosion. The disease is caused by a fungus known as Cephalosporium. Its course is terribly rapid; trees usually die within a few weeks after they are attacked. There is no known cure or preventive. It is quite possible that all the persimmons of America may join the chestnut trees, wiped out by the chestnut blight several decades ago.

AMERICA'S medical schools are in better shape now than ever before to educate medical practitioners, with the aid of intern training hospitals, according to a report of the council on medical education and hospitals of the American Medical Association. In the past five years, millions of dollars have been spent to improve organization, equipment and resources of medical schools. Among the 67 approved medical schools, 24 of the lower ranking schools have added more than a million dollars to their annual budgets, an average of $47,000 each. In 20 schools the cost of improved facilities for clinical teaching has aggregated $10,000,000. There are 734 hospitals approved for internships and 518 hospitals offering approved residencies and fellowships in specialties.

NORWAY gets undeserved blame when it is named as the original home of the Norway rat, the biggest and most aggressive of man's undesired house guests. Researches of Dr. Ernst Schwarz, of the Smithsonian Institution, indicate that it was first heard from in southeastern China, but even that may not have been its point of origin. The black rat, which the bigger Norway rat bullies and persecutes, originated in a species of wild rat in the Malay region. It "adopted" man in the New Stone Age, as a house pest in India. It followed its unwilling hosts to the shores of the Mediterranean and spread thence over Europe, and to all lands where European ships have gone. Other rats being traced by Dr. Schwarz include the lesser Malay rat and the East African Negro rat, which have more restricted distribution, mainly in the tropics. Another uninvited housemate of man is the Indian musk shrew. Although this animal looks something like a mouse it belongs to an entirely different and even more primitive class of animals, the insectivores.

NEW help in tracing the family tree of the American Indian in Asia was announced by Dr. Franz Weidenreich, of the Peiping Union Medical College. His study of the bones of a family of seven, who lived in a cave at Choukoutien, near Peking, in the latter part of the Old Stone Age reveals that this family included oddly assorted types similar to types found not infrequently among America's Indians. One woman had a skull like a modern Melanesian's. Another woman's head was of modern Eskimo type. The old man of the family resembled a late Old Stone Age European, with a touch of Asiatic about him. Finding such varied types in one family in the Asiatic region from which the American Indian must have migrated, Dr. Weidenreich pointed out that "It seems no longer necessary to assume that there were immigrations differing widely according to the physical character of the immigrants and the regions they came from." In the family of seven, the woman with the Melanesian type of skull had an artificially deformed head, which leads Dr. Weidenreich to speculate that this custom may have originated in Asia. The late Old Stone Age, to which the cave family of seven belonged, lasted in Europe from about 100,000 to about 20,000 years ago.

NEW evidence that the climate in Texas was nearly the same ten million years ago as it is now can be found in fossil leaves described in a new publication on plants of Eocene geologic time, by Professor O. M. Ball, of the Agricultural and Mechanical College. The fossils described by Professor Ball were found in various locations in southern Texas, mostly in thin beds of clay. They had lain undisturbed for ages, since some long-gone autumn when they fell from the trees and bushes and were covered by the silt of a stream in flood, or settled into the muck at the bottom of a lake. Some of the best of them came from what is now a claypit for a brickyard.

# SCIENCE NEWS

*Science Service, Washington, D. C.*

## PAPERS BEFORE THE INTERNATIONAL CONGRESS OF MICROBIOLOGY



MAN'S chemical warfare against the germs that invade his body occupied a leading part in the opening session in New York City on September 4 of the Third International Congress for Microbiology. Especial prominence was given to the powerful new weapons, sulfanilamide and its related chemicals. Just how sulfanilamide acts against bacteria is still pretty much of a riddle, it was admitted by Drs. Eleanor A. Bliss and Perrin H. Long, of the Johns Hopkins Medical School. It has been known for some time that in the presence of small quantities of the chemical, germs of the group known as cocci are not killed outright but stunned or paralyzed, so that the body's own fighting forces can make an end of them. However, in the researches reported by Drs. Bliss and Long, it has also been shown that stronger concentrations of sulfanilamide kill the bacteria outright. Another point developed was that the effectiveness of certain compounds of sulfanilamide seems to be due to their chemical decomposition, releasing ''straight'' sulfanilamide in contact with the bacteria.

Experiments in which sulfanilamide and sulfapyridine were used, either alone or in combination with injections of immune sera, on mice exposed to infection with meningitis were reported by Dr. Sara E. Branham, of the U. S. Public Health Service: ''In general, it may be said that, weight for weight, sulfapyridine protected mice better than sulfanilamide, and that the combination of either sulfapyridine or sulfanilamide with serum gave better protection than either the drugs or the serum did alone.''

A whole family of serious diseases, including typhus fever, Rocky Mountain spotted fever and several even worse maladies from the tropics, was discussed. The diseases of this group are all caused by members of the genus Rickettsia, which are small, bacteria-like bodies of variable shape. They are usually carried about by ticks, but have also been found in the bodies of lice and other biting insects. Climate influences the virulence of three types of infection, as shown by experiments on guinea pigs and other rodents, was reported by Dr. R. E. Dyer, of the U. S. Public Health Service. Animals inoculated with the viruses of spotted fever, endemic typhus and the St. Louis strain of encephalitis showed most pronounced reactions in winter and least in summer. Some of the tests, repeated under conditions of artificially controlled air temperature, yielded confirmatory results. The Japanese representative in this family, known as tsutsugamushi disease, was the subject of a report by Professor Norio Ogata, of the Medical University of Chiba, Japan. It occurs in certain districts during the summer months, and is fatal in between 30 and 70 per cent. of all cases. Another Rickettsia-caused disease was the subject of a paper prepared by Professor Ugo Reitano, of the University of Rome. It is a form of typhus fever always present among the natives of Abyssinia, and only the most alert precautions of the Italian medical service keeps it from spreading among white troops now garrisoned there. The most effective means of combat is vaccination.

The smallest plants, no less than the largest animals, must have their vitamins, hormones and other minutely concentrated but physiologically powerful substances if they are to live and grow. Not less than a dozen such substances, according to Dr. William J. Robbins, of the New York Botanical Garden, who opened the session with a general statement. To a very large extent, microscopic plants and full-sized animals need and use the same growth-promoting substances. One such substance, only recently discovered, was given the name ''coenzyme R'' by Dr. Franklin E. Allison and Francis W. Minor, of the U. S. Department of Agriculture. It has been found indispensable for the growth of the nitrogen-fixing bacteria that live in the roots of clover, peas and related plants. The bacteria need very little of it; they would grow and multiply in solutions containing as weak a dilution as one part in a million. But that much at least they had to have in order to grow at all.

Other bacterial growth-promoting substances, necessary in equally minute minimal quantities, were described by Drs. P. W. Wilson and P. M. West, of the University of Wisconsin. They found the same substances present in yeast as well as bacteria. Another nitrogen-fixing bacterium, Azotobacter, that lives free in the soil instead of in plant roots, has been found to require minute traces of molybdenum, the same metal that is used in hardening modern high-grade steels, and even smaller quantities of tungsten, the metal used in electric lamp filaments. Researches establishing these facts were reported by Drs. Dean Burk and Kenneth Horner, of the U. S. Department of Agriculture.

Relationship between rheumatic fever and pneumonia has been traced by Drs. Homer F. Swift and Thomas MacPherson Brown, of the Rockefeller Institute for Medical Research, who reported on their findings. Exudates oozing from the tissues of sufferers with rheumatic fever were cultured in various ways, both in the lungs of mice and on the embryonic membranes of incubated eggs. On the membranes the cultures produced characteristic lesions and in the mice they caused pneumonia. Microscopic examination disclosed the presence of the extremely small microorganisms known as pleuropneumonia bodies, which seem to have a size between the smaller types of bacteria and the invisible filterable viruses. Indeed, under certain circumstances the pleuropneumonia bodies themselves will slip through the invisibly fine pores of porcelain filters.

Two other strains of filterable organisms of the pleuropneumonia type, found in mice, were reported on by Dr. Albert T. Sabin, also of the Rockefeller Institute. Strain

A, which thrives either in the brain or in certain other tissues of the body, produces a toxin that either kills outright or leaves the animal crippled with symptoms like those of chorea. Strain B "has an almost specific affinity for the joints, in which it gives rise to a chronic, progressive, proliferative, ankylosing arthritis which clinically and pathologically resembles rheumatoid arthritis in man."

From the Far East and the Near East came simultaneous reports of a bacteriological feat long considered impossible: the growing of the virus of rabies in glass laboratory flasks instead of in the brains of living animals. Professor K. Kanazawa, of the University of Tokyo, made the virus grow by feeding it minced brains of either rabbit or chick embryo. In experiments of Professor I. J. Kligler and Dr. H. Bernkopf, of the University of Jerusalem, it was grown on a medium consisting of coagulated human blood plasma and mouse embryo brain.

Cancer, at least of certain types, is caused by filterable viruses, and thereby joins a numerous and varied group of human ills, including smallpox, influenza and infantile paralysis. Three converging lines of evidence were presented by Drs. James B. Murphy and Albert Claude, of the Rockefeller Institute for Medical Research; by Drs. Jacob Furth and Elvin A. Kabat, of the Cornell University Medical College, and by Dr. F. Duran-Reynals, of Yale University. Fluids from malignant transplantable tumors of chickens were whirled in the ultra-centrifuge, passed through fine-pored filters, and otherwise treated after the manner of virus-containing fluids in known animal and plant diseases. Materials obtained from these cancer-fluid filtrates, injected into the tissues of healthy chickens, produced typical cancerous growths. In the researches reported by Dr. Duran-Reynals, chicks responded to doses of a tumor virus by developing fatal hemorrhages and degeneration of tissues, without the development of tumors. However, extracts obtained from such chicks produced the characteristic growths when injected into healthy adult fowls. Similar evidence for virus causation of cancers in rabbits was reported in communications by Dr. Jerome T. Syverton, of the University of Rochester, and Drs. John C. Kidd and Peyton Rous, of the Rockefeller Institute. A virus was indicated as the probable cause of kidney cancer in frogs, by Dr. Balduin Lucké, of the University of Pennsylvania.

African monkeys may become immune carriers of yellow fever without being bitten by mosquitoes, according to Drs. G. M. Findlay and F. O. MacCallum, of London. They introduced yellow fever virus artificially into the stomachs of monkeys and found that it retained its virulence. Other animals, including man, could not be thus converted into carriers. Apparently the high acidity of their gastric juices inactivated the virus. "If non-biting arthropods with a long life span carry yellow fever virus and are occasionally eaten by monkeys, a solution would be found of the continuance of yellow fever in dry seasons when mosquitoes are absent or rare. Attention is drawn to the survival of yellow fever virus in cockroaches."

## PAPERS BEFORE THE AMERICAN PSYCHOLOGICAL ASSOCIATION



CHALLENGING the idea that a head wound injuring the frontal lobes of the brain could leave the victim unimpaired in intelligence, Dr. Ward C. Halstead, of the Otho S. A. Sprague Institute of the University of Chicago, stated that such an injury would cause "fundamental alteration" to the personality. The report was made to the American Psychological Association meeting at Stanford University. Scientific men have recently claimed that surgical removal of even the whole frontal lobe area left patients with normal or improved I.Q. Such conclusions, according to Dr. Halstead, are "based on inadequate methods" or standards. One type of abstract thinking, involving the storing of objects into categories on an abstract basis, is "relatively unavailable," for the person who suffers a frontal lobe injury regardless of which frontal lobe is damaged. Dr. Halstead's conclusions are based on a four-year study at the University of Chicago Clinics. He pointed out that it is only recently that such experimental studies of brain injury effects have been undertaken, although analyses were made of World War gunshot brain injury cases.

Anger and other emotions can make your finger tips cold. Close links between such body changes and mental states were described by Drs. Bela Mittelmann and Harold G. Wolff, of the New York Hospital and Cornell University Medical College. As the investigators discussed with a patient the difficult situations of his life in a psychoanalytic interview, they also made measurements of his finger temperature and the behavior of his digestive system. Anger, fear, depression and elation all were accompanied by a chilling of the finger tips. Even when the patient hid his emotion from himself, it was betrayed by the body changes and by his speech. The greatest drop in finger temperature came when the patient was in a state of tension, anxiety or conflict. The maximum drop was 13.5 degrees Centigrade or about 24 degrees Fahrenheit.

Braille, the language of the blind, can open the door of the world of printed literature to those who are blind only in their inability to "see" words, was stated by Dr. Grace M. Fernald, of the University of California. In learning Braille, she found, the word-blind slightly surpassed the "control group." In all cases, word-blind subjects could then learn to read Braille with the use of only the eyes even when they were still unable to read printed words. Emotional instability is characteristic of all the word-blind individuals studied.

Rats scurrying away on hearing a warning signal, as human beings have learned to run to shelter at an air-raid siren, demonstrated the potency of relief from anxiety as a means for "stamping in" the learning of certain lessons. Psychologists have recognized how powerful fear is for inhibiting or restraining the frightened one. Escape from fear, according to Dr. O. H. Mowrer, of the Institute of Human Relations of Yale University, is also powerful in determining the course of new behavior. When the rats in Dr. Mowrer's experiments were given a warning of impending punishment and allowed to escape from its threat, they learned better than with the aid of the punishment itself. "Human beings can take either of two courses of action in a danger situation," said Dr. Mowrer in discussing the human implications of his research with a representative of Science Service. "They can act in such a manner as to reduce the danger, or they can act in such a way as to reduce only their perception of the danger, that is, their fear."

Noise and imprisonment, as well as the dilemma of trying to make a correct decision when there is no right way, may be contributing causes to nervous breakdowns in rats. And what is true for rats may be true for men. Dr. Norman R. F. Maier, of the University of Michigan, last winter gained recognition and a $1,000 prize for causing rats to have nervous breakdowns. An animal was forced to take some action when there was no right way to do it. The driving force used in his experiments with rats was a jet of air. Now Dr. Maier finds that the noise of the air jet is a contributing factor in the breakdown. When the rats were placed on a small table and keys were jingled, the noise produced violent activity in 85 per cent.; the sound of an air jet caused it in 64 per cent. In some cases convulsions accompanied the extreme activity. Confinement is also a factor. When the rats were placed during the experiment in a closed wooden box, they were affected more than in a transparent box. But Dr. Maier sticks to his original conclusion that only the theory that breakdown occurs when a conflict is faced from which there is no escape, but in which it is necessary to take action, is broad enough to cover all the cases.

## ITEMS

A 1500-YEAR-OLD pair of small iron horseshoes which probably once shod the hooves of a Swiss Lake Dweller's horse is now on exhibition at the Field Museum of Natural History. It represents the last cultural phase of the Lake Dwellers of Lake Neuchâtel. Iron horseshoes were known by the fifth century.

THE American Museum of Natural History wants a group of rare and valuable 25,000,000-year-old bird tracks just beyond reach. The museum can not afford to build scaffolding to reach up, or block and tackle to reach down, to a deposit of tracks found exposed two thirds the way up a Slim Buttes, S. D., badlands cliff, and the tracks can not be reached in any other way. A sample of what is in store for the museum and its visitors was placed on exhibition. About 100 footprints made by wading birds on the shores of lakes that vanished ages ago are included in specimens picked up at the foot of the cliff by Henry Lee, of Rapid City, S. D. They had dropped from a stratum above. Mr. Lee saw more in the stratum. It is these the museum wants.

NATURE is slowly rebuilding the Long Island beaches struck by the memorable hurricane of September, 1938, is reported by Dr. Arthur David Howard, of New York University. Last year, in a few hours, the hurricane moved back the highwater mark at Jones Beach from 300 to 400 feet, but already natural accretion of sand is repairing the damage. Airplane photographs show this repair. Many of the inlets driven through the Fire Island sand dunes have submarine bars across them already. Dr. Howard explains in the new issue of *The Geographical Review* that during calm weather sand bars pile up offshore. During a storm this sand is washed landward. Some of it goes onto the beaches and some of it goes to enlarge the submarine bars across inlet channels. Gradually the beaches will be restored.

RIGOLLET'S comet, named after the amateur French observer who "discovered" it in the constellation Taurus (July 27), is very probably identical with one found in 1788 by Caroline Herschel, sister of the great English astronomer, Sir William Herschel, herself an astronomer. This was reported by Leland Cunningham, of the Harvard Observatory, who has found that the orbit of the "new" comet checks at virtually every point with that computed by Miss Herschel for her comet. It is possible that the two are not the same, but they are definitely of the same family and very probably identical. If it is the same one, this is the first time that it has been seen since its discovery.

USE of the spectroscope to determine the molecular patterns of simple hydrocarbons and to follow the changes occurring in their photochemical decomposition was reported at the conference on spectroscopy at the Massachusetts Institute of Technology by Professor Emma P. Carr and Hildegard Stucklen, of Mount Holyoke College. They obtained experimental results on a series of simple organic molecules which are necessary for the testing of theoretical predictions. This work promises ultimately to lead to a better understanding of the energy relationships involved in a carbon carbon double bond, a problem with significant biological implications. More than 25 hydrocarbons have been examined in this research, including some containing as many as eight carbon atoms and even two double bonds. Several previously unknown relationships governing molecular structure were found.

THE compression ignition principle of the Diesel engine was invented by Malay natives at least a thousand years before it was invented in Germany. Herbert W. Krieger, curator of ethnology at the U. S. National Museum, supports this claim by showing one of the old high-compression fire lighting gadgets of the Malay Peninsula, considered probably the most efficient fire-making idea that primitive man ever thought of. It is a tightly wrapped plunger which is forced into a wooden cylinder by a blow of the hand. At the bottom of the cylinder is a bit of tinder, which lights when the blow compresses the air in the cylinder, thereby generating heat. Crediting primitive men with other brilliant inventions, Mr. Krieger says that the textile industry was saved millions of dollars of royalties when an invention for winding cord so that it could be unwound with even tension turned out to be similar to an old Fiji idea. A Fiji twine ball, in the National Museum, prevented patenting of the device.

# SCIENCE NEWS

*Science Service, Washington, D. C.*

## CHEMICAL REACTIONS WHICH OBEY THE LAWS OF CHANCE



A ''GAMBLING'' type of chemical reaction, new to science, promising important developments in America's $200,000,000 organic chemical industry, was announced at the Boston meeting of the American Chemical Society, which opened its ninety-eighth semi-annual convention on September 10. It may explain even the aging of wines and liquors. The new reaction, revolutionary in its fundamental concepts, obeys the laws of chance by which mathematicians can determine the odds in games like dice, poker and bridge.

One might call the new reaction a ''chemical dice game,'' said Dr. George Calingaert, director of chemical research of the Ethyl Gasoline Corporation, who describes the new discovery. It takes place between chemicals ordinarily considered inert to one another and without chemical affinity which is usually thought to produce chemical activity. So new is the discovery that its potentialities are as yet unrealized, but they are believed to be very important. By what is called the ''redistribution reaction,'' chemical compounds are found to redistribute themselves into a number of compounds in the presence of a proper catalyst. It is possible to predict by the mathematical laws of chance, or probability, just what the end distribution of these new compounds will be.

The new reaction may help to explain the reactions which occur during the aging of wine or liquors. These subtle changes do occur, for man's taste is able to detect the differences. But chemical tests are worthless to measure the changes. Why they occur is still more of a puzzle. ''It may well be that this aging is in fact a 'natural redistribution' among the esters which are known to constitute the flavoring portions of these liquids,'' Dr. Calingaert said. ''If such should prove to be the case, it seems likely that a better understanding of the nature of the aging process will soon lead to improvement in the technique of accomplishing this all-important result. Simple catalysts were used throughout the experiments. These catalysts weaken intramolecular attractive forces commonly considered to be quite firm. The groups of atoms, which break loose from the molecules, interchange purely at random with other similar groups. After these random interchanges have taken place long enough, a state of 'mathematical equilibrium' is reached in which the composition of the reaction mixture exactly equals that which can be predicted by the laws of chance.''

Dr. Calingaert's initial experiments were carried out in research on the nature of tetraethyl lead and related ''anti-knock'' compounds for gasolines. It is already known, however, that the new type of chemical reaction takes place between compounds which chemists say are inert to one another, such as gasoline and kerosene, or milk and cream. All customary signs of chemical reaction are absent. There is no formation of a solid precipitate, or a gas, or even the heat so common to many chemical reactions.

## THE CHEMICAL STRUCTURE OF VITAMIN K

THE chemical structure of vitamin K has been discovered. Behind that simple announcement at the meeting of the society is the story of more, better, healthier babies, cleaner operations by surgeons with less risk, and help for one group of sick people whose blood does not clot in normal fashion. Vitamin K plays an essential rôle in making blood clot. Without it every one would be in the dangerous position of people afflicted with hemophilia, who may bleed to death from a tiny scratch. Hemophiliacs, however, do not suffer from lack of vitamin K but from a different disorder of the blood-clotting mechanism.

Two research teams of outstanding chemists, working independently at Harvard University and St. Louis University School of Medicine, have both arrived at the same structural formula for vitamin K. Using different methods, the exactness of their agreement leaves little doubt of the certainty of their findings. At Harvard Dr. Louis F. Fieser, with William P. Campbell and Edward M. Fry, synthesized the vitamin and determined the structure. At St. Louis Drs. Edward A. Doisy and D. W. MacCorquodale, with S. B. Binkley and S. A. Thayer, who were the first to isolate vitamin K in pure form, carried out an independent determination of the vitamin's structure.

The synthesis of vitamin K by Dr. Fieser's method is said to be efficient and practical for manufacturing purposes and the pure vitamin will thus be available to medicine to prevent and control hemorrhages. Dr. Doisy has also evolved a synthesis for vitamin K and found, moreover, another compound, a naphthaldehyde which is about one eighth as active as the pure vitamin but which has shown excellent results in use at the Mayo Clinic. The structural formula of vitamin K is 2-methyl-3-phytyl-1, 4-naphthoquinone.

Because the blood of a new-born baby does not possess the ability to coagulate, or clot, rapidly until several days after birth, hemorrhages are among the causes of a great many injuries to infants at birth. Estimates indicate that 25 per cent. of the damages associated with birth are due to bleeding, usually through a slow seeping of the blood in the skull cavity caused by a compression of the infant's head. To prevent such hemorrhages will be one of the greatest contributions of vitamin K that now should be available widely by synthetic manufacture.

## THE COLDEST REFRIGERATOR

THE world's coldest refrigerator, operating at 450 degrees below zero Fahrenheit, is in prospect as the result of discoveries reported at the opening meeting of the American Chemical Society by Professor S. C. Collins, of the Massachusetts Institute of Technology. The new type refrigerator would operate on compressed helium, the light inert gas used to inflate airships. When liquefied, helium produces the coldest cold known to man, only a few degrees above absolute zero.

Professor Collins said: "One does not ordinarily think of a steam or a compressed-air engine as being a refrigerating machine, yet the well-known principle on which they operate consists of the withdrawal of heat from the working gas and its conversion into work. Any gas expanding against a working piston is cooled by expansion. For instance, the temperature of a sample of air originally at 70 degrees Fahrenheit will fall more than 100 degrees if allowed to double its volume in an engine cylinder."

The major trouble to be overcome in a compressed helium engine is the matter of lubrication, for at 450 degrees below zero Fahrenheit all lubricants are frozen solid. Professor Collins solved this difficulty by doing away with lubricants and replacing the conventional piston of an engine with a flexible diaphragm of stainless steel. This diaphragm is sealed at its edges by a copper gasket between two steel plates. The expansion of the helium occurs between the diaphragm and one of the plates.

Two or even three such engines will be used in consecutive stages in refrigeration, for it is not practical to try to reach the extreme low temperatures in one single jump down the temperature scale.—ROBERT D. POTTER.

## WORLD MAPS

THE Great Triangulation of India, most famous of all the world's mapping projects, will some day become a geodetic "Garden of Eden" for half the world's maps. This thought that the vast and careful mapping of India will be the center of origin of a far-flung network of coordinated maps for all of Asia, Europe, Australia and the Philippines was contained in the address prepared by Brigadier H. S. L. Winterbotham, mapping expert of Great Britain and general secretary of the International Union of Geodesy and Geophysics.

The address of Brigadier Winterbotham, who was recalled to England on account of the war, was read by Dr. William Bowie, formerly of the U. S. Coast and Geodetic Survey, who also took his place as general secretary.

While war will now temporarily stay the project, Brigadier Winterbotham stated that plans were being considered for pushing the century-old mapping work of India "to Australia, and the Philippines, to Moscow on the north and to Valentia (Ireland) and Casa Blanca (Morocco) on the west."

World maps, his address continued, rest on exactly known great arcs on the earth's surface which give stability and definiteness to maps as does a skeleton to a fish. Any one with competent knowledge, Brigadier Winterbotham's address stated, can carry out surveying of a small region, but it is only when each of these individual surveys can be "tied" to the general large-scale arcs of geodesy that all the little pieces will fit together exactly like parts of a huge jig-saw puzzle.

The "father" of the great mapping project in India was Sir George Everest, for whom Mt. Everest in the Himalayan Mountains was named. It was Sir George who as surveyor general of India in 1830 discovered the gravitational effect of large masses (like mountains) on plumb bobs whose timing helped determine gravity and the horizontal lines created by surveying levels. The near-by, giant Himalayan Mountains seemed at the time to circumvent Everest's astronomical observations by which he was determining latitude.

One of the great unfinished mapping projects of the world is the determination of the thirtieth meridian of longitude which runs from Cape Town to Cairo, through Africa, and later is to be extended to North Cape in Norway so that it will link the Arctic and Antarctic. Until this project is completed the mapping of Africa will be in the same stage of India at the time of Everest. "Until it is finished no lesser survey can hope to take its precise place on the map of Africa."—ROBERT D. POTTER.

## PLAGUES TO COME IN THE WAKE OF WAR

INFLUENZA is almost certain to be wide-spread again if there is a general war, was predicted by Dr. Thomas M. Rivers, of the Rockefeller Institute for Medical Research, president of the New York meeting of the third International Congress of Microbiology. No effective weapon yet exists for this plague. Dr. Rivers pointed out that microbes will play a tremendous part in the war that has now started in Europe. He said no one is going to start a war of microbes. That would be next to impossible. Epidemics of influenza, typhus fever, trench fever and dysentery, however, are sure to follow in the wake of this war as they did during the last world war. Meningitis and European sleeping sickness, technically termed epidemic encephalitis, may also appear.

Dr. Rivers pointed out that medical men are better equipped to fight some of these war-born plagues than they were in 1914. Sulfanilamide, the new disease-conquering chemical, will not prevail against influenza or typhus fever, but it cures meningitis and gas gangrene. Serums also have been developed for fighting these deadly ailments.

The idea of using germs as a weapon of war is out on two counts. In the first place it is almost impossible for man to start an epidemic deliberately by releasing germs among a group of people or putting them into water or food. Not even cholera could be spread this way. Many factors besides germs are needed to start an epidemic. Even in laboratories, where conditions can be controlled far better than in communities of men and women, it is difficult if not impossible.

The second reason why germs will not be used as a weapon of war is that such a weapon would boomerang on the nation starting it. If an epidemic really got going, it would be impossible to prevent its spreading to people in the nation starting it as well as among their enemies. Germs, Dr. Rivers said, neither recognize nor stop at the front line.

## NEW TREATMENT FOR CANCER

A NEW treatment for cancer has been introduced with considerable success in laboratory experiments. Almost 50 per cent. better results from x-ray or radium treatment of mouse cancers were obtained with a new "death-by-drowning technique," according to figures reported by Dr. Kanematsu Sugiura, of New York City, at the International Cancer Congress on September 12.

If human cancers react to the new treatment in the same way as the mouse cancers, the successful application of x-rays in treatment of cancer will be materially increased. Cancers so insensitive to x-rays that they can now only be killed by doses so large that the surrounding normal tissue would be damaged may some day be successfully irradiated by the new technique.

In the laboratory experiments, the mouse cancers are first bombarded with x-rays, gamma rays from radium, or the newer, faster neutron rays may be used. This increases the flow of fluid into the cell from the outside, according to one explanation of x-ray destruction of cancers. The cell swells up and its life essential chemicals are greatly diluted and eventually the cell may die.

To hasten the death-by-drowning, if that is what it is, sterile distilled water is injected into the cancer after the x-ray treatment. In mice a very small amount of the water was injected two to four times daily for three or four successive days after irradiation. Without the distilled water, an x-ray dose of 1,000 roentgens caused regression of the cancers in about 50 per cent. of the cases. The same x-ray dosage caused regression of cancers in 95 per cent. when the sterile distilled water was injected.—Jane Stafford.

## ITEMS

Solar activity has been rapidly increasing with the number of spots greatly augmented, according to new photographs taken at the U. S. Naval Observatory. There were, last week, 209 spots observed on the sun, divided into 16 groups. One large group has appeared in the sun's southern latitude and it may menace foreign short-wave radio reception because of its angry character. It is believed that the increased intensity of radiation poured out by the sun at such times creates ionosphere storms in the radio reflecting layers miles above the earth. These layers act as "mirrors" for long-distance radio waves. The effect of ionosphere storms appears to "break the mirror" and cause distorted reception or even radio blackouts in severe cases.

Leadership in chemistry throughout the world is now in possession of the United States, according to a report submitted to the American Chemical Society by Professor E. J. Crane, of the Ohio State University, editor of *Chemical Abstracts*. Germany, which ranked first during the World War period and even a decade ago, has now dropped to third place with Great Britain second. Russia and Japan show striking gains. English is predominantly the language of science, the United States and England accounting for 40 per cent. of all scientific periodicals published. The report is based on an analysis of 65,000 abstracts of chemical discoveries reported last year in *Chemical Abstracts*. Chemical patents account for much of the leadership of the United States. During the last five years U. S. chemical patents have increased fifteen per cent. in number over the preceding five years. During this same time British chemical patents have declined twelve per cent., French chemical patents have decreased twenty-three per cent. and German chemical patents have dwindled to thirty per cent. of their former number.

Anti-flea-bite vaccination has been tried with "encouraging results," according to Drs. L. S. Cherney, C. M. Wheeler and Alfred C. Reed, of the University of California and the Hooper Foundation for Medical Research, in a report printed in the *American Journal of Tropical Medicine*. A group of susceptible persons has been actively immunized against the bite of this insect, which is both irritating and dangerous, since it may carry the germs of serious ailments such as typhus fever and plague. It is pointed out that "If it is possible to induce 'immunity' against flea bites, it is probably likewise possible to 'immunize' against bites of other insects. If so, this would be an extremely valuable adjunct in the control of insect-borne diseases. Insect bites may result in plague, yellow fever, malaria and other often fatal diseases, if the biting insects are carrying the germs of such ailments. The flea was chosen rather than the mosquito for the first attempts at anti-insect vaccination because it is the most common blood-sucking insect encountered in the San Francisco region. While the results are encouraging, a certain number of relapses after the immunization against flea bites have occurred, and no acute cases have been treated as yet.

Plans for forest fire insurance are being perfected by economists attached to the U. S. Forest Service which should bring at least financial relief to the estimated $43,000,000 lost annually throughout the nation from this cause. "An unquestionably sound basis" for insuring standing timber against the menace of fire has been worked out in a report prepared by H. P. Shepard, of the division of forest economics, after a three-year study. The northeastern states and the Pacific Coast lumbering area have already been surveyed in the research study of the feasibility of the plan. A nation-wide expansion is believed possible. For the northeastern area it is estimated that premiums of only 13.5 cents per $100 of valuation would be needed to make the plan satisfactory.

Two new bacterial diseases have been discovered by Drs. P. H. DeBach and W. A. McOmie, of the University of California. But nobody is expected to be worried, much. For the only creatures they are known to kill are termites. One bacterial species turns the heads of the dead termites black. The other turns the heads and legs red. The red disease is more than twice as deadly to termites than the black. In two lots of fifty termites each, infected with the two diseases by laboratory feeding, there were twenty-five "red" deaths as against eleven "black" fatalities.

Norwegian and Italian chickens of the same breed differ markedly in temperament, according to Professor N. Jaensch, of the University of Marburg. Professor Jaensch's description of the behavior of northern and southern chickens reads almost like a popular statement of the difference between Nordic and Mediterranean human races. The northern fowl, he says, walks more proudly, goes quietly and directly on its intended course; the southern bird is more excited and agitated and dashes about moving its head continually. The Norwegian chicken eats until it has had enough and then quits; the Italian can be induced to overeat if it sees its fellow-fowls picking up grain.

# SCIENCE NEWS

*Science Service, Washington, D. C.*

## MASS PRODUCTION OF HEAVY CARBON ATOMS

*(Copyright, 1939, by Science Service)*

MASS production of heavy carbon, the isotope of the ordinary kind of carbon that is a basis of all living matter, was announced at the meeting of the American Chemical Society by Professor Harold C. Urey, of Columbia University.

By the chemical method of separating the heavy kind of carbon of mass 13, from ordinary carbon of mass 12, Professor Urey is now able to supply the needs of scientific workers all over the world with this valuable stable kind of carbon whose atoms can be used as tags to aid chemists in labeling parts of their atoms. By adding atomic tags at the proper places intricate reactions can be carried out and the movement, within the molecule, of the atomic tags can be deducted.

With the successful production of quantities of carbon of mass 13 (which, incidentally, you can buy at $400 an ounce) the elements hydrogen, carbon, oxygen and nitrogen are now available in their stable isotopic form for use as tags in research. These four elements are found in over 90 per cent. of all chemical compounds known, and are especially important in all biological problems.

The other way to produce tags on atoms to trace out chemical behavior is to bombard them in atom-smashing machines and render them radioactive. This radioactivity, or spontaneous disintegration, can then be detected with the proper instruments.

In an interview, Professor Urey said: "Much interest has been exhibited in recent years in artificially radioactive substances in solving important biological problems. But it really seems to me, at the present time, that most of these problems can be solved best by the use of the stable isotopes of the overwhelmingly important elements, hydrogen, carbon, oxygen and nitrogen which can only be supplied in quantity by the chemical method of the separation of isotopes. Fortunately it appears that the stable and radioactive isotopes complement each other in scientific investigation. The chemical method of separation of isotopes works best with the all-important elements, hydrogen, carbon, nitrogen and oxygen. The method of thermal diffusion and the artificially radioactive method of tagging elements works very well for the remainder of the elements in the periodic table."

While atom-smashing and the production of radioactive elements for biological and chemical experiments is the current trend in physical science there are a whole host of experiments which are lengthy ones, involving the feeding of experimental animals with isotopic materials. For all such experiments, many of them the most important in the realm of biology and physiology, it is essential to have stable isotopes and not radioactive ones which disintegrate quickly. The half life of radioactive carbon, the element found in all living matter, is only about twenty seconds. Experiments performed with radioactive carbon must be done quickly. Such haste, potentially, may lead to errors.

ROBERT D. POTTER.

## MAGNETISM OF THE NEUTRON

MAGNETIC strength of the neutron, the smallest known particle without an electric charge, is 2,000 times smaller than the magnetic strength of an atom of iron. Expressed in the ordinary magnetic unit, it would require more than 20 zeros behind the decimal point before the first significant digit. Yet the results are declared to be correct within one per cent.

These results were announced on September 17 by a joint research team representing the University of California and Stanford University, which has been using the big cyclotron at Berkeley. Physicists who have worked on the problem are Professors Felix Bloch and Norris E. Bradbury, of Stanford University, and Professor Luis W. Alvarez, of the University of California.

A stream of free electrons was shot from the cyclotron at a magnetized iron plate. Those that passed through were polarized, that is, their minute magnetic fields were arranged parallel with that of the iron plate. These polarized neutrons were then permitted to strike a second magnetized iron plate. If the magnetization of the second plate was along the same lines as that of the first, the maximum number of neutrons was found to pass through it. But if the second plate was turned around so that its north pole lay in the opposite direction to the first plate's north pole, then the least number of neutrons would pass through the second plate.

To measure the strength of the neutron magnets themselves, Drs. Bloch and Alvarez simply turned the neutrons around, instead of turning the second plate. This was done by creating between the plates a magnetic field which oscillated at a radio frequency of about two million times a second. The oscillating field caused the neutrons to turn somersaults.

When the frequency of oscillation was such as to cause the maximum number of neutron somersaults, then the minimum number of neutrons passed through the second plate. A delicate counter was used to determine the precise condition of minimum passage, and from the oscillation frequency under that condition the strength of the neutron magnet was determined. In the course of the experiments 50 million neutrons were counted.

## FUEL TANK EXPLOSIONS IN ENGLAND

*(Copyright, 1939, by Science Service)*

OUT of England's mystery of exploding gasoline storage tanks, which Scotland Yard first thought was the work of Irish terrorists, has come the amazing discovery of a species of bacteria which can live on kerosene and ferment it into ethane and methane fuel gases, just as ordinary bacteria can ferment sugar into alcohol.

At the Boston meeting of the American Chemical Society, the new discovery had chemists shaking their heads and speculating on this new-found way to let nature create for them these hydrocarbon gases which can be the starting point of a host of synthetic chemical compounds.

The new kerosene-fermenting organisms were first described informally, and totally unreported, at the meeting of the International Congress for Microbiology in New York recently. The eminent British bacteriologist, Dr. A. C. Thaysen, of the British National Scientific Laboratory at Teddington, who is now on the high seas hurrying back for military service, described the new discovery.

His story, as related by chemists who talked with him in New York, runs like this:

Scotland Yard for months has been puzzled by mysterious explosions in gasoline storage tanks holding their wartime precious fuel. Sabotage was suspected but unproved, for the terrific explosions brought complete catastrophe. Dr. Thaysen, as the government's expert on the generation of gases by bacteria, was also called in but could find no answer. Finally, and fortunately, a kerosene tank blew up. A quick examination after the explosion showed bubbles of gas rising from the layer of water at the tank's bottom on which the kerosene had been floating. Taking some of the water and sediment to his laboratory, Dr. Thaysen discovered his new kind of bacteria which can live in kerosene and ferment it into 10 per cent. ethane and 90 per cent. methane. He cultured this organism and then sub-cultured it and obtained a pure strain of bacteria that would grow and propagate. It was the explosive methane and ethane gas generated by these bacteria which caused the explosion. While he has not yet solved the gasoline explosions he is virtually certain that a similar action occurs there too.

Chemists who understand bacterial fermentation see no reason why the discovery is not true, for they know of organisms which will live in strange places and which can ferment phenols like carbolic acid and also benzoic acid.

Dr. Thaysen is well known in his field as a careful investigator. While the new discovery must, of course, be substantiated by other workers, chemists are giving credence to Dr. Thaysen's amazing discovery.—ROBERT D. POTTER.

## IMPROVED CHEMICAL TREATMENT FOR COMMON COLDS

(*Copyright, 1939, by Science Service*)

AN improved chemical advance in the fight against the common cold, one of the unconquered afflictions of mankind, was announced at the meeting of the American Chemical Society by a physician-chemist research team, Drs. Simon L. Ruskin and M. P. Fejos, of New York.

By the new method, drugs frequently used in treating the common cold, adrenalin, ephedrine and benzedrine, are reacted with vitamin C (cevitamic acid) to produce stable compounds of enhanced physiological action. Both the drugs for colds and the vitamin are, by themselves, unstable materials, losing their potency with relative quickness. In combination, however, they form compounds that retain their potency for over two years.

Ephedrine, used to decrease nasal secretions and "dry up" a cold, is improved by the action of vitamin C. Some of the undesirable effects of this drug—nervousness, palpitation and intestinal upset—are diminished by the vitamin C radical.

"The wide-spread use of ephedrine in the treatment of common colds," they stated, "makes the preparation of ephedrine cevitamate a definite advance in the chemistry of the treatment of the common cold and suggests a chemical rational for the wide-spread use of drinks rich in vitamin C. It similarly marks an advance in the treatment of asthma and hay fever."

The action of vitamin C on the new drug sulfanilamide is also being studied. A stable compound has been found to result from the combination. This compound has an increased solubility over ordinary sulfanilamide.

It is reported that "Investigation is proceeding on the use of sulfanilamide cevitamate for the prevention of the complications of the common cold."—ROBERT D. POTTER.

## DEBATE ON THE VIRUS CAUSE OF CANCER

(*Copyright, 1939, by Science Service*)

CAN cancer be caused by a virus, the kind of ultramicroscopic substance that causes infantile paralysis, influenza and other baffling ailments? The case for and against this theory of cancer cause was debated by leading English and American authorities on cancer and on viruses at the closing sessions of the third International Cancer Congress.

The idea should be given very careful attention, according to Dr. C. H. Andrewes, of London. He pointed out that viruses are now accepted as the cause of some tumors in animals. There is no proof yet, he stated, that viruses are concerned in the cause of cancer in general, but the viruses have properties which fit them for the rôle of cancer-causing agents and they should therefore be given further study in this connection.

On the other hand, Dr. James B. Murphy, of New York City, gave as his opinion that there is no justification for the idea that there is one "universal virus" which causes cancers. Investigation of the viruses which cause tumors in animals is, however, interesting and important. The chief point against the idea that human cancer is caused by a virus is the failure so far to find a filterable substance such as a virus in tumors of mammalian animals (mouse or man) which can cause tumors when injected into other animals. This point was stressed both by Dr. Murphy and Dr. Andrewes.

Whether or not viruses cause cancer in man, they may provide the best lead to discovering the nature of "directive factors" in the life processes of both normal and cancer cells, and thus perhaps to discovery of what directs a cancer cell to become cancerous. This suggestion was made by Dr. W. M. Stanley, of the Rockefeller Institute at Princeton, N. J., who succeeded in isolating some viruses in the form of crystalline, non-living protein matter. The viruses represent a key to abnormal tissue changes, he said, and because many viruses are now available in essentially pure form for study, investigation of them may give the key to the abnormal tissue change that is cancerous.

Until these problems of cancer causes and prevention are solved, the practical attack on cancer rests on established methods of treatment applied as early as possible. The importance of early treatment was stressed at another session of the congress, and was summed up in survey figures quoted by the president, Dr. Francis Carter Wood, of Columbia University, New York.—JANE STAFFORD.

## THE NEW ENGLAND HURRICANE OF A YEAR AGO

*(Copyright, 1939, by Science Service)*

HURRICANE blasts tore at New England's woods and farms and towns on September 21 a year ago, leaving hundreds of deaths and millions of dollars' worth of property loss in their desolate wake.

To-day, a glance in the direction of New England discloses a picture unexpectedly cheerful. A combination of New England grit and general American intelligence and efficiency (plus a good deal of plain, ordinary healing by nature itself) has made possible much salvage out of the wreck and a real measure of progress toward full recovery.

A survey by the U. S. Forest Service shows that 9,551 New England timber owners have nearly one and two thirds billions of board feet of timber under agreement for salvage. Actual deliveries, however, are not expected to reach much more than half that figure, for a number of reasons. Nevertheless, by next spring some 875,000,000 board feet will have been brought out of the woods, in marketable timber forms.

About two thirds of the job has already been completed. 560,401,000 board feet are already out and stored, either as logs in ponds or as sawed lumber in yards—209,120,000 board feet in the latter category alone. Something over $6,453,000, from the New England Timber Salvage Administration, has changed hands over the whole transaction. The U. S. Forest Service takes no part in the commercial transactions; its task has been to help protect the down-timber areas from fire and to facilitate handling generally.

A conspicuous factor in the success of the salvage program has been the close and effective cooperation of all parties concerned—federal and state agencies and the public at large—in preventing fire. Despite the unprecedented drought from which the entire Northeast suffered this summer, greatly aggravating the fire hazard, there have been only two fires in the whole area that exceeded 1,000 acres in extent. There were several thousand little fires—all promptly extinguished before they could spread.

The work has been carried on by an army of some 14,000 men, divided among three main agencies: 3,400 in the CCC, 7,700 in WPA and 3,064 in the New England Forest Emergency corps. There are 18 permanent camps of 50 men each, two camps of 100 men each; the rest of the workers commute to their jobs from towns and farms.

Replacement of New England's devastated woodlands is proceeding naturally. Seedlings and young saplings were not broken or uprooted by the storm, and they are already showing rapid growth. Also, last season's white pine cone crop was heavy, so there should be thick stands of seedlings of the year.—FRANK THONE.

## ITEMS

FALL begins officially at 5:50 P.M. Eastern Standard Time September 23, according to calculations made at the office of the Nautical Almanac at the U. S. Naval Observatory. At that instant the sun will be passing over the earth's equator on its southward journey which brings autumn to the northern hemisphere. September 23, too, is the day when the moon passes the planet Mars in the sky. This passing will occur at 3:05 A.M. Eastern Standard Time.

AN extremely rich and large deposit of iron ore which contains about half of the total world iron resources will begin in 1940 to yield ore at the rate of 300,000 tons a year. It is known as the Kursk magnetic anomaly because of the immense effect that it has on the magnetic needle. The Kursk ore carries up to 67 per cent. iron content and the ore layers average 200 feet thick.

HAY-FEVER pollens ride the winds over the Atlantic Ocean, but only for a relatively short distance off shore, was stated by O. C. Durham, chief botanist of the Abbott Laboratories, after examining vaselined glass slides exposed by Engineer J. W. Etchison, of the Pan-American Airways plane, *Yankee Clipper*, on a recent trip to Europe and return. Pollens were found at altitudes between 2,000 and 8,000 feet out to 275 miles off shore. Above 8,000 feet there were practically no pollens over either land or sea. Since the plane did not fly at lower altitudes when far off shore, the possibility still remains that pollens may be present "at the bottom of the air" farther out at sea than the slides showed.

CHROMOSOMES in growing grain have their numbers doubled when the seed is treated with a fungicide distributed under the trade name "Granosan," Dr. Dontcho Kostoff, of the Institute of Genetics at Moscow, has discovered. Seeds treated with the compound are not attacked by fungi, whereas seeds treated with colchicine are frequently killed by these parasitic forms.

TAKING the methods of major industries, the regional laboratories of the U. S. Department of Agriculture are installing pilot plants to determine the feasibility of new methods for creating industrial materials from farm products. The pilot plants will carry new developments through the doubtful stage where manufacturers, who depend on profits, are unwilling to venture. Often the laboratory shows that a certain process can be done in the test-tube stage, says Dr. W. W. Skinner, associate chief of the Bureau of Agricultural Chemistry and Engineering. What the pilot plant does is to prove the economies for potential large-scale, commercial production.

LETTING men and machines stand idle, while national consuming power cries out for the things they might produce, is a worse waste of national resources than stripped timberlands or soil erosion, according to a report of the National Resources Committee, under the editorship of Gardiner C. Means. "Manpower, potential work, is a perishable resource like water-power," the report points out. "Ten or fifteen million idle workers combined with idle machines can mean a tremendous loss in potential national income. In addition, the failure to use available manpower reduces the effectiveness of future production as idleness breeds frustration and loss of skills. The magnitude of losses from waste of manpower throws the wastes in the exploitation of natural resources into insignificance."

# SCIENCE NEWS

*Science Service, Washington, D. C.*

## THE EXPECTED METEOR SHOWER

Astronomers are hoping that there will be an extraordinary display of shooting stars or meteors on October 9 or 10, although they are trying not to raise anticipation too much by making definite predictions.

Just six years ago, on October 9, 1933, there was visible in Europe for a few hours the strongest meteor shower of this century. It was one of those heavenly performances that one is lucky to see once in a lifetime. Astronomers figured out that the earth had passed through the region of space occupied 80 days previously by the faint, short-period comet Giacobini-Zinner. The meteors were produced by bits of débris tagging along in the same orbit as the comet. Since the period of this comet is 6.6 years, it is again due in the vicinity of the earth. This year the earth precedes the comet to the point where their paths cross by 136 days. In 1940 the earth follows the comet by 229 days. In either case there is a chance that there will be a recurrence of the Giacobinid meteor shower.

Dr. Fletcher Watson, of Harvard Observatory, finds that the earth reaches a favorable position for a shower on October 9 or 10, if the comet has not varied too much from its previous path, which it may have done. He suggests that observers over the whole earth be alert during those evenings so that any display of meteors can be properly recorded.

Any careful, observant person can make useful records. Here is how to go about it. Get out in the country where street and house light will not blind you for the majority of the meteors will be faint. Record the magnitude or identity of the faintest star you can see. If the transparency of the sky changes appreciably during the observations, record the changes. Watch some definite region of the sky, such as the polar region or the zenith, directly overhead. Count the number of meteors seen during intervals of five minutes. At least once each hour, over intervals of not less than five minutes, count the number of meteors of each magnitude. Determine as closely as possible the position and size of the area from which the meteors seem to come. If low-power binoculars are available make observations of the number of meteors of various magnitudes seen through them. Send in a full record of your observations to Science Service, Washington, D. C., for transmission to astronomers who will study them.

An extraordinary display of the Giacobinid meteors may occur in 1946 because then the earth and the comet are expected to be only eight days apart in reaching the same position. But astronomy has not yet lived down the failure of a much-heralded Leonid shower in 1899, which just didn't happen. For that reason, while hopeful, astronomers are not being dogmatic about the chances of seeing the Giacobinid shooting star shower, either this year, next year or in 1946.

## RADIOACTIVE TRIPLE WEIGHT HYDROGEN

Hydrogen of triple weight variety has been made radioactive in atomic bombardment experiments with the University of California cyclotron. It is a strange kind of hydrogen of mass 3 with a long half-life period of radioactivity and a very short range for the radiation given off from it.

Drs. Luis W. Alvarez and Robert Cornog obtained the evidence as a follow-up on atom-smashing experiments that showed an unusual kind of helium of mass 3 instead of the usual mass 4 is stable. The research also showed mass 3 helium to be about 12 times as plentiful in helium obtained from the atmosphere as in helium extracted from gas wells.

The helium of mass 3 when used as a bombarding material induced radioactivity in ordinary silicon of mass 28, probably forming phosphorus of mass 30 which broke down into silicon of mass 30 with release of electrons. The radioactive mass 3 hydrogen was produced by bombarding deuterium (hydrogen of mass 2) with deuterons (hearts of mass 2 hydrogen) by means of the cyclotron.

Ordinary hydrogen is the simplest element of unitary weight or mass one. It is one of the components of water and almost all living and many non-living things. Helium is the next heaviest element, usually of mass 4, and only in recent years has it been available in quantity for use in airships, diving and medicine. The report is published in the *Physical Review*.

## AIR SANITATION

Medical science may be on the verge of conquering epidemics of respiratory diseases, such as influenza, colds, etc., by keeping the air clean. Just as typhoid and other water-borne ills were brought under control by successful sanitary measures of control, so the next great advance in disease prevention may be air sanitation.

At the University of Pennsylvania Medical School there is in progress a special investigation of air-borne infections. One result is the idea that it is not alone the droplets sprayed in the air by coughs and sneezes that carry diseases, but the nuclei of the dried droplets that float in the air.

Respiratory infections are must less frequent in spring and summer than in winter because open windows change the air 100 times an hour compared with below 10 overturns per hour with the closed doors and windows of winter. If air disinfection in winter can accomplish similar hygienic results, a long step may be taken in air-borne disease control.

One of the most promising methods of air disinfection is through use of ultra-violet lamps that create invisible screens of radiation barring and wiping out the germ-laden bits floating in the air. Already used in hospitals to barricade sickrooms against release or entrance of infection, they promise to have wider use, even in homes and public places.—Watson Davis.

## HEARTWORM INFESTATION OF DOGS

A new drug to combat the rapidly spreading heartworm infestation of dogs will shortly be made available to veterinarians. The drug, antimonial-III catechol thiosalicylic acid sodium, is the result of three years of intensive research by James A. Austin and Dr. Harold P. Brown, of Kansas City, Mo.

Heartworm infestation of the dog is a unique disease because living adult worms, *Dirofilaria immitis*, 8 to 12 inches long, situate themselves in the right heart. Under treatment the adult worms are slowly killed by gradually building up a concentration of trivalent antimony in the blood stream of the dog. The selective habitat of the adult worm in the right heart is a fortunate arrangement for the dog, for if the Dirofilaria were located in the left heart they would, upon being killed, pass into the aorta and its branches and the dog would succumb to a generalized embolism. Owing to the rich blood-supply of the lung, this organ is usually capable of coping successfully with the task of absorbing the dead filariae.

The ill effect of heartworm infestation upon the host is not entirely due to the presence of the adult worms in the heart. Larvae liberated into the blood stream also damage the dog. These larvae, or microfilariae, 0.2–0.3 millimeters in length, are worm-like in appearance, and move through the blood with a whipping motion.

One 27-pound dog with a fairly heavy infestation presented a count of 186,000 microfilariae per cubic centimeter of blood, or approximately 175,000,000 heartworm larvae in its entire blood stream. Laid end to end these microfilariae would stretch a distance of 30 miles. Upon autopsy, the right heart and pulmonary vessels were crammed full of the adult worms. A rough estimate of 100 adult worms would place the total length of worms in the heart and blood vessels at about 100 feet.

Heartworm infestation can not be transmitted directly from dog to dog, but must pass through an intermediate host. The mosquito has been indicted, and the tick, flea and other biting and sucking arthropods and insects are suspected. Treatment of the condition involves a series of graduated daily doses of the drug administered intravenously.

## ITEMS

ENGLAND is investing nearly $30,000,000 in a new plant for the production of petroleum by the hydrogenation of coal, it has been learned by *Industrial and Engineering Chemistry*. The plant, the second to be built in Great Britain, is to be financed by government capital with the Imperial Chemical Industries, Ltd., the management corporation. The I. C. I. already operates the large coal-hydrogenation plant at Billingsham-on-Tee for the production of gasoline.

ALL medical officers of the British Royal Air Force have been instructed that no one should be allowed to fly or to drive an automobile while taking sufanilamide or related chemical remedies. Derivatives of these chemicals, by producing methemoglobin or sulfhemoglobin, may interfere with oxygen exchange of the blood and so prove a danger by reducing oxygen supply to the pilot's or driver's brain. Peace-time experience shows that a full dose of one of these sulfanilamide derivatives taken shortly before flying lowers an aviator's "ceiling" by about 5,000 feet. Dr. E. P. Mackie, medical adviser of Imperial Airways, saw a pilot who was suffering from severe oxygen lack as a result of flying at only 13,000 feet. Investigation showed he had been taking full doses of sulfanilamide for tonsillitis. Similar cases have been observed in America and Germany. The British experience is reported by a correspondent of the *Journal* of the American Medical Association.

RUST fungi, among the worst parasitic enemies of wheat and other grains, may possibly give their host plants something in exchange for what they take. Dr. Branquinho d'Oliveira, of the National Agronomic Station at Lisbon, reports in *Nature* the results of experiments suggesting that rusts can capture and fix nitrogen from the air, as do the bacteria that live in the roots of plants of the pea and clover family. Dr. d'Oliveira grew wheat seedlings on laboratory media from which all nitrogen had been carefully excluded, so that the customary supply of this vitally necessary element could not be obtained through the roots. Then he inoculated part of the plants with spores of various species of rust. After a time he analyzed the plants. The infected ones proved to have a slightly but definitely larger nitrogen content than the control plants that had grown up free from rust.

BENEFITS of protection to migrating hawks and other useful birds of prey at Pennsylvania's famous Hawk Mountain are shown in the first annual report of the association formed to acquire and develop the critical two square miles of crest land, where gunners used to station themselves to shoot the birds "just for fun." Although the Hawk Mountain Sanctuary Association has been functioning officially for only one year, close counts on the migrating hawks and eagles have been kept up since 1934. They show fluctuations in numbers of particular species, but the net totals have climbed from 10,776 in 1934 to 17,024 in 1938. (The 1939 migration has not yet taken place.) The biggest increase has been in numbers of the broad-winged hawk, which preys chiefly on rodents, reptiles and amphibians. In 1934, 2,026 of this species were counted at Hawk Mountain; the 1938 count was 10,761. Hawks and eagles in general are useful birds, destroyers of rodents and other vermin, explains Mrs. C. N. Edge, through whose activity the sanctuary was established. Only a few species are chicken thieves and hunters of the game birds which man considers his especial prerogative.

AMERICAN chemists now have ready more than 500 dyes for tinting the new Nylon stockings, made from coal, air and water, which soon will be on the market, according to the report of P. H. Stott, du Pont chemist, to the meeting of the American Association of Textile Chemists and Colorists. Originally created for use on wool, silk and acetate rayons, the dyes work equally well on the new synthetic, silk-like fiber. The introduction of Nylon and its dyeing, Mr. Stott indicated, is in sharp contrast to the struggles of the then-new rayon industry during the World War. At that time the industry was completely dependent on German dye imports and had difficulty in getting good dyes after the conflict began.

# SCIENCE NEWS

*Science Service, Washington, D. C.*

## THE SCIENTIFIC AND EDUCATIONAL ORGANIZATIONS OF WARSAW



As the smoke of devastation slowly clears away from the ruins of Warsaw, the world of science and learning is anxious to learn what has happened to the centers of scientific research and education in what was once the capital of the Polish republic.

No word has come out, during all the days of the furious siege, of what was happening to the University of Warsaw, alma mater to 10,000 students, with its magnificent library of 800,000 volumes. Has it shared the fate of Louvain University in the World War, of the University of Madrid during the Spanish insurrection?

However, even if by some miracle it escaped total destruction by bombardment and fire, the university is certainly ruined, and with it the dozen or so other special and technical schools that brought the total academic population of Warsaw up to about 20,000. For research and education must have students and teachers and both faculties and student bodies must now be either dead or prisoners or in exile.

Although the University of Warsaw is only a little more than a century old it has had a checkered career. It was founded in 1816, only to be closed in 1831. Reopened in 1862, it ran for only half-a-dozen years before it was closed again in 1869. Reorganized as the Imperial University of Warsaw in the following year, and renamed simply the Polish University in 1915, it has continued in operation and grown rapidly since the end of the World War and the repulse of the Bolshevik invasion in 1920.

Similar disruption of activities must have been the lot of other Polish institutions, notably the ancient University of Krakow; although at that place there probably was no major destruction of physical equipment because of the quick capture of the city by the Germans.

Because Krakow was the ancient capital of Poland, the Polish Academy of Sciences had its headquarters there. This organization, corresponding to the National Academy of Sciences in the United States and the Royal Society in Great Britain, is another scientific casualty of the new war.—FRANK THONE.

## WEATHER FORECASTS IN EUROPE



WEATHER, which regularly migrates from west to east, is proving an ally of the Allies in the present war, as it did in 1914–1918. Britain and France know what the weather is going to be like over Germany before the Germans themselves know, and can plan their military operations accordingly.

The British and French have this private foreknowledge of German weather because they get the same weather first. Storm centers and areas of fair weather that eventually reach Germany cross Britain or France on the way, or at least some stretch of ocean patrolled by Allied warships and open to non-German commercial shipping, from all of which weather information can be obtained for Allied use but denied to Germany.

To be sure, German submarines may possibly be sending weather information home by radio, but that would be a risky procedure, with British and French destroyers and aircraft constantly on the alert to pick up any hint of a U-boat's whereabouts. And if the anti-submarine campaign succeeds completely, as the British Admiralty claims it will, even this slender source of weather information would then be lost to the Reich.

In the meantime, every effort is being made in Britain to deprive the Germans of any possible crumb of weather information. Publication and broadcasting of weather data are strictly forbidden; not even the occurrence of a local thunderstorm may be mentioned. Public forecasting in the islands has undergone a complete black-out, lest the enemy glean any helpful information from it.

Weather broadcasts are still being radioed from such places as the Azores, Greenland and of course the United States; but these are too remote to give German meteorologists any real help. And the coastal countries—Belgium, the Netherlands and Denmark—are too near and too small to be of any use.

Weather knowledge has become of immense value in war. Before a major offensive is launched the general staff wants to be assured that it will not bog down in mud. Before an air raid takes off, or a naval move is undertaken, the chances of storm, cloudiness, fog and high wind must be determined. Chemical warfare is notoriously dependent on wind and the chances of rain. Meteorologists have taken the place of the augurs and soothsayers who used to go with the armies of antiquity.

Accounts of the successful British air raid on the Kiehl Canal area indicate that it was timed on a knowledge of weather probabilities. The pilots' stories of taking off in clear weather, flying into rain and swooping out of clouds to loose their bombs on German warships and shore works all suggest rather strongly that English weather men knew where a helpful storm area might be centered.

The converse of this story is one from World War days, of a pair of Zeppelins that started from their German base in what looked like good flying and bombing weather, but ran into a storm of which they had no warning and were both lost in the North Sea.

In old sailing-ship days, a fleet about to go into battle sought to get the ''weather gage'' of its opponent, that is, to maneuver into a position to his windward. The geographic position of England and France would seem to give them a permanent weather gage of Germany.—FRANK THONE.

## THE NUTRITIONAL PROBLEMS OF GERMANY

GERMANY'S new brightly colored food cards limiting rations of meat and other staples are likely to spell malnutrition.

The new tightening of the belt imposed on the civil population—the second notch drawn in since the war started—means that Germans will have a diet less adequate in fats and milk than the subsistence diet worked out in America. Nutritionists here emphasize that the subsistence level of diet is for emergency only. It shows the

best apportionment of small funds to buy food, but may not maintain health over any protracted time.

The American subsistence diet calls for a pint of milk a day for children; and for adults, half a pint or more than two ounces of cheese such as American cheddar type. Germany now restricts its milk ration to children, allowing those under six a full pint and a half a day, those between six and 14, a half pint a day. Older teen age boys and girls whose bone formation is in rapid progress get no milk allowance. Like adults, they have only a cheese allowance, and that is a mere two ounces for a whole week. One egg a week is recommended on the subsistence diet by American nutritionists, and one egg a week is about what Germans can buy, although there is no ration card limiting purchase.

The protective foods, such as milk, green vegetables, oranges, tomatoes, are important in any diet for warding off malnutrition, and are included even in the most economical budgeting by American nutritionists. Germany's garden crops are something of a question mark here, but it is considered unlikely that farms and freight trains are supplying civilian markets with adequate amounts of green produce, though Germany's community gardening may help out.

Americans, while not faced with Germany's ration card problems and shortages, are increasingly interested in warding off malnutrition. Farmers' Bulletin 1757, which discusses "Diets to Fit Family Income," is a "best seller" of the Department of Agriculture's current publications. As a free document it is now exhausted and a new free printing is in the presses, but orders at five cents a copy are being received and filled at the Government Printing Office. This is the publication of 1936 in which Dr. Hazel Stiebeling worked out four diet levels for American guidance: the emergency or subsistence diet, the minimum diet (not recommended for America, but the best apportionment of money at the lowest level to maintain health), the moderate diet and the liberal or more attractive and expensive diet.

## CANALS LINKING THE ATLANTIC AND THE PACIFIC



IF plans for the Nicaraguan Canal, now revived, actually get to the digging stage, America will have achieved three out of four much-talked-of canals for linking the Atlantic and Pacific.

The four main canal routes which have at various times been considered by American engineers are: *First,* the Panama route, now a 25-year-old reality. *Second,* the route across southern Nicaragua, linking in the San Juan River and Lake Nicaragua. Planned as far back as 1825, this project is now being studied in conference by the Nicaraguan Government and its neighbor Costa Rica, while American engineers are again at the task of surveying the ground problems. *Third,* the route across the narrowest part of Mexico, the Isthmus of Tehuantepec. A canal at this point, so much nearer the States than Panama, would bring Honolulu more than 1,200 miles closer to New York. *Fourth,* a route farther south than any of these, across Colombia near its Panama border. This route actually has once been dug—dug and practically forgotten. It was America's first achievement in joining the oceans, undertaken with no thought of this significance, by a Spanish monk, Antonio de Cereso, and Indian laborers back in 1788.

Recent discovery of an old map showing this canal is reported by the WPA historical records survey. Premilas F. Becnel, going over historic documents at Tulane University's Department of Middle American Research, unearthed this map, and realized its historic value. Continuing the search for more records of the Canal of Raspadura, as it was called, Mr. Becnel and a research student assistant have since found eight more maps showing the canal and have traced its history. It joined the San Juan River, which has an outlet on the Pacific, with a tributary of the Atraro River, which flows into the Gulf of Darien on the Atlantic side.

America's first ocean-to-ocean canal was dug, not for trade, but to settle a boundary argument between two families. It was a shallow ditch, but during periods of high water Indians began to find the route handy in their canoes, thus unknowingly becoming first to take a short-cut water route from one coast of America to the other. Cacao beans for Indians and white people were the early commercial cargoes that crossed the continent *via* this canal.

A Philadelphia engineer in 1852 found the Raspadura ravine route so filled up that even his light-draft canoe had to be dragged through a canyon on dry land before he could get to the San Juan River and the Pacific.—EMILY C. DAVIS.

## THE TREATMENT OF INSOMNIA

VITAMINS are replacing sleeping medicines in the newest treatment of insomnia or sleeplessness, reported by Dr. Louis J. Karnosh, Western Reserve School of Medicine, in the *Journal* of the American Medical Association.

The vitamin treatment may, in fact, be looked on as a cure, since it attacks an underlying cause of the condition, whereas the sleeping medicines are palliative. The physician using this treatment, however, does not rely on a glass of fruit juice at bedtime to put his patient to sleep. The vitamins are given like medicine, sometimes injected into veins, and in large doses, rather than merely as part of the diet.

$B_1$, the anti-beriberi vitamin of yeast, and C, or ascorbic acid, the citrus fruit and tomato juice vitamin, are the ones particularly recommended in this report of the newest ways of attacking both ordinary sleeplessness and the insomnia that accompanies certain diseases, including delirium tremens.

"Vitamin $B_1$ should be looked on as the perfect sedative for delirium tremens," Dr. Karnosh declared. Ascorbic acid, the vitamin C principle, is a serious rival of vitamin $B_1$ as the "ideal sedative" for exhaustive states, such as occur in patients with the severe thyroid disease or goiter known as thyrotoxicosis. Ordinary insomnia, irrespective of its cause, also yields to large doses of this vitamin. This treatment produced a "sound and normal sleep," there were no undesirable after-effects and in some cases a normal sleep rhythm was established for a week or more, Dr. Karnosh says, summing up a report of another physician who treated more than 100 insomnia sufferers with the C vitamin.

# Inorganic Analysis
# *with* Organic Reagents

SPEED, convenience, accuracy, and selectivity characterize the analytical methods in which organic reagents are employed for the determination of metals. A choice of procedures—gravimetric, colorimetric, or volumetric—is available for most of the common metals.

If inorganic analyses are an important part of your routine, write for the list of free abstracts describing the use of Eastman Organic Chemicals. . . . Eastman Kodak Company, *Chemical Sales Division*, Rochester, N. Y.

**EASTMAN ORGANIC CHEMICALS**

## PerfeKtum R
## AMPOULES

**(Made in Hungary of Hungarian glass tubing)**

*THOROUGHLY ANNEALED*
*ALKALI-RESISTANT*
*SHOCK-PROOF*

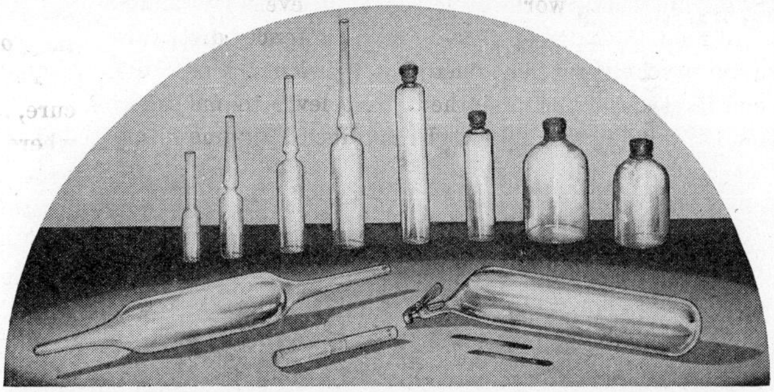

The distinguishing characteristics of PerfeKtum R Ampoules are as follows: Glass thoroughly annealed to obviate strains and stresses, during fusing or sterilizing, which weaken the ampoules and cause premature breakage. The Hydrogen Ion Concentration of the glass is recorded as pH-6.7, which is equal to that of the best resistant glass known on the market. Easy to seal due to comparatively low melting point. High thermic quality. Special composition of glass enables it to withstand a temperature of 260°C. without cracking. PerfeKtum R Ampoules fully comply with all official specifications in regards to chemical reactions. Complete stock of all items available for immediate shipment.

*Send for FREE Sample Case of Ampoules*

Quotations supplied upon request

Inquiries solicited for special requirements

**PERFEKTUM PRODUCTS COMPANY**

300 FOURTH AVENUE NEW YORK, N. Y.

Dr. Karnosh advises treatment with both vitamins $B_1$ and C to ward off the insomnia incidental to hardening of the brain arteries and senile decay, particularly because old people are likely to be short on vitamins. Rather than giving large and continued doses of ordinary sedatives, Dr. Karnosh believes vitamins should be used to treat sleeplessness in heart disease, in the weakness following infections and in all exhaustion states which deplete the nervous system.

## THE CHEMO-SCORE

AT Kansas State College, where a new system of examination grading is in vogue, if the student's answer is wrong it turns red; if it is correct the answer turns blue.

This method of grading, known as the Chemo-Score, was invented by two brothers, Dr. H. J. Peterson, of State Teachers College, Hattiesburg, Miss., and Dr. J. C. Peterson, of Kansas State College. Printed with two moisture-sensitive black inks, the correct and incorrect answer spots are initially indistinguishable, but when moistened they change color immediately. The student records his choice of answers by touching with a fountain pen which contains water instead of ink, or with a moistened paper clip, the spot which represents his chosen answer to each question. If his choice is correct the answer spot turns blue, if incorrect, it turns red.

A transparent answer sheet is used in correspondence work. To develop the answer spots on such a sheet the student dips a roughened pin in water, thrusts it through the sheet at the desired location and works it up and down a few times. The pin is removed and the perforated spot pressed between the thumb and forefinger. This causes the color to spread.

This self-instructor type of lesson calls for no writing whatsoever on the part of the student. For a three-hour course in psychology, the student works out 10 sets of problems and questions, using 10 accompanying self-instructor cards to record and check the answers.

After studying the assignment, the student takes up the problems one by one and checks his answers on the self-instructor cards. If his first answer is wrong, he will be informed of that fact by the red color reaction which issues from the spot. Directions call for him to re-read the relevant text material, study more intensely than before, and make another trial answer. The student continues until he gets the blue color reaction, signifying the correct answer. The uniqueness of the method compels and holds interest.

A "Play Your Way Reader" utilizing the same principle, has also been prepared by the Peterson brothers. With practically no assistance the child eagerly "plays his way" into a reading acquaintance with 120 common words. Each line in the book contains a problem and consists of a picture and four words, one of which names the pictured object. The word in each line which names the pictured object turns red and the others turn blue. Thus, the child can test his own solution to each problem.

This immediate check-up on every response serves to intensify interest and hold attention. It presents to the child, just when the word and its meaning are most vividly associated in his mind, the assurance that they belong together, or, if his choice is erroneous, he sees his mistake. This assurance, accompanied by the interest it creates, is probably the most powerful factor in learning that is known to psychology.

## ITEMS

THE number of World War soldiers who are patients in hospitals for mental disease is still going up and will continue to increase, it is estimated, for another eight years. In 1929, a decade after the war, 18,393 veterans were hospitalized for mental disease. Now, another decade later the number has gone up to 29,000. By 1947, it is estimated by the U. S. Veterans' Bureau, the peak will be 40,000. This figure does not include a much larger number suffering from mental and nervous diseases, but who are kept out of hospitals. The total number of World War veterans receiving compensation for neuropsychiatric disease on January 1, 1929, was 54,785. It is now 89,119, of which 67,366 cases are directly traceable to the war.

A NEW departure in weather forecasting is being tried at the district office of the U. S. Weather Bureau at the Kansas City airport. If it works out satisfactorily it may be extended to other Weather Bureau stations throughout the country. The new procedure, which went into operation on October 1, consists of making aviation and general weather forecasts at the same station, by the same staff. Hitherto, aviation weather forecasts have been made by special staffs working at airports, while the general forecasts were made independently at the old downtown Weather Bureau offices. The new system, it is hoped, will save expense through elimination of duplicate equipment and through a better scheduling of the time of the personnel. A possible drawback, which must be avoided if the new system is to function properly, might be simultaneuos demands for both aviation and general forecasts.

GLOWING colors in autumn leaves are due mainly to three kinds of pigment. Reds and purples come from a substance called anthocyanin, in solution in the cell sap. This is the same coloring matter present in beets, red cabbage and most deep red flowers, like dahlias and cannas. Yellow tones come from tiny solid pigment bodies made up of either xanthophyll or carotin. These are always present in the leaves, but during the summer are masked by the stronger hue of the green chlorophyll. When the latter pigment breaks down and becomes colorless the yellow hues come into their own.

WILT-RESISTANT alfalfa varieties, developed under a long-range breeding program by the U. S. Department of Agriculture, will be available to limited distribution in 1942. The new alfalfas are being produced by crossing resistant strains, brought from Turkistan by H. L. Westover, with varieties already established in the United States. Alfalfa wilt began to become a serious problem in this country about 15 years ago. Up to that time, a good stand of alfalfa could be counted on to last from 6 to 12 years without reseeding, but lately the wilt organism has been wiping out alfalfa fields in from two to four years.

# SCIENCE NEWS

*Science Service, Washington, D. C.*

## THE DISTANCE OF THE STARS



MORE than 5,000 stars nearest to the earth are only a half or a third as far away as astronomers have previously believed, is announced by Professor Jan Schilt, head of the department of astronomy of Columbia University. By analyzing thousands of determinations of distances of the "nearer" stars, made by the method of parallaxes, Professor Schilt has found a small systematic error which changes the calculated distances by a factor of from two to three.

Parallax is the method by which the distances of the nearer stars are computed, particularly those of the earth's galaxy. The parallax method is based on sighting the angle of the star in the sky at intervals six months apart and then computing its distance by trigonometry.

By examining the stellar parallaxes obtained through many years by many astronomers, Professor Schilt has determined small correction factors which occur systematically. Although it is only a working hypothesis, Professor Schilt suggests that the tides in the earth's atmosphere, caused by the pull of the moon, change the bending ability of the air for the light from the star and make the determinations of position slightly in error.

It is also suggested that the effect of sunlight passing through the air about the earth would warm it slightly and hence create "waves" that might change its bending ability. A combination of the moon and sun effect is believed to produce the errors. For any individual measurement the systematic error thus introduced is much smaller than the error of observation. Only by taking large numbers of observations and analyzing them statistically can the systematic error be detected.

While the new findings tend to shrink the known limits of the galaxy of stars containing the sun and earth, the discovery does not mean that the limits of the universe are likewise decreased. This is because the distances of remote stars are not determined by the parallax method but by means of the luminosity law which relates their brightness with their distance.

The new knowledge is expected to take the galaxy of stars to which the sun belongs out of the special category in which it has been placed. Because the new findings "move in" the stars, the number of them to be found in a cubic volume of the galaxy is increased. Previously it has been supposed that the sun's galaxy was "thinner" and had fewer stars per unit volume than other island universes out in space. The new discovery brings the sun's galaxy more in line with the characteristics of other galaxies.

It will be necessary to recompute the distances of all stars for which the method of parallaxes has been employed since the method was first introduced by the German astronomer, Friedrich W. Bessel, in 1838. Because of the systematic nature of the new correction, only recalculation will be needed without taking new observations on each star.

## A NEW KIND OF EARTHQUAKE WAVE DISCOVERED

A NEW type of earthquake wave, which is expected to alter radically now-accepted seismological theories and the allied concepts of building quake-proof structures, has been discovered by Dr. L. Don Leet, director of the Seismograph Station of Harvard University. The find is also expected to be of special military importance, since it will probably vitally affect the use of the seismograph in army artillery observation, which employs earth tremors as guides to the sites of heavy enemy guns. They are also used to check the accuracy of the army's own firing. Both the discharge of a cannon and explosion of a shell start underground vibrations which can be traced on earthquake recording instruments.

The new wave-form was detected after a ten-year study of man-made earthquakes, touched off by high-power dynamite explosions. Dr. Leet said that the new type vibration, entirely unpredicted in earthquake theory, is the fifth fundamental type known to science.

The four forms previously known have been recognized for about forty years and it was surprising to find a new type, especially since in many types of explosion-shocks the new form is dominant, registering strongly on the instruments while the other four forms hardly leave their marks. The new form is a sort of surface wave which travels through the upper 200 miles of the earth's crust, in contrast to the deeper waves which travel directly through the earth's core. It is the third fastest of known earthquake waves. Those through the earth's center are the speediest, and they impart a push-and-pull motion to particles in the path. Another internal wave, which shakes the particles from side to side of the wave-path, is second-fastest.

Then comes the new wave, which drives particles at a diagonal to its path, followed by another surface wave, with a side-to-side motion, and finally, the slowest wave of all, a surface wave which drives the particles in a curious sort of elliptical rotation. Dr. Leet has timed the new wave going about 2,500 feet a second when set off by dynamite in sandy ground, but he pointed out that this speed might be considerably different under other conditions. Thus far the new wave form has been observed only on dynamite-explosion records, not on natural quake-charts, but Dr. Leet said it is "almost certain" that it will eventually be found among natural tremors. In all other respects, he pointed out, natural and artificial quakes are similar.

An important problem arising from discovery of the new wave, and one which Dr. Leet is now investigating, is how much damage this new type of wave does. If it is mingled with the waves close to the sources of earthquakes, which cause heaviest damage, it may be necessary to change the design of quake-proof structures to withstand the ground conditions set up by the new wave.

The discovery may also have important implications for the science of geology, for many of the assumptions which

geologists have made concerning conditions deep in the interior of the earth are based on studies of earthquake waves. The fact that certain waves travel faster under the Pacific Ocean than under a continent, for example, has been interpreted to indicate differences in rock structure under oceans and continents. With a new concept of quake-waves, however, many of these conclusions may have to be reexamined.

## PAPERS READ BEFORE THE AMERICAN ACADEMY OF OPHTHALMOLOGY AND OTOLARYNGOLOGY

AT the Chicago meeting of the American Academy of Ophthalmology and Otolaryngology held on October 9, 10 and 11 the rare case of a patient whose eyesight was affected by a waterlogged condition of his cornea, relieved by a draining operation, was reported by Drs. R. O. Rychener, of Memphis, and D. B. Kirby, of New York. The cornea is the transparent tissue in front of the eye through which we see. Sometimes it is pushed forward into a cone shape instead of its usual flattened curve under the eyelids. The condition is caused by abnormal stretching of and high pressure within the eye. Vision in such cases is usually very poor. In this case of waterlogging the inside of the cornea was stretched so that the water fluid within the eye worked its way into the layers of the cornea, causing a diffuse cloudiness. By cutting the cornea and draining off some of the excess fluid, thus reducing the pressure, the condition was relieved and the patient had better vision than before the waterlogging complication set in. Only eight other cases of this condition have been reported in medical literature.

THAT diabetic patients whose vision has been impaired by bleeding into the retina of the eye have been helped by large doses of vitamins B and C, was reported by Dr. Jonas S. Friedenwald, of the Johns Hopkins University and Hospital. In these patients the tiny veins and arteries of the retina have very fragile walls and consequently bleed easily. Ordinarily, vitamin C, the scurvy-preventing vitamin of citrus fruits and tomatoes, makes these fragile blood vessel walls sturdier, thus controlling the bleeding tendency. Tendency to bleeding from tiny blood vessels because of deficiency of vitamin C is one characteristic of scurvy itself. Diabetic patients, however, apparently do not always utilize vitamin C normally, so even when given large doses of it, their eye condition does not improve. But when vitamin B, the vitamin found abundantly in yeast and liver, is given with vitamin C, the resistance of the small blood vessels in the eyes of diabetics is restored to normal. Dr. Friedenwald reported "marked improvement" in the eye condition of a small group of diabetic patients who were given the double vitamin treatment. Vitamin B is made up of a number of different vitamins which scientists have recently been separating. Which part of the B complex is responsible for the improvement in the eye condition is being investigated.

VITAMINS, or at least a diet with plenty of vitamins to build up the patient's general health, are a necessary eyesight-saving addition to treatment of syphilis of the brain and nervous system, it appears from the report of Dr. William M. Muncy, of Providence, R. I. High degrees of artificial fever plus powerful arsenical drugs are used in treating this kind of syphilis, but the combined treatment was found to cause inflammation of the optic nerve in a number of patients who had no previous eye trouble. Vitamin deficiency was believed responsible. Dietary building-up restored to normal the vision of a number of these patients, after which they were able to stand repeated doses of the necessary arsenical treatment for the syphilitic condition without further symptoms of visual disorder.

Two surgical hole-drilling operations, one of them brand-new, for relief of deafness were reported by Dr. O. Jason Dixon, of Kansas City. The new operation is for relief of deafness due to abnormal inward pressure of the ear-drum on the chain of tiny bones in the middle ear. To relieve this pressure, Dr. Dixon makes a hole behind the ear through the mastoid, connecting with the ear-drum from behind. The hole is lined with grafted skin and remains permanently open. Dr. Dixon reported that several patients who had this operation showed considerable improvement of hearing. The other operation for deafness discussed was described by Dr. Edward H. Campbell, of Philadelphia. It is applicable only to one type of chronic progressive deafness, characterized by a roaring in the ears. In this operation a hole is drilled into the outermost semicircular canal back of the ear, making a tiny window into the ear. Successful results depend on the window remaining permanently open. There is a tendency for the surrounding bone to grow rapidly and to close the window. The operation can not be performed if the patient is extremely deaf, or if he can not hear through the bones of the skull, or if he is dizzy or has other signs of imperfect balancing mechanism.

A NEW kind of sinusitis was reported by Lieutenant Colonel J. E. Ash, curator of the Army Medical Museum in Washington. The condition may feel like the same old sinus trouble to the patient, but Colonel Ash discovered that the lining of the sinus in one case showed a type of inflammation like that seen in chronic bladder inflammation. This, apparently, is the first time the condition has been reported. Sinus disease is due either to germs, to an allergy like hay-fever or to a combination of the two.

THE recently discovered danger of serious lung trouble from nose drops can be avoided if the drops are made with vegetable oils instead of mineral oils, according to Dr. Frank J. Novak, Jr., of Chicago. The danger arises when the nose drops or spray accidentally get into the bronchial tubes, which is especially likely to happen in babies and small children. Vegetable oils, unlike mineral oils, can be absorbed by the body tissues and disposed of without harm, whereas non-absorbable mineral oils accumulate and sometimes cause damage.

A RARE kind of eye trouble, in which the eye protrudes from its socket and beats or throbs in time with the heart beat, was reported by Drs. S. J. Meyer and H. Saul Sugar, of Chicago. Skull fractures from automobile accident injuries or other hard blows on the temple may cause the condition, but it is most often due to rupture of the carotid artery, the big artery running up the side of the neck, at the place where it passes through the large venous channel behind the eye. Besides the severe deformity of the eye, the patient hears the disagreeable noise of the blood rushing from the artery into the vein. The physician can hear this by listening through his stethoscope applied at the temple, and a whirring sensation is felt through the eyelid. For relief of the condition it may be necessary to tie the internal carotid artery.

Warning that glaucoma with loss of vision may follow the use of large doses of x-rays or radium in treatment of cancer of the cheek or tumors of the eye was sounded by Dr. Louis Bothman, of Chicago. In glaucoma the eye hardens because of changes that interfere with the normal escape of fluid from the eye. The condition is fortunately a rare complication of the life-saving cancer treatment and can be guarded against in most cases by careful screening of the eye against the rays.

Dr. William T. Davis, of Washington, reported that children with the kind of squint in which one eye turns in may be helped to overcome the condition by careful training plus the use of strong-lensed eye glasses. These children, Dr. Davis said, should be trained to use the squinting eye by covering up the good one. Such children squint when they see sharply, he explained, but the eyes become straight when the vision is blurred, either by strong lenses or by training. When the child learns to relax the muscles, glasses may be discarded. This type of squint is entirely different from that arising from muscular weakness or paralysis, which may require both glasses and operation for correction.

## ITEMS

A major epidemic of influenza is predicted for February, 1941, with a "Phase 2 outbreak of some severity" likely to occur in February, 1940. The two-phase theory of influenza occurrence on which these predictions are based has been developed by an English physician, Dr. J. H. D. Webster. It is brought to the attention of American physicians and health authorities through an editorial in the *Journal* of the American Medical Association. Analyzing 'flu epidemic history for the past 49 years, Dr. Webster finds that Phase 1, accounting for influenza outbreaks every 33 weeks, is the major phase in the influenza cycle. Phase 2, the intermediate, covers outbreaks occurring about 16 weeks after Phase 1. This phase has led to a number of serious outbreaks such as those in February-March, 1924, January-March, 1932, and the first and third world-wide epidemics of 1918–1919.

Very great solar activity is now speckling the sun's face, it is shown on photographic plates taken at the U. S. Naval Observatory. The rise in solar activity coincides with increase in magnetic disturbance which is forecast by the Department of Terrestrial Magnetism of the Carnegie Institution of Washington. On September 29, the U. S. Naval Observatory photographed 273 spots on the sun's disk. On the next day the number was substantially the same.

A new water-repelling chemical which becomes part of the fiber on which it is applied and which can not be removed by any known solvent was announced at the meeting in Boston of the American Association of Textile Chemists and Colorists. The new material, a long-chain quarternary ammonium compound, known as Zelan, gives a permanent water-repellent finish to clothing which laundering and dry cleaning will not remove. Use of the chemical for coating the clothing of armies is seen as one potential use, for the clothing will not become heavy with rain or perspiration. Yet at the same time the chemical does not close the pores of the clothing and allows the evaporation of perspiration which helps keep the body cool. George A. Slowinske, du Pont chemist, said that for flags, pennants and sailcloth the chemical was already showing excellent service. There is no need to dry out the sails to prevent mildew (the time-honored chore of yachtsmen).

At thirty-eight miles above the earth's surface the temperature is 100 degrees Centigrade, the boiling point of water, Dr. Fred L. Whipple, astronomer of Harvard University, told the meeting of the International Union of Geodesy and Geophysics. Dr. Whipple's discovery was accomplished with a new type of "meteor speedometer" which uses the appearance of shooting star tracks in the sky to tell temperatures in the stratosphere far beyond the reach of man. With his new apparatus Dr. Whipple obtains very accurate measurements of the height, brightness, velocity and deceleration of meteors which flash briefly in the area about 30 to 60 miles above the earth. At heights of 70 miles above the earth the temperature is found to be 20 degrees Centigrade, ordinary room temperature. The basic principle of Dr. Whipple's apparatus is to revolve a fan blade in front of a telescope-camera lens in such a way that if a meteor flashes down across the field of view, its fiery path is broken at measured intervals. This gives an indication of speed and deceleration. There is one such thermometer at Harvard Observatory in Cambridge, while the other is at Harvard's Oak Ridge station, 24 miles away.

Beams of piercing neutron particles are now being produced at the department of physics at Cornell University in an experimental advance which will be of great aid to the study of the transmutation of matter, artificial disintegration, etc. Professor R. F. Bacher, of Cornell, and Dr. D. C. Swanson, now at the University of Florida, report in *The Physical Review* that by placing a thick wall of water around a source of neutrons and then putting a "hole" through the water by means of a tube they have achieved a distinct collimation of their neutrons into a beam. Neutrons, because they lack electrical charge, easily penetrate into any atoms with which they come in contact. Previous attempts to produce a beam of them have only been partially successful. And yet such beams have been greatly needed to improve the geometry of many nuclear experiments in which scattering occurs, and cross sections of atoms for neutrons of different energies can be determined.

# SCIENCE NEWS

*Science Service, Washington, D. C.*

## BLIND LANDING FOR AIRPLANES



EXTREMELY difficult is the decision facing the committee of the National Academy of Sciences assigned to select a standard American system of blind landing for airplanes. In the interests of economy, efficiency and national defense, President Roosevelt has asked the academy for this decision.

This committee, as yet unselected, must choose from at least seven different blind landing systems which have been developed since Major James H. Doolittle, ten years ago, made the first blind instrument landing at Mitchell Field, L. I. The seven systems which have gone beyond the paper stage of development into actual airport installations include those of Air Track, Army, Bendix, I.T.D., Lorentz, M.I.T.-Metcalf and the Navy. The committee will examine impartially the claims, merits and tried performance of these systems and others and recommend accordingly. The fundamental question is whether it is wise now, after only the relative short time of ten years of development, to standardize on any one blind landing system.

The first of serious attempts to land an airplane with instrumental aid alone was that of the National Bureau of Standards in Washington in 1928. This method used a radio range beacon signal to mark the line of the runway and a marker radio beacon at the end of the field for longitudinal guidance. It was this system that Lieutenant Doolittle used in making the first successful blind landing in 1929. Later in 1929, at College Park Airport, Md., a glide path was added to the system by radio beams which provided the pilot with a positive and continuous indication of his vertical and lateral position. The marker beacons at the end of the airport gave indication of longitudinal position. The first landing on the complete system was made by M. S. Boggs on September 5, 1931. This was followed early in 1933 by landings at Newark.

Following publication of the Bureau of Standards work, the Lorentz Company in Germany developed a commercial system along similar lines. This system is in operation at several European airports and was tested at Indianapolis in 1937. During 1932 and 1933, the U. S. Army developed its own system of blind landing, which involved the use of a sensitive altimeter to give indication of the height above the ground. This system was quite easy to fly and required only a short pilot-training period, but failed to interest commercial aviation greatly because of lack of a finite course down the runway.

Essentially all the systems, with the exception of the Dingle system backed by the Navy, utilize very short radio waves to obtain sharp directional signals. The Navy in contrast employs very long wave-lengths. Standard practise is to detect with instruments in the plane the line of equal signal intensity between two directional radio beams. If the beams originate on a landing field, the equal-intensity line will furnish the pilot with the line of the runway. In the Army's newer system the direction is determined by direction finders on two radio stations.

## COLOR VISION

THE first explanation of the chemistry underlying color vision in an animal was reported at the Lake Placid meeting of the Optical Society of America by Dr. George Wald, of the Harvard University Biological Laboratories. Dr. Wald has isolated and identified three color pigments found in the cones of the chicken eye, the color-seeing receptors. These pigments, he said, probably act as color filters in much the same sort of arrangement used to take color photographs.

The pigments are astacene, which is responsible for the color of boiled lobsters; xanthophyll, the pigment of egg yolk, and a carotene, a pigment giving carrots their characteristic color. The color "film" of the chicken eye, on which the filtered light falls to start the seeing process, contains a violet, light-sensitive pigment which Dr. Wald has named iodopsin. It is the first light-sensitive pigment ever found in the cones of the eye.

Dr. Wald, winner of this year's Eli Lilly prize of the American Chemical Society for his outstanding research on the chemistry of vision, gave his explanation of chickens' color vision during a paper in which he massed experimental evidence to prove that many of the complicated phenomena of seeing, a process involving man's highest mental powers, can be explained on a basis of relatively simple chemical and physical reactions which take place in the eye. More and more, he said, scientists are learning that many of the properties of vision are derived directly from the properties of various substances in the retina of the eye, the photographic plate on which images of the outside world are formed. As an example Dr. Wald reported the direct chemical analysis of retinas which show that rhodopsin, a rose-colored, light-sensitive pigment found in the rods, is manufactured by the body from two different precursors, either retinene or vitamin A.

This discovery has afforded a physico-chemical explanation of varying rates of the adaptation of the eye to darkness, for the synthesis from retinene is much more than that from vitamin A and the speed of the adaptation depends entirely on which precursor is being used. It also explains why a deficiency of vitamin A results in night-blindness, the inability to see in dim light, he reported. Without the vitamin there just isn't enough rhodopsin being formed.

In studies of experimentally induced night-blindness in human subjects, conducted by Dr. Selig Hecht and his colleagues at Columbia University and Dr. Wald, it was found that not only the rods but also the cones of the eye are affected by a faulty diet, a discovery which implies that vitamin A may be the precursor of the light-sensitive material of the cones as well as of rhodopsin.

Dr. Wald has found that visual sensitivity may decrease markedly within 24 hours on a vitamin-deficient diet. It

can be cured, however, in as short a time as 20 minutes with a single dose of vitamin A or the provitamin, carotene.

## ATOMIC ENERGY OF URANIUM UNDER NEUTRON BOMBARDMENT

(*Copyright, 1939, by Science Service*)

FROM eight pounds of uranium enough atomic energy can be released by neutron bombardment to drive a giant ocean liner like the *Queen Mary* across the Atlantic.

This calculation, showing the potency of atomic energy in contrast to fuel oil used by the Atlantic liners, can be made on the basis of new experiments just reported to the American Physical Society by Dr. Malcolm C. Henderson, of Princeton University, who has measured the heating effect of the atomic energy in uranium splitting by neutrons.

Dr. Henderson exposed 13 grams of metallic uranium to intense beams of slow neutrons generated at the great cyclotron of the University of California. Inside the uranium sample he placed a resistance thermocouple and measured the rise in temperature. From this he found that each uranium atom being split liberates 175,000,000 electron volts of energy.

From this figure calculations show that, if uranium energy could be applied:

1. Eight pounds of uranium would drive the *Queen Mary* across the Atlantic, as a substitute for the 6,300 tons of fuel oil her bunkers now carry.
2. Splitting 155,000,000,000 uranium atoms would warm one gram of water one degree Centigrade.
3. Only a little over a half-pound of uranium would warm a ton of water to 3,860,000 degrees Centigrade; or convert 386,000 tons of ice water into boiling water.

## GIANT PROPELLERS

(*Copyright, 1939, by Science Service*)

THE world's largest propellers for airplanes, designed for the super-giants of the air, are now being made at the Riverdale, Md., laboratories of the Engineering and Research Corporation. Unique are these newest blades, for they are of composite structure and contain light wood, hard wood, plastics and metal. Fed E. Weick, chief engineer of the Engineering and Research Corporation, described the new propellers at the meeting of the Washington Section of the Society of Automotive Engineers.

The largest blades yet made by the composite process measure 17.5 feet from tip to tip, but engineers see no size limitation to the method. The large propellers of the Pan American "clippers," now flying the Atlantic, measure 14 feet. The new composite blades are easily produced, are 33 per cent. lighter than comparable metal propellers, are strong and have low cost. The blades consist of a core of laminated light wood which merges into a root of impregnated and compressed hard wood. This, in turn, is threaded into a controllable pitch propeller hub. The whole blade is covered with a heavy coating of reenforced plastic and the leading edge is protected by a flush strip of metal.

As aeronautical engineers have sought to get greater and greater power for airplanes they have been forced to go to larger propellers, for the greater the power the greater must be propeller diameter to retain equal efficiencies. While much progress has been made in speeding up engines so that they turn over more rapidly, there is a limit in this direction, for the propeller tip must not move at speeds comparable with those of sound, about 740 miles per hour. Interest in lighter propellers comes because as the size of a propeller increases its weight goes up faster in proportion than does the power it will deliver. This gives a light but strong propeller a sizable edge in utility.

## THE INVENTION OF A THERMAL PUMP

(*Copyright, 1939, by Science Service*)

AN ingenious "pump" that can compress gases, create vacuums or transfer heat against its normal direction of flow and thus be useful as a refrigerating mechanism, has been invented by the president of the Carnegie Institution of Washington, Dr. Vannevar Bush. A patent just issued (No. 2,175,376) describes the new apparatus which Dr. Bush developed while at the Massachusetts Institute of Technology in collaboration with Edwin L. Rose, chief engineer of the Waterbury Tool Company.

In contrast to other devices doing a similar job, Dr. Bush's machine uses not mechanical energy but heat energy to accomplish its "pumping" of either gas or heat. Patent rights have been assigned to the Research Corporation, non-profit corporation of New York City, founded to control the proper exploitation of important scientific discoveries.

When used to compress a gas, or transfer heat from a lower to a higher temperature, a substantially constant volume of gas is alternately heated and cooled, thereby alternately raising and lowering its pressure, says the patent.

"In the case of a compressor," continues the patent, "these fluctuations in pressure are utilized to effect the transfer of gas between two regions of different pressure by admitting gas to the system from a region of low pressure when the pressure is low and ejecting gas from the system to a region of high pressure when the pressure is high. In the case of the thermal pump, the fluctuations in pressure are utilized to effect corresponding fluctuations in pressure in another but communicating body of gas from which heat is ejected to a region of high thermal potential when the pressure is raised and which is caused to absorb heat from a region of low thermal potential when the pressure is lowered."

Heating of the working substance (a gas) is accomplished by a small burning flame. The system contains a blower to make the working substance flow in the proper directions at the proper times, but the patent emphasizes that this blower is used only to control the thermal cycle and does not do mechanical work in compression.—ROBERT D. POTTER.

## FOLSOM MAN

(*Copyright, 1939, by Science Service*)

Two decorated beads worn by Folsom Man or his wife are new evidence that America was no savage, uncouth place at the end of the Ice Age.

The bone "costume jewelry" is among discoveries reported by Dr. Frank H. H. Roberts, Jr., of the Bureau of American Ethnology, who has returned from excavating at the earliest American home yet found—a camp site of Folsom hunters near Fort Collins, Colo.

It is becoming clear, according to Dr. Roberts, that America's earliest known culture must have compared favorably with Europe's Stone Age cave society existing at the same time. Geologists who have studied Folsom Man's only known home pronounce the relics to be as old as the last glacial period in America, usually timed from 12,000 to 25,000 years ago.

Folsom hunters, so-called because their favorite and peculiar stone dart-points first came to light at Folsom, N. Mex., followed big game such as mammoth and bison. But far from spending all their time roving like savages and eating just to live, these early pioneers had home and community life. They enjoyed artistic decorations as shown by the beads, and also by the red and yellow paint found by Dr. Roberts.

They made the beads of long bones of some small animal, smoothing the rough edges and marking simple patterned lines on the surface. Their specialty in stone was the grooved Folsom point, beautifully made, but Dr. Roberts has unearthed a variety of tools and weapons which they contrived, including some new knives and scrapers first discovered this year.—EMILY C. DAVIS.

## THE TREATMENT OF DETACHED RETINA

ELECTRICAL spot-welding in the eye for restoring sight to patients threatened with blindness due to a detached retina was stated by Dr. Samuel J. Meyer, of Chicago, at the Philadelphia meeting of the American College of Surgeons, to be effective in a number of cases.

The retina is the light-sensitive part of the eye which transmits images to the brain through the optic nerve. It may be compared to the photographic film or plate in a camera. It depends for its nourishment on tissue called the choroid. When, because of injury or disease, it becomes detached from the choroid, it can not function properly and the patient feels as if a curtain were falling over part of his eyes. If not treated, the retina as a rule will eventually all peel off the choroid, like wallpaper off a wall, and total blindness results. Modern eye surgeons treat this condition by a kind of electrical spot-welding. Tiny needles carrying an electric current are applied to the choroid without puncturing it. The electric cauterization produces an adhesive inflammation between the choroid and the retina, causing the retina to become reattached.

This method is only 11 years old, but increasingly good results are obtained. More than one out of three patients operated on at the Illinois Eye and Ear Infirmary since 1934 had reattached retinas with vision ranging from normal to one tenth normal.

## ITEMS

THE skull of an evolutionary link between reptiles and mammals, that lived in South Africa many millions of years ago, has been studied in detail at the Walker Museum of the University of Chicago by the Reverend Harold W. Rigney, missionary-scientist now stationed at Accra, Gold Coast, West Africa. The animal, known to geologists as *Galesaurus planiceps*, belonged to the extinct order called cynodonts—the name means "dog-tooth." Although unquestionably reptiles, cynodonts resemble primitive mammals in some details of skull structure.

THE strangest fluid in the world might well be the title for liquid helium, which turns from a gas to a liquid only at the temperature of a few degrees above absolute zero. Dr. J. O. Wilhelm, low temperature expert of the University of Toronto, says that liquid helium, for equal volumes, weighs only one seventh as much as water. It has the ability to conduct heat as well as metallic copper, and it is so lacking in viscosity that it can be regarded as a gas.

AMERICAN corn fields potentially can produce fibers with wool-like properties, it appears from research reported by L. C. Swallen, chemist of the Corn Products Refining Co., at Argo, Ill. From a bushel of corn a pound of zein, a by-product of corn processing, can be obtained. Zein is a protein with uses, in many cases, like those of casein derived from cow's milk. It can be made into plastics, into water-proof wrappers, quick-drying printing inks and into films and fibers.

BOTANISTS and biochemists of the University of California have discovered in the juice of milkweed an active substance that can tenderize meat as successfully as can papain, extracted from the tropical plants, papaya, now used on a large scale for the purpose. The quantity of the new-found substance is small, but it is believed that large-scale and intensive cultivation of the plant might make its production profitable. At present, papaya imports amount to half a million pounds a year, costing several million dollars. The active principle of the milkweed has been named asclepain, from the botanical name of the plant, Asclepias, by analogy with the formation of the word papain from the plant name Papaya.

A NEW and simplified electron microscope, suitable for use in research institutions, was perfected in Germany by the great electrical firm Siemens and Halske A. G. shortly before the outbreak of war. Earlier models of this instrument, which uses streams of electrons in a vacuum tube to make visible minute structures and details not detectable by any microscope using beams of light, required the services of technicians specially trained in the handling of high vacuum and electrical instruments, which made operation too expensive for most research purposes. The new instrument obviates the necessity for these extra attendants.

THAT ultra-violet radiation, deadly to cells if administered in certain doses, proves a stimulant to growth in the same kind of cells if given in doses of two thirds the lethal magnitude, has been demonstrated in experiments at the Smithsonian Institution, performed by Dr. Florence E. Meier. Dr. Meier used cultures of the one-celled alga or water plant, *Stichococcus bacillaris*. Some were rayed, others were left unrayed, as controls. The cultures that were given the stimulative raying not only showed the response in their own generation but passed on the habit of rapid cell-multiplication to their descendants for many generations.

# SCIENCE NEWS

*Science Service, Washington, D. C.*

## THE GIACOBINI-ZINNER COMET

(*Copyright, 1939, by Science Service*)

The Giacobini-Zinner comet, periodic comet absent from the region of the sun and earth for 6.6 years, has again been sighted and the amazing meteor shower which Europe saw in 1933 may still have a chance to be repeated. Dr. George Van Biesbroeck, of the Yerkes Observatory of the University of Chicago, has discovered the comet whose crossing of the earth's orbit in 1933 caused the memorable meteor shower.

Astronomers had calculated that in 1933 the earth passed through the region of space occupied 80 days earlier by the Giacobini-Zinner comet. This region was still "dusty" from specks of matter carried along in the same orbit as the comet. As these specks struck the earth's atmosphere they flashed as "shooting stars." Astronomers had thought possibly that on October 9, 1939, this same happening might occur again.

The rediscovery of the Giacobini-Zinner comet occurred at a position almost precisely that predicted by astronomers. This means that its orbit has been disturbed only slightly, if at all, during its absence of 6.6 years from the region of the earth. Preliminary calculations prior to the comet's discovery suggested that the earth should precede the comet by some 136 days, to the point in space where their orbits crossed. Astronomers still hope for a meteor shower in 1940, when the Giocobini-Zinner comet passes ahead of the earth by 229 days.

The position of the Giacobini-Zinner comet, at the time of its discovery by Dr. Van Biesbroeck on October 15, was at right ascension 16 hours, 21 minutes and 7 seconds, while its declination was plus one degree, 18 minutes and 53 seconds.

While its magnitude is so faint (15th) that only telescopes can see it, astronomers will be able to detect it about half way up to the zenith in the northwestern sky shortly after sunset. It is near the center of the triangle formed by the widely separated bright stars, Vega, Arcturus and Antares.

## THE EFFECT OF SUB-OPTIMAL DIET

At the Pittsburgh meeting of the American Public Health Association Drs. Henry Borsook, professor of biochemistry at the California Institute of Technology, and Wilton L. Halverson, health officer of Pasadena, Calif., reported a survey showing that families on sub-optimal diets—less than the best—were no less healthy than families having adequate food intakes.

"Families on sub-optimal diets," they declared, "were not found by the measures employed to have a greater degree of ill health than those having adequate food intake. A study of a larger number of families over a period of years utilizing more exact measures of ill health will be necessary to show the alleged harmful effects of a suboptimal diet."

The diets of 50 families, 151 adults and 72 children, in economic levels from relief to those with annual incomes of $3,000 were studied. Clinical examinations were made of 80 persons in 25 of these families, including height, weight, evidence of rickets, heart, lungs, skin texture, hair texture, teeth and blood tests for anemia. No correlation between defects and dietary insufficiencies were found.

These families spent from $0.89 to $4.80 per person per week for food. Practically all families spending as much as $2.08 per person per week were eating adequately, and so were some spending as little as $1.50 per person per week.

Only about half the families got enough to eat as measured in calories. They were low on protein but got enough fat and starches and sugars. As to the important minerals and vitamins: They all got enough iron, according to present nutritional standards, but about half of them did not get enough calcium or lime. Almost all the families went short on vitamin A rations, only one getting more than the recommended amount. About a third of the families got less than enough vitamin B. All of them, however, received enough vitamin C from their diets.

## THE PREVENTION OF INFLUENZA

(*Copyright, 1939, by Science Service*)

Lieutenant-Colonel A. Parker Hitchens, M.C., professor of public health at the University of Pennsylvania, speaking at the meeting of the American Public Health Association, called attention to the fact that two weapons, a vaccine and a germ-fighting lamp, are ready for trial in the next great influenza epidemic. Either or both of them may emerge from such a trial as a practical means of preventing influenza. At least three institutions in America and one in England have already vaccinated small groups of people. If these groups come through the next epidemic without having influenza, the value of the vaccines will be shown. The institutions are all guarding their vaccination work, because they are not ready yet to vaccinate the entire population, even in the event of an epidemic. Under such conditions they could not get the accurate information necessary for a real appraisal of the vaccines. But they are ready and waiting for the results with the groups already vaccinated to show whether the entire population of a nation can be protected against influenza.

The influenza-fighting lamp, designed by Professor William F. Wells and Dr. Mildred Weeks Wells, of the University of Pennsylvania, is designed to fight any disease like influenza whose germs travel through the air, by letting down a curtain of ultra-violet rays to keep the germs out of a room and to kill any that may already be in the room. Similar lamps are being used in many operating rooms throughout the country to keep germs out of open wounds.

Schools and hospitals are already, in a few places, using the Wells lamp to protect children from germs of influenza, measles and similar infectious diseases. English, French and Canadian medical authorities, hearing about it at the

recent Congress of Microbiology in New York, are considering use of the lamp in dormitories to protect children, especially where there is crowding due to evacuation of children from London, Paris and other large cities.

## THE SUPPLY OF VANADIUM

URAVAN in Colorado, a new city, sounds as if it might be a Soviet settlement in the Urals, but it is instead a glowing achievement of American private enterprise, and a symbol of the reasons why the United States can never again be cut off from a supply of the essential silver-like alloy, vanadium.

Uravan is almost as remote as if it were in the Urals, at that. It is 115 miles from the county seat, Montrose; 60 miles from the nearest railroad, at Placerville. It is just east of the Utah line in southwestern Colorado, as wild and lonely a section as there is in the United States.

A few years ago Uncle Sam ranked a distant last among producers of vanadium, a strategic metal both in war and peace. In 1936 only 63 tons were produced here. By 1938 that production had leaped to 732 tons, an increase of more than 1100 per cent. The United States has in this short time become the producer of a third of the world supply.

This is especially important because, with the exception of Mexico, a minor producer, the centers of vanadium mining were in Northern Rhodesia, Southwest Africa and Peru—all far away.

Vanadium by increasing the toughness and "springiness" of steel has become well-nigh indispensable in the manufacture of autos and other vehicles, besides having many direct uses in war.

The Vanadium Corporation of America, a subsidiary of the Union Carbide and Carbon Corporation, developed the mines and the town. It is said that there is enough ore to keep the plant going for a hundred years.

This is not the first mining in the area. Instead it was the scene of one of the most important and romantic ventures in the history of American mining. Here was found the world's first major supply of radium, only a few years after it was discovered. The Standard Chemical Company and the Flannery interests of Pittsburgh worked thousands of tons of the carnotite ore for a thimbleful of radium. When the women of America gave Madame Curie a gram of radium it came from Colorado. Then the rich deposits of the Belgian Congo were discovered and the American mines became unprofitable. Those carnotites, and the vanadium ores which the radium miners threw over the dump, are among those now being worked at Uravan.

Both radium and uranium are being produced again, but now as by-products of the vanadium production. In 1938 the mines produced 7,811 milligrams of radium, against 3,141 in 1937.

As for vanadium, Colorado produced 1,382,000 pounds of concentrates in 1938. This was more than the whole United States production in 1937, and the total United States production in 1938 was only 1,613,000 pounds. In other words Colorado produced more than 80 per cent.

The company payroll runs about $50,000 to $60,000 a month, there are between 200 and 250 working, and the production is about 250 tons of ore daily. The town is completely company-owned, and such necessities as coal are brought in—from its own mines—by the company. Beef and vegetables are raised in the near-by Paradox Valley—so called because the Dolores River takes its stubborn way right across the waist of the valley instead of flowing down it as a well-conducted river should—but staples must be trucked in from Montrose or Grand Junction.

## ALASKA AND EUROPEAN REFUGEES



OPENING the door of Alaska to European refugees and United States immigrants, is a proposal now taking on a new and favorable angle.

While international conferees have been discussing the fate of several hundred thousand refugees, the United States' leading possibility for helping to resettle some of the homeless in Alaska needs Congressional action. The Department of the Interior advocates that private development corporations be permitted to open up suitable areas in Alaska, to offer opportunities for selected refugees and immigrants also from the states.

Since this view was reported, in August, the Department of the Interior, in cooperation with the State, Commerce and Labor Departments, has been putting finishing touches on a bill to provide a practicable way for admitting foreign settlers to Alaska. The favored plan is to provide a new quota-exempt class, exempting from quota provisions Alaska settlers as long as they are engaged in the corporate ventures, in the same way that students and certain other classes are admitted to the United States without conforming to quota requirements. The foreign settlers would not be permitted to enter the United States from Alaska except under quota provisions.

Alaskan industries, according to one advocate of the planned colonization project, are the type to be stimulated by war. Alaska has the only tin resources under United States control, and these are not fully developed. We still import 99 per cent. of our tin. Platinum, copper and gold are being produced on a limited scale and there are unworked deposits of coal, nickel, asbestos and gypsum.

Southeastern Alaska's forests offer Sitka spruce lumber as well as pulpwood sufficient to print one fourth of the news in the United States. Since the United States depends on foreign supplies, chiefly Canada, Finland and Sweden, for three fourths of its newsprint, the assurance that Alaska not only can supply timber but has the water power for running pulp and paper mills is more important now than it was two months ago.

Fish is always a food product in demand in wartime, and Alaska offers fishing opportunities, not so much perhaps in the salmon industry, which is already well developed, as in the herring industry. The United States imports almost all of its herring from Scandinavia and Great Britain and the pack of salted and pickeled products is likely to be diverted toward European needs.

The project for developing Alaska differs from most proposals to aid refugees and others seeking new opportunity in that Alaska's possibilities are industrial as well as agricultural. Those favoring planned pioneering to develop Alaskan resources point out, also, that the climate in many regions suitable for industry is no more rigorous than in Washington or in New York, and that a number of the present settlers are of southern European origin.

Individual pioneering in Alaska, or almost anywhere else, is over, it is argued by those who have been investigating Alaska's prospects. The new era of pioneering is seen as necessarily a planned economy, in which industrial development would be balanced and directed toward actual market needs.—Emily C. Davis.

## STAINLESS STEEL

*(Copyright, 1939, by Science Service)*

A new way to prevent corrosion of stainless steel in salt water, long an Achilles heel of an otherwise excellent structural material, was described at the opening meeting of the American Institute of Mining and Metallurgical Engineers at Chicago as part of the giant National Metals Congress now in session.

Dr. H. H. Uhlig, research associate of the Massachusetts Institute of Technology, described long-continued research to seek the causes and the prevention of the corrosion of stainless steel in salt water. It has been this handicap which has, in the past, led the U. S. Navy to regard, with only mild approval, the use of stainless steel on naval vessels where it is subjected to sea water.

Dr. Uhlig's research, supported by grants from the Chemical Foundation, shows that if stainless steels are exposed to air for some hours, or if they receive treatment by an oxidizing solution directly after the pickling operation, they will be corrosion-resistant in salt water.

Dr. Uhlig has worked in a cooperative research at the Massachusetts Institute of Technology, which has resulted in a number of important patents on ways of increasing the ability of stainless steels to resist corrosion. Those who have taken part in this research include John C. Wulff, Albert L. Kaye, and Professor Robert S. Williams.

Among the discoveries is the use of small amounts of the chemical that produces smoke for warfare, titanium tetrachloride, to give stainless steel a lustrous and extra smooth new surface which is especially resistant to pit corrosion. This surface has such luster that it can be fabricated into beautiful jewelry, rivaling precious metals in appearance.

They have also found that minute amounts of silver, as little as .42 per cent., can cut down the salt water corrosion of stainless steels more than 80 per cent. The silver, moreover, greatly improves the rolling and machining properties of the metal.

## ITEMS

Rainfall for the month of October thus far ranges from half normal or less in the western Prairie region, through one fourth to one third in the Ohio valley, 10 per cent. normal in Tennessee, down to almost zero in parts of the Gulf states and in western Kansas. This, following an abnormally dry September, creates a serious situation.

Diphtheria threatens to become wide-spread and severe in the South and there is no assurance that it will not do the same in the North. Diphtheria germs found in different parts of the country vary considerably in their disease-causing ability, according to a report made by Dr. Martin Frobisher, of The Johns Hopkins University, Baltimore, to members of the American Public Health Association. In the South, particularly in Virginia and Alabama, a more virulent, dangerous kind of germ has been prevalent within the last two years. During this same period there have been more cases of diphtheria. In the North, where diphtheria cases have declined enormously in the past ten years, a different type of germ is found. These facts suggest that health authorities, by studying the kind of germs in their locality, can predict the coming of an epidemic or of more severe cases of diphtheria. Not enough information is available yet, Dr. Frobisher said, to be sure whether such predictions can be made accurately, but he stressed the need for further studies along these lines.

Completion of a breeding program to produce chrysanthemums as brilliant and showy as most of the greenhouse varieties now in use, but able to survive winters as far north as Michigan and Wyoming, has been announced recently by the U. S. Department of Agriculture. The new chrysanthemum varieties, of which there are a dozen, all bearing Indian names, were developed by F. L. Mulford, who recently retired, after long service in the Bureau of Plant Industry. Mr. Mulford let nature do the selecting for hardiness and earliness. Late bloomers he ruthlessly discarded, and he let winter cold kill off non-hardy seedlings. The Department of Agriculture does not have any plants for free distribution, though it does have a free bulletin (Circular 528) describing them. The plants have been put into mass propagation by several leading commercial firms.

Experiments concluded at the Massachusetts Institute of Technology show that old-fashioned molasses is about the best food known for treating nutritional anemia, the kind of anemia due to improper diet. Spinach as a source of iron was thoroughly debunked by the research conducted by Dr. Robert A. Harris, Dr. John W. M. Bunker and L. Malcolm Mosher. Whereas molasses has 6.1 parts of usable iron per 100,000 parts by weight, spinach has only 0.5. Beef liver has 5.6; oatmeal, 4.6; apricots, eggs and raisins following in that order. Usable iron was computed, not total content, for only that iron which the body can use to manufacture hemoglobin is valuable. Both chemical and biological tests on rats were used. It is also reported that recent medical studies indicate that nutritional anemia is far more prevalent than had been suspected. More than 40 per cent. of infants have it and the figure for adult women is as high as 70 per cent. It is also fairly wide-spread among growing children.

There are autumnal migrations of bats as well as of birds. Much less is known, however, about bat migrations. Some of them appear to be for considerable distances, but many species only travel to some cave especially well adapted for comfortable and secure hibernation, which is not used as summer sleeping quarters. Other bat species do not migrate at all, but find their summer roosts good enough for the long winter sleep as well. No bats, however, remain active throughout the cold season as do some species of birds.

# SCIENCE NEWS

*Science Service, Washington, D. C.*

## ADVENTURES IN SCIENCE[1]

*Announcer:* "Adventures in Science" . . . with Watson Davis, director of Science Service. What's new in science to-day, Mr. Davis?

*Mr. Davis:* The National Academy of Sciences is meeting here in Providence, R. I., to-day, and I want to tell about some of the important scientific discoveries that were announced before it this morning and afternoon.

*Announcer:* What were some of them, Mr. Davis?

*Mr. Davis:* I was very much interested in the paper by Dr. Hudson Hoagland, Clark University physiologist, who has found that breathing of your brain cells sets the pace for your mental activity.

New understanding of paresis, or brain syphilis, one of mankind's major mental diseases, may result from this discovery.

Electric waves from the brain itself signal to scientists the nature of this chemical control.

Each cell in your brain, as a by-product of respiration, builds up electric potential. The cell walls have electric resistance. The electricity is discharged whenever the respiration process builds up potential and loads the capacities of the cell walls to their critical firing point. This electrical discharge forms the brain waves—electrical signals direct from the brain. Thus brain cell respiration creates the brain waves.

Thanks to brain waves, too, science's inquiring finger can now point more accurately to the parts of the cortex of the brain that discriminate sensation, or feeling, in various parts of the body. This is an achievement reported by Dr. J. G. Dusser de Barenne, of Yale University.

The electrical brain waves, generated in the brain itself, can be made to signal the location and the extent of the area of the sensory cortex.

The shape of man's body hints how he may die. The shape and proportions of a man, still in good health and a long way from his funeral, give fairly definite indication of how and when he may be expected to die. This is a find by Professor Raymond Pearl and Dr. W. Edwin Moffett, of the Johns Hopkins University.

Professor Pearl made a study of the histories of 2,332 men, all dead, representing the longest-lived and shortest-lived groups out of a much larger number. Information about their bodily constitution had been placed on file years before, when they were all in good health, with no indications of onset of the various diseases that finally killed them. He divided them into two classifications, long-lived and short-lived.

He found short-lived men who died of heart and kidney ailments were bigger around the body, in both chest and abdominal girth, than long-lived men who died of the same groups of diseases.

This condition was reversed in the case of men who later died of cancer and pneumonia: the skinny men were shorter lived than the stouter type.

[1] Radio program presented on Monday, October 23, under the auspices of Science Service, over the Columbia Broadcasting System.

In those eventually dying from cancer and from diabetes the average body weight was also greater in the short-lived than in the long-lived group. The difference here, however, was too small to justify any very definite conclusions.

Height apparently had nothing to do with length of life. Talls and shorts were scattered at random through all the disease groups, among both long-lived and short-lived.

Pulse rate was more rapid among all groups of the short-lived than it was among the long-lived groups.

Production of atomic projectiles of more than 100,000,000 electron-volts energy was forecast when Professor E. O. Lawrence, of the University of California, inventor of the atom-smashing cyclotron, told the academicians that building of a 120-inch, 2,000-ton cyclotron, double the size of his world's largest, is entirely feasible.

His new 60-inch cyclotron, weighing over 220 tons, has just gone into service. Gratifying results cause Professor Lawrence to look forward to a still more powerful machine for impressing large energies upon tiny fragments of matter.

By bombarding bismuth and lead with 32,000,000-volt helium ions, Professor Lawrence has obtained large yields of new radioactive substances that produce alpha particles, which are also emitted from natural radium.

These, or other cyclotron radiations, promise to prove useful in treatment of cancer and for other medical purposes.

The National Academy of Sciences is the leading scientific body of the nation before which are read and discussed scientific reports, as is being done here at Brown University this week. But that is only one of its functions. It is Uncle Sam's scientific consultant as well. As a body it is adviser to the United States Government on things scientific. Quietly, without much fanfare of publicity, the academicians give freely of their expert knowledge and opinion when the need arises. As senior scientific body of the nation the academy also cooperates closely with hundreds of other scientific groups in solving problems and conducting research of immense importance to all of us. Our Adventures in Science guest to-day is the president of the National Academy of Sciences, Dr. Frank B. Jewett. He is one of our leading engineers, president of that fruitful cradle of new industries, the Bell Telephone Laboratories. Dr. Jewett will tell us how science could be mobilized, and, indeed, is being mobilized, in the United States.

In time of war, Dr. Jewett, the mobilization of science would be as necessary as the mobilization of the Army and Navy.

*Dr. Jewett:* Yes, it is. War always brings emergency problems for the scientists of a nation. But we ought not to let this overshadow the fact that in a country like the United States science is always mobilized to a considerable extent. Our government always has problems—for example, those of public health, which deserve continuous study and which in wartime may be accentuated. Likewise, the Army and Navy have innumerable problems of so broad a character that they extend beyond the scope of

the organized forces and their specialized laboratories, and in the solution of which they ask the assistance of the nation's outstanding specialists. In the handling of such long-range problems it is apparent that we must take time by the forelock; adequate preparedness presupposes more or less continuous focusing of the nation's best scientific talent upon these problems of defense. Such problems arise not only in the newer developments, such as flying, but are equally numerous in the older services.

*Mr. Davis:* As I understand it, Dr. Jewett, the National Academy of Sciences, which serves the government in peace time, would have responsibilities placed upon it in time of war.

*Dr. Jewett:* That is correct, Mr. Davis. The National Academy of Sciences had its inception during the Civil War. It was created by an Act of Congress at the suggestion of Abraham Lincoln. Notable extensions have taken place in the meantime. The body which President Lincoln's administration created was called, and to-day is called, the National Academy of Sciences. I should like to read a portion of Section 3 of the Act of Incorporation:

". . . the Academy shall, whenever called upon by any department of the Government, investigate, examine, experiment, and report upon any subject of science or art, the actual expense of such investigations, examinations, experiments and reports to be paid from appropriations which may be made for the purpose, but the Academy shall receive no compensation whatever for any services to the Government of the United States."

*Mr. Davis:* And subsequently, Dr. Jewett, this National Academy of Sciences has been augmented by other organizations?

*Dr. Jewett:* Yes, and by one in particular. In 1916 President Wilson asked the academy to organize a subsidiary body of broader membership as a measure of national preparedness. This body, called the National Research Council, accomplished such important results in organizing research and in securing cooperation of military and civilian agencies before and during American participation in the last war, that on May 11, 1918, President Wilson issued an executive order establishing the National Research Council as a permanent body. Perhaps the best way to illustrate the functions of the council, and at the same time minimize words, is to list its divisions. They are nine in number, as follows: Foreign Relations, Educational Relations, Physical Sciences, Engineering and Industrial Research, Chemistry and Chemical Technology, Geology and Geography, Medical Sciences, Biology and Agriculture and, finally, a division for Anthropology and Psychology.

*Mr. Davis:* Won't you explain briefly, Dr. Jewett, how the proper personnel is selected from among the scientists of the country?

*Dr. Jewett:* In the first place, I ought to state that the 300 men and women who constitute the membership of the National Academy are elected on the basis of outstanding eminence in their field of science. The academy is divided into sections corresponding to the various sciences. Thus, there is a section for chemistry, another for mathematics, one for engineering, etc. Each section, of course, has a chairman who is, himself, preeminent in that field. Further, it is safe to say that the circle of acquaintanceship of the members of any section extends outward to include practically every person in the country who can qualify as well informed in the subject-matter of the section.

The National Research Council is likewise divided along lines of the various sciences. It has its permanent committees or divisions with chairmen who are selected for knowledge, experience and business ability. These chairmen, on the one hand, are naturally well acquainted with the officers of the government departments whence the problems and questions arise—and, on the other, are well acquainted with the nation's outstanding experts, whether connected with universities or with private industry. Thus, it will be seen that the National Research Council is a sort of business organization which derives its guidance from the academy and has behind it the prestige of the nation's leading scientists. Through its numerous working committees, the National Research Council is made up of many hundred scientists and engineers.

*Mr. Davis:* I think it might help us, Dr. Jewett, if you could say a few words about some of the problems which the academy and its council have studied or are studying for the government. Of course, I realize that many of these problems may be confidential, but doubtless there are others which are not secret.

*Dr. Jewett:* Well, one problem which comes to my mind is that of highway research. The council has cooperated over a period of years with the United States Bureau of Public Roads and has done effective work in coordinating information and in encouraging investigations upon the planning, building and operation of highways. During the past year, at the special request of the Bureau of Public Roads, the council has devoted particular attention to the problem of highway safety. These studies have been carried on in cooperation with the highway organizations in a number of states and comprise such topics as: Non-uniformity of state motor-vehicle traffic laws; skilled investigation at the scene of the accident needed to develop causes; inadequacy of state motor-vehicle accident reporting; official inspection of vehicles; case histories of fatal highway accidents; the accident-prone driver.

Another program of a long-time nature, and one which very definitely relates to public welfare, although not particularly to military activity, is research upon narcotics. In the first place, much has been added through this work to our knowledge of the chemistry and pharmacology of narcotic substances. From over three hundred new alkaloid substances produced experimentally, several have been found which promise medical uses. Much of the clinical work has been done at the United States Public Health Service Hospital in Lexington, Kentucky. Another important phase of narcotics research has been the development of means for the control of these new drugs.

These are but single instances. Since the academy's organization over one hundred major problems, covering practically all fields of science, in addition to a host of lesser ones, have been submitted to the academy by the Federal Government. One of the earliest, and presumably it arose as a result of the building of the iron gunboat *Monitor* during the Civil War, was to study the magnetic

compass with a view to compensating for the magnetic effect of ships built wholly or partly of iron. The findings arrived at by the academy are, I believe, standard even to this day.

*Mr. Davis:* Such problems are certainly of fundamental importance to the nation, Dr. Jewett. What are some of the current problems before the Academy and the Research Council?

*Dr. Jewett:* The most recent government request has to do with what kind of blind landing system should be adopted for American airplanes. Numerous systems have been demonstrated and the government has asked the academy to examine the evidence and advise as to a system which can be installed at all airports and on all airplanes.

Two other projects involve aviation. We are cooperating in aircraft production planes, both current and with a view to future developments. Also our psychologists are advising the Civil Aeronautics Authority on tests that can be used in connection with the training of thousands of college boys and girls to be airplane pilots. Not long ago the academy conducted for the government an extensive inquiry into lighter-than-air aircraft.

*Mr. Davis:* Many of the projects do not have a direct military bearing.

*Dr. Jewett:* That is true. For instance, the National Research Council is sponsoring research in aerobiology and scientists are flying aloft sampling the spores, bacteria, insects and other living things that the winds carry from place to place. Our program in endocrinology has achieved significant results that will not only add to knowledge but eventually save human lives. A conference called by the council this summer at the request of the government lent scientific aid to the United States Antarctic Expedition about to set forth. The Chemistry Division is just now surveying chemical research facilities in leading universities, and the council as a whole has undertaken to make a complete survey of the nation's industrial research facilities—both human and material.

*Mr. Davis:* How are these investigations paid for, Dr. Jewett?

*Dr. Jewett:* In part, expenses of investigations are paid by the department of the government posing the problem, but in part there are large expenses which we may call "going" expenses connected with organizations like the academy and the council—expenses which in private business would be analogous to "loading"—and these can not be billed to the government. To defray these and also to make possible many subsidiary lines of research, the academy has been very fortunate in attracting donations and gifts, the income from which amounts to about $200,000 per year. Private sources supply in large part, therefore, the funds which the academy and the council require, just as private sources form the chief support of the fundamental research programs of our universities.

*Mr. Davis:* It seems to me one of the most important contributions that has been made to American science is the training of leaders in research that has resulted from the National Research Council fellowships administered over a period of years.

*Dr. Jewett:* Yes, twelve hundred young scientists have been able to continue research training beyond the usual Ph.D. degree, and these splendidly equipped scientists are in many cases forging to the forefront of American science. I think, Mr. Davis, that the question of scientific mobilization for problems of national importance, whether of peace or war, can be summed up by saying that in the National Academy of Sciences and National Research Council the United States has an active operating agency which covers every field of fundamental and applied science. Further, that it is an agency which can bring to bear on any problem the best talent which the nation possesses.

*Mr. Davis:* Thank you, Dr. Jewett, for this insight into how science can be mobilized to aid our government and nation in times of peace and war.

## ITEMS

SULFAPYRIDINE, the chemical remedy that has been saving lives threatened by pneumonia, has been given to seven patients with tuberculosis in the hope that it would be equally useful as a remedy for this ailment. This hope was aroused by reports of previous use of the chemical for treating guinea pigs with tuberculosis. Unfortunately, the remedy failed to help any of the human patients, Drs. Stanton T. Allison and Robert Myers, of New York, report to the *Journal* of the American Medical Association. Both sulfapyridine and its chemical relative, sulfanilamide, are proving useful in treating another condition, the usually fatal blood poisoning due to staphylococcus infection. Cases in which these drugs are believed to have helped patients recover are reported in the same issue of the *Journal* by Drs. William A. Thornhill, Jr., Howard A. Swart and Clifton Reel, of Charleston, W. Va., and Samuel L. Goldberg and Allan Sachs, of Chicago.

A NEW rival for the carbon-arc searchlights has appeared in a 25,000,000 candlepower searchlight, using three tiny water-cooled mercury arcs, which has been developed by the General Electric Company. While present-day searchlights need an attendant to adjust the carbons for best illumination, the new searchlight does not wear out, needs no adjustment and is designed for lights in inaccessible places. Ninety gallons of water an hour are pumped through the cooling containers of the mercury arcs and then passed to an automobile-type radiator where the fluid is cooled for recirculation. Though more convenient, the new searchlight is still below the present high-intensity searchlights in beam candlepower and effectiveness.

DELIBERATELY knocking out front teeth was a youthful fashion in Indian days, it appears from an investigation of Dr. Aleš Hrdlička, of the Smithsonian Institution. He recently returned from anthropological study in the Soviet Union, where he found for the first time evidence indicating that America's Indians and Siberia's New Stone Age natives both widely practised the ceremony of knocking out front teeth of young boys and maidens. The custom provides a new bond showing origin of the American Indian in Asia. In adult skulls from both countries, Dr. Hrdlička explained, there may be back teeth missing from abscesses or other conditions, but in many skulls there are front teeth which show signs of having been extracted long ago, with indications that it was done in youth. The condition is prevalent even now among Australian and African natives and with them it is done generally as a sacrifice or a test of endurance.

# SCIENCE NEWS

*Science Service, Washington, D. C.*

## PAPERS READ AT THE SYMPOSIUM ON TEMPERATURE OF THE INSTITUTE OF PHYSICS



A symposium on "Temperature, Its Measurement and Control in Science and Industry," was held on November 2, 3 and 4 at the Hotel Pennsylvania, New York City, under the auspices of the American Institute of Physics, with the cooperation of the National Bureau of Standards, the National Research Council and officers and committees of scientific and technical societies. The symposium, the largest in its field to be held during the past twenty years, has gathered engineers, physicists, chemists and medical men from all over the country. Representing all fields of investigations, 127 scientific reports were presented, showing how temperature affects man directly or can be used to do new things and disclose new knowledge.

That athletes in severe muscular exercise can show body temperatures that normally would mean high fevers, was stated by Dr. Eugene F. DuBois, of the Russell Sage Institute of Pathology, Cornell University Medical School. He showed that the familiar 98.6 degrees Fahrenheit the clinical thermometer registers normally, is only one single spot between internal temperature and skin temperatures of 93.2 and lower. In severe exercise the temperature may run up to 104 degrees Fahrenheit. Just as the earth has broad zones of temperature, so, too, does the body have its temperature levels or zones. The torrid zone in man might be classed as that with temperatures of more than 105.2 degrees F., which can only be obtained by artificial fevers or when the body's temperature-regulating mechanism fails. Just below this, in what might be called the semi-tropics, is the familiar "fever" zone that is higher in temperature than normal and which comes from illness. With fever the skin temperature is warm. Here, too, come the higher temperatures of severe exercise which are accompanied, however, by cool skin. The body's normal temperature zone, corresponding to the temperate zone on the earth, is fairly wide. Below it come those body temperatures which are restored to normal values by shivering. And finally, analogous to the polar region on earth, is the body's zone of semi-hibernation where temperature regulation fails.

By turning their cells into a kind of living "glass" some microorganisms are able to withstand immersion into liquid air at temperatures of 190 degrees below zero Centigrade, was reported by Professor Basil J. Luyet, professor of biochemistry at St. Louis University. He stated that matter can exist in four physical states: as a gas, as a liquid, as a crystal and as a glass. Death by freezing comes because the temperature is lowered slowly. If an organism can be dipped into liquid air and pass on to the so-called vitreous state, some living tissues can be returned to a degree of vitality by quick warming to make them pass again through the danger stage of crystallization. Professor Luyet reported that he and his collaborators had used this rapid cooling to chill tissues from the epidermal cells of plants, moss leaves, frog's spermatozoa, isolated muscle fibers and myxamoebae. All these regained vitality on rewarming. He said: "Other protozoa or tissues experimented upon did not survive. One of the reasons for the lower resistance of the latter seems to be their too-high water content and the impossibility of sufficiently dehydrating them. These observations and those of other investigators . . . favor the theory that the structure required for vital activities is such that it is not destroyed by a lowering of molecular motion while it is destroyed by the withdrawal of some water molecules as when crystallization takes place."

Professor Otto Rahn, of Cornell University, pointed out that temperature is one of the three greatest physical factors controlling all life on earth. Not only are growth and synthesis speeded up by high temperature but also the processes of old age and decay. In all climates there is a balance between life and death and between development and deterioration. He said: "While the laws of temperature are inexorable, the ever-active powers of evolution have found a way around these laws by the creation of one of the great marvels of nature, the warm-blooded mammals and birds. All plants and all animals which can not control their body temperature display three cardinal points in regard to temperature: the optimum at which they thrive best, the maximum, which is the highest temperature at which they can still live, and the minimum or the lowest temperature at which existence is possible. Besides these three cardinal points . . . other temperatures are frequently mentioned, namely the temperatures at which an organism is killed either by excessive heat or by excessive cold. Neither of these points is very definite. At maximal temperature, the organism ceases to grow, but absence of this function does not mean death. If the temperature is raised slightly above the maximum, injury will set in very slowly, but the organism is capable of recovery for a long while. The higher the temperature, the sooner is the repairable stage passed, but the length of exposure will always remain a factor. With death by freezing, so many possibilities are open that general statements are entirely impossible. Death may be due to chemical causes, to solidification of lipids in the plasma membrane preventing diffusion, to a mechanical tearing of cells or tissues through ice formation, to a change of the colloid state of the protoplasm or to still other causes. Very rapid freezing causes 'vitrification' of the cell moisture with serious injury. Microorganisms can be cooled in liquid air to −190 degrees Centigrade without being killed, while they may die during slow freezing at −2 degrees C. Thus, life as well as death is intimately dependent upon temperature because the rate of most chemical and physical reactions is controlled by temperature. Though we can not explain all the observed facts, and though especially the causes of inhibition by low temperature are still obscure, we have no reason to assume that they will always remain unexplained."

Drs. M. Nielsen, W. H. Forbes, J. W. Wilson and D. B. Dill, of Harvard University, described Harvard's four trained dogs, which will lie quietly on a net in a cold room at temperatures of from 32 to 53 degrees Fahrenheit and wear oxygen masks. Exact physiological studies were made of their body activity. Skin temperatures, respiratory rate, pulse rate were tested and blood tests were made. Three of the four dogs withstood the chilling tests well. They lay quietly, though not narcotized, in a semi-conscious condition most of the time. At these low temperatures the dogs shivered moderately while breathing room air and thus increased their heat production and maintained their body temperature. When they breathed gas mixtures with lowered oxygen content through their masks the shivering soon stopped and their metabolism returned to the basal level and the body temperature fell about two degrees Centigrade per hour. The greatest total drop in temperature was six degrees Centigrade. The temperature fell gradually until the dogs were switched over to breathing the air in the cold room. Then the body's metabolism suddenly increased four times and within a half hour the body temperature was back to normal. It is concluded that "The ability of the dog to withstand low oxygen depends more on the toughness of his central nervous system than on an unusual ability to take oxygen in the lungs."

Homeothermy, the ability to maintain an even temperature in the body within the range of optimum biological activity, is the major mark of superiority of the higher animals, according to Dr. H. G. Barbour, of the Yale School of Medicine. The hypothalamus and endocrine glands are actively concerned with heat production and control in the body, he said. The mechanisms for enabling the body to lose heat become effective later than those of heat production, he added. At birth or hatching neither heat production nor heat-losing mechanisms appear to be present in the mouse or pigeon. In rabbits, man and cats heat production means is present but no means of losing heat. In guinea pigs and in chickens both mechanisms are present at the start. The body uses water to store and transport heat because of its high heat capacity. Water too appears to have insulation value against cold when blood is withdrawn from the surface of the body down into the deeper regions as in digestion of food in the stomach.

The difficulties of measuring the temperatures of stars was described by Dr. G. P. Kuiper, of the University of Chicago. By knowledge of the laws of radiation the relation between the color of a star and its effective temperature can be obtained. This is the amount of radiation leaving the star per unit area of surface. "For less than a dozen stars" are the basic assumptions of this way of getting stellar temperatures fulfilled. For the very hot stars with temperatures of over 10,000 degrees absolute the ionization of stellar gases and the resulting spectra enable ideas of star temperatures to be obtained. The complications of this method are so great that only when the temperatures are over 10,000 degrees K. can the necessary simplifying conditions be introduced into the calculations.

THE traditional explanation of the skin's sensitivity to heat and cold was discounted by new findings reported by Dr. William Leroy Jenkins, instructor in psychology at Lehigh University. The thought that temperature sensitivity of the skin was concentrated in small warm and cold spot receptors arose from the discovery that the locations of these spots could be mapped with a small stimulator. Dr. Jenkins has carried forward the mapping technique and by the process of seriatim, or repeated mapping, has found that the single warm and cold spots do not exist. "Seriatim mapping," Dr. Jenkins stated, "reveals hills and valleys of sensitivity. Warm and cold spots are found only in clusters, and mapping with smaller and smaller sizes does not resolve these clusters into discrete units; they simply disintegrate without being resolved." As a new and better way to explain the temperature sensitivity of the skin, Dr. Jenkins proposes a "concentration hypothesis," which suggests that the sensitivity depends primarily upon the concentration of the receptors. Where the receptors are highly concentrated, the skin's sensitivity is high. Where they are sparse, the sensitivity is low. According to this view, the traditional warm and cold spots are merely peaks of sensitivity and do not mark the locus of individual receptors.

Strong emotions like anger are found to make the fingers cold, according to Drs. Bela Mittlemann and H. G. Wolff, of the New York Hospital and the Cornell University Medical School. Temperature differences of more than 12 degrees Centigrade were noted in some cases.

That the fingers and arms are one of the body's first means of maintaining comfort was reported by Drs. Charles Sheard, Marvin M. D. Williams and Bayard T. Horton, of the Mayo Clinic and the Mayo Foundation. Studies of skin temperature under various environmental conditions show that the enlargement of the blood vessels, known as vasodilatation, helps to bring more blood to the surface of the body and aids in its cooling if the temperature becomes too warm. As the temperature on the test subjects was increased step by step it was found that vasodilatation occurred first in the fingers and upper extremities and then later a similar action began in the feet, toes and lower extremities.

A method of oil prospecting by measuring temperatures in the earth at depths of 100 to 200 feet was described by Melvin C. Terry. It is not necessary to take the temperature measurements at extreme depths because the intrusion of high conductivity materials will disturb the pattern of normal temperature gradients. Working over the ground of producing Texas oil fields at Hastings and Friendswood, it was found that the line of constant temperature at 23 degrees Centigrade ran about 100 feet higher over the oil salt domes than it did in the region between them.

The world is getting warmer. There appears to be a trend to higher temperature, according to J. B. Kincer, of the U. S. Weather Bureau, Washington, D. C. He stated "That there have been major changes in geologic climate has long been known, but that climatologists have considered historic climate as a rather stable thing, with short period variations of considerable magnitude, but without especially significant secular trends covering long periods of time. However, since the turn of the century there has been such a persistent trend to higher temperatures, world-wide in scope, as to suggest that the orthodox conception of the stability of climate needs some revision at least.'' Mr. Kincer cited as examples the records at Portland, Ore., where 17 of the past 20 years have been warmer than normal. And at Washington, D. C., 17 years in the last 20 have been warmer than normal and every year since 1926 above normal. Capetown, South Africa, has had 19 of its last 20 years warmer than normal. The world's lowest naturally occurring temperature yet observed is minus 90.4 degrees Fahrenheit measured in Siberia in the month of February, 1892. The highest temperature ever recorded on the earth's surface was observed in Tripolitania in September, 1922, when the thermometer reached 136.4 degrees Fahrenheit.

Skin temperatures of women are higher in warm atmosphere and lower in the cold than are those of men, according to a report made by Drs. James D. Hardy, A. T. Milhorat and E. F. DuBois, of the Russell Sage Institute of Pathology, New York Hospital and Cornell University Medical College. This is one of the first investigations to be made on heat production in women. Most prior work on this question has been done on men. The temperature difference at the higher temperature is accounted for both by the level of skin temperature required to induce sweating and by the amount of sweat. ''The women did not begin to sweat until the calorimetric temperature was two degrees above the threshold for sweating in the men, and the amount of sweating was less. The lower skin temperature of the women in the cold is apparently due to a thicker insulating layer of superficial tissue.'' Up to temperatures of about 81 degrees Fahrenheit, the heat production of the body for both men and women was essentially the same. Above that temperature the women showed a significant decrease in heat produced by their bodies.

How blocks of different metals are being used to help to control high temperatures with thermostats was described by Drs. C. L. Thomas and Gustav Egloff, of the Universal Oil Products Company. These blocks are used for temperatures above 200 degrees Centigrade. A hole is drilled in the block and a porcelain rod is inserted. The differential contraction and expansion between the rod and the metal block creates a tiny motion which, by levers, throws on and off switches that control temperature. Aluminum blocks are used for temperatures up to 500 degrees Centigrade, while aluminum bronze works up to 800 degrees. Stainless steel (18 per cent. chromium and 8 per cent. nickel) is used for temperatures up to 1,000 degrees Centigrade.

## ITEMS

SCIENTIFIC research has become so important to American industry that it is something to advertise instead of an activity that is kept hidden, Dr. Harrison E. Howe, editor of *Industrial and Engineering Chemistry*, the journal of the American Chemical Society, told the Ohio State University Research Foundation's Fourth Industrial Research Conference on November 4. In the past twenty-five years research has produced so many new products and earned so much money for important industries that now some chemical concerns invest 7 per cent. of their gross sales in hiring brains and equipment to renew continuously their business. About $100,000,000 is spent annually in America for industrial research, Dr. Howe estimated. If the cost of development of research findings into commercial processes and products were included, this figure would probably be doubled. Now there are over 2,000 laboratories doing industrial research, compared with a hundred or so a couple of decades ago.

THE San Francisco and the New York World's Fairs have enabled science to make its greatest analysis of deafness among the population ever undertaken, H. C. Montgomery, of the Bell Telephone Laboratories, reported to the meeting of the Acoustical Society of America at Iowa City on November 4. Over half a million people took the hearing tests at the telephone exhibits of the fairs. The largest previous survey on deafness was that of the U. S. Public Health Service in 1936, which studied the results on 9,000 persons. If the World-Fair visitors are a fair sample of the population, then eight people out of every thousand you meet have difficulty in hearing direct conversation. Forty people out of a thousand have trouble hearing in auditoriums. Only one in 400 will have difficulty in hearing over a telephone.

MORE food value per potato, per egg, per any-food-unit will be the objective of a new program of basic research initiated by the U. S. Department of Agriculture, to be centered on land adjacent to Cornell University, and to be conducted under the supervision of Dr. L. A. Maynard, professor and head of the laboratory of animal nutrition at Cornell. Hitherto, researches aimed at increasing agricultural production have striven primarily to boost the quantity of plant or animal material to be obtained from a given acreage. The new program will have as its first objective the improvement in quality, in terms of availability in human digestion and nutrition. First thing to be undertaken, according to the new plan, will be an investigation of soil minerals as they affect the yield and quality of crops. Scheduled for examination are not only the major mineral nutrients, like phosphorus, but also the so-called trace elements like cobalt, manganese and boron, which are necessary for good plant and animal health, but which need be present in only a few parts per million of the soil water.

''CRAZY TOP,'' a recently discovered disease of corn, has been found afflicting stalks in the wetter parts of fields in Iowa, Illinois and Indiana, Dr. Benjamin Koehler, of the Illinois Agricultural Experiment Station, reports in *Phytopathology*. The disease, cause of which is still unknown, changes the normal tassel at the top of the stalk into a mass of small, branching stems and leaves. Sometimes the ear is affected as well. Search for a possible causal organism has been hampered by the fact that the abnormal stalks were not noticed until late in the season.

# SCIENCE NEWS

*Science Service, Washington, D. C.*

## CENTRIFUGE FOR TESTING MINES AND BRIDGES IN NEW COLUMBIA SCHOOL OF ENGINEERING RESEARCH

AT Columbia University's School of Engineering, celebrating its seventy-fifth anniversary, a centrifuge method of engineering testing will be demonstrated publicly for the first time on November 10.

Professor Philip B. Bucky, of the Columbia School of Mines, and his students have built an enormous centrifuge in which can be placed models of the underground workings of a mine or models of bridges built to scale using transparent bakelite plastic. These structures are whirled faster and faster in the centrifuge merry-go-round, and as they whirl the centrifugal force stresses them and thus tests them. A force of 2,000 times gravity is created.

In the case of the mine structure, the problem is to find just how far miners can go in cutting holes in the rock they are mining. Holes might cause the rock to smash to bits under the thousands of tons of other rock pushing down from above. The stress built up in the centrifuge substitutes for the real stress that might be encountered under actual working conditions. The miniature block of rock collapses when the speed is high enough, just as the real mine would under the force of gravity. Professor Bucky can thus tell the mining engineers in a real mine how far they dare have the miners go with safety.

Light is used to measure the stress in the whirling bridge models. Polarized light, light that vibrates in one direction only, from a powerful mercury arc lamp, is flashed on and off so rapidly in exact synchronism with the centrifuge that the transparent model bridge is seen as though it were standing still. Bands of light and dark move through the model and these photo-elastic fringes enable the Columbia engineers to calculate just how and where a real bridge of that same design will be stressed in actual service.—WATSON DAVIS.

## FLICKERING SEARCHLIGHT BEAM FOR THE STUDY OF THE ATMOSPHERE

THE piercing, puzzling searchlight beam which mystified residents of northwest Washington last summer on moonless, dark and clear nights was explained on November 12 at the meeting of the Philosophical Society of Washington by Ellis A. Johnson, of the Carnegie Institution of Washington.

No ordinary searchlight beam was that seen by Washingtonians. Its brilliant beam flickered ten times a second and identified it, for scientific research, so that its scattering at heights of as much as 24.8 miles could be detected.

The experiments, Mr. Johnson reported, seek to probe the upper atmosphere for its secrets of temperature, density, presence of clouds and other important information at heights which are beyond the reach of stratosphere flights with balloons. Moreover, the new searchlight experiments tap that region of space lower than the radio reflecting layers in the ionosphere. The new technique thus investigates the "no man's land" of the atmosphere.

While the current experiments have been preliminary, seeking mostly to show the feasibility of the method, they indicate that studies can be carried out on the height of water vapor in the atmosphere, the amount of turbulence, the winds, dust, fluorescence and absorption of these upper altitudes up to nearly 20 miles. Actual measurements have been carried out at this height and it was found that the beam itself could be detected up to 40 kilometers, or about 24.8 miles.

In outline the searchlight experiment is simple. The beam of a great searchlight was directly upward and made to flicker (modulate) about ten times a second by an automatic Venetian blind type of shutter. Some three and a half miles away was placed a large mirror, containing at its focus a photoelectric cell. This mirror pivoted upward and caught light scattered from the beam in the sky. The photoelectric current generated by this scattered light was amplified in a special radio amplifier developed by Mr. Johnson, which is so sensitive that it can detect currents of only .000,000,000,000,000,032 amperes. From the geometry of the searchlight and the receiving mirror the altitudes at which the beam is studied can be calculated. The modulated, flickering nature of the light makes it possible to differentiate it from the general background light of the night sky. Even so, it was necessary to work only on clear nights without moonlight and at times when there was little haze at low altitudes. The experiments indicate that with a 60-inch searchlight and a 60-inch mirror as a receiver, the study of the upper atmosphere could be pushed to 90 kilometers, or nearly 56 miles.

## THE TRANSMUTATION OF PLATINUM INTO GOLD

THE ancient alchemists used to talk of transmuting base metals into gold, but in results accomplished little. Investigators at Columbia University, as a demonstration stunt, achieved a transmutation of the elements which results in gold. The starting point was not base metals but precious platinum.

The occasion was the seventy-fifth anniversary of Columbia University School of Engineering, which was founded as the first School of Mines in the United States. The modern alchemists were Dean George B. Pegram, of the Columbia Graduate Faculties, and Professor John R. Dunning, of the department of physics.

The method was to place platinum for some hours near a long glass tube containing a small amount of radium which emitted atomic particles that, by bombardment, turned platinum of atomic weight 195.25 into gold of atomic weight 197.2. The radioactive gold in turn emitted particles which alone made possible the detection of the transmutation.

Other demonstrations included: The detection of radioactive sodium in the human body and its circulation by

the blood; the collapse of a model subterranean mine roof structure by whirling it in a centrifuge to simulate the force of gravity in a real mine; the crushing of an eight-foot brick masonry pier in the compression testing machine of the school of engineering; the demonstration of water seepage under power dams and through various types of soil structures; a demonstration of the manufacture of isotopes by Professor Harold C. Urey.

## SOLAR RADIATION

TRAPPING the heat of the sun as it falls on the roof of a house and storing it in the basement for future use is to be attempted at the Massachusetts Institute of Technology soon, as part of a long-range program on the possibilities of using solar radiation as a direct source of energy.

An experimental house, which it is planned to heat during the winter, air condition during the summer and possibly even supply with power, all with the energy of sunlight, has already been constructed and the research is expected to begin at once.

One of the major features of the house is a large, well-insulated water storage tank which is to be used in ironing out the fluctuations in heat which are inevitable with a source as variable as the sun. The heating system is based on a method of forcing air either over the hot surface of the tank or through the coils of a refrigeration system which is also to be run on energy stolen from the sun.

Professor Hoyt C. Hottel, who is in charge of the program, plans to try several types of "heat traps," or energy collectors, during the research. First attention will be devoted to a shallow, box-like device which will be placed in a recess in the building's roof. For a bottom this box has a thin sheet of metal, painted black to absorb as much of the sun's heat as possible. Firmly fixed to this bottom is a series of small, thin-walled metal tubes which are to be heated by contact with the sheet and which will then pass this heat on to water circulating through them. This box has a series of glass covers, separated by dead air, through which nearly all the sunlight can pass but through which little heat can escape back to the outside. The sunlight, as it strikes the metal sheet, is converted into heat and the whole arrangement has a layer of mineral wool beneath it to prevent heat escape in that direction. The warm water in the coils is then piped, through carefully insulated tubes, to the well-insulated storage tank where the engineers expect to keep it hot anywhere from a few weeks to six months, depending on the size of the tank.

The best size for these units, the most heat-absorbent paint, the most effective number of glass plates and the best angle at which to slope the roof are among the problems to be investigated. Professor Hottel emphasized that he and his colleagues are well aware that the amount of solar heat in New England would make domestic heating by solar radiation uneconomical in comparison with other heat sources, but there is sufficient sunshine in this region to test the efficiency of heating systems for those localities where the climate is less rigorous.

The research is one of several projects planned at the Massachusetts Institute under the terms of a gift of nearly $650,000 from Dr. Godfrey L. Cabot, of Boston, "for research on the utilization of solar radiation for the tasks of man."

## INSULATION AND HEAT LOSS

ADEQUATE insulation of a house against heat loss can cut the fuel bill nearly in half, E. S. Draper, director of the department of regional planning studies of the Tennessee Valley Authority, reported at the meeting in New York on November 6 of the Committee on Hygiene of Housing of the American Public Health Association.

Mr. Draper announced at the same time that a simple heater practical for central heating of small houses, improved after tests in a TVA house at the Gilbertsville Dam construction community, is now in production for the open market.

The insulation studies were carried out in two identical four-room houses in the Hiwassee Dam construction community. Installation of electrical heaters made it possible to record with great accuracy the heat loss in the two houses. One of them was insulated throughout by wool bats in the walls and over the ceiling and an insulation board under the floor joists. Both houses had both doors weatherstripped. Both families were held to the same schedule of window-opening in bedrooms at night, windows closed by day, and the heaters were turned on and off at the same time. The reduction in total heat loss in the insulated house was 44.75 per cent. Cost of insulation, including labor and materials, was about $200.

The simple heater described by Mr. Draper was designed to effect a reduction in the capital cost of central warm air heating over that of installing the warm air furnaces then available on the market. The object was to have a primary heat source (without provision for air filtering or humidification) placed in an exceptionally small first floor heating chamber centrally located so that it might service all rooms of a small house without the usual extensive system and basement.

## COMETS

THE discovery of a new and unexpected twelfth magnitude comet on November 1 by Clarence L. Friend, of Escondido, Calif., brings to twelve the number of comets which so far have been sighted by astronomers during 1939. Seven of these comets have been of the periodic type which return to the region of the sun and earth at regular intervals which astronomers can calculate accurately. As might be expected, professional astronomers working in large observatories rediscovered all these returning comets.

Of the five new and unexpected comets found so far this year, two have been found by amateur astronomers, two jointly by an amateur and a professional and one by a professional astronomer alone.

The significant mark of the new Friend comet is its rapid motion. From its originally discovered position in the "keystone" of Hercules near right ascension 16 hours, 52.9 minutes and declination plus 34 degrees, three minutes, it is moving rapidly east and south.

The first comet of 1939 was the unexpected one found

independently on January 19 by Kosik, professional observer at Tashkent Observatory, U.S.S.R., and Leslie C. Peltier, Delphos, Ohio, an amateur who has discovered seven comets.

The second comet of the year was the return of the Pons-Winnecke comet found on March 17 by Dr. H. M. Jeffers, of Lick Observatory. This is comet 1939 c.

On March 17, too, Dr. Y. Vaisala, director of the observatory at the University of Turku, Finland, reported the discovery on asteroid photographic plates of a new comet. The Vaisala comet was granted designation 1939 b.

On April 18 was found comet 1939 d, a new comet and one of the "most discovered" of all the year. First reported by a professional observer, Hassel, at Oslo, Norway, it was later found that two Russian amateurs, Jurlof and Achmarof, had discovered it just ahead of him. A triple name, the Jurlof-Achmarof-Hassel comet, was thus assigned. Many observers all over the world reported independent discoveries of this comet for some days following.

The reappearance of the Kopff periodic comet (1939 e) was announced by Professor G. Van Biesbroeck, of Yerkes Observatory of the University of Chicago, on April 22.

The periodic Schwassmann-Wachmann comet (1939 f) was found anew by the professional observer Jackson, at Johannesburg, S. A., on June 12.

Periodic comet Brooks II (1939 g) was found by Dr. H. M. Jeffers, at Lick, shortly afterward.

On July 28 the new comet 1939 h was discovered by the French amateur astronomer Roger Rigollet, a variable star observer.

On July 31 came the one comet discovery of the year which has not yet been confirmed. This was the announcement of a seventh magnitude comet by the professional observer Kaminsky at Tashkent Observatory, U.S.S.R. While reported seen from Italy, also, the comet could not be located by astronomers elsewhere, and it has not yet been given a number designation.

Periodic comet Tuttle reappeared on August 14 when Dr. H. M. Jeffers, of Lick Observatory, found it on a photograph taken with the 36-inch Crossley reflector. It has received designation 1939 i.

September was without comet discoveries, but on October 14 Professor G. Van Biesbroeck, of Yerkes Observatory, announced the reappearance of the Giacobini-Zinner comet. This is comet 1939 j.

On the same astronomical announcement card listing the new Friend comet is the reported rediscovery of the Faye periodic comet by Dr. H. M. Jeffers, of Lick Observatory, on November 3.—Robert D. Potter.

## ITEMS

Completely successful operation of the experimental apparatus was obtained by the substratosphere expedition of the University of Chicago on October 23, according to Professor Arthur H. Compton, of the university. Rising to 29,000 feet, while scientists breathed oxygen, the airplane bore aloft a Wilson cloud chamber apparatus to make visible the tracks of the cosmic ray particles. Dr. Compton said that "Preliminary findings show the presence of cosmic ray tracks for every expansion of the cloud chamber at altitudes of over 20,000 feet as compared with the rate occurrence of the tracks at sea level." The major effort of the expedition was to find and study "slow" mesotron particles, the heavyweight charged particles, some 160 times as massive as ordinary electrons. The rate of mesotron production near 30,000 feet was very greatly increased. Professor Compton directed the flight by radio from the ground. In the plane, running the apparatus, were his assistants, Drs. Gerhardt Herzog and Winston Bostwick.

Warm-blooded animals can be sent into hibernation artificially by injecting insulin, or a combination of insulin and magnesium chloride, into their veins, according to Dr. Paavo Suomalainen, of the Helsinki Biochemical Institute. Working with European hedgehogs, Dr. Suomalainen found that the injections caused a drop in blood sugar content to less than half normal, and produced the cold-blooded state characteristic of warm-blooded animals in hibernation. The animals remained asleep as long as he kept them in a refrigerator, at temperatures around freezing point. When he removed them to a warm room, at a temperature of from 70 to 75 degrees Fahrenheit, they awoke and returned to the normal warm-blooded state.

Bacteria have been shown to be able to change the eye color in Drosophila, or fruit flies, in experiments reported by Dr. Edward L. Tatum, of Stanford University, who has been working on a project financed by the Rockefeller Foundation. Such changes have hitherto been considered to be a monopoly of genes, or hereditary units within the cells of the insects themselves. The change, from white to brown color in the eyes, is brought about by a hormone produced by the bacteria, working in conjunction with tryptophane, an amino acid which is part of the flies' diet. The bacteria-produced hormone seems to be identical with a hormone produced by the flies, under certain conditions. Dr. Tatum made his discovery when the tryptophane used in feeding his fruit flies became contaminated with a still unnamed species of bacterium.

Para rubber trees are being tried out in three nurseries at different altitudes in the Ethiopian highlands, in the hope of eventually making Italy independent of foreign sources of rubber. The plantings at the lowest altitude, at Gambela (2,000 feet above sea-level), have been most successful; the seedlings have reached a height of about two feet in the first year after sowing.

Dinosaurs may have died out because the world got too hot for them, not because it became too cold as commonly conjectured. This reversal of the usually accepted theory of dinosaurian extinction is suggested by Dr. Raymond B. Cowles of the University of California at Los Angeles. Dr. Cowles bases his theory on the known facts about present-day reptiles, distant cousins of the dead giants of the Mesozoic. Reptiles become sluggish when chilled, but when over-heated they die outright, even the lizards that are supposed to be happiest on a hot rock, he says. Any temperature above 98.6 degrees Fahrenheit is bad for them.

# SCIENCE NEWS

*Science Service, Washington, D. C.*

## MESOTRONS



MESOTRONS, the fiercely energetic particles generated by cosmic rays far up in the stratosphere, "commit suicide" on their way to earth.

They dash in uncountable hordes from their high birthplace toward sea-level, but on the way more than half of them disappear. That much was known. What was not known was whether they died from collisions with the atmosphere or from some other cause.

An elaborate series of experiments conducted all the way from Chicago to the top of 14,259-foot Mount Evans, where the world's highest laboratory is situated, has established that the mesotrons disintegrate according to a fixed schedule or life-span which seems largely independent of outside conditions.

Their suicidal impulse resembles that of the disintegration of radium, which is subject to no outside conditions possible for man to establish.

Dr. Bruno Rossi, the Italian physicist now a research fellow of the University of Chicago, and head of the party that made the experiments, computes the average life-span of a mesotron, dashing toward earth at a speed approaching that of light, as 27/10,000,000th of a second. He plans to return to the mountains with more equipment next summer, for further investigation into the nature of mesotrons and of cosmic rays. He and his party, which included Professors J. Barton Hoag, Winston Bostick and O. E. Polk, of the University of Chicago, and Professor Norman Hilberry, of New York University, brought an ordinary old school bus from Chicago to Mount Evans.

On its floor was installed a ton and a half of equipment. It included three cosmic-ray counters, with five inches of lead on top to insure that only the powerful mesotrons would get through. Boxes contained several hundred pounds of powdered graphite.

Observations were taken at Chicago, elevation 580 feet; Denver University campus, 5,200 feet; Echo Lake, west of Denver on the flanks of Mount Evans, 10,816 feet, and at the top of the mountain at the cosmic ray laboratory of Denver University, 14,259 feet. At Chicago, the counters clicked at the rate of 5 a minute; at Denver, 7; at Echo Lake between 9 and 10, and at the top of the mountain, 12. This only confirmed previous observations, which showed more mesotrons at high atmospheric levels.

When the last count had been checked and re-checked at the top of the mountains, the observers heaped graphite, in deep trays, on top of the counters until there was a layer 55 centimeters thick or obout 20 inches. This thickness was calculated to represent the same amount of mass as that contained in the air blanket, 3,641 feet thick, between the top of the peak and the altitude of Echo Lake.

Now, to reach the counters, the mesotrons would have to pass through the same mass, but they could pass in much less time. If the number of mesotrons now registered remained more numerous, it would show that many mesotrons passed successfully through the mass. But it would also show that many of them disintegrated in the greater time—short as it seems by ordinary measurements—that it takes them to travel through 3,641 feet of air rather than 20 inches of graphite.

The clicks at the mountain-top decreased to about 11 a minute, but there were still more than the 10 a minute registered at Echo Lake. Some mesotrons, therefore, "commit suicide" without outside impulsion, on the way down to earth.

## THE CAUSE OF SPRUE



A NEW theory of the cause of sprue, serious disease of the tropics which also occurs in the United States and other temperate regions, was announced by Dr. Edward B. Vedder, of the George Washington Medical School, at the opening session on November 21 of the American Society of Tropical Medicine, meeting at Memphis.

Sprue, Dr. Vedder believes, is caused by a failure of the tiny but powerful pituitary gland at the base of the brain. This little gland produces a number of hormones, among them one called prolactin, which stimulates milk secretion, and which also has an effect on the digestive tract. It is lack of this hormone which Dr. Vedder believes causes sprue, and he would like physicians to try the hormone as a remedy for their sprue patients. Most effective remedies for sprue at present are liver extract or some other source of the vitamin $B_2$ complex, but Dr. Vedder believes the gland hormone would prove a better remedy.

Sore mouth, anemia and digestive disorder are characteristic symptoms of sprue. The digestive disorders set up a vicious cycle, because the sprue patient, already unable to absorb enough of the B vitamins, has more and more trouble getting enough of these vitamins which he needs to remedy his illness. In severe cases they must be given by hypodermic injections. A number of investigators have concluded that the digestive disorder and vitamin deficiency were important parts of the picture, but no satisfactory explanation for what starts the vicious cycle has hitherto been forthcoming.

The start of the digestive disorder, Dr. Vedder believes, is the failure of the anterior pituitary gland to produce enough prolactin to keep the digestive tract functioning smoothly. Tropical service, he suggests, precipitates the pituitary gland failure in some persons, but such gland failure may occur without the precipitating effect of long periods of tropical heat, which may explain the nearly two hundred cases of non-tropical sprue in medical records.

## GERM-FREE SURROUNDINGS FOR INFANTS



PROTECTION for babies in maternity hospitals and infants' homes, from the germs they unwittingly give each other, is a leading topic in the two-day colloquium on newest progress in bacteriology now in progress at the University of Notre Dame.

Two principal systems to obtain this protection have been developed. In one, brought to its highest point by Professor James A. Reyniers, of Notre Dame, emphasis is placed on the complete isolation of all babies, brought about by keeping each one in a tiny room or cubicle, kept as germ-free as all imaginable precautions will insure.

The other system, developed by Professor William F. Wells, of the University of Pennsylvania, depends on floods of ultra-violet radiation across doorways and other critical areas in the hospital, which massacre the germs as they float through the air. Both systems are now under full-scale practical test at a well-known home for babies.

Animals and plants brought into the world without the contamination of germs, which is the fate of all ordinary living things, and kept germ-free throughout their lives, have been produced in Professor Reyniers' laboratory, and adaptations of his technique, as well as other methods, are now in use by a number of research workers. In his method, the young guinea pigs or other laboratory animals are born by Caesarian operation under completely aseptic conditions, within big tank-like cages where they are kept as long as necessary, receiving only sterile food, water and air. He has brought up guinea pigs, chickens and other animals from infancy to full growth, without their ever being invaded by a single discoverable germ.

Getting germ-free plants is usually a simpler job, according to Dr. Philip R. White, of the Rockefeller Institute laboratories at Princeton, N. J. The internal tissues of plants are usually naturally germ-free; it is a question simply of getting seeds out of a pod, or cutting tissues out of the inside of a stem or root, without their becoming contaminated. Many kinds of seeds have coats so resistant that they can be washed in effective antiseptic solutions without injuring the embryo plants which they contain. Dr. White described the method by which he obtains germ-free cuttings of roots, which he grows in flasks of nutrient fluid, maintaining them indefinitely without connection with any stems. In such cultures of non-green plant tissues he has proved that a little iron is as necessary to them as it is to the chlorophyll-containing leaves and green shoots. One part of iron in 10,000,000 of solution makes all the difference between life and death to simple tissues.

Other uses of germ-free techniques were set forth by Dr. R. W. Glaser, of the Rockefeller Institute, and by Dr. Oram Woolpert, of the Ohio State University. Also discussed at the colloquium were exceedingly delicate mechanical devices, which make it possible to insert a single germ, or a germ-size dose of a drug or virus, into a single living cell, to study results on this smallest of all experimental bases. Applications of these techniques have been made to many practical problems in diseased conditions of plant and animal cells, as well as to cells in normal states of life and growth.

## RELATION OF QUARTZ DUST TO SILICOSIS



MEDICAL men are now attacking the problem of silicosis by attaching a small transparent "window" to the ears of rabbits, it was reported to the meeting of the Air Hygiene Foundation by Dr. Eliot R. Clark, professor of anatomy of the University of Pennsylvania, and Darrow E. Haagensen.

A tiny sterile microscope viewing window, designed by Dr. R. G. Williams, associate professor of anatomy at the University of Pennsylvania, was attached last April to a rabbit's ear. Inside is a space only 1/333 of an inch thick in which the tissue of the ear could grow normally. Last June minute specks of silica ranging in size from one to seven microns (a micron is 1/25,000 of an inch) were placed on the tissue. A few particles up to 30 microns were also present. The cover was then placed over the microscope chamber, and the tissue cells as they sought to live in the same environment with the silica have been photographed daily.

While the important research must be continued much longer before final conclusions can be determined, it already appears that:

1. A relatively stationary grouping has developed among living cells called macrophages which have ingested, or taken in, the smaller particles of silica.

2. The silica laden cells tend to be very sluggish but seem to move slightly from day to day. They show grouping tendencies with occasional slow scattering and regrouping. Some of the larger particles from 15 microns and up in size appear to lie outside the cells and are not influenced by the tissue fluids.

3. Connective tissue has grown into the chamber and completely covered the observational area. As far as can be determined the lymphatic capillaries are normal as is the rich blood vessel plexus. Not even a mild inflammatory condition has appeared.

In a separate report Dr. Clark described the history of the use of observational "windows" placed over living tissues and showed that the tail of the tadpole, the bat's wing and the web of the frog's foot have all been used at one time or another for research.

Professor Philip Drinker, of Harvard University, chairman of the Foundation's Preventive Engineering Committee, describes studies seeking to learn what size of silica particles seem to have the most rapid effect in producing cell changes. Ground flint, consisting of 99.7 per cent. silica, was carefully separated into four sizes of 3.30, 1.65, 1.04 and 0.62 microns. Sterile suspensions of these fractions were injected into ear veins of rabbits twice at three-month intervals, and the animals were killed and autopsied periodically. Examination of the liver sections indicated that the fine particles were taken up more rapidly than the larger ones. There appears to be no striking effects for the larger size particles, while it seems, in these preliminary studies, that the smaller sizes produce the greatest changes.

The knowledge obtained will be useful to engineers in designing ventilation and filtering systems for mines and other places where silica dust is prevalent, and will also be of greatest use in the design of dust respirators.

## PNEUMONIA CONTROL

THE latest aid in the fight to save lives threatened by pneumonia, especially among children, is a new, speedy diagnostic technic which can shorten to six hours or less the time before starting effective treatment. Details of the new technic are reported by Dr. Franklin D. Poole and Miss Mildred D. Fousek, of the Orphan Asylum at New Haven and Yale University School of Medicine, in the *Journal* of the American Medical Association.

Rapid typing of pneumonia germs found in the patient's sputum, in order to determine which type of anti-pneumonia serum should be used in treatment, has already been accomplished, but often in children and sometimes in adults delay still occurs because of difficulty in obtaining sputum for the test. At Yale University the difficulty has been surmounted by applying the usual speedy typing technic to material obtained by swabbing the patient's nose. The method is valuable, it is pointed out, even though many pneumonia patients are now treated with the chemical, sulfapyridine, instead of with anti-pneumonia serum, because it is desirable for the doctor to know whether the pneumonia is caused by a pneumonia germ or by the streptococcus.

Small doses of sulfapyridine given for a short time in treatment of pneumonia in children are recommended by Drs. Charles Hendee Smith and Rosa Lee Nemir, of New York, in a report of their results with sulfapyridine treatment in 93 cases of pneumonia in children, which appears in the same issue of the *Journal.*

The value of sulfapyridine in saving lives, especially from Type III pneumonia for which serum treatment does not have as good a life-saving record as it does in other types, was stressed in another report to the *Journal* by Drs. Norman Plummer and Herbert K. Ensworth, of New York. Among 270 sulfapyridine-treated patients at New York and Bellevue Hospitals there were only 34 deaths. Of these, 11 died within 24 hours of the beginning of treatment, which reduces the death rate in this group to 8.5 per cent. Serum treatment was used in addition to sulfapyridine in 102 of the cases. In serum-treated pneumonia cases a death rate of about 18 per cent. to 20 per cent. has previously been reported from Bellevue Hospital. Besides reducing the death rate, sulfapyridine shortens the period of fever and sterilizes the blood stream.

## ITEMS

THE earthquake that jarred several Eastern cities on November 14 had its epicenter in New Jersey, about 15 miles southeast of Wilmington, Del., according to a first approximation by the U. S. Coast and Geodetic Survey, based on data obtained telegraphically by Science Service. Time of origin was 9: 53.9 P.M., EST. Geographic coordinates were latitude 39.7 degrees north, longitude 75.4 degrees west. This is the fifth earthquake felt in New Jersey within a decade. Most recent was one on August 23, 1938, near Mt. Holly, followed by a couple of light aftershocks. Other New Jersey earthquakes were recorded on May 31, 1937, on the sea coast; January 24, 1933, near Trenton, and January 26, 1931, in the Moorestown-Rivertown neighborhood.

SEATTLE'S earthquake, that cracked windows and pavements on November 13, had its epicenter about 60 miles southwest of the city, according to a provisional determination by seismologists of the U. S. Coast and Geodetic Survey, based on data collected telegraphically by Science Service. The spot lies a little to the south of Mount Olympus National Monument, in a rugged, mountainous, almost uninhabited region. Geographical coordinates were given as 47.5 degrees north latitude, 123.5 degrees west longitude. Time of origin was a quarter of an hour before midnight, Pacific time, or 2:45.8 A.M., EST.

DUST storms may swirl again unless something happens to break the grip of the severe drought, which still continues unrelieved as autumn merges towards winter. The U. S. Weather Bureau states that "In the southwestern Plains, especially western Kansas, the soil is dry, loose, and subject to drifting by high winds." Light rains over parts of the northern central valley, particularly in the Great Lakes region, brought temporary relief, but the moisture is confined to the topsoil, for immediate benefit of fall-sown grains. Deep wells are being put down, seeking water for thirsty livestock. Over the greater part of the principal crop-producing regions, however, it is still too dry for fall seeding. Indeed, farmers in the Corn Belt are complaining that it is not only impossible to plow, but that they can't even mend their fences because the soil is so dry and hard that they can't dig post-holes.

BENJAMIN FRANKLIN wanted the turkey, not the eagle, to be the national bird of the United States. Yet not quite: for the turkey that graces our tables on Thanksgiving Day is not the native American bird that Franklin had in mind. The tame turkey of the barnyard is not the same species as the wild turkey that once roamed all the eastern woods. It is a tropical cousin, brought up by indirect route from below the Rio Grande.

WOUNDS incurred by persons working in the Russian Arctic are said to heal more rapidly than usual if they require stitching, but more slowly if they are left open. Paradoxically, both effects are credited to the relatively germ-free Arctic air. Germs in closed-up wounds cause inflammation and suppuration, but on minor, open wounds they stimulate the natural self-closing and healing processes.

THERE are lambs on the outskirts of Washington whose sires have never been east of Idaho; lambs in Idaho whose sires live in the pastures of the U. S. Department of Agriculture station at Beltsville, Md. Airplanes carried the prize rams' semen that made these long-distance breedings possible. This animal parentage at a range of a couple of thousand miles is only the most spectacular aspect of the rapid development of the technique of artificial breeding in this country. A little over a year ago, it was well established in only one state, New Jersey. Now there are artificial breeding associations in fifteen states, either actually operating or in process of formation. The territorial range covered is literally from Maine to California. Artificial breeding enables a farmer or rancher to have his new stock sired by the choicest animals available, regardless of distance, at fees so moderate that it becomes unnecessary for him to maintain sires on his own place or to patronize near-by owners of male animals of possibly less desirable qualities.

## NEW BOOK AND INSTRUMENT CATALOGUES

**ALLIS COMPANY, LOUIS**, Milwaukee. *Adjusto-Spede; an Entirely New Principle for Altering Current Adjustable Speed Motors. Bulletin No. 611.* Pp. 8. Illustrated.

**BAKELITE CORPORATION**, New York. *Bakelite Review; October, 1939.* Pp. 15. Illustrated.

**BAKER AND COMPANY, INCORPORATED**, Newark. *Platinum Metals and the Chemical Industry.* Pp. 16. Illustrated.

**BAUSCH AND LOMB OPTICAL COMPANY**, Rochester. *Bausch and Lomb Magazine; Vol. XV, No. 3.* Pp. 22. Illustrated.

**BURKE AND JAMES, INCORPORATED**, Chicago. *Catalog 939.* Pp. 79. Illustrated.

**BUSINESS NEWS PUBLISHING COMPANY**, Detroit. *1939 Catalog: Air Conditioning and Refrigeration Publications.* Pp. 31. Illustrated.

**CALIBRON PRODUCTS, INCORPORATED**, West Orange, New Jersey. *Calibron Notebook, July, 1939.* Pp. 24. Illustrated.

**CENTRAL SCIENTIFIC COMPANY**, Chicago. *Cenco News Chats, October, 1939.* Pp. 22. Illustrated.

***Readers are requested to mention* SCIENCE *when they write for catalogues.***

# SCIENCE NEWS

*Science Service, Washington, D. C.*

## THE SEPARATION OF ISOTOPES

Hydrogen cyanide, HCN to chemists, is perhaps the deadliest chemical known. Yet this poison is being used by Dr. Harold C. Urey, of Columbia University, in his latest separation of varieties of elements, called isotopes. By demonstrating that there actually existed a kind of hydrogen double in mass the ordinary sort, by producing heavy water whose hydrogen was of this deuterium of mass 2, Professor Urey won the Nobel prize. Then high concentrations of heavy oxygen were obtained. Later he separated heavy nitrogen of mass 15 from the ordinary nitrogen of mass 14.

Now he is accomplishing a separation of heavy carbon of mass 13 from the much more abundant and common carbon of mass 12, using a complex apparatus of glass through which, night and day, large amounts of hydrogen cyanide are flowing. Tall columns of chemicals, totaling 65 feet in length, worked upon by vacuum pumps, make possible the separation, which depends upon the fact that the cyanide gas contains more of the heavier carbon than the sodium cyanide in water solution.

Thus it is possible to obtain sodium cyanide, a white powder, a quarter of the carbon atoms of which are mass 13. A mere pinch, a tenth of a gram, a three hundredth of an ounce, is manufactured each 24 hours, but Professor Urey's stock of the precious stuff is growing steadily until now he can display about 10 grams.

This unusual sort of carbon may very well unlock some of the secrets of life and industry. Carbon is one of the universal elements of all living things, all fuels, and almost everything else, ranking with hydrogen and oxygen. In carbon of mass 13 Professor Urey has carbon atoms that are effectively tagged or labeled. They can be distinguished from the ordinary kind. That is why they are precious.

Some of the heavy carbon will be used to discover important facts about how food is utilized in the human body. Other tagged heavy carbon atoms may be used to trace the part they play in puzzling combustion effects. This chemical pioneering promises to pay handsomely in new knowledge.—Watson Davis.

## TESTING TELESCOPE MIRRORS

(*Copyright, 1939, by Science Service*)

A new way of testing the accuracy of grinding for giant telescope mirrors, that saves two thirds of the cost, labor and time necessary for this vital operation, has been developed by Dr. Enrique Gaviola, astrophysicist of the National Observatory at Cordoba, Argentina. The discovery, believed one of the most important in the century in the construction of telescope mirrors, allows a parabolic surface to be ground on a great glass disk directly and tested continually during the grinding. For years astronomers have been grinding parabolic mirrors in a three-stage, tedious and costly process. From their original flat disk, as made in a glass works, they grind a spherical concave surface. Next they take another piece of glass and grind it to an optically flat surface. And finally they use the "flat" to test the spherical surface as they slowly grind and figure it into the desired parabola.

"The amount of work, time and money necessary for this three-stage operation," says Dr. Gaviola, "is about three times the amount demanded by the parabolic mirror itself. All three surfaces have to be figured, tested and corrected independently, and the optical flat has to be ground more accurately than the accuracy expected in the final parabolic mirror."

Dr. Gaviola, in a recent visit to the laboratories of the Mount Palomar Observatory, where the great 200-inch diameter mirror has been in the process of grinding since 1936, explained the methods to astronomers there. They appreciated its ingenuity but explained that they are so far advanced in their grinding, by time-tried methods, that they will continue to construct their mirror along the routine lines. At the most optimistic estimate it may be completed next year. If the method had been available and proved successful five years ago, the Mount Palomar mirror might now be in service, and the giant telescope could have been constructed at a much lower cost.

Dr. Gaviola was led to the discovery of the new method, which uses a fine wire instead of a knife edge for testing, by sheer necessity. In 1936, while at La Plata Observatory in Argentina, he set to work to correct noticeable errors in the 82-centimeter Cassegrain mirror at the observatory. "As we had no plane mirror of that size and no possibility of making either a flat or a Hindle spherical of 82-centimeter (over 2.7 feet) diameter it became necessary to find a new, simple method of testing the Cassegrain, using only the available equipment. After some experiments a satisfactory method was devised," Dr. Gaviola explains.

As described in a joint report with Ricardo Platzeck, of La Plata Observatory, to the *Journal* of the Optical Society of America, Dr. Gaviola says the new testing method works on the basic idea that to test an optical surface an arrangement is needed that will form an image of some kind. If the image is good, a study of it tells the quality of the optical surface.

If the image is not good, as it naturally will not be in a new mirror just being ground, it is subdivided into a number of good images by decomposing the main optical surface into sufficiently small parts or zones by the use of screens. The image is usually a so-called "artificial star," a bright point of light, or light from a narrow slit.

The common method is to observe the diffraction of light reflected off the telescope mirror as it passes by a sharp knife edge. The new method uses a fine wire as the diffracting object and the diffraction pattern is symmetrical on each side of it. The diffraction pattern from the various zones of the telescope mirror (secured by suitable screens with carefully cut holes in them) are observed. From these observations the curve of the mirror

surface can be calculated and the "high" or "low" spots, lying outside permissible accuracy, can be ascertained.

It is possible to obtain accuracy only 1/100 the wavelength of light by the method, which is not only applicable to parabolic mirrors but to optical surfaces which depart considerably from a spherical shape.—ROBERT D. POTTER.

## SULFANILAMIDE AND MALARIA

*(Copyright, 1939, by Science Service)*

HUMAN subjects as well as monkeys have been used in tests of the possible malaria-curing power of the widely used new chemical remedy, sulfanilamile, reported by Dr. L. T. Coggeshall, of the Rockefeller Foundation's International Health Division, to the American Society of Tropical Medicine meeting in Memphis.

These subjects were suffering from paresis, or general paralysis of the insane. Malaria is given such sufferers from the results of syphilis and frequently the malaria checks the mental deterioration. Some of these patients were resistant to one kind of malaria germ or parasite, *Plasmodium vivax,* but they volunteered for doses of another malaria parasite, called *Plasmodium knowlesi,* following which they were given sulfanilamide. They promptly got well of the malaria, just as did monkeys infected with the same kind of malaria parasites. This, however, apparently does not mean that sulfanilamide is a good remedy for malaria. In fact, Dr. Coggeshall stated that "when this drug was tried as a therapeutic agent against human malaria, there was no apparent effect."

The studies showed, however, that in testing any anti-malaria drug, the oxygen consumption and metabolism of the malaria germ should be taken into account. Sulfanilamide, both in monkey malaria and in test-tube experiments, was more effective against one kind of malaria parasite than against another less virulent one. The drug cured the *knowlesi* malaria in monkeys but had no effect on *Plasmodium inui* malaria. In the test-tube, similarly, it had no effect on *inui,* but markedly paralyzed the respiration or breathing of the *knowlesi* parasites.

No anti-malaria drug should be discarded, said Dr. Coggeshall, on the basis of its failure to cure one kind of malaria, but neither should the fact that it cures one kind of malaria lead to its being proclaimed as a universal remedy in malaria.

## PROBLEMS OF FOREST OWNERSHIP

*(Copyright, 1939, by Science Service)*

AMERICA'S forest lands: should they be publicly or privately owned; should there be much or little governmental regulation? These and other questions of forest policy were discussed at the opening meeting of the Society of American Foresters in San Francisco, and diverse solutions were proposed by well-known speakers.

Outright government ownership of all forest lands, excepting only farm woodlots, was advocated by George M. Peterson, associate economist of the Giannini Foundation. Upon the initial premise that a healthy and stable nation is most surely built on distributism, that is, the private ownership of a little property by every person, Mr. Peterson developed nineteen reasons for government ownership of all large timberland areas.

Ownership of vast forest holdings by wealthy individuals or large corporations is contrary to good public policy, he stated, because such ownership does not get full value out of the forests in either felled timber, grazing, recreational uses, wildlife protection and soil conservation. Large-scale private ownership, he argued further, commonly does not give adequate fire protection and is too apt to dodge taxes and indulge in unsound financing. Better to cut this Gordian knot and go all the way for public ownership and management.

Admitting the existence of many evils in American forest economy, C. S. Martin, forester of the Western Pine Association of Portland, Ore., traced them to other causes and proposed a less drastic remedial procedure. Lack of a well-developed forest policy embracing both private and public lands is a prime cause of present troubles, Mr. Martin held, and he pointed out that even the relatively limited steps toward industrial self-regulation that have been taken in recent years have produced encouraging results, especially in fire control, reforestation, selective cutting and the adoption of sustained yield programs.

Voluntary cooperation, resulting in part from consistent education of public and industry, was seen as a potent remedy by Stephen N. Wyckoff, director of the Pacific Northwest Forest and Range Experiment Station. The viewpoints to be reconciled are the public feeling that great social values are involved in the forest policy, and the private owners' resistance to any changes that would infringe upon traditional right to do as they please with what is their own.

Mr. Wyckoff set up five premises, acceptance of which he held to be necessary if a workable "middle way" is to be found. He called for simultaneous recognition of social values and the need for profits, for management to protect these social values, for private ownership on a sustained-yield basis wherever practicable, for public payments to defray extra costs of safeguarding social values, and finally for contractual guarantees from private owners whenever they receive public aid in management of their lands. Lands that can not yield a money profit and yet have intangible values to the public, Mr. Wyckoff concluded, should be publicly owned.

## REGISTER OF SCIENTIFIC MEN BY THE ROYAL SOCIETY

BRITISH scientists have been indexed and classified, but not regimented.

A voluntary register, containing upward of 80,000 names, has been prepared, giving qualifications and type of work for which the specialists are best fitted. This register was begun by the Royal Society and by various scientific and technical associations and has now been taken over and amplified by the National Service Department of the Ministry of Labor. It is available to the War Department who notify their requirements for trained personnel to appropriate committees in charge of the register. Industrialists in need of specially trained men can also apply.

"British science is in a very much stronger position now than in 1914, especially as regards the number of trained men," according to Professor J. C. Philip, acting head of the Imperial College of Science and Technology of the University of London and chairman of the Industrial Chemistry Section of the Central Register of Scientists.

Although there is a surplus over present requirements, nevertheless the government has decided not to repeat the mistake of 1914 when brilliant young scientists were allowed to join the fighting forces indiscriminately. Physicists still remember with regret the loss of Moseley, whose brilliant career in x-ray research was cut short at Gallipoli.

Scientists and research workers are considered to be in reserved occupations and those not engaged in war work may continue their usual activities. At the same time, while full freedom is allowed to the individual, steps have been taken to inform research workers of the type of urgent problems that await solution. Some of these are of long duration, others have arisen since the war.

The "blackout" has called for scientific development. For instance, more effective phosphorescent substances were needed for use in underground shelters. Suitable "light filters" that would allow daylight in while preventing artificial light from passing outwards are being sought. Similarly gasoline restrictions make important devices for increasing miles per gallon, and alternative types of fuel are being exploited.

The Chemical Society has formed an advisory Research Council under the chairmanship of Sir Robert Robinson, to advise research workers in universities and other research institutions concerning general war problems needing investigation.

Another set of problems, which for the time being are left to the initiative of unofficial groups like Political and Economic Planning and the Engineers' Study Group, are those likely to arise at the end of the war. Large surplus capacity for the production of light metals, explosives, etc., will exist at the end of the war, and this, as well as the workers engaged in those industries, will have to find other utilization if industrial dislocation is to be prevented.

British industry has at present a considerable reserve of trained personnel in the Germans, Austrians and Czechs who have sought refuge in Great Britain. They have so far been employed in their particular lines of work only to a slight extent. During the last war it was a "non-Aryan" chemist, Dr. Fritz Haber, who enabled Germany to fight a prolonged war by his development of a synthetic process for the manufacturing of ammonia and nitrates, essential in the manufacture of explosives. Haber died in Switzerland, an exile from Nazi Germany.

Have scientists any surprises in store in the present war? Faced with this question, Professor Philip smiled and replied: "It is not a question that I could very well answer; however, this much I can say: during the last war it was the chemist who produced some of the most unpleasant innovations, such as the use of the poisonous gases. It may be the physicists' turn now."—VICTOR COFFMAN.

## ITEMS

A NOTE on the supply of vanadium, printed under Science News in the issue of SCIENCE for October 27 describes the operations of the United States Vanadium Corporation at Uruvan, Colorado, but it is referred to as property belonging to "Vanadium Corporation of America, a subsidiary of Union Carbide and Carbon Corporation." As a matter of fact, the United States Vanadium Corporation is a unit of the Union Carbide and Carbon Corporation, and a competitor of the Vanadium Corporation of America, whose vanadium resources are in Peru.

THE number of fatal pneumonia cases in the Civilian Conservation Corps, whose members have been given anti-pneumonia vaccine, dropped this year to a rate one third that of the preceding five years. How much of this and of the reduction in total number of pneumonia cases is due to use of the vaccine can not yet be stated with certainty, according to Robert Fechner, director of the corps.

CHEMISTS of Egypt have been studying explosions which have been occurring in earthen molasses storage basins. The explosions turn the molasses into a hard carbonaceous material that makes a good fuel with properties somewhat like coke. The explosions occur between June and November when the dark-colored molasses is exposed to the hot tropical sun. Spontaneous combustion is believed to be the cause.

A TURKEY-LIKE bird with a three-inch horn growing out of its forehead, which was discovered in the jungles of Bolivia, has been announced by James Bond and Rodolphe Meyer de Schauensee, curators of birds of the Academy of Natural Sciences of Philadelphia. They call it the unicorn bird, *Pauxi unicornis* to the scientist. The bird resembles the new stream-lined Thanksgiving bird which was recently developed by the Department of Agriculture, in its size, which is about eight to ten pounds in weight. The horn which suggested its name is grayish-blue, while the feathers on the nape of the neck and back of the head are tightly curled and shiny. The new species was discovered by a collector for the academy, Mr. de Schauensee.

A MASS of bones, believed to be remains of nearly a hundred of Chief Powhatan's tribesmen, has been unearthed in an ossuary—ceremonial burial pit—beside the York River near West Point, Va. Dr. T. D. Stewart, of the Smithsonian Institution, was sent to investigate and excavate the bones, when residents notified the Smithsonian that high water had washed away the river bank, exposing human bones. The village of Chief Powhatan, father of Pocahontas, was presumably a short distance away, but Dr. Stewart reported finding no trace of it. A good deal of the shore has washed away. The burials, he said, represent an Algonquin Indian custom of digging up individual burials at stated times and re-burying them in mass, with ceremonies. Jesuit priests in Canada told of witnessing such ceremonies. Archeologists have previously found ossuaries as far south as the Potomac, but Powhatan's neighborhood represents a new southward limit for discovery of the custom.

# SCIENCE NEWS

*Science Service, Washington, D. C.*

## SOCIAL SCIENCE



DR. JULIAN HUXLEY, secretary of the Zoological Society of London, grandson of Charles Darwin's famous friend and champion, gave an address at a dinner at the Hotel Willard, Washington, D. C., on December 2.

Dr. Huxley, who will deliver one of the principal addresses before the Christmas meeting of the American Association for the Advancement of Science in Columbus, Ohio, spoke under the joint auspices of the Association, the Smithsonian Institution and *The Scientific Monthly.*

Some thinkers claim for Herbert Spencer, contemporary of Darwin and the elder Huxley, the distinction of being the first to point toward an eventual application of the findings and methods of objective science in the problems of human society, but Dr. Huxley relegated Spencer to a position analogous to that of one of the Hebrew prophets, rather than that of a direct precursor. ''He demonstrated that social science was an inevitable development,'' Dr. Huxley stated, ''but his notions of what form it would actually take and what methods it should employ were vague and essentially erroneous. Marx, on the other hand, developed a system directly based on social facts and directly applicable to them. He did not prophesy a Messiah, he indicated the Messiah. As natural scientists tend to undervalue Bacon because he himself did not make discoveries or work out experimental techniques, so social scientists tend to underrate Marx because his system is a dialectical one, ready-made and complete with answer to any problem, not sufficiently empirical and inductive for their scientific taste. It is doubtless true that, as occurred in the case of natural science, the social scientists must go their own way to work, regardless of doctrine or theoretical system; a precursor can not take the place of the Messiah or the gospel he indicates. But at least Marx, like Bacon, gave expression to a new outlook and a new method of attack, and helped materially to alter the intellectual climate so as to make it propitious for the scientific workers in his field.''

To the question why social science has taken so long to emerge into large-scale operation, Dr. Huxley returned two answers. First, the method of the controlled experiment, beloved tool of natural science, is impossible when working with human society. There are no societies among lower organisms sufficiently similar to human societies to serve as experimental material; man must be his own guinea pig in social experimentation. Moreover, nothing less than the whole of society will serve: results of experiments on limited groups of people, even in the most completely regimented state, would not yield dependable answers.

The second reason for the laggard state of social science offered by Dr. Huxley is the natural reluctance of the human mind to accept multiple causes for any phenomenon. No matter how complex the behavior of a human group, we always try to find ''the cause'' instead of seeking for a number of causes, of a complexity comparable to the results they produce. Also, man is always the victim of his own mental slant or bias; it is practically impossible for him to divest himself of inborn and acquired prejudices.

Methods will have to be worked out, especially by the application of mathematical analysis to the problems of multiple causation, and by the use of properly adapted propaganda for the overcoming of bias.

## THE CHEMICAL EXPOSITION



''CHEMISTRY catalyzes commerce'' headlines the exhibit of twenty new commercial products of chemical industry shown by the American Chemical Society at the Seventeenth Exposition of Chemical Industries in Grand Central Palace, New York, which opened on December 4.

Outstanding in interest are eleven synthetic and crystalline vitamins now available. This is the first time so large a group of these food essentials has been displayed. Included are vitamins A (carotene), $B_1$, $B_2$, $B_6$, C, $D_2$, E, K, riboflavin, nicotinic acid and ergosterol. Nine manufacturers have supplied these man-made duplications of essential body chemicals.

In the synthetic resin group are shown two new and totally synthetic fibers, Vinyon and Nylon. Hosiery and yarn made from both of these are displayed. Both are competitive with silk. Other products made from these materials include felt, filter cloth, thread, surgical sutures and fishing line.

Paint oil made from castor oil, domestically produced to compete with tung oil, and alkyd resins for making varnish from this source are also shown. Of interest in the paint and varnish industry in the American Chemical Society exhibit is a new hydrogenated rosin, ''Stabellite,'' of superior quality as to color and resistance to light and oxidation.

Other outstanding displays include:

Rubber filter cloth, and an all glass centrifugal pump for handling corrosive liquids.

High octane aviation fuels produced by new methods.

The ''threshold treatment'' for economically softening hard water for boiler use.

Resins and vanillin made from the waste of sulfite paper mills, now produced commercially.

A new type of rayon from ethyl cellulose in a variety of fabrics.

New chemicals exhibited are sulfamic acid and its derivatives, a collection of seventeen new nitroparaffins and new organic compounds of phosphorus.

Twenty-six companies are cooperating with the society to supply exhibit materials and a nearly equal number of others in supplying photographs for the photo murals forming the background of the exhibit.

## A NEW ELECTRICAL MICROMETER MEASURES

*(Copyright, 1939, by Science Service)*

A NEW and valuable kind of electrical micrometer, which uses a special radio tube to measure distances as small as five millionths of an inch, has been developed at the U. S. Naval Research Laboratory in Washington.

Dr. Ross Gunn, physicist and superintendent of the mechanics and electricity division of the laboratory, described the instrument at the meeting in Philadelphia of the American Society of Mechanical Engineers.

The electrical micrometer is a radio tube consisting of an electron-emitting filament and two tiny plates, insulated from one another and jointly supported by a rod which goes into an elastic diaphragm fixed in the bulbous part of the radio tube. Outside the tube, and attached to the diaphragm, is spot welded another small rod whose job it is to detect tiny displacements. Slight displacements of this rod are communicated through the diaphragm into the plates of the tube, which move very slightly from their normal positions. This motion brings one plate nearer to the filament and the other plate farther away, resulting in a decided difference in flow of electrical current within the tube. Normally the current to the two plates balances and zero current is obtained. With the slight shift of plate distance current flows in an amount proportional to the displacement. This current is put through a micrometer and the deflection of the needle of this instrument is a measure of original microscopic displacements.

Dr. Gunn stressed the compactness and stability of the new device as well as its great versatility to a variety of measurements. The electrical micrometer can be used to measure displacements at remote points, and these displacements may be due to tension, compression or torsion.

By attaching a small mass to the external detecting arm of the tube it can be converted into an accelerometer. By the use of elastic bellows fluid pressures can be measured. By using large calibrated proving rings, its range of measurement can be enlarged indefinitely and it has proved useful as an accessory to limit and tolerance gauges. Because it is able to follow vibrations up to 200 cycles a second it can be attached to an oscillograph and thus produce a visual pattern comparable to the motions of the tiny detecting rod.

## SOLAR RADIATION AND THE WEATHER

*(Copyright, 1939, by Science Service)*

POSSIBILITY of statistical error in the theory that there are significant periodic changes in the sun's radiation which predictably affect the earth's weather has been eliminated by a Harvard mathematician.

The findings, made by Dr. Theodore E. Sterne, lecturer on astrophysics at Harvard University, are believed to eliminate one of the major objections raised against the solar radiation-weather theory advanced by Dr. Charles G. Abbot, secretary of the Smithsonian Institution.

Dr. Abbot's deductions, based on years of solar radiation observations at stations spotted throughout the world, have been questioned as due to either statistical errors in analyzing the data or systematic errors of observation. The Harvard research removes this first objection.

In his findings, Dr. Abbot discovered evidence for changes in solar radiation in periods of 7, 8, 9¾, 11, 21, 25, 34, 39½, 46 and 68 months. Dr. Sterne believes that three of these periods may be due to statistical error—those of 7 months, 8 months and 34 months.

The other seven periods, Dr. Sterne has found, are not attributable to this and he has gone so far as to say that the odds against these seven periods being purely statistical error are about 30,000 to one, or even higher, running in some cases into the millions. He emphasized that his studies were concerned purely with the statistics of Dr. Abbot's researches and not at all with the question of observational technique.

The periods in question were worked out by Dr. Abbot during the fifteen years from 1920 to 1934 and are built on the average of solar radiation in many parts of the world three times each month. Dr. Abbot measured the amount of radiation received in calories per minute per square centimeter at right angles to the sun. The average during this 15-year period, he found, was 1.9410 calories per square centimeter per minute.

## THE AUTOGIRO

*(Copyright, 1939, by Science Service)*

THE important research finding, that autogiros with their whirling rotor blades have more inherent longitudinal stability (ability to react against a pitching motion in flight) than do normal airplanes, was announced at the concluding meeting in Philadelphia of the Philadelphia chapter of the Institute of Aeronautical Sciences by Professor Alexander Klemin, of New York University, in a scientific report with Lieutenant Victor Haugen, U. S. Army Air Corps, and S. B. Sherwin, first holder of the newly created Cierva Memorial Fellowship at New York University.

The new report contradicts some previous wind tunnel experiments and is in accordance with practical experience. The theoretical investigations show that the rotor with its flapping hinge placed at some distance from the center of rotation is definitely stable. In this the rotor is superior to the airplane wing, which has no inherent stability of its own.

The investigations also show that as the rotor is placed above the center of gravity of the machine with its axis of rotation somewhat behind the center of gravity, the autogiro will be stable without the intervention of the horizontal tail surfaces. Such inherent stability without horizontal tail action is impossible in the airplane. Furthermore, rotors of the direct control type are pivoted about a suitable point so that not only is it possible to secure longitudinal control without use of an elevator, but the rotor tends to change its inclination so as to increase stability. In the airplane, flying with free stick, the stability is less than flying with stick held in a fixed position. In the autogiro with pivoted rotor, on the other hand, there is a dual stabilizing effect. Thus from the point of view of horizontal static stability, the autogiro has distinct points of superiority over the airplane. To remove the discrepancy existing between wind tunnel data and theoretical and practical reasoning, Lieutenant Haugen will conduct an investigation into the stability of the rotor with offset hinge, systematically varying the position of the hinge.

One of the most interesting problems in the helicopter to-day is whether super-imposed air screws, as in the Breguet helicopter, or air screw placed on either side of the fusilage, as in the Focke helicopter, are more efficient. Mr. Sherwin has devised a special apparatus for investigating this point in the nine-foot wind tunnel of the Daniel Guggenheim School of Aeronautics of New York University.

## CHEMICALLY INDUCED PLANT TUMORS

CLUES to the mechanism of cancer production in man and other animals are now being sought in the plant world. Latest efforts to produce cancers in plants by the chemicals in tar which produce cancer in animals or by other chemicals were described by Dr. Michael Levine, Montefiore Hospital Biological Laboratory for Cancer Research, at a meeting of the Torrey Botanical Club in New York on December 5. Montefiore Hospital is the only hospital in the world which has a garden devoted to plant cancer studies.

Crown gall, the form of cancer which plants are known to harbor, is not analogous to human or other animal cancer, Dr. Levine said. Cancer-causing hydrocarbons, which produce cancer in animals, poison plants but fail to produce cancers in them. Certain other irritating chemicals, such as indole acetic acid, indole butyric acid, naphthalene acetic acid and a series of scarlet red dyes, when applied to the injured surface of a plant, produce roots together with small tumors. These tumors, however, are not, in Dr. Levine's opinion, analogous to human or other animal tumors, either. The plant tumor, he believes, is a part of a reparative and protective mechanism of the plant, analogous to inflammation in animals.

Dr. Levine expressed the hope that plants ultimately will be made to form tumors as a response to chemical substances. He implies that the plant cells will be so modified as to proliferate without limit, endowing them with a property now possessed by animal cancer. The production of malignant plant growths will throw light on the mechanism of cancer production in animals. The absence of blood and lymph streams and lack of diversity of tissue types make the plant a suitable subject for the study of this important problem.

## ITEMS

DR. KARL T. COMPTON, president of the Massachusetts Institute of Technology, pointed out at the seventy-fifth anniversary dinner of the Columbia University School of Engineering that the applications of scientific knowledge advance much more rapidly than the mere increase of knowledge. "There are two factors which account for the increasing rapidity in the development of new applications of science to human welfare," Dr. Compton said. "One of these is simply the fact that we are learning continually by experience how to make these applications more quickly and effectively. The second is that the possibilities for accomplishing our purposes increase somewhat as the square of the amount of knowledge which we possess." Thus if knowledge can be doubled in extent the applications can be increased four-fold.

How a four-lane highway was "jacked" apart to make a divided roadway and thus reduced fatal accidents over 83 per cent. was described at the meeting at Washington, D. C., of the Highway Research Board of the National Research Council by Arnold H. Vey, traffic engineer of the State of New Jersey. New Jersey took a popular four-lane highway and split it down the middle, jacking up separate concrete slabs and moving them sideways. Two roadways, separated by a dividing center strip, thus resulted. A study of accident figures on this road in 1933–34, before the division, and for 1937–38, after the division, showed that fatal accidents dropped 83.3 per cent. Non-fatal accidents decreased 48.5 per cent., and accidents involving property damage were cut 17.6 per cent. The reduction for accidents of all kinds was 40.4 per cent. Particularly valuable was the new divided highway at night, for accidents were then decreased by 47.2 per cent., while during the day they dropped only 31.4 per cent.

THE giant 608,170-pound locomotive, "American Railroads," which millions saw at the New York World's Fair, was the outstanding development of railroading for 1939, according to a report submitted to the meeting in Philadelphia of the American Society of Mechanical Engineers by its subcommittee. "American Railroads," while it stayed in one place, covered thousands of miles on rollers to thrill World's Fair crowds. Designed to haul 1,200-ton trains at speeds up to 100 miles per hour, it was the cooperative undertaking of the Baldwin, American and Lima locomotive companies.

ROTARY winged aircraft of the autogiro or helicopter type will usher in the third stage of growth in man's conquest of the air, according to Igor I. Sikorsky, pilot and designer, who spoke at the meeting of the Philadelphia chapter of the Institute of Aeronautical Sciences. Mr. Sikorsky forecast a brilliant future for planes with rotary wings, particularly in the field of private flying, to add to lighter-than-air and heavier-than-air transportation, the two earliest stages of man's aerial transport. By rotary wings, Mr. Sikorsky said, private flying can come into its own, for planes of this type overcome the main handicap of private flying to-day, which is lack of ability to take off and land in small spaces. It is this handicap, he feels, rather than lack of speed, lack of safety or even high cost of operation which has limited private aviation.

PLAIN ordinary water is now being used successfully as a lubricant for bearings in giant steel mill rolls and large ship propeller shafts through advances in the plastics industry, L. M. Tichvinsky, of the Westinghouse Research Laboratories, pointed out at the meeting of the American Society of Mechanical Engineers. Woven textile fabrics are impregnated with an organic binder and then treated by temperature and pressure to create these bearings, which require no oil or grease but perform efficiently when lubricated with water, which serves both as a cooling agent and as a lubricant.

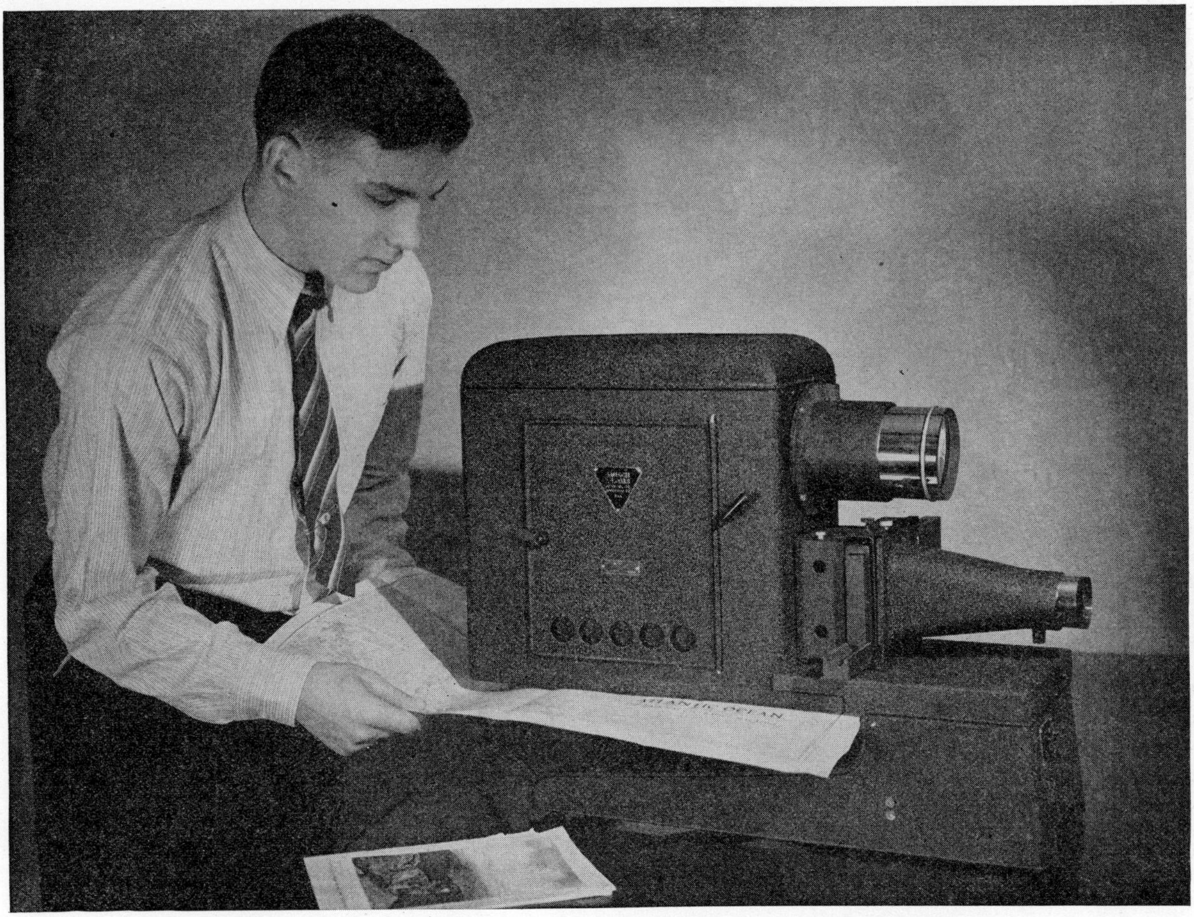

# SCIENCE NEWS

*Science Service, Washington, D. C.*

## SUPER-HEAVYWEIGHT STARS



THREE new super-heavyweights among stars, so solid that each cubic inch of their substance weighs not pounds but tons, are the latest discoveries made by Dr. G. P. Kuiper, using giant telescopes of McDonald Observatory at Fort Davis, Texas, and Yerkes Observatory at Williams Bay, Wis.

Known as white dwarfs, the newly found heavyweights are called Wolf 1516, the primary of the wide double star Wolf 672, Ross 640. This brings the number of white dwarfs known to 22, all stars relatively near the earth. Wolf 1516 is believed to have a diameter about four tenths that of the earth and such dense material that it weighs between 500 and 1,000 tons (1,000,000 and 2,000,000 pounds) per cubic inch. It has, however, not yet had its size and weight precisely determined, but it resembles an older one, A.C. 70 degrees 8247, that does have this amazing super-weight.

These two stars are the hottest white dwarfs known, with surface temperatures of over 30,000 degrees Centigrade. Only two other white dwarf stars, Wolf 457 and Wolf 219, are known to be similar to these stars. They are possibly even slightly heavier, at most about double in density. The other two new white dwarfs are probably less extreme. Dr. Kuiper has not yet finished his studies of them. Two other stars, Ross 22 and Wolf 923, are suspected of belonging to the same class and are also being investigated further.

More than half of all the white dwarfs known, 13 out of the 22, have a weight nearly the same as the famous companion of Sirius, about 3 tons per cubic inch, while the rest of them are heavier.

These very dense stars may be the result of a great stellar explosion, causing a collapse of a more ordinary star into smaller space. One idea is that they consist of stripped atoms, deprived of their electrons.

## A QUANTUM WORLD



AN amazing quantum world, where all elephants seem to have fur, where a tiger appears not as one animal but a whole group, and where a machine gun instead of a rifle would be needed to kill one of them, was described by Professor George Gamow, of the George Washington University, speaking before the Philosophical Society of Washington.

You could enter the quantum world if you could shrink down smaller than did Alice in Wonderland and become the size of an atom. Or you could do it, as did Professor Gamow, by increasing the magnitude of the quantum constant (which determines the uncertainty in position and motion of objects) so that it would have a noticeable effect on large objects.

If you went tiger-hunting in a quantum jungle, Professor Gamow explains, the elephant on which you would ride would appear to be covered with fur. This would only be the uncertainty in the size of the elephant, so that it appeared to have a fuzzy, furry outline.

The tiger for which you are searching would be the most baffling sort of animal. Instead of a single beast, it would entirely surround your elephant. To try and shoot it with a rifle by careful aiming would be useless. The chances would be many thousand to one that you would miss it. All you could do would be to use a machine gun and spray the landscape in the general direction of the "multiple" tiger. Eventually, and only by chance, would a bullet finally hit the tiger and finally kill it by direct impact.

Fantastic and imaginary as is Professor Gamow's tiger hunt, the happenings are similar to those which physicists now believe exist in the tiny world of an atom where individual particles are so minute that the quantum constant, determining the uncertainty of position, is a very real problem.

In experimental atomic physics the elephant corresponds to the heavy nuclei of atoms and the "multiple" tiger to the fuzzy, indeterminate position of an electron about the nucleus. The machine gun technique of hitting the "tiger" corresponds to attempts to bombard atoms in transmutation experiments where whole hosts of particle "bullets" must be fired in order to make a single hit.—ROBERT D. POTTER.

## ULTRA-VIOLET AND INFRA-RED RADIATIONS

ULTRA-VIOLET and infra-red radiation can have many uses on the electrified farm of the future, if only current becomes cheap enough and suitable equipment is developed, according to L. C. Porter, of the General Electric Company's incandescent lamp department in Cleveland, who spoke at the Chicago meeting of the American Society of Agricultural Engineers.

Infra-red rays are best known for their heating effects, Mr. Porter stated. Adaptations of the familiar dull-red-glowing electric heaters can readily be made for use in poultry houses, in barns to keep newborn animals warm and in the quick drying of hay. If their operation can be made cheap enough, their greater compactness and less fire risk will give them considerable advantage over present types of equipment.

Ultra-violet rays are known to have certain well-marked physiological effects, as in activating sterols to produce vitamin D and in keeping in check plants' growth in length. For producing well-proportioned plants in greenhouses, Mr. Porter suggested the use of a new kind of incandescent lamp, which has a globe permeable to ultra-violet as well as to visible rays. With these and other lamps in proper proportions, he stated, a close approximation to natural sunlight can be obtained, with control of duration and intensity not possible under natural conditions.

The well-known germicidal effects of ultra-violet rays still await a number of possible practical applications on the farm, Mr. Porter pointed out. They may be used in stables and dairy buildings as they now are in hospitals, to keep down the germ population of the air. They may be called on to control the spread of epidemics among farm animals, and to check the growth of molds and other fungi on hay, grain and other products. Their fluorescent effects may aid in diagnosing animal diseases and in examining vegetables and fruits.

With Dr. L. J. Buttolph, physicist of the General Electric Company, Mr. Porter will publish some of his suggestions in the forthcoming issue of *Agricultural Engineering*.

## THE DISCOVERY OF NEW OIL IN NEBRASKA



To the successful discovery of oil in Michigan and in Illinois can be credited the new discovery of petroleum in Nebraska at Falls City, near the Kansas border, according to a report of the U. S. Bureau of Mines.

The petroleum finds in Michigan and Illinois were based on geologic "basins" which look like some giant dinner platter with a corrugated bottom. Overlying the basin is surface material—in the case of Michigan, glacial drift—so that the ground level over the drift is not by itself indicative of the underlying depression in rock strata.

The new Nebraska finds have been based on two years of exploration of the Forest City basin, an area comparable to, though smaller than, the Michigan basin.

A typical procedure of geologists in searching for petroleum in a basin area is to follow "trends," the lines of the corrugations. A network of these corrugations is worked out and wells drilled at the intersections of the trend lines.

Production in the first Nebraska well is small, and it appears that the operators will have to push the well greatly to get sufficient oil to win the $15,000 prize offered by the state legislature for the first well which will produce 50 barrels daily for 60 days. In much greater production is the Mississippi discovery of oil, also recently reported, in Yazoo County. Over 700 drilling permits have been issued, but the possible extent of this field has not yet been determined.—Robert D. Potter.

## THE TREATMENT OF SYPHILIS

A new syphilis medicine, which can be taken in pills, has been developed by Dr. Paul J. Hanzlik and his assistants at the School of Medicine of Stanford University.

Success with exacting trials of the drug for over four years, in syphilis clinics in San Francisco and in Los Angeles, Cleveland and Philadelphia, has been reported. The council on pharmacy and chemistry of the American Medical Association in Chicago has accepted the new medicine as an anti-syphilitic agent.

Sobisminol is the name of the drug. It is a bismuth compound. Its great advantage is that it can be taken in pills, or capsules, at home, thus cutting down the number of visits to clinic or doctor's office and, of course, making unnecessary the hypodermic injections of bismuth which have been part of syphilis treatment.

The new medicine, however, is not a short-cut to a syphilis cure. It must be taken in combination with injections of arsphenamine or one of the other arsenical compounds. The total course of treatment still takes nearly two years, made up of alternating periods of six to 10 weeks of weekly arsphenamine injections and 10 to 20 weeks of taking the sobisminol capsules.

The new medicine will be sold on a physician's prescription only. Bismuth, the active ingredient, is a poison which is not safe for patients to prescribe for themselves. The new medicine is protected by patent held by Stanford University and the licensing agreements already made with three drug manufacturing firms restrict the sale of the drug without prescription and also forbid its exploitation to laymen by newspaper advertising, radio or window displays. Royalties will be used for further research in syphilis and related problems.

Sobisminol is said to produce prompt healing of syphilitic lesions and to have a killing effect on syphilis germs in the blood and tissues. Because of its ability to penetrate the brain and nervous system, it has been found to bring relief from pain in a high percentage of cases in the late stages of neurosyphilis. One physician who used it in treating patients reported that if used early in syphilis it "may prove to be of value in the prevention of neurosyphilis," the terribly destructive late stage in which the disease attacks the brain. The preventive action of the new medicine, however, can not be determined conclusively at this time, because neurosyphilis generally does not appear until 10 or 15 years after the first infection.

The production of a bismuth compound for oral treatment involved making a hypothetical chemical compound which had never been actually manufactured. This is triisopropanolamine, which is combined with sodium bismuthate and propylene glycol to make a bismuth compound that can be absorbed from the stomach into the blood, which is stable enough to withstand chemical action in the digestive system, and which prevents heat coagulation of the blood.

## A NEW TREATMENT FOR PNEUMONIA



A new chemical treatment for pneumonia, using a new drug, sulfathiazole, has been announced.

Physicians who tested it experimentally on human patients pronounce it even better than sulfapyridine, widely hailed in recent months as the chemical conqueror of pneumonia. The new drug is safer than sulfapyridine, and it does not make the patients sick. Nausea and vomiting, which have been a distressing feature of sulfapyridine treatment, are practically absent when sulfathiazole is given.

Developed in the Squibb Institute for Medical Research by Drs. H. B. van Dyke, R. O. Greep, Geoffrey Rake and C. M. McKee, the first report of the new drug is being published in the current issue of the *Proceedings* of the Society of Experimental Biology and Medicine.

Laboratory experiments on hundreds of mice show that the toxicity of sulfathiazole is much less than the toxicity of sulfapyridine except in doses far larger than are needed to cure pneumonia. In the body sulfapyridine is rather rapidly combined or conjugated with acetic acid. This unfortunately makes the drug quite inert and unless in its effect on the infection, only the uncombined form being active. The new drug, sulfathiazole, however, is combined with acetic acid to a much smaller extent, so that most of the drug given is effective until it is excreted. This means that doctors do not have to give as much sulfathiazole to treat a pneumonia patient. Chronic poisonous effects from accumulation of the drug in the body are much less apt to occur because sulfathiazole is excreted more rapidly than sulfapyridine.

Sulfathiazole is chemically related to sulfapyridine and sulfanilamide. It was prepared by several groups of scientists in the search for better chemicals with which to fight infections that threaten human life. The drug is given by mouth. In the mouse studies it had to be mixed with the food in order to make sure that all the drug given was being absorbed, so that comparisons between sulfapyridine-treated and sulfathiazole-treated animals would be on an exactly equal basis. For treatment of pneumonia patients, it is not necessary to mix the drug with the food.

## TRACHOMA ERADICATION

SULFANILAMIDE treatment of the blinding eye disease, trachoma, among American Indians has been so successful during its first year's trial that the Indian Service will launch a trachoma-eradication program next year.

Announcement of the success of the sulfanilamide treatment and of plans for a sharply expanded program, which it is hoped will bring this ancient scourge under control, was made by U. S. Commissioner of Indian Affairs John Collier in his report to Secretary of the Interior Harold L. Ickes.

The success of the new treatment will probably lead to its adoption in foreign countries, where trachoma is even more of a problem than it is here. Dr. R. Siri, a Siamese physician now in this country on a Rockefeller grant, plans to study the treatment on Indian reservations in the West before leaving for Siam in January. Out of Siam's population of 15,000,000, it is estimated that 3,000,000 persons are afflicted with trachoma.

Mr. Collier states that the disease has been eliminated completely by sulfanilamide treatment among the school children at Fort Apache, and trachoma in older Apaches is being rapidly cleared up. Of the more than 1,000 trachoma-afflicted Indians treated with sulfanilamide so far, 60 per cent. have improved to the point where physicians state the disease is "arrested." Since trachoma is caused by a germ and is largely limited to Indians in this country, it is believed that by arresting the disease in all patients, the spread of this eyesight-destroying scourge may be stopped. This would mean practical eradication of the disease. Quarantine regulations check its importation from foreign countries.

Sulfapyridine will be tried as well as sulfanilamide, according to Dr. J. G. Townsend, head of the Indian health service. The service is trying to determine which drug and what dosage will be most effective in arresting trachoma with greatest speed at least cost. One difficulty of the new treatment is in getting the Indians to take the medicine. Sulfanilamide is given them in the form of pills, and many of them can not understand why a pill should relieve an eye ailment. Nurses have found they must examine the children's mouths to be sure they swallow the pills.

Difficulty in checking trachoma in the past has been partly due to lack of sanitary facilities among the Indians. Many Navajos, Dr. Townsend pointed out, have to carry all their water, for drinking as well as washing, six or seven miles. Under such conditions, instructions about washing and the use of individual clean towels to prevent spread of germs are not too likely to be carried out.

## ITEMS

How America's flyers of to-morrow will be selected and trained was told by Dr. Dean R. Brimhall, assistant to the chairman of the Civil Aeronautics Authority, speaking as guest on Science Service's Adventures in Science program on Monday, December 11. A committee of nationally known psychologists is cooperating with Dr. Brimhall and the CAA in this work. Just as during the World War psychological tests were used to pick the proper jobs for soldiers, so in this new aviation activity psychology and other scientific methods are to be used in making the training most effective.

SEVEN billion or more young fish and eggs of four important commercial species—cod, haddock, pollock and flounder—have been planted in favorable spots along the North Atlantic coast of this country by the U. S. Bureau of Fisheries during the past year. The work was carried out by three marine hatcheries of the bureau in New England. The states of Maine and Massachusetts are also cooperating toward the repopulation of their offshore waters with lobsters.

A GREAT mass of living coral has been brought to St. Augustine, Fla., for the Marineland Studios by the fishing vessel *Porpoise*, which was fitted with a specially constructed well for the purpose. The coral tree was broken off its base, on the reefs near Walker City, Bahamas, and transferred into the ship without exposure to the air. Previous attempts to transfer living coral into aquaria have all ended in failure because even brief exposure to the air proved immediately fatal to the thousands of small polyp animals.

COTTON linings for irrigation ditches may be the new way to make a dent in the surplus cotton stock piles of the South, it was suggested to the National Reclamation Association meeting at Denver. The new utilization of cotton supplements the use of cotton fabrics as a binder for secondary highways and airport runways. W. H. Robinson, manager of an irrigation district in Idaho, described how a section of an irrigation canal was lined with a mixture of asphalt and gravel backed by heavy cotton fabric. Water losses in this section, which formerly ran from 20 per cent. to 30 per cent., have now been cut to about one and one half per cent. The standard method of lining irrigation canals is with concrete, which pays for itself despite high cost. The cotton-gravel-asphalt liner is cheaper.

# SCIENCE NEWS

*Science Service, Washington, D. C.*

## SCIENCE IN 1939

### Mathematics

A new generalization of the length of a curve made it possible in 1939 to determine the ''length'' of very general sets of points in a plane. Properties of several important subsets of well-known function spaces were studied.

Progress on the famous continuum problem, which concerns infinite numbers and whether there is any infinite number substantially smaller than the number of points on a line and substantially larger than the number of whole numbers, showed that there is no inconsistency in assuming that no such number exists, although it has not been proved that there is no such intermediate number.

The ergodic theorem was extended on the one hand to the study of homogeneous chaos; on the other hand, to the problems of diffusion gases, hydrodynamics and statistical mechanics.

The mathematical theory of the change in temperatures occurring in a non-homogeneous bar with discontinuous initial temperatures was studied.

Properties of very general spaces were investigated by means of related configurations called ''gratings.''

An application of elegant modern methods for elliptic functions and fields to the study of the more general Abelian fields was outstanding in abstract algebra.

### Chemistry and Physics

Atomic energy was released in 1939 by the splitting of uranium atoms under neutron bombardment. Originally discovered in Germany, uranium fission was quickly confirmed in America and elsewhere. Experiments indicated that for each uranium atom split there was released 175,000,000 electron volts of energy.

Thorium and protactinium were likewise found to split and release their atomic energy.

The fission of uranium was found to be accompanied by the emission of other neutrons in a delayed reaction which may be the link in a chain reaction that potentially would make possible the practical release of uranium's atomic energy.

Barium, krypton, antimony, tellurium, iodine, strontium, yttrium, lanthanum, xenon, caesium and rubidium are among the elements found to be created by the splitting of uranium with the release of large amounts of energy.

Experiments showed that the work of extracting an electron from tungsten (electronic work function) which usually is assumed to be a constant in classical theory actually varies with temperature amounting to an increase in energy of .00006 electron-volts for every increase of one degree Centigrade.

A new type of chemical reaction obeying the laws of chance and operating between compounds hitherto believed to be inert to one another, as cream and milk, was discovered.

The most sensitive current detecting device ever created was developed which can detect .000,000,000,000,000,000,001 amperes, or a current equal to a single electron passing down a wire every five minutes.

Density, temperature and other important facts about the atmosphere up to heights of 24.8 miles were determined by use of a flickering searchlight beam and photoelectric cell detectors.

The world's most powerful continuous magnetic field, with a strength of 100,000 gauss, was created.

An improved and simple way of producing thiodiglycol, starting material in the manufacture of mustard gas, was developed.

Hydrogen fluoride was discovered to be an excellent catalyst for many vital organic chemical reactions, improving the yield of many reactions and making possible some which have not previously been attained.

A new synthetic silk-like fiber made from polyvinyl acetal resin, and known as Vinyon, approached commercial production.

Optical glass having the highest index of refraction (light-bending ability) and the lowest dispersion ever attained was patented.

The speed of light, fundamental physical constant, was determined for the first time by a completely automatic method that makes the observations independent of the observer.

### Astronomy

The McDonald Observatory 82-inch telescope, second largest in the world, was put into use in 1939 on Mount Locke, Texas.

Television apparatus was devised to detect activity in the sun's corona without waiting for total eclipse, promising aid to forecasts of disruptions in intercontinental radio communication.

An unusual number of comets, 6 new and 7 returns of periodic comets found in previous years, were discovered: Kosik-Peltier, periodic Pons-Winnecke, Vaisala, Jurlof-Achmarof-Hassel, which came to naked eye brilliance, periodic Kopff, periodic Schwassmann-Wachmann, periodic Brooks II, Rigollet, Kaminsky, periodic Tuttle, periodic Giacobini-Zinner, Friend, periodic Faye.

Five more supernovae, tremendous super-exploding stars, were discovered in distant nebulae; occurrence of three such recent outbursts in one nebula within 16 years suggested that in some galaxies a tenth of the stars may explode in a time equivalent to the period since the earth's rocks cooled.

Solar activity remained at a high level during the year, with sun-spots totaling more than 200 on many days, auroral displays of unusual intensity and interference with long distance radio communication.

Mars made the closest approach to the earth in 15 years, Jupiter came nearer the earth than in 24 years, Saturn came closer to earth than in 20 years.

Two more extremely dense ''white dwarf'' stars, one with a weight of 9,000 tons per cubic inch, were the first discoveries made with the new McDonald Observatory telescope.

Harvard Observatory's 10,000th variable star was discovered.

A gigantic aura of stars was discovered enveloping our own universe of stars, the Milky Way.

### EARTH SCIENCES

A GOVERNMENT-SPONSORED American expedition to Antarctica set sail in 1939, equipped with planes and a specially built snow cruiser, to amass geologic, geographic and oceanographic data and collect zoological specimens and information.

A new method was developed for obtaining geologic data on the deep bottom of the ocean by means of TNT explosions.

A new type of "robot" unmanned observatory made possible the obtaining of weather data in remote and inaccessible places, like exposed mountain tops and the polar regions.

The U. S. Weather Bureau made two innovations: "breakfast time" radio broadcasts and combination aviation and general forecasts made at airfields.

A large iron meteorite was found in Modoc County, Calif.

There were more than 35 earthquakes of sufficient severity to be registered on the world-wide network of seismograph instruments.

After a nearly normal summer, an unprecedented autumn drought gripped most of the country.

The North Atlantic iceberg season was the longest on record.

The first submarine charts of the eastern coast showing depths out to some 10,000 feet with all sounding incorporated in submarine contours were issued.

A submarine peak, rising nearly two miles above the ocean bottom, was discovered in the Gulf of Alaska.

A new "deepest spot" for the Atlantic, 5.7 miles, was found in the Nares Deep, north of Puerto Rico.

### BIOLOGICAL SCIENCES

ONE of the big biological events of the century was the discovery, off the eastern coast of South Africa, of a large, deep-sea fish belonging to a group supposedly extinct since the days of the dinosaurs. The scaly monster, about five feet long and having huge blue eyes, has been given the scientific name *Latimeria chalumnae.*

Two human embryos, only eleven days old, were studied.

Light, either artificial or from the sun, serves to increase the ability of plants to withstand midsummer heat, experiments showed.

Undifferentiated plant tissue was induced to grow indefinitely in test-tubes.

A new genus of palm found on Cocos Island was named *Rooseveltia frankliniana* in honor of the President.

Oxygen requirement of a fertilized mammalian egg was found to be 0.00073 cu mm per hour.

A new method was devised for measuring soil moisture, by passing electric current through a buried block of gypsum.

A chemical necessary for the capture of carbon dioxide in food formation by plants was found.

Seedless watermelons were produced by chemical treatment of unpollinated flowers.

A plant growth-retarding substance was discovered.

A substance that makes plant wounds heal was discovered and named traumatic acid.

Legs were successfully cross-transplanted among embryos of chickens, turkeys and other fowl.

Colchicine was extensively applied in the breeding of new varieties of plants.

A new type of rubber cavity-filling for tree wounds was designed to provide an inexpensive treatment.

A new cooperative system for artificially inseminating cows, ewes and other farm animals was inaugurated in several states.

### ANTHROPOLOGY AND ARCHEOLOGY

AT Tanis, entering the tomb of Pharaoh Shishak I, plunderer of Solomon's Temple in Jerusalem, archeologists found the place undisturbed and the Pharaoh enclosed in silver and gold coffins. First discovery of Neanderthal Man in Central Asia was reported in 1939, the skeleton of an eight-year-old boy, unearthed near Tashkent, Turkestan.

The oldest known dated monument in America, the equivalent of 291 B.C. by one correlation, 31 B.C. by another, was discovered in Tres Zapotes, Mexico.

Nestor's Palace of Odyssey fame was found on the Promontory of Pylos, and in the ruins lay hundreds of archives in Cretan-like script.

The impressive ship grave of an Anglo-Saxon king, probably Redwald, who died about 620 A.D., came to light in Suffolk.

Measurements of 147,000 American children provided the clothing industry with its first scientific basis for sizing children's clothes.

Hailed as a new and important link between man and ape, a distinctive fossil tooth found at Sterkfontein, South Africa, was believed allied to remains of the man-ape of 50,000 to 100,000 years antiquity previously found in the same district.

An extraordinarily well-preserved Neanderthal skull with well-developed brain capacity was unearthed on the west coast of Italy.

Seven skeletons of "modern mankind" which had been found in the cave of Peking Man, China, were scientifically described and pronounced surprisingly varied with the inclusion of Indian-like types.

A village unearthed in Arctic Alaska revealed a form of prehistoric Eskimo life quite different from anything previously seen.

Beads and additional types of tools were found at the only known camp of Folsom Man in Colorado, clarifying the picture of earliest Americans as equal in culture to Stone Age Europeans of the same era.

Tree-ring technique of dating pueblo ruins in America was reported applicable to certain Viking and pre-Viking sites in Scandinavia; also to New England sites.

Life of refugees when Crete's civilization fell about 1100 B.C. was shown by excavation of a city of refuge on Mount Karphi, Crete.

Exploration of a royal chamber tomb of the Mycenaean

age in Athens showed that before the Trojan War era that city was rich and important.

### Psychology and Psychiatry

THREAT of European conflict and its reality stimulated research on the mental causes leading to war, effects of propaganda and war on the minds of belligerent and neutral peoples and means of protection from its influence.

Dentists, artists, engineers and teachers, not clergymen, church members, lawyers or domestic servants, were found to be more numerous in the cities rating highest in "general goodness of life."

Use of strychnine to vary the pattern of brain waves from the sensory cortex made possible the mapping of that area which was found to be very large with major subdivisions serving sensation in the face, arms and legs separately.

Idea of a strictly localized speech center in the brain came into further question when it was observed that some patients recover after loss of speech through brain injury.

The drug curare was found to depress the brain cortex or that part of the higher nervous system between the cortex and the spine so that learning can take place only through sub-cortical parts of the nervous system, explaining ability of the drug to produce "dual personality."

A special fund of more than $100,000 was set aside from the U. S. Government's civilian pilot training program to develop new and better methods for selecting and training pilots.

Brain wave study revealed that a chemical pacemaker controls the brain's activity through cell respiration, promising new understanding of brain syphilis.

Blood tests revealed that cell respiration in the brain is heightened during the fever treatment for the mental disorder paresis, brain syphilis, throwing new light on how the treatment benefits.

### Engineering and Technology

A PRACTICAL way of extracting the important metal manganese from low-grade ores was developed in 1939; also the use of small amounts of lead in steel to improve greatly its fabrication properties.

The U. S. Navy opened its new $4,500,000 towing tank at Carderock, Md.

Gas turbines which in wartime emergency can be buried underground with only fuel and air inlet and an electric cable outlet were developed in Europe and already several are in operation in the United States in industrial plants.

Commercial production was begun of high test gasoline, using sulfuric acid as the chemical catalyst.

The *S.S. America,* 30,000-ton passenger liner and largest ever built in America, was launched.

Commercial development was undertaken of frequency modulated radio transmission which makes possible transmission without interference from natural or man-made static.

The fulchronograph, a rotating magnetic lightning recording device, was developed, which successfully measured the maximum current of a direct lightning stroke and charted its complete wave shape.

By a new process of insulating telephone wires the number of wires which can be placed in present size cables was increased by 606 to a total of 4,242 wires.

Accurate values for the viscosity of steam up to pressures of 2,000 pounds and temperatures of 1,100 degrees Fahrenheit were established.

Scheduled television programs, after many years of laboratory experimentation, were inaugurated.

Shasta Dam, irrigation project in the Sacramento-San Joaquin Valley, Calif., was begun.

The Federal Government began the acquisition of strategic mineral stockpiles with a $10,000,000 purchase fund.

Iron 99.99 per cent. pure was made to serve as a spectroscopic standard.

### Medical Sciences

THE pneumonia case fatality rate was materially cut in 1939 by use of the new chemical remedy, sulfapyridine, while this and the related chemical, sulfanilamide, were reported promising in treatment of smallpox, primary peritonitis in infants, certain tropical diseases, infection with hemophilus influenzae (not virus influenza), tularemia, trichinosis, otitis media, gonorrhea, meningo-encephalitis of dogs, chronic ulcerative colitis; not useful in tuberculosis; and an effective vital stain for plant and animal tissues.

The National Cancer Institute at Bethesda, Md., was completed and occupied by its cancer research staff.

New buildings for Memorial Hospital for the Treatment of Cancer and Allied Diseases, in New York City, were completed.

A bill to extend medical and health services throughout the nation through a national health program was introduced into the Senate by Senator Robert F. Wagner, N. Y., and hearings were held and a preliminary report made, but the bill was not reported out of committee before Congress adjourned.

Refrigeration of human cancer patients to the point of artificial hibernation gave relief of intractable pain in more than 80 hopeless cases with regression of the tumor in some.

Cases of ulcerating x-ray and radium burns were cured with no recurrence during 10 years and probably prevented from becoming cancerous by treatment with alpha rays, beryllium and boron.

Treatment of cancer by neutron rays from the cyclotron was started.

"Cocktails" of radioactive sodium phosphate proved at least as effective leukemia treatment as x-rays in preliminary human trials of what is hoped will prove a "cure" for this fatal disease.

Vitamin K has been obtained in crystalline form and its chemical constitution has been determined as probably 2-methyl-3-phytyl-1, 4-naphthoquinone. Similar naphthoquinone compounds made synthetically exert the same influence in promoting the formation of prothrombin, one of the necessary factors in blood coagulation. They have been used successfully in treating certain diseases in which bleeding occurs from lack of prothrombin, such as obstructive jaundice and the bleeding of new-born infants.

# SCIENCE NEWS

*Science Service, Washington, D. C.*

## SUPER-EXPLOSIONS OF STARS IN DISTANT NEBULAE

*(Copyright, 1939, by Science Service)*

THE discovery by the collaborative efforts of astronomers at Mount Wilson, Palomar and Harvard Observatories of three gigantic stellar super-explosions within sixteen years in a distant system of stars like our own Milky Way, has been reported through the *Proceedings* of the National Academy of Sciences by Dr. Harlow Shapley, director of the Harvard Observatory, and leads to the speculation that these catastrophic star flare-ups are much more frequent than has been suspected hitherto, at least for one special type of stellar system.

It may be that in a system of stars similar to our own, a tenth of the stars explode in a time equivalent to that since the earth's oldest rocks cooled. Heretofore the accepted rate of occurrence of these supernovae, as they are called, has been one in 600 years for any one system.

Dr. Fritz Zwicky, of Palomar Observatory, and Dr. E. P. Hubble, of Mount Wilson Observatory, found two of the supernovae, one of which was also independently found on Harvard plates. The third was found on Harvard plates of 1921 by Miss R. Jones. This third supernovae actually exceeded at its peak brightness all other light from this northern nebula NGC 3184 in which it is but one of the 100,000,000 stars or more. In each of two other nebulae two supernovae have appeared, separated by intervals of thirteen years in NGC 4321 and twenty-two years in NGC 6946.

All these great aggregations of stars are nebulae of the most developed, and presumably older, type, labeled Sc in astronomical tabulations. They have the flat side of their spiral disc toward us. Most interesting from the viewpoint of earth dwellers is their probable similarity to the "island universe" or nebula in which our sun, with its planets, is an average star. The myriad of stars we see in the sky on a clear night are part of our nebula.

Although a nebula like NGC 3184 is so distant that it takes light 4,000,000 years to travel from there to here, what happens there is important because it may indicate what could happen in any well-developed stellar system.

Seven of the 30 supernovae discovered so far are in the three nebulae. One of the two supernovae that exploded in our own stellar system was the outburst observed by the Chinese in the year 1054. This supernovae can now be seen as the famous Crab nebula. It is not an external nebula but a different kind of cloud, not of stars, in our system.

Occasionally a star in our own nebula becomes very much brighter for a time and rises to naked-eye brilliance, only to fade away and become obscure again. Such a happening is called an ordinary nova. A supernova is many thousands of times more energetic. It is probably the greatest catastrophe that man's eye can witness.

On the basis of the three supernovae in NGC 3184, Dr. Shapley suggests that the light of perhaps 200,000 more are in transit from that nebula to earth, a phenomenon due to the long time (4,000,000 years) that it takes light to reach us from the immense distance of that nebula.

## CELLULOSE FROM THE AUSTRALIAN TREE CASUARINA

WOOD pulp for use in paper, guncotton, textiles and the other thousand uses of cellulose may be grown on "tree farms" of limited acreage in the warmer parts of the South, through the adoption of a fast-growing Australian tree, casuarina, is the belief of Professor Donald D. Bodé, of the department of chemistry of the University of Tampa.

Casuarina trees will grow 35 feet high with nine-inch trunks in six years; 56 feet high with 17-inch trunks in 12 years. They will produce from four to six cords per acre per year, as compared with one cord per acre per year for Southern jack pine. Moreover, a cord of casuarina wood is a fourth heavier than a cord of jack pine. The Florida State Forestry Service estimates that to supply a 200-ton mill with slash pine, 120,000 acres under forest management are needed. The same mill would be supplied by a 24,000-acre tract of casuarina.

Professor Bodé states that in fairly large-scale experiments he has produced 90 per cent. or better of alpha cellulose from casuarina pulp. Since ordinary commercial requirements for this purpose call for only 87 per cent., this would seem to be easily adequate. The pulp has been found good for book paper filler, but not as yet for newsprint. The best pulping process, so far as Professor Bodé's experiments indicate, is soda cooking. Considerably less bleaching compound is needed to produce good white alpha cellulose.

The tree can be grown on poor soil, down to the very edge of salt water. It should therefore thrive on the Florida keys and in the southern part of the peninsula, as well as elsewhere along the Gulf Coast. It must not be attempted, however, except where winter temperatures do not drop below a mean of 54 degrees Fahrenheit for the coldest month, and it must be carefully protected against fire, to which it is unusually sensitive.

The casuarina is a strange-looking but beautiful tree. It has no leaves; their place is taken by extremely slender, long, jointed green twigs, somewhat resembling the common horsetail or scouring-rush. It is sometimes called Australian pine, but it is not a pine; also beach she oak, but it is not an oak. It belongs to a botanical family unrepresented in the North American flora and named for the tree itself: the Casuarinaceae.

## VACCINE FOR PROTECTION AGAINST DISEASE CAUSED BY TICKS

*(Copyright, 1939, by Science Service)*

THE U. S. Public Health Service announces that a new vaccine for protection against a new and possibly widespread feverish ailment spread by ticks is ready for its first trials on human volunteers.

The new vaccine, successful in guinea pig trials, was prepared by Dr. Herald E. Cox and E. John Bell, of the Rocky Mountain Laboratory of the National Institute of Health at Hamilton, Mont. It was made from germs from infected ticks and also from the same kind of germs grown on developing chick eggs.

A member of the Washington headquarters staff of the National Institute of Health was the first recognized human case of the new disease, which has been named *Rickettsia diaporica.* He contracted it while observing the results of research during a visit to the Hamilton laboratories. He recovered after about a month's illness characterized by mild fever with chills, recurrent sweating and tender finger joints.

The ease with which the infection was picked up in the laboratory, plus the fact that the infection occurs naturally in ticks, suggests that there may have been other human cases. The disease is very similar to, if not the same, as the "Q" fever of Australia. The fact that two such similar diseases exist at points so geographically far apart leads health authorities to believe that other cases must be occurring in both countries and probably in many countries between here and Australia.

The germs of another ailment, relapsing fever, have been discovered in a tick by the name of *Ornithodoros hermsi,* by another of the Rocky Mountain Laboratory staff, Dr. Gordon E. Davis. Reporting his findings in the Public Health Reports, he states that this species of tick is undoubtedly a local agent for transmission of relapsing fever in Colorado.

## LEAF IMPRINTS IN SHALE NODULES



BEAUTY is sought and found in about the unlikeliest of all imaginable places—the waste-heaps of soft coal mines—by George Langford, of Joliet, Ill. For him it is not a profession but an absorbing avocation, for Mr. Langford makes his living as manager of a manufacturing plant in Joliet. His spare time he spends botanizing the forests of 250 million years ago, as represented by the fossil leaf-remains embedded in the nodules of hardened clay cast out with the shaly waste from the coal pits of central Illinois.

Finding fine leaf-imprints in shale nodules is not particularly new in itself. Thousands of them are in geological museums and in private collections. The real contribution of Mr. Langford is the method he has developed for bringing out their full color and beauty, something not accomplished by the kind of handling hitherto employed. Leaf-forms that ordinarily show dull and colorless take on almost the sheen of living flowers.

A shale nodule is a more or less elongated oval lump of stuff that looks like hardened clay. Indeed it is hardened clay, solidified around a leaf, or twig, or insect, or other object that fell into the mud and became embedded there, ages ago when coal was in the making. If you turn it edgewise and give it a sharp rap with a hammer it will split apart, showing the convex or positive side of the leaf-print on the face of one of the halves and the concave or negative side on the other.

That is all that has been done with leaf-nodules hitherto —just split them open to show the contents. But in that state the leaf-prints are dull and rather uninteresting, due to their being covered with tightly sticking tiny mineral particles—literally the dust of ages.

Mr. Langford undertook to get rid of this millennial dust. His technique is something between a jeweler's and a dentist's. He uses the small, keenly pointed and edged tools of a dentist, plus a variety of brushes, to dislodge the mineral particles, and then carefully burnishes each small detail of the cleaned-up design by hand. No buffing wheel, however fine, is permitted to touch one of his precious specimens.

Most people, when they first see a Langford leaf-nodule preparation, imagine that it has been painted or enameled. This is not the case. No artificial color of any kind is added, no varnish, no shellac. A little colorless burnishing fluid is the only aid he employs. The colors are those latent in the minerals composing the specimen itself.

Mr. Langford states: "The stone of the strip mine nodules is very variable. All of it contains more or less iron. In some places it is a buff-colored and rather soft shale. Occasionally it is sandstone. The stone best suited for fossil preservation is very close-grained and hard, in varying shades of fawn, gray, light blue and dark blue. Weathering converts the iron content into oxide, producing red, which, combining with the stone colors, results in orange, brown, purple and other colors. It remained for us to develop these colors by accentuating them in the plants and suppressing them in the surrounding stone. The result is a fine reproduction of the plant in color, and of surprisingly lifelike appearance."

The plant remains brought out by Mr. Langford's method are almost all leaves of ferns and fern-like plants, which were the highest forms of vegetation on the earth during the coal age. Higher flowering plants did not appear until much later. It is in the leaves, therefore, their delicate venation and smooth surface texture, that the greatest possible development of beauty must be sought.

## THE MEDICAL SCIENCES IN 1939

(*Continued from December 22*)

Prevention of 50 per cent. of deafness in adults is the future accomplishment expected from the discoveries that hyperplastic lymphoid tissue in and around the orifice of the eustachian tubes during childhood is the cause of middle ear deafness, that the condition can be detected by nasopharyngoscopic examination and that it can be checked by radium treatment.

Important development in the fight against infantile paralysis was the successful transmission of the virus to the Eastern cotton rat, which for the first time gives another animal than man or monkey for investigations looking toward a cure or preventive of the disease.

"Hormone banks," new technic in endocrine therapy evolved by English scientists and consisting of burying several months' supply of hormone in pellets under the skin, was successfully used in cases of Addison's disease and hypogonadism in both males and females.

Adrenal glands from animals were implanted under the skin of Addison's disease sufferers with more or less improvement in mild cases and improvements lasting 5 to 6 months in severe cases.

Male sex hormones were found to be of utility in treatment of reproductive-system disorders in women.

Tanning from exposure to sunlight was shown to be importantly dependent upon sex hormones.

Noma, serious human mouth ailment, was produced for the first time in monkeys by a deficient diet in studies indicating that dietary deficiencies rather than germs may be responsible for other human mouth and tooth ailments such as trench mouth.

A nation-wide drive to eradicate gonorrhea, second "hush-hush" plague, was started by the U. S. Public Health Service.

The American Museum of Health, first institution of its kind in the United States, was established in New York City.

Vitamins B and C were found useful remedies for retinal bleeding in diabetes.

Cultivation of rabies virus outside the brain of a living animal, once considered impossible, was accomplished and may make antirabies vaccine production easier.

New x-ray technic was developed for detecting placenta praevia by sixth month of pregnancy, thus allowing time to save both mother and baby from this often fatal complication.

Fluorine in drinking water, known to be the cause of mottled enamel of teeth, may act, according to some new observations, as a preventive of caries.

Apparent cure of hitherto incurable and rare scleroderma by parenteral treatment with an acid preparation known as Aciform II was announced.

The common gray house mouse was discovered to be a carrier of the causative virus of the human nerve disease, choriomeningitis.

Riboflavin, one of the B vitamins, is necessary for human nutrition, it was discovered from investigation of cases of ariboflavinosis, condition formerly confused with pellagra.

Partial sex determination by diet was achieved in rats, high protein diet fed the male parents and low protein to the female parents resulting in a sex ratio of 145 males to 100 females in the offspring.

Injections of the chemical, xanthine, were found to prevent jaundice and other liver damage in animals, a discovery believed useful for combatting human liver damage from solvents used in industries such as dry cleaning, plastics and certain manufacturing processes.

## ITEMS

ROCKS that form the crust of the earth have never been very hot—not more than 1,200 degrees Centigrade—in the opinion of Professor Norman L. Bowen, of the University of Chicago. He bases his assertion on the known melting and crystallizing points of crustal minerals. Some stones now at the surface have higher crystallization temperatures; diamonds, for example, but Professor Bowen points out, "We have no evidence that in their surface position diamonds were ever in any but crystal form." What temperatures were at great depths in the earth's earlier days, he adds, we do not know and probably never shall.

GLACIAL periods on the earth have been due to changes in the sun's radiation, according to an article by Sir George Simpson, the British meteorologist, in the annual report of the Smithsonian Institution. However, these big chills have come not when the sun, now known to be a variable star, was growing cooler, but when it was throwing out more heat. It works out this way: the increased heat causes increased evaporation from the oceans; this in turn produces greater precipitation. Near the Poles, this precipitation piles up as snow that packs and solidifies into ice—and the Ice Age is on the way. If the sun puts a damper on its radiation for a long period, evaporation slows down and the lands become dry. Sir George believes that we are living in such a cold, dry epoch now.

GLYCERINE has been turned to practical use in saving millions of young tomato and cabbage plants from dying in shipment through drying out of their roots. The method was worked out by Dr. R. N. Du Puis, industrial chemist of Chicago. Tomato and cabbage plants are grown in the South and shipped North by millions, their roots packed in moist sphagnum moss. It occurred to Dr. Du Puis to substitute a glycerine solution for the plain water, so that if the moss pack dried out there would still be a protecting layer of glycerine over the roots. Large-scale experiments gave encouraging results, and last season the method received a full-scale commercial workout. More than 75 million plants were shipped with glycerine-solution protection.

MORE, not less, vitamin A foods must be eaten as people get older, it appears from discoveries by Drs. J. T. Irving and M. B. Richards, of Rowett Research Institute, of Aberdeen, Scotland. The explanation probably is that the vitamin A needs of the body are related to body weight. Discoloration of rats' teeth gave the clue to the finding that the body needs more of this vitamin with increasing age. Changes elsewhere in the body seem to confirm this finding. Reporting their research to *Nature*, Drs. Irving and Richards point out that the increasing need for vitamin A with increasing age is in surprising contrast to requirements of other dietary factors, such as calcium and phosphorus. The need for these substances is not supposed to increase with age. Vitamin A is found in liver, particularly fish liver, and in green and yellow vegetables.

NEW kinds of soup, soup wafers, cheese and candies, made from dairy products by the Federal Bureau of Dairy Industry, are going to the Antarctic along with other supplies for the Byrd Expedition. The new foods are not yet on the market. They were devised to find ways of utilizing skim milk and whey. Whey powder was used in making the dried pea soup, which also contains split pea solids and fat. Potatoes, skim milk and salt make the soup wafers, which are said to be similar to potato chips except that they contain no fat and so will not turn rancid. Caramels and fudge for the expedition were made from a formula containing 25 per cent. whey solids. The American Cheddar cheese going on the expedition was made and packaged in valve-vented cans, a relatively new development in merchandising this type of cheese.

AN aviation-weather study, in which more than ten million separate observations at 239 major airports were used, will be published shortly by the U. S. Government. It will help airport planners to plan runway extensions and locate instrument landing systems. The work was done as a WPA project in New Orleans, more than 100 persons being employed. They extracted from the records of 239 airports data on visibility, wind direction and velocity, and other flying-weather factors and correlated it on punch cards for mechanical tabulation.

3/14